Neurological Rehabilitation

Neurological Rehabilitation

THIRD EDITION

Edited by

Darcy Ann Umphred, Ph.D., P.T.

Vice Chairman and Associate Professor
Graduate Program in Physical Therapy
University of the Pacific
Stockton, California;
International Lecturer, Consultant, Private Practitioner
Partners in Learning Clinic
Carmichael, California

with illustrations by Steve Schmidt and Ben Burton

with 50 contributors
with 362 illustrations

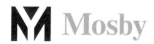 Mosby

St. Louis Baltimore Boston Carlsbad Chicago Naples New York Philadelphia Portland
London Madrid Mexico City Singapore Sydney Tokyo Toronto Wiesbaden

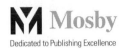

Mosby–Year Book, Inc.
11830 Westline Industrial Drive
St. Louis, MO 63146

Library of Congress Cataloging-in-Publication Data

Neurological rehabilitation / edited by, Darcy Ann Umphred ; with
   illustrations by Steve Schmidt and Ben Burton. — 3rd ed.
       p.   cm.
   Includes bibliographical references and index.
   ISBN 0-8016-7925-7
   1. Nervous system—Diseases—Patients—Rehabilitation.
  2. Exercise therapy. 3. Physical therapy. I. Umphred, Darcy Ann.
   [DNLM: 1. Nervous System Diseases—rehabilitation.   WL   100 N49466
1995]
RC350.E85N48   1995
616.8′0462—dc20
DNLM/DLC   94-44146

              99 / 9 8 7 6 5 4

Contributors

Leslie Allison, P.T., N.C.S.
Clinical Applications Specialist
NeuroCom International, Inc.
Clackamas, Oregon

C. Robert Almli, Ph.D.
Associate Professor of Occupational
  Therapy, Psychology and Neuroscience
Occupational Therapy Program
Washington University School of
  Medicine
St. Louis, Missouri

Myrtice B. Atrice, P.T.
Physical Therapy Supervisor
Department of Physical Therapy
Shepherd Spinal Center
Atlanta, Georgia

Johnny Bonck, M.S., O.T.R.
Alta Bates Medical Center
Berkeley, California

Gordon U. Burton, Ph.D., O.T.R.
Associate Professor
Occupational Therapy Department
San Jose State University
San Jose, California

Sharon A. Cermak, Ed.D., O.T.
Associate Professor
Department of Physical Therapy
Boston University
Boston, Massachusetts

Laurie Efferson, O.D., M.S., O.T.R.
Optometrist
Occupational Therapist
Department of Primary Eyecare
  Optometrics
San Lorenzo, California

Donna El-Din, Ph.D., P.T.
Distinguished Professor
Department of Physical Therapy
Eastern Washington University
Cheney, Washington

Debra Frankel, M.S., O.T.R.
Special Projects Manager
National Multiple Sclerosis Society
Massachusetts Chapter
Waltham, Massachusetts

Gertrude Freeman, M.A., P.T.
Retired
Galveston, Texas

Kathryn L. Gabriel, P.T.
Private Practitioner
Ann Arbor, Michigan

Maureen Gonter, P.T., M.S.
Physical Therapy Supervisor
Department of Physical Therapy
Shepherd Spinal Center
Atlanta, Georgia

Doris A. Griffin, P.T.
Coordinator, Outpatient Physical Therapy
Department of Physical Therapy
Shepherd Spinal Center
Atlanta, Georgia

Ann Hallum, Ph.D., P.T.
Associate Professor, Director
Graduate Program in Physical Therapy
University of California-San Francisco/
San Francisco State University
San Francisco, California

Susan R. Harris, Ph.D., P.T.
School of Rehabilitation Medicine
University of British Columbia
Vancouver, B.C.
Canada

Anne Henderson, Ph.D., O.T.
Professor Emeritus
Department of Occupational Therapy
Boston University
Boston, Massachusetts

Steven R. Huber, P.T., C.O.
Physical Therapist and Certified Orthotist
Huber Associates, P.A.
Physical Therapy and Orthotics
Auburn, Maine

Osa Jackson-Wyatt, Ph.D., P.T.
Associate Professor
Physical Therapy Program
School of Health Sciences
Oakland University
Rochester, Michigan

Martha J. Jewell, Ph.D., P.T.
Associate Professor and Chairperson
Department of Physical Therapy
Samuel Merritt College
Oakland, California

Kristin Krosschell, P.T.
Pediatric Clinical Manager
U.R.S.—Caremark Orthopedic Services
Oak Park, Illinois

Laura LeCocq, M.S., O.T.R.
Occupational Therapist
Department of Rehabilitation Services
Stanford University Hospital
Stanford, California

Marsha Mabry, M.Ed., P.T.
Physical Therapist, Administrative
  Support Services
Special Education
Houston Independent School District
Houston, Texas

Anne MacRae, Ph.D., O.T.R.
Assistant Professor
Occupational Therapy Department
San Jose State University
San Jose, California

Karen L. McCulloch, M.S., P.T., NCS
Clinical Assistant Professor
Division of Physical Therapy
University of North Carolina at Chapel Hill
Chapel Hill, North Carolina

Shari L. McDowell, B.S., P.T.
Physical Therapist
Department of Physical Therapy
Shepherd Spinal Center
Atlanta, Georgia

Marsha E. Melnick, Ph.D., P.T.
Clinical Professor
Graduate Program in Physical Therapy
University of California San Francisco and
San Francisco State University
San Francisco, California

Linda Mirabelli-Susens, P.T.
Physical Therapist
Sunbelt Physical Therapy Services, Inc.
Palm Harbor, Florida

Nancy M. Mohr, M.S., OTR/C
Instructor and Research Associate
Occupational Therapy Program
Washington University School of
   Medicine;
Pediatric Occupational Therapist
St. Louis Children's Hospital
St. Louis, Missouri

Sarah A. Morrison, P.T.
Physical Therapy Supervisor
Physical Therapy
Shepherd Spinal Center
Atlanta, Georgia

Gay M. Naganuma, M.S., P.T.
Rehabilitation Services
Kapiolani Medical Center for Women and
   Children
Honolulu, Hawaii

Charlene M. Nelson, M.A., P.T., ECS
Associate Professor, Emeritus
Division of Physical Therapy
University of North Carolina at Chapel Hill
Chapel Hill, North Carolina

Christine A. Nelson, Ph.D., O.T.R.
Cuernavaca, Morelos
Mexico

Roberta A. Newton, Ph.D., P.T.
Associate Professor
Director, Advanced Graduate Studies
Department of Physical Therapy
College of Allied Health Professions
Temple University
Philadelphia, Pennsylvania

Barbara S. Oremland, P.T., M.Ed.
Assistant Professor
Physical Therapy Program
University of Louisville
Louisville, Kentucky

Rebecca E. Porter, Ph.D., P.T.
Associate Professor
Department of Physical Therapy
Indiana University
Indianapolis, Indiana

Howell Runion, M.S., Ph.D., PA-C
Professor, Physiology-Pharmacology-
   Electrophysiology
School of Pharmacy
University of the Pacific
Stockton, California

Susan D. Ryerson, M.A., R.P.T.
Clinical Consultant and Lecturer: Partner,
   Making Progress
Alexandria, Virginia;
Adjunct Faculty
Massachusetts General Institute for
   Health Professions
Boston, Massachusetts

Jane W. Schneider, Ph.D., P.T.
Senior Physical Therapist-Children's
   Memorial Hospital;
Assistant Professor of Physical Therapy
Programs in Physical Therapy
Northwestern University
Chicago, Illinois

**Nina Newlin Simmons-Mackie, Ph.D.,
CCC-SP**
Private Practitioner
Speech-Language Pathology
New Orleans, Louisiana

Laura K. Smith, Ph.D., P.T.
Consultant
Post-Polio Clinic
The Institute for Rehabilitation and
   Research
Houston, Texas

Timothy J. Smith, R.Ph., Ph.D.
Assistant Professor
Department of Physiology and
   Pharmacology
University of the Pacific School of
   Pharmacy
Stockton, California

Bradley W. Stockert, M.S., P.T.
Assistant Professor
Physical Therapy
University of the Pacific
Stockton, California

Marcia W. Swanson, M.P.H., P.T.
Research Associate
Clinical Training Unit
Child Development and Mental
   Retardation Center
University of Washington
Seattle, Washington

Jane K. Sweeney, Ph.D., P.T., P.C.S.
Private Practitioner
Northwest Pediatric and Neurologic
   Rehabilitation Associates
Gig Harbor, Washington

Stacey E. Szklut, O.T.
Clinical Director-Occupational Therapy
   Associates;
Adjunct Professor
Department of Occupational Therapy
Boston University
Boston, Massachusetts

Wendy L. Tada, Ph.D., P.T.
University Affiliated Program
University of Hawaii
Honolulu, Hawaii

Darcy Ann Umphred, Ph.D., P.T.
Vice Chairman and Associate Professor
Graduate Program in Physical Therapy
University of the Pacific
Stockton, California;
International Lecturer, Consultant, Private
   Practitioner
Partners in Learning Clinic
Carmichael, California

Nancy L. Urbscheit, Ph.D., P.T.
Director
Physical Therapy Program
University of Louisville
Louisville, Kentucky

Gail L. Widener, Ph.D., P.T.
Assistant Professor
Department of Physical Therapy
Samuel Merritt College
Oakland, California

Patricia A. Winkler, M.S., P.T.
Owner and Physical Therapist
South Valley Rehabilitation;
President
Colorado Performance Lab, Inc.
Englewood, Colorado

TO

Gordon, Jeb, Benjamin, and my mother, Janet, whose love, patience, and understanding constantly gives me strength.

TO

All those special people whose insights, wisdom, guidance, and patience have helped to give each author in this book their unique gifts and talents, as well as their willingness to share their thoughts with all of you.

TO

A very dear friend, colleague, and past chapter author—Mary Jane Bouska. So many master clinicians and true leaders in the field of neurological rehabilitation have left us within the last 10 years. Mary Jane certainly fell into the category of clinical master and paradigm shifter and will be missed by all who knew her and were fortunate to call her a friend.

Preface

Fifteen years have passed since the conceptualization of this book. During that time the therapeutic management of clients with neurological dysfunction has transcended many stages of evolution. Efficacy based on research versus philosophy based on belief has become the choice of treatment procedures. A shift in paradigm from specific treatment approaches to a problem-solving systems model focus that looks at the impairment, functional limitations, and potential disability of the client seems to lead the flow of transformation that is inevitable if growth is reflected in a mirror of change. As these problem-solving approaches actualize, more effective, reliable, and valid therapeutic assessments and management strategies are being presented in the literature. Yet, our understanding of how man learns, relearns, or adapts is far from reaching closure. With so many unknowns and our belief in what is truly a known fact changing, the learner is left with the challenge of keeping his or her mind open to change and new learning while holding on to a flexible, not rigid, paradigm that allows that practitioner to comfortably evaluate and treat clients within a dynamic, ever-changing environment.

This book was designed to provide the practitioner and advanced therapy student with a variety of problem-solving strategies that can be used to tailor treatment approaches to individual client needs and cognitive style.

The treatment of persons with neurological disabilities requires an integrated approach involving therapies and treatment procedures used by physical, occupational, and recreational therapists, speech pathologists, and nurses. Contributors were selected for their expertise and integrated knowledge of subject area. The result is, we hope, a blend of state of the art information about the therapeutic management of the neurologically disabled person.

This book is organized to provide the student with a comprehensive discussion of all aspects of neurological rehabilitation and to facilitate quick reference in a clinical situation. Part One, "Theoretical Foundations for Clinical Practice," comprises an overview of integrated models, basic neuroanatomy and physiology, motor control theory, neurological development, psychosocial aspects of neurological disability, and treatment principles. Part Two, "Management of Clinical Problems," offers a clear description of the most common neurological disabilities encountered by physical and occupational therapists in general clinical practice and appropriate treatment strategies and techniques. Part Three, "Special Topics and Techniques for Therapists," is devoted to recent advances in the approach to treatment and rehabilitation, including oral, motor, speech, and visual perception, electrodiagnosis, pain management, balance, orthotics, and health education.

Special features of all three parts are evaluation tools and illustrated demonstrations of treatment plans.

A glossary of specific physical therapy terminology should be of equal value to students and practitioners.

During the conceptualization and preparation of the original manuscript many individuals gave time, guidance, and emotional support. To all those people I extend my sincere appreciation. My specific thanks go to:

- My many teachers, but especially Martha Trotter, Sarah Semans, Nancy Watts, and my father, who taught me to reach for the impossible and realize its actuality.
- The founders of the various treatment methodologies, whose conceptual ideas and flexibility created the foundation for development of an integrated problem-oriented approach to treatment.
- The numerous students, colleagues, and clients who taught me how to teach them.
- All the contributors who gave time, thought, and part of their lives to actualize this book.

During the reediting process of this book some additional individuals came to deserve special recognition.

- The editorial staff at Mosby, especially Martha Sasser, Kellie White, and Amy Dubin.

- Anne Gassett of Graphic World Publishing Services for her work in the production of this book.
- To all those teachers who have crossed my path in the last 15 years and who helped me continually realize that before we can find answers, unknowns must be identified and acknowledged.
- Special love and appreciation again goes to my family. Life's complexity is constantly evolving and the demands of each person close to me grows as does our bonds. Yet, each one in my family helped me relinquish precious time to meet the requirements necessary to complete this new manuscript.

- My two sons, Jeb and Benjamin, whose love and patience during the conception, gestation, and birth of this book far exceeded their age.
- Last, but certainly not least, my husband Gordon, who is the only one who truly knows what demands this book has made on me and everyone around me; yet his support has never dwindled.

This book was given birth to 15 years ago. It is growing with each author and each edition. We, as contributors, only hope that as the book grows, it will continually mature into a more integrated whole.

Darcy Ann Umphred

Contents

PART ONE

Theoretical Foundations for Clinical Practice

CHAPTER 1

Introduction and Overview

Multiple conceptual models:
frameworks for clinical problem solving

Darcy Ann Umphred

KEY TERMS

clinical problem solving
learning environment
systems model
disablement model

empowerment
visual analytical problem
  solving (VAPS)

LEARNING OBJECTIVES

After reading this chapter the student/therapist will:
1. Understand the concepts of an interlocking systems
   model.
2. Analyze each component of a systems model including
   cognitive, affective and motor subsections.
3. Synthesize the importance of the clinical triad and how
   each aspect of the triad affects the way the therapist
   interacts with the client and the environment.
4. Compare types of evaluation tools and realize their
   differences and similarities.
5. Analyze the difference between verbal and
   visual-analytical problem solving.

Although a physical therapist, occupational therapist, or other health professional may focus on a specific area of central nervous system (CNS) processing, a thorough understanding of the client as a total human being is critical for high-level professional performance. This book orients the student and clinician to the understanding and treatment of a variety of common neurological disabilities by a problem-solving approach. A secondary objective is the development of a theoretical framework that justifies the use of techniques for enhancing functional movement, enlarging the client's repertoire for movement alternatives, and creating an environment for procedural learning.

Evaluation and treatment methodology incorporate all aspects of the client's CNS, including overt and nonapparent integration. The role of specific disciplines with regard to the treatment of sensory processing, gross to fine motor performance, perceptual cognitive processing, and emotional-affective growth has not been defined. In the area of neurological disabilities, the overlap of basic knowledge and practical application of treatment techniques is so great that delineation of professional roles is often an administrative decision.

A problem-solving approach is used because it is logical and adaptable, and it is recommended by many professional studies during the last 25 years.[1,4,45,64] The concept of clinical decision making based in problem-solving theory has been stressed throughout the literature over the last few years and clearly identifies the therapist's responsibility to evaluate, analyze, and make decisions regarding possible goals and treatment alternatives.* Part One lays the foundation of knowledge necessary to understand and implement a problem-oriented approach. The basic knowledge of the human body is constantly enlarging and often changing in content, theory, and clinical focus; Part One reflects that change in both philosophy and scientific research. Part Two deals with specific clinical problems, beginning with pediatrics and ending with senescence. In Part Two each author follows the same problem-solving format to enable the reader either to focus more easily on one specific neurological problem or to address the problem from a larger perspective. Authors vary in their use of specific cognitive strategies or methods of addressing a specific neurological deficit. A variety of strategies for examining clinical problems is presented to enable the reader to see variations on the same theme and thus allow better adaptation to individual cases. Because clinicians tend to adapt learning devices to solve specific problems, many of the strategies used by one author apply to situations addressed by other authors. Readers are encouraged to use flexibility in selecting treatment with which they feel comfortable and to be creative when implementing any scheme.

Changes in evaluation methodology are reflected in many clinical problem chapters. Identification of objective measurement tools as well as a shift from a medical diagnostic to a contextual, impairment-function-disability construct is reflected in a variety of chapters. Change is inevitable and a problems-solving philosophy must reflect those changes.

Part Three of the text focuses on clinical topics that might be appropriate for any one of the clinical problems discussed in Part Two. Chapters have been added to reflect changes in focus of therapy as it evolves as an emerging flexible paradigm.

An appendix of evaluation tools presented throughout the text should help the reader easily identify the location of many objective measurement scales. The reader is reminded that although a tool may be discussed in one chapter, its use may have application to many other clinical problems. The same is true of treatment suggestions and problem solving strategies used to analyze motor control problems.

The study guide included in edition two has been deleted from the hardbound edition of the book but will be available as a paperback at publication.

CONCEPTUAL MODEL FOR EVALUATING AND TREATING NEUROLOGICAL DISABILITIES
Rationale for development of a model

Traditionally, both short-term and full-semester courses, as well as literature related to treatment of clients with CNS dysfunction, have been divided into units labeled according to a technique. Often, interrelation and integration among techniques have not been explored. As a result, **clinical problem solving** is impeded, if not stopped, when one approach fails, because little integration of theories and methods is achieved in the learning process. Learning is a sequential process in which the learner combines new information with previously acquired knowledge and integrates the whole.* Learning does not occur first by processing all information and then activating higher cognitive strategies. Rather, processing of available information and integrating that content into higher thought processes occur in an elliptical fashion. New input is constantly being retrieved from the environment while higher thought processes are integrating the information already present. Throughout life the individual is taking in new information, processing it, and storing the content appropriately for retrieval when needed for higher cortical and integrative functioning.[12,34,55]

It cannot be assumed that new information (input), when presented in fragmented units, will be integrated automatically with previously acquired information to become part of a functioning whole. This is especially true when identification of how those parts are linked to the total concept has not been made. Repetitive use of the sequencing pattern is necessary for memory. If the input (content) is totally new to the individual and thus previously stored material is not available for referencing, the new content is stored in fragmented units, but meaning is not applied. To assume the individual could use this fragmented content in flexible higher symbolic thought would be analogous to assuming that first graders, on initial introduction to concepts of addition, are ready for college calculus. The problem of introducing fragmented information has direct application to classroom learning and clinical performance. Clinicians may be bound to one specific treatment approach without the theoretical understanding of the step-by-step process, thus lacking the base for a change of direction when a treatment is ineffective. It is difficult therefore to adapt alternative treatment techniques to meet the individual needs of clients.

A conceptual model that incorporates all components of a client or all systems under the control of or that affect the client's thoughts and behaviors would potentially allow for integration of all treatment methods. It permits application of a variety of techniques because it is based on thorough understanding of the rationale or higher cognitive processing behind specific actions by the clinician and reactions by the

---

*References 13, 20, 30, 31, 43, 51, 60, 63, and 66.

*References 9, 15, 21, 34, 40, 41, 54, and 55.

client. This model or systems approach could look at motor behavior as the end product of all systems or at the motor system and all its subsystems. How a therapist conceptualizes his or her profession and its interlocking components determines and directs the paradigm and limits placed on that model.[6,20,51] How the therapist delineates any aspect of a subsection can determine the specificity or generality of his or her conceptual model.

Widely known and accepted theorists, with the empirical support of clinicians treating individuals with CNS damage, have identified a need for an upgraded, integrated approach to education, especially with regard to text and reference books. It is hoped that this book will continue to provide the background for such change. The conceptual models presented here are based on principles of neurophysiology, human movement and theories of motor control, and human interaction and learning both procedural and declarative. Such a conceptual framework gives therapists a foundation for future growth and change. Discussions of treatment strategies are also based on neurophysiological and learning principles. Identification of clinical problems and develop-

ment of treatment programs in terms of these concepts are the two major goals of each contributor.

The clinical triad: components of the conceptual model

The majority of techniques dealing with treatment of clients with CNS damage incorporate principles of CNS function, neuroplasticity, and evaluation and treatment principles based on control over functional behaviors and adaptation to various environmental contexts. Thus the basic science of central and peripheral nervous system function and behavioral analysis of movement must be included within the conceptual model.

Of considerable significance also is the client-therapist interaction, which is labeled the **learning environment.** This may be the critical factor in clinical success or failure. Fig. 1-1 illustrates the model as a conceptual triad. All aspects occur simultaneously, yet each component has unique characteristics and influences the clinical performance of the therapist. Although each component is explored separately in the following pages, the reader should retain the

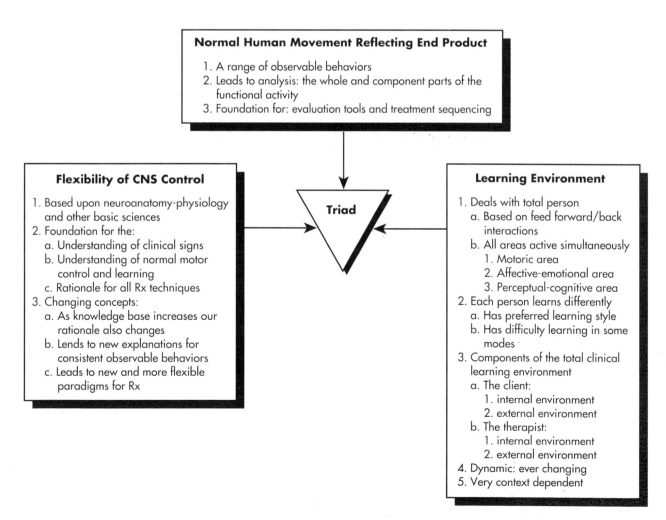

Normal Human Movement Reflecting End Product

1. A range of observable behaviors
2. Leads to analysis: the whole and component parts of the functional activity
3. Foundation for: evaluation tools and treatment sequencing

Triad

Flexibility of CNS Control

1. Based upon neuroanatomy-physiology and other basic sciences
2. Foundation for the:
   a. Understanding of clinical signs
   b. Understanding of normal motor control and learning
   c. Rationale for all Rx techniques
3. Changing concepts:
   a. As knowledge base increases our rationale also changes
   b. Lends to new explanations for consistent observable behaviors
   c. Leads to new and more flexible paradigms for Rx

Learning Environment

1. Deals with total person
   a. Based on feed forward/back interactions
   b. All areas active simultaneously
      1. Motoric area
      2. Affective-emotional area
      3. Perceptual-cognitive area
2. Each person learns differently
   a. Has preferred learning style
   b. Has difficulty learning in some modes
3. Components of the total clinical learning environment
   a. The client:
      1. internal environment
      2. external environment
   b. The therapist:
      1. internal environment
      2. external environment
4. Dynamic: ever changing
5. Very context dependent

Fig. 1-1. Clinical triad.

image of the entire model. This approach should help develop a gestalt—that is, picture of the client as a total human being even though a specific aspect of therapy may be the focus. When the client is not viewed as a whole being, the therapist often misses critical response patterns, such as movement in another body part, a grimace, or an autonomic response. These responses may be the key to successful goal attainment or client-therapist rapport.

Concept of human movement: a range of observable behaviors. As researchers continue to unravel the mysteries of brain function and learning, understanding of how children and adults learn initially or relearn following insult is often explained with new and possibly conflicting theories. Yet behavioral responses observed as functional patterns of movement, whether performed by a child, adolescent, young adult or aging person, are still visually identified by a therapist, family member, or innocent observer as either normal or abnormal.

Human beings exhibit certain movement patterns that may vary in tonal characteristics, aspects of the specific movement sequences, and even the sequential nature of development. Yet the range of acceptable behavior does have limitations, and variations beyond those boundaries are recognizable by most people. A 5-year-old child may ask why a little girl walks on her toes with her legs stuck together. If questioned, that same 5-year-old may be able to break down the specific aspects of the movement that seem unacceptable. From birth a sighted individual has observed normal human movement. Because the range of behaviors identified as normal has been established, the concept behind normal human movement can be considered a constant. This concept does provide flexibility in analysis of normal movement and its development. Some children choose creeping as a primary mode of horizontal movement, whereas others may scoot. Both forms of movement are normal for a young child. In both cases each child would have had to develop normal postural function in the head and trunk to carry out the activity in a normal fashion. Thus for the child to develop the specific functional motor behavior, the various components or systems involved in the integrated execution of the act would require modulation in a plan of action. Because the action must be carried out in a variety of environment contexts, the child would need the opportunity to practice those contexts, self-correct to regulate existing plans, identify error, and refine for skill development.[62] Thus each movement has a variety of complex systems interactions, which when summated are expressed via the motor pool to striated muscle function. The specifics of that function, whether fine or gross motor, total body or limb specific, still reflect the totality of the interaction of those systems. No matter the age of the individual, the motor response still reflects that interaction; and the behavior can be identified either normal and functional, functional but limited in adaptability, or dysfunctional and abnormal. Due to the simplicity or complexity of various movements and

the components necessary for modulatory control over various movement, therapists can (1) look at any movement pattern, (2) evaluate its components, (3) identify what is missing, and (4) incorporate treatment strategies that help the client achieve the desired function outcome. One can feel confident that no infant will be born, jump out of the womb, walk over to the doctor and shake hands, or say 'Hi' to Mom and Dad.

Instead, the infant must integrate the motor plans leading to normal rolling and head control. These plans will be modified and reintegrated along with other plans to develop normal motor control in more complex movement patterns. Each pattern and movement from one pattern to another requires time and repetition for mastery and CNS maturity.

Two very important aspects of the clinical problem-solving process emerge. First, the evaluation of motor function is based on the interaction of all the components of the motor system and the cognitive and affective influences over this motor system. Second, rehabilitation treatment strategies become clear when the therapist observes a client trying to perform specific functional behaviors and recognizes what aspects of the movement are deficient, absent, distorted, or inappropriate when cross-referenced with the desired outcome. These behaviors, although dependent on many factors, are consistent regardless of age. Certain aged clients may not have had the opportunity to mature to the desired skill, whereas others may have lost the skill due to changes within his or her CNS or disuse. In either case, the normal accepted patterns and range of behaviors remain the same. If an individual wishes to walk to the bathroom, falling will not lead to the desired outcome.

Evaluation. Before selection of an appropriate evaluation tool, the specific purpose for the request of evaluation and the model by which to interpret the meaning of the data must be identified (Fig. 1-2). Regardless of the tool selected, third-party payers are concerned with the statistics obtained through the assessment. If the therapist scores a number 12 one week and a number 14 the next and the payer knows a score of 16 means the individual's chance of falling is near normal, then the payer often permits additional visits. Those payers have little interest in the reasons why the client moved from a score of 12 to 14, only that the person is improving. This model might be considered a *statistical model* and is based on number crunching or gross quantitative measurements. If today's clinicians do not provide these types of quantitative measurements, payment for services often is denied.

Physicians use a *diagnostic model* for setting expectations of improvement or lack thereof. In patients with neurological dysfunction, physicians generally formulate their diagnosis based on complex, highly technical examinations such as magnetic resonance imaging (MRI), computed tomography (CT), positive emitting transaxial tomography (PETT), evoked potentials, and laboratory work. When abnormal results are correlated with gross clinical signs and patient

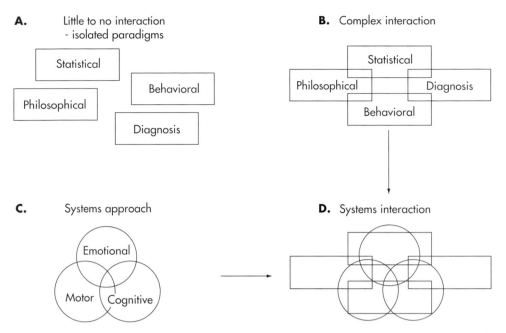

Fig. 1-2. Types of clinical models. **A,** Isolated paradigms. **B,** Complex interactive paradigms. **C,** Systems approach/paradigm. **D,** Systems interaction on traditional paradigms.

history such as high blood pressure, diabetes, or head trauma, a medical diagnosis is made along with an anticipated course of recovery or disease progression. This diagnostic model is based on an anatomical and physiological belief of how the brain functions and may or may not correlate with the *behavioral model* used by therapists. A *behavioral model* evaluates motor performance based on functional activities, which range from simple movement patterns such as rolling to complex patterns such as dressing, playing tennis, or using a word processor.

Traditional theorists such as Bobath, Brunnstrom, Feldenkrais, Knott, Rood, and Voss were keen observers of human movement and how movement distortions or limitations altered functional control. These individuals, as master clinicians, tried to explain what they were doing and why what they did worked. From their teachings developed a fourth model, which might be considered a *philosophical model*. This model is based on successful treatment procedures as identified through observation.

All four models can stand alone as acceptable models for health care (Fig. 1-2, *A*) or can interact or interconnect (Fig. 1-2, *B*). These interconnections should validate the accuracy of the data derived from each model. The concept of an integrated model, problem-solving model, or systems model does not depend on any one of the four previously mentioned models, but does identify the components that make up the client's world (internal and external) and how life and internal mechanisms affect the systems (Fig. 1-2, *C*).

The last model, *systems approach model,* can be overlaid on any other model separately or when they are interconnected (Fig. 1-2, *D*). A **systems model** is much more than

just motor and its components, or cognition with its multiple facets or the affective with all its aspects. The complexity of a systems model (Fig. 1-3), whether used for statistics, for medical diagnosis or behavioral analysis, cannot be oversimplified. As the knowledge bank of nervous and peripheral system function increases, the complexity of a systems model also enlarges. The reader must remember that each component has many interlocking subcomponents, and each of those components can be evaluated separately. Each component has many parts and each of those parts could be assessed quantitatively. Those quantitative and qualitative measurements related to specific areas of function are the guidelines therapists use to establish problem lists and treatment sequences. Those small yet critical components are of little concern within a general statistics model and may have little bearing on the medical diagnosis made by the doctor.

How the therapist evaluates for specifics necessary to establish a patient treatment protocol is based on the therapist's education, method of interpretation, and most important the evaluation tool selected by the job site. A variety of types of evaluation tools are mentioned in the following sections. How effectively the tool is used depends on the skill of the therapist and his or her problem-solving strategies and ability to extrapolate relationships between major and minor components of each system.

Sensory testing. Therapists traditionally have performed thorough peripheral sensory testing of the extremities and trunk. Whether the input is exteroceptive, as in light touch, discriminatory touch (sharp-dull, 2 point discrimination, etc.), pain, temperature, or texture, or proprioceptive (ten-

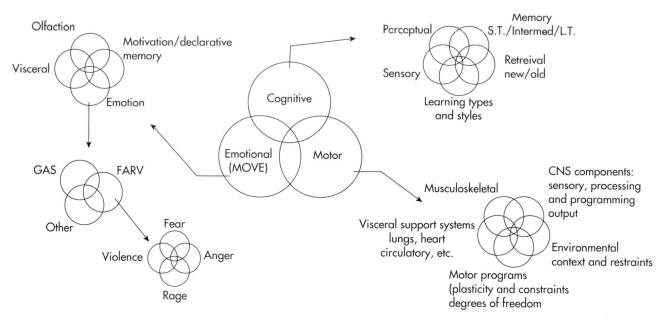

Fig. 1-3. Systems model: dynamic interactive subcomponents: whole to part to whole.

don, muscle or joint), therapists perform sensory testing to evaluate muscle, peripheral nerve, or CNS problems. Sensory testing of the vestibular system has been emphasized in balance deficits, learning disabilities, and a variety of cervical and brainstem problems. Other sensory systems such as auditory, visual, gustatory, or olfactory are often tested under cranial nerve assessments. Which tests are used and the extent of detail to which the evaluation is performed are patient dependent.

Motor performance evaluation. Some assessments have been designed to look specifically at children and evaluate whether the child is performing motor tasks that other similar-aged children are performing. Other assessments thought to be more appropriate for older children and adults were designed to look at activities these individuals perform during the day and have been labeled activities of daily living (ADL). The score for the ADL tests may or may not lead to a quantitative score which has been standardized to other individuals both of the same general age group and possibly the same diagnosis. Still others look at specific aspects of motor control such as balance, i.e., the likelihood of falling. This book presents many alternative assessments. Some assessments deal with age-specific areas, others deal with the cognitive/perceptual influence over motor control, and still others deal with activities considered necessary for independence in motor control. Which evaluation tool best meets the needs of the client and the therapist depends on many tangible and intangible variables. For the therapist to meet the demands of the third-party payer, part of that evaluation must have a quantitative, reliable, and valid measurement scale to meet the statistical model's paradigm for justification of payment. Yet, the evaluation tool must also provide enough delineated and specific information for the therapist

to understand the reasons for the list of problems and aids in guiding the direction of solution planning.

Many therapists extrapolate from what every form used, huge amounts of relevant data which is used to formulate the concept of the clinical problem of that particular client. Rood once stated that all you need to do is observe the child for a minute or two and you'll know everything there is to know. Her ability to observe, analyze movement, and extrapolate its clinical significance was truly remarkable and representative of a true master clinician. Today, many variables that therapists in past decades seemed to evaluate informally or intuitively, have been identified and can be assessed, recorded, and analyzed as separate yet interlocking components of the motor control system. As the therapeutic community integrates the research on motor control, new perspectives regarding evaluation may alter the methods and focus of assessment. The accompanying box summarizes many aspects of motor function that the therapist may choose to identify when implementing this type of assessment tool. Motor control theory (see Chapters 3 and 4) and its clinical application have opened up an avenue for new direction in analysis.

Many types of assessment forms exist and can be divided into the categories mentioned earlier. The reader must remember that all of these forms incorporate motor control variables, whether direct or indirectly assessed. Master clinicians automatically record data within their conceptual model of the client no matter the tool they use. Third-party payers to a large extent do not understand and thus do not care about the variables, but clinicians need to delineate these components to have the flexibility and insight into optimizing clinical decision making. Whether the evaluation incorporates the areas of reflex testing, aged-normed motor

---

Factors related to movement dysfunction: types of evaluation tools or questions needing attention*

A. Range of motion—differentiate joint from muscle limitations
B. Muscle strength—types of measurements
   1. Manual muscle test: MMT
   2. Dynamometer
   3. Isokinetic testing (controlled force production)
   4. ADL
C. State of the motor pool; presence of:
   1. Hypertonicity: location and extent
   2. Hypotonicity: location and extent
   3. Rigidity: location and extent
   4. Tremor (nonintentional): location and extent
D. Synergies (volitional or reflexive)
   1. What segments and in what order?
   2. Which muscles or joints does the client use to perform specific movements?
E. Postural integration
   1. Can the client hold in desired spatial positions?
   2. Can he control the proximal system or weight-bearing components while other segments are moving?
F. Balance (equilibrium)—need to determine:
   1. Sitting and standing static balance control
   2. Dynamic balance between various spatial positions, such as sitting-to-standing, walking, or higher-level activities
   3. Synergistic patterns: ankle to hip, hip to ankle
G. Speed of movement (assess quality)
   1. How fast can the patient move?
   2. What are the movement responses to speed demands?
   3. Is the rate of movement throughout the desired range appropriate for the task?
H. Timing
   1. Can the client start and stop a movement pattern appropriately, or are there delays in either initiation or stopping?
   2. Is the timing of muscle sequencing appropriate for the task?
I. Reciprocal movements
   1. Can the client change direction of a movement? If so, how easily is it performed, what rotatory components are present or absent, and are the patterns limited to only certain movement combinations?

2. What is the turnaround delay?
   a. Does the client smoothly change direction?
   b. Does the initial pattern come to a halt before the reciprocal pattern is begun?
J. Specific pattern or trajectory of the movement
   1. How smooth or jerky is the movement?
   2. What is the specific pattern of the trajectory, velocity, and acceleration curves.
K. Accuracy
   1. How accurate is the client in placement of the body or extremity in the specific desired location?
   2. Does the accuracy change as the distance or speed of the task increases or decreases?
L. Task content
   1. Is the task a new plan or retrieval of a previously learned activity?
   2. Is the difficulty of the total plan specific to one of the previous components or a combination of factors?
   3. Does the task have an emotional component that is affecting the motor outcome?
M. Endurance—differentiate disuse from cardiopulmonary function
N. Other
   1. Sensory organization intact, deficient, conflict
   2. Perception/cognition
      a. Systems
         1. Auditory
         2. Visual
         3. Kinesthetic
         4. Cross-modality
      b. Learning style performance
         1. auditory
         2. visual
         3. kinesthetic
      c. Environment context of activity
   3. Psycho/social environment
      a. Motivation
      b. Memory
      c. Autonomic stability
      d. Emotions [attitude, safety, trust, adjustment to disability]
   4. Task specificity: procedural vs. declarative

*Adapted from a presentation by Guiliani C: Motor control theory and application, informal presentation, Harmerville, PA, August, 1988, lecture notes.[26]

---

assessment, perceptual-motor planning abilities, and ADL information, all data should be consistent. At the same time, some tools emphasize additional aspects or qualities of movement, such as speed, timing, trajectory, and accuracy.

The perfect evaluation form will probably never exist. Each therapist or institution must select forms that give the staff the greatest comprehension of the client's global and specific strengths and deficits. What works best for one clinician may not work for the next. All assessments focus on behaviors, which reflect the sum total of all activities within the CNS. Motor output is like a hologram: Any aspect should give the therapist a complete picture of the patient. Some assessments are specific and others are general, yet it is the clinician's problem-solving ability that formulates the whole.

REFLEX TESTING. Fiorentino[16] developed a reflex test that can be used on both children and adults. Although her evaluation was based on the hypothesized hierarchical reflex integration within the CNS and that theory has not been shown to be valid, her evaluation of behavior and movement responses are still beneficial. The behavioral aspect of the stimulus-response pattern has been recorded for decades.[53] This reflex test is easy to administer. A therapist selects a spatial position, such as supine, elicits the stimulus, and records whether the response is present or absent and the degree of obligatory behavior. Once the assessment is completed, translating the results into meaningful information often creates a barrier for clinicians. If a client has an obligatory asymmetrical tonic neck reflex (ATNR), then many ADL are severely hampered and are not under volitional control of the motor system. An obligatory response reflects the state of the motor pool, the sensitivity of motor generators, and soft-wired motor plans and their interactions with sensory input. A reflex is not a hardwired, inflexible neurocircuit, which has lost higher center control, but rather a stereotypic system response to an environmental stimulus, which can generally be altered by many variables within the systems model. Understanding how these reflexes and reactions modulate normal activities is the key to determining whether reflex testing provides adequate evaluation data for a therapist. Fiorentino [17] discusses reflexes and their important clinical link to the analysis of CNS deficits in children. This link is also critical when looking at the adult CNS. The reader must remember that reflexes are only one aspect of the motor control system. This information alerts the clinician to important clinical elements affecting the motor behavior of the client. Whether the client is dominated by stereotypical plans, has volitional control over them, or has integrated the responses into refined and flexible motor plans are all critical aspects in analyzing the motor system and the client's level of function.

After a reflex assessment, the therapist could extrapolate range of motion (ROM), state of the motor pool, postural integrity, volitional and automatic movement, rate, trajectory, balance, etc. if those variables are part of the clinicians frame of reference when assessing the client. If according to the therapist the two conceptual ideas of reflex testing and motor control variables are separate, then little extrapolation will occur. In that case, a reflex test will not give the clinician the necessary information to either give quantitative data for justification of payment or delineated data for treatment planning.

PEDIATRIC AGE-RELATED MOTOR ASSESSMENT. A variety of norm-rated pediatric tests for infants and young children exist such as the Revised Gesell & Amatruda Developmental and Neurological Examination,[37] Bayley Scales of Infant Development,[5] and the Peabody Developmental Motor Scales.[19,61]

As researchers have improved their skills in assessment and children have accomplished tasks at earlier ages, the specific age norms for test items have changed; yet the concept has remained stable, and its popularity as an instrument for evaluating small children still persists. As with reflex testing, problems can develop in the interpretation of test results. A combination of reflex testing and age-related behavioral responses is often used with the neonate.[8,46] Understanding the tonal characteristic of in utero gestational ages seems critical when evaluating a premature or high-risk infant. This area of assessment is relatively new, and available literature is sparse.

The interaction of an age-normed test with predictive later motor performance is one way to bridge the difficult gap between assessment and expected outcomes after treatment. The Movement Assessment of Infants (MAI)[11] was designed to evaluate reflex integration, tonal patterns, volitional control, and automatic reactions over the first year of life. The test results have correlated with prediction of functional outcomes in children with cerebral palsy.[7,29]

FUNCTIONAL ACTIVITIES ASSESSMENTS. ADL evaluations are frequently used in adult testing, for example, after stroke or trauma. Forms for testing vary from clinic to clinic in specific tasks, number of test items, and emphasis on gross or fine motor skills required; but the formats have many consistent features. Categories are sequenced from basic motor skills, such as bed mobility, to complex motor plans, such as dressing.

The items within each category progress from simple to complex. Early ADL evaluations were designed through trial and error. Therapists realized that clients needed bed mobility skills, such as rolling, moving in bed, reaching for objects, and rising to a sitting position, before they were ready to achieve tasks such as transfers. Transfer skills normally precede walking activities. Achieving functional sitting and trunk stability is critical for addition of more complex upper-extremity and trunk skills, such as dressing and eating. Thus the sequential design of these tests developed through the success-to-failure ratio of the client's achievements.

Determining the reason a client cannot achieve bed mobility, including moving in bed, rolling, and coming to sit patterns, can be an important question. This individual might first need to modify and control some reflexes before attaining success. For example, if a client with head trauma were dominated by ATNR and tonic labyrinthine reflex (TLR), then rolling over and general bed mobility would be prevented. Depending on the movement patterns the client used to come to a sitting position, the two reflexes could also prevent that integrated motion. The ATNR would prevent the client from using a prone to crawling to side sitting to long sitting pattern because as the head turned, the arm closest to the skull would flex and be unable to support weight. The same problem would exist if a client used a side-lying, partial-rotation, coming-to-sitting pattern. The TLR, on the other hand, would stop the client from using a symmetrical supine-to-sit pattern, which requires neck and abdominal flexion in a supine position. These same and additional stereotypical motor plans could hamper transfers and disrupt more complex motor plans to be used as part of the ADL assessment. In addition, rotatory and postural skills used in bed mobility are foundation skills for transfers. Without these skills more complex activities, such as transfers or dressing, are impossible. Thus ADL forms have a motor control component base. Reflex testing and motor control components can be extracted from the results of an ADL test. Similarly, after evaluating a client with a reflex test or looking at motor control components during activities, a clinician should be able to deduce the majority of test item results on an ADL checklist.

Scales such as the Barthel Index,[44] the Katz,[35] and the Kurtzke[38,39] were developed to measure ADL skills on a quantitative scale to identify valid and reliable ways to measure functional change. Granger[25] developed the PULSES Profile, which again looked at ADL skills but incorporated additional factors such as support systems and other bodily functions interactions. As early as the 1970s people were verbally and in writing describing the relationship between functional outcomes and multiply systems interaction even though the words and terminology used to describe the behaviors have changed. In reality those interactions have always been present and may have laid the foundation for medicine in ancient times.

In the late 1970s and 1980s a variety of functional assessments were being developed. Certain assessments focused on specific clinical problems such as stroke,[10,23] whereas others looked at functional activities in relation to independence or lack thereof in daily life.[35,39,44]

The concept of outcome measurements and their relationship to independence, potential handicap, and cost to society have been intertwined with motor control and motor learning theory. The use of functional assessment that have a valid and reliable quantitative score has become increasingly more popular than earlier accepted measurement tools such as reflex tests and descriptive analysis.

An adaptation of the Functional Independence Measure (FIM) for pediatrics was introduced in 1988 called the Wee-FIM.[24] Haley and others[27] have gone one step further and developed the Pediatric Evaluation of Disability Inventory (PEDI), which has been standardized and normed on children from 6 months to 7 years of age.

Whether the functional assessment was designed for general use, for a specific age range, or a specific patient population, the items tested only give the therapist fragmented information regarding the totality of the patient. How the therapist interprets this information and intertwines the data with all other information obtained from or about the patient will determine appropriate goal setting and treatment planning. Tests that focus on smaller components of motor function such as balance, gait, reach, and potential falling, are used to assess specific functional movements and their components (see Chapters 13, 14, and 28). These specific

tests should be selected based on the specific needs of the client and therapist not on their generalizability for predicting all other aspects of daily activities.

PERCEPTUAL/COGNITIVE ISSUES IN ASSESSMENT OF PERFORMANCE. Psychologists and educators have stressed the importance of cognitive/perceptual issues when measuring motor performance.[3,18,22,57,68] The results not only provide data regarding gross and fine motor functioning but also focus on many specific perceptual and cognitive skills. A clear understanding of the normal development of declarative verses procedural learning and the influence on either system after CNS damage is vital in planning successful treatment of any client with a neurological deficit. Ayers[2,18] has been a principal leader in theory and implementation of perceptual-cognitive sequencing related to both physical and occupational therapy settings. Her research emphasis was in the area of learning disabilities, but her concepts and treatment sequences have far-reaching implications. As with the other forms of evaluation, interpretation of the results in each category is the most challenging aspect. Because of the complexity of higher-order problems encountered in this form of evaluation, interpretation of the reasons why a client may not be able to perform a specific test item may be overlooked. This interpretation and integration problem is significantly influenced by the medical-model approach to evaluation, in which a clinician identifies problem areas, evaluates only those problems, and then treats them. If instead therapists evaluate systems, they can then determine what perceptual strategies are functioning when the client performs successfully on a test item. Once analysis of intact systems and their component parts has been made, specific deficits in those systems can be identified and approached.

Summary. As with all assessments that have longevity, the use of the tool will change as the understanding of how and why the results obtained are truly reflective of CNS processing. As long as therapists are honest in their observation skill, evaluation batteries from the past will continue to be useful into the future, although the interpretations and predictive abilities may change as research clarifies confusion.

One of the characteristics of a highly skilled therapist is the ability to extract essential information from a variety of sources. The skilled therapist looks beyond the obvious interpretations for subtle clues to CNS dysfunctions.

As systems interactions become a comfortable part of therapeutic evaluation, regardless of the tests used to assess motor performance, all aspects of the individual will need to be considered to truly identify the clinical problems and predictive outcomes. Fig. 1-4 illustrates four clients with different systems involvement. Client A has a very low volitionally functioning motor system, but is highly motivated and cognitively aware of the problem. If the motor strategies are not regained or a form of motor expression established, the motivation of the client to continue trying

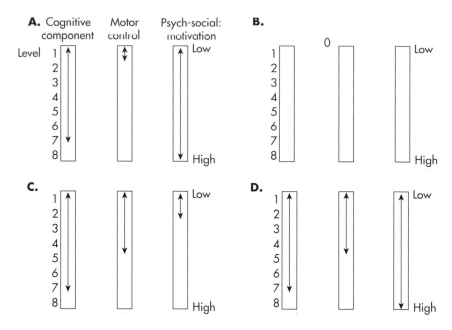

Fig. 1-4. Systems evaluation models of four clients.

may decrease. Client B has no motor function or has a locked-in syndrome. Many colleagues see these people in a vegetated state, but behaviorally the cognitive and affective components cannot be evaluated accurately. The emotional state can somewhat be assessed via the autonomic system, but that measure is very subjective. Clients C and D have the same functional control over their motor systems and the same cognitive ability, but represent different clinical problems. Client C is not motivated and unless the therapist can change the attitude, little functional change can be anticipated. Client D, who is highly motivated, will most likely adapt and modify the nervous system to maintain and regain functional control and empowerment over his or her quality of life.

This systems model easily integrates into behavioral models for evaluation and treatment of physical disabilities as presented by Nagi[49,50] and Wood.[67] As therapeutic emphasis is shifting from a medical model of diagnosis and prognosis to a **disablement model,**[58] the primary focus of evaluation and treatment is on the impairment (systems interaction) and how those systems interactions affect functional outcomes (Fig. 1-5). Whether the functional limitations and strengths lead to a disability or to adaptation and adjustment will determine the eventual quality of life and **empowerment** an individual will have over his or her life. Within each component of the disablement paradigm, risk factors occur that can be environmental, psychosocial, or CNS related. These risk factors can positively or negatively affect the process and eventual outcome.

As risk factors change so can the evolving process. For example, an individual with a spinal lesion may initially sequence through the schema and be considered moderately to severely disabled. The social environment is in shambles, the emotional system suicidal and the functional motor skills at various levels between dependent to independent. The financial risk to society is high. A year later this person meets a significant other who does not perceive this person as disabled. Instead, the significant other encourages the client to go back to school, start playing wheelchair sports, and father their children. The impairments still exist, but functional strength has increased. The client is adapting and no longer has a self-image as disabled. The quality of life is under the client's empowerment and the risk to society minimal. Thus this disablement process can be in a constant state of dynamic flux and can never be considered static.

Treatment planning. During the last 30 years treatment sequencing has often been associated with the term *developmental sequencing.* It was hypothesized that for a patient to gain motor control and learning over a specific functional activity, the patient needed to gain function over all movement patterns that a child practiced before developing that skill. Today, research has shown that the motor plans needed to carry out a functional activity are specific to that activity; to assume that one activity will automatically lead to another is no longer valid.[59,62,66] This change in treatment philosophy does not mean that individuals no longer need to practice rolling for bed mobility or coming to sitting to change spatial positions, or to use kneeling, half-kneeling to stand to get off the floor. It does mean that if independent sitting while eating, reaching, or dressing is a goal of treatment, the individual needs to practice that activity while sitting. The therapist would obviously evaluate sitting as an ADL task and needs to determine the motor control

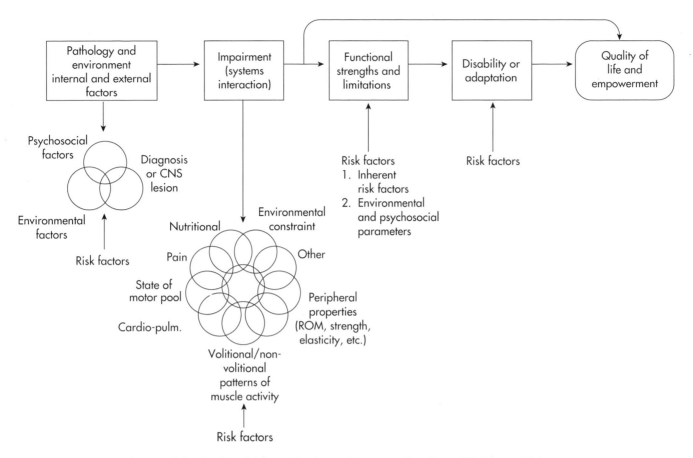

Fig. 1-5. Behavioral model for evaluation and treatment: based on a Disablement Schema.

components that might be missing. Differentiating lack of pelvic mobility or ROM from postural instability or from other motor control components would determine what specific procedural aspects of sitting were causing the difficulty. Once that diagnostic differentiation has been made specific, treatment alternatives can be selected that allow practice or modification of those particular components that are causing difficulty. That practice needs to have repetition with enough variance that the client can self-correct error in the specific activity.

It cannot be overemphasized that the context in which the client practices is a critical component to learning or relearning motor control.[28] If sitting balance has been determined to be the missing or a deficit component and the client needs to be able to sit independently in a chair in order to dress, then a specific environmental context has been identified. This context has interlocked with the deficit component to direct treatment. The therapist now knows that the patient needs to practice on a noncompliant surface while dressing, eating, talking, writing, etc. Sitting on a therapeutic ball or compliant surface would be out of context and not the primary choice of seated surface. If on the other hand the client wants to fish while sitting in his or her boat, then the environmental context has changed and a compliant surface

would be more appropriate. If time permits, obviously the therapist would like the client to be able to balance on all surfaces.

How to sequence specific activities has also shifted from a developmental perspective to outcome measurement concepts. If a goal of treatment is for a client to independently come out of a chair to standing and then sit back down, how a therapist progresses will again be variable specific. Coming out of a chair requires a plan of action, with the goal of stopping in a vertical position while weight bearing on both feet. Sitting back down, especially with control, also is a plan- or goal-directed activity. Thus the total activity may require a shift in plans between coming to standing, standing, and sitting back down. Which plan is practiced first is not as critical as the final sequential practice of the entire goal-specific task. Thus beginning in relaxed standing and working toward sit may modulate eccentric volitional control of the postural extensor system while working on strength, control over synergic patterns and coactivation, trajectory, rate, etc. and while being contextually accurate. Having the client begin to sit and then regain standing incorporates balance, change in postural set, change in plans, etc. Once the individual can sit down with control, he or she will already have the plan of coming to stand and stopping in standing because that was repetitively practiced while learning to sit.

Another critical variable to consider would be drawing cognitive attention off the task in order to practice the procedure as a procedure. This can be accomplished by talking to the patient or having the patient sit while holding something that might spill or drop. These contextually accurate activities are not new ideas or new tasks, just new words to describe master clinicians' visual observations.

Rood emphasized that the postural system needed to learn to hold against resistance, release the hold first in weight-bearing and then in non-weight bearing if appropriate.[52a] The previously described activity of stand-to-sit-to-stand clearly represents Rood's concept of a (1) shortened held-resisted contraction (volitional standing) and (2) mobility in a weight-bearing pattern (controlled eccentric lengthening toward sit and concentric control back to stand). Although Rood's neurophysiological explanation for why she thought a treatment sequence promoted motor learning may have been inaccurate, it does not negate the fact that the treatment may have worked. As the professions shift in terminology, philosophy, and paradigms, it is paramount that the successes of the past not be lost or unsuccessful treatment protocols be maintained for sentiment. Therapists will need to analyze treatment protocols from the past and determine their validity as they will need to do for all new ideas, philosophies, and treatment suggestions. Because someone says a procedure will promote motor learning or motor control does not and never has guaranteed its effectiveness. Its efficacy has to come from case studies and research and needs to have some quantifiable measurement to convince all individuals of its validity.

When the therapist and client identify functional activities that the client wishes to achieve, the therapist needs to determine whether the function is within the possibility of success by the client. Once those goals have been established and the functional outcome determined as much as possible, the therapist needs to analyze the movement activities in regard to motor control components. Table 1-1 illustrates how functional movement might be analyzed with regard to the movement patterns, softwired nervous system, cognitive-perceptual influences, and various motor control components. From these schema a clinician can determine what factors are interacting to assist in regaining motor control over the desired functional activity and which factors are preventing attainment of the functional goal. With this information the therapist should be able to determine how to go about establishing a treatment protocol that optimizes the client's potential to attain the desired goal. Example 2, coming to sitting, requires movement patterns made up of multiple component sequences. Given the complexity of so basic a movement pattern, it is no wonder that helping a client accomplish such activities as dressing, climbing on and off a bus, or achieving wheelchair independence may be frustrating to client and to health personnel. Therefore it is important for the therapist to explain that even though a task may seem simple, it is composed of many integrated parts that may be critical for a more complex activity.

Although only two activities are presented in Table 1-1, any functional activity can be analyzed by using the same factors. The specifics for each activity will vary and always have an environmental context component that is patient related. A therapist who understands normal movement patterns through observation can easily detect deviations from normal and degrees of abnormality. Gross to finite aspects of abnormal patterns can be identified by components.

Once identification has been made, goals for correction of those deviations can be established and treatment begun. Treatment should be based not only on observable behavior, but also on understanding of CNS function. For example, when analyzing a hemiplegic gait pattern, a therapist can identify the total movement pattern as one unit or can break down the pattern into components. Each aspect of the gait cycle—from heel strike, mid-stance, push off, to swing through, which consists of trunk, hip, knee, and ankle movement patterns—can be examined. If joint motion functions normally throughout the gait cycle, no intervention would be indicated. With deviations, such as the substitution of plantar flexion of the foot for dorsiflexion, treatment procedures to correct the difficulty can be selected. For example, a therapist might select a proprioceptive neuromuscular facilitation (PNF) pattern to facilitate dorsiflexion at push off, or tapping or vibrating with resistance of the dorsiflexors and evertors during swing phase. Although each joint action needs attention, the interaction of all joints during any phase of gait is even more critical. Consequently, once normal and deviant patterns have been identified, the combined responses of all muscles—and thus joint action—can be analyzed for each component of the cycle.

Combining total patterns of trunk and leg movement to correct deviations would be another important treatment protocol. Sequencing the treatment activity to a movement pattern less complex than a gait motion would be one way to recombine total patterns into normal movement sequences. For example, a client may be unable to go into dorsiflexion during stance phase, thus remaining in plantar flexion and altering the trunk, hip, and knee action. One treatment possibility is to work on half-kneel–to–stand or modified squat-to-stand over a bolster. These patterns maintain dorsiflexion while the hip and knee go into extension. This occurs for many physiological reasons. First, because total flexion inhibits extension, the client initially would be placed in flexion. In addition, heavy joint approximation, especially down through the heel, tends to facilitate a postural weight-bearing pattern and modify the positive supporting pattern elicited by pressure on the ball of the foot. Additional treatment procedures, such as quick stretch, resistance, tapping, and prolonged stretch, when

Table 1-1. Concept of sequential development as a treatment progression

Movement patterns	Softwired programs that assist	Softwired programs that prevent	Necessary perceptual concepts	Motor control components	Treatment sequences
Activity: horizontal movement—rolling					
1. Start at head a. Head flexion with rotation or head extension with rotation b. UE, trunk, and LE follow in appropriate sequential progress	Neck righting Optic and labyrinthine righting	Tonic labyrinthine reflex Asymmetrical tonic neck reflex	Limited at this level if therapist elicits response manually Complex if therapist expects client to perform from either auditory or visual cues	ROM Strength State of motor pool Postural integrity Balance Synergies Rate Trajectory Environmental context	Modify programs preventing behavior Elicit neck righting via any number of treatment techniques Use treatment techniques when appropriate, according to desired neurophysiological response
2. Start at LE a. Supine to prone—LE: flexion, adduction, internal rotation, followed by trunk and head in appropriate progression b. Prone to supine—LE: extension, abduction, external rotation, followed by trunk and head in appropriate progression					
Activity: Coming to sit from horizontal					
1. Roll to prone and push up a. Rolling patterns b. Postural tone in prone c. Movement patterns from prone to four-point to sitting d. Postural tone in sitting e. Balance in sitting					
2. Partial rotation a. Rolling patterns b. Head, trunk, and shoulder stability in asymmetrical pattern c. Balancing from side to sitting d. Asymmetrical patterns in LE and possibly UE e. Same as *d* and *e* in no. *1*					
3. Adult sitting a. Symmetrical head and trunk flexion, LE extension b. Balance from supine to sitting c. Same as *d* and *e* in no. *1* under coming to sit					

Comments: When would you encourage neck righting versus body on body on head righting and vice versa? *Why?* When would you encourage one coming-up-to-sitting activity versus another, and *why?* UE, Upper extremity; LE, lower extremity.

applied to the appropriate muscle groups or synergistic patterns, can further enhance a normal combination of muscle activity.

Once the client is able to initiate the desired plan or movement sequence, the therapist needs to remove the external/contrived treatment and allow the client to practice the activity with error and variations of the initial task. The movement needs practice in many environmental contexts to guarantee carry-over in normal daily living activities. The repetition needs to be on a feedforward plan and under inherent self-correcting modulatory control. (Refer to Chapters 3 and 4 for additional information.)

The concept of normal movement does not translate into a hierarchy of movement in which a patient must, for example, roll before sitting. Instead it presents the concept that all behaviors can be broken down into components. Each component may, in and of itself, be a separate behavior. How components combine and the number of component combinations needed in any one behavior determine the difficulty of the task. Prior learning versus new learning play significant roles in task difficulty. Familiarity with the spatial position in which the task is presented plays a key role in success. For example, eating while sitting and eating while side-lying are two totally different movement combinations, yet the task goal is the same. Side-lying may give greater support, but vertical positioning is more familiar.

To have higher-level motor control, a person needs the schemata and plans necessary to implement the behavior. Some behaviors are best practiced as a whole activity (coming to stand from a chair), whereas others can easily be learned as component parts (a tennis serve). To find the best learning environment, including how to teach tasks effectively, is the goal of all therapeutic techniques. Each instructor teaching a particular approach feels that his or her way is the most viable, and because so many colleagues with so many methods seem to create positive changes in client behavior, it might seem that all methods are viable. What will best fit each client may be client dependent and needs to be evaluated by the problem-solving clinician.

Concept of CNS control: a multicomplex control system. The concept of CNS control is based on a therapist's understanding of the CNS and how it regulates response patterns. This understanding, which requires in-depth background in neuroanatomy and neurophysiology, gives the therapist the basis for clinical application and treatment. Understanding the intricacies of neuromechanisms provides therapists with direction as to when, why, and in what order to use clinical treatment techniques. Behaviors are based on maturation, potential, and degeneration of the CNS. Each behavior observed, sequenced, and integrated as a treatment protocol should be interpreted according to neurophysiological and anatomical principles. Unfortunately, our knowledge of behavior is ahead of our understanding of the intricate mechanism of the CNS. Thus the

correlation of vital links between observed behavior and CNS processing is not always known

Because information about the functioning of the CNS is constantly increasing, the rationale for the use of certain treatment techniques may also change. This change can create frustration among therapists who desire solutions and treatment rationales that are reliable, valid, and constant. Because it is unrealistic to expect to know all the answers, therapists should keep abreast of the literature and be open to new ideas. The following example illustrates this need.

Assume I were to learn Rood's concept of cocontraction, which is based on the intricate neuromechanism of the interaction of the Ia and II sensory receptors within the muscle spindle. Rood's theory assumes that the II receptors are polysynaptic and facilitate the antagonist of the postural muscle. I then discover that some II receptors are monosynaptic,[18] which would put the validity of Rood's rationale in question. My clinical observations produce the same doubt. That is, while observing postural muscles after CNS insult in adults, I note two behaviors that contradict Rood's theory: first, a hypertonic postural muscle rarely facilitates antagonistic activity. Second, I note that a client who gains some voluntary control over the postural muscle, especially in the shortened range, is not necessarily able to facilitate coactivation. In fact, the postural muscle seems to function optimally in a movement pattern but has great difficulty holding in an isometric pattern. Further, even more frustration occurs when the therapist tries to elicit dynamic-automatic cocontraction. Both clinical problems suggest that the II receptors, at a spinal level, may not be the mechanism for cocontraction. In fact, it may not be the spindle receptors at all that modulate over postural function.

Thus I face a dilemma. I have two recourses. First, I can decide that Rood is wrong and thus her approach invalid, and I can discard all of the treatment procedures classified under that technique. Or, I could choose a second strategy knowing that Rood's method for developing coactivation has worked effectively on many clients, I can assume that the techniques or methods are reliable and viable treatment approaches but that the *reason* why they work can no longer be explained by Rood's theory. A new rationale might follow the assumption that postural control and dynamic coactivation are regulated at multiple levels within the CNS.

To program the function of dynamic coactivation, creating an environment conducive for learning that motor function would be important. The CNS would need to be placed in an environmental context that requires postural muscles to successfully carry out a functional task. First, the CNS would need to regulate the coactivation necessary for motor control components within the plan of action. Creating an environment where the system can control and practice that control seems consistent with motor control theory. If the control was first activated in the shortened range where (1) joint limitations help to stop the movement, (2) the postural muscles' afferent sensitivity would require CNS modulation, and (3) joint compression as weight-bearing would encourage the cerebellum to coactivate for peripheral stability, the shortened range would be the best place to begin treatment. Because the muscle's function is primarily to hold, asking the client to hold rather than move would again be consistent. To increase feedback to the CNS and develop better internal stretch and strength, resistance would also be indicated. Allowing the client to practice that holding while concentrating on a functional task that takes attention away from conscious holding and turns it into a procedural task would again be consistent with motor learning and motor control theory.

Thus I could conclude that Rood's concept of shortened, held, resisted contraction (SHRC) as well as her sequences are still valid treatment approaches. Although this new rationale would be based on current neurophysiological concepts, in time it might also be shown to be invalid. If so, a new mechanism would be sought to take its place if the behavioral responses remain consistent.

Our understanding of the brain is still fragmented and incomplete. The more we learn, the more we are astounded and frustrated by its complexity. The problem can be likened to the technological advances of recent years. This rapid influx of knowledge, often contradicting past beliefs, creates anxiety and confusion. Thus a clinician must try to keep abreast of current scientific concepts, research, and facts by either continuing education and focusing on neuroapplication, or by reading and applying advances from current textbooks. Without updated information, colleagues begin to feel that the CNS is beyond their grasp.

When a topic defies easy comprehension, people may create myths to make the complexity seem accessible. Although myths make people feel secure, they are constantly under attack. This again creates anxiety and, often, defensive behavior until a new, more acceptable myth can be established. Myths are found not only in highly technological fields but in all avenues of life. One of the best-established myths within the field of physical and occupational therapy is that the various approaches to treating children or adults with neurological impairment have no similarities or that traditional treatment philosophies have no basis in motor control theories as presented today.

A clinician often hears a colleague say, "The technique I am using is the only one that adequately treats the client according to a valid rationale." Another myth is the assumption that approaches developed to treat neurological conditions have no relevance in such specialties such as orthopedics, sports, or psychiatry. When someone attacks those beliefs, many clinicians become uncomfortable.

Before we discard the notion that commonalities may exist or that an integrated whole may be found, it might be advantageous to go back 40 or 50 years. At that time Berta Bobath, Margaret Rood, Signe Brunnstrom, Temple Fay,

Margaret Knott, Dorthy Voss, Moshe Feldenkrais, and others were working as clinicians trying to treat their clients with the most current techniques available. All of these colleagues were gifted in their clinical abilities. Over time they conceptualized strategies and treatment sequences, which they explained with available scientific knowledge. Their main goal was client care, not establishment of a dynasty. As these talented, intelligent pioneers tried to share their concepts with colleagues, many therapists had difficulty understanding the rationale, but they recognized that the technique worked.

Currently, it seems a dilemma has developed that has created havoc within the field. A clinician who is comfortable and successful with one approach and understands only its rationale (i.e., refuses to explore other approaches) reinforces the myth that this approach is far superior to all others or that it is the only valid approach. As large numbers of colleagues begin to accept such a myth, strong lines of defense are built. Lack of communication and growth very often results, which is in direct opposition to the objectives of those who created the techniques.

Clinicians in the 1990s may have been told that traditional approaches such as neurodevelopmental therapy (NDT), Rood, etc., were grounded in totally inaccurate theory. They were based on concepts of feedback not feedforward and hard-wired hierarchical CNS and used constant feedback, which meant that the neurophysiological inaccuracy would not help the client learn or relearn good motor control. From the verbal discussion, many colleagues believe that those traditional approaches should be abandoned and functional activities practiced. The question arises: Are colleagues just shifting paradigms and placing rigid structure around what they believe to be motor control treatment techniques? If so a new approach will have developed, which may be said to be as rigid and structured as older traditional methodologies.

Approximately 30 years ago a large number of colleagues met to try to dissolve barriers and regain the momentum of growth and understanding of the whole.[52] At this meeting various treatment approaches, based on neurophysiological and orthopedic principles, were presented. It was the intent of these colleagues to identify commonalities and develop integrated trends among the various methods. Some evidence strongly suggests that clinicians have come closer to a gestalt approach rather than become more fragmented and territorially defensive. Farber[14] and Randolf and Heiniger[56] published books emphasizing the importance of an integrated approach to client care based primarily on our understanding of the CNS. More and more courses at undergraduate and graduate levels are being offered that focus on clinical problems and alternative treatments. This is not to negate the importance of in-depth knowledge and training that may emphasize a specific philosophy toward client care. As long as clinicians strive toward a better understanding of the whole and avoid falling into the trap that one fragment is the whole, they and the professions they represent will continue to change, grow, and offer better services to the public.

In the early 1990s a second symposium was created to bring new theory and knowledge to colleagues, which would survey contemporary issues related to the treatment of children and adults with motor control disorders. Much debate, arguments, and territorial guarding were observed during the first half of the symposium. As commonalities were identified, differences accepted, and mutual unknowns acknowledged, colleagues began again to integrate their knowledge and tremendous growth pursued. Within the pages of this book links between both the past and the future reflect the fluid evolution of our professions. At no time will all colleagues be comfortably stationed at the same point, nor will we all be moving at the same speed or in the same specific direction. Nevertheless, growth is a key element to the continual maturation of all professions working in the area of motor control. Basic and applied science research will continue to change our ideas, theories, or practice. This change should improve the quality and efficacy of our treatments and eventually positively affect the quality of life of our patients.

In this book classifications of common treatment techniques, based on principles of neurophysiology, are presented to help the reader conceptualize the whole and develop an integrated treatment approach. (See Chapter 6 for additional information.)

Because this book focuses on a problem-oriented approach using a conceptualized model, a word of caution is in order. Our knowledge of the CNS is in its infancy; it is easy to identify myths from the past, but it is just as easy to create new myths. Although use of the concept of neurophysiology to explain clinical symptoms, treatment rationales, and observable behaviors is valid, details will change as our scientific knowledge grows.

Because of the plasticity of the nervous system and the multitract nature of any one response, the potential of the CNS to change seems great. All techniques are based on this assumption. If presented with an environment conducive to change, people will, theoretically, change. The importance of this principle leads us to the third concept of the model used in this book.

Concept of the learning environment. Critical to the clinical triad of our conceptual model is the concept of the learning environment. Clinicians spend a lifetime learning and teaching yet probably never intensively reflect on how they learn or how others learn from them. Understanding personal learning styles and how that leads to perceptions and responses helps the clinician understand why he or she behaves in certain ways. It also helps in becoming tolerant of clients and their variant cognitive, affective, and motor systems (CAM). By assessing the client for intact subcomponents of all three systems (CAM), the therapist-client will have a better understanding of (1) how the client best

learned, (2) whether those processes are still available, and (3) the potential for alternative learning mechanisms to access the motor systems. The master clinician seems to know how to manipulate the environment by both increasing and decreasing all variables, similar to the way in which a conductor modulates a large orchestra. It is beautiful to watch but difficult to grasp its complexity.

Awareness of and sensitivity to this learning process is vital. Gifted clinicians can be found in each field of the health care system. When these individuals are observed treating clients, it often seems as if the clients demonstrate marked improvement, show a high potential for future achievement and experience carry-over in learning. A phenomenon can be seen even in a short time spent observing clinician with client. The observing therapist may write down step by step what the master therapist does with the client and may formulate it into an optimal treatment plan. Yet the therapist may attempt the plan with a client and find that it does not work—that the client is unable to function at the high level expected and may indeed be successful only with those skills already acquired. This leaves the clinician frustrated and the client unable to achieve the desired level of function.

The question arises as to why the sequence worked effectively with one therapist on one day and not on the next with the other therapist. Many answers can be hypothesized. First, the gifted clinician has some "magic healing power." Second, the gifted clinician did not tell the observing group what was truly going on. Third, the second clinician's skills are inadequate for effective therapy. Fourth, the client did not practice; thus there was little carry-over. Fifth, the initial clinician used extrinsic feedback to correct the movement problems and there was little intrinsic carry-over. For most clients, tremendous carry-over occurred, but difficulty arose in making transitions to new functions not addressed by the master clinician and taught by the regular therapist. This carry-over suggests that the initial clinician did use treatment concepts (either consciously or intuitively) that reflect motor control and learning theory. Although any one of the five explanations come quickly to mind, a more accurate explanation may be found by analyzing the learning environment.

Each clinician, as well as each client, processes millions of bits of sensory data each second. How that information is processed and how appropriate response patterns are implemented constitute a unique characteristic of each individual. When two people are interacting, as in a client-therapist relationship, each person is responding to the moment-to-moment changes occurring within the environment. At no time is that environment the same. Thus the therapist has the responsibility of interacting dynamically with the client to create an optimal situation. An analogy might be made between the therapist and a multimillion channel biofeedback system. The more skillful the therapist, the more channels he or she is able to modulate. The therapist is responsible not only for processing information within his or her CNS, but also for directing the way the client processes within his or her CNS. This interaction is not just a sensorimotor exchange but incorporates the entire client-therapist interaction. Thus perceptual, cognitive, and affective channels must be established, and a method of processing the data flowing through those channels must be found. Master therapists seem to grasp this totality and create a treatment sequence that guides the client toward optimal independence. It does not seem to be the sequential steps themselves that are the clues to successful treatment but rather the dynamic interaction of the therapist and client taking those steps. Thus a different therapist using the same sequential steps with the same client might be unsuccessful. The difference in interaction may account for the failure or success of that treatment plan, carry-over, and long-term retention.

If indeed the learning environment must be client-therapist dependent, then regimented, preestablished treatment plans would not promote optimal learning for each client because they could not take into consideration individual differences. Clients need acute care, rehabilitation, or home health services, whether they have sustained a CNS insult or a severe orthopedic injury; they need to learn or relearn something, either a psychomotor skill or cognitive process. The individual who is relearning to walk after a stroke, a total hip replacement, or an amputation faces an environment that is different in place and time from the one in which that individual took his or her first steps. Additional problems of distorted and diminished sensory imput; processing of cognitive, perceptual, and affective data; and motor output may confound the relearning process. Seldom in a rehabilitation setting can a client be a passive participant while a clinician acts on that person. For this reason no matter what the therapist's background, knowledge, or clinical skill, both the client and the therapist are actively involved in what can be referred to as the clinical learning environment. Success within this area depends on the therapist's problem-solving abilities, flexibility in creating environments conducive to client learning, sensitivity to client needs, and various opportunities for the client to gain personal control over his or her life, both internally and externally.

The concept of the learning environment is the most abstract and complex of the three concepts in the theoretical model. For that reason it is by far the hardest to present in concrete terms. Both simultaneous and successive components formulate and maintain this environment. At any one moment multitudinous input events occur simultaneously and continuously. Thus a temporal ordering of successive events plays a role in the CNS response to the environment. To comprehend the dynamics of this interaction and be able to function with optimal success, the clinician must:

1. Understand the learning process to provide an environment that promotes learning.
2. Investigate the input, processing, feedforward, feedback, and output system as a vital servomechanism for higher-order learning.
3. Understand higher-order processing, procedural learning, practice scheduling, reinforcement concepts, and other motor control principles if carry-over of treatment into other environments, such as the home, is to be expected.
4. Differentiate how he or she learns from how the client learns. If these learning styles conflict, then the clinician needs to teach through the client's preferential systems or learning styles.
5. Be aware simultaneously of the motoric, affective, and cognitive aspects of an individual, no matter what the clinical emphasis might be at any one time.

Four distinct components of the learning environment must be identified and addressed: the internal and external environments of the client and the internal and external environments of the clinician (Fig. 1-6).

The client's internal environment is an obvious focus of all health care professionals. A lesion has occurred within the system and is affecting how the entire mechanism functions. If the lesion occurred before initial learning, then habilitation must take place. Although a learning style has not yet been established, the individual probably has a genetic predispo-

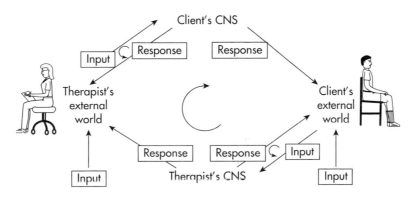

Fig. 1-6. Clinical learning environment.

sition. The therapist should test the inexperienced CNS by creating experiences in various contexts that require a variety of types of higher order processing to discover optimal methods of learning that best suit the CNS of the client. Then the therapist can focus treatment on the most effective strategies. If previous learning has occurred and preferential systems have been established, then the therapist needs to know what they are and whether they have been affected by the insult so that proper rehabilitation can be instituted. The use of preferential modes such as visual versus verbal or kinesthetic versus verbal does not mean that other modes are ineffective. Nor do all modes function optimally in any given situation.

One way to determine general preestablished preferential styles is by taking a thorough history. Leisure-time activities and job choice often give clues to learning styles. For example, a client who loved to take car engines apart or build model ships demonstrates preference to visual-spatial learning style, whereas another client, whose preference for pure enjoyment was sitting in a chair with a novel, demonstrates a probable preference toward verbal learning. Again, this does not mean both clients could not selectively use both methods, but it does illustrate preference. Both the position of the lesion and preferential learning styles can play a key role in matching the learner with a particular environment and in identifying potential. If a client has suffered massive insult to the left temporal lobe and before the trauma showed poor ability in using the right parietooccipital lobe, then spatial or verbal strategies may be ineffective in the relearning process. However, a client with the same lesion, who had high-level right parietooccipital function before the insult, will probably learn at a much faster rate if visual-kinesthetic strategies are used to promote learning.

The client's external environment is the second critical component. All external stimuli, including noise, lighting, temperature, touch, humidity, and smell, modulate the client's internal responses. This external input can invoke negative and positive influences on the internal mechanism and alter the client's ability to manipulate his or her world. Because a therapist should make every effort to be aware of what is happening to the client externally, knowing generally what is happening within and outside the hospital is important. Any behavioral change displayed by the client, such as mood, attitude, or muscle tone change, should serve as an indicator to the therapist that a change may have occurred. Following up that observation by determining what happened can help the therapist not only in understanding but in assisting the client to deal with environmental change or in obtaining additional professional assistance.

The clinician should also be aware of personal internal and external factors that influence patient responses. Everyone has preferential styles of teaching and learning, yet many may be unaware of what they are and how they affect outlook on life and interaction with other people. A common example of a mismatch of styles is what happens when two people are arguing opposing sides of a political issue. Although both individuals may process the same data, they may also have different learning strategies and come up with very different conclusions.

The interplay of learning styles occurs continually in an academic setting. A student, asked the question, "What do you want out of this course?" would probably say, "A good grade." Getting a good grade requires doing well on course requirements, including tests. High test performance usually requires not only demonstrating knowledge of materials presented but also integration of the concepts when the student addresses teacher-formulated questions. When the clinician relates the same concepts to a client, it is important that the clinician be aware of the client's behaviors and responses and adapt to the client rather than having the client adapt to the therapist.

This external-internal interaction concept brings up another important clinical consideration. As students, most of us probably "clashed" with one or two teachers with whose learning styles we could never identify. That is, we as learners probably cannot or will not adapt to all learning styles. For that reason there may be clients whom we cannot teach and who also cannot learn through our approach. When that seems evident, a shift of therapists is most appropriate for the rehabilitation process to succeed.

The fourth component of the learning environment is the clinician's external environment. It is generally expected that personal life should never affect professional work. To accept this assumption, however, may be to deny that emotions affect behavioral patterns (see Chapter 5). When an individual is feeling unwell, emotionally upset, or under stress, response patterns vary without cognitive awareness. For example, suppose that Mr. Smith, who has a hypertonic condition because of a cerebrovascular accident, comes down early for therapy each morning, has a cup of coffee, and chats while you write notes. If one day you are under extreme stress and do not feel like interacting as Mr. Smith rolls his wheelchair into your office, you might say, "Mr. Smith, I'll be with you in a few minutes. Go over to the mat, lock your brakes, pick up the pedals, and we'll transfer when I get there." Mr. Smith will quickly identify a change in your behavior. He believes you are a professional and that your personal life will not affect your job. Thus he may draw a logical conclusion—that he must have done something to change your behavior. When you go to transfer him, you notice he is more hypertonic than usual and ask, "Is something bothering you? You are tighter than usual," and so goes the interaction. Your external environment altered your internal state and thus normal response patterns. In turn you altered Mr. Smith's external environment, changing his internal balance, and created a change of emotional tone that resulted in increased hypertonicity.[47,48] If instead of interacting with Mr. Smith as if nothing were wrong, you informed him you were upset over something unrelated to him, you might avoid creating a negative environment. First, you let Mr. Smith know that there are days you are upset and have mood changes. As he accepts your changes as normal, you help him realize he can have similar "off" days. Second, you give him an opportunity to offer his assistance to comfort or help you if he so desires. Such behavior encourages interdependence and social interaction, long-term goals for all rehabilitation clients.

Although each client is unique and thus analysis of specifics related to the learning environment is difficult, certain basic learning principles can be formulated. Six clinically significant learning concepts have been selected from many that have been established.[12,32,33] Basic learning principles relevant to clinical performance may be summarized as follows:

1. Individuals need to be able to solve problems and practice those solutions if independence in daily living is desired.
2. Although assigned tasks must be challenging, there must be a possibility of success.
3. When tasks are difficult or unfamiliar (new problem), an individual will revert to safer or more familiar patterns or ways to solve the problem.
4. When working on learning within one area of the CNS, learning is occurring simultaneously in other areas.
5. Necessary to learning is motivation to try to experience the unknown and, simultaneously, success in learning in order to retain that motivation.
6. Clinicians need to be able to analyze an activity, to determine its components, and to use problem-solving strategies to design good individual programs. At the same time, if independence in living skills is an objective, the therapist needs to teach the client those same problem-solving strategies rather than teaching the solution.

Clients need to use intrinsic feedback systems to modulate feedforward plans. Although all six learning concepts seem simple, their application within the clinical setting is not always as obvious. Principles *1* and *2* are intricately linked with the appropriateness and difficulty of tasks presented to clients. If a client is asked to perform a task such as standing, rolling, relaxing, dressing, or maneuvering a wheelchair, a problem has been presented that requires a sequence of acts leading to a solution. To succeed, the client must be able to plan the entire task and modulate all motor control during the sequence of the entire activity. If steps are unmastered, if sequencing is inappropriate or absent, or if motor control systems are not modulated accurately, dependence on the clinician to solve the problem is reinforced.

If the clinician can differentiate missing components from functioning systems creating an environment that encourages and allows the CNS to adapt and learn ways to regain that control will lead to optimal self-empowerment of the client. More specifically, a client should not be asked to perform a task unless he or she understands what is expected and can obtain the objective with some degree of success. Error in practice in order to intrinsically self-correct is critical for motor learning. Error that always leads to failure does not help the client learn avenues of adaptation. Linked intricately with success is the challenge of the task. The greater its difficulty or complexity, the greater the challenge and consequently the greater the satisfaction of success.

There is a subtle interplay in degree of difficulty, challenge, and success. Selecting tasks that are age appropriate, clinically relevant, and goal related is a challenge to the therapist. For the patient to be successful, the therapist must be a creative problem solver and knowledgeable about the client's needs, abilities, and goals. If the tasks are too simple or if the client considers them unimportant, boredom will ensue and progress may diminish. If the tasks are too difficult, the client may feel defeated and turn away from them. In such cases a child tends to withdraw physically, whereas an adult usually avoids the problem. Being late to therapy, having to leave early, needing to go to the bathroom, and scheduling conflicting sessions are all avoidance behaviors that may be linked to inappropriate tasks.

A third learning principle describes a behavior inherent in all people: reversal. When confronted by a problem, we revert to patterns that produce feelings of comfort and competence to solve the problem. In Fig. 1-7, a 2½-year-old child is confronted with just such a conflict. The bridge he wants to cross is unstable. The task goal is to cross the bridge; how that is accomplished is not as relevant as the task specificity. Therefore the child chooses a 6-month-old behavior and thus scoots. On gaining confidence, the child sequences from scooting to four-point bunny hopping, then crawling, on up to cruising, and finally to reciprocal walking. The child's reversal lasted approximately 2 minutes. Although reverting to more familiar or comfortable ways of solving problems is normal, it creates constant frustration in the clinic if it is prolonged. For example, if a hemiplegic client has spent a week modifying and controlling a hypertonic upper-extremity pattern during a simple task and is now confronted with a more difficult problem, the hypertonia will most likely return. If another client has successfully worked to obtain the standing position and then is asked to walk, the strong synergistic patterns that had been controlled may return. The pattern or plan for standing is different than that of walking and the emotional implications of walking are very high. Returning to a more stereotypical pattern should be anticipated and the client prepared. Anticipating that less efficient patterns will usually return as the tasks demanded increase in complexity, the clinician can attempt to modify the unwanted responses. The key to comprehension of this concept is not the behavior itself; instead, it is the attitude of a therapist toward a new task presented to the client. If the clinician expects the client to be successful, the client will also expect success. If failure occurs, both parties will be disappointed and a potentially

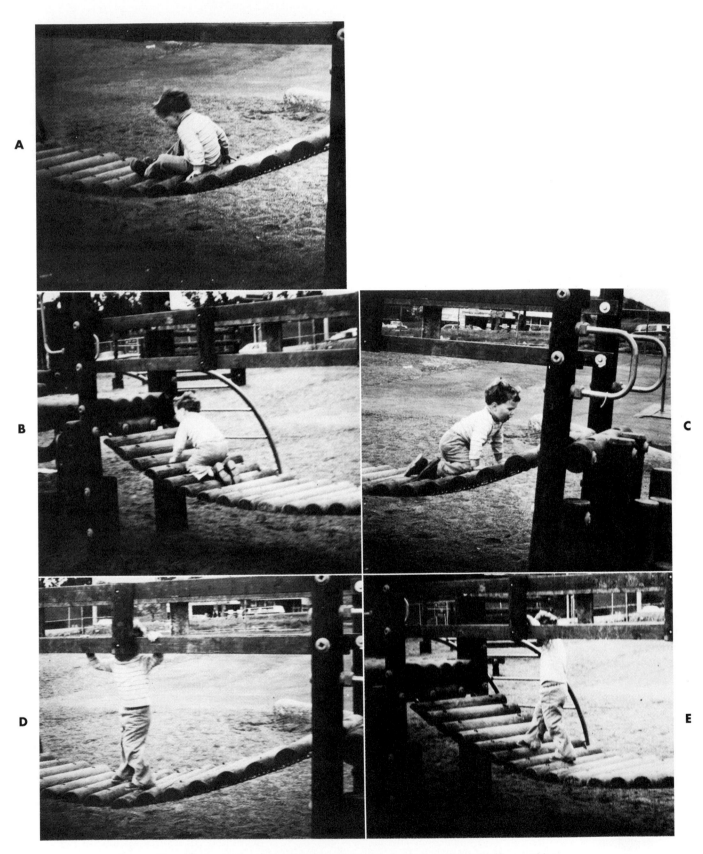

Fig. 1-7. Reverting to more comfortable behavior patterns when confronted with a problem.
A, Scooting. **B,** Bunny hopping. **C,** Crawling. **D,** Cruising. **E,** Walking.

negative clinical situation will be created; however, if the client succeeds, both will have expected the result and their attitude will be neither excited nor depressed. On the other hand, a clinician who expects the client to revert to an old behavior can prepare the client. If the client reverts, neither party will be disappointed; but if no reversion occurs, both will be excited, pleased, and encouraged by the higher functional skill. By understanding the concept, the clinician can maintain a very positive clinical environment without the constant negative interference of perceived failure when a client does revert.

The fourth learning principle deals with the totality of the client. Whether the area of emphasis is performance, emotional balance, or perceptual integration, all areas are affected. Therefore understanding and respect for all areas are important if optimal client function is a primary objective. This does not suggest that therapists should address each aspect of personality; however, integration of the client's physical, mental, and spiritual areas should be a responsibility of the staff. Awareness of possible adverse effects of one learned behavior on other CNS functions can help avoid potential problems. For example, if working on lower-extremity patterns creates extreme upper-extremity hypertonicity through associated patterns, the clinician is not dealing with the client as a whole.

The unknown creates fear as well as curiosity for most individuals, and the fifth concept points out that for most clients the unknown is all-encompassing whatever the degree of prior learning. For a client whose only difficulty

is a flaccid upper extremity, functional activities such as toileting, dressing, or eating will be troublesome and unfamiliar. Motivation is a critical factor for success. Fig. 1-8, *A* illustrates a child experiencing the unknown. He is walking off the bench as if the seat extended forever. He is confident, relaxed, and oblivious to the problem. Fig. 1-8, *B* and *C* show the child's surprise, his orientation to the task, motivation to succeed, and the ability to alter his preconceived feedforward motor plans to solve the problem. Obviously, instructing clients to walk off park benches is not the point. Maintaining motivation to try while ensuring a high degree of success is an important teaching strategy that tends to encourage present and future learning.

An additional comment regarding clients who lack motivation should be made. If a client wants to be totally dependent and has no need to become independent, then a therapist will probably fail at whatever task is presented. For example, Mr. Brown, a 63-year-old bank president with a wife, four children, and ten grandchildren, survives an operable brain tumor with residual right hemiparesis and minimal cognitive-affective deficits. The client's work history indicates that he was highly success oriented. Unknown to most persons is that for 63 years Mr. Brown desired to be a passive-dependent person, but circumstances never allowed him to manifest those behaviors. With the neurological insult he is in a position to actualize his needs. Until the client desires to improve, therapy will probably be ineffective. Thus motivating the client becomes critical and might be accomplished in a variety of ways. Knowing that

A   **B**   **C**

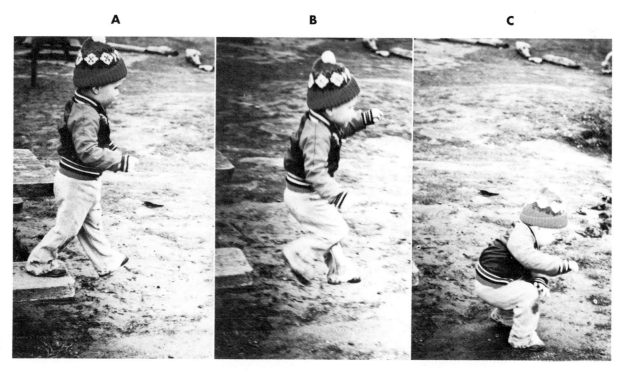

Fig. 1-8. A, Experiencing the unknown. **B,** Identifying the problem. **C,** Solving the problem.

Mr. Brown values privacy, especially with respect to hygiene, that he thoroughly enjoys dancing and bird watching in the forest, and that he ascribes importance to being accepted in social situations, such as cocktail parties, helps the therapist create a learning environment that motivates this client toward independence. Being independent in hygiene requires certain combinations of motor actions, including sitting, balance, and transfer skills. Being able to bird watch deep in an unpopulated forest requires ambulation skills, tolerance to the upright position for extended periods of time, and endurance. Being socially accepted depends to a large extent not only on grooming but on normal movement patterns, especially in the upper extremity and trunk. Creating a therapeutic environment that stresses independence in the three goals identified by the client will simultaneously create further independence in other areas. Whether the client decides to return to banking and other activities in conflict with his personality will need to be addressed later. Another way to motivate Mr. Brown is to place him in an environment in which he is not satisfied, such as a nursing home or his own home with an assistant rather than his wife to help him with his needs. Dissatisfaction with the current environment will generally motivate an individual to change. Obviously, creating a positive environment for change versus a negative one would be the method of choice.

Many supplemental learning principles from the fields of education, development, and psychology can be used. It is not expected that all therapists will intuitively know how to create an environment conducive to another's optimal potential. Yet all can become better at creating a maximal learning environment by understanding how people learn. This concept (see Fig. 1-6), which provides the final link between behavioral and scientific theory, adds the third element in the clinical triad (see Fig. 1-1).

The sixth and last concept in this section addresses the development of problem-solving strategies. The health care professions are stressing the importance of problem-solving skills, development of a problem list for patient and constant reassessment of the problem list, and patient progress during therapy. Schools are basing entire curriculum designs on problem-solving principles. Developing good problem-solving skills is paramount for high-level clinical performance. The clinician evaluates the client, establishes relevant goals with the client and then teaches the client the best solution to a specific problem. Unfortunately, teaching a solution to a problem can often be synonymous with teaching a splinter skill, that is, a skill that has no application to similar functional activities. For example, a therapist might identify that Janet needs to learn to perform a standing pivot transfer. They repeatedly practice the skill of transferring from a wheelchair to the toilet in the clinic. The independence that Janet achieves in this activity may not carry over to other transfer activities or even other toilets. Therefore teaching the client to solve problems in a variety

of environmental contexts while self-correcting errors within the motor plan must accompany skill acquisition if that individual is to reach optimal independence.

PROBLEM SOLVING

A theoretical model that integrates the traditionally separate cognitive subject areas of behavioral analysis, applied neuroanatomy and neurophysiology, and learning theory has already been presented. This section deals with a specific problem-solving format that can be applied to this model. This format serves as the basis for the clinical-problem chapters within Part Two of this volume. The second topic discussed here consists of additional suggestions regarding problem-solving strategies such as formulation of a client profile and visual-analytical problem solving.

Problem-solving format

Although cognitive strategies vary when a clinician approaches a specific clinical problem, an identifiable format is generally followed. The format has at least five areas: existence of the problem (component parts), evaluation procedures (analyzing components of the problem), goal selection (behavioral responses in terms of goals), treatment planning (choosing the best process to obtain desired goals), and specific psychological aspects and adjustment (modifying the solution to individual needs).

Before evaluating a clinical problem, an understanding of the general characteristics of the dysfunction is important. The neuroanatomical and physiological aspects of a problem and how they affect the client's general performance provide scientific understanding of the problem. Comprehension of typical clinical signs, as well as stages of recovery from acute to long-term rehabilitation, also provides vital background knowledge. Pharmacological considerations and medical management during various phases of recovery or progress can change the response to and direction of a treatment program. All of this background information, in addition to the client's individual characteristics, helps the therapist conceptualize the nature of the problem and formulate a problem list. Although the clinician needs to remain flexible and to accept clinical signs as they occur, grasp of a total concept of the problem provides direction for evaluation, goal setting, and treatment planning. Conceptualizing the clinical problem or observing the client's behavior leads the clinician to formulate questions that focus attention on both selection of evaluation procedures and direction of administration.

Once a clinical problem has been identified and a problem list has been formulated, evaluation procedures are selected. The selection of testing procedures may vary according to clinical preference, clinically established procedures, and client deficits, but it should be thorough and inclusive of all areas. Specific areas of evaluation have already been presented (see the discussion of the concept of normal human movement). Again, the choice of a specific evaluation form is not a critical issue. *How* the therapist extracts information from an evaluation is critical to the problem-solving strategy. Through experience clinicians learn to identify additional data not considered part of the test. For example, a therapist who is evaluating rolling and observes a strong shift in muscle tone as the head turns to the side that prevents rolling may decide that the client is incapable of rolling or cannot roll because of a strong tonal shift with head turning. The more observant and knowledgeable therapist, however, might conclude that the client has an ATNR or, even more accurate, that this reflex not only prevents rolling but affects many other ADL tasks. The therapist who identifies only that the client cannot roll has answered the test questions appropriately. The therapist who cannot only pinpoint the observed behavior but also recognize its manifest pattern and that it has the potential of affecting other functional activities can extract a large amount of pertinent, additional data that can be used when progressing to other functional tasks. These data provide direction for further evaluation procedures, goal establishment, and possible treatment protocol. Specific suggestions regarding development of these strategies for extracting additional information is discussed in the section dealing with visual-analytical problem solving.

Caution must be observed regarding conceptualization of a problem and evaluation procedures. Biasing findings of an evaluation to fit what is perceived as the problem is an issue all clinicians need to address. The clinician must allow the specific clinical signs of the patient to direct evaluation findings, goal setting, and treatment planning. Preconceptions based on familiarity with the medical diagnosis and general clinical problem can negate both the client's individuality and specific needs.

Although realistic goals and specific objectives are usually considered an end-product of therapeutic intervention, they need to be part of an ongoing evaluation process. Clinical signs often vary quickly. Observation of finite as well as gross changes plays a key roll in establishing and reestablishing goals. The process used to establish goals is based on the evaluation results and knowledge of the general progression the problem will take. Goals that seem appropriate for one phase of recovery or disease may need to change quickly as the phase changes. The clinician who uses high-level problem-solving strategies identifies finite clinical signs that indicate a phase change and therefore reestablishes new goals without losing precious time. For example, if a hemiplegic client has severe hypertonicity in the biceps and no palpable tone in the triceps, one goal might be to reduce tone in the biceps and facilitate triceps activity. A clinician would never isolate those two muscles without considering the rest of the client's arm, shoulder, and trunk, but for minimizing complexity, the following treatment focuses on the two identified muscle groups. Placing the biceps in extreme stretch will inhibit that muscle's action via its tendon organs (TO) (see Chapter 6). Simultaneously, the

tendon organs will facilitate the triceps. Tapping and vibration of the triceps during a weight-bearing pattern while the other arm is reaching for a cup or performing some functional activity should further facilitate this action. The assumption has been made that the biceps, as well as higher centers in the CNS, are inhibiting the triceps. Thus by inhibiting the biceps' function and using facilitative techniques, the therapist hopes that triceps activity will develop. Instead of low or normal tone development in the triceps, however, hypertonicity may ensue. If that is the case, the specific goal needs to be modified as soon as excessive tone is palpated. If not, triceps tone may become severe, causing additional problems.

Treatment procedures are established in terms of treatment objectives. Although the problem-solving protocol seems to follow a temporal, step-by-step sequence, in reality many aspects are occurring simultaneously as a system analysis. The focus may be on evaluation, but treatment is also intricately intertwined, and during treatment a reevaluation is ongoing. Understanding the neurophysiological processes being modulated during a treatment procedure should give the clinician flexibility to alter input strategies including type, duration, and amplitude to meet the dynamic needs of the client. Similarly, that knowledge also helps the clinician establish environments that encourage clients to self-correct, thus eliminating the need for extrinsic feedback from the therapist, and promotes greater carry-over in learning.

The last area generally affecting the problem environment and thus the strategies used by the therapist is specific psychosocial aspects and adjustment during various stages of recovery. An in-depth discussion of this area is presented in Chapters 5 and 7. Although most therapists focus their treatment on physical health and not on the social and adjustment aspects, the psychological state of the client affects the outcome of all other areas, including tone production.

Problem solving is continually implemented by therapists from the moment they learn they will be treating specific clients to the moment those clients leave the clinical environment. Gifted therapists are often thought to have intuition. Yet intuitive behavior is based on experience, a thorough knowledge of the area, sensitivity to the total environment, and ability to integrate the three and respond optimally. Intuitive abilities may be equated with high-level problem-solving skills. Refer to Chapter 5 for additional information on intuitive behavior. In that respect each clinician should, with learning and practice, become more skillful and thus a better problem solver. *One very important aspect of clinical problem solving is the ability of clinicians to ask pertinent questions as they evaluate, conceptualize about, and treat their clients.* How these questions are formulated and the answers recorded vary among therapists, but the result is the formulation of a profile for each client.

Problem-solving strategies

The client profile. A therapist reads charts to gain background information on a client before or at the initial meeting. In the past, emphasis was to get a "feeling for" the client. Instead, time might be better spent gathering useful information about specific areas: cognition, affect, and motor. Because these three areas are interwoven, the therapist needs to focus not only on each of them but on their interaction. To optimize treatment effectiveness, clinicians should ask questions whose answers will give them valuable information regarding the client's past, present, and potential status as well as provide indicators of the most effective learning environment.

Cognitive area. Perception and cognition cannot be separated. Perception lays the foundation for higher-level cognition, but there is also spiral overlapping that cannot be overlooked. It would appear that as perception develops, it lays the foundation for cognitive development, which, along with perception, matures and sequences to higher and higher levels. Within the cognitive domain four general areas are identified: sensory input, perceptual awareness and development, preferential higher-order cognitive systems, and level of cognition. All play important roles in the optimal function of the client within the cognitive domain. The box, below left, summarizes pertinent questions a clinician must answer with regard to the cognitive area of the client's profile.

Affective area. The client's level of cognition is directly influenced by the affective or emotional area. Simultaneously, all other cognitive domains can be affected by or

---

Cognitive area questions for client profile

A. Sensory input: awareness level
  1. What sensory systems are intact?
  2. Are any sensory systems in conflict with others?
  3. If conflict between systems is present, to which system does the client pay attention?
B. Perceptual awareness and development
  1. What specific perceptual processing deficits does the client have, and how would that affect motor performance?
  2. Do the perceptual problems relate to input distortion, processing deficits, or both? If input distortion is alleviated, is information processed appropriately?
C. Preferential higher-order cognitive system
  1. Was or is the individual's primary preferential system verbal or spatial?
  2. Is the client's preferential system different from yours? If so, can you work through the client's system?
  3. Is the client's preferential system affected by the clinical problems?
  4. Can the client adequately use nonpreferred systems?
D. Level of cognition
  1. Is the client functioning on a concrete, abstract, or fragmented level?
  2. Does the client's level of cognition change? If so, when and why?
  3. Is the client realistic? Does the client exercise judgment? If so, when? If not, when and why?
  4. Which systems or individuals are interfering with or distorting potential? (Systems within the individual and the environment around the client, such as the staff, the family, and the other patients, must be considered.)

Affective area questions for client profile

A. Level of adjustment or stage of adjustment to the disability
  1. At what level or stage of adjustment is the client with respect to the disability?
  2. At what level of adjustment is the family?
  3. Will the level of adjustment of the client or family affect treatment?
  4. If emotions are affecting treatment, what can be done to eliminate this problem?
B. Level of emotional control
  1. Can the client exercise impulse control?
  2. When does degree of emotional or impulse control vary?
  3. How did and does the client respond to stress?
  4. How did and does the client respond to perceived success and failure?
  5. What types of stresses outside of the specific physical disability are being placed on the client?
C. Attitude (attitude toward the disability is covered to some degree under level of acceptance, although additional information needs to be gathered)
  1. Before the onset of disability what was the client's attitude toward disabilities, and specifically, those related to his or her primary deficit?
  2. What is the client's attitude toward your professional domain?
  3. What is the family's attitude toward disabilities, especially those related to its family member?
  4. What is the family's attitude toward your professional domain?
D. Social adjustment
  1. At what social-developmental stage is the client's performance?
  2. Is the social interaction in alignment with cognitive and sensorimotor stages of development?
  3. Are the family's social interactions and expectations at the level of the client's performance?
  4. Is the client's level of social adjustment the same as the rehabilitation team's level of expectation?
  5. Is the client aware of his, her, or others' socially appropriate behavior?

affect the emotional factor and responses of the client. When considering the affective domain at least four general areas should be explored: level of adjustment to disability, level of emotional control, attitude, and social adjustment. Questions arise within each category that indicate the client's emotional status and how it will affect a therapeutic environment (see box at right on p. 26 and for additional information refer to Chapters 5 and 7).

Sensorimotor area. Commonly used sensory, age-related, developmental, and ADL evaluations assess both the

---

Sensorimotor area questions for client profile

A. Level of motor performance with respect to performance
   1. Is the client's level of motor performance or sensory and motor integration congruous with the staff's expected performance level?
   2. Is the client's level of motor control integration congruous with the family's expected performance level?
   3. Is the client's level of motor function congruous with his or her expected level of performance?
B. Functional skills
   1. What functional skills does the client perform in a normal fashion?
   2. What functional skills does the client perform in an abnormal manner?
   3. What functional skills has the client learned to perform that are reinforcing stereotypical patterns or hindering normal movement?
   4. What functional skills does the client and family consider of primary importance? Will splintering these skills hinder normal learning?
C. Abnormal patterns
   1. What patterns are present?
   2. When are these normal and abnormal patterns observed? Do they vary according to spatial positions?
   3. Is there ever a shifting or altering in degree of these abnormal patterns? If so, under what circumstances does this variance occur?
D. Degree of cortical override
   1. Does the client need to inhibit abnormal output by intentional thought, or does he or she use procedural adjustment through normal feedforward mechanisms?
   2. What amount of energy is being used to override abnormal output?
   3. Can the client use cognitive systems to control motor output?
   4. What amount of energy are you demanding the client to use when attending to the task? Are you asking the client to attend totally to the specific motoric task, or are you overloading the system to take away some cortical attending?

---

sensory and motor systems referred to as sensorimotor. Today those two systems are separate but interlocking. Specific questions need to be formulated to obtain information that will help guide the therapist into appropriate functional training activities with the client. Most therapists are more comfortable addressing both the sensory and the motor control areas than either the affective or cognitive systems. Four identifiable categories (see box at left) have been presented, although many additional focal areas could have been presented.

Summary. Linking the cognitive, affective, and sensorimotor domains is the key to providing a productive and satisfying clinical learning environment for both the therapist and the client. Identification of overlapping problems is important. The client's affective response at any one time will influence both cognitive processing and motoric performance. This affect may be extreme or mild, either positive or negative, and in many situations will need to be addressed for optimal performance. Cognitive-perceptual processing by the client will often determine the learning environment to be used, the sequences for treatment, and estimated time needed for therapeutic intervention. The motoric output area is a main system the client uses to express thoughts, feelings, and level of independence to family, therapists, and community. Although this motoric area can be evaluated effectively by itself, focusing on the cognitive-perceptual and the affective-emotional areas, identification of appropriate treatment progressions, potential for improvement, and estimated time for therapy can be of great value to all involved.

A clinical example is used here to help the reader through the various questions posed in the client profile. Mary H. is a 22-year-old client with closed head injuries who has been admitted to Jones Rehabilitation Hospital after a 6-month stay in an acute care facility following an automobile accident. At the time of insult Mary was a senior at X University. Her major was architectural engineering, and her primary interests were sports such as tennis, skiing, and track. She was to be married after graduation. The accident, which killed her fiancé, occurred on the way home from a beer party. The doctor reported that on admission to the rehabilitation hospital, Mary was awake and verbally responded to questions, but articulation and monotone difficulties made her responses almost incomprehensible. Her volitional motor skills were limited because of extreme hypertonicity. Mary seemed depressed and exhibited bursts of anger at seemingly insignificant problems.

Many of the questions on the client profile cannot be answered on initial evaluation. Answers to specific questions will also change as Mary's neurological condition changes. The FIM[36] presented in the conceptual model section is the evaluation form used at Jones Rehabilitation Center along with ROM and sensory test forms, and the Southern California sensory integration battery.[2]

When the therapist addresses the cognitive profile, certain

directional indicators can be identified. Mary's visual system has deficits that cause distortion in the perception of her spatial world. Her proprioceptive-vestibular system is intact, but her visual deficits override former sensory systems. Thus when sitting, Mary leans 30 degrees to the left with both head and trunk and perceives that she is in a vertical position. With her eyes closed, she still remains off vertical but can reposition herself to vertical when proprioceptive-vestibular cues are given. Knowing that one system is intact but overridden, a therapist can increase both temporal and spatial input through that modality to increase awareness. That increased awareness may help correct the deficit system. One way this might be accomplished would be asking the client to assume different positions in supine. The therapist instructs Mary to close her eyes and feel her position in space, adding approximation down through head and shoulders and quick stretch to appropriate muscle groups. Then the clinician takes Mary out of the position and asks her to reassume it. The goal would be accurate assumption of a totally symmetrical position. This first step toward reorientation to verticality is accomplished in a nonstressful position, thus eliminating anxiety, undue emotional tone, and conflicting input stimuli. Knowing that the client's preferential systems, based on her career choice and leisure-time activities, were visual-spatial and kinesthetic and that certain sensory systems critical to higher perceptual-cognitive performance in these areas are still intact reveals (1) which modality to use to introduce input and (2) which teaching strategies should be most beneficial to this client. That is, the client should be treated through spatial patterns rather than through verbal commands or visual demonstration of desired behavior, at least initially. Thus Mary's intact systems and her preferential modes of thought are tapped. Once an accurate form of communication has been established, other forms such as visual demonstration or verbal instruction can be presented. Then additional questions posed in the profile can be addressed.

As the clinician focuses on the cognitive-perceptual area, the affective area can also be explored. Most of the questions listed under level of emotional control in the affective area outline can be answered while evaluating cognitive-perceptual performance. Many other questions can be answered by spending a few minutes with Mary's family members. Getting at least two other individuals' opinions of Mary's level of adjustment, emotional control, and attitude helps eliminate individual bias. Thus it might be assumed that Mary highly valued her physical status, that she was always uncomfortable around anyone with a physical disability, and that she had a quick temper and was intolerant toward failure. The therapist can assume that these values and behavior patterns have not changed drastically. In fact, the clinician might expect that these attitudes may at times be exaggerated until Mary has adjusted to her disability, or they may even be retained forever. Her temper and intolerance toward failure need to be considered when establishing a treatment protocol. Success will be critical to motivate Mary in a rehabilitation setting, and her temper should help the therapist regulate the success/failure ratio and thus the task variation used during treatment.

Just as the affective domain influences and is influenced by the cognitive-perceptual systems, the sensorimotor area affects and is affected by the first two systems. The entire evaluation process may begin by using an ADL form. Answers can also be found to questions in the other areas of the profile. In actuality all areas should be addressed simultaneously while focus is placed on a specific topic, such as state of the motor pool, postural integrity, muscle strength, synergy dominance, etc. Perhaps Mary can be placed in total flexion when supine and can hold the position but is unable to reassume the pattern when placed in total extension. Thus she can assume aspects of the pattern but not in its entirety. If asked to position only her arms or legs, she succeeds. This would tell the clinician that Mary has the ability to inhibit certain reflexes, such as a dominant TLR or crossed extension reflex. The fact that Mary can remember a three-step sequence in the arms or the legs but not a six-step sequence of arms and legs together might suggest a temporal sequencing problem and that further evaluation is indicated to determine the degree of difficulty. Although this problem is perceptual-cognitive, it would severely hamper motor performance. If Mary were unable to perform a relatively simple perceptual-motor sequence as identified in the task of rolling over from a supine position, the frustration she would feel when asked to do a standing pivot transfer might be enormous. Although rolling in horizontal is a very different plan than the vertical stand-pivot transfer, the complexity of the transfer requires many more components of the motor system to interlock and function together. Rolling does not require the same degree of motor control even though in some patients it may be a more difficult plan. If Mary simultaneously was obligated to a reflex pattern such as an ATNR, she may have difficulty performing successfully either functional task. The interaction of a reflex such as the ATNR and Mary's poor temporal sequencing should limit the number of ADL tasks she would be asked to perform. Her intolerance to failure should alert the therapist to avoid test items in which there is a great likelihood for failure.

Answers to questions in the motor area of the profile should direct the clinician to areas in which Mary can succeed, areas in which she will definitely fail, and areas that are still doubtful. That is, Mary may be able to perform any three- or four-step sequence in prone and supine positions but will have difficulty changing positions because of the ATNR. Sitting activities are limited as a result of the visual-perceptual distortions of verticality and their influence over muscle tone in the vertical position. Standing, ambulation, and complex ADL tasks, such as dressing, should be considered extremely difficult because of tonal patterns dominance, that is, the ATNR in the lower extremity, the complex sequencing of the task, and the complex interaction of muscle function in all parts of the body during these complex activities. Selection of these tasks as treatment procedure to make the client feel more normal may in reality clearly identify her disability, may cause extreme frustration and anger, and may dissolve the client-therapist rapport.

Once the therapist has a clear understanding of the client's strengths and weaknesses, specific clinical problems can be identified and treatment procedures selected that allow flexibility in treatment sessions. Many treatment suggestions for various problems can be found in Chapters 8 through 32.

VISUAL-ANALYTICAL PROBLEM SOLVING

The last section of this chapter deals with a specific type of problem-solving strategy that has definite clinical significance: the area of visual-analytical problem solving.

Problem solving has become a major issue in professional development, and the question arises as to whether all problem-solving strategies are the same. Some strategies may be more appropriate for clinical performance and others more relevant to academic achievement. The answer is still hypothetical, for no empirical research has been found that addresses all these specific questions. However, at least one research study was undertaken to identify a particular problem-solving strategy that seems to have important clinical application.[65] This strategy is referred to as **visual-analytical problem solving (VAPS).** It is defined as the ability to look at a complex array of visual stimuli, identify the critical attributes, and then use appropriate strategies to solve simple to complex problems. The solution to those problems stems from the original visual information. The following is an example of the use of VAPS.

Mrs. J. sustained a closed head injury 4 months ago and has just been referred to your rehabilitation center. She was brought down in a wheelchair and placed against the wall in between two other clients (complex array of simultaneous visual stimuli). She first turns to the right to look at another client, then turns to the left (successive and simultaneous visual stimuli). You note as you are treating another client that, as Mrs. J. turns her head (critical attributes of the visual array), she has strong changes in muscle tone and that she has an obligatory bilateral ATNR. From that information you could determine many difficulties and failures that would occur if you gave an ADL test to this individual.

One problem encountered when making the transition from an academic to a clinical environment is having intellectual knowledge but being unable to associate that knowledge with the simultaneous and ongoing observation and palpation conducted in the clinic. Therefore many therapists believe that information learned in the classroom is irrelevant to the clinical environment. Another problem some students face is the frustration of working with a highly gifted therapist who cannot verbalize what is being done or why it works but can demonstrate the behavior or technique

extremely well. A plausible explanation for problems of transference is that part of the high-level problem solving needed in the clinic is based on a nonverbal strategy. To communicate this nonverbal, visual-analytical model, one must translate it into verbal language, and this is very difficult because visual-analytical thought is both simultaneous and sequential. For example, a therapist who pictures a client progressing through a transfer from the wheelchair to the bathtub might visualize the activity as if observing the client from the front, the side, the back, or even from above. In fact, visualizing the movement from all directions gives additional information regarding the behavioral aspect of the client's transfer abilities. There is no rule to tell the therapist from which direction to order such visualization. The combined visualizations make up the total picture, and it is the total picture that is important. Language, on the other hand, is dominated by rules. Those rules are specific and have very clearly defined temporal sequencing. Thus translating a simultaneous process occurring internally into a temporal sequence to discuss all components changes the consistency of the thought process. Reflecting back on the original problem, a student would need to translate theoretical knowledge that has definite temporal rules into a simultaneous process observed in the clinic. The student must recognize that many gifted therapists cannot explain *verbally* what they know *spatially*. Therefore when asked to explain the treatment procedure, they translate only fragments of the whole, which is often of little help to the student.

A similar example would be taking a picture of a beautiful sunrise over a huge mountain range while the photographer sits at the mouth of a large lake that is absorbed into the mountain landscape. The photographer is engrossed with the whole experience. The totality of the multisensory, three-dimensional emotional interaction needs to be caught forever in the picture. When the picture is developed, the photographer discovers that the camera was unable to capture the whole. In fact, it recorded only a small portion of the original scene. The disappointed photographer may try to explain to friends who are looking at the picture what was really occurring, which would probably lead to frustration and a comment such as, "Well, you just had to be there."

To perceive the clinical implications of visual-analytical problem solving, understanding of its sequential steps is paramount. Although this concept tends to use a nonverbal mode of thought, it is not suggested that language is omitted from this strategy. Indeed, language may be critical in storage and retrieval of these images from memory. Development of the sequence seems to be hierarchical, consisting of three general categories: visual recognition, spatial orientation, and spatial transformation.

The first step, visual recognition, implies the ability to recognize key attributes of the visual array and pull out those pieces of information necessary to begin to solve problems. Obviously, this means clinicians need to have mastery of visual information relevant to their professional responsibilities. Students often have difficulty generalizing information obtained at this level of visual recognition. An example would be a student who learns to evaluate the strength of the quadriceps muscle in a sitting position and thus assumes that this is the only position in which the strength of the muscle can be tested. Or, if students study a reflex such as the ATNR and visually learn the motor pattern, they often hold the visual image of a child in the ATNR pattern. That is, they are unable to recognize the ATNR in adults who demonstrate the same reflex. The student stores the visual recognition with tremendous restrictions and thus limits clinical application of that information.

If visual content in one spatial position has been mastered, the second phase of the sequence, spatial orientation, can be addressed. This strategy requires identification of the key visual elements in various spatial planes. For example, if the clinical problem required the therapist to recognize an ATNR in sitting, four-point, and standing positions, a spatial orientation strategy would be used, which can easily be applied in the clinic. For instance, a therapist may be giving an ADL evaluation and may ask Mrs. J. to transfer in and out of the tub to the right. She fails because she is unable to bend her hip and knee to clear the tub while she is looking at her knee or its placement in the activity. One therapist might identify only that Mrs. J. failed to transfer to the right, thus deciding that the best strategy would be to teach her to transfer to the left: a compensatory skill. A second therapist might realize that Mrs. J. failed because she has a dominant ATNR to the right. The second clinician not only identified that Mrs. J. failed but also *why* she failed. Knowing the reason gives the therapist freedom to select alternative treatment programs, such as teaching the client to modify the influence of the ATNR in tub transfer to the right, thereby eliminating the need for teaching a compensatory strategy. This would also be true in all ADL activities that require head turning, such as dressing, eating, and climbing into a car. Recognition of the ATNR in sitting position is a spatial orientation strategy because the therapist has gone beyond recognizing this reflex in the supine position. This second stage requires that the clinician visually recognize behavioral patterns in the three-dimensional external world. An important key to successful use of this strategy is allowing oneself the visual freedom to see what is actually present instead of preconceiving and then cognitively altering what one is seeing. Having predetermined *questions* relevant to specific clinical problems is an important aspect of problem solving. Having preconceived *answers* limits the flexibility of the clinician, decreases alternatives to treatment planning, and often limits the potential of the client.

The third stage, spatial transformation, requires a higher degree of spatial analysis. Up to this point, internalizing complex spatial or visual images was not necessary, although some imagery may have been used. That is, many people use compensatory verbal strategies to try to interpret what is being seen in the external world. Spatial visualization implies first that complex visual images are being manufactured within the mind of the observer. Then the individual must transpose one image on top of another or, while looking at one image, transform it (through the CNS), enabling the observer to view it simultaneously from a different position. For example, a woman may be looking at a picture of a lake in the mountains. If within her CNS she could form an image of that picture as if she were on the other side of the lake looking across the lake and at herself, that would be visualization transformation.

A clinical example of spatial transformation is knowing a client has an ATNR to the right from observing that individual's behavior in a sitting position and being able to transpose that behavior into a visual image of a transfer activity and determine at what point in the transfer the client would have difficulty or would fail. This could be accomplished before confronting the client with that task. If a therapist knows a client is going to fail, there is little reason to attempt the task. Thus an evaluation could be used to maintain an environment that provides positive reinforcement.

This type of spatial thought process involves visually breaking down the observed environment into its component parts and then progressing visually through each component. The clinician is also confronted with less complex clinical problems. If, simultaneously, a total picture of the client can be maintained, then a high-level clinical problem-solving strategy has been achieved. This manipulation of total-to-part to total-to-part is considered a highly integrated cortical function requiring both hemispheres.[47] An example is a clinician who recognizes that, as Janie walks across the floor, she is using a combination of the ATNR, symmetrical tonic neck reflex (STNR), positive supporting reactions, static postural tone, and moderate equilibrium reactions. The combination of tonal patterns creates a bizarre movement sequence that cannot be explained as a single act. Yet when the act is broken into components, the summative tonal response resulting from the combined influence of the various reflexes and reactions clearly explains the abnormal movement sequence. Treating each component problem separately and recombining the newly learned normal strategies lead to a more normalized gait pattern. That is, the whole is observed, the parts are detected and treated, and then the whole is reassembled in a new order to allow better function.

The development of visual-spatial strategies for use in visual-analytical problem solving is not specifically taught in schools. Yet these skills may provide an explanation of what is often called a therapist's intuitive gift. Academicians are beyond the point of accepting the premise that all problem-solving strategies are the same. Identifying in the next decade which problem-solving strategies lead to high-level clinical performance is a major objective for health care professionals. Learning such skills before entry into a clinical setting should ease the transition between the highly verbal environment of the classroom and the highly visual and kinesthetic environment in the clinic. How to develop this skill depends on the student's preferential learning styles and ability to change learning styles when necessary.

Some general suggestions can help all learners. The first step is to master visual content of normal movement and postural patterns. Pictures or slides, where the visual stimuli can be held for extended periods of time, help the learner identify specific patterns without the demand of recognizing the pattern in a movement sequence. Next, the visual strategy should be mastered during a movement pattern. This requires recognition of key visual elements while additional simultaneous and successive visual input are present. When this is accomplished in one spatial position, the same problems should be practiced in all spatial positions. This second strategy can be practiced by viewing videotapes or movies of individuals in a clinical setting.

The third strategy, visual transformation, requires the ability to internalize those images recognized in the first two stages. This can be practiced externally before the learner is asked to internalize two sequential images, place them on top of each other, and visualize the summative effect. Slide frames of a normal movement pattern can be taken and placed in front of the learner. A second visual input—such as the presence of a stimulus for the ATNR, as well as the response pattern—can be drawn, pictured on film, or discussed to help the learner visualize it internally. The end-product of the second pattern can then be overlaid on the first sequence. At some time the motor-response may coincide with the desired effect; at another time the stimulus for the second response may not be present in the first movement pattern. Finally, with the stimulus present, the desired response of the first pattern may conflict with that of the second, and thus the summative effect would cause deviation from normal movement. This strategy of summating externally two or more response patterns can then be practiced with internal visualization. The use of language to clarify visual images should help the learner make the transition from verbal to visual-spatial thought. Feeling and observing tonal changes in the client while visualizing what these total patterns look like should also help the learner begin to develop some of these higher-level visual-spatial strategies.

SUMMARY

This chapter has laid the foundation for an integrated problem-oriented approach to neurological disability. Three general areas were discussed: philosophy and rationale for the book; presentation of a conceptual model incorporating normal behavioral movement patterns, neurophysiology, and the learning environment; and general discussion of clinical problem solving. The concepts presented should not be taken as appropriate only for clients with CNS damage. Whenever change occurs, whether it be neurological, cardiovascular,

pulmonary, or orthopedic, a therapist's role is to structure the clinical environment in a way that promotes optimal healing and return of function. Individuals with neurological damage often have orthopedic, pulmonary, or cardiovascular problems. It has been my experience that orthopedic patients almost always have neurological change with respect to learning or awareness of movement at the involved site. As long as clinicians can retain the concept of the total client, the integrity of the person is maintained, and the potential for that client to reach optimal function is closer to fruition.

REFERENCES

1. American Occupational Therapy Association: Standards of practice for occupational therapy in schools, *Am J Occup Ther* 34:900-903, 1980.
2. Ayers AJ: *Sensory integration and learning disabilities,* ed 1, Los Angeles, 1972, Western Psychological Services.
3. Bayley N: *Manual for Bayley scales of infant development,* New York, 1969, The Psychological Corp.
4. Barr J, Coordinator: Curriculum Planning Workshop, Midwinter Combined American Physical Therapy Association Sections Meeting, Washington DC, 1976.
5. Bayley N: *Bayley scales of infant development,* ed 2, San Antonio, 1993, Psychological Corporation.
6. Beissner KL: Use of concept mapping to improve problem solving, *J Phys Ther Educ* 6(1): 22-27, 1992.
7. Brander R and others: Inter-rater and test-retest reliabilities of the movement assessment of infants, *Pediatr Phys Ther* 5(1): 9-15, 1993.
8. Brazelton TB: *Neonatal behavioral assessment scale,* Philadelphia, 1973, JB Lippincott Co.
9. Bruner JS: *The process of education,* New York, 1968, Vintage Books.
10. Carr JH, Shepherd RB, and Lynne D: Investigation of a new motor assessment scale for stroke patients, *Phys Ther* 65: 175-180, 1985.
11. Chandler LS: *Movement assessment of infants: a manual,* Rolling Bay, Wash, 1980, Chandler, Andrews & Swanson.
12. Cronback LJ and Snow RE: *Aptitudes and instructional methods,* New York, 1977, Irvington Publishers, Inc.
13. Des Marchais JE, Dumais B, and Pigeon G: From traditional to problem-based learning: a case report of complete curriculum reform, *Med Educ* 26: 190-199, 1992.
14. Farber S: *Neurorehabilitation: a multisensory approach,* Philadelphia, 1982, WB Saunders.
15. Farmer JA and others: Cognitive apprenticeship: implication for continuing professional education, *New Dir Adult Cont Educ* 55: 41-49, 1992.
16. Fiorentino MR: *Reflex testing methods for evaluating CNS development,* ed 2, Springfield, Ill, 1979, Charles C Thomas, Publisher.
17. Fiorentino MR: *A basis for sensorimotor development-normal and abnormal,* Springfield, Ill, 1981, Charles C Thomas, Publisher.
18. Fisher AG, Murray EA, and Bundy AC: *Sensory integration: theory & practice,* Philadelphia, 1991, FA Davis.
19. Folio MR and Fewell RR: *Peabody developmental motor scales and activity cards,* Allen, Tex, 1993, DLM Teaching Resources.
20. Foster MA: Family systems theory as a framework for problem solving in pediatric physical therapy, *Pediatr Phys Ther* 3(2): 70-73, 1992.
21. Freeman MK and Whitson DL: An overview of learning style models and their implication for practice, *J Adult Educ* 20(2): 11-18, 1992.
22. Frostig M, Lefever DW, and Whittlesey J: *Developmental test for visual perception,* Palo Alto, Calif, 1963, Consulting Psychologists Press.
23. Fugl-Meyer AR and others: The post-stroke hemiplegic patient, *Scand J Rehabil Med* 7:13-31, 1975.
24. Granger CR: *Guide for the use of the Functional Independence Measure (Wee FIM) of the uniform data set for medical rehabilitation,* Buffalo, 1988, Research Foundation, State University of New York.

25. Granger SV and Hamilton BB: Outcome of comprehensive medical rehabilitation: measurement by PULSES Profile and the Barthel Index, *Arch Phys Med Rehabil* 60: 145-154, 1979.

26. Guiliani C: Motor control theory and application. Informal presentation, Harmerville, Pa, Aug 1988, lecture notes.

27. Haley SM and others: *Pediatric evaluation of disability inventory: development, standardization, and administration manual,* Boston, 1992, New England Medical Center Hospitals Inc, & PEDI Research Group.

28. Haley SM and Binda-Sundberg K: Measuring physical disablement: the contextual challenge, *Phys Ther* 74(5): 443-451, 1994.

29. Harris SR: Early diagnosis of spastic diplegia, spastic hemiplegia, and quadriplegia, *Am J Dis Child* 143:1356, 1989.

30. Hayes KW, Sullivan JE, and Huber G: Computer-based patient management problems in an entry level physical therapy program, *J Phys Ther Educ* 1(5):65-71, 1991.

31. Hayes KW: The effect of awareness of measurement error on physical therapists' confidence in their decisions, *Phys Ther* 72(7): 515-525, 1992.

32. Hunt DE: *Matching models in education,* Ontario Institute for Students in Education Monograph Series No 10, Toronto, Ontario, 1974.

33. Joyce B and Weil M: *Models of teaching,* Englewood Cliffs, NJ, 1972, Prentice-Hall, Inc.

34. Kandel ER, Schwartz JH, and Jessell TM: *Principles of neural science,* ed 3, New York, 1991, Elsevier Medical Science Publishing.

35. Katz SFA and others: Studies of illness in the ages. The index of ADL: standardized measure of biological and psychosocial function, *JAMA* 185: 914-919, 1963.

36. Keith RA, Hamilton BB, and Sherwin FS: *The functional independence measure: a new tool for rehabilitation,* New York, 1987, Springer.

37. Knobloch H and others: *Manual of developmental diagnosis: the administration and interpretation of the revised Gesell & Amatruda developmental and neurological examination,* Houston, 1987, Gesell Developmental Materials.

38. Kurtzke JF: A new scale for evaluation disability in multiple sclerosis, *Neurology* 5: 580-583, 1955.

39. Kurtzke JF: Rating neurologic impairment in multiple sclerosis: an expanded disability status scale (EDSS), *Neurology* 33: 1444-1452, 1983.

40. Langer SK: *Philosophy in a new key,* Cambridge, 1942, Harvard University Press.

41. Lewis CB and Bottomley JM: *Geriatric physical therapy: a clinical approach,* Norwalk, Conn, 1994, Appleton & Lange.

42. Lister MJ, editor: *Contemporary management of motor control problems. Proceeding of the II STEP Conference,* Alexandria, Va, 1991, Foundation for Physical Therapy.

43. Magistro C and others: Diagnosis in physical therapy: a roundtable discussion, *PT Magazine* 1(6): 58-65, 1993.

44. Mahoney FI: Functional evaluation: the Barthel Index, *Maryland State Med J* 14, 61-65, 1965.

45. May BJ: An integrated problem-solving curriculum design for physical therapy education, *Phys Ther* 57:807-815, 1977.

46. Milani-Comparetti A: Routine developmental examination in normal and retarded children, *Dev Med Child Neurol* 9:631, 1967.

47. Moore JC: The limbic system, Workshop presented in San Francisco, Feb 1980.

48. Moore J: Neuroanatomical structures subserving learning and memory. In *Fifteenth Annual Sensorimotor Integration Symposium,* San Diego, July 1987.

49. Nagi S: *Some conceptual issues in disability and rehabilitation.* Washington, DC, 1965, American Sociological Association.

50. Nagi S: *Disability concepts revisited: implication for prevention,* Washington, DC, 1991, National Academy Press.

51. Norton BJ: Report on colloquium on teaching clinical decision making, *J Phys Ther Educ* 6(2): 58-66, 1992.

52. NUSTEP (Northwestern University Special Therapeutic Exercise Project): Proceedings: an exploratory and analytical survey of therapeutic exercise, *Am J Phys Med* 46(1), Feb 1967.

52a. Stockmeyer SA: An interpretation of the approach of Rood to the treatment of neuromuscular dysfunction. In *Am J Phys Med* 46(1):900-961, Feb 1967.

53. Peiper A: Cerebral function in infancy and childhood, New York, 1968, Consultants Bureau.

54. Piaget J: *Science of education and the psychology of the child,* New York, 1970, Onion Press.

55. Pribram KH: *Languages of the brain: experimental paradoxes and principles in neuropsychology,* Englewood Cliffs, NJ, 1971, Prentice-Hall, Inc.

56. Randolf S and Heiniger M: *Neurophysiological concepts in human behavior; the tree of learning,* St Louis, 1981, Mosby.

57. Roch EG and Kephart NC: *The Purdue perceptual-motor survey,* Columbus, Oh, 1966, Charles E Merrill.

58. Rothstein JM: Physical disability: special issue, *Phys Ther* 74(5):1, 1994.

59. Sahrmann SA: Movement science and physical therapy, *J Phys Ther Educ* 7(1): 4-7, 1993.

60. Schmidt HG: The psychological basis of problem-based learning: a review of the evidence, *Acad Med* 67: 557-565, 1992.

61. Schmidt LS and Crowe JK: Interrater reliability of the gross motor scale of the Peabody Development Motor Scales with 4- and 5-year-old children, *Pediatr Phys Ther* 5(4): 169-175, 1993.

62. Schmidt RA: *Motor control and learning: a behavior emphasis,* ed 2, Champaign, Ill, 1988, Human Kinetics.

63. Shipp KM: Clinical decision making: osteoporosis to manage fragility, *PT Magazine* 1(10): 70-77, 1993.

64. Umphred D: Teaching, thinking and treatment planning, Unpublished Master's Thesis, Boston, July 1971, Boston University.

65. Umphred D: Visual analytical problem solving, Unpublished doctoral dissertation, Syracuse, NY, 1978, Syracuse University.

66. Weinstein CJ: Movement science its relevance to physical therapy, *Phys Ther* 70:759-762, 1990.

67. Wood P: *International classification of impairments, disabilities & handicaps (ICIDH).* Geneva, Switzerland, 1980, World Health Organization.

68. Valett RE: *Valett developmental survey of basic learning abilities,* Palo Alto, Calif, 1966, Consulting Psychologists Press.

CHAPTER 2

Normal Sequential Behavioral and Physiological Changes Throughout the Developmental Arc

C. Robert Almli and Nancy M. Mohr

OUTLINE

Physical development of the human
    Prenatal physical development
    Postnatal physical development
Normal human nervous system development
    General principles of human nervous system development
    Nervous system development during embryonic, fetal, and early postnatal periods
    Normal sequential human nervous system development
    Prenatal and postnatal development of the brain
Behavioral and physiological characteristics of development
    Motor development
    Sensory development
    Language development
    Cognitive (learning and memory) development
Summary

KEY TERMS

nervous system

development

prenatal development

postnatal development

myelination

synaptogenesis

motor development

autogenic movement patterns (AMP)

LEARNING OBJECTIVES

After reading this chapter the student/therapist will:

1. Differentiate various stages of prenatal and postnatal development.
2. Identify various growth spurts and how those rapid stages of development affect behavior.
3. Compare various stages of motor development and identify what behaviors should be seen.
4. Differentiate the various sensory systems rate of development and how that affects motor behavior and learning.

The study of the development of relationships between the brain and behavior is interesting for people who want to know more about themselves. Such knowledge is also important as a background for understanding the anatomy and physiology of the **nervous system** and the behavior of human beings. Knowledge of neurological and behavioral ontogeny is also important for understanding the pathogen-esis of developmental neurological abnormalities, as well as for understanding the normal sequences of behavioral development.

The human developmental process is characterized by rather dramatic changes in both the physiology (e.g., nervous system) and the behavior (e.g., movement patterns) of the developing organism from conception through death at any age. In this sense the developmental process is lifelong. At present we have amassed considerable knowledge of the developmental process from conception through adulthood, and from adulthood through senescence and subsequent death.[38]

This chapter presents a survey of representative and critical characteristics of the human developmental process from conception through young adulthood, with greatest emphasis on the late prenatal through early childhood phases. These phases are particularly important because of the extremely rapid changes that take place in both the physiology and the behavior of the human organism and because of the organism's increased vulnerability to biological, environmental, and experiential influences. During these developmental phases, the normal sequential changes that occur in the central nervous system (CNS) and the behavior of the developing human organism are stressed.

The first section of this chapter presents a general discussion of prenatal and postnatal physical development of the human organism. In the next section the **development** of the human nervous system is presented, and the development of the brain is emphasized. The final section is a representative look at general motor, sensory, language, and cognitive development of the human organism.

Human development data are presented when available; otherwise data for lower animals are introduced. A basic knowledge of neuroanatomy is assumed of the reader. (Refer to chapter 3 for additional clarification.)

PHYSICAL DEVELOPMENT OF THE HUMAN
Prenatal physical development

Prenatal development is often divided into three basic phases: the germinal phase, the embryonic phase, and the fetal phase (Table 2-1). The germinal phase begins at the moment of conception, or fertilization, and lasts through approximately the first 2 weeks of gestation. The germinal phase is the period of rapid cellular division and implantation of the embryo into the wall of the uterus. The next phase, the embryonic phase, begins at this time and continues through approximately 8 weeks of gestation. The embryonic phase is a period of rapid growth and differentiation of the major body systems and organs. The final prenatal phase, the fetal phase, begins at about 8 weeks of gestation and lasts through gestation term (birth), at approximately 38 to 40 weeks after fertilization. During the fetal phase, rapid growth and changes occur in the body form of the fetus.

During prenatal development, the human organism displays a physical developmental sequence that proceeds in general rostral-to-caudal and proximal-to-distal gradients. Development proceeds from the head region to lower body parts, and from the central body parts out to the peripheral body parts. The averages and normative data presented in this chapter for the various growth measures are intended to communicate a general picture of growth and development

Table 2-1. Phases of the human development process

Phase	Time
Prenatal (conception to birth)	
Germinal	Conception to 2 weeks
Embryonic	2 to 8 weeks
Fetal	8 to 38-40 weeks
Postnatal	
Newborn (neonatal)	Birth to 2 weeks
Infancy	2 weeks to 1 year
Childhood	1 to 12-13 years
Puberty	
Females	12 to 15 years
Males	13 to 16 years
Adolescence	15-16 years to 18-25 years
Adulthood	18-25 years to ?
Senescence	? to death

of the human organism. The reader must keep in mind that these averages and norms vary considerably, and "normal" in most cases can only be broadly defined.

After fertilization, the fertilized ovum (zygote) begins division during the 3- to 4-day trip through the fallopian tube to the uterus. Upon arrival at the uterus, the future human is a fluid-filled sphere called a blastocyst. The cells around the edge of the blastocyst cluster to form the embryonic disk, from which the human organism will develop. The embryonic disk differentiates into two layers, the upper layer, or ectoderm, and the lower layer, or endoderm. A short time later a third layer, the mesoderm, or middle layer, develops. These three germ layers give rise to all tissues and organs of the body (Table 2-2). The ectoderm is the embryonic tissue from which the nervous system, sensory systems, and many other tissues develop (Fig. 2-1). The mesoderm differentiates into the muscles, skeleton, and other tissues, whereas the endoderm differentiates into the respiratory and digestive systems, as well as other tissues.[91]

At 3 to 4 weeks of gestation, the developing human is only a few millimeters long, yet morphogenesis is significantly advanced. The paraxial mesoderm of the embryo begins to divide into paired surface elevations, called somites, at about 20 days of gestation. Approximately 40 pairs of somites will develop shortly (occipital, cervical, thoracic, lumbar, sacral, and coccygeal), and these paired somites eventually give rise to most of the skeleton, musculature, and dermis of the head, trunk, and limbs. By about 24 to 26 days of gestation, the primitive mouth begins to form as the mandibular and hyoid brachial arches become distinct. The heart has developed to such an extent as to produce a bulge on the ventral surface of the embryo, and the primitive heart has begun to beat at approximately 65 beats/minute.[46] The upper limb buds and the otic pits (primordia of the inner ears) are recognizable by 26 days of

Table 2-2. Layers of the trilaminar embryonic disk and the tissues derived from the germinal layers

Germinal layers	Tissue and organ derivatives
Ectoderm	Central nervous system (brain and spinal cord); peripheral nervous system; sensory epithelia (eye, ear, nose); epidermis; hair; nails; mammary glands; pituitary gland; subcutaneous glands; tooth enamel; adrenal gland (medulla); pigment cells of the dermis; muscle, connective tissues, and bone of branchial arch origin; leptomeninges (pia-arachnoid)
Mesoderm	Bone, cartilage, and connective tissue; striated and smooth muscle; heart, blood, lymph vessels, and cells; kidneys, gonads (ovaries and testes), and genital ducts; serous membranes lining pericardial, pleural, and peritoneal body cavities; spleen; adrenal gland (cortex); microglial cells
Endoderm	Epithelial lining of the gastrointestinal, respiratory, urinary bladder, urethra, and auditory tracts and cavities; tonsils; thyroid, parathyroid, and thymus glands; liver; pancreas

gestation, followed by the lower limb buds and optic placodes (lens) at 28 days. During this period the primitive nervous system, kidney, liver, and digestive tract are continuing to differentiate (Table 2-2 and Fig. 2-2).

During the fifth week of gestation, the upper limbs are paddle shaped and the hand plates have formed. Formation of the lower limbs and feet follow within a few days. The nasal pits become prominent during this week and the optic cups and vesicles are present. The embryo has grown to approximately 8 mm long by the fifth week of gestation. Within the following week (sixth week of gestation) the upper limb buds have further differentiated and the elbow, wrist, and digital rays (fingers) are identifiable. The eyes have become obvious at this age, because of the appearance of retinal pigments. By the seventh week of gestation, the embryo has grown to approximately 16 to 18 mm long and the eyelids are now forming. The trunk of the embryo is elongating and straightening, and notches are appearing between the finger rays.[91]

The embryo continues to grow until it is approximately 2.5 cm long by 8 to 9 weeks of gestation. The face, mouth, eyes, ears, and nose are slowly becoming well defined, and the organism begins to resemble a very small baby. The arms, legs, hands, and feet have now become apparent and stubby fingers and toes can be distinguished.[45] Development of the sex organs and muscle tissues have already begun, and activation of muscles by neural input has achieved a functional, though primitive level. Associated with the tremendous development of the brain that is occurring at this time, the head is quite large in comparison with the rest of the body. The head makes up approximately one half of the total body length.

The development of the fetus extends from the end of the second month of gestation through gestation term. Development during the fetal period is characterized by growth and differentiation of the organs and tissues that have evolved during the embryonic period. The rate of body growth is especially rapid between the ninth and twentieth weeks. During the early part of the fetal period, the fetus begins to respond to tactile (touch) stimulation with flexion of the trunk and extension of the head.[55,134] From this age

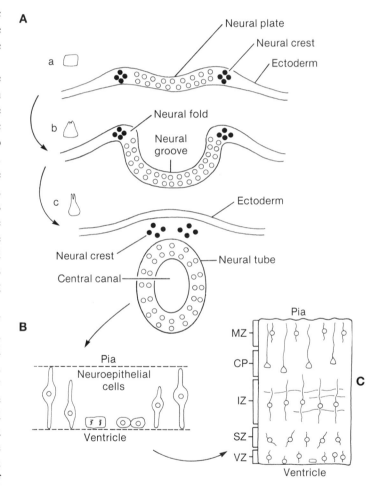

Fig. 2-1. Early development of the nervous system. **A,** Formation of the neural tube from the neural plate showing the relative positions of the ectoderm, neural crest, neural plate, neural folds, neural groove, neural tube, and central canal (ventricle). *a-c,* Relative changes in the shape of cells of the neural plate producing the neural folds and neural groove and ultimately, the neural tube. **B,** Cross section of the early neural tube showing the neuroepithelial or germinal cells at various stages of mitotic division. Postmitotic cells migrate out of this ventricular zone to form the intermediate or mantle zone. **C,** Cross section through the early forebrain showing the ventricular zone *(VZ),* subventricular zone *(SZ),* intermediate (mantle) zone *(IZ),* cortical plate *(CP),* and marginal zone *(MZ).*

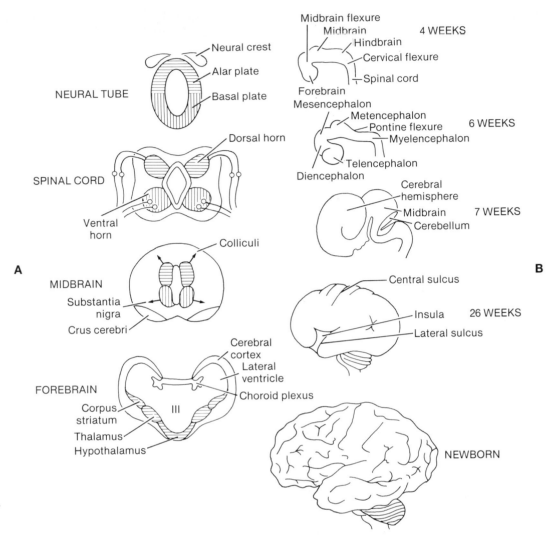

Fig. 2-2. Gross development of the nervous system. **A,** Cross sections through the early neural tube, spinal cord, midbrain, and forebrain. Horizontal cross-hatching indicates alar plate and vertical cross-hatching indicates basal plate. **B,** Lateral views of the developing nervous system from 1 month of gestation through gestation term (newborn). Noted are the brain flexures and the brain vesicles.

onward, motor functions of the human organism become increasingly complex and differentiated. The earliest movements of the fetus are generalized including the whole-body.

From 9 to 12 weeks of gestation the body length of the fetus doubles. The face is broad, the eyes are widely separated, and the ears are set low. The eyelids are now closed. By the end of 12 weeks, the upper limbs have almost reached their final relative lengths, but the lower limbs are less well developed and are still relatively short. The neck region of the fetus is now well defined and the early fingernails are differentiating.[91]

At approximately 12 to 13 weeks of gestation, the fetus has grown to about 7.5 cm long and weighs over 40 g. The muscles and the nervous system have greater connection and spontaneous generalized movements are made

with the arms and legs. The head of the fetus now makes up approximately one third of its total body length, and many organ systems are beginning to function. Further morphological differentiation of the fetus has occurred, and the lower limbs are increasing in relative length. The sex organs of the fetus can be identified by their external morphology, and the internal sex organs have primitive egg or sperm cells. During weeks 12 to 16 of the fetal period, the nervous system continues to differentiate and grow at a rapid rate, and motor behavior becomes more complex. The fetus is now displaying movements resembling breathing and is swallowing amniotic fluid. In addition, the fetus at this age displays movement of the legs, feet, arms, thumbs, and head. The mouth opens and closes, and the fetus makes squinting movements in response to tactile stimulation of the eyelids. Touching the palm stimulates a closing of the hand into a fistlike shape, touching the lip region stimulates sucking movements, and stimulating the sole of the foot elicits toe fanning. Still present at birth and for a period of time after birth, many of these reflexlike behaviors disappear during postnatal maturation. These are the primitive reflexes (Table 2-3).

By 16 to 17 weeks of gestation, motor movement of the fetus has achieved a magnitude that allows the mother to actually feel the fetus moving around inside her. The fetus at this age has grown to approximately 15 cm long and weighs approximately 170 g. The reflexes and motor movements of the fetus become more brisk with age as the nervous and muscular systems continue to mature.

At 20 weeks of gestation, the fetus is approximately 19 cm long and weighs about 400 g.[57] The mouth of the fetus shows all of the movements required for sucking, including opening, closing, and protrusion of the lips. The fetus also displays cyclical activity and quiet periods, which may signal the beginning of sleep-wake cycle development. During quiet periods, the fetus seems to display a "favorite" body position (or body lie) within the uterus. During active periods the fetus kicks, stretches, squirms, opens and closes the hands, and displays hic-cuplike spasms. The fetal heartbeat can be clearly heard, yet the respiratory system remains quite immature. The fetus at this age shows coarse hair on the eyebrows and eyelids and fine hair on the head. A woolly type of hair, called lanugo, covers most of the body and will disappear shortly before or after birth.

When the fetus is at approximately 24 weeks of gestation, it has grown to about 23 cm long and weighs about 800 g. Fat pads under the skin are developing, and the eyes are almost completely formed. The eyelids periodically open and close. Regular movements resembling breathing are seen, along with movements resembling crying. The grip of the hand has also increased in strength, and taste buds appear on the tongue.[19] A fetus born at this age has a good chance of survival with intensive care; however, the infant will likely have varying degrees of respiratory, medical, and/or developmental problems.

At 28 weeks of gestation, the fetus is approximately 27 cm long and weighs about 1200 g. At this age the nervous, circulatory, and other body systems have sufficiently matured to allow the fetus a good chance of surviving birth; however, special care would be required. The fetus now displays well-developed motor movements, reflex patterns, and breathinglike inspirations and expirations. Crying, swallowing, and thumb sucking are part of the frequently observed behavior patterns. The fetus displays reactions to changes in temperature of its surroundings somewhat like those of full-term infants, and if born at this age, they seem capable of differentiating the four basic tastes of sweet, sour, bitter, and salt.[21] These premature infants also display reactions to visual and auditory stimulation; and responses to

Table 2-3. The primitive reflexes and ages at which they disappear

Reflex	Age (months) reflex disappears
Rooting	9
Moro	3-6
Grasping	2-3
Swimming	6
Tonic neck	2-7
Babinski	6-9
Walking	4-8
Placing	1

painful stimulation are attenuated when compared to the responses of older infants.

At 8 months of gestation, the fetus is about 30 cm long and weighs about 2000 g. The movement of the fetus is somewhat decreased at this age, which may be related to the cramped quarters within the uterus. The fetus continues to accumulate body fat layers that will help in adjusting more readily to temperature decreases in the environment.

In the final month of gestation the fetus displays a general slowdown in body growth, especially within the final week. The final weight of the fetus is approximately 3400 g with a final length of about 50 cm. Males tend to be a little longer and heavier than females at birth. The various organs of the body have now sufficiently developed to allow the newborn to survive extrauterine life. Growth and differentiation, however, do not stop here; rather, tremendous growth continues through the postnatal period.

Postnatal physical development

Postnatal development of the human is often considered to progress by stages (Table 2-1). The newborn (or neonatal) period is the first 2 weeks after birth, and the infancy period is the first year after birth. During the infancy period, the whole body grows very rapidly. The childhood period extends from the end of the first year through 12 to 13 years and is a period of active ossification of the bones. Growth is rapid during the early part of this period and slower toward the end. Just before puberty, body growth accelerates during the prepubertal growth spurt. The puberty periods for girls (12 to 15 years) and boys (13 to 16 years) are signaled by development of secondary sexual characteristics (e.g., pubic hair). Adolescence is the 3- to 4-year period following puberty, extending from the earliest signs of sexual maturity until adulthood. In our culture, these periods are not sharply defined. Adulthood is the period when growth and ossification are virtually complete, beginning at approximately 18 to 25 years of age. Growth of the human during adulthood, through the senescence period, is considerably slowed.

Normal postnatal physical development follows a relatively strict course; however, the time at which individual infants reach specific milestones varies considerably. The first 3 years of postnatal life are characterized by tremendous body growth and change in body proportions. At birth neonates are approximately 19 to 20 inches long (50 cm) and weigh about 7 to 8 lb (3.5 kg). By the end of the first year of postnatal life, infants have grown to approximately 30 inches (75 cm) long and weigh about 20 to 25 lb (9 to 10 kg). At 2 years of age they are about 35 inches (85 cm) long and weigh about 27 lb (12 kg); at 3 years of age, they are approximately 38 inches (95 cm) tall and weigh about 35 lb (15 kg).[146]

During the first few days after birth, the neonate may lose up to 10% of body weight, primarily because of a loss of fluids. By the fifth postnatal day, body weight gains are seen and birth weight is usually reachieved by about 10 to 14 days of age.[43]

The newborn infant is rather pale and pinkish in color because of thin skin and possesses varying amounts of lanugo (body hair). The head makes up about one fourth of the total body size. It may be elongated and misshaped because of the molding that has occurred in utero and during the birthing process. The skull bones have not yet fused and the separations between skull bones (fontanels) are overlaid with a thick membrane. The fusion of the skull bones occurs approximately 18 months after birth.

The Apgar scale[11] was developed to give a general assessment of the medical status of the newborn shortly after birth. This scale continues to be widely used and is made up of five subtests. A score of 0, 1, or 2 is given to the newborn on the basis of appearance (color), pulse (heart rate), grimace (reflex irritability), activity (muscle tone), and respiratory (breathing) effort. The maximum score on the Apgar scale is 10 and scores are assigned at 1 and 5 minutes after delivery. For most normal deliveries (90%), an Apgar score of 7 or better is achieved. A score of 4 or less indicates that the infant requires immediate medical attention. Research has shown that low Apgar scores are fairly good predictors of later neurological problems.

Apgar scores at 1 minute after birth were correlated with performance on the Bayley Scales of Infant Development at 8 months of age. Infants scoring 0 to 3 on the 1-minute Apgar test tend to score lower on the Bayley Scales of Infant Development administered at 8 months of age than infants who scored from 7 to 10 on the Apgar test.[127] Thus retrieval of the Apgar score from an infant's or child's record may provide information about the relationship between a child's difficulties and perinatal status.

Because of the required adaptation to the extrauterine environment, newborns are often closely monitored. At birth the respiratory status of the newborn is of great concern: first because of the effect of anoxia on the still-developing brain and second because respiratory problems tend to be the major killer of newborns.[103,144] Many infants, especially those who are premature, develop a physiological jaundice (a yellowing of the eyeballs and skin) at 3 to 4 days after birth. This jaundice is usually related to immaturity of the liver. The premature infant also has less fat than the full-term infant and thus has greater difficulty in regulating body temperature. Full-term infants can usually regulate body temperature around a slight decrease in environmental temperature by increasing their activity.[53] Premature infants also have a higher incidence of various pathological conditions, including periventricular and intraventricular hemorrhage.[4,144]

During the various stages of the postnatal period, changes occur in the portions of the body displaying the most rapid growth. For example, from conception to birth, the head grows faster than any other body part and is approximately 70% of adult size at birth. From birth through 1 year of age, the trunk is the fastest growing body segment. Trunk growth represents 60% of the total body growth in the first year. From 1 year of age through adolescence, the legs are the fastest growing of body regions from adolescence through adulthood, comprising 60% of total body growth during this period.[142] Differential body growth during development has direct clinical implication. For example, because of these body growth spurts, orthotic devices may need to be reevaluated more frequently.

The pliable nature of the bones of infants is due to their lack of ossification. Different bone groups ossify at different times during development. The bones of the body are derived from cartilage tissue that becomes ossified or hardened by the deposition of minerals during development. The ossification process begins during the prenatal period and continues through adolescence. Some bones of the hand and wrist ossify by the end of the first year of life, and the six fontanels do not completely ossify until about 2 years after birth. Other bones ossify through late adolescence.[140]

Newborn infants essentially have their full complement of muscle fibers at birth; however, the muscle fibers are smaller than they should be even in relation to body size. There is a general rostral-to-caudal gradient in the development of muscle fibers, beginning in the head and neck region and extending to those of the lower limbs. Infant males already have a greater proportion of muscle tissue than females at birth, and this differential is maintained throughout life.[43]

Although males are generally larger than females, females develop faster. This sex difference begins during the prenatal period. As indicated earlier, the sexes also differ in body composition, with females having a greater proportion of fat and less muscle and water than males. Except during the prepubertal growth spurt, females tend to be lighter and shorter than males. Females are less variable than males in terms of physical growth characteristics, and physical growth of females is more stable over time. Skeletal development of a 2-year-old girl is a better predictor of future skeletal development than that of a boy at the same age.[1]

Physical growth increases rapidly during the preschool

years, with no significant differences between boys and girls. During this time, the muscular, nervous, and skeletal systems mature rapidly. As might be expected, factors such as nutrition and exercise can profoundly affect physical growth and development at these ages.[140]

During the middle childhood period, physical development is less rapid than earlier periods. Although boys are typically taller and heavier than girls at the start of this period, girls attain the adolescent growth spurt earlier than boys and thus, tend to temporarily exceed the height of boys. During the middle childhood period, the bodily and facial proportions of the child change a great deal, and it is now possible to predict future adult height relatively accurately for both boys and girls.

The adolescent period is a phase of rapid physical growth and maturation of reproductive functioning (primary and secondary sexual characteristics) associated with puberty. Both boys and girls show sharp growth in height, weight, muscular, and skeletal development—the adolescent growth spurt. The end of the adolescent period is diffuse rather than clearly demarcated, and it is often culturally specified. Growth during adulthood is complete, and body weight changes are typically related to changes in body fat.

NORMAL HUMAN NERVOUS SYSTEM DEVELOPMENT
General principles of human nervous system development

During growth and development, many impressive structural and functional changes take place within the human nervous system. These developmental changes are not homogeneous in rate throughout the nervous system and they do not occur in discrete stages. Rather, different neural regions develop at different rates and develop in a continuous fashion.[28,42] The development of the human nervous system can only be accurately characterized as a differential process over time. Each alteration in structure and function simultaneously represents the beginning, middle, and end of each preceding and each successive alteration. During human nervous system development, the more primitive neural regions tend to begin to form earlier than "higher" neural regions.[61] Regions of the nervous system that appear first in phylogeny tend to appear first in ontogeny, whereas more recently evolved neural structures arise later in ontogeny. For example, neurons of the most recently evolved layers of the cerebral isocortex (outer layers) are the last cortical neurons to be generated during ontogeny.[78] The age at which a neural region attains functional maturity, however, cannot be absolutely predicted by the age at which the neurons are derived during neurogenesis.[2] In addition, some neural regions (e.g., cerebellum) begin significant development relatively late in the prenatal period and, as a function of accelerated growth, achieve mature characteristics quite rapidly, whereas other neural regions (e.g., cerebral cortex) may have extremely elongated developmental peri-

ods. Thus the development of the human nervous system is not one of homogeneous accretion of substance, but rather a process of differential rates and differential timing of growth changes within and between the various neural regions. Understanding these growth changes and the average age span of their occurrence allows the clinician to identify functions that are most likely to be affected by neural trauma for clients at different ages.

The major events that occur during the development of the human nervous system are presented in the following sections. These events appear to be common to the development of the nervous system in all mammals and represent the basic processes for building a brain.

Major events in human nervous system development. The major events in the development of the human brain and the peak times of their occurrence are (1) formation of the neural tube from the neural plate (called neurulation) at 3 to 4 weeks of gestation, (2) cellular proliferation at 2 to 4 months of gestation, (3) cellular migration at 3 to 6 months of gestation, (4) cellular differentiation and organization at 6 months of gestation through many years after birth, and (5) **myelination** of neurons at birth through 10 or more years of age and continuing into adulthood. Each of these major events is described more fully later in this chapter.

The major events presented here may give the impression that brain development occurs in five stages or steps; however, this is not the case. First, there is considerable overlap of these events within and between neural areas. Second, neural regions are not homogeneous from the onset and duration of these events. Third, different types of neurons within a given neural region display different time courses for these events. The considerable overlap of these events reinforces the notion that development of the human brain is a continuous process over time. The various events, stages, steps, and phases presented within this chapter are for organizational purposes only and do not accurately reflect the process of neural development as it occurs in nature. The task of the reader is to keep in mind that these developmental processes are just that—continuous processes over time. An understanding of the general timetables for the various developmental events, however, should help the reader gain insight into those neural areas affected when insult to the CNS occurs at different times during development (Fig. 2-3).

The processes of neurulation, cellular proliferation, cellular migration, cellular differentiation and organization **(synaptogenesis),** and cellular myelination lead to the formation and development of the most complex and slow growing of human organs, the human brain and the remainder of the human nervous system. The vast complexity of the human brain is staggering when we merely consider one of its attributes, the number of neurons. The mature human brain contains approximately 100 billion neurons (100,000,000,000 neurons)! If this number is not sufficiently impressive, consider further that each of these

NEUROGENIC CYCLES

Neural induction: 3-6 wk G
Neuronal proliferation: 2-4 mo G
Glial proliferation: 2 mo G-yr P (?)
Neuronal migration: 3-5 mo G
Neuronal organization: 6 mo G-yr P (?)

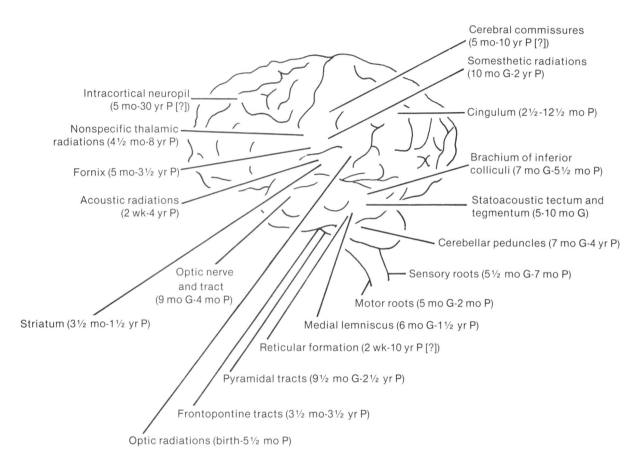

Fig. 2-3. Timetable of neurogenic and myelogenic cycles. Myelogenic cycles are detailed for selected neural areas showing the age at which myelination begins for that region and the age at which myelination is essentially complete for that neural area. Question marks *(?)* indicate that the maturation age is not determined. Gestation age *(G)* and postnatal age *(P)* are indicated.

100 billion neurons is capable of making literally thousands of functional contacts with other neurons. Because of the tremendous complexity of the mature brain, many scientists have been studying the development of the brain, perhaps under the assumption that during development we would have a "simpler" system. Yet during the 9-month prenatal period, neurons are being generated at an average rate of approximately 250,000 neurons per minute!

While it may seem as though precise scientific study of the human brain is futile, this is really not the case. Major technological advances (e.g., microelectrode recording techniques, biochemical analyses, autoradiography, and brain scanning such as magnetic resonance imaging [MRI] and positron-emission tomography [PET]) used by creative scientists are continuously unlocking some of the secrets of the brain and its development. Thus in spite of the complexity of human brain development, our knowledge of it is increasing rapidly.

Nervous system development during embryonic, fetal, and early postnatal periods

The development of the human nervous system during embryonic, fetal, and early postnatal periods is an awesome process that is as intriguing as it is complex.[105] From its embryonic beginnings, the human nervous system is dynamic and ever changing. During the embryonic and fetal periods, it grows from a strip of undifferentiated tissue to a recognizable brain that is distinctly human (Fig. 2-2). During the early postnatal period and continuing on for many years, the human nervous system displays further growth and development and is shaped in all of its detail into a mature organ capable of the highest human function. Basically, the embryonic and fetal periods show high rates of qualitative and quantitative growth, whereas the postnatal period is one of tremendous qualitative growth. Thus damage during any period of life, but especially the prenatal period, has the potential for producing drastic changes in CNS functioning.

Prenatal and postnatal development of the nervous system in humans can be characterized by nine major interactive and dependent processes.[28] Many of these processes, which are begun in the prenatal period, are continued through the postnatal period. The processes of building a human brain are (1) induction (formation) of the neural plate followed by formation of the neural tube (neurulation), (2) localized regional cellular proliferation of neurons and glia, (3) migration of neurons and glia to their final positions, (4) aggregation of cells into neural regions, (5) differentiation of immature neurons and glia, (6) formation of interneuronal connections as a function of dendritic and axonal growth and establishment of synapses, (7) selective neuronal death as a result of "overproduction" of neurons, (8) loss of some early interneuronal connections and stabilization of other interneuronal connections, and (9) myelination of axons. To varying extents, the fifth through the ninth processes are active throughout the postnatal life span (Fig. 2-3).

Formation of the neural plate and neural tube. At approximately 18 days after conception, the human embryo is only 1.5 mm long, yet differentiation of two germ layers, the ectoderm and mesoderm, has begun.[67] Induced by an interaction between the ectoderm and the mesoderm, the ectoderm thickens along the embryonic midline, as a function of migration of neuroepithelial cells (germinal cells), to form the neural plate. The neural plate is made up of approximately 125,000 neuroepithelial cells (Fig. 2-1). In the formation of the nervous system, the neural plate is the smallest substrate that can give rise to the complete CNS.[61]

Neurulation is the process of forming the neural tube from the neural plate. During formation of the neural tube, the number of cells in the neural plate does not significantly change; instead, the neural tube results primarily from changes in the shape of cells of the neural plate.[48,63,121] The cells of the neural plate are initially cuboidal in shape. At the onset of neurulation, cells along the lateral edges (or margins) of the neural tube, as well as those of the midline, begin to elongate and constrict at one end (their dorsal surface). This change from cuboidal to flask shape results in a raising of the neural folds and a midline depression called the neural groove. As more and more cells of the neural plate change to the flasklike shape, the lateral edges of the neural folds curve over to meet at the midline. The changes in cell shape appear to be mediated by intracellular microtubules and microfilaments.[61] During closure of the neural tube, the lateral ectoderm is pulled dorsally and medially over the neural tube, which then sinks under and breaks away from the ectoderm. Simultaneously, cells at the margin of the neural folds and lateral ectoderm move to the dorsal aspect of the neural tube to form the neural crest.[61,93]

The initial fusion of the neural folds of the neural tube occurs at the presumptive "low medulla-cervical" level at approximately 22 days of gestation for the human. The fusion then spreads in both rostral and caudal directions until the tube has fully closed.[44] The rostral (brain end) fusion of the neural tube (anterior neuropore) is complete at approximately 24 days of gestation, and the posterior fusion of the tube (posterior neuropore) is complete to the first and second lumbar segments (presumptive or future segments) by approximately 26 days of gestation. The more caudal aspect of the neural tube, the presumptive lower spinal cord, is formed later. The lumen of the neural tube develops into the ventricular system of the brain and the central canal of the spinal cord.[67] Discussion of neural tube abnormality can be found in Chapter 15.

The neural plate and neural tube are the embryonic precursors of the brain and spinal cord—the CNS (Table 2-2). This embryonic tissue is the source of neurons and macroglia (astroglia and oligodendroglia). Microglia are mesodermally derived and appear to enter the CNS via the vasculature.[80] The neural crest is the embryonic precursor of many cells intrinsic to the peripheral nervous system. Derived from the neural crest are cells such as the spinal dorsal root (sensory) ganglia, sensory ganglia of some cranial nerves, autonomic ganglia, Schwann cells, and cells of the pia-arachnoid (Figs. 2-1 and 2-2). The dura mater is formed by an ectodermal-mesodermal interaction.[61]

The neural tube of the human embryo is formed at 3 to 4 weeks of gestation. At the time of closure of the neural tube, cellular proliferation becomes rapid and averages 250,000 neurons per minute during the prenatal period. As a result of rapid cellular proliferation, the cephalic (or brain) end of the neural tube becomes enlarged, forming the three primary brain vesicles by 4 to 5 weeks of gestation (Fig. 2-2).[67,153] These vesicles are the prosencephalon (forebrain), which gives rise to the cerebral hemispheres and basal ganglia of the telencephalon, the mesencephalon (or midbrain), and the rhombencephalon (hindbrain), which give rise to the cerebellum and pons of the metencephalon and medulla of the myelencephalon. The caudal remainder of the neural tube develops into the spinal cord.

Cellular proliferation and migration. From the time of formation of the neural plate through formation of the neural tube at 3 to 4 weeks of gestation, the neural plate changes from a simple layer of neuroepithelial cells to a thick layer of cells whose nuclei lie at several levels (Fig. 2-1). Early in development, mitotic figures are confined to the layer of neuroepithelial or germinal cells lining the lumen of the neural tube.[61] The layer of germinal cells of the neural tube is called the ventricular layer (or zone). All of the cells of the ventricular zone are involved in cellular proliferation (mitotic activity), and the period of major proliferation of cells in the developing human brain is at 2 to 4 months of gestation.[31]

The germinal cells of the ventricular zone have cytoplasmic processes that extend from the lumen of the neural tube to its most superficial or peripheral extent. As neurogenesis proceeds, young neurons migrate out of the ventricular zone to form the mantle or intermediate zone.[124] The peripheral aspects of the cytoplasmic processes of germinal cells make up the outermost layer, the marginal layer or zone. Thus the early neural tube consists of the innermost ventricular zone, the intermediate or mantle zone, and the outermost marginal zone.[61]

The germinal cells of the ventricular zone are thought to give rise to both neurons and glial cells (Fig. 2-1). It has been suggested that a "common" germinal cell may give rise initially to young neurons and later to glioblasts (cells capable of further division). Glioblasts then give rise to all of the macroglia.[40]

The germinal cells are columnar in shape and extend from the inner to the outer surfaces of the neural tube (Fig. 2-1). The soma and nucleus are found within the ventricular zone. The nuclei of the germinal cells synthesize deoxyribonucleic acid (DNA), migrate toward the ventricular (luminal) surface, and divide (mitosis). The nuclei of the daughter cells then return to the outer surface of the ventricular zone and the cycle is repeated. This to-and-fro movement cycle is repeated for each occurrence of DNA synthesis and mitosis within the ventricular zone (Fig. 2-1). The number of proliferative cycles differs for cells destined to populate different neural regions and for different types of cells.[120] After a number of these proliferative cycles have been completed, cells destined to become neurons lose their capacity to synthesize DNA and migrate out of the ventricular zone or remain as ependymal cells.

Most neurons and macroglia in the CNS are generated from the ventricular and subventricular zones (a second germinal zone, to be discussed later).[61] Using DNA as a chemical correlate of cell number, Dobbing and Sands[31] have identified two major phases of cellular proliferation in the developing human brain. The first phase, from 2 to 4 months of gestation, is the phase of major neuronal proliferation. The second phase, from 5 months of gestation to 1 year or more after birth, is the phase of major glial proliferation (Fig. 2-3). There is some overlap in these two proliferative phases, especially in the cerebellum. It is also

interesting to note that proliferation of the vasculature within the brain corresponds to the phase of neuronal proliferation. Development of arteries typically precedes that of veins.[67]

As early development proceeds, there is first an increase in the number of germinal cells, as the dividing cells undergo mitosis repeatedly. Later, a steady state is reached for the number of germinal cells, as one daughter cell of each pair migrates out of the germinal zone. Still later, as germinal cells cease dividing, the population of postmitotic cells increases and the population of germinal cells decreases. Ependymal cells lining the ventricles may represent the final differentiation of the neuroepithelial cells.

In developing mammals, including humans, large neurons are typically generated before small neurons, and neurons are produced before their associated glial cells.[61] It is possible that neural proliferation may actually stimulate glial proliferation.[81] Most glial proliferation occurs during the phase of neuron growth and differentiation. The proliferative cycle or cell cycle of glioblasts is typically much longer than that of neurons, and for some neural regions may be five times as long.[41] Large neurons tend to be generated within the ventricular zone, whereas most small neurons and essentially all macroglia are probably generated in a second germinal zone, the subventricular zone.[61] The subventricular zone develops between the ventricular and intermediate (or mantle) zones of the forebrain (Fig. 2-1). This zone retains mitotic figures during adulthood, presumably for glial cells only.[91] Although most neuronal proliferation occurs during the prenatal period, postnatal neuronal proliferation sometimes occurs in the olfactory bulbs, hippocampal formation, brainstem nuclei, and cerebellar cortex in lower animals (e.g., rodents).[6,54,85,139]

During migration of a daughter cell out of the ventricular zone, the cell loses its basal or inner (ventricular) attachment and flows or is pulled into its external process as it migrates to the intermediate (mantle) layer. Differentiation of the cell proceeds within the intermediate layer. The remaining daughter cell prepares for another cycle of cell division.[120] In the telencephalon, the young neurons migrate to the intermediate (mantle) zone, which increases in size as a result of ingrowth of afferent axons and migration of cells. The dorsal portion of the intermediate zone forms the cortical plate (Fig. 2-1). As cells and fibers continue to invade this zone, the cortical plate of the telencephalon undergoes progressive differentiation to form the layers of the cerebral cortex.[61]

Most glioblasts and the neuroblasts destined to become small neurons migrate from the ventricular zone to a second germinal zone (located between the ventricular and intermediate zones) called the subventricular zone. The subventricular zone is found, among other places, in the forebrain.[108] The proliferating cells of the subventricular zone give rise to the smaller neurons of the cortex and deep structures of the cerebral hemispheres (such as the basal ganglia). Most of the glioblasts migrate to this subventricular zone, and after the period of major neuronal proliferation, the major period of glial proliferation begins. The macroglia retain their ability to proliferate throughout life.[6] Thus most glial cells are typically generated before the oligodendroglia. The astroglia tend to be the primary glial cells found within the gray matter (e.g., cortex); and the oligodendroglia, because of their role in myelination, are the primary glial cells found within the white matter (e.g., fiber tracts).

Culminating with humans, there appears to be an evolutionary trend for an increase in the ratio of Golgi type II neurons/Golgi type I neurons. Golgi type I neurons are large neurons that make up the major afferent and efferent pathways. Golgi type II neurons are smaller neurons that usually function as interneurons or local circuit neurons. Many of these smaller neurons are generated postnatally in lower animals, and thus they may be affected by the postnatal experience of the organism. The number of Golgi type I neurons in an organism's brain seems correlated with body mass, whereas the number of Golgi type II neurons is correlated with behavioral complexity.[60] In humans the ratio of granule cells (interneurons) to Purkinje cells (projection neurons) of the cerebellum is on the order of 1500:1.[17] There is also a phylogenetic trend for the glia/neuron ratio to increase up to humans.[39] These phylogenetic trends are primarily manifest in humans during the period of cellular proliferation.

Neuronal migration appears to be an actual ameboid-like movement of the cell out of the germinal zone to its final position within the nervous system. This migration process may take on different forms at different stages of neurogenesis.[61] Early in neurogenesis, when distances to be traveled are short, migrating cells appear to translocate via their attachment processes. Migrating cells have cytoplasmic attachment processes to both the inner (ventricular) and outer (pial) surfaces of the developing neural tube (Fig. 2-1). In this situation, the soma or nucleus is drawn or flows into the outer or leading process and the trailing process is withdrawn.[16] In later stages of neurogenesis, when there are long distances and complex "terrain" with which to contend, cells appear to use specialized glial guides (radial glia cells) for migration.[107,130] The radial glial guides (Fig. 2-4) are found as early as 10 weeks of gestation in the human brain and persist throughout the period of neuronal migration.[10] The radial glia are probably associated with the subventricular germinal zone and later differentiate into astroglia.[125]

In the human brain the period of major neuronal migration at 3 to 5 months of gestation overlaps and follows the period of major neuronal proliferation at 2 to 4 months of gestation. The two basic forms of migration are radial, as discussed earlier, and tangential. Tangential migration is found for both the cerebral and cerebellar cortex. Tangential migration is found for smaller neurons and glia of the superficial layers of the cerebral cortex, where cells of the subventricular zone migrate over the cortical surface, and then inward and down through the cortical layer. Tangential migration is also found for granule cells of the cerebellum, where proliferative cells migrate from the ventricular layer

in the alar plate of the medulla to the external granular layer. These germinal cells migrate over the surface of the cerebellum, then inward to give rise to granule cells of the cerebellum.[138] As might be expected, migration of cells to their final positions takes longer as development proceeds, especially for the cerebral and cerebellar cortices, where distances to be traveled are long and tortuous. Problems with neuronal migratory processes may result in ectopic neurons (neurons that migrate to the wrong neural regions) and/or neuronal disorientation (neurons with an improper axis), both of which may result in neurological dysfunction.

The proliferation and migration of cells in the human CNS follow some general patterns that differ for different neural regions. For example, the cerebral cortex, optic tectum, hippocampus, and substantia nigra (laminar structures) typically show an inside-to-outside developmental gradient.[61,130] An opposite, outside-to-inside (or lateral-to-medial) gradient of neurogenesis is found for the thalamus and hypothalamus.[9] Rostral-to-caudal, caudal-to-rostral, and ventral-to-dorsal gradients also occur in the development of the nervous system. In the cerebellar cortex, the various cells develop in the following order from first to last: Purkinje

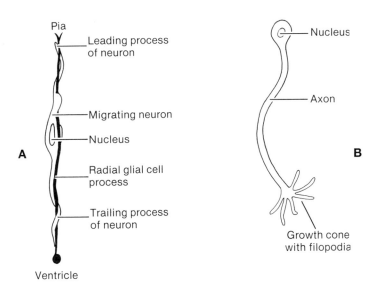

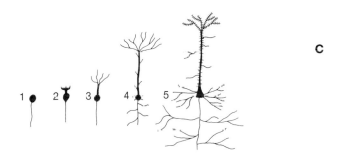

Fig. 2-4. Growth and migration of neurons. **A,** Schematic drawing of a neuron migrating along a radial glial guide. **B,** A growing axon with growth cone and filopodia. **C,** Sequence of development of the dendritic arbor of a pyramidal cell.

cells, Golgi type II, basket, stellate, and granule cells. In the cerebral cortex, pyramidal cells are generated first and granule cells are generated last.[8] The largest neurons, the ventral horn spinal motor neurons, are also generated first in the spinal cord.[42] Thus the timing of trauma sustained by different regions of the CNS will differentially affect large and small neurons and also neuronal migration patterns.

In the motor cortex, the thalamocortical afferent neurons arrive before and during cellular migration to the cortex (Fig. 2-5).[77] The first cells to appear in the cortex are cells of layer I, then Cajal-Retzius cells, then pyramidal cells of layers V and VI at 5 months of gestation, and then interneurons (such as cortical basket cells of layer IV) at 7 months of gestation. The pyramidal cells, first of layer III and second of layer II, reach their final positions at 7.5 months of gestation. The various Golgi type II and small neurons complete migration during late prenatal periods.[77] Cells may be dormant within the cortex for many months before further differentiation and synaptogenesis take place. By 20 to 24 weeks of gestation, the cerebral cortex seems to have gained the majority of its neurons.

This section has presented the major characteristics of neuronal proliferation and migration, and these are summarized as follows.[28,31,108,109] First, the time at which a cell ceases to synthesize DNA and ceases dividing (mitosis) appears to be genetically determined (Fig. 2-1). Second, the cessation of mitosis seems to trigger migration of the cell to its final destination. Third, large cells with long processes (Golgi type I neurons) are generated and migrate before small cells with regionally confined or local processes (local circuit or Golgi type II neurons). Fourth, the sequence and timing of cellular proliferation and migration are characteristic for a given neural region. Fifth, some glial cells are generated with neurons, but most glial cells are generated at high rates after neuronal proliferation has essentially been completed. Sixth, the number of neurons for a given region is determined by the duration of the proliferation period for that region (ranging from days to several weeks for different regions), the duration of cell mitotic cycle (a few hours per cycle early in development to 4 to 5 days per cycle later in development), and the number of germinal or precursor cells. Seventh, more cells are generated for a given neural region than are found in the mature neural region; this cell loss results from cell death due to the lack of establishment of functional synaptic connections. Finally, most neuronal migration involves postmitotic cells, except those cells of special germinal zones, such as the subventricular zone and the external granule layer of the cerebellar cortex.

Cellular differentiation and organization. Neuronal differentiation and growth are predominant events during the migration process, but more so after the neurons have reached their final positions. In these later phases of neurogenesis, the developing telencephalon consists of the ventricular zone; the subventricular zone (which persists after birth and contains mitotic figures for glial cells throughout adulthood); the intermediate zone, which differentiates into subcortical regions and the cortical plate (which further differentiates to form the layers of the cerebral cortex except layer I); and the marginal zone, which is sparsely populated by neurons and forms layer I of the cerebral cortex (Fig. 2-1).[61]

The final position in the brain occupied by a migrating cell is primarily determined by its position in the germinal zone when the cell is generated.[56] Final neuronal aggregation and orientation within neural regions is most likely related to trophic factors, some characteristics of cell surface molecules, and neuronal activity.[28] Molecules on the cell surface (cell ligands) may function as receptor sites and

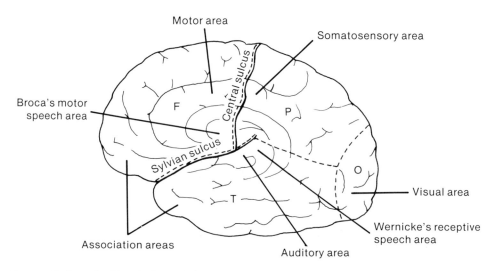

Fig. 2-5. Left cerebral hemisphere of the human brain with locations of sensory, motor, speech, and association areas. The occipital *(O)*, temporal *(T)*, frontal *(F)*, and parietal *(P)* lobes are indicated, as are the central and Sylvian sulci.

promote aggregation of cells. Different types of cells may have different ligands resulting in aggregation of like cells and exclusion of foreign cells. Disruptions of the neuronal aggregation process may result in ectopic or disoriented neurons and neurological dysfunction.

The peak period of neuronal differentiation and organization in the human brain occurs from 6 months of gestation through several years after birth (Fig. 2-3).[24] Development of the elaborate circuitry of the human brain is achieved through the following processes: the attainment of proper orientation and alignment of neurons such as seen in the cortical layers and columns, the elaboration of dendritic and axonal ramifications, the establishment of synaptic contacts, and the proliferation and differentiation of glia (Fig. 2-4). In addition, these organizational processes are influenced by developmental changes: a neuron's mode of transmission (e.g., to action potential from graded potential), the formation of chemical synapses rather than electrical synapses (gap junctions), the chemical transmitter finally utilized (e.g., norepinephrine or acetylcholine), and the major ion of the action potential (e.g., calcium in the immature versus sodium in the mature).

Most newly differentiated neurons have many short dendritic processes and thus are multipolar neurons, the most frequent type of neuron in the mature brain.[82] In addition, neurons typically generate their processes (axon and dendrites) after migrating to their final destination, although, exceptions are found. Recent studies suggest that the distinctive dendritic arbor of a neuron may be genetically determined, but that afferent input can influence the expanse of the arbor (Fig. 2-4). Axons are usually well developed and complete with terminals before dendritic growth and expansion occur. The time elapsing between the origin of a neuron and the time it is fully differentiated varies as a function of neuron type. Some neurons, such as Purkinje cells, originate early but have a long period of differentiation, whereas others such as cerebellar granule cells are generated relatively late and differentiate rapidly.[61]

Elongation of neuronal processes (axons and dendrites) is accomplished via the growth cones at the tips of growing processes.[61] Growth cones are enlarged areas of about 10 μm in diameter from which emerge fingerlike projections called filopodia, which are 0.15 to 0.30 μm in diameter and about 20 μm long (Fig. 2-4). Filopodia wave, expand, and contract within periods of seconds. They are the sites of adhesion between the growing process and the substrate and may also function as tactile and/or chemosensory agents that test the environment in which they are growing.[61] The growth cone is also the site of incorporation or acquisition of new material that has been transported to the growth cone from the soma. The growth cone is not only the site of new growth of a process, but also may be the site of process branching or bifurcation. Other processes may not have growth cones per se, but may grow along gradients, glial channels, or "pioneer" axons. Throughout the nervous system, axonal

process development tends to precede the development of dendritic processes.

The initial axon outgrowth appears to be genetically preprogrammed to aim in a particular direction. Later axonal growth and reaching the final destination(s) seem contingent on external forces, such as characteristics of the electrical, chemical, and physical substrate. Growth of the axon is at the tip, and the materials for growth have been transported outward from the soma. Once an axon has grown to its general destination, axonal branching may or may not be random, and contacts with other neurons that do not become functional may eventually be eliminated.[61]

Dendritic differentiation starts later than axonal differentiation and proceeds long after axonal differentiation has essentially been completed. The dendritic tree shape of a neuron is characteristic of that neuron, yet the dendritic expanse of the tree may be influenced by external factors.[51,61] Similar to the timetable for generation of neurons, dendritic development and elaboration seem to proceed first in large neurons and then in small neurons. Dendritic development occurs typically in a ventrodorsal or inside-to-outside sequence (Fig. 2-4); however, there are general exceptions to this trend. For example, Purkinje cells originate early and have a prolonged period of dendritic development, whereas cerebellar granule cells are generated late, yet show rapid dendritic differentiation. Within the cerebral cortex, dendritic expansion is first radial (vertical) and then tangential (horizontal) for both pyramidal cells and local circuit neurons (Fig. 2-4).

The dendritic tree of a "mature" neuron has 90% of its postsynaptic surface in the mature organism. Early in neural development, however, the dendrites are short, stout, varicose, and of uneven diameter (Fig. 2-4). Fine hairlike protrusions are evenly distributed along the young dendrite. With further growth, the proximal portions of the dendrites attain a more even diameter and the long hairlike protuberances remain. These hairs may be searching out growing axons. Further growth of the dendrites is associated with the formation of a substantial number of spines, some of which have dilated tips. As the dendritic tree reaches maturity, the number of spines gradually decrease and many of the early dendritic branches are lost or absorbed.

Understanding how the brain develops with all of its appropriate interneuronal connections is far from complete; however, we are currently gaining some insights.[28,61,106] As indicated earlier, cells generated at the same time from the same region of the germinal matrix tend to stay together throughout migration and differentiation. Like cells tend to aggregate and thus are more likely to interconnect; axons tend to grow with their neighbors. In addition, a number of trophic factors have been studied as possible guides for neuronal interconnections, such as nerve growth factor.[70] It has also been frequently observed that neurons tend to generate more processes and make more connections early in development than are found later in the fully mature neural region. Thus there seems to be a period of process retraction and connection (synaptic) elimination that contributes to neural organization during development. Finally, cell death seems to contribute to neural organization. More neurons are initially generated for a neural region than are found with maturation.[27,42] During the period of formation of neural connections, cell death may claim up to 85% of the neurons within a given region. The range of cell death varies from 15% to 85% of the neurons of regions studied to date. Cell death may be related to the size of the region innervated, the availability of functional contacts, or the amount of some trophic material.[28]

Synaptogenesis. Synaptogenesis within the human brain begins early in prenatal development and continues to some extent throughout the life span of the human organism. It may occur, for example, with learning and with repair phenomena associated with brain damage (Fig. 2-3). Synaptogenesis is the establishment of a chemically mediated functional contact between neurons. The development of a synapse requires specialization of the presynaptic and postsynaptic membranes and neurotransmitter synthesis, release, storage, and inactivation. There are numerous known and putative neurotransmitters within the nervous system, for example acetylcholine and dopamine. Synaptogenesis is a prerequisite for communication and functional interaction between neurons.

While synaptogenesis in the human brain begins early in gestation, the highest rates of synaptogenesis occur during the early postnatal period.[61] It must be kept in mind, however, that the rates of synaptogenesis differ for the various neuron types, both within and between neural regions. Chemical indices of synaptogenesis show a rapid increase in synapse formation from 2 months before birth to 2 years after birth. The increase in synapse formation from birth through 2 years of age is approximately threefold.

The process of developing a synapse (e.g., axodendritic synapse) requires the growth of an axon at the growth cone (filopodia), such that contact is made with a potential postsynaptic membrane, a dendrite for example. When a filopodia makes contact with a dendrite, filopodia activity ceases for about 30 minutes. The filopodia will then frequently resume its activity, either leaving the contact intact or breaking contact. If contact is preserved, a postsynaptic specialization begins to appear within a few hours, and this specialization elongates with time. The synaptic cleft widens within about 2 days to achieve the normal adult distance of approximately 18 nm. Parallel with the postsynaptic specialization, a presynaptic dense projection develops. By approximately 1 day after initial contact, synaptic vesicles can be seen within the presynaptic terminals, and the number of vesicles continues to increase with time. While synapse formation appears to depend heavily on an interaction of presynaptic and postsynaptic membranes and intercellular contacts, the events associated with synapse formation do not seem to depend totally on functional activity per se.[93]

In the development of a synapse, the postsynaptic membrane may be sensitive to putative neurotransmitters before the synapse has fully developed. In fact, postsynaptic specializations may even develop before any interneuronal contacts are made.[111] Thus in most cases, the postsynaptic system interacts with the neurotransmitter showing a simultaneous development; however, this can occur even before the development of neurotransmitter synthesis in the presynaptic terminals have reached adult levels. At the early or immature synapse, the receptors are few and sparse, and there are low levels of synthesis and release of neurotransmitters. At this time, there are very few recognizable synaptic structures or specializations. Later, rudimentary synaptic structures develop, and there is a rapid increase in the number and density of postsynaptic receptors. Still later, biochemical maturation of presynaptic and postsynaptic components for synthesis, transport, and inactivation of neurotransmitters is achieved. Finally, all synaptic structures are present.[61]

The early appearance and maturation of neurotransmission in the absence of a morphologically and biochemically mature presynaptic apparatus seem to be a general developmental phenomenon for synaptogenesis. This may indicate that early synapses function under different and more primitive conditions than in the adult. A low release of neurotransmitter from an immature presynaptic terminal may be sufficient to trigger the process of neurotransmission and subsequent phases of synaptogenesis.

Synaptogenesis proceeds in an orderly sequence in various brain regions. The development of functional synapses, however, appears to be different between neuron types and between neural regions. For example, synapses can be found in the human cerebral cortex as early as 8.5 weeks of gestation.[90] These synapses are found above and below the cortical plate, never within the cortical plate. At 8.5 weeks of gestation, the density of synapses is low (5 per mm^2); then the number of synapses increases rapidly with age. The earliest synapses within the cortical plate are found at 23 weeks of gestation. The development of synapses in the cortical plate at this age may be associated with a second wave of axonal input to the cortex in conjunction with the development of dendrites of neurons within the cortical plate. All of these cortical synapses are presumably the axodendritic variety. At these early ages, many of the presynaptic elements have vesicles, but presynaptic vesicles are fewer in number than in mature presynaptic terminals. This layering of synapses in the developing cortex, first above and below the cortical plate, then within the cortical plate, is an indication that development of synaptic strata may be a characteristic feature of the immature cortex. This stratification may result from the fact that thalamocortical fibers reach the presumptive cortical layers before the migrating cortical neurons.[77]

Potential presynaptic and postsynaptic membranes may not appear morphologically different from other areas of the cell surface. Spines of postsynaptic neurons tend to be associated with synapses, however, and this might indicate that areas of the spine surface membrane have a special capacity to initiate synaptic contacts. Because dendritic spines are a prevalent site of synapse formation, the number of dendritic spines on a neuron may be used to estimate the number of synapses. In addition, increases in dendritic length may be associated with increased numbers of spines and thus increased synapse formation.[61]

In the developing cerebrum, there is a large prenatal and postnatal increase in total dendritic length, suggesting an increase in the number of synapses.[61,83] However, there is a general trend for the number of spines and synapses to increase during development, with a subsequent loss or regression of spines and synapses, as nonfunctional synapses are eliminated. In the visual cortex of the human brain, the maximum rate of spine development occurs from 25 to 32 weeks of gestation.[106,143] In the hippocampus, the maximum rate of spine development occurs earlier, at 20 to 28 weeks of gestation, and the full complement of spines is achieved by approximately 6 months after birth.[96,97,104]

While change in the sensitivity of the presumptive postsynaptic membrane may be important for the development of a functional synapse, it may not be the only regulator of synaptic development. Synaptic development may also be regulated by some characteristic of afferent input.[61,111] For example, in the visual system, deafferentation results in a 50% decrease in the surface area of dendritic spines. It is also known that axons form contacts with large numbers of neurons in their projection field, but the final distribution of contacts depends in part on competition with other axons for a limited number of synaptic sites on the receptor cell. Axons normally in the vicinity of a receptor cell tend to form synapses preferentially with that cell. If those axons were destroyed, the receptor sites would be available to axons from other normally foreign neurons. Finally, the pharmacology of a synapse may be relatively flexible during development. For example, some neurons can become noradrenergic or cholinergic, depending on the types of postsynaptic membranes with which they come into contact.[61]

Myelination. The period of myelination within the human nervous system begins prenatally and extends well into adult life.[151,156] The period of most rapid myelination within the human brain is after gestation term (Fig. 2-3). It is thought that myelination of neurons improves coordinated behavior via an increase in neuronal conduction velocity. Myelinated fibers propagate impulses approximately six times faster than nonmyelinated fibers, and conduction velocity of myelinated fibers in humans increases threefold from birth to adulthood. Although myelination is considered to be an important characteristic of neural development, it should be remembered that neurons are capable of carrying impulses before myelination. In other words, functional characteristics of neurons appear before myelin; however, myelination is often considered to be an index of total neuronal maturity.

Immediately preceding and overlapping the onset of myelination is a period of rapid proliferation of glial cells (presumably an increased proliferation of oligodendroglia that are associated with the processes of myelination) within the CNS (Fig. 2-4). This burst of cellular (glia) proliferation occurs at 20 to 30 weeks of gestation, a time that follows most of the neuronal proliferation.[31] From 30 weeks of gestation to gestation term, there is a twofold increase in cells and a further twofold increase of cells from birth to 8 months of age. Smaller increases in cells continue for many years after birth.

Myelin formation is the major source of growth of the white matter in the CNS. Myelination begins close to the soma of a neuron and spreads distally. Myelin accumulates in two forms. It increases in thickness as it circles an axon, and it increases as the axon elongates during development. It has been suggested that myelin formed early in development differs in some chemical characteristics from myelin formed later in development.[61,156] The accuracy and potential significance of this suggestion are unknown. In the mature brain, myelin represents approximately 25% of total brain weight.[61]

Myelination of neurons occurs generally in the same order as neuronal generation and differentiation, and for a given level of the neuraxis, large neurons myelinate before small neurons.[156] The first myelination occurs in neurons of the peripheral nervous system when axons attain a diameter of approximately 1 to 2 μm. In general, axons generated earliest tend to be largest and those tend to myelinate earliest. The earliest myelinating axons are the ventral (motor) roots of the spinal cord, which begin myelination at approximately 4 months of gestation. Next to myelinate are the dorsal (sensory) roots of the spinal cord, which begin at 5 months of gestation and continue to develop for many months after birth (Fig. 2-3).

In the human nervous system, myelination tends to follow a general caudal-to-rostral gradient; however, different neurons within a neural region may myelinate at different rates. Homogeneous nerves and fiber bundles tend to myelinate as a group and display a relatively short cycle for myelin completion. More heterogeneous nerves and fiber bundles tend to take longer to complete myelination. The sequence of myelination within the nervous system parallels phylogenetic trends of regional neural development.[156]

Within the developing CNS, gradients occur in the process of myelination. Myelination progresses from the lower lamina of the cortical plate to the outer lamina of the cortical plate, and from the intracortical plexus of vertical fibers to the plexus of horizontal fibers. Myelination of fiber systems mediating sensory input to the thalamus and cortex generally precedes myelination of fiber systems mediating integration of sensory input into motor output (efferents). For example, myelination of the medial and lateral lemniscus, trapezoid body, brachium of the inferior colliculus, optic chiasm, optic tract, and optic radiations begins earlier than myelination of the pyramidal tract, corticospinal tract of the midbrain and pons, superior cerebellar peduncle, and frontopontine tract. Within the cerebral hemispheres (especially within the association areas, intracortical neuropil, and cerebral commissures) the process of myelination persists over decades of postnatal life (Fig. 2-3).[156]

One of the earliest myelinating systems in the brain is the vestibulocochlear system, which shows myelination in the tegmentum and tectal region by the end of the fifth month of gestation (Fig. 2-3), about 2 weeks earlier than myelination of the medial lemniscus (somatosensory function). The vestibulocochlear system at the brainstem level completes myelination before gestation term, whereas myelination of the medial lemniscus is not complete until approximately 1 year after birth. In the forebrain, the first myelin appears at approximately 7 months of gestation, and myelination becomes rapid in the thalamus, subthalamus, and pallidum during the last trimester of gestation.[156]

There is little myelin within the white matter of the cerebral hemispheres until about the last month of gestation. In the precentral gyrus (sensorimotor function), myelination begins at approximately 2 to 3 months after birth. It is interesting that, similar to the commissural and association fibers of the cerebral cortex, the fibers of the reticular formation show little myelin at gestation term and a very long postnatal period of myelin formation (Fig. 2-3).

Brainstem fibers of the vestibular and acoustic sensory systems (medial longitudinal bundle, lateral lemniscus) myelinate early, and myelination is well advanced by gestation term.[156] The brainstem fibers (medial lemniscus, inferior cerebellar peduncle, and brachium conjuctivum) of the proprioceptive and exteroceptive sensory systems begin myelination later than the brainstem fibers of the vestibular and acoustic sensory systems. In addition, the duration of the period of myelin formation is elongated. In the forebrain the projections from the thalamus to the geniculocalcarine (optic), postcentral (somesthetic), and precentral (propriokinesthetic) cortices display rapid myelination during the first year after birth, whereas the thalamic projections to the geniculotemporal (auditory) cortices have a protracted period of myelination beyond the first year. With the exception of the latter, myelination of the thalamocortical projections precedes that of the corticofugal fiber systems of sensorimotor integration.

Interestingly, the prethalamic levels of the vesticuloacoustic system begin and complete myelin formation early compared with the somatosensory, optic, and corticofugal fiber systems. At the cortical end, however, the optic system rapidly myelinates during the first year of postnatal life, whereas the auditory system of the temporal lobe displays a protracted period of myelin formation beyond the first year

of postnatal life. This sequencing of myelination suggests very early development of brainstem levels of vestibuloacoustic function, as compared to other sensory systems.

Normal sequential human nervous system development

The development of the human nervous system begins with the formation of the neural groove and neural plate at about 18 days of gestation (Figs. 2-1 to 2-5). This is followed, at 3 to 4 weeks of gestation, by formation of the neural tube, which is composed of the ventricular (innermost), mantle, and marginal (outermost) layers, and by formation of the neural crest. The neural tube differentiates into the CNS (brain and spinal cord), and the neural crest gives rise to most of the peripheral nervous system (cranial, spinal, and autonomic ganglia and nerves). The neural tube is the site of the four fundamental embryonic zones (ventricular, subventricular, intermediate, and marginal zones) involved in cellular proliferation and migration. The germinal zones involute or disappear with maturation. At this time, the three primary vesicles of the brain are beginning to form: the prosencephalon or forebrain, the mesencephalon or midbrain, and the rhombencephalon or hindbrain. By the fifth and sixth weeks of gestation, the telencephalon, diencephalon, mesencephalon, metencephalon, and myelencephalon are beginning to differentiate and the cerebral hemispheres are bulging. The three primary flexures (cervical, pontine, and midbrain) of the brain are represented, nerves and ganglia are present, and sympathetic ganglia are forming segmental masses (Fig. 2-2).

The paired cerebral hemispheres, corpus striatum, thalamus, and hypothalamus are rapidly increasing in size at 7 weeks of gestation. In addition, the pituitary gland is recognizable, and the choroid plexuses of the ventricle are appearing. At 8 weeks of gestation, the cerebral cortex begins to acquire its typical cells and the olfactory bulbs are visible. The dura mater and pia-arachnoid are distinct by this time. By 10 weeks of gestation, the spinal cord has attained its internal structure (Fig. 2-2).

At 12 to 14 weeks of gestation, the hemispheres are readily recognized, the thalamus is enlarged, and the cerebellum has begun to develop. At this age, the brain attains its general structural features, the spinal cord shows cervical and lumbar enlargements, and the cauda equina and filum terminale are appearing. The lateral ventricles of the brain are separated and connect the third ventricle via the interventricular foramen (of Monro), the cerebral hemispheres are not yet showing fissures, and neuroglia are beginning to differentiate (Fig. 2-2).

The cerebral hemispheres have bulged and lie over much of the brainstem at 16 weeks of gestation. The lateral (sylvian) fissure now separates the temporal lobe from the other neural lobes (frontal, parietal, and occipital), which are also recognizable at this time (Fig. 2-5). The cerebellum assumes some prominence at this age and the corpora quadrigemina (superior and inferior colliculi) are appearing. By 20 weeks of gestation, the major brain commissures are in place and myelination of the spinal cord has begun. At 25 weeks of gestation, the cerebral cortex begins to show its typical layering pattern, and at 28 to 30 weeks of gestation the fissures (central, calcarine, and parietooccipital sulci) and convolutions of the cerebral hemispheres are appearing rapidly (Figs. 2-2 and 2-5). By 8 months of gestation, the precentral and postcentral gyri are prominent and the lateral sulcus remains wide, exposing the insula. Essentially all primary and secondary cortical sulci are represented at this age, as are some tertiary cortical sulci. During the final month of gestation, myelination of the brain becomes rapid. The frontal, temporal, and occipital lobes are stubby or blunt and the lateral sulcus is still wide. Most of the cerebral gyri are broad and plump and the fissures are shallow (Fig. 2-2).

At gestation term, the regions of the cerebral hemispheres posterior to the central sulcus are more developed than those regions anterior to the central sulcus (Fig. 2-5). The frontal and temporal poles are still short; however, the closure of the lateral sulcus almost covers the insula. Few tertiary sulci are on the cerebral cortex. The subcortical white matter is not yet completely myelinated, and the brain has a soft gelatinous consistency. By 2 years of age, the brain proportions are similar to those of the adult. Myelination of the brain is now quite advanced, the cerebral hemispheres show many tertiary sulci, and the brain is of a firmer consistency.[67,122,154,155]

The brain of the typical full-term newborn human infant weighs approximately 350 g, which represents approximately 10% of the newborn's total body weight. By 1 year of age the brain has increased in weight to about 1000 g.[31] At puberty the female brain weighs approximately 1250 g and the male brain weighs approximately 1375 g. The brain of a female generally grows more rapidly than that of a male up to the third year of age; thereafter, the brain of a male grows faster than that of a female. The human adult brain weighs approximately 1500 g and represents only 2% of adult body weight. Thus it is clear that the major increase in absolute size and weight of the human brain occurs postnatally. The increase in brain size is twofold to threefold during just the first 12 months of postnatal life! This rapid brain growth period begins after the final neuronal number has been largely achieved (by midgestation) and is a function of glial multiplication, dendritic and axonal growth, establishment of synaptic connections, and myelination.[31]

In comparison to the remainder of the brain (forebrain and brainstem), the cerebellum shows a delay in reaching its peak period of cellular proliferation and weight increase. In spite of the delay, however, these measures reach adult values sooner in the cerebellum than in the forebrain or brainstem.[31]

Spinal cord and peripheral nervous system. In the portion of the neural tube that will become the spinal cord, two alar plates develop dorsolaterally and two basal plates develop ventrolaterally (Fig. 2-2). These plates (columns) are connected by roof and floor plates and separated by the

sulcus limitans. The basal plate will contribute elements to motor units and does not appear to extend beyond the mesencephalon rostrally. The alar plate contributes to development of the telencephalon and diencephalon in addition to lower structures (Fig. 2-2).[67,122]

The basal plate gives rise to the ventral horn cells and cells of the intermediolateral cell column of the spinal cord. These cells will eventually make up the preganglionic sympathetic neurons, the intermediate motor neurons, the ventral motor neurons, and the motor neurons of certain cranial nerve nuclei. The alar plate gives rise to relay and internuncial (interneuron) neurons in the spinal cord. Peripheral sensory neurons are derived from the neural crest.[61] Fibers leaving the alar plate and found as early as the fifth week of gestation are for intersegmental connections.

Up to 3 months of gestation, the spinal cord fills the entire vertebral column. With differential rates of growth between the spinal cord and the vertebral column, the end of the spinal cord is at the third lumbar vertebra at gestation term and at the first to second lumbar vertebra in the adult. This allows low lumbar punctures to be made without danger of spinal cord injury.

Cell bodies in the alar plates form the dorsal or posterior horns of the spinal cord gray matter. Likewise, cell bodies of the basal plates form the ventral (anterior) and lateral gray horns. Axons of the ventral horn cells grow out of the spinal cord to innervate somites, and the axons acquire myelin sheaths from Schwann cells (which are derivatives of neural crest cells). These axons form the ventral roots of the spinal nerves. The dorsal roots of the spinal nerves are formed by unipolar neurons whose cell bodies reside in the dorsal root ganglia. These neurons are derived from neural crest cells. Some axons of these neurons enter the spinal cord and make synapses, whereas others ascend the spinal cord up toward the brain.[29]

The peripheral nervous system develops as follows (Table 2-2). Sensory ganglion (dorsal root) neurons are derived from the neural crest. Lower motor neurons are derived from the basal plate, and their axons emerge through the ventral root to innervate muscles and glands. Neuroblasts of the neural crest and basal plate migrate peripherally to form the autonomic nervous system ganglia. The outgrowths of the neural crest and basal plate form early and invade the adjacent somites. As the somite differentiates and migrates to its final location in the body, the initial neuronal connections are maintained and carried away with the migrating somite. Because the number of nodes of Ranvier are fixed early in development, the carrying of the axon by the somite results in an elongation of the internodal segments of the axon.

A reciprocal relation exists between a peripheral nerve and peripheral tissue. For example, an uninnervated muscle cell is receptive to becoming innervated, but once innervated it will not usually accept any additional innervation, thereby sparing muscle cells potentially antagonistic axonal inputs.

Because of the branching capacity of nerve fibers, however, a single axon may branch repeatedly and thus innervate many muscle cells (a motor unit). This process of axonal branching increases the probability that all muscle cells will receive axonal input.

Evidence suggests that neural crest cells may be pluripotent; that is, they differentiate according to the sites in which they settle. The cells of the spinal sensory ganglia form compact cell aggregates under the influence of somites. Somites appear to be required for appropriate growth of spinal sensory neurons (Fig. 2-2).[61]

Cerebellum. The cerebellum develops from symmetrical thickenings of the dorsal parts of the alar plates, which eventually fold over the fourth ventricle (Fig. 2-2). At 9 to 10 weeks of gestation, the Purkinje cells move out of the ventricular zone to initiate the cerebellar cortex.[110] By 10 to 11 weeks of gestation, the external granule cells of the subventricular zone have migrated to the outer surface of the cerebellar cortex. At this time, the cerebellar cortex already has many afferent inputs. From 16 to 25 weeks of gestation, the Purkinje cells enlarge and form apical dendritic trees.[157] Also at this time, the first granule cells appear in the cerebellar cortex followed by the appearance of basket cells. The normal maturation of the Purkinje cells is influenced by contacts with climbing fibers. All lobules of the cerebellar vermis can be identified as the major fissures develop at 15 weeks of gestation, and the fissures continue to develop up to 2 years of age.[74]

The two sources of neurons for the cerebellum are the ventricular-subventricular zones and the rhombic lip. The neurons migrate to form the cerebellum via radial and tangential migration (Fig. 2-1). Neuroblasts migrate to the mantle layer of the cerebellar plate and the mantle layer evolves into two strata. These strata are (1) the deep stratum, which differentiates to the deep cerebellar nuclei (fastigii, globose, emboliform, and dentate nuclei) and (2) the superficial stratum, which differentiates into the Purkinje and Golgi type II cells. Germinal cells of the rhombic lip migrate over the surface of the cerebellar cortical plate to form the external granular layer (another germinal zone). This layer gives rise to the granular cells of the granular layer and the stellate and basket cells of the molecular layer.[139]

While the Purkinje cells are forming their dendritic trees within the molecular layer, the granule cells are migrating down from the external granular layer through the molecular layer to the granular layer along the preexisting processes of Bergmann glial cells (a radial glial cell). The interaction between the migrating granule cells and the Purkinje cells results in the formation of the parallel fibers of the granule cells, the normal differentiation of the Purkinje cell dendritic tree, and the specific synaptic connections between these two neuron types. The timing of these developmental phenomena is remarkable. The final cerebellar development is complete within about 2 years after birth, with the differentiation and

growth of Golgi type II cells, stellate cells, basket cells, climbing fibers, and mossy fibers.[61]

Cerebral cortex. The neurons of the six-layer neocortex are derived from the ventricular and subventricular zones of the neural tube, and cells migrate to successively more peripheral layers. The first sign of neocortical development is a narrow plate of neuroblasts immediately beneath the marginal zone in the lateral wall of the presumptive hemisphere, dorsolateral to the presumptive corpus striatum in the vicinity of the presumptive central sulcus. This cortical plate can be identified at approximately 8 weeks of gestation and progressively thickens by the addition of migrating cells (Fig. 2-1).[130]

Cells migrating to the cortex are simple, typically bipolar neurons with a 200 μm leading process. These neurons appear to attain their final positions via radially oriented glial guides. The presumptive cortex is already rich in afferent neurons from the thalamus as it gains in cells. The final positioning of cortical cells is a function of interactions of migrating cell processes with the processes of other cells.

In the motor cortex, thalamocortical afferent neurons arrive before and during cellular migration (Fig. 2-5). The first cortical cells to appear are the cells of layer I (an exception to the inside-to-outside gradient of neurogenesis), followed by the Cajal-Retzius cells and the pyramidal cells of layers V and VI at approximately 5 months of gestation. At approximately 7 months of gestation, the cortical basket cells (interneurons) appear in layer IV, and at 7.5 months of gestation, the pyramidal cells have arrived in layers III and II. The various Golgi type II cells and other small neurons appear later during the prenatal and possibly the early postnatal periods.[77] The final appearing neurons in the cortex are intrinsic interneurons (stellate cells), neurons for lateral interactions (horizontal cells), interhemispheric callosal cells, and secondary extrinsic afferent neurons (association neurons).

During the development of individual pyramidal cells of the cortex, the apical dendrites appear first, followed by the basal dendrites (Fig. 2-4). The apical dendrites develop primarily during the late prenatal period, and the basal dendrites develop primarily during the first year of postnatal life.[89] Axonal sprouts begin to leave the cortex after 8 weeks of gestation and are directed toward the diencephalon and lower centers. Many of the axons terminate within or dissect the corpus striatum, whereas others project through the internal capsule and on through the crus cerebri and pyramid to enter the spinal cord.

The mature human cerebral cortex contains approximately 5 to 10 billion neurons. In addition to gaining neurons during development, the characteristics of the cortex change dramatically during the early growth periods. For example, in layer III of the midfrontal gyrus, there is a fivefold decrease in cell packing density from birth through 1 year of age. During the same 1-year period, there is a fourfold increase in cell body volume, a fivefold increase in dendritic branching, and a 16-fold increase in total dendritic length (Fig. 2-5). Between 1 year of age and adulthood, each of these measures shows a further change of approximately twofold (Fig. 2-4).

The cortex develops in a basic inside-to-outside and caudal-to-rostral gradient. The laminar structure of the six-layer neocortex is (at least partially) a function of these neurogenesis gradients. The radial (vertical) pattern of neurogenesis is reflected in the cortical layers and also is apparent for the cortical columns. For at least the basal dendrites of the pyramidal cells of layers V, IV, III, and II, there is an inside-to-outside pattern of basal (lateral) dendritic formation of pyramidal cells within and across layers.[89] The tangential (horizontal) organization of cortical dendrites in humans persists through 2 years of age.[123] Tangential cortical development also is apparent for dendrites of Golgi type II cells and other small neurons with later-appearing dendrites.[92]

The synaptic input to the cortex also appears to develop in strata. A direct route of axons from the thalamus is through the presumptive corpus striatum in the outermost zone of the hemisphere wall. The thalamic projections separate into a deep and a superficial sheet around the cortical plate at approximately 8 weeks of gestation. A third stratum projects to the cortical plate, forming synapses at approximately 23 weeks of gestation. Cortical cells typically form synapses at the time they reach their final positions; however, some cortical cells may be dormant for weeks or months before developing interconnections.

Changes in cortical thickness have been frequently studied and provide important data on human brain development.[106,153] In the presumptive hand area of the precentral gyrus (sensorimotor cortex), the increase in cortical thickness is rapid from 8 months of gestation through gestation term (Fig. 2-5). From birth to 6 years of age, the increase in thickness of the cortex is slow and then is rapid again from 6 years through adulthood. In the presumptive motor area for speech (Broca's area), the thickness of the cortex increases rapidly from 8 months of gestation to about 1 month after birth. Further increase in cortical thickness is slow through 4 years (Fig. 2-5), and little change in cortical thickness takes place after 4 years of age. In the presumptive orbital-frontal cortical area (higher cognitive function), the cortical thickness increases rapidly from 8 months of gestation through 2 years of age; from 2 years of age through adulthood, the increase in cortical thickness is slow and steady (Fig. 2-5). Although these developmental changes in cortical thickness tend to parallel behavioral development, the correspondence is not exact for these representative areas.[106]

The cerebral convolutions (sulci and gyri) appear in humans during the fifth month of gestation and continue to develop postnatally (Fig. 2-2). This time period corresponds to the period of maximal increase in volume of the cerebral cortex. The primary convolutions are the first to appear developmentally and are relatively constant in location, configuration, and relationship to cortical architectonic fields. The constancy of the primary and secondary cortical sulci may result from regional differences in growth of dendrites and thalamocortical projections to functionally distinct regions (Fig. 2-5). The cortex on the gyrus tends to get strong thalamic projections, whereas the cortex at the bottom of the sulcus gets weak thalamic projections. The major gyri also tend to receive heavy thalamic projections from distinct peripheral regions, which represent a functional mapping into the cortex.[149] The tertiary convolutions begin to develop during the third trimester of gestation and mature postnatally. The tertiary convolutions appear random in their form and anatomic relationships and may be produced by intracortical forces, that is, mechanical forces generated by differential growth of the various cortical layers.[113]

None of the cortical convolutions make their appearance during neuronal proliferation; rather, convolutions begin to appear during the phases of glial production, growth of neuronal processes, and myelination. This is the period of the most rapid growth and increase in volume of the cortex. An earlier theory proposed that convolutions develop as a function of more rapid growth of the flexible cortex, relative to the slower growth of the more rigid subcortical structures.[66] The more recent theory (presented in the preceding paragraph) is that convolutions are a result of relative growth differences within the cortex itself, that is, between layers and regions. The three outer cortical layers grow faster than the three layers of cortex, and different cortical regions grow at different rates as a function of the growth of their thalamic projections.[113]

Prenatal and postnatal development of the brain

Brain growth spurts. Postnatal development of the human brain results primarily from growth of neurons and elaboration of their axonal and dendritic processes, glial proliferation, synaptogenesis, and formation of myelin. Among the principal features of growth of an individual neuron during the postnatal period are enlargement of the cell body, increase in the number of Nissl's granules (ribonucleic acid, RNA), formation of neurofibrils, increase in numbers of mitochondria, branching of axons and increased axonal diameter, elaboration of the dendritic tree, increased numbers of axon terminals, and elaboration of myelin.[61] This neuronal growth produces developmental changes in characteristics of various neural regions. For example, because of the growth of neurons, cortical width increases with age, and concurrently, neuronal density decreases because of the relative expansion of the neuropil. At birth, cell bodies occupy approximately 14% of the volume of the cerebral cortex; in the adult, cell bodies occupy only 6% of the volume (Fig. 2-3). While each of these processes are active during the prenatal period, they are all accelerated during the early postnatal period.

The late prenatal period extending through the early postnatal period is a time of rapid brain growth, which Dobbing and Sands[31] called the "brain growth spurt." The brain growth spurt in the human is a transient period of rapid brain growth that begins when the final number of neurons has already been largely achieved.[31,152] The human brain growth spurt begins at approximately midgestation, and the onset of this spurt is correlated in time with the enormous multiplication of glial cells, not neurons. The later phase of the brain growth spurt is a function of elaboration and growth of axons and dendrites, increase in synaptogenesis and myelination, as well as growth in neuron size. The deceleration of the brain growth spurt parallels the decrease in the rate of myelin formation. The brain growth spurt per se ends at approximately 2 to 4 years of age; however, subsequent brain growth continues through adulthood, at an attenuated rate (Fig. 2-4).[31]

These results reinforce the notion that significant human brain growth takes place during the postnatal period. This period of extremely high rates of growth begins during midgestation and continues through the first 2 to 4 years. It is worth noting that at least five sixths of this brain growth spurt occurs postnatally. At the time of gestation term, the human brain has achieved only 27% of the adult value for weight and cell number.[31] The human brain growth spurt may be a period of increased brain vulnerability to extraneous influences, for example, malnutrition, drugs, or trauma.

Epstein[33-35] has taken the concept of brain growth spurts a step further and uses indirect data to support the hypothesis that postnatal brain development occurs as a series of growth spurts and plateaus through at least the young adult years. He suggested that brain growth spurts occur for the human brain at 3 to 10 months, 2 to 4 years, 6 to 8 years, 10 to 12 or 13 years, and 14 to 16 or 17 years of age. During the intervening years, the brain displays essentially no growth, that is, a plateau. The total increase in brain weight that occurs during these five brain growth spurts is approximately 35% of the total adult brain. Each of these brain growth spurts (e.g., increase in myelin or neuropil) contributes to an increase in complexity and speed of interneuronal communication, leading to more complex and more reliable neural networks. The individual brain growth spurts appear to be correlated in time with developmental phenomena such as Piaget's stages of cognitive development, the growth of mental age, development of language, sensory growth, and electroencephalogram (EEG) changes.* These brain growth spurts appear to be related to total brain weight only, and no obvious brain regions show similar spurts. It is highly possible, however, that telencephalic structures may be

displaying growth corresponding to these postnatal brain growth spurts. This notion has interesting implications for education and therapy.[52]

Development of hemispheric lateralization and specialization. The existence of hemispheric specialization or lateralization has been known for many years. The left hemisphere of most right-handed individuals has a special role in language and the control of complex voluntary movement, whereas the right hemisphere has special functions associated with analyses of visuospatial dimensions of the world (Fig. 2-5). Functional lateralization of the hemispheres is relative, not absolute, however, and females appear to have less functional hemispheric asymmetry than males. Lenneberg[68] concluded from his research on brain-damaged developing humans that lateralization of function in the brain begins at the time of language acquisition and is complete by puberty; however, anatomical, electrophysiological, and pathological data indicate that hemispheric lateralization may be manifest prenatally.

Considerable evidence indicates that hemispheric morphological asymmetries are present in utero and can be attributed to differential growth patterns of the two hemispheres.[88] For example, one of the major indices of hemispheric asymmetry in adults, a larger planum temporale on the left hemisphere, is also found in fetal brains. The planum temporale incorporates the auditory association area known as Wernicke's area, an area important for receptive language abilities. An asymmetry in the size of Broca's area (important for expressive language abilities), which is larger in the left hemisphere, is also found in fetal brains. Because these brain areas are important for language function, their prenatal asymmetrical presence in the left hemisphere may indicate a biological predisposition for the acquisition of language in humans. Other anatomical hemispheric asymmetries present in utero include a wider and more protruding right frontal pole and a corresponding wider and more protruding left occipital pole.

There is also evidence of a right-to-left gradient in the embryological development of the cerebral hemispheres, in addition to other well-known gradients including anterior-to-posterior and ventral-to-dorsal gradients.[88] Interaction of these multiple gradients over time requires a 3-dimensional conceptualization of the complex embryonic hemispheric growth. Evidence for the right-left hemispheric gradient includes the development of the primary fissures in the right hemisphere at approximately 1 to 2 weeks earlier than in the left hemisphere. The left hemisphere may have a growth advantage for earlier embryonic/fetal development of the tertiary sulci and gyri. This pattern may indicate that frontal motor and premotor areas, as well as primary sensory areas, develop at earlier ages in the right hemisphere. Support for this pattern is obtained from studies showing a right hemispheric advantage for discrimination of musical notes by 2 months postnatal, along with no advantage for the left hemisphere in discrimination of speech syllables until 3

*References 13, 62, 68, 100, 129, and 147.

months of age. Earlier development, however, does not necessarily mean that mature function is achieved earlier. For example, although children begin reading (left hemisphere) at around 6 years of age, they do not develop the ability to process complex geometric patterns and faces (right hemisphere) until around 10 years of age. The issue of hemispheric and functional lateralization is further complicated by the early effects of hormones on brain development and the well-known gender and handedness differences seen in various developmental disabilities (e.g., males and left-handers showing a greater incidence of cerebral palsy and mental retardation).[88]

The evidence in favor of early hemispheric specialization and lateralization is quite strong across a variety of other behavioral systems, including sensorimotor systems. Hemispheric specializations are not necessarily fixed, however, and can change during infancy and childhood. In most individuals, the development of a right-hand preference is thought to indicate a left cerebral hemisphere specialization. However, if the frequency of reaching behavior is used to measure hand preference, infants at 4 to 5 months of age typically reach with their left hands. A switch to the right hand for reaching typically occurs at about 6 to 9 months of age, and this preference is strengthened through approximately 8 years of age. In contrast, grasp duration as an index of hand preference shows a right-hand preference as early as 1 month of age. Further, there is increased right-hand gesturing during speech, reduced speed of right-hand finger tapping when talking, a stronger right hand, a right-foot stepping bias, and preference for head positioning to the right, all being displayed by 3 years of age or earlier.[135]

Hemispheric lateralization is also apparent for sensory functions. Results of dichotic listening, evoked potential, and electroencephalographic research suggest hemispheric asymmetry in the auditory system of infants only a few weeks old. These infants exhibited lateralized preference for phonemes (left hemisphere) and notes or tones (right hemisphere). For the visual system, hemispheric asymmetry develops between birth and 6 years, depending on the measures used. For rhythmical visual stimuli, a right hemisphere specialization is found for newborn infants. Finally, head turning to the right predominates when perioral tactile stimulation is applied. These results suggest that tests of hemispheric lateralization of sensory or motor function may be used in the evaluation of neurological development and pathology.

BEHAVIORAL AND PHYSIOLOGICAL CHARACTERISTICS OF DEVELOPMENT
Motor development

The acquisition of movement and motor skills occurs in a definite order during development, proceeding from the generalized and simple movements of the fetus, to the highly specific and complex volitional movements of the mature human organism.[65,117] With **motor development,** there is greater control and specificity of movement, spreading from the trunk to the arms, hands, and then fingers. The earliest movements of embryos are generalized whole body movements, which appear to develop into specific movements. A variety of these specific movements each become individually differentiated; then all of the differentiated movements are integrated into a complex behavior pattern. For example, individual leg, foot, and arm movements are ultimately integrated into the walking pattern. This represents a hierarchical integration, or the integration of individual movements into more complex movements.[150]

Motor systems. The anatomical systems critical for the control of movement and tone begin their development during the early prenatal period, and the developmental process continues for many years postnatally (Fig. 2-5). Because the fetus has essentially a full complement of nerve and muscle cells before birth, the later development of the neuromuscular system is primarily a function of cellular growth, establishment of intercellular connections, and myelination. The establishment and development of neuromuscular circuits are required for regulating muscle contractions, and these circuits are basically established during the prenatal and early postnatal periods. Muscle contraction (spontaneous or stimulated) appears to be essential for normal motor development to proceed during both the prenatal and the postnatal periods.

The major neuronal systems controlling motor movement via the lower motor neuron are the (1) primary motor efferent system, comprising the corticospinal and the corticobulbar tracts (pyramidal system); (2) basal ganglia; (3) cerebellum; (4) the rubrospinal, reticulospinal, vestibulospinal, tectospinal, and long spinal tracts; and (5) segmental reflex pathways. The corticospinal tract is concerned with movement of the axial and appendicular musculature (refined voluntary movements), whereas the corticobulbar tract is concerned with movements of muscles innervated by cranial nerves. The basal ganglia (caudate, putamen, globus pallidus, subthalamic nucleus, and substantia nigra) influence muscle power, tone, and movement primarily through effects on cortical motor neurons. The cerebellum is concerned with coordination of motor activity, muscle tone, posture, and equilibrium. The other three tracts are concerned with muscle tone and flexor muscle groups (rubrospinal tract), muscle activity and tone (reticulospinal tract), and extensor muscle tone (vestibulospinal tract). The development of each of these systems appears to be associated with corresponding development of motor behavior. For example, the development of the rubrospinal tract may be related to the flexor posture (flexor tone) in the limbs of a full-term newborn. The reticulospinal system may mediate changes in muscle tone of newborn infants during changes in levels of alertness. The vestibulospinal tract may mediate the reflex activity associated with vestibular input and extensor muscle activity, as displayed by the tonic neck and Moro reflexes (Table 2-3).[144]

The development of muscle in the human organism goes

through eight phases beginning in the first 5 weeks of gestation through gestation term.[14] Axonal terminals contact the developing muscle cells as early as the eleventh week of gestation, and motor endplates begin to appear by the fourteenth week of gestation. From 15 to 20 weeks of gestation, the nuclei of muscle cells migrate to the periphery of the myotube, and from 20 to 24 weeks of gestation early histochemical differentiation occurs. By 38 weeks of gestation the mature myocytic stage begins, which continues through approximately puberty.[20]

During development the motor neuron appears to play a role in the determination of the muscle fiber type.[64] Thus not only do muscle fibers require motor innervation for normal growth, but the motor neuron influences the type of muscle fiber that eventually develops. In this fashion type I fibers (slow, sustained activities) and type II fibers (rapid burst activities) are determined.

Because the axon increases in diameter and the myelin increases in thickness during development, nerve conduction velocities are faster in adults than in newborns. Thus the changes in motor competence that occur during development are a function of changes in muscle, changes in neural input to muscles, changes in higher level inputs to lower motor neurons, and changes in these biologic processes related to movement experience itself.

Prenatal motor development. The earliest movements of the human fetus in utero occur at least as early as 6 to 7 weeks of gestation with smooth, wormlike movements of the body. At 8 weeks of gestation, rapid irregular wormlike movements of the body can be measured, as well as quick flexion and extension movements of the trunk. Asymmetric movements of the whole body and trunk flexion and extension are present at 9 weeks of gestation. The head and limbs begin to extend during the tenth week of gestation. At 11 weeks of gestation, limb movements are wider and the fetus tends to jump and jerk; at 12 to 13 weeks of gestation the head rotates. Leg and arm movements are frequently in opposite directions, and the hands are often brought up to the face. Rotations of the head and trunk result in body position changes within the uterus.

At 13 to 14 weeks of gestation reciprocal and symmetric limb movements become evident. Mouth and breathing movements begin at this age, and the lower limbs may extend and cross. At the fifteenth week of gestation, the fetus may suck the fingers, turn the head, open the mouth, and swallow. At 16 weeks of gestation there is good coordination of the limbs, the hands grasp, and the hands "explore" the uterine walls. Full body extension from one side of the uterus to the other occurs at this age. During the eighteenth and nineteenth weeks of gestation, the fetus displays simultaneous breathinglike and swallowing movements, and "explores" its own body with the hands. By 20 to 21 weeks of gestation, isolated movements of the fingers, feet, eyelids, and mouth are observed. Hiccuplike movements are displayed by the fetus at 22 weeks of gestation. At 24 to 25

weeks of gestation, mechanical stimulation provokes head rotation; and by 26 to 28 weeks of gestation, a sound will stimulate a startle reaction or trunk and head rotation.[58]

From 16 weeks of gestation through term, the fetal motor repertoire increases in complexity and diversity. The fetus kicks, squirms, rolls, stretches, breathes, and hiccups.[141] Through the last trimester of pregnancy the fetus appears to be moving much of the time. There are fast and slow jerks, and more sustained slow movements. The twisting and rolling of the fetus can produce a total change in body position within the uterus. Even the very young fetus is capable of a rich repertoire of movement that is occurring as soon as neuromuscular connections are made during development.

Sontag[132] has classified fetal movements into three basic types. The first is sharp kicking or punching movements of the extremities. These movements increase in frequency and amplitude from 6 months of gestation through birth. The second type of movement is squirming or a slow writhing movement, which is displayed most often during the sixth and seventh months of gestation. The third type of movement is sharp convulsive movement, which resembles a hiccup or spasm of the diaphragm. It has been suggested that fetal movement is a relatively good predictor of later activity, such that active fetuses tend to display advanced motor development at 6 months after birth.[112] Decreases in fetal movements, and/or changes in patterns of fetal movement, may signal fetal distress.[114]

Spontaneous (autogenic) movement patterns. The most prominent behavior displayed by embryos, fetuses, and neonates of a wide variety of species is movement.[3,5,26] Although movement in young fetuses can be elicited by sensory stimulation (e.g., vibration, sound), much of the movement displayed by fetuses appears to be spontaneous/autogenic, i.e., movement that is endogenously generated by the nervous system and is not linked to any known form of internal or external stimulation.[26] Neuroembryologists have theorized that early **autogenic movement patterns (AMP)** play a significant role in neural circuitry modeling, and thus in functional neurobehavioral development. Across species, the ubiquity and neurogenic nature of AMP during periods of nervous system immaturity indicate that the display of AMP during early prenatal and postnatal development may indicate functional nervous system status or integrity.[3,5]

One of the most notable characteristics of AMP is that it is cyclical in nature; that is, bursts of movement activity recur every 1 to 3 minutes. AMP cyclicity in the 1 to 3 minute range has been described for embryos, fetuses, and neonates of a wide variety of vertebrate species, including humans.[3,5,26,131] AMP cyclicity appears to be one of the many rhythmical/cyclical phenomena (e.g., circadian, sleep-wake, behavioral state, rest-activity, kicking-stepping) common to biological systems.

AMP may play a significant role in developmental neuronal modeling by influencing synaptogenesis, neuronal death, and synaptic elimination processes. AMP may represent an overt behavioral manifestation of spontaneous bursting patterns of motor neurons, which is important for the development of sensorimotor neural circuitry patterns. Similar relations between spontaneous neuronal bursting activity and the development of neural circuitry patterns are seen in the development of ocular dominance columns in the visual system. In utero (and in ovo) AMP may facilitate structural and functional development of muscles and joints, as fetal akinesia is often associated with joint contractures and muscle maldevelopment. Thus spontaneous neural activity influences on functional development may be a general principle of neurobehavioral development.

Neurobehavioral continuity of AMP, from prenatal to postnatal life in humans, is indicated by its putative presence from the first trimester of pregnancy and through early postnatal periods. Comprehensive long-term postnatal studies of AMP development in humans are not available; thus it is unclear how (or when) AMP may be integrated, inhibited, or otherwise changed during subsequent postnatal development. Embryonic/fetal/neonatal AMP may contribute to the later development of more mature rest-activity cycles and/or sleep-wake patterns.

Neural control of AMP appears to develop from the spinal cord to brainstem and to forebrain.[3,26] During early embryonic development, endogenous bursting patterns in the ventral horn neurons appear to generate AMP; however, these neurons appear to come under the influence (control?) of brainstem, and subcortical and/or cortical structures, as development proceeds through the later embryonic, fetal, and neonatal periods.[3,119] Relatively early supraspinal influence on AMP is supported by in utero and postnatal studies of fetuses and neonates with abnormal brain development or damage. Hypoxic-ischemic encephalopathy, anencephaly, encephalocele, and myelomeningocele may be associated with relatively normal reflexes, but abnormal spontaneous movement patterns. These results indicate that the AMP measure may be quite sensitive to early nervous system injury or dysfunction.[3,5]

Present research indicates that the cyclicity of AMP is a robust and stable movement pattern during periods of nervous system immaturity. AMP cyclicity appears to be continuous from approximately the first trimester of pregnancy through the early postnatal period, indicating stability across different levels of early nervous system development.[3] AMP cyclicity also appears to be relatively independent of the absolute level (amount) of motor activity. High or low numbers of movements can be associated with similar AMP periodicities at 1 to 3 minutes for fetuses and neonates. In addition, newborn premature infants do not differ for AMP periodicity when measured in supine or prone positioning, in spite of fewer movements displayed in prone position.[3,5] AMP periodicities also appear to persist throughout various waking and nonwaking behavioral states in neonatal, preterm, and full-term infants; however, some

evidence indicates that AMP periodicities may elongate developmentally and therefore relate to developing behavioral state transitions, rest-activity cycles, and sleep-wake patterns. AMP periodicities also do not appear to be disrupted by tactile stimulation (touch, pressure, and/or brush) in newborn preterm infants or by auditory stimulation of newborn full-term infants. Finally, evidence suggests that disruption of neonatal AMP in premature infants is predictive of feeding difficulties at the initiation of oral feeding and performance on standardized behavioral assessments (e.g., Bayley Scales) at 1 to 3 years of age.

Thus AMP appears to be a reliable, robust, and ubiquitous characteristic of neuromotor functioning during embryonic, fetal, and early neonatal periods. The display of AMP may be uniquely sensitive to nervous system injury or dysfunction during early periods of nervous system development. Prechtl[102] has proposed the concept of "quality of movement" to emphasize the importance of characteristics of AMP for assessing nervous system function. Attending to an infant's spontaneous or autogenic movement patterns will likely be an important adjunct to reflex testing for assessing neurobehavioral function of very young infants.[3,5]

Aborted fetuses: Analysis of motor development. Studies of aborted fetuses have generally focused on sensory stimulation-induced movements. Aborted fetuses at 8 weeks of gestation have been reported to display unilateral body flexion in response to stimulation of the primitive mouth region. At 9 weeks of gestation, similar stimulation produces bilateral body flexion. The fetus may extend its trunk at 10 weeks, and the fingers may flex in response to touch at 11 weeks of gestation. Some changes in facial expression may be displayed at 14 weeks of gestation, and the fetus may close and grip the hands. A head turn at 20 weeks of gestation often produces ipsilateral arm movements, and at 25 weeks of gestation, shallow rhythmic respiratory movements are often displayed.[47]

Reflex development. Many of the reflexlike behaviors that are displayed by fetuses in utero will also be seen in newborn, preterm, and full-term infants for several months after birth. These reflexlike behaviors are often referred to as the primitive reflexes (Table 2-3). It is thought that these primitive reflexes are mediated by subcortical neuromuscular systems that are already quite mature, even during the prenatal period. Disappearance of these primitive reflexes during the normal course of neuromuscular maturation is attributed to functional maturation of "higher" forebrain or cortical mechanisms. Presence of these primitive reflexes beyond certain ages of development is considered a signal of possible neurological dysfunction.

Basic primitive reflexes are elicited in the premature and full-term infant at birth (Table 2-3). The rooting reflex is produced by stroking the cheek, which causes the infant to turn the head toward the side of stimulation and opening the mouth. This primitive reflex disappears around 9 months of age. The Moro reflex is also a primitive reflex whereby infants first extend their arms, arch their back, and extend their legs, followed by a total flexor pattern. This reflex can be elicited by a sudden dropping of the head into extension, and the reflex typically disappears at 3 to 6 months of age. The primitive darwinian or grasping reflex, which consists of a strong fist and grip that allows the infant to carry its own weight, is a response to stroking the palm of the hand. The grasping reflex disappears at about 2 to 3 months of age. The swimming reflex consists of well-coordinated swimming movements, in response to placing the infant's face in water. This primitive reflex disappears at approximately 6 months of age. The asymmetrical tonic neck reflex is the adoption of a "fencer" position while the infant lies on the back with the head turned to one side. The limbs on the side of the face extend, while the opposite limbs flex. This primitive reflex disappears at about 2 to 7 months of age. The Babinski reflex is a primitive reflex where the foot twists in (inversion) and the toes fan out in response to a sharp stroke down the sole of the foot. The Babinski reflex drops out at about 6 to 9 months of age. The primitive walking reflex is a series of steplike motions of the infant's legs when held under the arms and with the feet in contact with a surface. This reflex disappears at approximately 4 to 8 weeks of age.

It is thought that primitive reflexes are subcortically mediated and eventually disappear with maturation of cortical/forebrain inhibitory mechanisms. Bower,[18] however, has suggested that many of these primitive reflexes are repetitive processes that reenter the infant's behavioral repertoire at some later stage of development. For example, the primitive walking reflex disappears at approximately 4 to 8 weeks of age, and returns at about 1 year of age when the child begins to walk independently. It also has been shown that if the primitive reflexes are exercised they may not disappear. For example, the walking reflex does not disappear if the infant is repeatedly exercised with it, and exercised infants walk unassisted earlier than nonexercised infants.[158] This characteristic may not apply to all primitive reflexes, however, especially those that appear to have no clear functional significance, such as the Babinski reflex.

Muscle tone in the premature or full-term infant is typically assessed by careful observation of spontaneous posture and passive manipulation of the limbs with the head placed in midline.[45,47] Maturation of tone follows an approximate caudal-cephalic and distal-proximal progression, particularly for flexor tone. By 28 weeks of gestation, the limbs show minimal resistance to passive manipulation in any direction. At 32 weeks of gestation, the lower extremities display distinct flexor tone. Flexor tone has become prominent in the lower extremities by 36 weeks of gestation, and flexor tone is palpable in the upper extremities at this age. The full-term infant displays a flexor posture in all limbs. These indices of tone are apparent in the quiet infant's flexor posturing. It must be noted, however, that at all gestational ages, postures change frequently.[144] Related to muscle tone is the measure of muscle power. Neck flexor

and extensor power are minimal in the infant born at 32 weeks gestation, as indicated by the complete head lag during the pull-to-sit test.[144] In an infant born at 36 weeks of gestation, however, neck extensor power can be observed. In the term infant, neck extensor power has improved and neck flexor power is apparent. The full-term infant can usually hold the head upright for several seconds.[45,47]

It is apparent that considerable motor development has been achieved during the prenatal period, and subsequent motor development after birth appears to be an integration and refinement of the basic movement patterns already established in utero. As put forth by developmentalists, the embryonic organism is active before it reacts to stimulation (i.e., autogenic movements before reflex movements), and partial motor patterns differentiate from total patterns.[67]

Postnatal motor development. Newborn infants display autogenic movement patterns and respond to sensory stimulation.[7] The initial spontaneous movements of the newborn are relatively generalized kicking of the legs and flailing of the arms and are under subcortical regulation. As more refined and specific movements emerge at around 4 months of age, maturation of cortical regulation of movement may be responsible. From this age onward, voluntary movements become more frequent and precise, and balance and posture rapidly improve over subsequent months and years. Thus precision of movement and balance appears to be associated with vestibular, cerebellar, and cerebral maturation; and movement evolves from autogenic through reflexive through voluntary movements during late fetal and early postnatal development.

The general postnatal development of the human infant is an ever-expanding sequence of precision of individual and integrated movement patterns. Newborn through 1-month-old infants are typically capable of turning their heads from side to side while lying in a supine position and are also capable of lifting their heads to some extent while lying prone. The newborn demonstrates a variety of reflexes such as the grasp reflex.[25] In the second month after birth, the infant can lift the head up for a few seconds while in prone. The 3- and 4-month-old infant can lift up the head and chest while prone and can kick the legs. At 4 months of age, the head can be held erect, and the infant can roll from prone to supine.[94] By 6 months of age, infants can raise themselves on their wrists while in prone position, and they can sit in chairs with support. At 7 to 8 months of age, the infant can sit independently, and can stand with the hands held.[128] The 7-month-old infant is also capable of a hook-grasp pattern (hand grasp without thumb opposition).[25] The 9- to 10-month-old infant can turn around on the floor and can creep and crawl.[94] The infant can also stand when holding onto furniture and can walk when handheld.[94,128] The 9-month-old infant also displays a full hand grasp.[25] At 11 to 12 months, infants can pull themselves up to a standing position and can stand alone by 13 to 14 months of age.[128] The 15-month-old child can walk alone and can climb stairs when held. Walking while pushing toys is accomplished at about 16 months, and picking up toys from the floor while standing is displayed at 17 months of age. At 18 months the child can climb into a chair and sit and can run. The 19-month-old child can climb up and down stairs and at 20 months the child can jump.[94] Children can walk up stairs alone at 22 months of age, seat themselves at the table at 23 months of age, and walk up and down stairs alone at 24 months of age.[25]

The developmental sequencing of motor behaviors can also be seen during evaluation of spontaneous postures and movement of the arms and legs. At birth, the spontaneous posture of the arms and legs is predominantly a flexor pattern, which predominates for the first few weeks of life. Over the next few months the pattern evolves through semiflexion, extension, and finally, posture without a predominant pattern. This final pattern is achieved by approximately 6 to 7 months for the arms and 13 to 14 months for the legs. This developmental sequence parallels the development of goal-directed motility, and the progression through the sequence is most rapid for the arms. Likewise, the development of spontaneous motility of the arms and legs of infants progresses through a series of stages from (1) a stereotyped alternating flexion-extension pattern, (2) predominantly asymmetrical movements, (3) predominantly symmetric movements, (4) symmetrical and voluntary movements, and finally, (5) predominantly voluntary movements.

The newborn alternating flexion-extension pattern for the arms is displayed for about the first month. The arms show predominantly asymmetrical and symmetrical patterns at 2 to 4 months. The symmetrical and voluntary pattern of arm movements is displayed through approximately 7 to 11 months, and the voluntary arm movement pattern is displayed by 11 to 12 months. Infants tend to watch and play with their hands and grasp for objects at the same time that symmetrical motility patterns of the arms become manifest. This progression shows how movement patterns become incorporated into goal-directed activities during development. The development of leg motility follows a similar sequence (asymmetrical pattern at 2 to 7 months, symmetrical pattern at 4 to 12 months, and voluntary pattern at 16 to 17 months); however, the developmental time course is elongated.[25]

The development of the grasp reflex of infants also shows a clear developmental sequencing. At 1 to 2 months of age, stimulation between the thumb and index finger produces adduction and flexion of these segments, representing the beginning of the development of the true grasp reflex. The true grasp reflex develops by 3 to 4 months of age, when a stimulus to the medial palm produces sustained flexion and adduction of the fingers. The infant now begins to reach for things and uses a crude palmar grasp. At 4 to 5 months, stimulation of the hand causes supination or an orienting response of the hand, followed by groping for the retreating

stimulus. By 8 to 10 months, the hand gropes after the stimulus, adjusts, and grasps the object; this is the instinctive grasp reaction. It is now possible to fractionate the grasp reflex, that is, produce flexion in a single digit. When the grasp reflex can be entirely fractionated, a true pincer grasp with opposition of thumb and index finger characterizes the voluntary prehension of the infant.

The development of arm and leg posturing, motility, and hand grasp each show a sequencing pattern, whereby each successive developmental component represents an integration and elaboration of each previous component. These behaviors progress from essentially stereotyped automatisms in the newborn through voluntary movements within the first year of life. Each of these behaviors also influence one another during development. Arm and leg posturing advances appear to directly influence the development of goal-directed or voluntary arm and leg movements, and voluntary arm movements appear to directly influence voluntary prehension patterns of the infant. This sequencing continues during the development of eye-hand coordination and through complete maturation of all sensorimotor function.

It is easy to see from the preceding developmental sequence that motor development in the human infant tends to proceed in a general proximal-to-distal (heads-to-hands) and rostral-to-caudal (head-to-legs) fashion. As postural and balance systems mature, the infant attains greater and greater control of locomotor skills. Prewalking locomotor behavior evolves through the crawling (wiggle or belly), hitching and scooting, bear walking, and creeping (on hands and knees) phases before development of bipedal locomotor skills.

Compared to basic locomotor skills, precise hand manipulation tends to develop late and over a relatively long time course. According to Corbin,[25] eye-hand coordination develops in four sequential stages. The first stage, from birth through 16 weeks of age, is the period of static visual exploration when infants look at their hands. From 17 to 28 weeks of age, during the period of active and repeated visual exploration, infants study objects with their eyes—a sort of ocular "grasping." The arms are flung toward the object in a crude attempt to grasp it. The period of initiation of grasp and/or manipulation lasts from 28 to 40 weeks of age, and arm movements are corrected to enable the grasping of objects. In the final stage of refinement and extension, the infant visually explores and grasps objects. This period begins at 40 weeks of age and continues for years, with further development of grasp precision, manipulation, and speed.

During the preschool years motor development improves vastly. Children show tremendous progress in large muscle, small muscle, and eye-hand coordination. These children are usually more advanced in gross motor skills relative to fine motor skills. The middle childhood period is one of improved motor development and coordination. By adolescence, boys tend to exceed girls in physical achievement.

This sex difference may be related to interactions between social and physical factors and does not always favor boys, for example, in endurance and fine motor skills.

Sensory development

A considerable amount of research has been conducted on sensory function with prenatal humans, especially with the tactile and auditory systems (see the preceding section on motor development). Less is known about visual, vestibular, gustatory, and olfactory systems. Anatomically, however, research suggests that most sensory receptors are morphologically mature before birth in humans. Although morphologically mature receptors suggest sensory receptivity, such maturity may not be essential for early reflex responses for some sensory systems, such as the tactile system.[55] Nevertheless, the available data suggest that the tactile (1 to 6 months of gestation), taste (3 months of gestation), vestibular (4 to 6 months of gestation), auditory (6 months of gestation), and visual (mostly complete at birth) receptors mature morphologically while the human fetus is in utero. If these receptors are indeed functional, the developing human fetus must have the ability to monitor its surroundings while in utero.[87]

The sensory systems most likely stimulated within the prenatal environment are the gustatory, tactile, temperature, auditory, and vestibular systems. Fetal responses to stimulation of each of these modalities has been demonstrated in utero; however, although the fetus responds to these stimuli, such responses do not imply that the fetus can "perceive" such sensory stimuli. It is not until approximately 3 months after birth that the sensory receiving areas of the cerebral cortex begin their accelerated maturation (Fig. 2-5).[24]

Thus fetal receptors may mature in utero to prepare for function after birth, and the intrauterine environment may be ideal for sensory development based on the level and quality of stimulation. Optimal stimulation of developing fetal receptors may influence the subsequent formation of optimal neural connections in sensory pathways. This reaction indicates that normal sensory stimulation prenatally, like that postnatally, is essential for normal sensory development. It is also possible that prenatal sensory function allows the fetus to monitor its environment and thus adapt to that environment by making adjustments in behavior and position. For example, vestibular stimulation may be involved in changes in fetal positioning within the uterus, and gustatory stimulation may be a regulator of prenatal swallowing behavior. It is not known how these systems are affected by premature birth, although a considerable number of questions are now being generated.

Development of the visual system. Development of the visual system begins when the optic vesicle invaginates to the optic cup at 5 weeks of gestation. At 7 weeks of gestation the optic nerve fibers grow up the optic stalk from the retinal ganglia cells. These fibers reach the base of the brain at the optic chiasm. At 9 weeks of gestation the eyeball is about 1

mm in diameter, and the precursor muscle fibers are present. The optic tracts of the brain are being laid down at 10 weeks of gestation, and the macula is distinguishable at 11 weeks of gestation. Rods and cones are differentiated by about 4 months of gestation. At birth, the eye is fairly well developed, except for the photoreceptors in the foveal region. Myelin has reached the optic disk, but there is little if any within the brain visual tracts (Fig. 2-4). During the first 4 months after birth, the foveal cones are differentiating and the optic radiations are becoming myelinated. Differentiation of the occipital cortex is also nearly complete at this age (Fig. 2-5).

The newborn infant appears to have 20/150 vision, with a fixed focus of about 20 cm and displays little accommodation. Accommodation is good by 4 months of age. Pupil light and blink reflexes are present by 29 to 31 weeks of gestation, and by 33 weeks of gestation there is a positive response to soft light. At 1 day after birth, the newborn infant displays visual fixation and visual following.

Newborn humans blink to a bright light shown into the eyes and will shift their gaze to follow a moving light.[71] On the day of birth, the infant will also follow a moving target,[115] and neonates seem to prefer curves and corners over straight contours, suggesting that the neonate's visual world is selective.[36] At 1 month of age, infants can recognize their mothers based on visual information, and they display good depth perception by 6 months of age.[79,145] Evidence also suggests that visual fixation ratings for newborns are better predictors of IQ at 3 to 4 years of age than are newborn neurological ratings.[86]

Color vision is demonstrable in infants of at least 2 months of age,[98] and preference for facial patterns develops between 10 and 15 weeks of age. A 1-month-old infant will actually imitate facial gestures.[84] The reader can refer to Chapter 25 for more in-depth review of visual-perceptual systems.

Development of the auditory system. The development of the auditory pontomedullary junction begins at the mid-hindbrain level at about 20 days of gestation, with the initiation of the otic placodes. By 3 to 4 weeks of gestation, the invaginations are closed, forming the otic vesicles (otocysts). The otic vesicle shows rapid development beginning at 4 weeks of gestation. By the fifth week of gestation, the endolymphatic appendage, cochlear duct, utricle, and semicircular canals are all showing their beginnings. The development of the organ of Corti (auditory receptor) progresses rapidly and smoothly from 8 to 24 weeks of gestation. The internal and external hair cells (receptors) are differentiated by about 4 months of gestation, and all peripheral auditory structures appear present by 6 months of gestation. Central auditory structures mature postnatally (Figs. 2-4 and 2-5). Between 6 and 7 months of gestation, the fetus displays responses to external auditory stimulation.

As early as the thirteenth week of gestation, the human

fetus may respond with convulsive movements to extreme auditory (vibratory) stimulation.[132] Newborns may experience heart rate acceleration in response to increasing sound intensity. Such responses have been observed as early as 29 weeks of gestation with differential responses to different tones.[15,133] Newborns show a response threshold to sounds of 40 decibels in intensity.[137]

Using habituation design (decreased responding to repeated stimuli), newborn infants seem capable of sound localization and auditory-visual integration.[12,69] By 3 to 5 days of age, infants are capable of auditory discrimination based on intensity, pitch, and rhythm of sounds. These results suggest that cortical function is achieved very early in development based on the temporal discrimination involved in rhythm of sounds. It must be remembered, however, that auditory cortex myelinates quite late after birth (Figs. 2-3 and 5-5). Intensity and pitch are thought to be at least partially mediated subcortically. Although total myelination occurs later, speech phonemic sounds are discriminated by infants as early as 1 month of age.[32] For additional background in speech and language development, see Chapter 26.

Development of the vestibular system. The vestibular system is one of the most well-advanced sensory systems at birth, in terms of both morphology and function. At birth the vestibular apparatus has achieved the same configuration, size, and position as that of the adult. Early functional development of the vestibular apparatus is also indicated by vestibular responses to low threshold stimulation and vestibular responses, which are proportional to the intensity of the stimulus. These functional characteristics are already present at birth.

The vestibular system is embryologically and anatomically associated with the peripheral auditory system. The otic vesicle gives rise to the three vestibular end organs (the utricle, saccule, and semicircular canals and their specialized epithelial cells), which begin to differentiate during the fourth week of gestation. These end organs are innervated by the sensory endings of the vestibular portion of the eighth cranial nerve. The peripheral vestibular apparatus essentially completes morphogenesis by approximately 45 days of gestation; however, there is some continued development of the semicircular canals at later ages.[91] The late prenatal and early postnatal development of the vestibular system is primarily concerned with the elaboration of central connections. The vestibular system is made up of vast interconnections within the CNS, especially the spinal cord, cerebellum, and oculomotor nuclei. Many of the vestibular projections are the earliest fiber systems to myelinate within the brain, at approximately the fifth month of gestation (Fig. 2-3).[156]

One function of the vestibular system is the stabilization of body and eye positions for precise goal-directed movements.[122] This system is also involved in the control of muscular activity, balance or equilibrium, and position sense. Because of the advanced development of the vestib-

ular system during the early prenatal period, this system may be quite functional in the fetus and may be related to the frequent changes in position of the fetus within the uterus.[87]

Indices of vestibular function are widely used in infant neurological examinations because vestibular function appears essential for maintenance of the body and head in space.[144] A majority of neonates produce active eye movements contrary to the direction of axial rotation while in supine suspension (doll's-eye phenomenon). This reaction is produced in infants as early as 30 weeks of gestation, then disappears or becomes latent with age. The Moro reaction (see Prenatal Motor Development and Table 2-3) assesses vestibular function and is present at birth and disappears by 3 to 6 months of age. Extension of the legs during the positive supporting reaction may also assess vestibular function. By 5 to 11 months of age, most infants produce leg extension and bear their body weight on their legs for a few seconds.

A more direct measure of vestibular function is obtained by assessing postrotatory nystagmus. Developmental studies indicate that postnatal maturation of vestibular function does take place to some extent, in spite of precocious morphological maturation of this system.[144] A more intense postrotatory nystagmus is found in younger children than in older children. The high amplitude responses of younger children may result from low-level reactions of central mechanisms to the vestibular sensory impulses, that is, immaturity of central systems that inhibit vestibular function.

Development of the somatosensory system. The somatosensory system includes the skin senses (touch, pressure, pain, temperature, itch, vibration, and tickle) and the body senses (joint position and movement, muscle length and tension) (Fig. 2-5). This system has a wide variety of receptors, most of which appear to mature during the prenatal period.[87] For example, pacinian corpuscles, though immature, are found in the sole of the foot and thumb of the hand by approximately 20 weeks of gestation. Muscle spindles begin to differentiate at 12 to 20 weeks and become morphologically complex by 22 to 26 weeks of gestation. Mature receptors in the hand are found at 4 months (Merkel's) and 6 months (Meissner's and pacinian) of gestation. The functional development of the somatosensory system, as indicated by myelination (Figs. 2-3 and 2-5), proceeds from the dorsal roots (5 months of gestation), to the medial lemniscus (5 months of gestation through the first year after birth), and then to the cortical projections (1 or more years after birth).[156]

Somatosensory-evoked responses have been studied in premature infants. In infants as young as 29 weeks of gestation, somatosensory-evoked responses of the median nerve (wrist) show constant primary waveform components. The response pattern equivalent to that of the mature newborn is reached by infants at 37 to 38 weeks of gestation. These somatosensory responses appear a few weeks earlier than the comparable visual evoked potential. Both types of evoked potentials (somatosensory and visual) display a linear decrease in response latency, as a function of increasing gestational age.[144]

The development of receptive fields for tactile stimulation occurs initially in the perioral region and spreads down the trunk region. The earliest responses to tactile stimulation are generalized, and the responses appear to be avoiding or withdrawal responses. The earliest fetal (aborted) responses to tactile stimulation (touch) are from the perioral region at about 7 ½ weeks of gestation. The receptor fields for touch then spread to the nose and chin regions (8 to 9 ½ weeks); the eyelids and palms of the hand (10 weeks), the soles of the feet (11 weeks); the face, upper chest, thighs, and legs (11 to 12 weeks); the tongue and back (14 weeks); and finally the abdomen, buttocks, and inner thigh (32 weeks of gestation).

The premature infant of 28 weeks gestation appears to discriminate touch from pain.[144] Touch stimulation produces alerting and slight motor activity, whereas painful stimulation produces withdrawal and crying reactions. Thresholds for painful stimulation become lowered as the infant ages. The rooting reflex in response to tactile stimulation of the perioral region is well established by 32 weeks of gestation.[144] Other details of somatosensory system development have been presented in the sections on motor, auditory, and vestibular system development.

Development of the olfactory and gustatory systems. The olfactory epithelium is differentiated before 2 months of gestation and then matures over the next prenatal months. In atricial species, such as humans and rats, a considerable amount of maturation of the olfactory system (bulb and projections) may occur postnatally.

Research with humans has shown early development of olfactory function. Infants as young as 32 weeks of gestation respond with sucking, arousal, or withdrawal to the odor of peppermint.[118] Newborn infants differentially respond to onionlike odors or anise oil, as well as other substances.[72] Infants can also discriminate the odor of a breast pad belonging to their own mother from that of other mothers.[76]

The development of the gustatory system also begins early in the prenatal period. In the human fetus, the presumptive taste buds (receptors) are present on the tongue as early as the first to second month of gestation and are mature at about 3 months of gestation.[19] By 8 months of gestation, the fetus responds to unpleasant stimuli within the amniotic fluid by decreasing its swallowing. The newborn infant is quite responsive to variations in taste of substances and can make relatively subtle gustatory discriminations. The newborn infant can discriminate among sweet, salty, and bland solutions.[73,148]

As olfactory and gustatory development coincides closely with primitive protective responses, it may play a protective or alertive role in neonatal development. Stimulation of the olfactory or gustatory systems may be used as a treatment technique to arouse infants or young children who are delayed or nonresponsive to visual or auditory modes of stimulation.

Language development

The development of language and cognitive (thinking, reasoning, memory, problem solving, and planning) processes is obviously interrelated and interactive (Figs. 2-4 and 2-5). Language allows a form of communication of information (cognitive) that is uniquely human. During the second year of life, the infant already understands much of another's speech, and now the infant begins to speak the language; however, little agreement is found between the various theories of language development.

The development of language has been studied for many years. Children learn to understand language before they can speak it. Shortly after birth, neonates can determine the direction from which a sound comes and can discriminate different sounds, in particular, the mother's voice. By 2 weeks of age, they can recognize the differences between voices and other sounds, and by 2 months of age, they can recognize different human voices. By the end of the first year, human infants can make fine discriminations between individual words.[68]

Before the acquisition of speech, infants display the following expressions of sound. First is undifferentiated crying, which may be a reflexive form of communication, followed at 1 month of age by differentiated crying, which appears to communicate different need states. At about 6 weeks of age, simple cooing sounds are made, which evolve into babbling at about 3 to 4 months of age. Infants display lallation or imperfect imitation during the second half of the first year and imitate many of their own sounds. During the ninth and tenth months, the infant imitates the sounds of others (echolalia). By the end of the second year of life, the child has developed a form of speech (a string of words) that is not yet completely communicative.

At approximately 1 year of age, the child is capable of using one word sentences ("dada"), which expand into two-word sentences ("me go") at about 2 years. These one- and two-word sentences are true language, because this telegraphic form of speech contains words that carry true meaning. By the age of 3 years, the child has a vocabulary of approximately 900 words and the sentences become longer. By 4 to 5 years of age children are capable of using full, complex, adultlike sentences that demonstrate near mastery of the rules of grammar in their speech. By 6 years of age, most children have amassed a vocabulary of about 8000 to 14,000 words.

The preschooler's speech is of two main types: egocentric and socialized. Egocentric speech is used to guide the child's behavior, and socialized speech is intended to communicate with others. The younger the child, the more egocentric speech is used. The environment of the preschool-aged child can strongly influence the subsequent development of language. The school-aged child up to about 9 years of age displays an increased understanding of more complex syntax. Egocentrism is diminishing at this time and communication is increasing.

Two frequently studied theories of language development are the learning and the biological theories. The learning theories stress that language is acquired through reward and punishment, or imitation; however, psycholinguists typically disagree with these theories. The biological theories propose that humans possess a built-in neural system that enables a child to process language (see Development of Hemispheric Lateralization and Specialization and Fig. 2-5).[22,23] Piaget favors an interactionism theory, which acknowledges the mutual influences of heredity, maturation, and environmental stimulation.[99-101]

Cognitive (learning and memory) development

Although it seems intuitive that neonates and infants are capable of learning, the type and extent of learning in infants have been the subject of much controversy. Evidence suggests, however, that even very young infants are capable of several types of learning, including habituation, imitation, classical conditioning, and operant conditioning.

Piaget[59,99-101] has classified cognitive development into three basic stages. The sensorimotor stage of cognitive development is from birth to 2 years of age. The preverbal infant exhibits intelligent (adaptive) behaviors during this stage. The infant evolves from a primarily reflexive individual to one who is capable of rudimentary foresight, and the infant develops the concept of object permanence. The preoperational stage of cognitive development lasts from 2 to 7 years of age. During this stage, symbolic function develops, which allows children to represent and reflect on their environments. Thought is gradually becoming more flexible, but the child still cannot deal with adultlike abstractions. Symbolic function is manifest through language, deferred imitation, and symbolic play. The child is still egocentric and has difficulty with reversibility of events. The stage of concrete operations ranges from 6 to 11 years. Here, the child now uses symbols (mental representations) to carry out operations. The child becomes increasingly proficient at classifying and ordering objects and events, dealing with members, and perfecting the reality of conversation. The constraint of egocentrism on thought processes is diminishing at this time. The adolescent years are the stage of formal operations, during which the child develops the ability to think abstractly. Thus the child can now solve problems, test hypotheses, and engage in hypothetical, deductive reasoning. The environment is of crucial importance during this stage, and thought progresses from extreme rigidity to flexibility. The changes in cognitive processing that occur between birth and adolescence are clearly under biological and environmental influences. Current research has focused on the development of different types of learning and memory processing abilities, and the neurology of memory.

Research conducted with a variety of species, including humans, indicates that there are at least two types of memory processing, referred to as declarative/configural or procedural/elemental by different authors.[75,126,136] The configural versus elemental memory terminology will be used here because it does not rely on language per se. Configural memory relates to disambiguation of stimuli, where the meaning of a stimulus changes as a function of relational, contextual, or configural cues, i.e., "knowing what." Elemental memory relates to simple stimulus-response associations, such as found in classical conditioning, i.e., "knowing how." Evidence suggests that configural memory abilities depend on functioning of the temporal lobe, whereas elemental memory is more diffusely encephalized in widespread spinal cord and brain areas, including the cortex, the basal ganglia, and the cerebellum. The frontal lobes are involved in short-term (i.e., "working") memory, attention, and response inhibition, all of which are important for cognitive functioning.[49,95]

The development of memory processing abilities is of interest for both practical (e.g., educational) and theoretical reasons (e.g., memory neurology), and it is clear that profound changes take place in memory processing abilities during development of humans and other species.[30] The phenomenon of infantile amnesia displayed by children younger than approximately 4 years of age is suggestive of significant changes in memory processing that occur during early development. Issues of infantile amnesia and formal schooling readiness strongly indicate that there are qualitative changes in memory processing abilities from infancy through childhood. Ontogeny of these memory systems appears to display a differential developmental time-course, with early functional maturation of the elemental memory system, and later functional maturation of the configural memory system.

During the late fetal, neonatal, and early infancy periods, rats, nonhuman primates, and humans appear capable of elemental memory processing (e.g., habituation and simple associative conditioning). However, development of configural memory processing abilities appears to be prolonged or delayed until later stages of development. Children do not appear to be able to process configural memories until approximately 3 to 5 years of age,[50,116] a period that appears to parallel (and may underlie) the late abatement of infantile amnesia and the late onset of school readiness at 4 to 5 years of age. This phenomenon may be related to the prolonged postnatal development of the temporal and/or frontal lobes. Not only do frontal and temporal regions show prolonged postnatal development, but also the degree of development of both regions can be influenced by environmental enrichment.[37] Thus the relatively late development of the frontal and temporal lobes, combined with their sensitivity to environmental stimulation, may underlie the well-known influences of the environment on cognitive development in children.

With regard to the preceding discussion, it is interesting to note that many children may have academic problems in school, although their performance on standardized assessments (e.g., intelligence tests) may be within the normal range. This observation may indicate that standardized developmental and intelligence assessments are not sufficiently sensitive to identify subtle cognitive impairments that may hinder future school performance, especially standardized assessment of cognitive functions of children before 2 to 3 years of age. In this age group test items are limited to simple recognition memory and overlearned routines and skills. Further, standardized assessments, especially those used with younger children, do not directly measure the learning/memory process itself. Thus the learning and memory processing skills that are mediated by the frontal and temporal lobes appear to be important for academic success in school; more specifically for response inhibition, frequent memory updating, problem solving, and relational and contextual concept formation. These cognitive functions are not strongly evaluated by most standardized assessments of the preschool child. As our knowledge of cognitive and nervous system development increases, it is anticipated that more rational biologically and environmentally based assessments of cognitive abilities will become available for accurate early prediction of later learning/memory impairments and academic success.

SUMMARY

This chapter presented the basic characteristics of the development of the human organism from the time of conception through adulthood. In each aspect of development, whether morphological, physiological, or behavioral (psychological), the pattern of development is clear: a series of interdependent and interactive structure-function processes over time (i.e., neural and behavioral fine-tuning). This pattern is seen in the development of the nervous system, motor systems, sensory systems, and cognitive and language processes.

Each phase of nervous system development depends on each preceding phase, thereby allowing ever greater complexity of structure-function interactions. Although many developmental changes reach a peak during the prenatal phase of development, most are active postnatally as well. Considerable evidence suggests that myelination of the nervous system continues beyond the middle years of life in humans; and additional evidence exists for axonal, dendritic, and synaptic changes associated with postnatal experience. In this context we are only beginning to appreciate the true extent of postnatal development of the nervous system. The frequently used concept of "neural plasticity," as applied to the "mature" nervous system, may reflect nothing more than continuation of early developmental processes. More research is obviously needed in this area to increase credibility for relating postnatal neural developmental concepts to learning and therapy intervention practices.

Knowledge and awareness of neural and behavioral developmental processes are important for a complete understanding of normal ontogeny through the developmental arc, and such knowledge is important for an understanding of developmental neural-behavioral abnormalities. Although development is generally characterized as a period of growth and building, periods of rapid development are also periods of increased vulnerability to biological, environmental, and experiential influences. These influences may or may not be pathogenic in nature. Pathological consequences of development are presented in other chapters of this volume.

The development of the human organism is a truly complex process that begins at conception and proceeds essentially throughout the total life span. At each phase of development, a unique behavioral-biological substrate is achieved. Thus the behavioral capacity of the human at any point in time is a function of the past and current biological substrate interacting with past and current environmental experiences. Each phase of human development depends on each preceding phase of structure-function interaction; thus humans are forever developing and adapting.

REFERENCES

1. Acheson RM: Maturation of the skeleton. In Faulkner F, editor: *Human development,* Philadelphia, 1966, WB Saunders.
2. Almli CR: The ontogeny of feeding and drinking behaviors: effects of early brain damage, *Neurosci Biobehav Rev* 2:281, 1978.
3. Almli CR: Influence of perinatal risk factors (pre-term birth, low-birth weight, and oxygen deficiency) on movement patterns: an animal model and premature human infants. In Anastasiow NJ and Harel S, editors: *At-risk infants: interventions, families, and research,* Baltimore, 1993, Brooks.
4. Almli CR and Finger S, editors: *Early brain damage: research orientations and clinical observations,* vol 1, New York, 1984, Academic Press.
5. Almli CR and Mohr, NM: Born too soon: intervention theory and research with premature infants in the NICU. In Vergara E, editor: *Foundation for practice in the neonatal intensive care unit and early intervention,* Rockville MD, 1993, American Occupational Therapy Association.
6. Altman J: Autoradiographic and histological studies of postnatal neurogenesis. II. A longitudinal investigation of the kinetics, migration and transformation of cells incorporating tritiated thymidine in infant rats, with special reference to postnatal neurogenesis in some brain regions, *J Comp Neurol* 128:431, 1966.
7. Amiel-Tison C: *Neurological assessment during the first year of life,* New York, 1986, Oxford University Press.
8. Angevine JB Jr: Critical cellular events in the shaping of the neural centers. In Schmitt FO and Melmechuck T, editors: *The neurosciences,* New York, 1970, Rockefeller University Press.
9. Angevine JB Jr: Time of neuron origin in the diencephalon of the mouse, *J Comp Neurol* 139:129, 1970.
10. Antanitus DS and others: The demonstration of glial fibrillary acidic protein in the cerebrum of the human fetus by indirect immunofluorescence, *Brain Res* 103:613, 1976.
11. Apgar V: A proposal for a new method of evaluation of the newborn infant, *Curr Res Anesth Analg* 32:260, 1953.
12. Aronson E and Rosenbloom S: Space perception in early infancy: perception within a common auditory-visual space, *Science* 172:1161, 1971.

13. Banks MS and others: Sensitive period for the development of human binocular vision, *Science* 190:675, 1975.

14. Battaglia FC and Meschia G: *An introduction to fetal physiology,* New York, 1986, Academic Press.

15. Bernard J and Sontag LW: Fetal reactivity to sound, *J Genet Psychol* 70:205, 1947.

16. Berry M and others: The pattern and mechanism of migration of the neuroblasts of the developing cerebral cortex, *J Anat* (London) 98:291, 1964.

17. Blinkov SM and Glezer I: *The human brain in figures and tables,* New York, 1968, Plenum Press.

18. Bower TGR: Repetitive processes in child development, *Sci Am* 235:38, 1976.

19. Bradley RM and Stein IB: The development of the human taste bud during the fetal period, *J Anat* 101:743, 1967.

20. Brooke MH and Engel WK: The histographic analysis of human muscle biopsies with regard to fiber types. 4. Children's biopsies, *Neurology* 19:591, 1969.

21. Carmichael L: The onset and early development of behavior. In Carmichael L, editor: *Manual of child psychology,* ed 2, New York, 1954, John Wiley & Sons.

22. Chomsky N: *Syntactic structures,* The Hague, 1957, Mouton Press.

23. Chomsky N: A review of verbal behavior by B.F. Skinner, *Language* 35:26, 1959.

24. Conel JL: *The postnatal development of the human cerebral cortex,* 6 vols, Cambridge, 1939-1960, Harvard University Press.

25. Corbin C: *A textbook of motor development,* Dubuque, Iowa, 1973, William C Brown.

26. Corner MA: Sleep and the beginnings of behavior in the animal kingdom-studies of ultradian motility cycles in early life, *Prog Neurobiol* 8:279, 1977.

27. Cowan WM: Neuronal death as a regulative mechanism in the control of cell number in the nervous system. In Rockstein M, editor: *Development and aging in the nervous system,* New York, 1973, Academic Press.

28. Cowan WM: The development of the brain. In *The brain, a Scientific American Book,* San Francisco, 1978, WH Freeman.

29. Detwiler SR: Observations upon migration of neural crest cells, and upon the development of the spinal ganglia and vertebral arches in amblystoma, *Am J Anat* 61:64, 1937.

30. Diamond A: *The developmental and neural basis of higher cognitive functions,* New York, 1990, New York Academy of Sciences Press.

31. Dobbing J and Sands J: Quantitative growth and development of human brain, *Arch Dis Child* 48:757, 1973.

32. Eimas PD and others: Speech perception in infants, *Science* 171:303, 1971.

33. Epstein HT: Phrenoblysis: special brain and mind growth periods. Human brain and skull development, *Dev Psychobiol* 7:207, 1974.

34. Epstein HT: Phrenoblysis: special brain and mind growth periods. II. Human mental development, *Dev Psychobiol* 7:217, 1974.

35. Epstein HT: Correlated brain and intelligence development in humans. In Hahn ME et al, editors: *Development and evolution of brain size,* New York, 1979, Academic Press.

36. Fantz R and Miranda S: Newborn infant attention to forms of contour, *Child Dev* 46:224, 1975.

37. Finger S and Almli CR, editors: *Early brain damage: neurobiology and behavior,* vol 2, New York, 1984, Academic Press.

38. Finger S and others, editors: *Brain injury and recovery: theoretical and controversial issues,* New York, 1988, Plenum Press.

39. Friede RL: The relationship of body size, nerve cell size, axon length and glial density in the cerebellum, *Proc Natl Acad Sci USA* 49:187, 1963.

40. Fujita S: An autoradiographic study on the origin and fate of the subpial glioblasts in the embryonic chick spinal cord, *J Comp Neurol* 124:51, 1965.

41. Fujita S: Application of light and electron microscopic autoradiogra-phy to the study of cytogenesis of the forebrain. In Hassler R and Stephan H, editors: *Evolution of the forebrain,* New York, 1966, Plenum Press.

42. Fujita H and Fujita S: Electron microscopic studies on neuroblast differentiation in the central nervous system on domestic fowl, *Zeit Zellfor Mikroskop Anat* 60:463, 1963.

43. Gain SM: Fat, body size and growth in the newborn, *Hum Biol* 30:265, 1958.

44. Geelen JAG and Langman J: Closure of the neural tube in the cephalic region of the mouse embryo, *Anat Rec* 189:625, 1977.

45. Gesell A: *The embryology of behavior,* New York, 1945, Harper & Row.

46. Gesell A and Amatruda CS: *Developmental diagnosis: normal and abnormal child development.* New York, 1941, Harber.

47. Gesell A and Amatruda DS: Normal and abnormal child development. In Knobloch H and Pasamanick B, editors: *Developmental diagnosis,* New York, 1974, Harper & Row.

48. Gillette R: Cell number and cell size in the ectoderm during neurulation, *J Exp Zool* 96:201, 1944.

49. Goldman-Rakic PS: Cellular and circuit basis of working memory in prefrontal cortex of nonhuman primates, *Prog Brain Res* 85:325, 1990.

50. Gollin ES and Schadler M: Relational learning and transfer by young children, *J Exp Child Psychol* 14:219, 1972.

51. Greenough WT and Volkman FR: Pattern of dendritic branching in occipital cortex of rats reared in complex environments, *Exp Neurol* 40:491, 1973.

52. Guralnick MJ and Bennett FC: *The effectiveness of early intervention,* New York, 1986, Academic Press.

53. Hey EN: Thermal regulation in the newborn, *Br J Hosp Med* 8:51, 1972.

54. Hinds JW: Autoradiographic study of histogenesis in the mouse olfactory bulb. I. Time of origin of neurons and neuroglia, *J Comp Neurol* 134:287, 1968.

55. Humphrey T: The development of trigeminal nerve fibers to the oral mucosa, compared with their development to cutaneous surfaces, *J Comp Neurol* 126:91, 1966.

56. Hunt RK and Jacobson M: Neuronal specificity revisited. In Moscona A and Monroy A, editors: *Current topics in developmental biology,* vol 8, New York, 1974, Academic Press.

57. Hurlock EB: *Child development,* New York, 1950, McGraw-Hill Book Co.

58. Ianniruberto A and Tajani E: Ultrasonographic study of fetal movements, *Semin Perinatol* 5:175, 1981.

59. Inhelder B and Piaget J: *The growth of logical thinking from childhood to adolescence,* New York, 1958, Basic Books.

60. Jacobson M: Development and evolution of type II neurons: conjectures a century after Golgi. In Santini M, editor: *Golgi centennial symposium,* New York, 1975, Raven Press.

61. Jacobson M: *Developmental neurobiology,* New York, 1978, Plenum Press.

62. John ER: *Functional neuroscience,* Hillsdale, NJ, 1977, Lawrence Erlbaum Associates.

63. Karfunkel P: The mechanisms of neural tube formation, *Int Rev Cytol* 38:245, 1974

64. Karpati G and Engel WK: "Type grouping" in skeletal muscles after experimental reinnervation, *Neurology* 18:447, 1968.

65. Krasnegor NA and others, editors: *Perinatal development,* New York, 1986, Elsevier Publishing Company.

66. Le Gros Clark WE and Medavar PB, editors: *Essays on growth and form,* London, 1945, Oxford University Press.

67. Lemire RJ and others: *Normal and abnormal development of the human nervous system,* New York, 1975, Harper & Row.

68. Lenneberg EH: *Biological functions of language,* New York, 1967, John Wiley & Sons.

69. Leventhal AS and Lipsitt LP: Adaptation, pitch discrimination and

sound localization in the neonate, *Child Dev* 35:759, 1964.

70. Levi-Montalcini R and Angeletti PV: Nerve growth factor, *Physiol Rev* 48:534, 1968.

71. Lightwood R and others: *Paterson's sick children,* London, 1971, BailliŠre Tindall.

72. Lipsitt LP and others: Developmental changes in the olfactory threshold of the neonate. *Child Dev* 34:371, 1963.

73. Lipsitt LP and others: Effects of experience on the behavior of the young infant, *Neuropadiatrie* 8:107, 1977.

74. Loeser JD and others: The development of the folia in the human cerebellar vermis, *Anat Rec* 173:109, 1972.

75. Lynch G and others, editors: *Neurobiology of learning and memory,* New York, 1984, Guilford Press.

76. MacFarlene A: Olfaction in the development of social preferences in the human neonate. In *Parent-infant interaction, CIBA Foundation Symposium,* New York, 1975, CIBA.

77. Marin-Padilla M: Prenatal and early postnatal ontogenesis of the human motor cortex: a Golgi study. I. The sequential development of the cortical layers, *Brain Res* 23:165, 1970.

78. Marin-Padilla M: Prenatal ontogenetic history of the principal neurons of the neocortex of the cat (Felis domestica): a Golgi study. II. Developmental differences and their significances, *Z Anat Entwicklungsgesch* 136:125, 1972.

79. Mauer D and Salapatek P: Developmental changes in the scanning of faces by young children, *Child Dev* 47:523, 1976.

80. Maxwell DS and Kruger L: Small blood vessels and the origin of phagocytes in the rat cerebral cortex following heavy particle irradiation, *Exp Neurol* 12:33, 1965.

81. McCarthy KD and Partlow LM: Neuronal stimulation of {3H} thymidine incorporation by primary cultures of highly purified non-neuronal cells, *Brain Res* 114:415, 1976.

82. McMullen NT and Almli CR: Cell types within the medial forebrain bundle: a Golgi study of preoptic and hypothalamic neurons in the rat, *Am J Anat* 161:323, 1981.

83. Meller K and others: Synaptic organization of the molecular and outer granular layer in the motor cortex in the white mouse during postnatal development: a Golgi and electron-microscopical study, *Z Zellforsch Mikrosk Anat Abt Histochem* 92:217, 1968.

84. Meltzoff AN and Moore MK: Imitation of facial and manual gestures by human neonates, *Science* 198:75, 1977.

85. Miale IL and Sidman RL: An autoradiographic analysis of histogenesis in the mouse cerebellum, *Exp Neurol* 4:277, 1961.

86. Miranda S and others: Neonatal pattern vision: predictor of future mental performance? *J Pediatr* 91:642, 1977.

87. Mistretta CM and Bradley RM: Taste and swallowing in utero, *Br Med Bull* 31:80, 1975.

88. Molfese DL and Segalowitz SJ, editors: *Brain lateralization in children: developmental implications,* New York, 1988, Guilford Press.

89. Molliver ME and Van der Loos H: The ontogenesis of cortical circuitry: the spatial distribution of synapses in somesthetic cortex of newborn dog, *Ergeb Anat Entwicklungsgesch* 42:7, 1970.

90. Molliver ME and others: The development of synapses in the cerebral cortex of the human fetus, *Brain Res* 50:403, 1973.

91. Moore KL: *The developing human,* Philadelphia, 1977, WB Saunders.

92. Morest DK: The growth of dendrites in the mammalian brain, *Z Anat Entwicklungsgesch* 128:290, 1969.

93. Morest DK: A study of neurogenesis in the forebrain of opossum pouch young, *Z Anat Entwicklungsgesch* 130:265, 1970.

94. Nelson W and others: *Textbook of pediatrics,* ed 10, Philadelphia, 1975, WB Saunders Co.

95. Obrzut JE and Hynd GW: *Child neuropsychology, theory and research,* vol 1, New York, 1986, Academic Press.

96. Paldino AM and Purpura DP: Branching patterns of hippocampal neurons of human fetus during differentiation, *Exp Neurol* 64:620, 1979.

97. Paldino AM and Purpura DP: Quantitative analysis of the spatial distribution of axonal and dendritic terminals of hippocampal pyramidal neurons in immature human brain, *Exp Neurol* 64:604, 1979.

98. Peeples DR and Teller DY: Color vision and brightness discrimination in two-month-old human infants, *Science* 189:1102, 1975.

99. Piaget J: *The origins of intelligence in children,* New York, 1952, International Universities Press, Inc.

100. Piaget J: *Psychology of intelligence,* Totowa, NJ, 1969, Littlefield & Co.

101. Piaget J and Inhelder B: *The psychology of the child,* New York, 1969, Basic Books, Inc, Publishers.

102. Prechtl HFR: Qualitative changes of spontaneous movements in fetus and preterm infant are a marker of neurological dysfunction, *Early Human Dev* 23:151, 1990.

103. Purpura DP: Stability and seizure susceptibility of immature brain. In Jasper HJ, et al, editors: *Basic mechanisms of the epilepsies,* Boston, 1969, Little, Brown & Co.

104. Purpura DP: Dendritic differentiation in human cerebral cortex: normal and aberrant development patterns. In Kreutzberg GW, editor: *Advances in neurology,* New York, 1975, Raven Press.

105. Purvis D and Lichtman JW: *Principles of neural development,* Sunderland, Mass, 1984, Sinauer Press.

106. Rabinowicz T: Some aspects of the maturation of the human cerebral cortex, *Mod Probl Paediatr* 13:44, 1974.

107. Rakic P: Mode of cell migration to the superficial layers of fetal monkey neocortex, *J Comp Neurol* 145:61, 1972.

108. Rakic P: Timing of major ontogenetic events in the visual cortex of the Rhesus monkey. In Buchwald NA and Brasier MAB, editors: *Brain mechanisms in mental retardation,* New York, 1975, Academic Press.

109. Rakic P and Sidman RL: Supravital DNA synthesis in the developing human and mouse brain, *J Neuropathol Exp Neurol* 27:246, 1968.

110. Rakic P and Sidman RL: Histogenesis of cortical layers in human cerebellum, particularly the lamina dissecans, *J Comp Neurol* 139:473, 1970.

111. Rees RP and others: Morphological changes in the neuritic growth cone and target neuron during synaptic junction development in culture, *J Cell Biol* 68:240, 1976.

112. Richards TW and Nelson VL: Studies in mental development: II. Analyses of abilities tested at six months by the Gesell schedule, *J Genet Psychol* 52:327, 1938.

113. Richman DP and others: Mechanical model of brain convolutional development, *Science* 189:18, 1975.

114. Roberts AB and others: Fetal activity in 100 normal third trimester pregnancies, *Br J Obstet Gynaecol* 87:480, 1980.

115. Rosenblith JE: The modified Graham behavior test for neonates, test-retest reliability, normative data and hypotheses for future work, *Biol Neonate* 3:174, 1961.

116. Rudy JW, Keith JR, and Georgen K: The effect of age on children's learning of problems that require a configural association solution, *Dev Psychobiol* 26:171, 1993.

117. Saint-Anne Dargassies, S: *The neuro-motor and psycho-affective development of the infant.* New York, 1987, Academic Press.

118. Sarnat HB: Olfactory reflexes in the newborn infant, *J Pediatr* 92:625, 1978.

119. Sarnat HB: Do the corticospinal and corticobulbar tracts mediate functions in the human newborn?, *Can J Neurosci* 16:157, 1989.

120. Sauer FC: Mitosis in the neural tube, *J Comp Neurol* 62:377, 1935.

121. Saxen L and Toivonen S: *Primary embryonic induction,* London, 1962, Logos Press.

122. Schade JP and Ford DH: *Basic neurology,* Amsterdam, 1973, Elsevier Scientific Publishing.

123. Schade JP and others: Maturational aspects of the dendrites in the human cerebral cortex, *Acta Morphol Neerl Scand* 5:37, 1962.

124. Schaper A: The earliest differentiation in the central nervous system

of vertebrates, *Science* 5:430, 1897.

125. Schmechle DE and Rakic P: Arrested proliferation of the radial glial cells during midgestation in rhesus monkey, *Nature* 277:303, 1979.

126. Scoville WB and Milner B: Loss of recent memory after bilateral hippocampal lesions, *J Neurol Neurosurg Psychiatry* 20:11, 1957.

127. Serunian S and Broman S: Relationship of Apgar scores and Bayley mental and motor scores, *Child Dev* 46:696, 1975.

128. Shirley MM: *The first two years: a study of twenty-five babies,* monograph, Institute of Child Welfare, Minneapolis, 1933, University Minnesota Press.

129. Shuttleworth FK: The physical and mental growth of girls and boys, age six to nineteen in relation to age at maximum growth, *Monogr Soc Res Child Dev* 4:1, 1939.

130. Sidman RL and Rakic P: Neuronal migration, with special reference to developing human brain: a review, *Brain Res* 62:1, 1973.

131. Smotherman WP and Robinson SR, editors: *Behavior of the fetus,* Caldwell, NJ, 1988, Telford Press.

132. Sontag LW: Implications of fetal behavior and environment for adult personality, *Ann NY Acad Sci* 134:782, 1966.

133. Sontag LW and Wallace RI: Changes in the heart rate of the human fetal heart in response to vibratory stimuli, *Am J Dis Child* 51:583, 1936.

134. Speidel CC: Studies of living nerves. VII. Growth adjustments of cutaneous terminal arborizations, *J Comp Neurol* 76:57, 1942.

135. Springer SP and Deutsch G: *Left brain, right brain,* San Francisco, 1993, WH Freeman.

136. Squire LR and Lindenlaub E: *The biology of memory,* Stuttgart, 1990, FK Schautter Verlag.

137. Steinschmeider A: Developmental psychophysiology. In Brackbill Y, editor: *Infancy and early childhood: a handbook and guide to human development,* New York, 1968, The Free Press.

138. Taber-Pierce E: Histogenesis of deep cerebellar nuclei studied autoradiographically with thymidine-H3 in the mouse, *Anat Rec* 157:301, 1967.

139. Taber-Pierce E: Time of origin of neurons in the brain stem of the mouse, *Prog Brain Res* 40:53, 1973.

140. Thompson H: Physical growth. In Carmichael L, editor: *Manual of child psychology,* New York, 1954, John Wiley & Sons.

141. Timor-Tritsch I and others: Classification of human fetal movement, *Am J Obstet Gynecol* 126:70, 1976.

142. Valadian I and Porter D: *Physical growth and development,* Boston, 1977, Little, Brown.

143. Voeller K and others: Electron microscope study of development of cat superficial neocortex, *Exp Neurol* 7:107, 1963.

144. Volpe JJ: *Neurology of the newborn,* Philadelphia, 1987, WB Saunders.

145. Walk RD and Gibson EJ: A comparative and analytical study of visual depth perception, *Psychol Monogr* 75:170, 1961.

146. Watson EH and Lowrey GH: *Growth and development of children,* ed 5, Chicago, 1967, Year Book Medical Publishers.

147. Wedenberg E: Auditory training of severely hard-of-hearing preschool children, *Acta Otolaryngol Suppl* 110:7, 1954.

148. Weiffenback J and Thach B: Taste receptors in the tongue of the newborn human: behavioral evidence, Paper presented at the biennial meeting of the Society for Research in Child Development, Denver, 1975.

149. Welker WI and Campos GB: Physiological significance of sulci in somatic sensory cerebral cortex in mammals of the family Procyonidae, *J Comp Neurol* 120:19, 1963.

150. Werner H: *Comparative psychology of mental development,* Chicago, 1948, Follett.

151. Weston JA: The migration and differentiation of neural crest cells, *Adv Morphogen* 8:41, 1970.

152. Winick M: Cellular growth of cerebrum, cerebellum and brain stem in normal and marasmic children, *Exp Neurol* 26:393, 1970.

153. Yakovlev PI: Pathoarchitectonic studies of cerebral malformations. I. Arrhinencephalies (halotelencephalies), *J Neuropathol Exp Neurol* 18:22, 1959.

154. Yakovlev PI: Anatomy of human brain and the problem of mental retardation. In Bowman PW and Mautner HV, editors: *Mental retardation, Proceedings of the first conference on mental retardation,* New York, 1960, Grune & Stratton.

155. Yakovlev PI: Morphological criteria of growth and maturation of the nervous system in man, *Ment Retard* 39:3, 1962.

156. Yakovlev PI and Lecours AR: The myelogenetic cycles of regional maturation of the brain. In Minkowski A, editor: *Regional development of the brain in early life,* Oxford, 1967, Blackwell Publisher.

157. Zecevic N and Rakic P: Differentiation of Purkinje cells and their relationship to other components of developing cerebellar cortex in man, *J Comp Neurol* 167:27, 1976.

158. Zelazo NA and others: Walking in the newborn, *Science* 176:314, 1972.

CHAPTER 3

Overview of the Structure and Function of the Central Nervous System

Martha J. Jewell

KEY TERMS

posture	goal-oriented movement
homeostasis	higher cortical processing

LEARNING OBJECTIVES

After reading this chapter the student/therapist will:
1. Identify the four major classes of CNS function and their relationships.
2. Recognize that all CNS function is expressed through the motor system.
3. Analyze how feedback can alter or modify movement through CNS synthesis of that information.
4. Identify the general roles of afferent neurons, interneurons, and efferent neurons in homeostasis, posture, goal-oriented movement, and higher cortical processing.

This chapter provides the reader with a conceptual model or framework of nervous system function. It is hoped that the reader will be able to use this framework as an initial platform from which to implement a problem-solving approach in the evaluation and treatment of the patient with neurological dysfunction. Other chapters in this book will lend more detail to the reader's understanding of nervous system function.

NERVOUS SYSTEM FUNCTION

Simply stated, the function of the nervous system is to receive, integrate, and act on information. We begin the development of the model with a simple reflex arc consisting of an afferent neuron, interneuron, and efferent neuron, whose respective functions are reception, integration, and action (Fig. 3-1). Integration is the summation of all input to that particular neuron. This model is relatively simple, but is only a "stylized representation" of the nervous system and therefore may be too simplistic for some readers. As you read this chapter you may want to seek more detailed information in neuroscience texts and research articles. Some additional readings are listed at the back of this chapter.

Afferent or sensory neurons in the peripheral nervous system conduct impulses (carry information) to the central nervous system (CNS). Efferent or motor neurons innervate glands and muscle (smooth, cardiac, or skeletal). Some efferent neurons (preganglionic autonomic neurons) innervate postganglionic autonomic neurons. All other neurons are interneurons.

A primitive, single segmented organism receives information from its internal organ(s), integrates that information, and acts on that information. It also needs to receive information from its external environment and to protect itself from external danger. The model as described in Figure 3-1 can only receive and react to stimuli on one side of the organism. The model is expanded in Fig. 3-2 to include a collateral of an interneuron and in Fig. 3-3 to include a second interneuron, which spreads information to the opposite side. This second interneuron is called a commissural fiber. Commissural fibers are axons that link right and left halves of the CNS.

The model is still too simple. If several segments are placed together in a stack or column, more complex functions could be possible. To function as a unit, however, information received at one segment must be disseminated to all other segments. This is accomplished by two modifications of the basic model. An afferent fiber can enter one segment and send collaterals to adjacent segments, and/or interneurons can link several segments (Fig. 3-4). Interneurons linking several segments in a rostral or caudal direction are called projection fibers.

The model is now several segments long, receives information from all segments, integrates that information, and produces appropriate actions. The appropriate action might require the coordinated activity of efferent neurons at multiple levels. Some projection fibers might be involved in the integration of afferent information from multiple segments, whereas other projection fibers might be involved in coordinating activity of efferent neurons at multiple levels. Ascending pathways (projection fibers) generally carry sensory information, and descending pathways (projection fibers) generally are involved in coordinating efferent activity. As the complexity of the interneuronal integration increases, there is a need to centralize integration of similar activities to increase efficiency (Fig. 3-5). Therefore regions of the CNS become somewhat specialized to integrate certain activities. Centers in the spinal cord, brainstem, diencephalon, and telencephalon can be conceptualized as groups of interneurons that are involved in the integration of

information received from various segments and in contributing to the production of appropriate actions. For example, as this model of the nervous system becomes large enough to be influenced by gravity, integration centers must be included that respond to externally or internally generated perturbations in the base of support. Simply stated, a key function of the CNS is anticipating internal and external perturbations, for example, to keep or return the body's center of mass over its base of support. To perform this function, existing circuits in the spinal cord and brainstem are used to produce muscle activity aimed at maintaining or returning to an upright **posture.** No new segmental wiring is necessary. Interneurons involved in the integration of agonist and antagonist activity already exist at the segmental level.

To reiterate, the nervous system consists of afferent neurons, interneurons, and efferent neurons. A few specific examples are given in Table 3-1, and many others can be found in neuroscience textbooks. The nervous system functions to receive information by way of afferent neurons and to integrate that information through simple to extremely complex series of interneurons; it also functions to produce activity. The activity must be appropriate, adaptive, and timely. It is important to understand that appropriate activity may present itself to the outside observer as no activity or as a modification or cessation of a concurrent activity. Therefore it is easier to generalize and say that groups of interneurons function to produce and/or regulate activity.

Nervous system function is often observed and measured clinically by noting the results of nervous system activity, often in response to an external stimulus, for example by observing reflex behaviors. Skeletal muscle contraction is observed most commonly and may be as simple as a flexor withdrawal reflex or as complex as postural adjustments. Other results of nervous system activity that can be observed

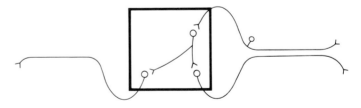

Fig. 3-2. An interneuron with a collateral to the opposite side.

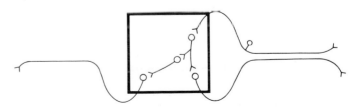

Fig. 3-3. An interneuron synapses on the second interneuron, which crosses to the opposite side.

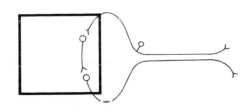

Fig. 3-1. A basic model of the nervous system.

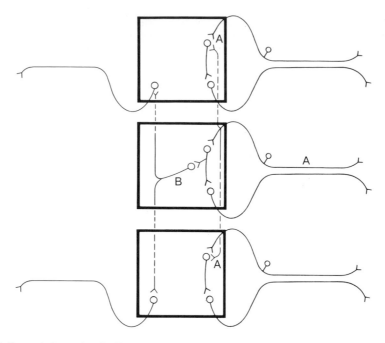

Fig. 3-4. Afferent information is disseminated to segments above and below by afferent collaterals *(A)* and interneurons *(B)*.

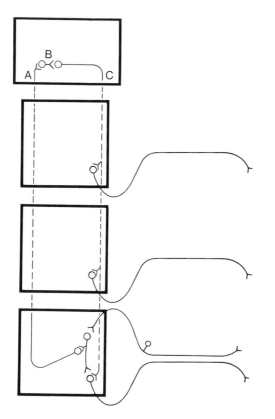

Fig. 3-5. A centralized integration center for segments. *A,* Ascending projection fibers. *B,* The integration center. *C,* The descending projection center.

include contraction of smooth and cardiac muscle and the secretion of glands. These functions are also extremely useful for a clinician to observe and measure.

Another way to conceptualize and discuss CNS function is in relation to evolution. The first, most primitive nervous system functioned to provide internal **homeostasis.** Primitive organisms also needed to protect themselves from their environment. To do this they needed to sense potential danger and withdraw or defend themselves. In humans "fight or flight" reactions, flexor withdrawal, and blink reflexes are examples of protective activities. The hypothalamus and other areas throughout the CNS that are considered part of the autonomic nervous system regulate internal homeostasis in humans. As organisms evolved in size they were influenced by gravity. They needed mechanisms to maintain their position or posture and to return them to that position if disturbed, to maintain their center of mass over their base of support. Righting and equilibrium responses are examples of these postural mechanisms.

As animals continued to evolve, they moved about in their environment, exploring and seeking food. This necessitated the production of **goal-oriented movement** and was dependent on sensory systems capable of providing discriminative information, not only about the environment (exteroception), but also about the musculoskeletal system of the animal itself (proprioception). The animal must localize the source of the stimulus more precisely and respond to it more discretely. The more discrete the input received, the more precise the possible responses. Information from internal and external sources, from general to detailed, must be integrated,

Table 3-1. Examples of afferent neurons, interneurons, and efferent neurons

Afferent neurons	Interneurons	Efferent neurons
Somatic		
Cutaneous 1. Receptors: touch, pain pressure, etc. 2. Fibers: spinal nerves and cranial nerves V, IX, X	1. Synapse: dorsal horn and trigeminal nucleus 2. Projection fibers: spinothalamic, spinoreticular, spinotectal, trigemino-thalamic, and propriospinal	Ventral horn and cranial nerve nuclei III, IV, V, VI, VII, IX, X, XI, XII; plus visceral preganglionics (see below)
Proprioceptive 1. Receptors: muscle, tendon, joint 2. Fibers: spinal nerves and cranial nerves III, IV, V, VI, X, XI, XII	1. Synapse: dorsal horn and mesencephalic nucleus 2. Projection fibers: dorsal column—medial lemniscus, spinocerebellar tracts	Same as above plus visceral preganglionics
Vestibulocochlear 1. Receptors: labyrinth and organ of Corti 2. Fibers: cranial nerve VIII	1. Synapse: vestibular nucleus, cochlear nuclei, inferior colliculus, medial geniculate 2. Projection fibers: lateral lemniscus, geniculotemporals (projection fibers for vestibular system not well traced at this time) 3. Descending tracts: vestibulospinal and tectospinal	Same as above plus visceral preganglionics
Visual 1. Receptor: retina 2. Fibers: cranial nerve II	1. Synapse: superior colliculus, pretectal nucleus, lateral geniculate 2. Projection fibers: geniculocalcarines 3. Descending tracts: tectospinals	Same as above
Visceral		
General 1. Receptors: pain, distention, pressure 2. Fibers: spinal nerves, splanchnic nerves, and cranial nerves VII, IX, X	1. Synapse: dorsal horn and solitary nucleus 2. Projection fibers: spinoreticular, propriospinal 3. Descending tracts: reticulospinal	1. Preganglionics; lateral horn T1-L2, 3; ventral horn S2, 3, 4; cranial nerve nuclei III, VII, IX, X 2. Postganglionics: collateral ganglia such as ciliary, celiac, otic, mesenteric, etc. plus somatic efferent neurons (see above)

Special
1. Gustatory
  a. Receptors: tastebuds
  b. Fibers: cranial nerves VII, IX, X
	1. First synapse: solitary nucleus
	2. Projection fibers: solitary tract
	3. Descending tracts: reticulospinal
		Same as above (somatic and visceral)

2. Olfactory
  a. Receptors: olfactory epithelium
  b. Fibers: cranial nerve I
	1. First synapse: septal area, amygdala, insula, etc.
	2. Projection fibers: hypothalamus, etc.
	3. Descending tracts: reticulospinal
		Same as above (somatic and visceral)

interpreted, and responded to in a timely manner. For the animal to respond appropriately the nervous system must attend to changes in information, not just the status quo. The nervous system therefore must have some mechanism(s) to detect change and alert the rest of the nervous system to that change (reticular activating system). Integration now must include processing information from multiple sources and at different times. Therefore the nervous system must be

capable of memory, learning, association, and recall. The ability to generalize, to use symbols, to anticipate, to predict, and to plan are all CNS functions that are relatively new in evolution and that are certainly complex. Even these functions, however, have afferent, interneuron, and efferent components.

Later sections of this chapter address four major classes of CNS function: homeostasis, posture, goal-oriented movement, and **higher cortical processing,** always using the afferent neuron, interneuron, and efferent neuron model to explain function. It must be emphasized, however, that in reality the nervous system does not function as four separate units. Therefore the interrelationship among the four functions must be considered, each of which is represented and therefore integrated in some way throughout the different anatomic areas of the CNS. All four functions are expressed by accessing the same spinal and brainstem circuits, which are involved in integrating efferents. Muscle contraction is the final printout of motor control systems; therefore, the basic unit of behavior is the motor unit.[5]

All observable somatic behavior is expressed through what has been called the "final common path," the alpha motoneuron and the muscle cells it innervates. What the nervous system controls is partially defined by the properties of the system it controls, the musculoskeletal system. When describing a movement from a kinesiological and biomechanical framework, factors such as speed, acceleration and deceleration, force, distance, complexity, accuracy, and internal versus external stops to the movement must be considered.

The speed of a movement influences how and when the movement can be modified. Balistic movements such as pitching a baseball are too fast for the nervous system to use feedback from the movement to modify the movement while it is in progress. These fast movements are referred to as open loop or feedforward with regard to the use of afferent information. Fast movements require information gained from prior experience. Slower movements such as lifting a half-filled paper cup allow time for the nervous system to compare the actual feedback from the movement in progress to the feedback that was predicted and make adjustments during the activity. This is referred to as a closed loop movement and requires feedback if the movement is to occur smoothly.

All the characteristics of a movement must still be reduced to a basic code, to parameters expressed through motor units. The only parameters that can be varied are the number of motor units firing; the frequency of firing of each motor unit; the sequence in which motor units are recruited; and the onset, duration, and cessation of motor unit activity. From these few variables we can achieve accurate force generation to hold an egg or lift heavy weights, fine coordinated manual movements of a skilled craftsperson, or accurate high velocity movements of a baseball pitcher. Somehow the nervous system converts duration of motor unit activity into distance. How does the nervous system calculate the distance and then produce a movement that is exactly that distance? Somehow the nervous system converts the number of motor units and frequency of firing of those units into the accurate generation of force. The force a muscle generates, however, also depends on the length of the muscle when the movement starts and during the movement.

Perhaps the nervous system "knows" about length-tension curves. Force is also inversely related to the velocity of the movement. The nervous system must "know" something about force-velocity curves; and the nervous system must "know" about mass, the weight of the various segments of the body, inertia, and gravity. The movements produced are not produced by single muscles but by groups of muscles, and each muscle contributes a part to the movement in some predetermined ratio. Motor control from a biomechanical frame of reference then might be conceptualized as controlling degrees of freedom, such as numbers of joints and directions of joint movement, length-tension, or stiffness across those joints.

NERVOUS SYSTEM DYSFUNCTION

Hughlings Jackson believed that nervous system lesions produced no new functions; that they could be explained as too much function (positive signs) or too little function (negative signs).[12] This view works extremely well for understanding peripheral nervous system signs and symptoms where efferent neuron loss results in weakness to paralysis and weak to absent reflexes. Afferent neuron loss results in abberent to absent sensation and weak to absent reflexes. Jackson's model does not work as well to explain dysfunction secondary to CNS lesions. Are clinicians observing the malfunction of centers that have definitive functions in motor control? Systems control theory (see Chapter 4) would not support this hypothesis. Are we observing the nervous system's attempt to adapt to external and internal events given its remaining integrative abilities? If so is our role to facilitate the nervous systems adaptation to a new set of external and internal parameters in a way that is most energy efficient for that individual?

HOMEOSTASIS

As stated earlier in this chapter, homeostasis can be divided into two subfunctions: regulation of the internal milieu and protection of the organism from its environment, that is, internal and external survival.

Regulation of the internal milieu

Anatomical substrates. Part of the afferents for the autonomic nervous system includes sensory fibers that carry information from the walls of blood vessels and viscera, including the entire gastrointestinal, genitourinary, and cardiopulmonary systems. This information includes tissue damage, distention, pressure, vibration, and various forms of chemical information, such as airborne (olfactory sensation) and dissolved (gustatory sensation, oxygen tension, hydrogen ion concentration) chemicals. The afferent information is carried to the CNS in both somatic and visceral afferent neurons found in peripheral nerves from the limbs and body wall, in splanchnic nerves, and in cranial nerves I, VII, XI, and X. In addition, somatic afferent fibers (especially cutaneous, but also visual, auditory, and vestibular) can be involved in visceral reflexive function. The interneurons in the CNS *most directly* associated with afferent visceral information are those of the dorsal horn of the spinal cord (visceral afferent nucleus), the solitary nucleus in the brainstem (which is associated with cranial nerves VII, IX and X), the cardiovascular and respiratory centers (also in the brainstem), and the hypothalamus. Many other centers are involved in integrating visceral afferent information, including the cerebellum, thalamus, and cerebral cortex. The cell bodies of the efferent fibers in the autonomic nervous system (preganglionic visceral motor neurons) are located in the lateral and ventral horns of the spinal cord (T1 to L2 or L3, and S2 to S4, respectively) and in nuclei associated with cranial nerves III, VII, IX, and X (Edinger-Westphal, lacrimal, salivatory, and dorsal vagal nuclei, respectively). Therefore preganglionic efferent fibers are found in spinal nerves T1 to L2 or L3 and S2 to S4 and in cranial nerves III, VII, IX, and X. The craniosacral outflow is the peripheral component of the parasympathetic nervous system, and the thoracolumbar outflow is the peripheral component of the sympathetic nervous system. This information is summarized in Table 3-2. Refer to gross and neuroanatomy textbooks for further details.

Dysfunction. For this discussion we will return to the basic model of nervous system function and dysfunction. If the afferent and/or efferent limb of the reflex is damaged, there is decreased or absent function. A peripheral nerve lesion results in decreased sympathetic regulation of vascular tone in the body part innervated by that nerve. Signs might include trophic skin changes and lack of temperature regulation of the part. (Review physiology textbooks to explore smooth muscle response to denervation and circulating epinephrine.) There is also a loss of autonomic responses associated with somatic sensation from the denervated part (see the previous example of a noxious stimulus and the withdrawal reflex). Peripheral components of the autonomic nervous system are often surgically destroyed. For example, the vagus nerve may be cut to decrease gastric acid secretion. The other functions of the vagus nerve below the lesion are also lost (gut motility, etc.). Occasionally, sympathetic ganglia (usually the stellate ganglion) are surgically or pharmacologically destroyed to decrease sympathetic vasomotor tone. This results in decreased sympathetic function in the head and neck (Horner's syndrome) with ptosis, miosis, endophthalmos, and anhydrosis.

Autonomic function may also be decreased by lesions involving the central component of the afferent or efferent limb. For example, lesions of the dorsal or ventral-lateral horn of the spinal cord or cranial nerve nuclei, where cell bodies of visceral afferent neurons are located, may also result in signs of an autonomic nervous system lesion. If interneurons are damaged, there may be decreased function and/or inappropriate function. For example, spinal cord lesions often result in inability to voluntarily initiate emptying of bowel or bladder, and orthostatic hypotension. Reflexive voiding may be viewed as an adaptive response secondary to loss of regulation of an intact reflex arc by interneurons above the level of the lesion. Taken to extremes, extensive brainstem damage may destroy cardiovascular and respiratory centers, resulting in death. Less profound brainstem lesions may result in inappropriate or uncoordinated function, such as apnea and other inappropriate breathing patterns and even cardiac arrhythmias.

The hypothalamus is an interesting grouping of interneurons in that there are areas that appear to function in direct opposition to other areas. For example, one area decreases

Table 3-2. Examples of afferent neurons, interneurons, and efferent neurons in the autonomic nervous system

Afferent neurons	Interneuron		Efferent neurons
General			
1. Aδ and C fibers carry information on stretch, pain, and pressure in spinal and splanchnic nerves	Visceral afferent nucleus; spinoreticular and propriospinal tracts		Lateral horn T1 to L2 or L3 Ventral horn S2 to S4 Edinger-Westphal nucleus Lacrimal nucleus Salivatory nucleus
2. Aδ and C fibers in cranial nerves VII, IX, and X	Solitary nucleus; solitary tract; reticulospinal tract	Hypothalamus	Dorsal vagal nucleus
Special			
1. Gustatory in cranial nerves VII, IX, and X	Solitary nucleus; solitary tract; reticulospinal tract		Same as above
2. Olfactory in cranial nerve I	Septal area, amygdala, insula		Same as above

body temperature and another increases it. Here we are presented with the first of many semantical problems. If the first area is damaged, is the client's problem inability to decrease body temperature or inappropriate body warming? Hyperthermia is a fairly common sign in clients with head injury.

The autonomic and somatic sensorimotor systems function together in the client and, in fact, often use the same afferent and efferent neurons. Body temperature is raised in part by shivering, which requires somatic motor neurons and skeletal muscle. Shivering may be elicited by a cool breeze on the skin. Any somatic sensorimotor act has an accompanying autonomic activity. Increased muscle activity results in and is paralleled by autonomic activity: increased heart and respiratory rate and decreased gut motility. These two systems do not function in isolation, and they have profound effects on each other. The cerebral cortex also has a profound effect on autonomic interneurons. The treatment environment, through interpretation by interneurons, can influence the autonomic nervous system. Anxiety, fear, and anger enhance sympathetic nervous system response along with somatic and emotional responses (refer to Chapter 5).

External survival

Anatomical substrates. For an organism to survive in a potentially hostile environment, it must be able to sense external danger. Obviously, humans are capable of sensing potential danger that comes in contact with the body; but humans are also capable of seeing, hearing, smelling, and tasting potential danger. Therefore the afferent limb of this arc includes high-threshold cutaneous mechanoreceptors, thermoreceptors, and chemoreceptors whose information is conducted over predominantly Aδ and C fibers in spinal nerves and in cranial nerves V, IX, and X. These high-threshold receptors are often referred to as nociceptors. The noncutaneous information arrives by way of cranial nerves I, II, VII, VIII, IX, and X. The afferent neurons then synapse on interneurons in the dorsal horn of the spinal cord, in the trigeminal nuclear complex and the solitary and cochlear nuclei of the medulla and pons, in the superior colliculus of the midbrain, and in the olfactory areas of the telencephalon. Through a series of interneurons, information finally reaches efferent neurons. To survive in a hostile environment, a person must be able to withdraw from a harmful stimulus. This might include withdrawing a limb from a pinprick or hot stove, blinking and ducking away from a flying object, or spitting out certain strong-tasting foods when you were rather young. The magnitude of the response may vary in relation to the intensity of the stimulus. Therefore the efferent neurons may vary from stimulus to stimulus. In each preceding example a somatic response was elicited; however, each somatic activity is also accompanied by an autonomic (usually sympathetic) response. Not only does the organism withdraw from a stimulus, but the organism also

Table 3-3. Examples of protective reflexes

Stimulus	Afferent neurons	Interneurons	Efferent neurons	Response
Pin prick to index finger	Aδ and C fibers; median nerve; brachial plexus; C6 or C7 root; dorsal horn	Spinal: Association: spread within level Commissural: to opposite side Projection: spinothalamic, spinoreticular and spinotectal; tectospinal, reticulospinal, and tectobulbar	Alpha and gamma motor neurons and adjacent levels Visceral motor neurons Cranial nerve III Cranial nerves VII, X, XII	Withdrawal of finger and possibly whole limb Vasodilation Pupillary dilation "Ouch"
Dust in eye (corneal reflex)	C fibers by way of cranial nerve V to pons	Trigeminal nucleus	Alpha motor neurons in facial nucleus (VII) Lacrimal nucleus: visceral motor fibers by way of VII	Blink Tear
Fast-moving object	Rods and cones; cranial nerve II	Superior colliculus Pretectal nucleus Lateral geniculate Tectobulbar Tectospinal	Alpha motor neurons in facial nucleus (VII) Alpha and gamma motor neurons; cervical ventral horn Visceral motor neurons; upper thoracic cord	Blink Duck head Increase heart rate

prepares internally with increased heart and respiratory rate. Some animals, including some humans, by choice or by instinct will not withdraw from certain threatening stimuli (situations) but will prepare to fight; however, the autonomic response is the same. Some examples of protective reflexes are given in Table 3-3.

Dysfunction. Disturbances in the peripheral nervous system, such as a peripheral nerve lesion, may affect the afferent neuron or efferent neuron (usually both) of a protective response and result in the absence of function. Loss of the blink reflex to visual or tactile stimuli, loss of a startle response, or loss of withdrawal of a body part to noxious cutaneous stimulus may result from the loss of afferent neurons (cranial nerves II, V, VIII, spinal or peripheral nerves, respectively) or of efferent neurons (facial nerve or appropriate spinal and peripheral nerves, respectively).

Disturbances in the CNS may result in an absence of function or inappropriate or adaptive responses. Loss of function might include decreased or absent sympathetic responses, resulting from lesion of the lateral horn of the cord or involvement of the reticulospinal tract or hypothalamus. Loss of function might also include loss of awareness of the existence of the stimulus and inability to localize or identify the stimulus. A structure, path, or nucleus produces a function; a lesion in that structure, path, or nucleus will result in loss of that function. Adaptive signs might include spread of the reflex to the whole limb and to the opposite limb with a relatively mild stimulus. An example is the client with a spinal cord injury who reflexively goes into total body flexor withdrawal when sheets are drawn across the legs. Here, interneurons responsible for regulating the reflex are damaged. Therefore adaptive signs include hypersensitivity or overreactivity to the stimulus, that is, some type of inappropriate response. Tactile defensiveness may be an overreaction of the protective mechanisms to cutaneous stimuli, in fact to nonthreatening stimuli. It can then be conceptualized as the result of decreased function or an imbalance in input to the interneurons that regulate protective mechanisms. When regulatory interneurons do not regulate production, interneurons tend to overproduce and/or to produce inappropriate responses to normally inadequate stimuli. One group of interneurons omitted from the previous tables is the group having to do with affective behavior (the limbic system). In addition to producing a parallel somatic and autonomic response, sensory stimuli also elicit an affective response, an emotional interpretation of the situation. This "emotional tone" has a normal resting level, just like "muscle tone." In CNS damage, however, affective tone may be hyperactive and, like all other systems, it can affect all systems. In fact, it would be more practical and functional to look at sensorimotor responses as three parallel responses: somatic, visceral (autonomic), and affective (emotional). This "affective tone" influences somatic function dramatically, as exemplified by the client whose muscle tone increases with emotional level or the client who becomes more tactilely defensive with increased stress.

POSTURE
Anatomical substrates

As the size and mobility of an organism increases, so does the influence of gravity on that organism. The organism must be able to maintain itself, keeping its rostral end upright and its receptors in a position to search for food and danger. Humans attempt to keep the head upright and the eyes level. Once disturbed, humans, like other organisms, must be able to right themselves. Three sensory systems provide information regarding "uprightness" or the lack of "uprightness," that is, position in relation to gravity and the surrounding environment: the vestibular, proprioceptive, and visual systems. The vestibular system provides information regarding the position of the head in relation to gravity and the linear and rotatory movement of the head. Proprioceptors, especially those associated with axial joints and muscles, provide information about movement of the body segments on each other. The visual system provides information about the body's position in relation to the external environment. Once the vertical position is learned, the motor programmers' feedforward postural function will only change the plan when either the intent to change occurs or the feedback from peripheral receptors mismatch with what is expected.

The interneurons in these systems are involved in the production of appropriate postures. The word *postures* tends to bring forth pictures of rigid poses. But postures produced by the intact nervous system (appropriate postures) are very dynamic. They change constantly with very slight perturbations. They also change from segment to segment and limb to limb. One influences the other. Two examples may make the point clearer. First, consider the vertebral column during gait. If the subject rotates the pelvis to the left during swing, the lumbar spine will rotate to the right to keep the face and trunk facing forward. If the upper trunk is to stay in the frontal plane and if the opposite arm swing is to occur in the sagittal plane, the thoracic spine must be stabilized on the moving lower trunk. For the second example, stand with your arms at your side, then lift your arms straight out in front of you. Just before lifting your arms forward, your trunk and lower extremity muscles moved you slightly posterior in anticipation of the change in your center of mass. This is an example of a feedforward mechanism.[4] Adjustments are also made in the upper trunk and proximal upper-extremity musculature to provide a stable base on which the movement of the limb can occur. Again, "stable" does not mean fixed or immovable. Stability and posture are words that should be prefaced by dynamic, not static.

The terms *posture, a posture,* or *postural control* mean different things to different readers. In this section posture refers to the motor activities whose goals are to maintain or regain upright positions in relation to gravity.

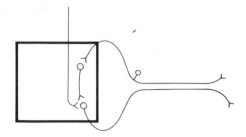

Fig. 3-6. A descending interneuron influences the motorneuron directly.

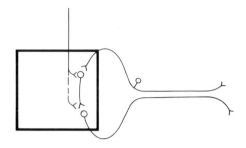

Fig. 3-7. A descending interneuron influences the motorneuron through another interneuron.

Referring back to our basic nervous system model (Fig. 3-5), we can see that it can be applied to the control of posture. The afferent neuron may be part of the visual, vestibular, or proprioceptive systems. The interneurons could be in the tectum of the midbrain, the vestibular nuclei, or the spinal cord. The efferent neurons are alpha and gamma motor neurons to muscles of the trunk and limbs. We wish to reinforce a critical concept at this point. There are basic wiring diagrams at segmental levels. These consist of afferent neurons, several interneurons, and efferent neurons. It makes little difference what the afferent or efferent neurons are for now. It is more important to understand that *all* systems effect output through these basic pathways. The most direct route is monosynaptically through the alpha motor neuron (Fig. 3-6). In fact, much of vestibular control is expressed through this route. The most common way of effecting output is through one or more segmental interneurons (Fig. 3-7). Additionally, control can be exerted through the afferent neuron itself (Fig. 3-8).

A second critical concept is that the influence or effect produced may be facilitory *or* inhibitory. Any synapse represented in Figs. 3-6 to 3-8 could be facilitory or inhibitory. Possibly the single most important concept in understanding neurological function is that *each event, each neuronal firing, produces an effect (facilitation or inhibition) on the postsynaptic neuron, but in most cases no single synapse is adequate to fire the next neuron.* It is the *sum of all the synaptic events,* both facilitory and inhibitory, at any point in time, that determines whether the next neuron will fire. In other words, what we observe clinically reflects the sum total of synaptic events on those alpha motor neurons that respond. Unfortunately, this is all we can observe, record, or measure. This is *not* to say, however, that if there is no observable response there was no effect. Rather, there was no *observable* effect.

All responses are produced ultimately through alpha motor neurons, and it most often involves alpha motor neurons to antigravity muscles such as the gastrocnemius, soleus, and quadriceps (refer again to Figs. 3-5 to 3-8). Reticulospinal and vestibulospinal tracts have both a direct (monosynaptic) and an indirect (via segmental interneuron)

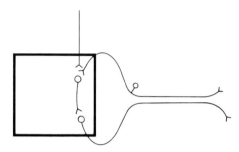

Fig. 3-8. A descending interneuron influences the motor neuron by affecting the afferent neuron.

effect on somatic efferent neurons. All other systems involved in regulation of posture and in production of movement (except corticospinal tracts to hand intrinsics) have an indirect influence on alpha motor neurons. The monosynaptic group Ia reflex, the "quick stretch reflex," was thought to contribute to fine adjustments in standing posture when, for example, the gastrocnemius/soleus is stretched with anterior sway at the ankle. But Nashner[7] has demonstrated that the latency of this reflex response to quick ankle dorsiflexion in standing humans is 120 msec, and H-reflex studies at the knee have shown that the electrically induced reflex response is 30 msec. Therefore the Ia input probably has an "influence" but does not produce the postural response by itself. Nashner[7] postulated that the postural response was the function of a long spinal reflex based on the latency of the response. Nashner also showed the suppression of the response when the response would be inappropriate to the motor program goal and staying upright.

As we examine organisms higher in the evolutionary scale, we can see that more and more functions become controlled by higher centers, especially at the level of the cerebral cortex. A spinalized cat (one whose spinal cord has been severed for experimental purposes), if suspended and stimulated properly, can be made to walk. A cat with chronic decerebrate posturing can stand if placed and may even right itself if knocked over. The basic wiring necessary to produce locomotion is present in the spinal cord. Locomotion can be

Table 3-4. Examples of reciprocal innervation

System	Afferent neurons	Interneurons	Facilitates	Inhibits
Spinal cord				
Cutaneous	In skin over extensor muscle	In gray matter of cord	Underlying extensors	Antagonists
	In skin over other muscles	In gray matter of cord	Flexors	Antagonists
Proprioceptors	Joint afferents (traction)	In gray matter of cord	Flexors	Antagonists
	Muscle spindle (quick stretch)	In gray matter of cord	Motor neurons to muscle stretched	Antagonists
Brainstem				
Vestibular	Cranial nerve VIII	In vestibular nucleus, vestibulospinal tracts, gray matter of cord	Extensors, especially in stance phase of gait	Antagonists
Reticular	All types of sensory information feed into this system	In brainstem reticular nuclei, reticulospinal tracts, ascending reticular activating system	Extensors	Antagonists
Red nucleus	Receives from other CNS interneurons such as cerebellum, basal ganglia, cerebral cortex	In rubrospinal tract, gray matter of cord	Flexors, especially during swing phase of gait	Antagonists
Telencephalon				
Sensorimotor cortex	Mostly exteroceptive and proprioceptive information from cord and brainstem	In lateral corticospinal tract, gray matter of cord	Flexors or extensors	Extensors, flexors

triggered with limb movement in a spinalized cat that is also treated with dopamine.

Why then can't a spinalized primate be made to produce locomotor movements? Primates, especially humans, are the beneficiaries and the victims of *encephalization*. The basic segmental wiring diagrams are probably the same, but the control, the "on-off" switch, is at higher centers. By control we mean the establishment of background activity in the wiring so that it can be triggered by afferent input. *Control* may be the production of a function, or it may be the regulation of a function produced elsewhere. Using the vestibular system as an example, extensor or antigravity tone is produced primarily by the vestibular system and contributed to by the reticular system. Extensor tone can be modified at the spinal cord level by those joint and cutaneous afferent neurons that tend to produce flexor responses, or it can be modified by descending systems, such as the corticospinal tracts, which are capable of inhibiting extensor activity. Extensor tone can be modified from the brainstem by influencing the vestibular nuclei and thus indirectly modifying the activity at spinal levels. In cats with decerebrate posturing this is demonstrated by the further increase in extensor tone when a lesion is also placed in the anterior lobe of the cerebellum or by a decrease in extensor

tone when the intact anterior lobe is stimulated electrically. The gait pattern of the severe, chronic alcoholic with cerebellar damage may be caused in part by the loss of cerebellar regulation (inhibition in this case) of vestibular function. Also, chronic cerebellar stimulation has been used as an invasive method of modifying hypertonicity in humans.[9]

Another basic concept in CNS function that must be understood is Sherrington's concept of reciprocal innervation.[11] This is best explained by examples. The vestibular system, specifically the lateral vestibulospinal tract, tends to exert its facilitation on extensors or antigravity muscles. Actually this tract facilitates motor neurons to antigravity muscles and inhibits motor neurons to progravity muscles. Table 3-4 lists common examples of reciprocal innervation.

Dysfunction

Disturbances in posture occur whenever there is damage to structures whose functions are to produce, modify, or control posture. Lesions that affect structures that produce posture result in a clinical picture of too little posture or postural hypotonicity. Referring back to the model of nervous system function, too little function, in this case too little posture, could result from damage to afferent neurons, efferent neurons or interneurons involved in the production of postural tone. Bilateral vestibulocochlear nerve damage would remove vestibular afferent neurons and result in postural hypotonicity, especially with the eyes closed. Damage to peripheral nerves to extensor muscles or to their motor neurons directly, as in Guillain-Barré syndrome or polio, results in decreased postural control. It also results in decreased movement because it does not selectively effect motor neurons to antigravity muscles. Postural hypotonia is also seen in cerebellar and central brainstem lesions.

More commonly CNS damage results in postural instability and leads to hypertonicity. Rigidity is commonly produced when interneurons that regulate posture or that regulate other interneurons involved more directly in producing posture are damaged. Too much posture is observed when the interneurons that produce posture are not controlled by other interneurons. The example cited earlier involved the cerebellar regulation of the vestibular nuclei and therefore the control of posture indirectly. Another example is the cerebral cortex, which has a powerful inhibitory influence on brainstem and spinal postural mechanisms. The corticospinal tracts send collaterals (probably more correctly called *corticobulbar fibers*) into the brainstem reticular formation. These collaterals help regulate the reticular formation's role in the production of posture. Therefore the corticospinal tracts facilitate progravity muscles and inhibit antigravity muscles directly at cord levels and indirectly at brainstem levels. Thus when these fibers are damaged in the internal capsule, a common site of cerebrovascular accident, the combined loss of regulation of antigravity mechanisms results in a patient who has difficulty inhibiting antigravity postures and facilitating movement. Admittedly, this is stated simplistically, but treatment that uses systems that facilitate movement and inhibit posture will benefit such clients. Refer to Chapter 6 for specific examples of afferent input that could be used to increase posture in the hypotonic or decrease posture in the hypertonic client.

VOLUNTARY: GOAL-DIRECTED MOVEMENT
Anatomical substrates

Movement is the result of muscle contraction. Muscle contraction is controlled by motor neurons. Motor neurons are influenced by interneurons. Interneurons are influenced by other interneurons and by afferent neurons. Therefore movement must be produced and regulated by interneurons and afferent neurons. Although motor programs are not initiated by afferent input per se, afferent data are necessary for programming the movement, for feedback to assess the progress of the movement, and for learning new movements and developing skill.

Let us assume that there are several different groups of interneurons at different levels of the neuroaxis that are "movement generators." At the segmental level there is a generator for flexion and a reciprocal generator for exten-

sion. This generator can be triggered by an afferent neuron or by an extrasegmental interneuron. If the flexion generators of several adjacent segments are linked, a flexor pattern generator for that limb is created. If the flexor pattern generator of one limb is linked to the extensor pattern generator of the other limb, a reciprocal limb movement could be produced. If the flexor pattern generator of the lower limb were linked with the flexor pattern generator of the contralateral upper limb, reciprocal arm and leg movement could be produced. Such generators have been hypothesized based in part on Orlovsky's[8] experiments on spinalized cats. The central pattern generators of upper and lower limbs could then be linked to interneurons driven by neck proprioceptors to produce tonic neck reflexes, or they could be linked to interneurons driven by labyrinthine afferent neurons to produce tonic labyrinthine reflexes.

The point is the spinal cord and brainstem have all the preexisting wiring necessary to produce rather complex but stereotyped movements. With just the wiring in the spinal cord and brainstem, an organism could withdraw from danger, seek food, and maintain itself in relation to gravity. But evolution did not stop there. Not only are we able to protect ourselves and maintain ourselves in relation to gravity, but we are also able to explore our environment and to seek and process information. This ability is made possible in part by our ability to discriminatively process information. No longer is gross touch, heat, and cold adequate information. To explore our environment we need receptors that are capable of providing information in small increments, that is, two-point discrimination, and small distances between sources of reflected light. We need afferent fibers that conduct rapidly and interneurons that are capable of integrating information from multiple sources. We need interneurons capable of integrating recent and past information, that is, memory, learning, and association. Finally, we need a motor system capable of producing more discrete, finite movements by isolating movement at distal segments.

This motor system is built on and is a refinement of preexisting wiring. It uses motor units at segmental levels to produce muscle contraction just as the withdrawal, labyrinthine, and righting reflexes do. One difference between higher-order or goal-directed movements and protective or postural movements relates to variety, flexibility, and versatility. Although a withdrawal reflex may vary in amplitude, latency, and duration, it always looks like a withdrawal reflex, and it can only be modified during the reflex by amplification or damping. *What makes one movement program simple and another complex is the amount of modification made on the program while the program is in progress.* The flexor withdrawal reflex can be increased or decreased, but once initiated it is carried through to completion at an amplitude determined by events before its initiation. Simple locomotion is also a fairly stereotyped movement pattern. Suprasegmental, vestibular, and rubral control is exerted by increasing the amplitude or duration of muscle activity but not the sequential relation of muscles in that phase. In other words, a locomotor pattern exists that can be increased or decreased in speed, but the program itself is not normally modified. Apparently, more complex patterns can be generated by centers above the brainstem. Grillner[3] and others have postulated something like a motor program generator that is capable of producing both ballistic and slow movements. *Ballistic movements* are movements that are too fast to be modified while in progress. The subthalamic nucleus may play a role in the regulation of the production of ballistic movements, as evidenced by subthalamic lesions resulting in ballismus. A likely place for the motor program generators is the basal ganglia (see Chapter 21).

If central program generators exist outside the cerebral cortex, what then is the role of the cerebral cortex in movement? The motor cortex is the executor for the program generators. It carries out the orders and controls the speed and force of movements by regulating recruitment order and repetition rate. To this control the cerebellar hemispheres add order (synergy and coordination) and distance (see Chapter 23). The cerebellum controls the distance the limb traverses by regulating the time (duration) of motor unit activity. In other words, given a constant force and speed of muscle shortening, if the muscle contracts for a longer *time,* the limb will move a greater *distance.* This, of course, is not all the cerebral cortex, cerebellum, and basal ganglia do; but it is enough to use in our model for now.

To summarize the movement model to this point, we have segmental wiring (spinal cord and brainstem) originally designed for homeostasis and modified by linking segmental program generators in different patterns to produce postural responses and "whole organism" protective responses, such as the startle response or "blink and duck" reflex. We then add central program generators to this model: a cerebellum to coordinate and time movements and a motor cortex to regulate force and speed as it carries out the coordinated order of the spinal program generator.

These orders are carried out, not by creating new wiring at the segmental level, but by regulating, modifying, *facilitating,* or *inhibiting* the ongoing activity in existing wiring. The cerebral cortex can influence the spinal cord wiring directly through the corticospinal tract. However, only a very small percentage of that influence is expressed directly onto motor neurons. The majority of the cerebral cortex's influence is through interneurons, influencing the background neuronal activity within segmental wiring. Both corticospinal and rubrospinal tracts tend to facilitate progravity muscles (movement) and inhibit antigravity muscles (posture).

Not all of the regulation of movement occurs at the segmental reflex arc. As mentioned earlier, the corticospinal tract also influences brainstem centers involved especially with regulation of posture. Therefore the cerebral cortex facilitates movement in at least two ways: by facilitating progravity muscles at the segmental level and by inhibiting brainstem level centers that facilitate antigravity muscles.

The cerebellum and the basal ganglia influence movement through the cerebral cortex. The cerebellum receives information regarding ongoing segmental activity (in part via spinocerebellar tracts) and regarding the motor program generators' intentions via corticopontocerebellar paths. The cerebellum then monitors the program (via spinocerebellar input) to determine whether the movement is according to intent regarding distance, force, etc. and signals other centers to make adjustments if necessary. Again, because the cerebellum has no direct connections to the motor units, it must work with and through the other systems to produce modifications in the movement.

Dysfunction

If a lesion can result in loss of function, then in this system a loss of movement or weakness should be observed. This loss of movement is different from the loss of movement seen at spinal cord levels, where, for example, a peripheral nerve injury causes weakness and loss of reflexes. Loss of function in the systems involved in producing motor programs results in problems with planning and initiating the movement. Signs include akinesia, apraxia, and perseveration. Adaptive responses may be expressed as too much movement (athetoid or chorea-form movements and hypertonicity). The involuntary movements appear to be parts of motor programs no longer under control of the regulatory centers. Adaptive responses may also be expressed as uncoordinated movement, such as past-pointing, ataxia, dyssynergia, or the inability to resolve conflicting sensory input.

The CNS lesion most commonly seen in older adults is ischemia secondary to cerebrovascular accident. This commonly involves the white matter in the internal capsule, including the corticospinal and corticobulbar tracts. The resulting sign is an inability to perform skilled movements, especially those of distal segments. These clients, however, also often have hypertonicity, which may be an adaptive response to the loss of peripheral stability and systems input to motor programmers. With a lesion of the corticospinal and corticobulbar fibers, there is a loss of cortical inhibition of postural mechanisms at brainstem levels, a loss of facilitation of progravity muscles (movement) at segmental levels, and the concomitant loss of reciprocal inhibition of antigravity muscles (posture).

Studies have shown that the movement disorder in the client with spastic hemiplegia is not the result of hypertonicity preventing movement but of the inability to recruit motor units in the proper timing and sequence.[10,13] Other evidence indicates that eventually there may also be a lower motor neuron component to the weakness seen in clients with hemiplegia.[2,6,14]

In other types of CNS lesions involuntary movement is seen. In this situation there may be an instability in a movement generator, there is a loss of regulation of that generator, and parts of movements are expressed without apparent purpose. Examples include athetosis, chorea, and ballismus. Tremor, although certainly an involuntary movement, may be a loss of control of the inherent oscillation within the sensorimotor system.

Because a major function of the cerebellum is the regulation or coordination (not production) of movement, cerebellar lesions manifest themselves as problems of incoordinated movement. In the case of cerebellar tremor, there may be an apparent loss of the damping of the inherent oscillation in the sensorimotor system so that there is "too much" oscillation during attempted movement. Or it may be an inability to "hold" a postural position.[1]

As in previous sections the model can be applied to evaluation and treatment. First, it must be determined whether signs such as weakness are the result of a lesion of the afferent neuron, interneuron, or efferent neuron. If afferent neurons are involved, other afferent neurons must be found to provide similar information, for example, substitute visual for proprioceptive information or use joint approximation to increase proprioceptive input. If efferent neurons are involved, other motor units must be brought in to substitute for the weak or absent functions. To recruit more motor units the clinician may use afferent input to enhance output. Biofeedback is a less obvious example of using afferent input (usually auditory or visual) to enhance motor output.

If the interneurons are the source of the clinical signs and symptoms, the therapist must first attempt to determine where in the motor programming the problems lie. Is the problem ideation, motivation, generation of programs and subprograms, accessing programs, coordinating and sequencing programs, or executing programs? Then the therapist's challenge is to find alternate ways of producing motor output and/or facilitating the client's nervous systems. Are there other ways to access the remaining programs? Is the client to learn programs as if they were new? Are there other strategies to perform the same task? Can the programming be augmented, facilitated, or accessed by afferent input as the client's nervous system attempts to adapt to remaining systems control? For example, some apraxic clients can imitate a motor task but cannot perform the task if only given verbal commands. If interneurons are the source of abnormal or adaptive signs, such as involuntary movement and uncoordinated movement, the therapist must determine whether other systems remain intact that may be used to regulate, override, or inhibit the unwanted movement programs or determine whether this is an adaptive response that is most efficient for the client given the circumstances. This is probably the most difficult task for the therapist. Control systems for movement are newer, more susceptible to damage, and fewer in number than control systems for lower-level functions. Pharmacological intervention has provided some assistance but may be more detrimental than beneficial in the long run.

HIGHER CORTICAL FUNCTIONS
Anatomical substrates

Although the integration that occurs in the cerebral hemispheres is infinitely more complex than a segmental reflex, it can still be compared to that reflex arc. Cerebral cortical activity still involves, at least in part, the receipt of information from inside and outside the body. This information is carried to the CNS by way of afferent neurons—all afferent neurons (interoceptive, proprioceptive, and exteroceptive) eventually influence the cortex. Once the information reaches the CNS, it is conducted to the cortex by way of interneurons. These would include projection fibers such as spinothalamics, the medial lemniscus, specific and diffuse thalamocortical projections, geniculocalcarine fibers (visual), and geniculotemporal fibers (auditory). Information is further processed by interneurons in the thalamus, hypothalamus, basal ganglia, and cerebral cortex. Other interneurons may carry the information from gyrus to gyrus or lobe to lobe (association fibers). Still others carry information from side to side (commissural fibers). Finally, an appropriate response must be executed. This requires descending projection fibers, such as the corticospinals and corticobulbars, to carry information to motor neurons. We now have come full circle (or arc) to our motor output. Perhaps some examples of higher cortical function will make this clearer.

Earlier in this chapter segmental reflexes in response to cutaneous stimuli were examined. We will now examine what else happens along with that segmental reflex. If someone sticks your index finger with a pin, besides the flexor withdrawal response, possibly a brainstem-mediated "ouch," and pupillary dilation, you *perceive* the stimulus. This requires interneurons carrying the information to the cortex by way of the thalamus. The information first reaches the appropriate primary sensory cortex, and then the information is carried to the sensory association cortex via association fibers (more interneurons). Besides knowing you were stimulated, you also know where, how much, what shape, based on past experience, and by what object. You also have made a decision as to how threatening the stimulus was and whether you should flee, fight, or stay neutral. This decision involves reviewing your past experience and putting an emotional value or weight on the situation. The action you take in this situation requires descending pathways, such as the reticulospinals, for the sympathetic response (cardiovascular) and corticospinals for removing the pin with which you were stuck.

Now instead of being stuck with a pin, you are shown a picture of a sunset in the wilderness of Alaska and asked to tell about what you see. The afferent neurons are in the retina. Interneurons carry the visual information from the retinas to the primary visual cortex (with stops in such places as the tectum and the lateral geniculate). You see the picture. Interneurons carry information to visual association areas. You recognize the picture as a sunset in the wilderness. Your memory is searched. You do not recognize the specific picture. Interneurons carry information to the parts of the brain that have to do with emotional tone (see Chapter 5). You become apprehensive. Now you tell the person showing you the picture that you see a sunset in the woods. You begin to fidget in your chair because when you were a child you were nearly attacked by a bear while camping with your parents.

Hemispheric specialization can be thought of as a division of labor between interneurons. To be more efficient, interneurons process information differently in the two hemispheres. It is *not* that some information is processed only in one hemisphere but that each hemisphere analyzes the afferent input for different content. In most humans the left hemisphere analyzes the sequential content of an event, whether auditory, visual, tactile, or proprioceptive, and the right hemisphere analyzes the spatial content of the event. The left hemisphere counts the trees; the right hemisphere identifies it as a dense forest. Each hemisphere also contributes to the response. The left hemisphere is involved in the production of speech, a *sequence* of sounds. The right hemisphere adds the tone and rhythm of voice, the spatial content. The left hemisphere is involved in the *sequencing* of motor acts. The right hemisphere is more involved in whole body, body in space types of integration.

Dysfunction

A lesion of the cerebral hemispheres can result in both loss of function and adaptive responses. If, when asked what you saw in the picture, you did not answer, is it caused by decreased afferent input? You either did not *hear* the question or you did not *see* the picture—or perhaps you heard and saw but did not understand the question or could not formulate the answer. Or perhaps it is the result of a lesion in interneurons responsible for executing the motor command (corticospinals and corticobulbars), or the result of a loss of efferent neurons, motor neurons, as might be seen in bulbar polio or laryngeal nerve palsy. Is the inability to perceive a pin prick the result of a loss of afferent neurons, projection fibers, thalamus, or primary sensory cortex? Or is it caused by an inability to orient to a stimulus? Hemispatial neglect appears to be an inability to orient to a stimulus rather than an agnosia, as seen in right parietal lesions. Adaptive responses to loss of higher cortical function might include inappropriate responses, such as emotional lability, hyperactive behavior, jargon speech, and perseveration.

In assessing the client with hemispheric damage, the clinician may need the assistance of other members of the rehabilitation team. Does the client have an afferent lesion, that is, auditory, visual, proprioceptive, cutaneous sensation? If this is the source of the sign, then other sensory systems may be substituted. Does the client have an efferent lesion, that is, motor neuron loss? If so, then treatment may involve recruiting functioning motor units. Does the client have an

interneuronal lesion, and if so, is it in production of function or regulation of function? If the interneurons produce the function, there may be few treatment alternatives because there is much less duplicity with higher cortical functions. There is another hemisphere that does the same function with a different strategy. If only some of the interneurons that produce the function are damaged, then appropriate afferent input can be used to enhance their function. The client with visual perceptual problems may be helped with added proprioceptive input, for example. If the dysfunction is caused by loss of regulatory interneurons, then other regulatory centers may be recruited. In some instances less is better. In the hyperactive child who cannot regulate (filter) and focus on the task at hand, decreasing afferent input by controlling the environment assists the child's nervous system to regulate function.

SUMMARY

Regardless of the systems involved and the severity of the lesion, the therapist must evaluate, identify the problems of, and treat the client with a neurological dysfunction. Many evaluation procedures include testing the intactness of the afferent neuron, interneuron, and efferent neuron. All reflex testing is based on this arc. The clinician may also need to consider testing gait, coordination, functional performance, and higher cortical functions. The clinician is attempting to determine whether there is adequate and appropriate afferent information, whether it is integrated appropriately, and whether an appropriate and/or adaptive response is produced. Treatment is then determined based on the same model. The clinician must find a way to provide adequate and appropriate afferent input to facilitate integration and the production of an adaptive response. In Chapter 6 categories of afferent input can be found that may be used in treating the neurological client.

For a greater in-depth analysis of the motor control and limbic systems, the reader is referred to Chapters 4 and 5, respectively. The goal of this chapter was to present an overview of the role and function of the CNS. The nervous system must be understood as a whole, for no part functions in isolation. Once a comfortable whole has been achieved, an in-depth study of or focus on one area should widen the reader's comprehension of the whole. The path to learning is exciting but complicated. As long as an understanding of the whole is maintained, the reader will always be able to find the way back to comprehension whenever he or she becomes lost.

ACKNOWLEDGMENT:

The author would like to thank Gail Widener, Ph.D., P.T. for her valuable contribution to this chapter.

REFERENCES

1. Aschoff JC and Kornhuber HH: Functional interpretation of somatic afferents in cerebellum, basal ganglia and motor cortex. In Kornhuber HH, editor. *The somatosensory system.* Stuttgart, 1975, Thieme.

2. Chokroverty S and others: Hemiplegic amytrophy, *Arch Neurol* 33:104, 1976.

3. Grillner S: Locomotion in vertebrates: central mechanisms and reflex interaction, *Physiol Rev* 55:247, 1975.

4. Horak FB and Nashner LM: Central programming of postural movements: Adaptations to a lifted support surface configuration, *J Neurophysiol* 55:1369-1381, 1986.

5. Kandel ER, Schwartz JH, and Jessell TM: *Principles of neural science,* New York, 1991, Elsevier Publishing Co.

6. McComas AJ and others: Functional changes in motoneurons of hemiparetic patients, *J Neurol Neurosurg Psychiatry* 36:183, 1973.

7. Nashner LM: Fixed patterns of rapid postural responses among leg muscles during stance, *Exp Brain Res* 30:13, 1977.

8. Orlovsky GN: The effect of different descending systems on flexor and extensor activity during locomotion, *Brain Res* 40:359, 1972.

9. Penn RD and Etzel ML: Chronic cerebellar stimulation and developmental reflexes, *J Neurophysiol* 46:506, 1977.

10. Rosenfalck A and Andreassen S: Impaired regulation of force and firing pattern of single motor units in patients with spasticity, *J Neurol Neurosurg Psychiatry* 43:970, 1980.

11. Sherrington CS: *The integrative action of the nervous system,* New Haven, 1906, Yale University Press.

12. Walshe F: Contributions of John Hughlings Jackson to neurology: a brief introduction to his teachings, *Arch Neurol* 5:119, 1961.

13. Whitley DA and others: Patterns of muscle activity in the hemiplegic upper extremity, *Phys Ther* 62:641, 1982 (abstract).

14. Young JL and Mayer RF: Mechanical properties of single motor units in short-term hemiplegia, *Neurology* 29:609, 1979.

ADDITIONAL READINGS

Brooks VB: *The neural basis of motor control,* New York, 1986, Oxford University Press.

Bruggencate G ten: Functions of extrapyramidal systems in motor control. I. Supraspinal descending pathways, *Pharmacol Ther* B1:587, 1975.

Bruggencate G ten: Functions of extrapyramidal systems in motor control. II. Cortical and subcortical pathways, *Pharmacol Ther* B1:611, 1975.

Bruggencate G ten and Lundberg A: Facilitory interaction transmission to motoneurons from vestibulospinal fibers and contralateral primary afferents, *Exp Brain Res* 19:248, 1974.

Burke D: A reassessment of the muscle spindle contribution to muscle tone in normal and spastic man. In Feldman RG et al, editors: *Spasticity: disordered motor control,* Chicago, 1980, Year Book Medical Publishers, Inc.

DeLong MR and Strick PL: Relation of basal ganglia, cerebellum and motor cortex units to ramp and ballistic limb movements, *Brain Res* 71:327, 1974.

Desmedt JE, editor: Spinal and supraspinal mechanisms of voluntary motor control and locomotion, vol 8, *Progress in clinical neurophysiology,* Basel, 1980, S Karger.

Desmedt JE, editor: Motor unit types, recruitment and plasticity in health and disease, vol 9, *Progress in clinical neurophysiology,* Basel, 1981, S Karger.

Eyzaguirre C and Fidone SS: *Physiology of the nervous system,* Chicago, 1975, Year Book Medical Publishers, Inc.

Feldman RG and others: *Spasticity: disordered motor control,* Chicago, 1980, Year Book Medical Publishers, Inc.

Grillner S: Locomotion in vertebrates: central mechanisms and reflex interaction, *Physiol Rev* 55:247, 1975.

Grillner S and Hongo T: Vestibulospinal relations. Vestibular influences on the lumbosacral spinal cord. In Brodal A et al, editors: *Basic aspects of central vestibular mechanisms,* Amsterdam, 1972, Elsevier Publishing Company.

Hongo T and others: The rubrospinal tract. II. Facilitation of interneuronal transmission in reflex paths to motoneurons, *Exp Brain Res* 7:365, 1969.

Kuypers HGJM: The descending pathways to the spinal cord: their anatomy and function, *Prog Brain Res* 11:178, 1964.

Landau WM: Spasticity: What is it? What is it not? In Feldman RG and others, editors: *Spasticity: disordered motor control,* Chicago, 1980, Year Book Medical Publishers, Inc.

Lundberg A and Voorhoeve P: Effects from the pyramidal tract on spinal reflex arcs, *Acta Physiol Scand* 56:201, 1962.

MacLeon PD: The triune brain in conflict, *Psychother Psychosom* 28:207, 1977.

Miller S and Scott PD: Spinal generation of movement in a single limb: functional implications of a model based on the cat. In Desmedt, JE, editor: *Progress in clinical neurophysiology,* vol 8, Basel, 1980, S Karger.

Sarnat HB and Netsky MG: *Evolution of the nervous system,* New York, 1974, Oxford University Press, Inc.

Williams PL and Warwick R: *Functional neuroanatomy of man,* Philadelphia, 1975, WB Saunders Co.

Willis WD and Grossman RG: *Medical neurobiology,* ed 3, St Louis, 1981, Mosby.

CHAPTER 4

Contemporary Issues and Theories of Motor Control

Assessment of movement and balance

Roberta A. Newton

LEARNING OBJECTIVES

After reading this chapter the student/therapist will:

1. Identify the difference between motor control based theory and reflex/hierarchical based theory.
2. Identify and analyze the parameters of motor control and interlocking subsections.
3. Compare the various elements of motor control and identify how each factor might affect balance and movement.
4. Recognize how this theory can be applied to assessment of clients with neurological dysfunction.

KEY TERMS

neurological assessment   motor control theories

Foundation sciences fundamental to **neurological assessment** physical therapy and occupational therapy assessment and treatment are motor control, motor learning, and motor development. Therapists are interested in how the brain controls movements, how movement patterns or motor behavior is learned, and how motor behavior changes across the life span. Therapists need to understand how the brain controls movements in persons with deficits in posture and movement and also in healthy individuals. As information about motor control becomes available, therapists reexamine principles that form the bases for assessment and treatment and replace older, outmoded notions with newer principles of motor control. The newer ideas arise from many disciplines including neuroscience and motor learning.

This chapter has two purposes. First, it provides the reader with a review of current models used to represent neural regulation of posture and movement. Second, it describes some deficits of motor control using these models, and the ways in which therapists can use this schema to evaluate patients with neurological dysfunction.

A model is a schematic representation of a theory: in this case, of how the brain regulates motor behavior. Various models are created because researchers use different approaches to develop and test theories. All models have limitations and are constantly changing as researchers gain new information and as technological advances are made. A theory that is constantly being tested and undergoing change is better than an outdated theory or no theory. Early researchers used techniques such as visual observation and palpation to develop models of motor control. Today researchers use techniques and tools that include electromyography, film analysis, force plates, electron microscopy, and cerebral blood flow studies to develop hypotheses about motor control. Finally, models may portray only a small part of the nervous system; for example, a model of spinal cord control mechanisms would not include higher-center control processes. Other models may be more holistic; for example, a systems model may be used to describe and to investigate the interrelationships among various brain centers and the spinal centers.

Models of **motor control theories** used as a basis for predicting motor responses during patient assessment and treatment should have a broad scope. A therapist using a spinal level reflex model, for example, may inaccurately predict motor behavior because this model does not consider motor behavior regulated by higher centers. Selecting and using a proper model is important for the analysis and treatment of individuals with posture and movement dysfunction.

A CLASSICAL MODEL OF MOTOR CONTROL

The term *motor control* refers to the regulation of movement and dynamic postural adjustments. Described here is the hierarchy, the bases for traditional neurological therapy. A description of the hierarchy, its application to pathophysiology, and its limitations are included.

The hierarchy model proposes a commander, a higher center, which plans and delegates the motor program to subordinate centers for execution (Fig. 4-1). This model implies that the motor program is developed at the highest level and is not influenced by peripheral feedback during execution of the movement. Feedback loops are included in more contemporary models depicting hierarchical motor control. In these later modifications of the hierarchy, information about the internal and external environment before and after movement is available to the commander. The commander, however, does not need to use the information during execution of the movement.

When disease or injury damages the highest center, dissolution of the whole nervous system occurs.[11] The more stable lower and evolutionarily older nervous centers control movement. Movements represented at the lower levels are reflexive; that is, stereotypical and not capable of modification when the external or internal environmental conditions necessitate a change. Damage to nervous tissue in the highest centers leads to either destruction or instability of movement. Pathophysiology can also lead to over-readiness of the nervous system to become active.

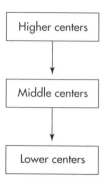

Fig. 4-1. Model of a hierarchy of motor control.

In this theory the highest center contains all the information necessary for movement, and the "commander" may or may not use external or internal feedback to regulate movement. Further, the levels do not communicate with one another. Rather they serve as subordinates carrying out a series of commands generated by the highest center.

The hierarchy model for motor control represents the state of science from the middle of the nineteenth century to the early twentieth century. Although this model has limitations, it was the basis for development of the disciplines of neurology and neurological physical therapy. Since the incorporation of the hierarchy model into physical therapy theory, researchers have developed other theories for the regulation of posture and movement. The hierarchical model is useful for examining motor activity that occurs without feedback; however, this model is of limited use when trying to understand the interrelationships of brain centers for planning and initiating motor activity.

CONTEMPORARY MODELS OF MOTOR CONTROL

Researchers adopted the term *systems* from engineering terminology to describe the relationship of various brain and spinal centers working together with the use of feedback (Fig. 4-2). Sensation is the process whereby receptors receive information relative to the internal and external environment. The receptors encode the information for transmission to various areas of the nervous system. The central nervous system (CNS) receives and interprets the sensations based on present experiences, the present state of the internal and external environment, and memory of similar situations. This procedure is termed *perception*. Processing the information leads to the development of a movement (and postural) strategy. This operation is termed *response selection*, that is, choosing the most contextually appropriate movement strategy to meet the needs of the individual. The response is then executed (response execution) by the muscles and joints. The observable motor behavior is the result of the processing, selecting, and executing the selected motor and postural response.

Researchers have garnered principles and concepts from

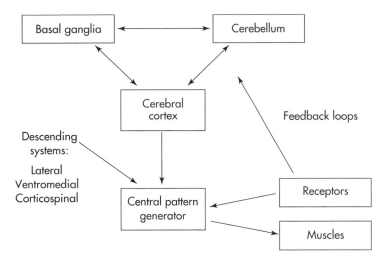

Fig. 4-2. Systems model of motor control.

different disciplines to develop the systems approach to motor control, for example, neuroscience theory, principles of nonlinear phenomena in physics, and Bernstein's work on degrees of freedom. Some of the principles and concepts included in systems theory are described later. The concepts presented in this section are representative of systems theory and dynamical action theory, and by no means are inclusive of all the concepts included in these multifaceted and complex theories. Comprehensive discussions of these theories are found elsewhere.[3,7,14,23,26]

Principles and concepts related to contemporary motor control theories

As mentioned earlier, contemporary motor control models have a similar set of assumptions and concepts, yet each model contains additional assumptions and concepts. Described in this section are elements from the various contemporary theories that are useful for the description of motor and postural control in the patients with neurological dysfunction, as well as in healthy individuals. These elements themselves may be considered components of a theory, as well as represent theory themselves. They do not stand alone to explain motor control in the healthy individual or the individual with neurological dysfunction. Rather, they interact and interrelate. The interaction of these various elements produces the emergent motor and postural behavior exhibited by the individual in response to the environmental and task demands of the situation.

Central pattern generator or reflex. Traditionally, in the hierarchical model, the basic spinal level unit is the reflex. If a particular stimulus activates receptors, a single stereotypical motor response results. In systems theory developed from a neuroscience perspective, the basic spinal level unit is the central pattern generator (CPG).[15,6] If a single stimulus activates a CPG, a series of motor responses occurs (Fig. 4-3). Spontaneous activation of the neural network can also occur. For example, spontaneous activation

A. A single response per stimulus

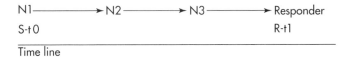

Time line

B. Emergent property: more than one response

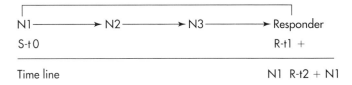

Time line   N1   R-t2 + N1

Key:
N = neuron
S-t0 = start time
R-t = response 1; response 2, etc.

Fig. 4-3. Emergent property.

occurs in the sinoatrial (SA) node of the heart. This node is considered a neural network. The SA node fibers are extremely permeable to sodium ions. When increased membrane permeability causes an influx of sodium ions into the nodal fibers, depolarization and excitation of the SA node fibers occur, which in turn leads to excitation and contraction of atrial muscle fibers.

Information processing. The configuration of the systems model lends itself to many methods to process information. Serial processing denotes a specific order of processing (Fig. 4-4) of information by various centers. Information proceeds lockstep through each center. Parallel processing denotes processing of information by more than one center simultaneously or nearly simultaneously, and that information can be used for more than one activity.

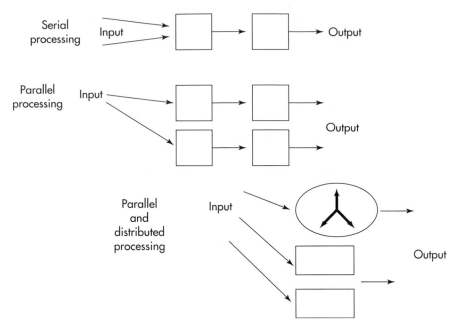

Fig. 4-4. Methods of information processing.

A third and more flexible type of processing of information is parallel-distributed processing.[17] This type of processing combines the best attributes of serial and parallel processing. That is, when the situation demands serial processing, this type of activity can be conducted. At other times, parallel processing is the mode of choice. For optimum utilization of information from various regions of the brain combined with immediate internal and external sensory information, a combination of both parallel and serial processing may be the most efficient way to handle the variety of information. The type of processing used depends on factors such as the time needed to react to a particular situation or whether the processing occurs during learning of a particular movement strategy.

Adaptive behavior. Although the brain is capable of producing a generalized pattern of motor activity via central pattern generators, this concept may not be sufficient to explain the variability of movement patterns. The system needs to be organized so that it can adapt and respond to constraints in the external environment, metabolic constraints, and internal constraints associated with the various physiological systems of the body (i.e., musculoskeletal and cardiovascular systems). The musculoskeletal system, by nature of the architecture of the joints and muscle attachments can be a constraint on the movement pattern. An individual with a functional contracture may be able to bend a joint only so far into the range. Another constraint on the formation of the behavior is the constraints of the task. Certain requirements of the task need to be met to accomplish a task. For example, dorsiflexion of the foot needs to meet a critical degree of toe clearance during gait. The movement pattern is influenced by environmental

demands or constraints. For example, posture and gait may be altered when a person walks on a moving walkway compared to a stable support surface.

To review, the nervous system needs to respond to many types of internal and external constraints to develop and execute motor behavior that is age appropriate and efficient to accomplish the task. Efficiency can be examined in terms of metabolic cost to the individual, type of movement pattern used, the preferred or habitual movement ("habit") used by the individual, and time to complete the task.

Movement patterns arising from self-organizing subsystems. A coordinated movement pattern is developed from the dynamic interaction of subsystems to accomplish the task in relation to internal and external constraints. Therefore the movement pattern is contextually appropriate and arises as an emergent property of subsystem interaction. Several principles relate to self-organizing systems.

Reciprocity. Reciprocity implies information flow between two or more neural networks. These networks can represent specific brain centers, for example, the cerebellum and basal ganglia. Or, the neural networks can represent interacting neuronal clusters located within a single center (Fig. 4-2). Information is modified as it flows between centers because each center is involved in the processing of the information.

Distributed function. Distributed function presupposes that a single center or neural network has more than one function. Distributed function also implies that several centers share the same function. For example, in generating one movement task, a center may serve as the coordinating unit. In another movement task, the center may serve as a pattern generator to continue to produce the activity. An advantage of distributing function among groups of neurons or centers is that many centers have overlapping or redundant functions. Neuroscientists believe redundancy is a safety feature. If a neuronal lesion occurs, other centers can assume critical functional roles.

Consensus. Instead of a single brain center serving the role of a commander, several centers work together as a command center. For an activity to occur, a majority of neurons or centers must become active. When centers reach a critical threshold, they act. This consensus function filters information that may not necessarily need immediate attention. If a novel stimulus enters the system, however, it carries more weight and immediate action occurs. A novel stimulus may be a stimulus that is new to the system or may be a stimulus reflecting a potentially harmful situation.

Emergent properties. The concept of emergent properties may be understood in the adage "the whole is greater than the sum of its parts." It implies that brain centers work together and that no single center produces movement alone. An example of the emergent properties concept is the concept of continuous repetitive activity (oscillation). In Fig. 4-3, *A*, a hierarchy is represented by three neurons arranged in tandem. The last neuron ends on a responder. If a single stimulus activates this network, a single response occurs. What is the response if the neurons are arranged so that the third neuron sends a collateral branch to the first neuron in addition to the ending on the responder? In this case (Fig. 4-3, *B*), a single stimulus activates neuron no. 1. Neuron no. 1 activates neuron no. 2 and no. 3, causing a response as well as reactivating neuron no. 1. This neuronal arrangement produces a series of responses rather than a single response. This function is described as endogenous activity (oscillation).

Another example of an emergent property is the production of motor behavior. Rather than having every motor program stored in the brain, an abstract representation of the intended goal is stored. At the time of motor performance, various brain centers use present sensory information, with past memory of the task accomplishment to develop the appropriate motor strategy. This concept negates a hard-wired motor program concept. If motor programs were hard-wired and if a motor program existed for every movement ever performed, the brain would need a huge storage capacity.

Controlling the degrees of freedom. The body contains a large number of degrees of freedom that contribute to movement, for example joints and muscles. A system with a large number of degrees of freedom is called a high dimensional system. For a contextually appropriate movement to occur, these degrees of freedom need to be constrained. Bernstein[5] suggested one way to reduce the number of degrees of freedom is to have muscles work in synergies; for example, the muscles and joints of a limb are coupled into a functional synergy pattern. The functional unit of motor behavior then is the synergy, also called coordinative structure. By reducing the degrees of freedom,

a high dimensional system becomes a low dimensional system, that is, a system with fewer degrees of freedom. For example, a functional synergy pattern for the lower extremity can be a step. Functional synergies can be linked together with functional synergies from other limbs to form interlimb coordination, for example, walking.

Sequence or order of muscle activation is a method to control the degrees of freedom. For example, muscle A is activated before muscle B, and so on. If muscle activation occurs out of sequence, the movement appears jerky or uncoordinated. Coordinated movement is defined as an orderly sequence of muscle activity necessary to produce appropriate motor behavior. Other methods to control degrees of freedom are to express movement parameters such as force and duration in terms of fix and relative ratios.

Duration of muscle activity that occurs in a particular movement pattern can be expressed as a ratio. If muscle A is active for 10% of the duration of the motor activity and muscle B is active 50% of the time, the ratio of A/B is 1:5. The overall duration of the movement pattern is considered a relative parameter. If the movement is performed very slowly, the time for the entire movement pattern increases and the relative muscle duration increases proportionally. Writing your name on a blackboard very slowly or very fast yields the same results—your name.

Force production is also expressed as a ratio. If muscle A and muscle B have a ratio of 1:2, then muscle A will generate one-half as much force as muscle B. If the overall force of the movement increases or decreases, force production of each muscle proportionally increases or decreases in relation to one another and with respect to the fixed ratio. Writing your name on a blackboard in very large or very small letters yields the same results—your name. If muscle A had a delayed onset and the same duration, however, then the movement would not appear to be smooth. Or if muscle B had a longer duration that continued into the time of the activation of the antagonistic muscle, then the motor behavior could appear stiff. These are just two examples of the effects of altered muscle timing, i.e., onset and duration, that can influence motor behavior.

Fixed ratios such as amplitude and timing that are built into a synergy decrease the degrees of freedom. The relative parameters provide the flexibility or adaptability of the system for the task to be accomplished; however, the movement pattern may be self-limiting or limited by constraints imposed by the environment or the body. The amplitude of writing on a blackboard is limited by the height of the blackboard, the length of the arm, or the overall height of the person stretching to make the letter larger.

These functional synergies are not hard-wired but represent emergent properties. They are flexible and adaptable to meet the needs of the task and the environment constraints. They can be described in terms of timing, for example, timing of the flexion and extension phases, and in terms of phasing, that is, when the flexion and extension phases occur in relation to one another. The movement can also be described in terms of the positional relationship between joints. These descriptors of motor behavior have been termed *order parameters.* In summary, the nervous system is organized so as to limit the degrees of freedom to accomplish the task. Limiting the degrees of freedom to accomplish a task also implies that a finite number of strategies are available to accomplish the goal.

Preferred, not obligatory, movement patterns. An individual uses preferred movement patterns that are stable yet flexible to meet the ever-changing environmental conditions. These are *preferred,* not *obligatory,* movement patterns. That is, the individual can choose to use another movement pattern to accomplish the task. An obligatory or stereotypical movement pattern suggests that the individual does not have the capability to adapt to a new situation or cannot use a different movement pattern to accomplish the task. This inability may be due to internal constraints that are functional or pathophysiological. The patient who had a cerebrovascular accident has CNS constraints that limit the number of different movement patterns that can emerge from the self-organizing system. With recovery, the patient is able to select and use additional movement strategies. The ability to learn may also limit the number of movement patterns available to the individual and the ability of the subject to use new or different movement patterns.

When change occurs in one or more of the subsystems, a new movement pattern emerges. The element that causes change is called a *control parameter.* For example, when we are late to a meeting or a class we begin to walk faster. We increase the speed of walking until we reach a period when we are uncertain whether to walk or run. When a critical speed and a critical degree of hip extension is reached, we begin to run. In this example, speed of walking is the control variable. When this variable is removed, we shift back to the preferred movement pattern. In our example, when we decrease speed we begin to walk. The control parameter then shifts the individual into new patterns of behavior.

This concept underlies theories of development and learning. Development and learning can be viewed as moving the system from a stable state to a more unstable state. When the control variable is removed, the system moves back to the early more stable state. As the control variable continues to push the system, the individual spends more time in the new state and less time in the earlier states until the individual spends most of the time in the new state. When this occurs, the new state becomes the preferred state. Moving or shifting to the new preferred state does not obviate the ability of the individual to use the earlier state of motor behavior. Therefore new movement patterns occur when critical changes occur in the system due to a control parameter. Control parameters are not just confined to movement parameters, but may also come from the environment.

Role of sensory information. The CNS uses sensory information in a variety of ways in the process of motor control. Before movement is initiated, information about the position of the body in space, body parts to one another, and environmental conditions is obtained from sensory receptors. This information is used in the selection and execution of the movement synergy. During movement, various brain centers use feedback from receptors to determine whether the actual motor behavior is the same as the intended motor behavior. If the actual and intended motor behaviors do not match, an error signal is produced, and alterations in the intended motor behavior occur. In some instances, the control system anticipates and makes corrective change before the detection of the error signal. This anticipatory correction is termed *feedforward control.*

Ballistic movements do not rely on sensory feedback loops to modify the program as it is being executed because the execution phase occurs very quickly. For example, a baseball pitcher throws a fast ball in a relatively short time and does not rely on feedback to control the movement during execution.

Another role of sensory information is to revise the reference of correctness before executing the motor program again. For example, a young gymnast is learning to stand on a balance beam with the feet close together and falls off the balance beam. An error signal occurs because the intended motor behavior and the actual motor behavior differ. If the performer knows that the feet were too close together when the fall occurred, then the next time the gymnast will space the feet farther apart. The information about what happened, falling or not falling, is called knowledge of results (KR). The CNS can store KR and use it when planning movement strategies for balancing on any narrow object, whether a balance beam or a log.

Several researchers have investigated whether peripheral feedback is necessary for the regulation of movement as it takes place.[13,24] Rothwell and others[19] studied a patient with a unilateral deafferented upper extremity. The deficit was caused by a peripheral sensory neuropathy. The individual could write sentences with the eyes closed and drive a car with a manual transmission without watching the gear shift, but had difficulty with fine-motor tasks, such as buttoning a shirt and using a knife and fork. The patient was unable to sustain a muscle contraction using a pincer grasp when asked to perform the task with eyes closed and could not learn to drive a new car with a manual transmission. Based on these observations, continued peripheral feedback may not be necessary when executing a learned motor behavior. However, peripheral feedback is necessary during the acquisition or learning of new motor behaviors that are not inherent.

Errors in motor control. Sometimes the actual motor behavior does not match the intended motor behavior. When this phenomenon happens, one or several errors working alone or in combination may be the cause of the problem. This section describes several kinds of errors.

One type of error is selecting the wrong movement strategy. For example, a person is unexpectedly and forcefully pushed. The individual selects a motor program, sway about the ankle to maintain upright stance. If the person falls, we can postulate the individual selected the wrong movement strategy. Although sway about the ankle is a proper strategy for maintaining balance, it is inappropriate for this situation because the person fell.

Selecting the wrong movement strategy can also occur when there is sensory conflict in the environment. For example, a person stopped at a red light is looking forward; peripheral vision picks up a car rolling backward. The individual slams on the brakes and sheepishly realizes that his car is not rolling backwards. What happened? Input from peripheral vision identified movement, but information from the vestibular receptors was not used in response selection. An error in assessing initial conditions occurred. The resultant motor behavior is correct for the visual information, but it is not correct for the situation if both visual and vestibular information were assessed.

An individual may select an appropriate motor program but use inappropriate relative parameters. A classic example is lifting a box full of textbooks. The CNS has stored in motor memory a previous experience of lifting textbooks. One characteristic stored is the concept that textbooks (particularly those for physical therapy) are heavy. As a result, the CNS adjusts the relative amplitude for the movement strategy for lifting heavy books. The person lifts the box and almost throws it in the air because the box is so light. The individual used the correct movement strategy for lifting; however, the amplitude was inappropriate.

Errors also occur when unexpected factors disrupt the execution of the program. For example, an individual walks on a moving sidewalk. When the individual steps off the sidewalk, a disruption in walking occurs. The individual's first few steps are not smooth. The individual is still using the movement strategy developed for a moving support surface. As a result, an error occurs when the individual steps onto the stationary support surface.

Errors can occur in the selection of the program, selection of the variable parameters, or in the response execution. Errors in selection and execution of the motor program in patients are generally the result of a neurological deficit. An assessment of motor deficits in patients should include analysis of these types of errors.

All individuals, both healthy individuals and those individuals with CNS dysfunction, make errors in motor programming. These errors are assessed by the CNS and are stored in past memory of the experience. Errors in motor programming are extremely useful in learning. Learning can be viewed as decreasing the mismatch between the intended and actual motor behavior. This mismatch is a measure of the error. A decrease in the degree of the error can be viewed as learning. Errors then are a very important part of the rehabilitation process. The ability of the patient to detect an error and correct it to produce appropriate motor behavior is one key to recovery.

Summary. The above components of contemporary motor control theories are interrelated. Movement is an emergent motor behavior that arises from the cooperative working of many centers to assess information from the internal and external environment, to process that information with past memories, and to produce a movement strategy that is appropriate to the situation and accomplishes the task. The movement has appropriate amplitude and duration and appropriate sequencing of muscle activity. The movement pattern selected may be a preferred movement pattern for that particular task but is not an obligatory motor pattern. The movement pattern is efficiently executed, both in terms of metabolic efficiency and movement efficiency. Movement efficiency in terms of energy expenditure relates to the appropriate controlling of the multiple of degrees of freedom at the various joints to accomplish the movement. The movement is accomplished with the flexibility and adaptability to be modified if new constraints occur as the movement is being executed. The movement pattern used by the individual is the preferred movement pattern selected by that individual to accomplish the task. Once the task is accomplished, elements of the task are stored in motor memory. The representation of the movement pattern that is stored may be modified as a result of learning and development.

Balance strategies

In terms of balance strategies, a finite number of movement responses are available for response selection. Although individuals appear to use a variety of movements to maintain balance due to an internal or external perturbation, all balance strategies appear to have common elements of three identifiable strategies. Horak and Nashner[9] identified three balance strategies available to the person when the person was unexpectedly perturbed. A person maintains balance after a small unexpected linear perturbation by executing a movement strategy that first activates muscles at the ankle and temporally spreads to more proximal musculature. This strategy is termed *ankle strategy*. If the linear perturbation is greater or unexpected rotation about the ankle occurs, a different movement strategy is used—a hip strategy. If the perturbation is such that the hip and ankle strategies are not successful, then the individual takes a step to prevent falling. The time the individual has to react to maintain balance and prevent falling is extremely short. Coupling muscles together into functional synergies decreases the time for response selection. The parameters that assist in response selection include the conditions of the perturbation, the initial conditions of the individual, the environmental conditions, past experiences, and the goal. Conditions of the perturbation include the amplitude, velocity, and direction of the perturbing force. Initial conditions of the individual are the position of the individual in space and the relationship of the person's body parts to each other. This also includes the biomechanical, neurological, and general physiological status of the individual. Environmental conditions include not only the support surface, but other objects in the environment and the condition of the lighting. The goal to be achieved in this particular scenario is to maintain or regain the center of mass over the base of support so the individual does not fall (see Chapter 28).

ASSESSMENTS BASED ON CONTEMPORARY MOTOR AND BALANCE CONTROL THEORIES

Many of the assessments used to examine motor behavior in patients with neurological dysfunction are typically used in the clinical setting. The evaluation differs according to the way in which the therapist uses and interprets the data in light of the contemporary theories of motor and balance control.

Evaluation procedures are designed with an understanding of how the individual's physical, mental, and cognitive status affects motor abilities. Further, evaluation procedures are designed to determine functional outcome. A custom-designed evaluation approach is used because the mechanism of injury or disease, secondary brain damage, recovery rate, and functional outcome differ in every individual. One strategy to the assessment of the patient with neurological dysfunction is to assess the individual's previous and present activity levels.

Activity level

Unobtrusive evaluation at bedside or in the clinic provides an excellent opportunity to examine functional activity level and compensatory or preferred movement strategies used by the individual. Another unobtrusive observation period can be "staged," for example, having the patient assist the clinician to move objects off and on a low mat table or when the patient is asked to remove shoes and socks. During these observation times, the patient is not "performing" a motor task and a more natural pattern of motor behavior may be observed. A patient may sit on the floor to remove shoes and socks because the floor is more stable than sitting on a low mat table. In this instance, the therapist observes the movement the patient uses to reach the floor, the mobility and stability patterns the patient uses when shoes and socks are being removed, and the movement strategy used to get up from the floor.

Items incorporated in an assessment of activity level vary depending on the age of the patient;[30] severity of complaints; observational analysis before beginning the evaluation; and the physical, cognitive, and behavioral status of the individual. For example, an elderly patient with CNS dysfunction may have preexisting movement and balance dysfunction due to the aging process.[16,29] Activity level, however, should not be based solely on the assumption that elderly persons are more inactive than younger adults. Inactive elderly and inactive college-aged individuals have lower functional patterns for righting reactions when coming to standing from supine than their active cohorts.[27] Assessment of activity level involves employment status including type of work (sedentary or active); participation in leisure activities, both organized or solo (sports, choir, bridge, walking, gardening); and the effect of the preexisting and existing dysfunction on current activity levels in terms of assistance with activities of daily living, work, and leisure activities.

It is also important to identify activities the individual believes he or she can no longer perform due to the motor control problem or due to loss of confidence. Tasks used in the evaluation should be similar to those activities the patient can perform and those activities that are familiar to the individual. Inability to perform a new task may be due to CNS damage or the inability of the individual to understand and carry out an unfamiliar task. Tasks can incorporate transitional movements including rolling on a compliant surface, moving from supine to sit, bending down and reaching for something on the floor, and moving from stand to sit. Functional activity permits analysis of motor and postural control, interplay between individual and the environment, and the ability of the individual to function safely in everyday home and work environment.

Physical deconditioning decreases general flexibility, endurance, and strength and predisposes the individual to movement instability. Biomechanical factors such as the degree of motion between the head and neck, intersegmental rotation of the trunk, and degree of movement in the lower extremities are examined as the individual performs a functional activity. A decrease in range of motion could be due to a functional biomechanical loss or to a motor control problem such as alteration in the timing of the movement. For example, a patient with a cerebrovascular accident may exhibit foot drop. Initially, the foot drop is due to alteration in the movement pattern due to the loss of CNS control for timing and sequencing of interlimb muscle activity. If the foot drop persists, however, a biomechanical change of the ankle in relation to the lower extremity occurs and contributes to the deficit in the lower extremity movement pattern.

Another element to consider is metabolic changes or a reduced exercise capacity. That is, if the individual develops changes in the cardiovascular and pulmonary systems due to inactivity, the ability to sustain activity or perform activities for a period of time decreases. In addition inefficient oxygen consumption affects oxygen utilization by the musculoskeletal system.[25] The resulting decline increases stress on these physiological systems when the patient is asked to perform a task. A task as simple as walking up several steps can cause the individual to exceed his or her exercise capacity. When the decreased aerobic capacity is coupled with alterations in the CNS or biomechanical system, a cycle occurs in which a reduced exercise capacity leads to an increase in inactivity, which further reduces exercise capacity. This cycle can also cause a loss of self-confidence.

Finally, the motor and postural control systems are assessed according to the ability of the individual to perform the activity smoothly and efficiently. A more detailed discussion follows.

CASE 1 ▼   Person with Parkinson's Disease

When evaluating motor control deficits in the patient with Parkinson's disease, the severity of the disease, the activity level of the person, and the medication schedule are important considerations. Described here are some motor control deficits that may be evident in this patient population. Fig. 4-4 can be used to guide the evaluation.

The Get Up and Go Test can be used to assess both gait and transition phases. Alterations in stride length, speed, and frequency produce changes in the gait pattern in the person with Parkinson's disease. The person may demonstrate a gait pattern with decreased amplitude or duration of the gait cycle, decreased trunk rotation and arm swing, and a festinating gait in which the patient appears to be trying to catch up with the center of gravity. A decrease in righting and equilibrium reactions also contributes to instability in gait. Whenever the preferred speed and frequency parameters are altered in any movement, they can increase metabolic costs and alter the ability of the individual to safely complete the functional movement with appropriate coordination of postural and motor control. In fact, any gait deficit increases metabolic costs.

Another characteristic to examine is force. Force implies the ability to generate the appropriate amount and rate of force. Persons with Parkinson's disease generate appropriate force when performing an isometric task, but are unable to increase or decrease force at an appropriate rate.[22,28]

Another deficit in motor control is difficulty in initiating movements. This deficit can be assessed at three different times in the Get Up and Go Test: when the person rises from the chair, when the person turns at the end of 3 meters, and when the person turns and then sits down in the chair. Although researchers have demonstrated that clients with Parkinson's disease are able to prepare the motor strategy and use advance information, the primary problem is the slow onset of execution of movement.[21]

To illustrate the multiple motor control deficits, imagine a patient performing the Get-up and Go Test. The patient is asked to stand up from a chair, walk a specified distance, turn around, walk back to the chair, and sit down. The patient may have difficulty accelerating and decelerating to turn around and may have difficulty decelerating when approaching the chair and sitting down. The motor control deficits exhibited in the patient are numerous and intertwined. As mentioned earlier, the patient cannot appropriately control the increase and decrease in the rate of force production, which is evident in the acceleration and deceleration phases of the movement. If the rate of force production is altered, amplitude of force production may also be affected.

The person may have decreased ability in prediction, that is to predict and prepare the motor pattern for turning before the actual turn. There appears to be a slow initiation of the turning task. This phenomenon could be due to the inability to sequence the motor behavior as a whole. Several researchers have observed that the person completes one movement before starting the next movement in the sequence rather than executing a smooth, ongoing movement pattern.[2,20] Another reason for the decrease in the ability to perform this task smoothly is the patient's dependence on visual feedback. Relying more heavily on visual feedback to accomplish a task slows down the movement.[4]

The movement deficits observed may also be due to the inability to effectively coordinate movements such as that observed between postural and movement components of the task.[12] Postural strategies may be classified on a continuum that includes postural preparations, postural accompaniments, and postural reactions.[5] The patient with Parkinson's disease may not predict and make appropriate postural adjustments before the movement and may also have deficits in postural reactions, i.e., righting and equilibrium reactions. When patients are externally perturbed, some researchers have noted a simultaneous activation of two balance strategies occurs[10], whereas others have noted a decrease in functional activation of muscles, particularly around the ankle.[1,18] In the case of the Get Up and Go Test, movement and balance strategies are assessed when the client stands up and sits down. If the client does not use a controlled descent into the chair, but rather flops, what are the possible causes for the sudden descent? The individual's preferred pattern may be to flop into the chair; the individual may not be able to predict the time and force needed to activate the muscles for a smooth descent; the individual may be deconditioned and does not have the strength or endurance to perform a smooth descent; or the individual may not have the balance strategies required to perform this maneuver.

In summary, to assess the patient with Parkinson's disease or any other neurological deficit, all aspects of motor control need to be examined as the individual executes a variety of functional tasks. The patient may have multiple motor and postural control deficits; only a few were examined in the example. It is not the scope of this section to present all the motor and postural control deficits but to highlight the complexity of patients with neurological pathophysiology. A more accurate identification of motor control problems in patients will assist in the development of effective treatment goals and plans and will be discussed throughout Section 2.

USE OF MOTOR CONTROL PARAMETERS TO ASSESS POSTURE AND MOVEMENT DEFICITS IN PATIENTS WITH NEUROLOGICAL DISEASE OR TRAUMA

Patients with neurological disease are unable to generate "normal" motor behavior because the CNS deficit has altered the integrative capability of the brain. Biomechanical and metabolic factors are also altered. The movement pattern executed by the patient is considered a functional movement pattern used to accomplish the goal. Depending on the pathophysiology of the trauma and secondary complications, the pattern may not be efficient in terms of neurological, biomechanical, or metabolic costs to the system. Nevertheless, the pattern is the preferred pattern (emergent property) arising from a self-organizing system that permits the individual to function. This preferred pattern is a result of the constraints imposed on the individual by the neurological condition, as well as the constraints imposed by the environment and the task. The use of assistive devices may further increase the costs to the system.[8] For example, a person using a walker will have altered gait pattern and increase in metabolic costs, and prolonged use of the walker will alter the biomechanical and neurological relationship for postural alignment and location of the center of mass.

Evaluation and treatment should focus on those movement parameters that have been altered and the way in which the individual can optimally function in a particular task. To guide the evaluation of posture and movement, several general questions can be addressed. For example, what is the activity level of the person? Is the person able to safely function in the everyday environmental home and work setting? Does the person have the capability to generate movement strategies, and is the person capable of learning new motor strategies?

Another guiding factor is the life span developmental status of the person. A young child with cerebral palsy has a reference of correctness about movement that is based on the constraints imposed from the condition. An adult with an acute CNS deficit may have either a preinjury reference of correctness or a postinjury reference of correctness that may or may not be compatible with the new constraints imposed by the acute neurological condition. For example, a client with a cardiovascular accident may exhibit a list to the involved side while sitting but perceives that he or she is sitting upright.

Specific questions relative to motor control also guide the assessment. For example, is the individual appropriately processing sensory information? Is the person generating an appropriate motor response? Can the individual modify the motor response to accomplish the task, or does the person use limited or obligatory motor patterns? Is the person selecting the appropriate motor strategy, but parameters such as amplitude, timing, phasing are not appropriate? The clinician identifies inappropriate parameters of motor control. The therapist then develops a hypothesis(es) pertaining to alter-

ations in the motor control system, in the physiological system, or in the biomechanical systems and uses this hypothesis(es) as a basis for treatment. Treating the patient and assessing the outcome are the means to test the hypothesis.

These examples are only a few examples of the guiding questions that can be asked relative to motor and postural control. Once the therapist observes the patient, the therapist can formulate hypotheses as to what factors are contributing to the deficits in motor behavior. Observational analysis can be used to focus the remainder of the evaluation in a more contextually appropriate manner. The more focused questions can be used to test the hypotheses. Often, a single factor does not produce the motor deficit, but rather an interaction of present and past constraints. The satisfying part of an evaluation is to be able to test and rule out hypotheses. Theoretically, by ruling out hypotheses, the treatment program can become more focused and effective. A list of a large variety of assessment tools can be found in Chapter 1 and those located within this text identified in the appendix at the back of the book.

REFERENCES

1. Allum JHJ and others: Disturbance of posture in patients with Parkinson's disease. In Amblard B, Bertha A, Clarse F, editors: *Posture and gait: development, adaptation, and modulation,* New York, 1988, Elsevier Science Publications.
2. Benecke R and others: Simple and complex movements off and on treatment in patients with Parkinson's disease, *J Neurol Neurosurg Psychiatry* 50:296-303, 1987.
3. Bernstein N: *Coordination and regulation of movement,* New York, 1967, Pergamon Press.
4. Flowers FA: Visual closed-loop and open-loop characteristics of voluntary movements in patients with parkinsonism and intention tremor, *Brain* 99:269-319, 1976.
5. Frank JS and Earl M: Coordination of posture and movement, *Phys Ther* 70:855-863, 1990.
6. Grillner S: Control of locomotion in bipeds, tetrapods, and fish. In Brooks VB, editor: *Handbook of physiology* (section 1), The nervous system, vol 2: Motor control, part 2, Bethesda, 1981, American Physiological Society.
7. Heriza C: Motor development: traditional and contemporary theories. In *Contemporary Management of Motor Control Problems. Proceedings of the II STEP Conference,* Fredericksburg, Va, 1991, Foundation for Physical Therapy.
8. Holt KG: Toward general principles for research and rehabilitation of disabled populations. *Phys Ther Practice* 2(2): 1-18, 1993.
9. Horak FB and Nashner LM: Central programming of postural movements: adaptation to altered support surface configurations, *J Neurophysiol* 55:1369-1381, 1986.
10. Horak FB, Nashner LM, and Nutt JG: Postural instability in Parkinson's disease: motor coordination and sensory organization. *Soc Neurosci Abstr* 10:634, 1984.
11. Jackson H: The Croonian lectures on evolution and dissolution of the nervous system. lecture 2. *Br Med J* 660-663, 1884.
12. Johnels B and others: Measuring motor function in Parkinson's disease. In Benecke R, Conrad B, Marsden CD, editors: *Motor disturbances,* I. San Diego, 1987, Academic Press.
13. Marsden CD, Rothwell JC, and Day BL: The use of peripheral feedback in the control of movement. In Evarts EV, Wise SP, Bousfield D, editors: *The motor system in neurobiology,* Amsterdam, 1985, Elsevier Biomedical Press.

14. Newell KM and Corcos DM, editors: *Variability and motor control,* Champaign, Ill, 1993, Human Kinetics Publishers.

15. Newton R: Current perspectives on neural control. *Proceedings of the Tenth International Congress of the World Confederation for Physical Therapy.* Sydney, Australia, 1987, W.C.P.T.

16. Newton RA and Deo AV: Standing balance in elderly adults with and without hearing impairments. *Proceedings of the World Confederation for Physical Therapy.* 11th International Congress, London, 1991, W.C.P.T.

17. Pribram KH: Holonomic brain theory: *cooperativity and reciprocity in processing the configural and cognitive aspects of perception.* Hillsdale, NJ, 1988, Erlbaum.

18. Rogers MW: Motor control problems in Parkinson's disease. In *Contemporary Management of Motor Control Problems. Proceedings of the II STEP Conference.* Fredericksburg, Va, 1991, Foundation for Physical Therapy, Bookcrafters, Inc.

19. Rothwell JC and others: Manual motor performance in a deafferented man, *Brain* 105:515-542, 1982.

20. Shimizu N, Yoshida M, and Hagatsuka Y: Disturbance of two simultaneous motor acts in patients with parkinsonism and cerebellar ataxia, *Adv Neurol* 45:367-370, 1987.

21. Stelmach GE and Phillips JG: Movement disorders—limb movement and the basal ganglia, *Phys Ther* 71:60-67, 1991.

22. Stelmach GE and Worringham CJ: The preparation and production of isometric force in Parkinson's disease, *Acta Physiologica Scand* 26:93-103, 1988.

23. Schoner G and Kelso JAS: Dynamic pattern generation in behavioral and neural systems, *Science* 239:1513-1520, 1988.

24. Taub E: Movements in nonhuman primates deprived of somatosensory feedback, *Exerc Sport Sci Rev* 4:335-374, 1976.

25. Thompson RF, Crist DM, and Marsh M: Effects of physical exercise for elderly patients with physical impairments, *J Am Geriatr Soc* 36:130-135, 1988.

26. Tuller B, Turvey MT, and Fitch HL: The Bernstein perspective: II. The concept of muscle linkage or coordinative structure. In Kelso JAS, editor. *Human motor behavior: an introduction.* Hillsdale, NJ, 1982, Erlbaum.

27. VanSant AF: Life-span motor development. In *Contemporary Management of Motor Control Problems. Proceedings of the II Step Conference.* Fredericksburg, Va, 1991, Foundation for Physical Therapy.

28. Wing AM: A comparison of the rate of pinch grip force increases and decreases in parkinsonian bradykinesia, *Acta Physiologica Scand* 26:479-482, 1988.

29. Woollacott MJ: Age-related changes in posture and movement. *J Gerontol* 48(Special Issue):56-60, 1993.

30. Woollacott M and Shumway-Cook A, editors: *Posture and gait: a lifespan perspective,* Charleston, 1989, University of South Carolina.

CHAPTER 5

Limbic Complex

Influence over motor control and learning

Darcy Ann Umphred

LEARNING OBJECTIVES

After reading this chapter the student/therapist will:
1. Identify the complexity of the limbic complex and its influence over behavioral responses.
2. Differentiate between limbic motor control responses and cerebellar/basal ganglia motor regulation.
3. Identify different emotional or limbic responses and their influence on the spinal and brainstem motor generators.
4. Differentiate between declarative and procedural learning.
5. Analyze client's functional responses to environmental demands and determine if the limbic complex has negatively or positively influenced the observable behavior.

KEY TERMS

limbic system or complex
hippocampus
declarative memory
amygdala

F^2ARV (Fear/Frustration, Anger, Rage, Violence) continuum
emotional behavior
reverberating loops or circuits

As stated at the end of Chapter 3, the understanding of the nervous system is based on viewing it as a total entity made up of many interlocking parts. The puzzle may initially consist of 5 to 10 pieces that fit together, but when joined give the student a feeling of accomplishment and intellectual mastery. The process of unlocking and reassembling the puzzle while either subdividing each original puzzle piece or adding new pieces is the journey a student begins in school and can, if so chosen, continue throughout life.

The traditional way to analyze and study brain function is to first approach the hard-core science (i.e., anatomy and physiology). Then the learner studies normal function as it relates to anatomy and physiology. At this level, behavior patterns expressing the specific functions might be introduced. Finally, dysfunction is presented. The study of dysfunction often relates animal studies to potential function in humans. The validity of these correlations is always questionable.

The complexity of the anatomy, physiology, and neurochemistry of the limbic complex baffles the minds of basic science doctoral students. Yet a therapist deals on a moment-to-moment functional level with the limbic system of clients throughout the day. This chapter helps the reader to combine basic neuroscience (Chapters 3 and 4) with psychosocial theory (Chapter 7). Fig. 5-1 illustrates the interlocking/co-dependency of all major central nervous system (CNS) components with the environment. At no time does any system stand in isolation. Thus from a clinical perspective the therapist should always maintain focus on the whole environment and all major interactive components within it, while directing attention to any specific component.

This chapter was initially written using a traditional educational and textbook presentation. When put together as a whole, the complexity of the limbic system became overwhelming. It became apparent that colleagues would drown in the basic science presentation before they reached the application. Thus, a nontraditional presentation has been used in this chapter. An overview of the limbic system is followed by a section on functional application, including limbic lesions and their influence on the therapeutic environment. The later sections introduce the anatomy and physiology. The goal of this chapter is to help the student recognize how limbic function drastically affects the clinical environment and why motor behavior can be dramatically changed with limbic dysfunction or imbalance. Once acceptance of the primary objective is achieved, it is hoped that the reader will be enticed to study further the basic science sections to understand more fully the true function of the limbic system.

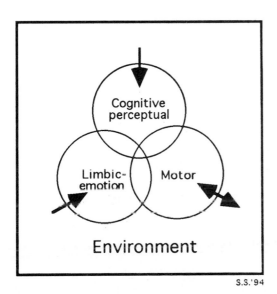

Fig. 5-1. Interlocking/co-dependency of all major CNS systems.

THE LIMBIC SYSTEM: ITS FUNCTIONAL RELATIONSHIP TO CLINICAL PERFORMANCE
Overview: the limbic system's role in motor control, memory, and learning

It is not easy to find a generally accepted definition of the **"limbic system or complex,"** its boundaries, and the components that should be included. Mesulam[47] likens this to a fifth century BC philosopher's quotation: "the nature of God is like a circle of which the center is everywhere and the circumference is nowhere." Brodal[10] suggests that functional separation of brain regions becomes less clear as we discover the interrelatedness through ongoing research. He sees the limbic system reaching out and encompassing the entire brain and all of its functional components and sees no purpose in defining such a subdivision.

Though the anatomical descriptions of the limbic system may vary from author to author, the functional significance of this system is widely acknowledged in defining human behavior and behavioral neurology.

Brooks[11] divides the brain into the limbic brain and the nonlimbic sensorimotor brain. The sensorimotor portion is involved in perception of nonlimbic sensations and motor performance. The limbic brain is primitive, essential for survival, sensing the "need" to act, and thereby initiating need-directed motor activity for survival. The limbic brain also has the capability for memory and can select what to learn from experience. Brooks also defines the two brain systems functionally and not anatomically, because their anatomical separation according to function is almost impossible and changes with the task (Fig. 5-2).

Kandel and others[32] state that behavior requires three major systems: the sensory, the motor, and the motivational or limbic. When analyzing a seemingly simple action, such as swinging a golf club, we recruit our sensory system for visual, tactile, and proprioceptive input to guide the motor systems for precise, coordinated muscle recruitment and postural control. The motivational (limbic) system does the following: (1) provides intentional drive for the initiation, (2) integrates the total input, and (3) plays a role in motor expression. The motivational system plays a role in control of the two motor systems: the autonomic system and the somatic sensorimotor system. It thereby plays a role in controlling both the skeletal muscles through input to the frontal lobe and brainstem and the smooth muscles and glands through the hypothalamus, which lies at the "heart" of the limbic system (Fig. 5-3). Noback and others[52] state that "the limbic system is involved with many of the expressions that make us human, namely emotions, behaviors and feeling states." That humanness also has individuality. Our unique memory storage, or variable responses to different environmental contexts and our control or lack thereof over our emotional sensitivity to environmental stimuli, all play roles in molding each one of us. Due to this uniqueness, each therapist and each client need to be accepted for their own individuality.

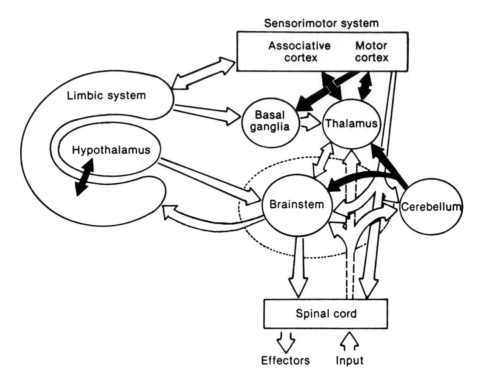

Fig. 5-2. Divisions and interconnections between the limbic and nonlimbic (sensorimotor) cortex.

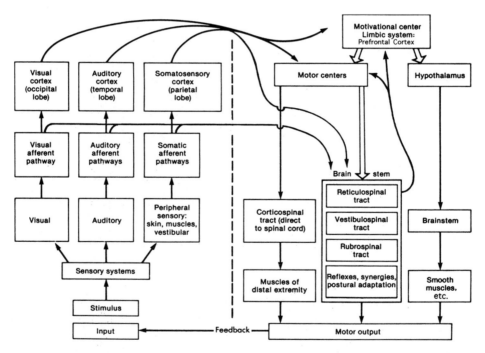

Fig. 5-3. Motivational systems influence over the sensorimotor and autonomic nervous systems. (Adapted from Kandel ER, Schwartz JH, and Jessell TM: *Principles of neural science,* ed 3, New York, 1991, Elsevier Medical Science Publishing.)

Broca[9] first conceptualized the anatomical regions of the limbic lobe as forming a ring around the brainstem. Today, neuroanatomists do not differentiate an anatomical lobe as limbic, but rather refer to a complex or system that encompasses cortical, diencephalon, and brainstem struc-

tures.[32] This description is less precise and encompasses, but is not limited to, the orbitofrontal cortex, **hippocampus,** parahippocampal gyrus, cingulate gyrus, dentate gyrus, amygdaloid body, septal area, hypothalamus, and some nuclei of the thalamus.[6,32] Anatomists stress the importance of looking at interrelated segments or loops within the limbic region and include fiber bundles such as the fornix, mamillothalamic fasciculus, stria terminalis, medial forebrain bundle, and the stria medullaris as part of the system.[6,13,15] These multiple nuclei and interlinking circuits play crucial roles in behavioral and emotional changes,[12,18,20] **declarative memory,**[3,72] and motor expression.[31] The loss of any link can affect the outcome activity of the whole circuit. Thus damage to any area of the brain can potentially cause malfunctions in any or all other areas, and the entire circuit may need reorganization to restore function.

Researchers do not ascribe a specific single function to CNS formations, but see each become a part of a system, participating to various degrees in the multitude of behavioral responses (see Chapters 2, 3, and 4 for additional information). Therefore the loss of any part of higher centers or limbic system may not be clearly definable functionally, and the return of function is not always easy to predict.

Recovery of function after injury may involve mechanisms that allow reorganizing of structure and function of cortical, subcortical, and spinal circuits. In very young infants, areas within opposite hemispheres may "take over" function, whereas in more mature brains reorganization of existing systems seems to be the current accepted hypothesis within expanding knowledge of neuroplasticity.[21] For complex behavior, such as in motor functioning requiring many steps, the limbic system, cortex, hypothalamus, basal ganglia, and brainstem work as an integrated unit, with any damaged area causing the whole system to malfunction. A loss of function or a change in behavior cannot necessarily be localized as to the underlying cause. A lesion in one area may cause a malfunction of an area that is not actually damaged.

The complexity of the limbic system and its associative influence over both the motor control system and cortical structures are enormous. A therapist dealing with a client with motor control or learning problems needs to understand how the limbic system affects behavioral responses. The knowledge base not only focuses on the client's deficits, but also on the integrative function of the therapist. This understanding should lead to a greater awareness of the clinical environment and the factors within the environment that cause change.

The limbic system's influence on behavior: its relevance to the therapeutic environment

Levels of behavioral hierarchies: where does the limbic system belong? Strub and Black[68] view behavior as occurring on distinct interrelated levels, which represent behavioral hierarchies. Starting at level one, a state of alertness to the internal and external environment must be maintained for motor or mental activity to occur. The brainstem reticular activating system brings about this state of general arousal by relaying in an ascending pathway to the thalamus, the limbic system, and the cerebral cortex. To proceed from a state of general arousal to one of "selective attention" requires the communication of information to and from the cortex, thalamus, and the limbic system and its modulation over the brainstem and spinal pattern generators.[31,32]

Level two of this hierarchy lies in the domain of the hypothalamus and its closely associated limbic structures. This level deals with subconscious drives and innate instincts. The survival-oriented drives of hunger, thirst, temperature regulation, and survival of the species (sex), and the steps necessary for drive reduction are processed here, as well as learning and memory. Most of these activities relate to limbic functioning.

On level three, only cerebral cortical areas are activated. This level deals with abstract conceptualization of verbal or quantitative entities.

Level four behavior is concerned with the expression of social aspects of behavior, personality, and life-style. Again, the limbic system and its relationship to the frontal lobe are vital here.

The interaction of all four levels leads to the integrative and adaptable behavior seen in humans. Our ability to become alert and protectively react is balanced by our previous learning, whether it be cognitive-perceptive, social, or affective. Adaptability to rapid changes in the physical environment, in life-styles, and in personal relationships results from the interrelationships or complex neurocircuitry of the human brain. When insult occurs at any one level within these behavioral hierarchies, all levels may be affected.

The limbic system MOVEs us. Moore[51] eloquently describes the limbic system as the area of the brain that moves us. The word *move* can be used as a mnemonic for the functions of the limbic system.

Limbic system function*

Memory/motivation: drive
1. Memory: attention and retrieval
2. Motivation: desire to learn, try, or benefit from the environment

Olfaction (especially in infants)
1. Only sensory system that does not go through the thalamus as its second-order synapse in the sensory pathway before it gets to the cerebral cortex

Visceral (drives: thirst, hunger, temperature regulation, endocrine functions)
1. Sympathetic and parasympathetic reactions
2. Peripheral autonomic nervous system (ANS) responses that reflect limbic function

Emotion: feelings and attitude
1. Self-concept and worth
2. Emotional body image
3. Tonal responses of motor system
4. Attitude, social skills, opinions

* Adapted from a lecture by Moore JC, Fifteenth Annual Sensorimotor Integration Symposium, San Diego, July, 1987.[50]

As seen in this outline, the "M" depicts the drive component of the limbic system. Before learning, an individual must be motivated to learn, to try to succeed at the task, to solve the problem, or to benefit from the environment. Without motivation the brain will not orient itself to the problem and learn. However, once motivated the individual must be able to pay attention and process the sequential and simultaneous nature of the component parts to be learned, as well as the whole. The limbic **amygdala** and hippocampal structures and their intricate circuitries play a key role in this aspect of memory. Once learned, the information is stored in cortical areas and can be retrieved at a later time.

The "O" refers to the incoming sense of smell, which exerts a strong influence on alertness and drive. This is clearly illustrated by the billions of dollars spent annually on perfumes, deodorants, mouthwashes, and soap. This input tract can be used effectively by therapists who have clients with CNS lesions, such as internal capsule and thalamic involvement. The olfactory system synapses within the olfactory bulb and then with the limbic system structures and then may go directly to the cerebral cortex without synapsing in the thalamus. Although collaterals do project to the thalamus, unlike all other sensory information, olfaction does not use the thalamus as a necessary relay center to access the cortical structures. Other senses may not be reaching the cortical levels, and the client may have a sensory-deprived environment. Olfactory sensations, which enter the limbic system, may be used to calm or arouse the client. The specific olfactory input may determine whether the person remains calm or emotionally aroused.[7] Pleasant odors would be preferable to most people.

A comatose and seemingly nonresponsive client may respond to odor. The therapist needs to be *acutely* aware of the responses, for they may be autonomic instead of somatomotor.

The "V" represents visceral or autonomic drives. As noted earlier, the hypothalamus is nestled within the limbic system. Thus regulation of sympathetic and parasympathetic reactions, both of the internal organ systems and the periphery, reflect ongoing limbic activity. Obviously, drives such as thirst, hunger, temperature regulation, and sexuality are controlled by this system. Clients demonstrating total lack of inhibitory control over eating or drinking or manifesting very unstable body temperature regulation may be exhibiting signs of hypothalamic/pituitary involvement and/or direct pathways from hypothalamus to midbrain structures.[19,32]

Less obvious autonomic responses that may reflect limbic imbalances often go unnoticed by therapists. When the stress of an activity is becoming overwhelming to a client, he or she may react with severe sweating of the palms or an increase in dysreflexic activity in the mouth area rather than heightened motor activity. A therapist must continually monitor this aspect of the client's response behaviors to ascertain that the behaviors observed reflect motor control and not limbic influences over that motor system.

If the input to the client is excessive, the limbic system will not function at the optimal level and learning will diminish. The client may withdraw physically or mentally, lose focus or attention, decrease motivation, and become frustrated or even angry. The overload on the reticular system may shut down the limbic system and not the limbic system itself, although it is part of the loop system. All of these behaviors may be expressed within the hypothalamic/autonomic system as output, no matter where in the loop the dysfunction occurs. The evaluation of this system seems even more critical when a client's motor control system is locked, with no volitional movement present. Therapists often try to increase motor activity through sensory input, however, they must cautiously avoid indiscriminately bombarding the sensory systems. The limbic system may demonstrate overload while the spinal motor generators reflect inadequate activation. Although the two systems are different, they are intricately connected, and the concept of massively bombarding one while ignoring the other does not make sense in a learning framework.

"E" relates to emotions, the feelings and attitudes unique to that individual. This refers especially to the amygdaloid aspect of the limbic system and orbitofrontal activity within the frontal lobe.[70] This is a primary emotional center, and it regulates not only our self-concept, but our attitudes and opinions toward our environment and the people within it.

Self-concept is the emotional aspect of body image. For example, assume that one morning I looked in the mirror and said, "The poor world, I will not subject it to me today." I then go back to bed and eat nothing for the rest of the day. The next day I get up and look in the same mirror and say, "What a change, I look trim and beautiful. Look out world, here I come!" In reality my physical body has not been altered drastically, if at all, but my attitude toward that body has changed. That is, the emotional component of my body image has perceptually changed.

A second self-concept deals with my attitude about my worth or value to society and the world and my role within it. Again this attitude can change with mood, but more often it seems to change with experience. This aspect of client/therapist interaction can be critical to the success of a therapeutic environment. Two examples will be given to illustrate this point, with the focus of bringing perceived roles into the therapeutic setting:

1. Your client is Mrs. S., a 72-year-old woman with a left cerebrovascular accident (CVA). She comes from a low socioeconomic background, and was a housekeeper for 40 years for a wealthy family of high social standing. When addressing you (the therapist) she always says "yes, ma'am" or "no, ma'am," and does just what was asked, no more and no less. It may be very hard to get this client to assume responsibility for

self-direction in the therapeutic setting. Her perceived role in life may not be to take responsibility or authority within a setting that may, from her perception, have high social status, such as a medical facility. She also may feel that she does not have the power to assume such responsibilities. Success in the therapeutic setting may be based more on changing her attitudes than on motor control. That is, the concept of empowerment may play a crucial role in regaining independent functional skill and control over her environment.

2. Your client is a 24-year-old lumberjack who suffered a closed head injury (CHI) during a fall at work. It is now 1 month since his accident, and he is totally alert, verbal, angry, and has moderate to severe motor control problems. During your initial treatment you note that he responds very well to handling. He seems to flow with your movement, and with your assistance is able to practice much higher level motor control; although at times he needs your assistance, you try to release that control whenever possible to empower him to control his body. At the end of therapy he sits back in his chair with much better function. Then he turns to you (the female therapist) and instead of saying "That was great," he says, "You witch, I hate you." The inconsistency between how his body responded to your handling and his attitude toward you as a person may seem baffling, until you realize that he has always perceived himself as a dominant male. Similarly, he perceives women as weak, to be protected, and in need of control. If his attitude toward you cannot be changed to see you in a generic professional role, he will most likely not benefit as much from your clinical skills.

Preconceived attitudes, social behaviors, and opinions have been learned by filtering the input through the limbic system. If new attitudes and behaviors need to be learned after a neurological insult, the intactness, especially of the amygdaloid pathways, seems crucial (see the section on anatomy). Damage to these limbic structures may prevent learning, and thus socially maladaptive behavior may persist, making the individual less likely to adapt to the social environment.

As our feelings, attitudes, and values drive our behaviors both through attention and motor responses, the emotional aspect of the limbic system has great impact on our learning and motor control. Placing too little value on a motor output often leads to complacency and lack of learning. On the other hand, placing an extremely high value on a motor output or learning skills, such as in a cognitive test situation, can overload the system and decrease function.

Motivation and reward. Moore[51] considers motivation and memory as part of the MOVE system. Stellar and Stellar[67] link motivation with reward and help, illustrating how the limbic system learns through repetition and reward. They state that the concept of motivation includes drive and satiation, goal-directed behavior, and incentive. They recognize that these behaviors maintain homeostasis and ensure the survival of the individual and the species. Although the frontal lobe region appears to play an important role in self-control and execution activities, these functions seem to require a close interlocking neuronetwork between cognitive representation within the frontal regions and motivational control provided by limbic and subcortical structures.[70]

Motivated behavior is geared to reinforcement and reward. Repeated experience of reinforcement and reward lead to learning, changed expectancy, changed behavior, and maintained performance.[36] Repetition with the feeling of success (reinforcement) is a critical element in the therapeutic setting, and consistently making the task more difficult just when the client feels ready to succeed will tend to decrease reinforcement/reward and thus lessen the client's motivation to try. With the pressure placed on therapists to produce changes quickly, repetition and thus long-term learning are often jeopardized, and this may have a dramatic effect on the quality of the client's life and the long-term treatment effects once he or she leaves the medical facility. Motor control theory (see Chapters 3 and 4) coincides with limbic research regarding reinforcement. Inherent feedback within a variety of environmental contexts and allowing for error lead to greater retention. Repetition or the opportunity to practice a task (motor or cognitive) in which the individual desires to succeed will lead to long-term learning. Without practice or motivation the chance of successful learning is minimal to nonexistent.

Integration of the limbic system as part of a whole functioning brain. Motivation, alertness, and concentration are critical in motor learning because they determine how well we pay attention to the learning and execution of any motor task. These processes of learning and doing are inevitably intertwined: "we learn as we do, and we do only as well as we have learned."[11]

Both motivation or "feeling the need to act" and concentration are contributed by the limbic system. As discussed later in the neuroanatomy portion of this chapter, the amygdaloid complex with its multitude of afferent and efferent interlinkages is especially adapted for recognizing the significance of a stimulus, and it assigns the emotional aspect of feeling the need to act. These neuroanatomical loops have tremendous connections with the reticular system. Hence, some authors call it the reticulolimbic system.[32,50] The interaction of the limbic system and the motor generators of the brainstem and ultimate modulation over the spinal system lead to need-directed and therefore goal-directed motor activity. It also filters out the significant from the nonsignificant information by selective processing and storing the significant for memory, learning, and recall.

Goal-directed or need-directed motor actions are the result of the nervous system structures acting in an

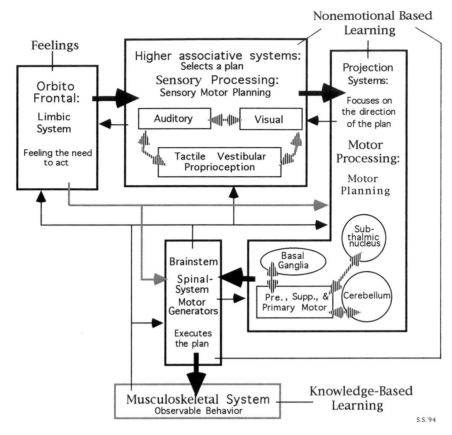

Fig. 5-4. Functional and dynamic hierarchy of systems based on both limbic and motor control interactions. (Adapted from Brooks VB: *The neural basis of motor control*, New York, 1986, Oxford University Press.)

interactive system, which is also a functional, dynamic complex based on systems interacting together. In this system (Fig. 5-4), the most important level is represented by the limbic system and its cortical and subcortical components. In response to stimuli from the internal or external environment, the limbic system initiates motor activity out of the emotional aspect of feeling the need to act. This message is relayed to the sensory areas of the cerebral cortex, which could entail any one or all association areas for visual, auditory, tactile, olfactory, gustatory, or proprioceptive input. These areas are located in the prefrontal, occipital, parietal, and temporal lobes, where they analyze and integrate sensory input into an overall strategy of action or a general plan that meets the requirements of the task. Therefore these cortices recognize, select, and prepare to act as a response to relevant sensory cues when a state of arousal is provided by reticular input. The limbic cortex (uncus, parahippocampal gyrus/isthmus, cingulate gyrus and septal nucleus) has even greater influence over the sensorimotor cortices via the cingulate gyrus, both directly and indirectly through association areas. The thalamus, cerebellum, and basal ganglia contribute to the production of the specific motor plans. These messages of the general plan are relayed to the projection system. The limbic structures via the cingulate

gyrus also have direct connections with the primary motor cortex. This certainly has the potential to assist in driving fine motor activities via corticobulbar and corticospinal tracts. The thalamus, cerebellum, basal ganglia, and motor cortices (premotor, supplementary motor, and primary motor) contribute to the production of the specific motor plans.[32] Messages regarding the sensory component of the general plan are relayed to the projection system where they are transformed into refined motor plans. These plans are then projected throughout the motor system to modulate motor generators throughout the brainstem and spinal system.[32] Limbic connections with (1) cerebellum, basal ganglia, and frontal lobe[32] and (2) the motor generator within the brainstem[31] enable further control of limbic instructions over motor control or expression.

Within these projection and motor planning complexes, the specifics are programmed and the tactics are given a strategy. In general, the "what" is turned into "how" and "when." The necessary parameters for coordinated movement are programmed here as to intensity, sequencing, and timing to carry out the motor task. These programs which incorporate upper motor neurons and interneurons are then sent to the brainstem and spinal motor generators, which in turn via lower motor neurons send orders regarding the specific motor tasks to the musculoskeletal system. (See Chapters 3 and 4 for more specific in-depth discussion.) The actions performed by each subsystem within the entire limbic/motor control complex constantly loop back and communicate its actions to all subsystems to allow for adjustments of intensity and duration and to determine whether the plan remains the best choice of responses to an ever-changing three-dimensional world.

In summary, the limbic complex generates need-directed motor activity and communicates that intent throughout the motor system.[31] This step is vital to normal motor function and thus client care. Clients need the opportunity to analyze correctly both their internal environment (their preset and feedforward plans and their emotional state) and the external world around them requiring action on a task. The integration of all this information should produce an appropriate strategy for the present activity. These instructions must be correct and the system capable of carrying out the motor activity. If the motor system is deficit, lack of adaptability will be observed in the client. If the limbic complex is faulty, the same motor deficits might present themselves. The therapist must differentiate what is truly a motor system problem verses a limbic influence over the motor system problem.

Schmidt[60] stresses the significance of "knowledge of results feedback" as being the information from the environment that provides the individual with insights into task requirements. This insight helps the motor system correctly select strategies that will successfully initiate and support the appropriate movement for accomplishing the task. This knowledge of results feedback is required for effective motor learning and to form the correct motor programs for storage. The following example is presented to help the reader understand the limbic role in this motor programming.

You are sitting in your new car. The dealer has filled the tank with necessary fuel. The engine mechanism is totally functional with all its wires and interlocking components. The engine will not perform without a mechanism to initiate its strategies or turn on the system. The basal ganglia/frontal lobe motor mechanism plays this role in the brain. In a car you have a starter motor. Yet, the starter motor will not activate the motor system without your intent and motivation to turn the key and turn on the engine. The limbic complex serves this function in the brain. Once you have turned the key, the car is running and ready for your guidance. Whether you choose reverse or first gear usually depends on prior learning unless this is a totally new experience. Once the gear is selected, the motor system will program the car to run according to your desires. It can run fast or slow, but to change the plan both a purpose and a recognition that change is necessary are required. The car has the ability to adapt and self-regulate to many environmental variables such as ruts or slick pavement to continue running the feedforward program, just as many motor systems within your CNS play that function. The limbic system may emotionally choose to drive fast while your cognitive judgment may choose otherwise. The end result will drive your peddle and brake pressure and ultimately regulate the car. The components discussed play a critical role

in the total function of the car just as all the systems within your CNS play a vital role in regulating your behavioral responses to the environment.

Brooks[11] distinguishes insightful learning, which is programmed and leads to skills when the performer has gained insight into the requirements, from discontinuous movements, which need to be replaced by continuous ones. This process is hastened when clients understand and can demonstrate their understanding of what "they were expected to do." Improvement of motor skills is possible by using programmed movement in goal-directed behavior. The reader must be cautioned to make sure the client's attention is on the goal of the task and not on the components of the movement itself. The motor plan needs programming and practice without constant cognitive overriding. The limbic/frontal system helps drive the motor toward the identified task or abstract representation of a match between the motor planning sequence and the desired outcome.

Without the knowledge of results, feedback, and insight into the requirements for goal-directed activity, the learning is performing by "rote," which merely utilizes repetition without analysis, and little meaningful learning or building of effective motor memory in the form of motor holograms will occur.

Schmidt[60] suggests that to elicit the highest level of function within the motor system and to enable insightful learning, therapy programs should be developed around goal-directed activities. These activities direct the client to analyze the environmental requirements (both internal and external) by placing the client in a situation that forces development of "appropriate strategies." Goal-directed activities should be functional behavior and thus involve motivation, meaningfulness, and selective attention. Specific techniques such as proprioceptive neuromuscular facilitation (PNF), neurodevelopmental therapy (NDT), Rood, and Feldenkrais can be incorporated into goal-directed activities in the therapy programs as can any treatment approach as long as it identifies those aspects of motor control and learning that lead to retention and future performance.[60] With insights into the learned skills, clients will be better able to adjust these to meet the specific requirements of different environments and needs, using knowledge of response feedback to guide them. The message then is to design exercise or programs that are meaningful and need-directed, to motivate clients into insightful goal-directed learning. Thus understanding the specific goals of the client is important. A therapist cannot assume that "someone wants to do something." The goal of running a bank may seem very different from that of bird-watching in the mountains, yet both may require ambulatory skills. If a client does not wish to return to work, then a friendly smile and stating, "Hi, I'm your therapist and I'm going to get you up and walking so you can get back to work," may lead to resistance and decreased motivation. In contrast, by knowing the goal of the client, a person highly motivated to ambulate may be present in the clinic every day to meet the goal of bird-watching in the mountains.

Clinical perspectives

The client's internal system influences observable behavior. At least once a year almost any local newspaper will carry a story that generally reads as follows:

> Seventy-nine-year-old, 109-pound arthritic grandmother picks up car by bumper to free trapped 3-year-old grandson.

All of us read these articles and at first doubt their validity and then question the sensationalism used by the reporter. I would also question such news reporting if, at age 13, I had not seen three teenage boys pick up a 1956 Chevrolet and put it back in the garage in its correctly parked position. The boys had moved the car because they feared that if they did not put the car back into its original parked position, their parents would find out that they had driven the car without a license or permission. That elderly lady picked up the car out of fear of severe injury to her grandchild. Emotions can create tremendous high tonal responses, either in a postural pattern such as in a temper tantrum or during movement strategy such as picking up a car.

F²ARV (Fear/Frustration, Anger, Rage, Violence) continuum. One sequence of behaviors used to describe the emotional circuitry of the amygdala is called the **F²ARV (Fear/Frustration, Anger, Rage, Violence) continuum**[50] (Fig. 5-5). This continuum begins with fear, often exhibited as frustration by children. If the event inducing the fear/frustration continues to heighten, anger will often develop. From anger the person may go next into rage and finally violence. How quickly any individual will progress from fear to violence depends on many factors. First, the initial wiring or genetic predisposition will influence their behavioral responses. Second, their soft-wired or conditioned responses resulting from environmental influences and reinforcement patterns will determine output. For example, it is commonly known that abusive parents were usually abused children; they learned that anger quickly leads to violence, and that the behavior was acceptable. Third, the stimulus and its intensity will determine the level of response.

The neurochemistry within the individual's CNS, whether inherent or brought into the system, will have great influence on the plasticity of the existing wiring.[22] When the chemistry or wiring becomes imbalanced due to damage, environmental stress, learning, or other potentially altering situations, then the control over this continuum may also change.[21,32]

Anger itself creates tone through the amygdaloid's influence over the basal ganglia, sensory and motor cortices, and their influence over the motor control system. This is clearly exhibited in a child throwing a temper tantrum (Fig. 5-6) or an adult putting his fist through a wall. How far a client or a friend will progress through the F²ARV continuum depends on a large number of variables. From observation, it is clear that clients do not want to lose control and progress to rage or violence, which often causes embarrassment. This fear, in and of itself, may be frustrating and trigger the continuum. When a client loses that control the therapist must first determine whether the therapist forced the client beyond his or her ability to control. If so, changes within the therapeutic environment need to be made to allow the client opportunities to develop control and modulation over that continuum. Creating opportunities to confront frustration/fear or even anger in real situations while the client practices modulation will lead to independence or self-empowerment. The client simultaneously needs to practice motor control without these emotional

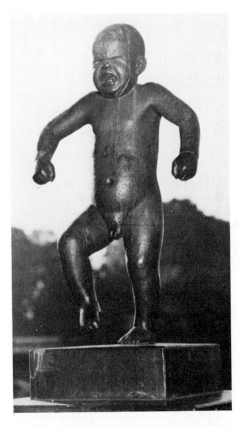

Fig. 5-6. Behavior responses caused by anger. ("Angry Boy," Vigelund Sculpture Grounds in the Frogner Park, Oslo, Norway. Adapted from photo by Normann.)

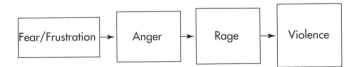

Fig. 5-5. Fear/Frustration, Anger, Rage, Violence: F²ARV continuum.

overlays. In time, practicing the same motor control while confronted with a large variety of emotional situations should be a therapeutic goal.

Similarly, being unaware of a client's anger may lead the therapist to the false assumption that that individual has adequate inherent postural tone to perform activities such as independent transfers. If the client is angry at the therapist and performs the transfer only to "get the therapist off his or her case," when the client is sent home he or she may be unable to create the postural extension to do the transfer. This transfer skill is not independent because it is based on limbic/frontal influence over the extensor system. The client needs to learn how to do the activity without the emotional overlay. When a therapist is unwilling, unaware, or unable to attend to these variables, the reliability or accuracy of functional test results become questionable.

Therapists need to be acutely aware of this continuum in clients who have diffuse axonal shearing (DAS) within the limbic complex. DAS most commonly is seen and reported in research on head trauma. As a result of lesions within the limbic structures may result in an individual who progresses down this continuum at a rapid speed.[12]

Grief or depression. Emotions such as grief or depression can be expressed by the motor system.[32] The behavioral responses are usually withdrawal, decreased postural adaption, and often a feeling of tiredness and exhaustion (Fig. 5-7). (See illustration, right.) Sensory overload, especially in the elderly, can create the same pattern of response of flexion, internal rotation, and adduction. Again, it is hypothesized that these motor responses are the result of the limbic system's influence over motor control.[31] Learned helplessness is another problem that therapists need to avoid. When patients are encouraged to become dependent, their chances of benefiting from services and regaining motor function are drastically reduced.[37,42]

Relaxation and bonding. Because of the potency of the limbic system's connections into the motor system, a therapist's sensitivity to the client's emotional state would obviously be a key factor in understanding the motor responses observed during therapy. In Fig. 5-8 an entire spectrum of motor responses can be observed in the four statues. A client who feels safe can relax and participate in the learning without strong emotional reactions. The woman being held in Fig. 5-8 is safe and relaxed. The man and woman are interacting through touch with warmth and compassion that is often observed when colleagues watch a "master clinician" treating a client. The client and clinician seem to flow together during the treatment as one motor system. When looking at the man and woman, it becomes obvious that the two figures could not be separated, for they are one piece of art. On the other hand, the statue on the left of the two men could represent two pieces of art. Those two

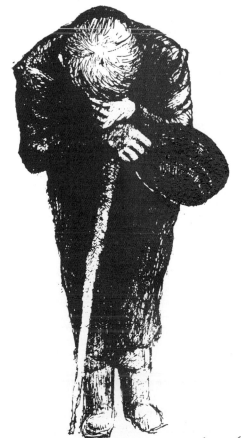

Fig. 5-7. Behavior responses elicited by concern, pain, grief. (Vigelund Sculpture Grounds in the Frogner Park, Oslo, Norway. Adapted from photo by Normann.)

S. Schmidt 69

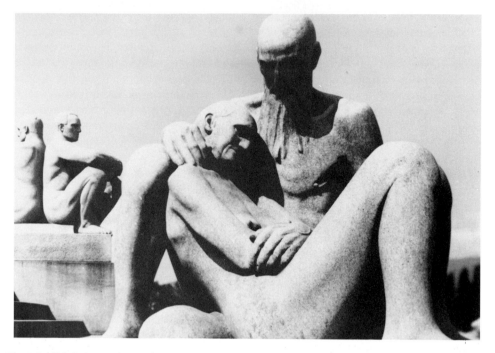

Fig. 5-8. Grief, depression and compassion responses are seen in the center figures, and rigid, stoic, distancing behaviors are observed in the left two male statues. (Vigelund Sculpture Grounds in the Frogner Park, Oslo, Norway. Adapted from photo by Normann.)

men have no bonding. In fact, the closer they would get, the more they would repel each other.

These pictures illustrate therapist/client interactions. If an artist can clearly depict the tonal characteristics of emotion, certainly the therapist should be able to recognize those behaviors in the client. If a client is frustrated or angry and simultaneously has rigidity, spasticity, or general high tone, then a therapist might spend the entire session trying to decrease the motor response. If the client could be helped to deal with the anger or frustration during the therapy session and thus release the emotion, then the specific problems could be treated effectively. Differentiating the limbic system component from the motor control system and establishing treatment protocols for each may not be within the spectrum of a therapist's skills. Thus, working simultaneously with another professional such as a psychologist, social worker, or neuropsychologist may be an acceptable alternative approach. This cotreatment will allow all aspects of the client to be addressed simultaneously. Carry-over of procedural learning (motor learning; see discussion of neurobiology of learning and memory for details) into adaptive motor responses needs to be practiced with consistency.[32] The influence of the limbic system when the client is oscillating according to large mood swings may drastically dampen the procedural learning and limit the success of the therapeutic setting.

Limbic concepts that influence therapist/client interactions. How a clinician reacts at any given moment during a therapeutic session depends on both the client's and the clinician's declarative problem-solving skills and their procedural motor skills (see discussion of neurobiology of learning and memory). The limbic complex drives our motor responses; therefore the sensitivity and specific level of attention of the therapist toward the responses of the client depend on the clinician's limbic system.

In an analysis of what differentiates a truly gifted or master clinician from a group of highly skilled and talented colleagues, the following philosophical concepts may be expressed:

1. That person has a rare gift.
2. That person seems to intuitively know what to do or what the client needs.
3. When that clinician treats a client, the two seem to flow together in their movements.
4. The client seems to totally trust that clinician; I have never seen that before.
5. I cannot believe that the client accurately did that with that clinician; before, the client was too afraid.

Many factors in an interactive setting, such as therapy, cannot be identified, but certain limbic/emotional factors may play a role in that gifted clinician's skill.

Trust/responsibility.[39] Trust is a critical component of a successful therapeutic session. The therapist gains the client's trust by his or her actions. Honesty and truth lead to trust.[39] Telling someone you will not hurt them and then continually ranging a joint beyond a pain-free range is neither honest nor truthful and will not lead to trust. That trust

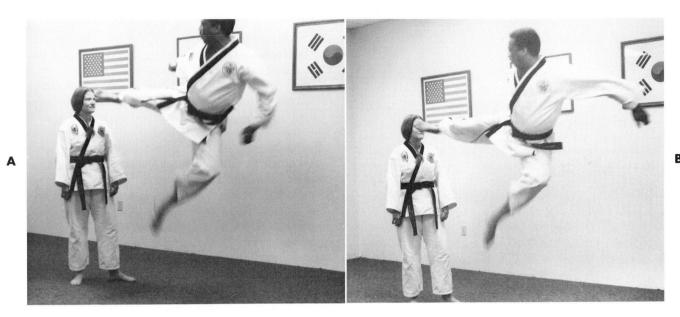

Fig. 5-9. Trust relaxes the limbic system's need to protect. **A,** The skill of the teacher is obvious. **B,** The student trusts that she is in no danger.

can be earned by stopping as soon as the client verbalizes pain or shows pain with a bodily response such as a grimace.

Once a client gives his or her trust, a clinician can freely move or move with a client and little resistance because of fear, reservations, or need to protect self will be felt or observed. Trust does not mean lack of awareness of potential danger; it means acceptance that although the danger is present, the potential of harm, pain, or disaster is very slight and the expected gain is worth the risk. In Fig. 5-9, A and B, the student's trust that the instructor will not hurt her can be seen by her lack of protective responses and by her calm, relaxed body posture. The student is aware of the potential of the kick, but trusts her life to the skills, control, and personal integrity of the teacher. Those same qualities are easily observed when watching a gifted clinician treat clients. The motor activities in a therapeutic setting are less complex than in Fig. 5-9, but in no way are they less stressful, less potentially harmful, or less frightening from the client's point of view.

Therapists must trust themselves enough to know that they can effect changes in their clients. Understanding their own motor system; how it responds; and how to use their hands, arms, or entire body to move someone else is based partly on procedural and partly on declarative learning (see Neurobiology of learning and memory on p. 112). Trusting that they have the skill to implement that motor response has a limbic component. If a therapist has self-doubts, it will change his or her motor performance, which will alter input to the client. This altered input can potentially alter the client's output and vary the desired responses.

Very close to the concept of trust is the idea of responsibility. Accepting responsibility for our own behavior seems obvious and is totally accepted as part of a

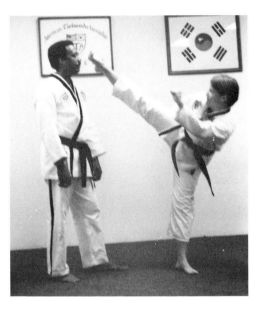

Fig. 5-10. The teacher relinquishes the task to the student, and the student trusts the teacher is right even if self-doubt exists.

professional role. Accepting and allowing the client the right to accept responsibility for his or her own environment are also key elements in creating a successful clinical environment and an independent person. Fig. 5-10 illustrates the concept through the following example:

The teacher (or therapist) asked the student (or client) to perform a motor act. In the figure, the act was to perform a kick to the teacher's head. The kick was to be very strong or forceful and completed. The student was told not to hold back or stop the kick in any way, yet the kick was to come within a few inches of the teacher's head. This placed tremendous responsibility on the student. One inch too far might dangerously hurt the instructor, yet one inch too short was not acceptable. The teacher knew the student had the skill, power, and control to perform the task and then passed the responsibility to the student. She was hesitant to assume the responsibility, for the consequence of failure could have been very traumatic, but the student trusted that the teacher would not ask for the behavior unless success was fairly guaranteed. That trust reduced anxiety and thus gave her more control over the act. Once the task was completed successfully, the student gained confidence and could repeat the task with less fear or emotional influence while gaining refinement over motor control.

Although the motor activities described in this example are more complex than those required by therapists and clients, the dynamics of the environment relate consistently with client/therapist roles and expectations. A gifted clinician knows that the client has the potential to succeed. When asked to perform, the client trusts the therapist and assumes the responsibility for the act. The therapist can facilitate the movement or postural pattern, thereby ensuring that the client succeeds. This feeling of success stimulates motivation for task repetition, which ultimately leads to learning. The incentive to repeat and learn becomes self-motivating and then becomes the responsibility of the client. The limbic complex and its interwoven network throughout the nervous system play a key role in this behavioral drive. The task itself can be simple, such as a weight shift or a holding pattern, or as complex as climbing onto and off of a bus. No matter what the activity, the client needs to accept responsibility for his or her own behavior before independence in motor functioning can be achieved. Although the motor function itself is not limbic, many variables that lead to success, self-

motivation, and feelings of independence are directly related to limbic and prefrontal lobe circuitry.

Dedication to reality. Another component of a successful clinical environment deals with learning on the part of the therapist. A truly gifted therapist sees and feels what is happening within the motor control output system of the client. That therapist does not get stuck with what he or she has learned only because it was what was taught. Instead, learning is constantly related to past memories. Each client is a new map, sketchy at the beginning, that needs to be constantly revised as the terrain (client) changes. Similarly, the therapist will be able to transfer one motor activity into another spatial position. That is, the therapist can let go of an outdated map or treatment technique and create a new one as the environment and motor control system of the client changes. This transference or letting go of old maps or ideas is true for both the client and therapist. If a position, pattern, or technique is not working, then the clinician needs to change the map or directions of treatment and let the client teach the therapist what will work. The ability to change and select new or alternative treatment techniques is based on the attitude of the therapist toward selecting alternative approaches. Willingness to be flexible is based on confidence in oneself, a truly emotional strategy or limbic behavior.

Fig. 5-11 depicts a map with a beginning and a terminal goal. The parameters of the map illustrate the boundaries of that therapist's experience and education. The clinician, through training, can identify what would seem to be the most direct and efficient way or path toward the mutually identified goal. When the client becomes a participant within

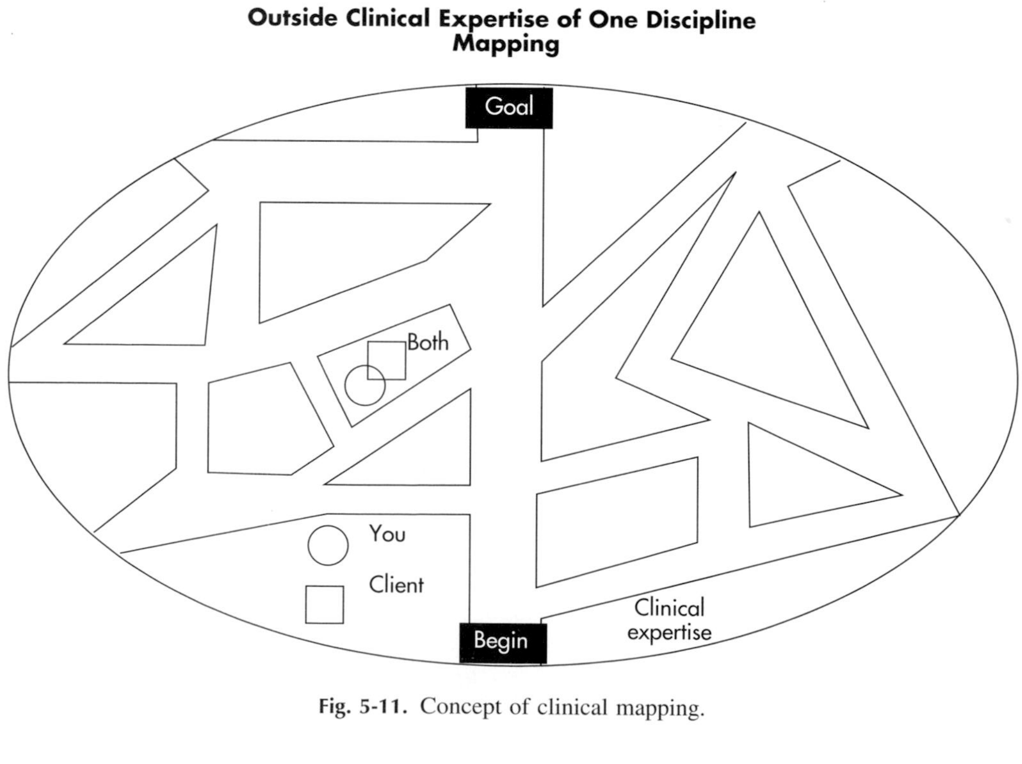

Fig. 5-11. Concept of clinical mapping.

the environment or map, what would seem like a direct path toward a goal may not be the easiest or most direct for the client. If empowerment of the client leads to independence, then allowing and encouraging the client to direct therapy may provide greater variability, force the client to problem solve, and lead to greater learning. The therapist needs to recognize when the client is not going in the direction of the goal. For example, the client is trying to perform a stand-pivot transfer and instead is falling. If it is important to practice transfers, then practicing falling is inappropriate and the environment (either internal or external) needs modification. Falling can be learned and practiced at another time. Once both strategies are learned, the therapist may place both in the map and allow the client to practice transfers and, if the client starts to fall, allow for the change in required motor behavior. In that way the client is gaining independent control over a variety of environmental contexts and outcomes.

Vulnerability. To receive input from a client, a therapist has to be open to that information. If a clinician believes that he or she knows what each client needs and how to get those behaviors before meeting the client, then the client falls into a category of a recipe for treating the problem. Using the recipe does not mean the client cannot learn or gain better perceptual/cognitive, affective, or motor control, but it does mean that the individuality of the person may be lost. A more individualized approach would allow the clinician to identify through behavioral responses the best way for the client to learn, how to sequence the learning, when to make demands of the client, when to nurture, when to stop, when to continue, when to assist, when to have fun, when to laugh, or when to cry. An analogy might be going to a fast food restaurant versus a restaurant where each aspect of the meal is tailored to one's taste. It does not mean that both restaurants are not selling digestible foods. It does mean that at one eating place the food is mass produced with some choices, but individuality with respect to the consumer is not an aspect of the service.

To be open totally to processing the individual differences of the client, the clinician must be relaxed and nonthreatened and feel no need to protect himself or herself from the external environment. The clinician is highly vulnerable because he or she is open to new and as yet unanalyzed or unprocessed input. Being open must incorporate being sensitive to not only the variability of motor responses, but also the variability of emotional responses on the part of the client. This vulnerability leads to compassion, understanding, and acceptance of the client as a unique human being.

Limbic lesions and their influence on the therapeutic environment. Many lesions or neurochemical imbalances within the limbic system drastically affect the success or failure of physical, occupational, and other therapy programs. This chapter does not discuss in detail specific problems and their treatment, but instead it is hoped that identification of the limbic involvement may help the reader develop a better understanding of specific neurological conditions.

Stress and sensory overload. The autonomic responses to stress have been identified as following a specific course of behavioral changes and are referred to as the general adaptation syndrome (GAS).[6,41,62] The sequential stages of this syndrome directly relate to limbic imbalance and can play a dramatic role in determining client progress. This stress can be caused by pain, illness itself, ramification of the illness, confusion, sensory overload, and a large variety of other potential sources. Initial reaction to stress or neurochemical imbalance creates a state of alarm and triggers a strong sympathetic nervous system reaction. Heart rate, blood pressure, respiration, metabolism, and muscle tonus will increase. At this stage the grandmother lifts the car off the child. If the overstimulation or stress does not diminish, the body will protect itself from self-destruction and trigger a parasympathetic response. At this time, all the symptoms reverse and the client exhibits a decrease in heart rate, blood pressure, and muscle tonus. The bronchi become constricted and the patient may hyperventilate and become dizzy, confused, and less alert. As the blood flow returns to the periphery, the face may flush and the skin may become hot. The patient will have no energy to move, will withdraw, and again exhibit signs of flexion, adduction, internal rotation, and lack of postural tone.

This stress or overstimulation syndrome is characterized by 70 common symptoms. If the acute symptoms are not eliminated, they will become chronic and the behavior patterns much more resistant to change.

GAS is often seen in the elderly, with various precipitating health crises,[41] and also in infants (see Chapter 8), head trauma victims, and other clients with neurological conditions. What causes the initial alarm can range from internal instability and minimal to mild external stress, to minimal internal instability and severe external sensory bombardment. Head traumas, inflammatory problems, and tumors often create hypersensitivity to external input such as noise, touch, or light. Normal clinical environments may create a sensory overload and trigger this general adaptation syndrome.

In the elderly, stresses such as change of environment, loss of loved ones, failing health, and fears of financial problems can each cause the client's system to react as if overloaded. Our elderly clients usually have two or more of these issues to deal with while trying to benefit from a therapeutic setting that demands their full attention for effective functioning. No wonder so many older clients shut down, withdraw from the therapeutic environment, and eventually from the entire world and become resistant and confused.

It is logical to assume that because of the autonomic responses that this syndrome evokes, strong interactions exist with the hypothalamus and limbic system. Stress, no matter what the specific precipitating incident (confusion, fear, anxiety, grief, pain), has the potential of triggering the first steps in the sequence of this syndrome. The clinician's sensitivity to the client's emotional system will be the therapeutic technique that best controls and reverses the acute condition. Decreasing stimulation versus increasing facilitation may lead to attention, calmness, and receptiveness to therapy. When the client feels control over his or her life has been returned or at least the individual is consulted regarding decisions, resistance to therapy or movement often is released and stress reduced. Even semicomatose clients can participate to some extent. As a clinician begins to move a client, resistance may be encountered. If slight changes are made in rotation or trajectory of the movement pattern, the resistance is often lessened. If the clinician initially feels the resistance and overpowers it, total control has been taken from the client. Instead, if the clinician moves the patient in ways his or her body is willing to be moved, respect has been shown and overstimulation potentially avoided.

No single input causes these reactions, nor does one treatment counteract its progression. Being aware of clinical signs is critical. Another important therapeutic skill is not prejudging withdrawn clients by assuming that they need more stimulation to regain function. The specific techniques appropriate for treating this syndrome are tools all therapists possess. How each clinician uses those tools is a critical link to success or failure in clinical interaction.

Alcoholism/drug abuse. The anterior temporal lobe (especially the hippocampus and amgydala) has a lower threshold for epileptic seizures than other cortical structures.[19,32] This type of epilepsy is produced by use of systemic drugs such as cocaine and alcohol. This type of seizure is often accompanied by sensory auras and alterations in behavior, with specific focus on mood shifts and cognitive dysfunction.[64] Obviously, the precise association between behavior and emotions or temperolimbic and frontolimbic activity is not understood, yet the associations and thus their impact on a therapeutic setting cannot be ignored.[1,6]

Whether street bought, medically administered, or ingested for private or social reasons, as in alcohol consumption, drugs and alcohol can have dramatic effects on the CNS. Korsakoff's syndrome, caused by chronic alcoholism and its related nutritional deficiency, is identified by the structural involvement of the diencephalon with specific focus on the mammillary bodies, and the dorsal medial and anterior nucleus of the thalamus[32] usually shows involvement (see the anatomy section and Fig. 5-12). This syndrome is not a dementia, but rather a discrete localized pathological state with specific clinical signs. The most dramatic sign observed in a client with Korsakoff's syndrome is severe memory deficits. These deficits involve declarative memory and learning losses, but the most predominant problem is short-term memory loss. As the disease progresses, clients generally become totally unaware of their memory loss and are unconcerned. Initially, confabulation may be observed, but in time most clients with a chronic condition become apathetic and somewhat withdrawn and are in a profound amnesic state. They are trapped in time, unable to learn from new experiences because they cannot retain memories for more than a few minutes, and are unable to maintain their independence;[19,42] many become street people.

The use of alcohol affects not only adults but also children and adolescents. Still another population of children suffering from alcohol abuse is just surfacing as a specific clinical problem. These children are infants who suffer from the effects of fetal alcohol syndrome (FAS). A variety of researchers have investigated the effects of alcohol and other toxic drugs on neuromotor and cognitive development.[16,30,54,57,61]

Alzheimer's disease (see Chapter 25). In Alzheimer's disease, the hippocampus and nucleus basalis are the most severely involved structures, followed by neurofibrillar degeneration of anteriotemporal, parietal, and frontal lobes.[6,19,42]

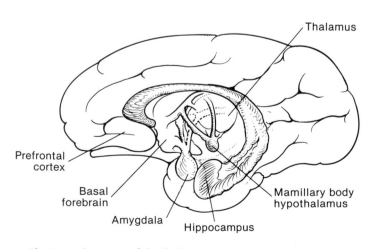

Fig. 5-12. Anatomy of the limbic system: schematic illustration.

Initially, the symptoms fall into several categories: emotional, social, and cognitive. Usually the symptoms have a gradual onset. Depression and anxiety often are seen during the early phases because of the neuronal degeneration within the prefrontal lobes and limbic system.[56] During the second stage, the emotional, social, and intellectual changes become more marked. Clients have difficulty with demands, business affairs, and personal management. Their memory and cognitive processing continue to deteriorate while their awareness of the problem is often still insightful, causing additional anxiety and depression. The third phase manifests itself with moderate to severe aphasic, apraxic, and agnostic problems. Object agnosia, the failure to recognize objects, is a typical sign of advancing Alzheimer's disease. Distractability and nonattentiveness are also common signs of this third stage. The final stage is marked by an individual who is noncommunicative, with little meaningful social interaction and who often takes on the features of the Klüver-Bucy syndrome. Thus they exhibit emotional outbursts, inappropriate sexual behaviors, severe memory loss, constant mouth movements, and often a flexor type postural pattern. In this latter phase, the client is virtually decorticate and clinically indistinguishable from other dementias.

The continual degeneration of the limbic system is a key distinguishing factor in Alzheimer's disease.[68] Many clients are misdiagnosed as having other problems such as intracranial tumors, normal-pressure hydrocephalus, multi-infarct dementia, or alcoholic/chronic drug intoxication.[4] Similarly, many clients with tumors, multifaceted dementias, alcoholism, or heart attacks resulting in hippocampal damage may be diagnosed with Alzheimer's disease. When the disease is correctly evaluated and diagnosed, however, it becomes obvious that the limbic-cortical area involved from phase one through the last phase is overlaying and constantly affecting the behavioral patterns of the patient.

Head injury

Traumatic injury

SHEARING.[2,5] One potentially severe limbic problem that can be present following traumatic closed head injury is diffuse axonal injury (DAI). The long associative bundles or fibers that transverse the cortex on a curved route can be sheared by an impact or a blow to the head. One of these long associative bundles is the uncinate fasciculus, which coordinates the amygdala and hippocampal projections to and from the prefrontal cortex. Many basic perceptual strategies, such as body schema, hearing, vision, and smell are linked into the emotional and learning centers of the limbic system through the cingulate fasciculus. Thus, declarative learning through sensory/cognitive processing can become impossible. If the pathways to and from the hippocampus and amygdala are sheared bilaterally, total and permanent global anterograde amnesia can be present.[28,68] If destruction of both tracts on one side occurs, but the contralateral is left intact, the individual can compensate, but learning will be slower or the rate of processing delayed.[50] If only one tract

on one side is damaged, such as the tract to and from the hippocampus, the amygdaloid system on the same side will compensate, but be slower than without the lesion.[50] Thus the specific degree of involvement will vary and depend on the extent of shearing. Those people with total shearing on both sides will usually be in a deep coma and will not survive the injury.[5] Those individuals with less severe insult will show signs ranging from total amnesia to minor delays in declarative learning.[5]

CONTUSIONS. Cerebral contusions (bruises) have long been a primary sign of traumatic head injury.[53] Regardless of impact, the contusions are generally found in the frontal and temporal regions. The regions most frequently involved are orbitofrontal, frontopolar, anterotemporal, and lateral temporal surfaces.[5] The limbic system's connection to these areas would suggest the potential for direct and indirect limbic involvement. The greater the contusion, the greater the likelihood that the limbic structures might simultaneously be involved. Impulsiveness, lack of inhibition, and hyperactivity are a few of the clinical signs associated with orbitofrontal–limbic involvement. The dorsomedial frontal region, involved in the hippocampal-fornix circuit (once referred to as Papez circuit), when damaged, seems to induce a pseudodepressed state, including slowness, lack of initiation, and perseveration.

Nontraumatic head injuries: anoxic/hypoxic brain injury. Lack of oxygen to the brain, regardless of the cause, seems not only to have a dramatic effect throughout the cortex, but also selectively damages the hippocampal regions.[5] The loss of hippocampal declarative memory systems bilaterally would certainly provide one reason for the slowness in processing so commonly observed in head injury. A hypothesis could also be made regarding the limbic systems interrelation with other cortical and brainstem structures. In cases of hypoxia, many structures feeding into the limbic system are potentially affected, so information sent to the limbic system may be distorted. These distortions could cause tremendous imbalances within the limbic processing system, with not only attention and learning problems but also hypothalamic irregularity often seen in head trauma.

Summary. The behavioral sequelae following any head injury reflect many signs of limbic involvement. In both pediatric and adult studies,* behaviors of impulsiveness, restlessness, overactivity, destructiveness, aggression, increased tantrums, and socially uninhibited behaviors (lack of social skills) are frequently reported. These behaviors all reflect a strong emotional or limbic component. After discussion of Moore's concept of a limbic system that MOVEs us and the F²ARV continuum regarding emotional control over noxious or negative input, it is no wonder so many clients have difficulty with personal and emotional control over their reactions to the therapeutic world. If the imbalance is within the client, then the external environment would be one possible way to help center the client emotionally. This centering requires that the therapist be sensitive to the emotional level of the client. As the client begins to regain control, an increase in external environmental demands would challenge the limbic system. If the demand is excessive, the client's emotional reaction as expressed by motor behavior should alert the therapist to downgrade the activity level.

Head injuries affect many areas of the CNS. A client with spasticity, rigidity, or ataxia may exhibit an increase in those motor responses when the limbic system becomes stressed. Learning to differentiate a motor control problem from a limbic problem that influences the motor control systems requires that the therapist be willing to address the cause of the problems and their treatment. Each client is so different and in each moment has the potential of affecting the limbic system with great variance. Thus the therapist needs to give undivided attention to the client at all times and be willing to make moment-to-moment adjustments within the external environment to help the client maintain focus on the desired learning.

Cerebrovascular accidents. The most common insult results in occlusions with tributaries of the middle cerebral artery.[32] When this occlusion is in the right hemisphere, studies have shown that clients are often confused and exhibit metabolic imbalance.[59] The primary problem of this confused state is inattention. After brain scans, it has been shown that focal lesions existed both within the reticulocortical and limbic cortical tracts, suggesting direct limbic involvement in many middle cerebral artery problems.[47]

Many clients with a CVA do not have direct limbic involvement, yet the stresses placed on the client, whether external or internal, are often reflected in the limbic system's influence over the motor control systems. Everyday existence, as well as performance of the motor task required during therapy, is usually valued highly in the client's life. This value or stress placed on the limbic system overflows into the motor system and never allows it to relax, as observed by noting the increase of tonus in the nonaffected leg. The client is usually unaware of this buildup of tonus, but can release it once attention is drawn to it. If attention is never directed toward these tension buildups, a therapist trying to decrease tonus in the affected arm or leg will always be interacting with the associated patterns from the less-involved extremities.

Tumor. Any brain tumor, whether or not directly affecting the limbic structures, will certainly arouse the limbic system because of the stress, anxiety, and emotional overlays of the diagnosis. The degree of emotional involvement will obviously affect the declarative learning of the client as well as the limbic system's influence over motor response.

Tumors specifically arising within limbic structures can cause dramatic changes in the client's emotional behavior and level of alertness, especially with hypothalamic tumors.

The behaviors reported include aggressiveness, hyperphagia, paranoia, sloppiness, manic symptoms, and eventual confusion.[32] Tumors within the hypothalamus cause not only behavioral abnormalities, but also autonomic endocrine imbalances, including body temperature changes, menstrual abnormalities, and diabetes insipidus.[68]

When the tumor is located within the frontal and temporal lobes associated with limbic structures, psychiatric problems may manifest themselves, ranging from depression to schizoid psychosis.[68] Amnesia has been reported in tumor patients with dorsomedial thalamus, fornix, midbrain lesions, and reticulolimbic pathway lesions. This again reinforces the importance of the limbic system's role in storage.[68]

Ventricular swelling following spinal defects in utero, CNS trauma, and inflammation. Although the effects of ventricular swelling following trauma, inflammation, and in utero cerebrospinal malformations are not discussed in great detail in the literature with respect to limbic involvement, the proximity of the lateral and third ventricle to limbic structures cannot be ignored. It is common knowledge that most people, when exposed to hot, humid weather and thus begin to swell, become more irritable, less tolerant, moody, and may complain of headaches. Some people become aggressive, others lethargic. All these behaviors are linked to some extent with limbic function. Thus ventricular swelling causing hydrocephalus, whether caused by trauma, inflammation, or obstruction, would potentially affect the limbic structures. Reported behavioral changes such as seizures, memory and learning problems, personality alterations, alertness, dementia, and amnesia can be tied to direct or indirect limbic activity.[32]

It is easy to identify limbic problems when the behaviors deviate drastically from normal responses. It is much more difficult to determine subtle behavior shifts in clients. The therapist should be sensitive to these minor mood shifts, for they may represent early signs of future problems. Similarly, noting that a particular client is always irritable and has difficulty learning on hot days should help direct the therapist toward establishing a treatment session that regulates humidity and temperature to optimize the learning environment.

BASIC ANATOMY AND PHYSIOLOGY OF THE LIMBIC SYSTEM
Anatomy and physiology

Basic structure and function. The limbic system can best be visualized as consisting of cortical and subcortical structures with the hypothalamus in the central position (Figs. 5-12 and 5-13). The hypothalamus is surrounded by the circular alignment of the subcortical limbic structures vitally linked with each other and the hypothalamus. These structures are the amygdaloid complex, the hippocampal formation, the nucleus accumbens, the anterior nuclei of the thalamus, and the septal nuclei (Fig. 5-12). These structures are again surrounded by a ring of cortical

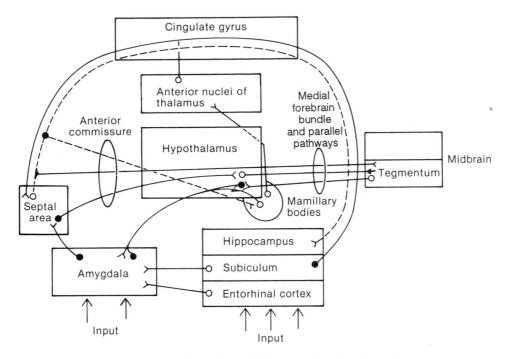

Fig. 5-13. Limbic system circuitry with medial forebrain bundle and parallel connections.

structures collectively called the "limbic lobe," which includes the orbitofrontal cortex, the cingulate gyrus, the parahippocampal gyrus, and the uncus. Other neuroanatomists also include the olfactory system and the basal forebrain area (Fig. 5-13). Vitally linked and often included in the limbic system as the "meso-limbic" part is the excitatory component of the reticular activating system and other brainstem nuclei of the midbrain. Some consider components of the midbrain a very important region for emotional expression.[20] Derryberry and Tucker found that attack behavior aroused by hypothalamic stimulation is blocked when the midbrain is damaged, and that midbrain stimulation can be made to elicit "attack behavior" even when the hypothalamus has been surgically disconnected from other brain regions. This "septo-hypothalamic-mesencephalic" continuum, connected by the medial forebrain bundle, seems to be vital to the integration and expression of emotional behavior. The linking of other brain structures to emotions comes from the work of Papez[55] who proposed the so-called Papez circuit (Figure 5-14). This loop is now referred to as the hippocampal-fornix circuit. This circuit starts at the mammillary bodies (nuclei of the hypothalamus), extends to the anterior nuclei of the thalamus (via the mammillothalamic tract), and then on to the cerebral cortex and cingulate gyrus, where the feelings reach the level of "conscious, subjective emotional experiences." Further projections reach the hippocampus for integration to be relayed back to the hypothalamic mammillary bodies. Papez saw this as a way of combining the "subjective" cortical experiences with the emotional hypothalamic contribution. Earlier, Broca[9] labeled the

cingulate gyrus and hippocampus "circle" as "the great limbic lobe." These concepts were combined by Maclean[44] into the construct of the limbic system.

Other regions then were added, such as the amygdaloid complex located in the temporal lobe. In their studies on monkeys, Klüver and Bucy[34] removed the anterior half of the temporal lobes bilaterally and reported the following changes in behavior, which were subsequently specifically linked with loss of the amygdaloid complex and anterior hippocampus input: (1) restless overresponsiveness, (2) hyperorality of examining objects by placing them in their mouths, (3) psychic blindness of seeing and not recognizing objects and the possible harm they may entail, (4) sexual hyperactivity, and (5) emotional changes characterized by loss of aggressiveness. These changes have been named the Klüver-Bucy syndrome.[6,13,19] A myriad of connections link the amygdala to the olfactory pathways, the frontal lobe and cingulate gyrus, the thalamus, the hypothalamus, the septum, and the midbrain structures of the substantia nigra, locus ceruleus, periaqueductal gray, and the reticular formation. The amygdala receives feedback from many of these structures it projects to by reciprocal pathways.

At the heart of the limbic system is the hypothalamus, which oversees many functions. The specific nuclei relating to the limbic functions are the mammillary bodies and the lateral and ventromedial nuclei. The hypothalamus, in close reciprocal interaction with most centers of the cerebral cortex, the amygdala, hippocampus, pituitary gland, brainstem, and spinal cord, is a primary regulator of autonomic and endocrine functions and controls and balances homeostatic mechanisms. Autonomic and somatomotor responses

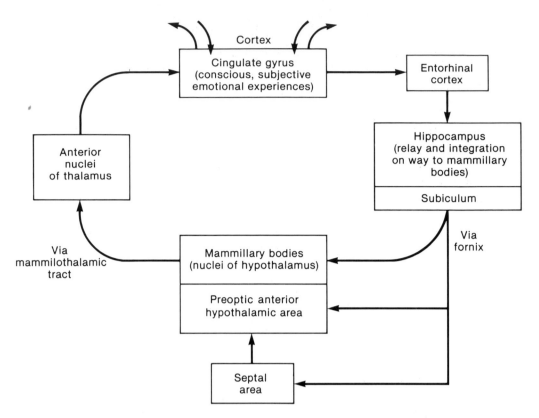

Fig. 5-14. Hippocampal-fornix circuit (Papez circuit) (Adapted from Kandel ER, Schwartz JH, and Jessell TM: (*Principles of neural science,* ed 3, New York, 1991, Elsevier Medical Science Publishing.)

controlled by the hypothalamus are closely aligned with the expression of emotions.

In the temporal lobe, anteromedially, are the amygdaloid complex of nuclei, with the hippocampal formation situated posterior to it. The hippocampal formation consists of the horn of Ammons, the subiculum, and the dentate gyrus. Located medial to the amygdala is the substantia innominate. This region contains the basal forebrain nuclei, which receive afferent neurons from the reticular formation, the hypothalamus, and the limbic cortex. From this basal forebrain efferents project to all areas of the cerebral cortex, the hippocampus, and amygdaloid body, providing an important connection between the neocortex and the limbic system. These nuclei represent the center of the cholinergic system, which supplies acetylcholine to limbic and cortical structures involved in memory formation (see the neurochemistry section). Depletion of acetylcholine in clients with Alzheimer's disease relates to their memory loss.[6]

Interlinking the components of the system. The limbic system has many reciprocating interlinking circuits between its component structures, which provide for much functional interaction and also allow for ongoing adjustments with continuous feedback (Fig. 5-15).

The largest pathway is the fornix. It has a C-shaped configuration that is almost circular. Its fibers arise from the hippocampus, for which it is the main efferent pathway extending to the hypothalamus and through its commissural portion to the contralateral hippocampus. The fornix fibers terminate in the mammillary bodies where they synapse with the neurons of the mammilothalamic tract heading for the anterior nuclei of the thalamus and eventually reach the cingulate gyrus of the limbic lobe and mammilotegmental tract to midbrain tegmentum or reticular formation. This circuit, called the hippocampal-fornix circuit (Fig. 5-14), runs from the hippocampus via the fornix to the hypothalamus (mamillary nucleus) and on to the cingulate gyrus via the thalamus. The circle is completed by fibers to the entorhinal cortex and back to the hippocampus.

Another limbic pathway is the stria terminalis, which originates in the amygdaloid complex and follows a course close to the fornix to end in the hypothalamus and septal regions. The amygdala and the septal region are also connected by a short direct pathway called the diagonal band of Broca. A third pathway, the uncinate fasciculus, runs between the amygdala and the orbitofrontal cortex.[32]

The medial forebrain bundle (MFB) and other parallel circuits (Fig. 5-13) are considered important connections of the limbic system. These pathways connect the septal region and the nucleus accumbans with the preoptic area and the amygdala. These course through the lateral hypothalamus

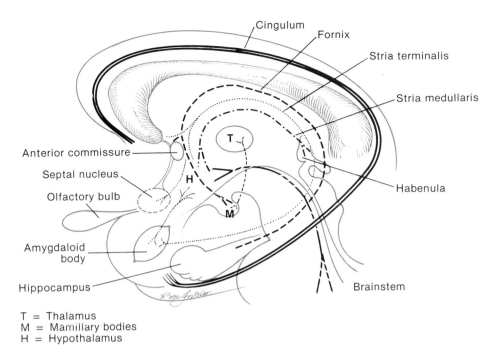

Cingulum
Fornix
Stria terminalis
Stria medullaris
Anterior commissure
Septal nucleus
Olfactory bulb
Habenula
Amygdaloid body
Hippocampus
Brainstem

T = Thalamus
M = Mamillary bodies
H = Hypothalamus

Fig. 5-15. Interlinking neuron network within the limbic system. (Adapted from Kandel ER, Schwartz JH, and Jessell TM: *Principles of neural science,* ed 3, New York, 1991, Elsevier Medical Science Publishing.)

and terminate in the cingulate gyrus in its ascending limb and in the reticular formation of the midbrain in its descending part. These links enable the limbic system itself and the nonlimbic associated structures to act as one neural task system. It is important to realize that no portion of the brain, whether limbic or nonlimbic, has only one function.[32] Each area acts as an input-output station. At no time is it totally the center of a particular effect, and each site depends on the cooperation and interaction with other regions.

During the last decade new anatomical pathways have been identified that are descending motor tracts that terminate in the caudal brainstem and spinal cord.[31] These new pathways help modulate the activity level of somatic and autonomic motor neurons. Some of these tracts receive direct and indirect afferent information from the periphery and are part of the interneuronal projection system to motor neurons. They are found in the caudal brainstem, spinal cord, and between the two and may play a role in the generation of fixed action patterns such as biting and swallowing. Some of the new pathways are linked with the ventromedial and lateral systems identified for many years as part of both the proximal/axial and distal motor control system modulated by a variety of structures. The last tracts are the most recently discovered. They connect the limbic system to the brainstem and spinal neuronal pools. These tracts do not seem to synapse on what would be considered true motor nuclei of the brainstem (e.g., red nucleus, vestibular nuclei, lateral reticular nuclei, interstitial nuclei of Cajal, or inferior olive). However, these new pathways do connect with raphe nuclei and

locus coeruleus. The medial components of these new tracts originate within the medial portion of the hypothalamus, and the lateral portion originates in the limbic system (lateral hypothalamus, amygdala, and bed nucleus of the stria terminalis). The prefrontal area may be the master controller over this regulatory system, but that is yet to be determined.

The functional implication of these tracts is determined by whether the fibers project as part of a medial or lateral system. The medial system, via the locus coeruleus and raphe spinal pathways, plays a role in the general level of activity of both somatosensory and motor neurons. Thus the emotional brain or limbic system has an effect on both somatosensory input and motor output. These fibers can alter the level of excitation to the first synapse of somatosensory information, thus altering the processing or importance of that information as it enters the nervous system. Similarly, it can alter the level of motor generators involved in motor expression, which may account for the extension with anger and flexion with depression. The lateral system seems to be involved in more specific motor output related to **emotional behavior** and may explain some of the loss of fine motor skill when placed in an emotional situation such as competition.[31] To differentiate whether the tonal conditions of a client are due to limbic imbalance or problems within the traditionally accepted motor system, the clinician would need to observe the emotional state and how it changes within the client. If the abnormal state consistently alters with mood shifts, then limbic involvement causing motor control disturbances would be identified.

Neurobiology of learning and memory
Functional applications for an intact system

"Ultimately, to be sure, memory is a series of molecular events. What we chart is the territory within which those events take place."[50]

The brain stores sensory and motor experiences as memory. In processing incoming information, most sensory pathways from receptors to cortical areas send vital information to the components of the limbic system. For example, extensions can be found from the visual pathways into the inferior temporal lobe[32,48] (limbic system). Visual information is "processed sequentially" at each synapse along its entire pathway, in response to size, shape, color, and texture of objects. In the inferior temporal cortex, the total image of the item viewed is projected. In this way the sensory inputs are converted to become "perceptual experiences." This also applies to other sensory stimuli such as tactile, proprioceptive, and vestibular. The process of translating the integrated perceptions into memory occurs bilaterally in the limbic system structures of the amygdala and the hippocampus.

Before delving into the limbic system's impact on learning and memory, a clear understanding of what is meant by these functions is needed.

Current theories support a "dual memory system" using different pathways in the nervous system. Terms such as verbal and nonverbal, procedural and declarative, and habit versus recognition have been given to these two memory systems. These systems do not operate autonomously, and many therapeutic activities seem to combine these memory systems to achieve functional behavior.

For this discussion, two specific categories of learning, declarative and procedural, will be used. Declarative knowledge entails the capability to recall and verbally report experiences, whereas the procedural counterpart is the recall of "rules, skills, and procedures."[32]

Procedural learning is vital to the development of motor control. A child first receives sensory input from the various modalities via the thalamus, terminating at the appropriate sensory cortex. That information is processed and relayed to the motor cortex. From there, it is sent to both the basal ganglia and the cerebellum to establish plans for postural adaptations; refinement of motor programs; and coordination of direction, extent, timing, force, and tone necessary throughout the entire sequence of the motor act. Storage and thus retrieval of memory of these semiautomatic motor plans are thought to occur throughout the motor control system.

The basal ganglia and cerebellum are critical nuclei for changing and modulating existing programs. Many interlocking neuronetworks establish pathways allowing for the conceptualization of research on motor theory concepts of reciprocity, distributed function, consensus, etc. (see Chapters 3 and 4).

Procedural learning and memory do not necessitate limbic system involvement as long as value is not placed on the task; it deals with skills, habits, and stereotyped behaviors. This system is involved in developing procedural plans used in moving us from place to place or holding us in a position when we need to stop.

Declarative learning and thus memory (unlike procedural) require the wiring of the limbic system. This type of thought deals with factual, material, semantic, and categorical aspects of higher cognitive and affective processing. A strong emotional and judgmental component is linked with declarative thought. *Thus as soon as a motor behavior has value placed upon the act, it becomes declarative as well as procedural, and the limbic system may become a key element in the success or failure of that movement.* Most tasks or activities asked for in a clinical setting have value attached to them.

The two **reverberating loops,** or **circuits,** within the limbic system most intimately involved in declarative learning are: (1) the amygdaloid–dorsomedial thalamic–nucleus cortical pathways, and (2) the hippocampal–fornix–anterior thalamic nucleus–cortex.

The hippocampus may be more concerned with sensory and motor signals relating to the external environment, whereas the amygdala is concerned with those of the internal environment. They both contribute in relation to the significance of external or internal environmental influences.[65,66]

The amygdaloid circuits seem to deal with strongly emotional and judgmental thoughts, whereas the hippocampal circuits are less emotional and more factual. The amygdala may be more involved in emotional arousal and attention, as well as motor regulation, whereas the hippocampus may deal with less emotionally charged learning. These limbic circuits seem crucial in the initial processing of material that leads to learning and memory. Once the thought has been laid down within the cortical structures, retrieval of that specific intermediate and long-term memory does not seem to require the limbic system, although new associations will need to be run through the system.

A third component in the memory pathway involves the medial diencephalon, a structure that contains the thalamic nucleus. When this region is destroyed by strokes, neoplasms, infections, or chronic alcoholism, as in Korsakoff's syndrome, global amnesias result because of the destruction of the amygdala and hippocampus. The amygdala and hippocampus send fibers to specific target nuclei in the thalamus, and the destruction of these tracts also causes the same amnesic effect. It appears that the limbic system and the diencephalon cooperate in the memory circuits. The medial diencephalon seems to be another relay station along the pathway that leads from the specific sensory cortical region to the limbic structures in the temporal lobe to the medial diencephalic structures and ending in the ventromedial part of the prefrontal cortex (Fig. 5-16).[26]

According to Fig. 5-16, memories may be stored in the sensory cortex area where the original sensory input was

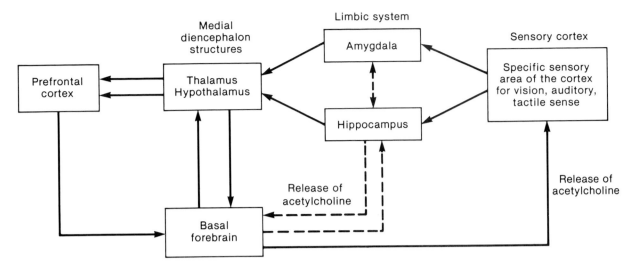

Fig. 5-16. The basal forebrain closes the circuit and causes changes in sensory area neurons, which could lead to correct perception and stored memory.

interpreted into "sensory impressions." Today, concepts regarding memory storage suggest that declarative memory is stored in categories similar to a filing system. Those categories or files seem to be stored in several cortical areas bilaterally depending on the context.[24] This system allows for easy retrieval from multiple areas. Memory has stages and is continually changing. Thus to go from short-term to long-term memory, the brain must physically change its chemical structure (a plastic phenomenon). Memory first begins with a representation of information that has been transformed through processing of perceptual systems. The transferring of this new memory into a longlasting chemical bond requires the neuronetwork of the limbic complex. Due to the multiple tracts or parallel circuits in and out of the limbic system and throughout neocortical systems, clients, even with extensive lesions, can often learn and store new information.[32] This may also explain why damage to the limbic system structures does not destroy existing memory nor make it unavailable, since it is actually stored in many places throughout the neocortex. The circular memory circuit illustrated in Fig. 5-15 shows only one system. The reader must remember that many parallel circuits function simultaneously. The circular memory circuit shown reverts back to the original sensory area after activation of the limbic structures to cause the necessary neuronal changes that would inscribe the event into retrievable stored memory. This information can be recognized and retrieved by activation of storage sites anywhere along the pathway.

The last station or system to be added to the circuit is the "basal forebrain cholinergic system," which delivers the neurochemical acetylcholine to the cortical centers and to the limbic system with which it is richly linked. The loss of this neurotransmitter is linked to memory malfunctioning in Alzheimer's disease. Performance of visual recognition memory can be augmented or impaired by administration of

drugs that enhance or block the action of acetylcholine.[35]

It has also been shown that the amygdala and hippocampus are both interchangeably involved in recognition memory. The hippocampus is vital for memory of location of objects in space, whereas the amygdala is necessary for the association of memories derived through the various senses with a specific recognition recall. For example, a whiff of ether might bring to mind a painful surgical experience, or the sight of some food may cause a recall of its pleasant smell. Removal of the amygdala brings out the behavior shown in Klüver-Bucy syndrome. For clients with this neurological problem, familiar objects do not bring forth the correct associations of memories experienced by sight, smell, taste, and touch and relate them to objects presented. Association of previously presented stimuli and their responses appear to be lost. Animals without amygdaloid input had different response patterns that ignored previous fears and aversions. Thus the amygdala adds the "emotional weight" to sensory experiences.[49] Loss of the amygdala also loses the positive associations and reward and thereby alters the shaping of perceptions that lead to memory storage.

When stimuli are endowed with emotional value or significance, attention is drawn to those possessing emotional significance, selecting these for attention and learning. This would give the amygdala a "gatekeeping" function of selective filtering. The amygdala may enable emotions to influence what is perceived and learned by reciprocal connection with the cortex. Emotionally charged events will leave a more significant impression and subsequent recall. The amygdala alters perception of afferent sensory input and thereby affects subsequent actions.

Long-term potentiation: the key to limbic function. As discussed in the introduction, limbic functions may not be localized in specific structures or regions, but may be associated with "circuit interactions," and the structures

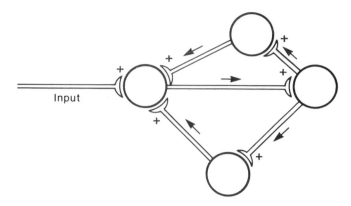

Fig. 5-17. Schema of a reverberating circuit, brief excitatory input could produce long-lasting neural activity.

themselves can influence the resulting effector activity. This can best be demonstrated by the concepts of reverberating circuits (Fig. 5-17) or oscillatory circuits. These circuits operate on positive feedback within the neuronal pool, which is arranged in a circular fashion. In this way the neuronal pool can feed back to reexcite itself in the circular circuit, and activity might be sustained for periods of time by repetitive discharges.[27,32] The mechanism of reverberating circuits may be used to "encode short-term memory" with brief excitation that can cause neural activity of long duration, producing memory traces.[32] These reverberating circuits could easily be demonstrated in the circular pathways of the limbic system, in pathways such as were suggested by the hippocampal-fornix circuit.

Slightly longer-term memory could be mediated by posttetanic potentiation. First, there must be a persistant train of high-frequency tetanic facilitary stimulation. This facilitation could last for hours, especially if it occurs in reverberating circuits. The chemical reaction to this continual volley of input creates a larger than normal influx of calcium into the presynaptic terminal during the initial stimulation. This leads to increased release of transmitters from the terminals, causing larger than normal excitatory postsynaptic potentials (EPSPs). These potentials enhance synaptic transmission for an extended time.

This maintained excitation or processing is referred to as "the simplest kind of memory." The neuron remembers the increased train of impulses that increased the amount of calcium, and each action potential playing on this memory causes an increased amount of transmitter to be released, which will repeat the process in this posttetanic potentiation.[32]

In humans, memory functioning has been associated with the phenomenon of long-term potentiation (LTP) observed in hippocampal pathways.[26] This potentiation of synaptic transmission, lasting for hours, days, and weeks, occurs after brief trains of high-frequency stimulation of hippocampal excitatory pathways.[6] Whether this phenomenon is caused by alteration at the presynaptic or postsynaptic terminals has

not been established. The question remains whether there is an increased amount of neurotransmitter released presynaptically (glumate)[26] or whether the expected amount is producing a heightened postsynaptic response. Or, are both sites involved?[32]

Learning and memory evoke alterations in behavior that reflect neuroanatomical and neurophysiological changes.[32] These include the phenomenon of LTP as an example of such changes. The hippocampus demonstrates the importance of input of LTP in associative learning. In this type of learning, two or more stimuli are combined. Tetanizing of more than one pathway needs to occur simultaneously. When only one pathway is tetanized, the effect is decreased synaptic transmission. LTP, requiring the cooperative action of numbers of coactive fibers, is engendered and formed by the "associative" interaction of afferent inputs. Thus LTP could serve as a model for understanding the neural mechanism for associative learning.

Learning/memory problems following limbic involvement. For initial declarative learning and memory, the combination of hippocampus and amygdala of the limbic system is required.[32] For memory formation to occur, there must be a storing of the "neural representation" of the stimuli in the association and the processing areas of the cortex. This storage occurs when sensory stimuli activate a "cortico-limbo-thalamo-cortical" circuit.[32] This circuit serves as the "imprinting mechanism," reinforcing the pathway that activated it. On subsequent stimulation, a stimulus recognition or recall would be elicited. In associative recall, stored representations of any interconnected imprints could be evoked simultaneously.

A vital processing area for all sensory modalities is located in the region of the anterior temporal lobe. This area is directly linked with the amygdala and indirectly with the hippocampus. The hippocampus and amygdala are also linked both structurally and functionally to each other and to specific thalamic nuclei. Clients with temporal epileptic seizures and whose temporal lobes have been surgically removed developed global anterograde amnesia; that is, amnesia developed for all senses and no new memories could be formed. Experimental removal of only the hippocampus does not bring about these changes, although processing is slowed down. When both the hippocampus and the amygdala are removed bilaterally, the amnesia is both retrograde and global. It is postulated that the amygdala is the area of the brain that adds a "positive association," the reward part to stimuli received and passed through processing. In this way, stimulus and reward are associated by the amygdala, and an emotional value is placed on it.[28]

It appears that limbic involvement in the declarative memory creates a chemical bond that allows cortical storage of "stimulus representation" necessary for subsequent recognition and recall of the information.[32]

When analyzing declarative and procedural learning from a clinical reference, a separation of functional mediation can be observed. Clients with brain lesions localized in the limbic system components of the amygdala and hippocampus have the ability to acquire and function with "rule-based" games and skills, but have lost the capacity to recall how, when, or where they gained this knowledge, or to give a description of the games and skills learned. Relating this to clinical performance, clients may develop the skill in a functional activity but not the problem-solving strategies necessary to associate danger or other potentially harmful aspects of a situation that may develop once out of the purely clinical setting.[8,17,25,45,69] Similarly, if a client needs to learn a procedural task such as walking, transfers, eating, etc., it may be extremely important to direct the attention off the task while the task is being practiced procedurally.

Neurochemistry

Discussion of the limbic system's intricate regulation of many neurochemical substances is not within the scope of this chapter; yet therapists need to appreciate how potent this system can be with respect to neurochemical reactions.

The hypothalamus, the physiological center of the limbic system (see Figs. 5-2 and 5-13), is involved in neurochemical production and is geared for passage of information along specific neurochemical pathways. Guyton[27] considers it the major motor output pathway of the limbic system, which also communicates with every part of this system. Certain nuclei of the hypothalamus produce and release neuroactive peptides that have a long-acting effectiveness as neuromodulators. As such, they control the levels of neuronal excitation and effective functioning at the synapses. By their long-lasting effects, they regulate motivational levels, mood states, and learning. These peptide-producing neurons extend from the hypothalamic nuclei to the autonomic nervous system components and to the nuclei of the limbic system, where they modulate neuroendocrine and autonomic activities.[27]

Lesions in the medial hypothalamus affect hormone production and thus alter regulation of many hormonal control systems.[32] For example, clients with medial hypothalamic lesions may have huge weight gains because of the increase of insulin in the blood, which increases feeding and converts nutrients into fat. Similarly, this weight gain may be caused by hyperphagic responses resulting from the loss of satiety. General hyperactivity and signs of hostility after minimal provocation can also be observed. These problems are often encountered in patients with head trauma.

Lesions in the lateral hypothalamus lead to damage of dopamine-carrying fibers that begin in the substantia nigra and filter through the hypothalamus to the striatum. Lesions, either along this tract or within the lateral hypothalamus, lead to aphagia and hypoarousal. Decreased sensory awareness contributing to sensory neglect is also present in lateral hypothalamic lesions. The decreased awareness may be caused by a decrease of orientation to the stimuli versus awareness of the stimuli once they are brought to conscious attention. These lesions cause the client to exhibit marked passivity with decreased functioning.

As noted earlier, depression is clearly identified as a limbic function. A functional deficiency in monoamines, especially serotonin, is hypothesized to be a primary cause of depression.[58] The serotonin systems originate in the rostral and caudal raphe nuclei in the midbrain. Ascending serotonergic tracts start in the midbrain and ascend to the limbic forebrain and hypothalamus; they are concerned with mood and behavior regulation. Damage with direct or indirect limbic involvement results in the client exhibiting depression. Descending pathways to the substantia gelatinosa are involved in pain mechanisms and have also been linked through a complex sequence of biochemical steps to the increased sensitization of the presynaptic terminals of the cutaneous sensory neurons leading to a hyperactive withdrawal reflex or hypersensitivity to cutaneous input.[32] This would account for the behavior patterns seen in clients with head trauma, where the therapist sees a flexed posture with a withdrawn or depressed affect yet with an extremely sensitive tactile system.

It is hypothesized that the underlying pathophysiology of one form of schizophrenia involves an excessive transmission of dopamine within the mesolimbic tract system.[32] The dopaminergic cell bodies are located in the ventral tegmental area and the substantia nigra. Some of these neurons project to the limbic system. These projections go to the nucleus accumbens, the stria terminalis nuclei, parts of the amygdala, and to the frontal entorhinal and anterior cingulate cortex. It is the projection to the nucleus accumbens that seems critical, because of its influence over the hippocampus, frontal lobe, and hypothalamus. This nucleus may act as a filtering system with respect to affect and certain types of memory, and the dopaminergic projections may modulate the flow of neural activity.[32] The flat affect seen in clients with Parkinson's disease and the paranoid/schizophrenic behaviors observed in some clients with CNS damage may directly reflect back to these mesolimbic dopaminergic systems.

The specific roles of the noradrenaline pathway are numerous and affect almost all parts of the CNS. The center for the noradrenaline pathways is located within the caudal midbrain and upper pons. Its nucleus is referred to as locus ceruleus. This nucleus sends at least five tracts rostally to the diencephalon and telencephalon.[32] Of specific interest for this discussion are the projections to the hippocampus and amygdala. The axons of these neurons modulate an excitatory effect on the regions where they terminate.[14] Thus the activation of this system will heighten the excitation of the two nuclei within the limbic system intricately involved in declarative learning and memory. Hyperactivation may cause overload or the lack of focus of attention. Decreased activity may prevent the desired responses. Attention to task may depend on on-going noradrenaline stimulation. These tracts from the midbrain rostrally play a key role in alertness. The correlation of alertness and attention to performance of motor tasks as well as to learning can be demonstrated.[32]

More than 200 neurotransmitters have been identified with the nervous system.[32] How each transmitter and the interaction of multiple transmitters on one synapse affect any portion of the CNS is still unknown. Certainly, some relationships have been identified. Novelty-seeking behavior of the limbic system seems to be dopamine dependent,[46] whereas melatonin receptors seem to coordinate circadian body rhythm.[43] Adrenal steroids modulate hippocampal long-term potentiation.[23] The specifics of the total complexity are still beyond the grasp of human understanding.

In conclusion, the neurochemistry of the limbic system is intricately linked to the neurochemistry of the brain. All systems within the limbic circuitry seem to be interdependent, with the summation of all the neurochemistry being the determinants of the specific processing of information. Similarly, the interdependence of the limbic system to almost all other areas of the brain and the activities of those areas at any time reflect the complexity of this system.

SUMMARY

The complexity and interwoven neurological network of the limbic system may seem overwhelming. A reader who tries to grasp all parts on first study will feel lost and defeated, a true limbic emotion. Thus this chapter was presented in two parts. The first part introduces the system and its potential clinical application. This section, in and of itself, has many interwoven components, for nothing in the limbic system functions in isolation. Yet the mysteries of this complex neurological network when solved may hold the answers to many clinical questions regarding the art and gift of a master clinician. The second part introduces in more detail the basic anatomy and physiology of the limbic system. It is hoped that once the student/clinician has been drawn to the conclusion that this system may be a key to clinical success, he or she might be willing to delve into the science of the system. This path of exploration is challenging, difficult, and frustrating at times, but certainly worth the effort once understanding is achieved.

ACKNOWLEDGMENT

With great appreciation for editorial contributions by Josephine C. Moore, Ph.D., O.T.R. and for illustrations by Steve Schmidt, M.S., P.T. Marlene B. Appley is also acknowledged for her contribution to the second edition.

REFERENCES

1. Adamec R: Kindling, anxiety, and limbic perspectives. In Wada JA, editor: *Advances in behavioral biology,* New York, 1990, Plenum Press.
2. Adams JH and others: Diffuse axonal injury due to nonmissile head injury in humans: an analysis of 45 cases, *Ann Newal* 12:557-563, 1982.
3. Aggleton JP and others: Removal of the hippocampus and transection of the fornix produce comparable deficits on delayed non-matching to position by rats, *Behav Brain Res* 5 2(1):61-71, 1992.
4. Appel SH, editor: *Current neurology,* vol 6, Chicago, 1986, Mosby.
5. Auerbach SH: Neuroanatomical correlates of attention and memory disorders in traumatic brain injury: an application of neurobehavioral subtypes, *J Head Trauma Rehab* 1(3):1-12, 1986.
6. Barr ML and Kiernan JA, editors: *The human nervous system: an anatomical viewpoint,* ed 6, Philadelphia, 1993, JB Lippincott.
7. Bell IR, Miller C, and Schwartz GE: An olfactory-limbic model of multiple chemical sensitivity syndrome: possible relationships to kindling and affective spectrum disorders, *Biol Psychiatry* 3 2(3):218-242, 1992.
8. Blais C: Concept mapping of movement: related knowledge, *Percept Mot Skills,* 7 6(3):767-774, 1993.
9. Broca P: Anatomie comparie des circonvolutions cerebrales. Le grand lobe limbique et la scissure limblique dun la serie des mammiferes, Rhone Antropologie, I.385, 1878.
10. Brodal A: *Neurological anatomy in relation to clinical medicine,* ed 5, New York, 1992, Oxford University Press.
11. Brooks VB: *The neural basis of motor control,* New York, 1986, Oxford University Press.
12. Burns LH, Robbins TW, and Everitt BJ: Differential effects of excitotoxic lesions of the basolateral anygdala, ventral subiculum and medial prefrontal cortex on responding with conditioned reinforcement and locomotor activity potentiated by intro-accumbens infusion of D-Amphetamine, *Behav Brain Res* 5 5(2):167-183, 1993.
13. Burt AM: *Textbook of Neuroanatomy,* Philadelphia, 1993, WB Saunders.
14. Cai Z: The neural mechanism of declarative memory consolidation and retrieval: a hypothesis, *Neurosc Biobehav Rev* 1 4(3):295-304, 1990.
15. Carpenter MB: *Core text of neuroanatomy,* ed 4, Baltimore, 1991, Williams & Wilkins.
16. Conry J: Neuropsychological deficits in fetal alcohol syndrome and fetal alcohol effects, *Alcohol Clin Exp Res* 14:650-655, 1990.
17. Courchesme E: Neuroanatomic imaging in autism, *Pediatrics* 87(5):781-790, 1991.
18. Davis M: The role of the anygdala in fear and anxiety, *Annu Rev* 15:333-375, 1992.
19. deGroot J: *Correlative neuroanatomy,* Norwalk, Conn, 1991, Appleton & Lange.
20. Derryberry D and Tucker DM: Neural mechanism of emotion, *J Consult Clin Psychol* 60(3):329-338, 1992.
21. Dobkin BH: Neuroplasticity: key to recovery after central nervous system injury, *West J Med* 159:56-60, 1993.
22. Falls WA, Miserendino MJ, and Davis M: Extinction of fear-potentiated startle: blockage by infusion on an NMDA antagonist into the amygdala, *J Neurosci* 12(3):854-863, 1992.
23. Filipine D and others: Modulation by adrenal steroids in limbic function, *J Steroid Biochem* 39(2):245-252, 1991.
24. Gabrieli JD: Disorders of memory in humans, *Curr Opin Neurol Neurosurg* 6(1): 1993.
25. Glisky EL: Acquisition and transfer of declarative and procedural knowledge by memory-impaired patients: a computer data-entry task, *Neuropsychologia* 3 0(10):899-910, 1992.
26. Greenberg DA, Aminoff MJ, and Simon RP, editors: *Clinical neurology,* Norwalk, Conn, 1993, Appleton & Lange.
27. Guyton A: *Basic neuroscience: anatomy & physiology,* Philadelphia, 1991, WB Saunders.
28. Haist F, Shimamura AP, and Squire LR: On the relationship between recall and recognition memory, *J Exp Psychol Learn Mem Cogn* 18(4):691-702, 1992.
29. Haley SM and others: Head trauma in children: application to assessment and treatment of patients with neurological disorders or dysfunction. In Lister MJ, editor: *Contemporary management of motor control problems,* Alexandria, Va, 1991, Foundation for Physical Therapy.
30. Harris SR and others: Effects of prenatal alcohol exposure on neuromotor and cognitive development during early childhood: a series of case reports, *Phys Ther* 73(9):608-617, 1993.

31. Holstege G, editor: *Descending motor pathways and the spinal motor system: limbic and non-limbic components,* New York, 1991, Elsevier Science Publications.

32. Kandel ER, Schwartz JH, and Jessell TM: *Principles of neural science,* ed 3, New York, 1991, Elsevier Medical Science Publishing.

33. Kato S, Hayashi H, and Yagishita A: Involvement of the frontotemporal lobe and limbic system in amyotrophic lateral sclerosis: as assessed by serial computed tomography and magnetic resonance imaging, *J Neurol Sci* 116:52-58, 1993.

34. Klüver H and Bucy PC: Preliminary analysis of functions of the temporal lobes in monkeys, *Arch Neural Psychiatry* 42:979, 1939.

35. Knopman D: Long-term retention of implicitly acquired learning in patients with Alzheimer's disease, *J Clin Exp Neuropsychol* 13(6):880, 1991.

36. Kostandov EA: Organization of human higher cortical functions with different forms of reinforcement, *Neurosci Behav Physiol* 19(2):93-102, 1989.

37. Lachman HM: Alterations in glucocorticoid inducible RNAs in the limbic system of learned helpless rats, *Brain Res* 609(1-2):110-116, 1993.

38. Leahy P: Head trauma in adults: problems, assessment, and treatment. In Lister MJ, editor: *Contemporary management of motor control problems,* Alexandria, Va, 1991, Foundation for Physical Therapy.

39. Leonard G: *The silent pulse,* New York, 1981, Bantam Books, Inc.

40. LeVere TE, Almli RB, and Stein DG, editor: *Brain injury and recovery: theoretical and controversial issues,* New York, 1988, Plenum.

41. Lewis CB: *Aging: the health care challenge,* Philadelphia, 1990, FA Davis.

42. Lewis CB and Bottomley JM: *Geriatric physical therapy: a clinical approach,* Norwalk, Conn, 1994, Appleton & Lange.

43. Lindross OF, Leinonen LM, and Laakso ML: Melatonin binding to the anteroventral and anterodorsal thalamic nuclei in the rat, *Neurosci Lett* 143(1-2):219-222, 1992.

44. Maclean PD: Role of transhypothalamic pathways in social communication. In Morgane PJ and Panksapp J, editors: *Handbook of the hypothalamus,* vol. 3, part B, New York, 1981, Marcel Dekker Inc.

45. McKee RD and Squire LR: On the development of declarative memory, *J Exp Psychol Learn Mem Cogn* 19(2):397-404, 1993.

46. Menza MA and others: Dopamine-related personality traits in Parkinson's disease, *Neurology* 43(3 pt 1):505-508, 1993.

47. Mesulam MM: *Principles of behavioral neurology,* Philadelphia, 1985, FA Davis.

48. Mishkin MA and Appenzeller T: The anatomy of memory, *Sci Am* 256:680, 1987.

49. Mishkin M and others: An animal model of global amnesia. In Cashin S editor: *Alzheimer disease: a report of progress,* New York, 1982, Raven Press.

50. Moore JC: Neuroanatomical structures subserving learning and memory. In Fifteenth Annual Sensorimotor Integration Symposium, unpublished manual, San Diego, July, 1987.

51. Moore JC: Review of neurophysiology as it relates to treatment, Personal notes, San Francisco, 1980.

52. Noback CR, Strominger NL, and Demarest RJ: *The human nervous system: introduction and review,* ed 4, Philadelphia, 1991, Lea & Febiger.

53. Ommaya AIC and Gennarelli TA: Cerebral concussion and traumatic unconsciousness, *Brain* 24:1181, 1974.

54. Osborn JA, Harris SR, and Weinberg J: Fetal alcohol syndrome: review of the literature with implication for physical therapists, *Phys Ther* 73(9):599-607, 1993.

55. Papez JW: A proposed mechanism of emotions, *Arch Neurol Psych* 38:725, 1937.

56. Reding M and others: Depression in patients referred to a dementia clinic, a three-year prospective study, *Arch Neurol* 42:894, 1985.

57. Rosenthal M and others, editors: *Rehabilitation of the adult and child with traumatic brain injury,* Philadelphia, 1990, FA Davis.

58. Ruat M and others: Molecular cloning characterization and localization of a high-affinity serotonin receptor activating cAMP formation, *Proc Natl Acad Sci USA* 90(18):8547-8551, 1993.

59. Schmidley JW and Messing RO: Agitated confusional states in patients with right hemisphere infarctions, *Stroke* 15:883, 1984.

60. Schmidt RA: Motor learning principles for physical therapy. In Lister MJ, editor: *Contemporary management of motor control problems,* Norman, Okla, 1991, Foundation for Physical Therapy.

61. Schneider JW and Chasnoff IJ: Motor assessment of cocanin/polydrug-exposed infants at age 4 months, *Neurotoxicol Teratol* 14:97-101, 1992.

62. Selye H: *The stress of life.* New York, 1959, McGraw Hill.

63. Siesjo BK: Basic mechanism of traumatic brain damage, *Ann Emerg Med* 22(6):959-969, 1993.

64. Spiers PA: Temporalimbic epilepsy and behavior. In Mesulam MM, editor, *Principles of behavioral neurology,* Philadelphia, 1985, FA Davis.

65. Squire LR: Memory and the hippocampus: a synthesis from findings with rats, monkeys, and humans, *Psychol Rev* 99(2):195-231, 1992.

66. Squire LR: The medial temporal lobe memory system, *Science* 253(5026):1380-1386, 1991.

67. Stellar JR and Stellar E: *The neurobiology of motivation and rewards,* New York, 1985, Springer Verlag.

68. Strub RL and Black FW: *Neurobehavioral disorders: a clinical approach,* Philadelphia, 1988, FA Davis.

69. Thompson RF: Are memory traces localized or distributed, *Neuropsychologia* 29(6):571-582, 1991.

70. Tucker DM and Derryberry D: Motivated attention: anxiety and the frontal executive functions, *Neuropsychiatry Neuropsychol Behav Neurol* 5(4):233-252, 1992.

71. Vietze P and Vaughan H, editors: *Early identification of infants with developmental disabilities.* San Diego, 1988, Grune & Stratton.

72. Zola MS and others: Damage to the perirhinal cortex exacerbates memory impairment following lesions to the hippocampal formation, *J Neurosci* 13(1):251-265, 1993.

CHAPTER 6

Classification of Treatment Techniques Based on Primary Input Systems

Inherent and contrived feedback/loop systems and their potential influence on altering a feedforward motor system

Darcy Ann Umphred

KEY TERMS

input systems or modalities   patterned responses
neuromechanisms   modulation
multiple system interactions   adaptation

LEARNING OBJECTIVES

After reading this chapter the student/therapist will:

1. Develop an appreciation for the complexity of motor responses and the multitudinous ways to influence those behaviors.
2. Recognize the large amount of soft wired programming within the central nervous system (CNS) and the various ways to affect those programs.
3. Differentiate feedback systems and therapeutic procedures to delineate variables that may affect both positively and negatively complex motor responses.
4. Analyze how to differentiate extrinsic from intrinsic feedback as a contrived verses a functional therapeutic procedure.
5. Identify procedures and sequences that might be added or deleted from an environment to allow the client to develop adaptable behaviors.
6. Analyze why the client has selected various procedures. Base his or her understanding on the function of the CNS and current research.

Before discussing therapeutic treatment procedures, the therapist must identify the *learning environment* within which the client will perform. As discussed in Chapter 1, that environment is made up of the therapist and the client, including both the internal central nervous system (CNS) mechanisms and the external restraints of the world. Using current motor control/learning theories (Chapters 3 and 4) and systems models, the therapist must determine the flexibility or inherent control the client may have when executing a functional activity. Then the therapist will need to break down the components of movement and determine, which if any, are causing distortions or inefficient execution of the overall plan. That is, after the therapist evaluates range of motion (ROM), muscle strength, state of the motor pool or pattern generators, synergies (volitional and reflexive), postural integrity, balance, rate, timing, trajectory, environmental context, ethnic and social factors, sensory intactness, and processing and learning abilities of the client functional goals must be established that lead to the client's control over his or her environment and lead to a higher quality of life.

Some treatment alternatives require little if any hands-on therapeutic manipulation of the client during the activity. For example, the patient practices transfers on and off many support surfaces with stand-by guarding only. Thus the client self-corrects or uses inherent feedback mechanisms to self-correct error and refine the motor skill. This ultimate empowerment of the client allows that individual to adapt and succeed at self-motivated and identified objectives. Often, allowing the client to try to succeed enables the therapist to evaluate what components of the task the client can control and what components are not within the client's adaptable capabilities, especially if normal fluid, efficient, and effortless movement is the desired outcome. In this case, the therapist may use hands-on or adaptive aids, which would be considered contrived or noninherent feedback.

Such contrived techniques make up a large component of the therapist's "bag of tricks." The difference between contrived and functional or intrinsic might be the need for the therapist to be part of the client's external environment in order for the client to succeed at the task. The therapist must recognize that as long as the therapist is part of that environment, the client is not functionally independent. Thus any contrived therapeutic technique must be at some time transferred to the client's ownership in order for that individual to achieve full empowerment and to resume control over the environment. Fig. 6-1 illustrates this concept of functional versus contrived and must be constantly considered throughout any treatment session. At times, selecting functional activities without the use of contrived procedures will not help the patient achieve the desired outcome. Thus contrived techniques are often the early choices of treatment. Once the client has the ability to perform without contrived methods and does so in func-

tional, efficient plans, those contrived techniques need to be selectively eliminated.

A problem-oriented approach to treatment of any disability implies that flexibility is a key element. That flexibility, however, is not random, disjointed, or without parameters. It should be based on methods that provide the best combination of available treatment alternatives to meet individual needs and differences. This flexibility is achieved through development of a clinical knowledge bank that incorporates as many alternatives as the therapist is capable of both understanding and implementing. A professionally educated therapist no longer bases treatment on identified recipes, although the ingredients for those recipes may be alternative treatment tools if, and only if, the client needs them. Treatment is based on an interaction between therapist and client.

Within this environment, the client needs to learn efficient motor behaviors. The client needs to direct the therapist's decision-making strategies by the plans selected as motor responses to a given task. If the response is effortless, efficient, and noninjurious to any part of the body and meets the client's expectations and goals, then the therapist knows the strategies selected were effective. If the response does not meet the desired goal for any reason, then the therapist must determine why. Many correct solutions may answer the question "why." Which solution is best, may be more client- than approach-dependent. Yet, if flexibility means that the therapist selects any component of any method that helps the client reach an objective, then the therapist is confronted with hundreds—if not thousands—of various treatment procedures. If the treatment procedures used introduce information to the client through sensory systems, then from a neurological perspective, a limited number of **input systems or modalities** are available. The myriad of treatment procedures are transduced into chemical and electrical transmissions that must travel along a limited number of pathways. Thus many treatment procedures must produce the same types of neurotransmission. The temporal and spatial sequencing or timing of the input will vary according to the technique and specific application. The clinician has little basis for decision making without a comprehensive understanding of the neurophysiology of: (1) the various techniques, introduced as input systems, (2) the potential interactions that information will have with various areas within the CNS, (3) the individual's prior learning and ability for new learning, and (4) the client's willingness to adapt.

Appropriate selection of specific techniques can be overwhelming unless a classification schema is developed that helps categorize these treatment techniques. The primary goal of this chapter is to help the reader develop such a classification system: a system based on the *primary* input modality used when introducing a stimulus. A discussion of the physiology of each sensory modality is presented. In-depth discussion of some basic treatment strategies, in addition to explanation of less familiar techniques, is also included. Those treatment strategies

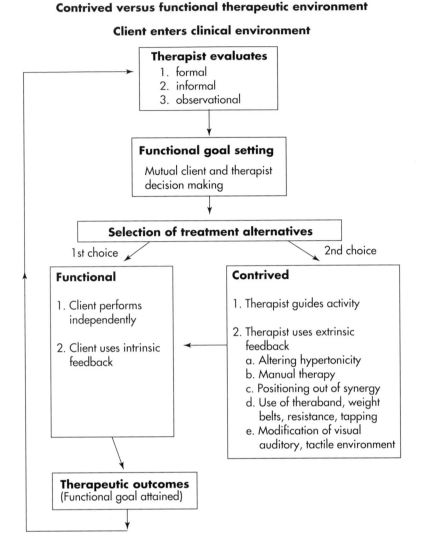

Fig. 6-1. Contrived versus functional therapeutics (Modified from the original work of Jan Davis, OTR, San Jose State University.)

frequently practiced and whose physiology is commonly known are included only in the tables and lists. Although only the primary input system is identified, at no time do we suggest it is the only input system affected. For example, when a proprioceptor is introduced, tactile input is simultaneously firing. If there is a noise component (such as with vibration), then auditory input has been triggered. There is also evidence that a given sensory modality may "cross over" or fuse with a completely different modality, helping in the synthesis of motor responses. These responses may occur in a modality that does not appear to be related. For example, olfaction may improve the tactile sensitivity of the hand. This concept is called *cross-modal stimulation* or *synesthesia.*[67,94] Yet a classification schema based on a primary modality promotes flexibility because the therapist can select from available treatment procedures that theoretically provide similar information to the CNS and thus help in the organization of appropriate motor responses. The motor system and its various motor programmers adapt to

the environment to achieve functional motor output toward a goal. Feedback is critical for adaptability and change. Feedback in this chapter is considered a mechanism to help the client's CNS optimally learn adaptability *not* the facilitation of a hard-wired reflexive response. Therapists must realize that even if the primary goal may be to facilitate or dampen a motor system response through multiply interlooping tracts, diverging pathways may also connect with endocrine, immune, and autonomic systems. Thus the clinical picture may be only a small aspect of numerous molecular and systemic reactions to environmental changes.

Therefore this type of classification system is based on identified input, observed responses, hypothesized **neuromechanisms,** current research on the function of the central nervous system (CNS), and the various systems involved in control and modification of responses. An understanding of normal processing of input and its effect on the motor system helps the clinician evaluate and use the client's intact system as part of treatment. When response to certain stimuli does

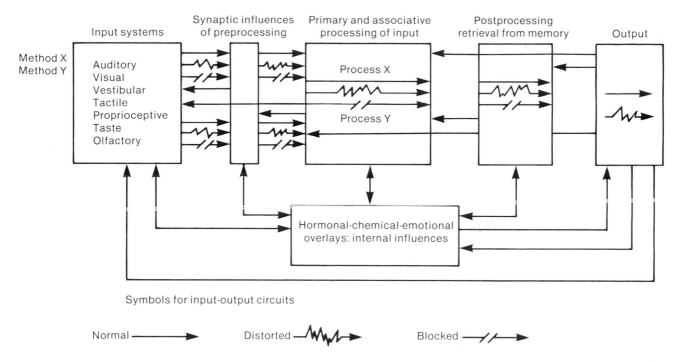

Fig. 6-2. Model of possible interactive effects among methods of treatment, input systems, processing and output systems, internal influences and feedback systems.

not help the client select or adapt a desired motor response, then the classification schema provides the clinician with flexibility to select additional options. This can be done by spatially summating input, such as using stretch, vibration, and resistance simultaneously, or temporally summating input, such as increasing the rate of the quick stretch. Many factors can influence motor behavior, such as method of instruction or the resting condition of the nervous system before introducing feedback, synaptic connections, cerebellar/basal ganglia or cortical processing, retrieval from past learning, motor output systems, or internal influences and balance. Fig. 6-2 illustrates this total system. Its clinical implications are more clear if the therapist retains a visual image of the client's total nervous system, including afferent input, processing, and efferent response and their multiple interactions on each other. At any moment in time multiple stimuli are admitted into client's input system. Before that information reaches a level of primary processing, it will cross over at *least* one synaptic junction. At that time the information may be inhibited, it may be changed or distorted, or it may be allowed to continue without modification. If the information is inhibited, then no response will be observed, even if it were considered reflexive. If it is changed, then the processing of the input will vary from the one normally anticipated. The end product after **multiple system interactions** will either be close to or further away from the desired motor pattern. Furthermore, sensory processing can take place at many segments of the nervous system. Although the CNS is not hierarchical with one level in total control over another, certain systems are biased to effect

various motor responses. At the spinal level the response may be phasic and synergistic. Brainstem mechanisms may evoke flexor or extensor biases depending on various motor systems and their modulation. Cerebellar, basal ganglia, and cortical responses may be more adaptive and purposeful. Thus the therapist must try to discern where within the system the feedback or feedforward is being short-circuited.

The same three alternatives—inhibiting (dampening), distorting, or normal processing—can occur anywhere in the system. Finally, motor output is programmed and a response observed. If the response is normal, the clinician knows that the system is intact with regard to use of the input and processing. If the response is distorted or absent, little is known other than there is lack of the normal processing somewhere in the CNS. Internal influences also need to be considered because they affect each aspect of the system. Once normal processing is identified, understanding of deficit systems and potential problems can be analyzed more easily. To reiterate, this requires awareness of the totality of the individual, that is, the client's personal preference of stimuli and uniqueness of processing and internal influences. A systems model requires simultaneous processing of multiple areas with interactions relaying in all directions. A client's CNS and peripheral nervous system (PNS) is doing just that, and the therapist must develop a sensitivity to a client as a whole while interacting with specific components. (Refer to Chapters 3, 4, and 5 for additional information.)

It is the therapist's responsibility to select methods most efficient for each client's needs. This viewpoint, based on a variety of questions, leads to a problem-oriented approach to treatment. Because the output or response pattern is based on alpha motor neuron discharge and thus extrafusal muscle contraction, the first question is posed: What can be done to alter the excitatory state of the alpha motor neuron? Second, what input systems are available, either directly or through adaptation of the motor system, that will change this motor neuron's level of excitation? Third, which techniques use these various input systems as their primary modes of entry into the system? Fourth, what internal mechanisms need modification or adaptation to produce a desired behavior response from the client? Fifth, which input systems are available to alter the internal mechanism? Sixth, what combination of input stimuli will provide the best internal environment for the client to learn and rehearse a more optimal response pattern? For example, assume that a client with a residual hemiplegia due to a middle cerebral artery problem has a hypertonic lower extremity that produces the pattern of extension, adduction, internal rotation of the hip, extension of the knee, and plantar flexion inversion of the feet. The answers to the first two questions are based on the knowledge that the proprioceptive and exteroceptive systems can drastically affect spinal central pattern generators and that these input systems are intact at a spinal, brainstem, cerebellar, and thalamic level and may even project to the cortex.

Appropriate selection of specific techniques—such as prolonged stretch using the tendon organ to modulate the hypertonic pattern, quick stretch or light touch to the antagonistic muscle, or any other treatment modality within the classification schema—provides viable treatment alternatives. Awareness that the client's response pattern is an inherent synergistic pattern and that it is further elicited by pressure to the ball of the foot leads to a better understanding of the clinical problem. Knowing that the client is unable to combine the alternative patterns, such as hip flexion and knee extension, needed for the latter aspects of swing through and early aspects of heel strike in gait, the therapist can use the other inherent processes to elicit these and other patterns. Finally, techniques such as combining standing and walking with application of quick stretch, vibration, or rotation or having the client reach for a target or follow a visual stimulus while walking provide a variety of combinations of therapeutic procedures to help the client learn or relearn normal response patterns. Further, this approach gives the clinician a choice of various procedures and promotes a learning environment that is flexible, changing, and interesting. The therapist must make the transition from applying contrived therapeutic procedures during functional tasks to allowing the client to practice the task without the therapist interceding with external feedback. In that way the client uses inherent feedback to self-correct. This self-correction leads to independence and adaptability. (Refer to Chapter 1 regarding contrived versus functional therapeutics.)

CLASSIFICATION ACCORDING TO SPECIFIC SENSORY MODALITIES

A variety of nerve fiber classification systems have been accepted by physiologists, neuroanatomists, and therapists. To avoid confusion about which nerve fiber is being discussed, the two primary methods of classification, along with a description of the functional component, have been included in Table 6-1 for easy referral.

Table 6-1. Classifications of peripheral nerves according to size[103,115,158]

Gasser-Erlanger	Lloyd	Motor (functional component)	Sensory (functional component)
A fibers: large myelinated fibers with a high conduction rate			
Aα	Ia	Large, fast fibers of the alpha motor system (large cells of anterior horn to extrafusal motor fibers)	Muscle spindle: primary afferent endings, (primary stretch or low threshold stretch; Ia tonic responds to length, Ia phasic responds to rate)
	Ib		Golgi tendon organ for contraction: responds to tendon stretch or tension
Aβ	II		Muscle spindle: secondary afferent endings—tonic receptors responding to length
			Exteroceptive afferent endings from skin and joints: respond to light or low threshold stretch
Aγ 1 and 2	II	Gamma motor system (small cells of anterior horn to intrafusal motor fibers)	Bare nerve endings: joint receptors, mechanoreception of soft tissues—exteroceptors for pain, touch, and cold (low threshold)
AΔ	III		
B fibers: medium-sized myelinated fibers with a fairly rapid conduction rate			
Bβ		Preganglionic fibers of autonomic system (effective on glands and smooth muscle; motor branch of alpha): unknown function	
C fibers: small, poorly myelinated or unmyelinated fibers having the slowest conduction rate; augmentation and recruiting occurs within the nervous system after stimulation of these fibers has ceased			
	IV	Postganglionic fibers of sympathetic system	Exteroceptors: pain, temperature, touch

Proprioceptive system

Proprioception as an input system has direct effect on program generators at the spinal level.[121] Due to its importance in motor learning and motor adaptation to new or changing environments, however, proprioception also has significant connections to the cortical and cerebellar neuronetworks. That its divergent pathways have synapses within both the brainstem and diencephalon, as well as the spinal system, demonstrates how a systems model functions. Proprioceptive input can potentially influence multiple levels of CNS function, and all those levels can potentially modulate the intensity or importance of that information through many mechansims such as presynaptic and postsynaptic activity, neuropeptides, and collateral inhibition.[31,121]

Muscle spindle. The muscle spindle consists anatomically of efferent and afferent, noncontractile tissue, and striated intrafusal muscle. This entire feedback mechanism, which includes afferent and efferent fibers from the muscle structure to and from the spinal cord, is called the gamma loop or the fusimotor system[183] (Fig. 6-3). Varied in function, the system plays an important role in ongoing modulation of the alpha motor neurons innervating the extrafusal muscle within which it is located. Spindle afferents also facilitate polysynaptically agonistic synergies while dampening antagonistics and their synergies. Information is then sent via ascending pathways to the ipsilateral cerebellum and contralateral parietal lobe. Consequently, the spindle system seems to play an important role as an ongoing peripheral feedback mechanism to various centers within the CNS. These centers in turn regulate the continuous neuroexcitation at the brainstem and spinal cord level. Gamma innervation regulates the degree of internal stretch on the noncontractile portion of the spindle. Internal stretch, along with the external stretch of gravity, positioning, and therapeutic procedures, in turn help modulate the efferent responses.

The afferent or sensory receptors are divided into Ia tonic and phasic, once referred to as annulospinal or primary endings; the II receptors are often called flower-spray or secondary endings. Ia tonic and II receptors are length receptors and respond to length changes placed on the noncontractile portion of the spindle. This length change can result from a mechanical external force, such as positioning or stretch to the muscle, or from an internal mechanism caused by intrafusal muscle contraction. Spinal motor generators and supraspinal influences modulate both the alpha and gamma motor neuron activity to produce flexibility in regulation over patterns of striated muscle contraction. As long as the spindle has enough internal sensitivity, any therapeutic technique that creates a length change to the spindle has the potential of firing the Ia tonic receptors. If the intensity is great enough (such as increased range), the II receptors, which have a higher threshold, will also discharge. Their exact connections have not yet been fully identified. The Ia phasic receptors respond to rate versus length change. Techniques such as quick stretch, vibration, and tapping cause a rapid rate change within the spindle and thus

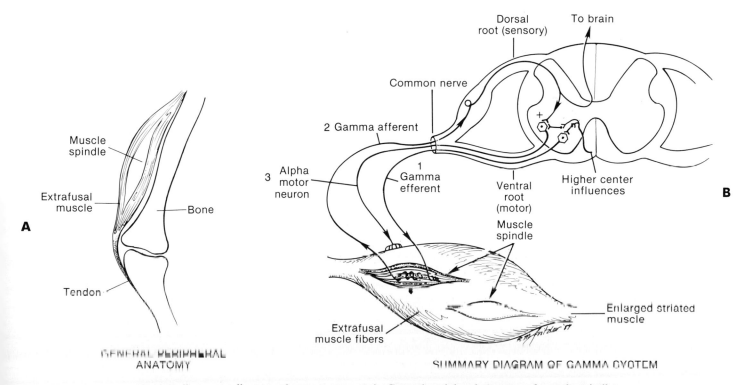

Fig. 6-3. Summary diagram of gamma system. **A,** General peripheral anatomy of muscle spindle, joint, and bone. **B,** Enlarged striated muscle and spinal cord with gamma system neuroconnections: (1) γ efferent (motor); (2) γ afferent (sensory); (3) αMN (motor).

potentially facilitate the Ia phasic receptors. The importance of muscle spindle afferent input as a treatment technique may lie in its ultimate influence over the cerebellum and basal ganglia to change existing programs permanently. Its direct influence over the spinal system is most likely short lived and has little long-term effect, although neuroplasticity within the spinal cord is possible. Cerebellar and basal ganglia/frontal lobe influence over ventral medial and lateral motor nuclei in the brainstem and their modulation over alpha, gamma I, and gamma II and interneurons within the spinal pattern generators should lead to change of existing patterns if change is either needed or within the potential of the available system (Fig. 6-4).

Table 6-2 lists a variety of treatment procedures believed to use the proprioceptive muscle spindle system as a primary mode of sensory stimulation. The varying intensity, amount of tension, or rate of the stimuli, in addition to the original length of the muscle fiber before application of the stimulus, will determine which sensory receptor within the spindle is firing. When the Ia phasic or tonic receptors are excited, one response at the spinal level will be monosynaptic facilitation

of the agonist. This important neurological connection at a behavioral level is referred to as "the monosynaptic stretch reflex." Simultaneously, polysynaptic, long-chain circuitries are triggered that may (depending on the intensity and duration of the stimulus) lead to facilitation of agonistic muscles and dampening of the antagonist and antagonistic synergies (Fig. 6-5). The representation is at a spinal level only to demonstrate the complexity of the spinal system. Remember: afferent information is projecting to many areas above the spinal system, and the ultimate effect will be regulation or modulation of and from all areas and their effect on efferent activity.[121]

Resistance. Striated muscle has a unique ability to contract and thereby perform mechanical work. The physiology of muscle contraction includes a complex chain of neurological, histological, and chemical processes.

Resistance is often used to facilitate intrafusal and extrafusal muscle contraction. Resistance can be applied manually, mechanically, and by the use of gravity in an activity. Resistance also recruits more motor units. Although muscles can contract both in an isometric and isotonic

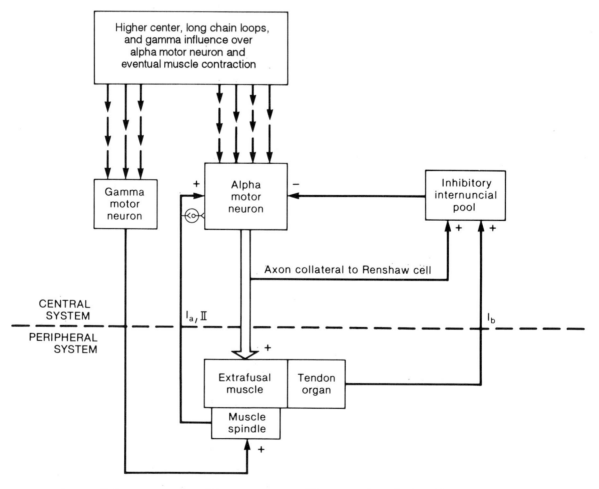

Fig. 6-4. Influences over the alpha motor neuron. The summation of all facilitory and inhibitory activity on the αMN will determine the response of the muscle.

fashion, most contractions are a mixture of the two. Certain muscle groups, such as the flexors, benefit from both isometric and isotonic, and eccentric and concentric exercise. Under normal circumstances, the flexors are used for repetitive or rhythmical activities. The extensors, on the other hand, usually remain contracted in an effort to act against the forces of gravity. Therefore the extensor groups benefit best from isometric and eccentric resistance.[121a]

When resistance is applied to a voluntary muscle, spindle afferent fibers and tendon organs fire in proportion to the magnitude of the resistance. The motor response is also contingent on the amount of contraction needed to withstand the resistance force. Light resistance will activate a small number of motor units to develop a proportional amount of muscle tension. An increased load or resistance will generate more tension and require more motor units (recruitment) to respond with the appropriate amount of contraction.

Resistance is more facilitory to an isometrically contracted muscle than to an isotonic contraction.[6] As isometric resistance to isometric contraction continues, more motor units are recruited, thereby increasing the strength of extrafusal contraction.[183]

Isotonic contraction of muscles can be either concentric or eccentric. Concentric muscle contraction refers to shortening of muscle fibers while the joint is moving against gravity or resistance. Eccentric isotonic contraction refers to the lengthening of muscle fibers to resist force, as in lowering the arms while holding a heavy object. Eccentric contraction uses less metabolic output and promotes strength gains in less time.[183] However, all types of muscle contraction will promote increased strength. Isokinetics is a type of isotonic exercise that mechanically controls the rate of movement and resistance.

Resistance is an important clinical treatment.[196,204] Theorists have used resistance in different fashions. Brunnstrom[30] uses resistance in conjunction with traction and joint compression to excite muscle synergies. Rood[180] used resistance and joint approximation greater than body weight to promote co-innervation. Kabot[124] used resistance and stretch to facilitate difficult volitional motor responses.

Tapping. Three types of tapping techniques are commonly used by therapists. Tapping of the tendon is a fairly nondiscriminatory stimulus. The tendon is tapped, which in turn causes the Ia phasic to discharge, causing a response similar to quick stretches of the entire muscle. Physicians use this technique to determine degree of stretch sensitivity of a muscle. A normal response would be a brisk muscle contraction. Because of the magnitude of the stimulus and the direct effect on the alpha motor neuron, this technique is not highly effective in teaching a client to control or gradiate muscle contraction. Instead, tapping of the muscle belly, a lower-intensity stimulus, is more satisfactory, because it allows the motor programming system to adapt and respond to the environment with new programs. Reverse tapping, a less frequently described technique, is often used. The extremity is positioned so gravity promotes the stretch, instead of the therapist manually tapping or actively inducing muscle stretch. Once the muscle responds, the therapist taps or pas-

Table 6-2. Proprioceptive muscle spindle system

Receptor	Stimulus	Nature of response
Ia tonic	Length	Monosynaptic and polysynaptic facilitation of agonist
Ia phasic	Rate of change in length	Polysynaptic inhibition of antagonist and antagonistic synergy
		Polysynaptic facilitation of agonistic synergy
		Input to cerebellum
		Input to opposite parietal lobe
		Specific responses open for question:
II	Length	Monosynaptic facilitation of agonist
		Polysynaptic facilitation of specific muscle groups, depending on muscle function of tissue where II originates
		Transmittal of information to higher centers

Possible treatment alternatives:

Resistance
Quick stretch to agonist
Tapping: tendon and muscle belly
Reverse tapping: gravity stretches; tapping agonist into shortened range
Positioning (range)
Electrical stimulation
Pressure or sustained stretch
Stretch pressure
Stretch release
Vibration within a facilitory frequency
Gravity as a prolonged stretch
Active motion

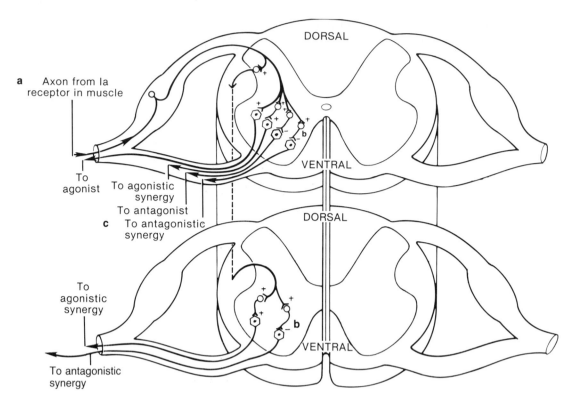

Fig. 6-5. Myo-tatic stretch reflex and relationship to muscle in synergy and agonists. *a,* Primary sensory afferent Ia (tonic and phasic) from muscle spindle. *b,* Interneurons: + = facilitory; – = inhibitory. *c,* Alpha (α) motor neurons going back to muscle tissue. If the interneuron at its synapse excites the alpha motor neuron, then the potential for firing has been heightened. If the interneuron inhibits the αMN, then potential for firing has been dampened. Note the Ia facilitates the αMN going back to the primary agonist via internuncials. The Ia has the potential of: (1) facilitating agonistic synergies both at the level it enters the cord as well as other segments, and (2) inhibiting the antagonist at the level it enters and antagonistic synergies both at the entry level and other segments. *Remember,* this only represents a spinal level activity. Collateral projections are occurring off all incoming afferent and relay this information to cortical and cerebellar neuronetworks.

sively moves the muscle or a bony prominence to help the muscle obtain a shortened range. For example, assume the client is in a kneeling position and the therapist is kneeling behind the client. Instead of tapping the gluteus maximus to assist in hip extension, the therapist allows the client to momentarily drop out of full extension. This quick lengthening of the gluteus maximus is caused by gravity pulling the client toward the floor, which is a normal inherent feedback to the system and helps the motor areas to learn appropriate responses. As the muscle begins to contract, the therapist can apply a quick tap to the gluteus maximus to assist in obtaining a shortened range. Another example would be reverse tapping the elbow when the client is bearing weight on extended elbows. Gravity quick stretches the triceps. Then the therapist taps the elbow into full extension. This tapping is usually performed at the elbow.

Positioning (range). The concept of submaximal and maximal range of muscles is highly significant to clinical application. Bessou and LaPorte[16] monitored the neuronal firing of muscle spindles at different ranges of motion. Their finding contributed to the understanding that manual stretch-

ing of muscles causes the Ia endings to discharge at specific submaximal ranges; the secondary endings begin to fire near the maximum physiological length. It is important to note that upper motor neuron lesions can alter the sensitivity of the spindle afferent reflex arc fibers by not using presynaptic inhibition to normally dampen incoming afferent activity.[50,51] As a result, the afferents modulate at their highest frequency and the reflex arc becomes supersensitive to stretch. Therefore ROM should be carefully assessed on an individual basis to determine what is maximal or submaximal range for an individual.

For example, normal elbow range of motion extends up to 130 degrees. The submaximal range would be about 90 degrees of flexion or extension. The last 20 degrees of flexion or extension would place maximal range of stretch, and the secondary afferent fibers would begin to discharge. A client with upper-extremity hypertonicity resulting in a flexion contracture may be left with 30 degrees of motion. The submaximal range for this individual may be 10 degrees. Anything beyond 10 degrees of flexion or extension would place the extremity in maximal range, causing the secondary ending to fire. This would be counterproductive if the goal is to reduce tone in the biceps muscle. Additional stimulation of the secondary endings probably would cause further contraction of the biceps muscle, resulting in diminished range of motion. As an alternative, the therapist should position the joint and muscle in the submaximum range while stimulating the antagonist muscle(s).[125,131,208]

Electrical stimulation. For in-depth discussion of the use of electrical stimulation (ES) both as an evaluation and a treatment modality (see Chapters 29 and 30). Electrical stimulation is not generally identified as a muscle spindle facilitation technique. However, when any mixed nerve is stimulated, not only is the alpha motor neuron affected but both gamma efferent neurons and spindle afferent neurons are also stimulated. Afferent firing helps to increase the sensitivity of the alpha motor neuron for further firing. The gamma efferent system causes intrafusal contraction, afferent firing, and thus continued biasing of the alpha motor neuron. Thus electrical stimulation has the potential for being an excellent muscle spindle facilitory technique, especially if additional therapeutic tools, such as resistance, are used. The additive effect when the techniques are applied for a period of time helps the motor system learn and thus reprogram (see Chapter 30).

Stretch pressure. The muscle belly is the stimulus focus of stretch pressure. The thumb, fingertips, or palm of the hand is used. First, quick stretches are applied, followed by briefly maintained pressure. Both Ia phasic and tonic receptors have the potential of being stimulated. When the muscle is placed 30 to 50 degrees beyond midrange in a normal muscle, the II receptors should also fire. The Ia phasic receptors are the focus of the technique until enough motor activity within the spinal level has developed to fire the striated muscle. This approach would obviously not be used on a hypertonic muscle because it would increase the tone, but it could be used on the antagonist muscle to inhibit a hypertonic agonist.[67,83]

Stretch release. This technique is performed by placing the fingertips over the belly of larger muscles and spreading the fingers in an effort to stretch the skin and the underlying muscle. The stretch is done firmly enough to temporarily deform the soft tissue so the cutaneous receptors and Ia afferent fibers may produce facilitation of the target muscle.

Manual pressure. Manual pressure can be facilitory when applied as a brisk stretch or frictionlike massage over muscle bellies. The speed and duration at which the manual pressure is applied determine the extent of recruitment from receptors. Volitional effect allows for motor learning.

Vibration. Bishop[17,18] wrote an excellent series of articles on the neurophysiology and therapeutic application of vibration. High-frequency vibration (100 to 300 hertz [Hz] or cycles per second) to the muscle or tendon elicits a reflex response referred to as the tonic vibratory response (TVR). Each cycle of vibration elicits stretch to the muscle spindle and causes selective firing of the Ia afferent receptors.

Tension within the muscle will increase slowly and progressively for 30 to 60 seconds and then plateau for the duration of the stimulus.[133] Certain researchers found that at cessation of the input, the contractibility of the muscle was enhanced for approximately 3 minutes.[133,212] Others found vibration to have a short duration period, lasting only as long as the stimulus was applied. The discrepancy in the research may reflect the way the individual is using the input, both from a motor generator perspective as well as supraspinal modulation over the importance of the input from learning.

By facilitation of the Ia afferent receptors through vibration, a variety of neurophysiological responses can be produced. Agonist facilitation and antagonistic inhibition, also called reciprocal innervation, are physiological responses that have significant clinical application. To facilitate a hypotonic muscle, the muscle belly is first put on stretch and then vibratory stimuli are applied.[99] To inhibit a hypertonic muscle the antagonistic muscle could be vibrated.[17,99] The use of vibration can be enhanced by combining it with additional modalities, such as resistance, position, and visually directed movement. Vibration also simulates cutaneous receptors, specifically the pacinian corpuscles and thus can be classified as an exteroceptive modality.[191] This is especially true with vibration of 60 cycles per second. Because of its ability to decrease hypersensitive tactile receptors via supraspinal regulation, vibration is considered an inhibitory technique; it is also discussed in the section on exteroceptors—maintained stimulus (see Table 6-4, p. 137).

Farber[67] summarized the use of vibration and clearly identified precautions that must be taken. Again, frequencies of 100 to 300 cycles per second can be used to effectively elicit the tonic vibratory response. We have observed, however, that in a hypertonic muscle the resting threshold of the Ia afferent is lower (biased) and the normal inhibitory mechanisms are not present. As a result, 60 Hz is an adequate stimulus to cause contraction of superficial mobilizer muscles. Frequencies over 200 Hz can be damaging to the skin. We have found frequencies over 150 Hz to cause discomfort and even pain. Thus it is recommended that vibrators registering 100 to 125 Hz be used. Most battery-operated hand vibrators function at 50 to 90 Hz.[71] Frequencies below 75 Hz are thought to have an inhibitory effect on normal muscle.[133] For that reason it is recommended that batteries be replaced when the frequency begins to drop. A common error is applying additional pressure to the muscle with the vibrator when the batteries begin to lose their charge. This additional pressure causes resistance and further decreases the frequency of the vibration. Cutaneous pressure is also known to cause inhibition, so if it is combined with vibration, it can only serve to cancel out the desired effects.

Amplitude or amount of displacement must also be considered when analyzing vibration as a modality. High-amplitude vibration has the potential of causing skin breakdown. An understanding of various responses and their neurophysiological explanation should be part of a clinician's background. Because of the potency of vibration as a treatment technique, its indiscriminate use should be highly discouraged. It has been reported that this technique causes adverse effects, especially in clients with cerebellar dysfunction[18]; thus keen clinical observation strategies should always be employed whatever the anticipated response. Vibration is not recommended for infants because their nervous system is not yet fully myelinated, and it might cause too much stimulation. The reader is also cautioned about using vibration over areas that have been immobilized due to the underlying vascular tissue potential for clotting. Vibration on or near these blood vessels could dislodge a clot, causing an embolism. Vibration also needs to be used cautiously over skin that has lost its elasticity and is very thin, for the friction itself from the vibration can cause tearing. Therapists have reported that vibration over acupoints can modulate localized pain syndromes. It seems to trigger A-delta exteroceptive fibers, which in turn dampen the effect of C-fiber. (Refer to Chapters 30 and 31 for more information on treatment of pain.)

The tendon organ. The tendon organ (TO) is a specialized receptor located in both the proximal and the distal musculotendinous insertions. In conjunction with the muscle spindle, the TO plays an important role in the mediation of unconscious proprioception.[44,113,145]

The principal role of the TO is to monitor muscle tension exerted by the contraction of the extrafusal muscles. Originally, it was believed that the TO had a high threshold to stretch and low threshold to contraction. The high-threshold organs are usually located in the insertions of the muscles. They are thought to be a protective mechanism designed to prevent structural damage when extreme tension is put on muscles and tendons. However, the TO is much more than a protective device. Recent research has demonstrated that the tendon organ is highly sensitive to tension and acts conjointly with the muscle spindle to inform higher centers of ongoing environmental demands to modulate or change existing plans, which in turn regulate tonicity and compliance of extrafusal muscles.[44,121]

TOs are innervated by Group Ib afferent fibers. Because the TO adapts slowly, it provides continuous information about extrafusal muscle contraction. Physiological studies have shown that, once activated, the TO discharges rapidly and then settles down to fire at a rate nearly proportional to the muscle tension. The TO (Ib) is signaling not only tension but also rate of change of tension and provides the sensation of force as the muscle is working.[98]

Perhaps a better understanding of the TO can be achieved if it is compared and contrasted with the muscle spindle. A fundamental difference between the two proprioceptors is that the muscle spindle detects length, whereas the tendon organ monitors tension and force. Motorically, the muscle spindle and the TO spinal effect are the exact opposite.[44,82,136] The muscle regulates reciprocal inner-

vation, whereas the TO modulates autogenic inhibition.

In multiarthrodial muscles (superficial flexors and adductors), small-range repeated contractions will reduce hypertonicity in hypertonic muscles.[58,113] This is accomplished by synaptic connections to inhibitory interneurons in the spinal cord, which in turn produce a dampening effect on the alpha motor neurons from which the stimulus was derived. This is thought to occur due to flexor reflex afferent activity along with higher center adaptation and modulation over those afferents.[50]

Clinically, this phenomenon is seen in clients with upper motor neuron lesions. Usually the patient has some degree of hypertonicity. As the hypertonic extremity is passively moved through range of motion, resistance is felt and then suddenly "melts away," allowing more freedom of movement. The exact mechanism that dampens the hypertonicity is not known. It appears that other joint and cutaneous receptors could be sending signals to supraspinal centers, as well as TO, and it most likely is an accumulative effect.[121]

There appears to be a delicate balance between the inhibitory loops and the excitatory loops of the fusimotor system. These systems provide feedback control mechanisms to inform the CNS about the length, speed of movement, and contraction of a given muscle. Therefore this balance of excitatory and inhibitory feedback mechanisms is basic to control of fine movements, as well as to decision making when feedforward plans need changing to adapt to the environmental demands. Table 6-3 lists a variety of known treatment approaches that use the TO to inform higher centers regarding needed change and regulation over spinal generators.

Inhibitory pressure. Pressure has been used therapeutically to alter motor responses. Mechanical pressure, such as cones, pads, or the orthokinetic cuff developed by Blashy and Fuchs,[19] provides continuous pressure (force). Pressure on tendinous insertions activates deep receptors called *pacinian* corpuscles, which are rapidly adapting receptors. Vallbo and others[210] describe the pacinian corpuscle as the largest, most studied, and most highly structured end organ in cutaneous and tendon tissue. These receptors are usually found in the deep subcutaneous layers of skin in the palms of the hands, soles of the feet, mesentery, periosteum, tendon sheaths, and intramuscular connective tissue.[63,151] Tuttle and McClearly[203] studied the pacinian corpuscles in the mesentery of cats. They postulated that the pacinian corpuscle is a baroreceptor initiating vasomotor reflexes in the skin and muscles. Pertovaara,[167] studying the modification of pain thresholds in seven healthy adults, found that the pacinian corpuscles were activated by vibrotactile stimulation when the subjects were exposed to painful electrical stimuli. The pacinian corpuscles probably suppress other sensations in the receptor field.[212] This may be done at a spinal level and/or by higher center modulation.

This inhibitory pressure technique also works when pressure is applied across the longitudinal axis of a tendon.

Table 6-3. Proprioceptive tendon organs and joints

Receptor	Stimulus	Response
Tendon organ lb	Tension on extrafusal muscle	Polysynaptic inhibition of agonist, facilitation of antagonist spinal level circuitry: supraspinal regulation

Possible treatment suggestions

1. Extreme stretch
2. Deep pressure to tendon
3. Passive positioning in extreme lengthened range
4. Extreme resistance: more effective in lengthened and shortened range
5. Deep pressure to muscle belly to put stretch on tendon
6. Small repeated contractions with gravity eliminated

Type of joint		Stimulus	Response
I	6-9 μ	Static and dynamic joint tension: muscle pull	?: Facilitates postural holding: joint awareness
II	9-12 μ	Dynamic: sudden change in joint tension	?: Facilitates agonist and awareness of joint motion: range
III	13-17 μ	Dynamic: linked to GTO traction; activates in extreme range	?: Inhibits agonist
IV	2-5 μ ≤ 2 μ	Pain	?: Inhibits agonist

Possible treatment alternatives

1. Manual traction (distraction) to joint surfaces to facilitate joint motion
2. Manual approximation (compression) to joint surfaces to facilitate cocontraction or postural holding
3. Positioning: gravity used to approximate or apply traction
4. Weight belts, shoulder harnesses, and helmets to increase approximation
5. Wrist and ankle cuffs to increase traction
6. Wall pulleys, weights, manual resistance
7. Manual therapy[134]
8. Elastic tubing to provide compression during movement

The pressure is applied across the tendon with increasing pressure until the muscle relaxes. Constant pressure applied over the tendons of the wrist flexors may also dampen the hypertonicity as well as elongate the tight fascia over the tendenous insertion.

Pressure over bony prominences has modulatory effects. A common example is pressure on the medial aspect of the calcaneus, which dampens calf muscles and allows contraction of the lateral dorsiflexors muscles, whereas pressure over the lateral side of the calcaneus also dampens calf muscles to allow for contraction of the medial dorsiflexor muscles.[180] Localized finger pressure applied bilaterally to acupuncture points has been shown to relieve pain and reduce muscle tone.[138,139,186] This technique has also been found to be particularly effective when used in a low-stimuli environment and when combined with deep breathing.

This combination of pressure, environment demands (low), and parasympathetic reactions (slow relaxed breathing) illustrate the various systems interacting together to create the best motor response. The real world requires the client to respond to many environmental conditions while relaxed or under stress. Thus once a client begins to demonstrate adaptable motor responses, the therapist needs to change the conditions and the stress level to allow the client to practice variability. That practice should incorporate motor error, especially error or distortions in the plan, yet still achieve the desired goal. As the client self-corrects, greater demand and variability should be introduced.[181]

The joint. A joint may be described as the articulating surfaces between two or more bones. Joints are usually classified according to the degree of movement they allow. On the basis of this interpretation, three types of joints are recognized: synarthrosis, amphiarthrosis, and diarthrosis.[177,216] Synarthrotic joints are relatively immovable and make up the sutures of the skull. Amphiarthrodial joints are partially movable because the adjacent bones are separated by a thick layer of cartilage—for example, the intervertebral joints and the pubic symphysis of the pelvic girdle. Diarthrosis refers to a joint in which there is a separation (cavity) between adjacent bones that allows them to be freely movable. The joint is encased in a ligamentous capsule. The inner layer of the capsule, except for the articular surfaces, is lined with the synovial membrane. This membrane generates synovial fluid, which lubricates and nourishes the joint. Diarthrodial joints are subdivided according to shape and the type of movement the joint performs.

From a neurophysiological standpoint, joint movement provides the cerebellum and cortical sensory and motor nuclei with constant information about position and movement.[54] It would appear that the diarthrodial joints contain the greatest number of receptors with the capacity to respond to the slightest change of angle between two bony articulations. In other words, joint receptors are arranged so that any change in the joint angle causes maximal discharge of designated receptors monitoring that degree of angle. Thus as a joint is moved through range of motion, each degree of movement activates a division of overlapping receptors sensitive to certain zones of movement. This arrangement of overlapping sensitivity zones is called *range fractionation*. Most important, the CNS receives continuous information about minute changes in joint positions; however, receptors have been shown to have a certain amount of specificity. That is, some receptors are specifically sensitive to one form of energy. Receptor specificity is related to interaction of mechanical, chemical, electrical, and thermal energy tranduction. With the exception of some pain receptors, all joint receptors are mechanoreceptors. They signal mechanical distortion. They also give information about opposing ranges, such as abduction and adduction, based on the side of the joint on which they are found.

Numerous physiological studies have been conducted to determine the exact functions and threshold levels of joint receptors. To date many questions have been left unanswered, but from a clinical standpoint, the joint receptors are most amenable to treatment techniques.*

The awareness of movement and position requires the integration of many receptors. Any detection of joint movement in the gravitational field causes the discharge of receptors in the somatic, visual, and vestibular afferent systems. Some joint receptors have absolute thresholds for specific ranges of motion, the sense of movement, and position. In addition a host of peripheral skin and muscle afferent fibers sense the movement.

Four major types of joint receptors are described in the literature. Anatomically, these receptors are localized in the joint capsules and ligaments. They include the Golgi-type endings, Golgi-Mazzoni corpuscles, Ruffini's corpuscle, and free nerve endings.[31,121] In general, the joint receptors are slowly adapting receptors. That is, they do not adapt completely but continue to send impulses to the CNS as long as the stimulus is present. With the exception of the free nerve endings, the joint receptors are subserved by well-myelinated type A alpha-neurons. Joint receptors have different thresholds for the rate of movement and the degree of angulation and thus play a key role in providing information about movement and position.[4,198] These impulses project to many areas involved in both perception of the body in space and motor control over the body. Feedback to many areas is not crucial unless the existing environment does not match the predetermined feedforward motor plan.

If input matches existing expectation, it is erased. When the input does not match with what is expected from the predicted motor behavior, a change or modification in motor output or plan is needed to meet the desired goal. At this time feedback is critical and without it, the client will not have adequate adaptive mechanisms to rapidly change to environmental demands. How the motor programmer adapts, learns and changes is discussed in Chapters 3-5.

Type III, Golgi-type endings, are found primarily in the ligaments around the joints. These are the largest joint receptors and appear to be similar to the TOs in appearance. Their location in joint ligaments allows them to be stimulated very strongly by rate of joint movement and the force of gravity. Subsequently, the Golgi-type ending fires rapidly when the joint is first moved and then discharges at a steady lower rate. This slowly adapting joint receptor may also provide the brain with information about joint position.[31,44,136]

Type II, Golgi-Mazzoni corpuscles (paciniform corpuscles), resemble pacinian corpuscles in physical appearance. They are small, encapsulated receptors found sparsely in tendon surfaces and joint capsules. In comparison with the other joint receptors, Golgi-Mazzoni corpuscles are rapidly adapting. Higher concentrations have been found in the connective tissues of the hands. These corpuscles function principally as a detector of rapid joint movements. They have also been found to discharge under deep pressure and vibration stimulus.[198]

Type I, Ruffini's corpuscles, are exclusively joint receptors found in the fibrous joint capsules. These receptors have a lower threshold to stimulation than the Golgi-type ending. However, both receptors respond vigorously with a volley of impulses at the beginning of joint movement and taper off to a steady state of firing at different angular positions. Ruffini's corpuscles monitor both the rate and direction of joint movement. These receptors also discharge when touch pressure is applied to joint surfaces.[31,195]

Free nerve endings are widely distributed throughout the body's soft tissues. Morphologically, they are more primitive than the encapsulated joint receptors. Moreover, the free nerve endings are contiguous with unmyelinated group IV or C fibers. The actual role the free nerve endings play in joint reception has not been identified. However, it has been speculated that they provide a crude awareness of initial joint movement and the signaling of joint pain.[72,136,210]

There is some question about the specificity of these afferent receptors when functioning in the totality of the body. Although laboratory studies have analyzed these receptors in isolation when functioning together with all other input and regulatory systems, it is believed that they operate more like an orchestra whereby various rates of firing patterns are determined by both internal and external mechanisms. Thus when treatment is considered, the therapist needs to consider the system as part of a whole, not as an isolated receptor whose rate of firing can be modified.

Thus although joints play a role in awareness of joint position and movement, studies[85] have been conducted in

---

* References 4, 16, 41, 64, 136, and 180.

which joint receptors have been selectively anesthetized in an effort to determine their exact function. The studies revealed that an unidentified set of muscle afferent fibers and cutaneous receptors also contribute to the sense of movement and position.[136] Hence it may be safe to say that the somatosensory system works cooperatively as a unit.[85]

Because joint receptors are stretched and compressed during joint movement, they are in a good position to transmit signals regarding joint position, direction, and velocity of movement, but not force. Force sensations seem to be mediated by the receptors of the muscles and TOs.

The joint receptors lend themselves well to treatment techniques. As already stated, the joint receptors are both slow and fast adapting. They exert strong influences on the motor system and ultimately on musculature. Although the histological properties of the joint receptors are not entirely clear, certain techniques elicit predictable responses. Joint receptors are sensitive to movement, position, traction, compression, and palpation. Further studies to delineate the properties of individual receptors may not prove fruitful because the somatosensory system works as a whole. For clinical purposes, a variety of potential treatment approaches focus on the joint receptor (Table 6-3).

Combined proprioceptive techniques. Many techniques succeed because of the combined effects of multiple input. Some approaches that seem to combine two or more proprioceptive modalities are:

1. Jamming
2. Ballistic movements
3. Total positioning
4. Proprioceptive neuromuscular facilitation (PNF) patterns
5. Postexcitatory inhibition with stretch, range, rotation, and shaking
6. Heavy work patterns
7. Feldenkrais[69,70,119]
8. Manual therapy[33,134]

Jamming. Jamming is usually applied to the ankle and knee with the intent of dampening plantar flexion while facilitating postural cocontraction around the ankle. The client can be placed in side-lying position, can sit on a chair or mat, or can be positioned over a bolster with the hip and knee in some flexion. This flexion dampens the total extension pattern, including the plantar flexor muscles. With release of plantar flexion these muscles are placed on extreme stretch to maintain the modulation. At this time intermittent joint approximation of considerable force is applied between the heel and knee. If the client is sitting, this approximation can easily be applied by pounding the heel on the floor and controlling a counterforce at the knee. Once cocontraction is minimally palpated, the clinician should initiate a movement pattern such as partial weight-bearing to further encourage the CNS to readapt with postural control. This technique can also be used to dampen dorsiflexion of wrist and fingers by focusing on appropriate upper-extremity

patterns, modulating the flexor reflex afferent activity, and applying a large amount of joint approximation between the heel of the hand and the elbow.

Ballistic movement. Ballistic movements or pendular exercises are effective because of their combined proprioceptive interaction. The client is asked to initiate a movement, such as shoulder flexion while prone over a table with the arm hanging over the side. As the muscle approaches the shortened range, the amount of ongoing gamma afferent activity decreases. Thus the agonist alpha motor neuron bias and the inhibition of Ia and II receptors of the antagonistic alpha motor neurons decrease. Simultaneously, the antagonistic muscle is being placed on more and more stretch. This stretch, as well as the lack of inhibition on the antagonistic alpha motor neurons, will encourage the antagonistic muscle to begin contraction and reverse the movement pattern. The TOs also play a key role in ongoing inhibition. As the muscle approaches the shortened range and tension on the tendon becomes intense, the TO increases its firing, thus inhibiting the agonist muscle in the shortened range while facilitating the antagonistic muscle. This technique is highly movement oriented, and the traction applied to the shoulder joint while swinging the arm further facilitates the movement. These ballistic movements are part of the program generators within the spinal system and are certainly more complex than a reflex response. Supraspinal influence over a preprogrammed activity also plays a role in the effectiveness of this treatment.

The clinician using this technique must exercise caution. ROM can easily be obtained through pendular movement. If limitation of motion is caused by superficial splinting of muscles whose function is to move (which now protects torn muscles), the technique will encourage the splinting muscles to relax; it will inhibit the postural patterns by traction and thus have the potential of tearing the muscle further by the pull and weight of the arm. Consequently, the clinician must always determine before therapy the reasons for specific clinical signs and whether the total problem will be corrected through an activity such as a ballistic movement. If only one component of the problem is alleviated, such as limitation of range, while lack of postural tone or joint stability possibly increases in severity, then additional techniques must be combined with this treatment modality. For example, assume the rotator cuff muscles were slightly torn and the movers of the shoulder are superficially splinting to prevent further tearing. Instructing the client to hold the humerus in the glenohumeral joint by active contraction of the rotator cuff muscles will facilitate postural holding and strengthen the torn muscles. Having the client simultaneously perform a ballistic movement with the arm will expedite shoulder movement, thus preventing unnecessary splinting and possible limitation of joint range.

Total body positioning. Total body positioning implies the use of *reflex-inhibiting postures* and gravity to dampen afferent activity on the alpha motor neurons.[165] Today the rationale for why relaxation of striated muscle occurs after this treatment would imply that the effect of the flexor reflex afferents are being dampened by a combination of input and interneuronal activity. These changes in the state of the muscle tone should revert back to the original problem unless motor learning and adaptation within the system occur simultaneously. Thus for this treatment to effect change, a vast number of sensorimotor systems need to occur such as autogenic inhibition, reciprocal innervation, labyrinthine and somatosensory influences, and cerebellar regulation overtone.[122] Changing the degree of flexion of the head also alters vestibular input and state of the motor pool.

Proprioceptive neuromuscular facilitation patterns. To analyze and learn the patterns and techniques that constitute proprioceptive neuromuscular facilitation, a total approach to treatment, refer to the texts by Kottke[125] and Sullivan and others.[196] This approach is being used extensively in orthopedic problems, and the research on this method has been studied more in lower motor neuron and musculoskeletal problems than in upper motor neuron lesions[33] (see Chapter 12).

Postexcitatory inhibition with stretch, range, rotation, and shaking. The concept of postexcitatory inhibition (PEI) is based on the action potential or electrical response pattern of a neuron at the time of stimulation, as well as the entire phase response until the neuron returns to normal. At the time of stimulation the action potential will build and go through an excitatory phase. The neuron then enters an inhibitory phase or refractory period during which further stimulation is not possible. This is referred to as the postexcitatory inhibition phase or postsynaptic afferent depolarization (PAD).[67] After the second stage an increase of excitation above resting level ensues, followed by return to a normal neuronal activity. These phase changes are extremely short and, in normal muscle, asynchronous with respect to multiple neuronal firing. In a hypertonic muscle more simultaneous firing occurs; with an increase of range, and thus tension, more fibers will be discharged. It is hypothesized that if the hypertonic muscle is placed at the end of its spastic range and a quick stretch is applied and held, then total facilitation followed by total inhibition will occur because of postexcitatory inhibition. As the inhibition phase is felt, the therapist can passively lengthen the spastic muscle until the facilitory phase sets in repolarization. At that time the clinician holds the lengthened position. Increased tone will ensue, followed by inhibition and continued lengthening. Holding the range (or not allowing concentric contraction during the excitatory phase) is critical. If shortening is permitted, higher centers adapt to the demand of the environment, the muscle readapts to the new position, and the therapist will find that the hypertonic muscle quickly becomes more hypertonic. In contrast, if the muscle is held as the tone increases, the resistance and stretch are then maximal and probably further facilitate the inhibitory phase.

At a certain point in the range, the hypertonic muscle will become dampened and tone will disappear. It is thought that at this time either the TO activity takes over and maintains inhibition or flexor reflex afferents are modified, thus creating an inhibitory range where antagonistic muscles can be more easily initiated and controlled by the client. If this technique is performed in a pure plane of motion, the clinician will find it a time-consuming procedure. Range can be achieved quickly by integrating a few additional techniques—that is, incorporating rotatory patterns of movement. For example, if the spastic upper extremity is positioned in the pattern of shoulder adduction, internal rotation, elbow flexion, wrist pronation, and finger flexion, then a pattern in the exact opposite direction can be incorporated to include external rotation of the shoulder and supination of the wrist. Every time the clinician begins to lengthen the spastic extremity, those rotatory patterns should be used. This should be done both on initial stretch and hold and during the inhibitory phase. Rotation seems to lengthen the inhibitory phase and allows additional range. If the clinician adds a quick stretch to the antagonistic during the inhibitory phase of the agonistic muscle, then further facilitation of antagonist muscle will occur. Because the agonistic muscle is in an inhibitory phase, movement in and out of its spastic range should not affect it. Yet the quick stretch facilitation of the antagonistic muscle inhibits the spastic agonistic muscle and again lengthens the inhibitory phase. This entire procedure occurs quite quickly. An observer might say that the clinician shakes the spasticity out of the arm. The shaking action is thought to be the quick stretch as well as joint oscillations. The degree of success depends on the therapist's sensitivity to the tonal shifts or phase changes occurring in the client. These tonal shifts are automatic and not under the client's conscious control. The technique does not teach the client anything and should be used to maintain range of motion and to create an optimal environment to encourage the client to initiate normal antagonistic control.

Rood's heavy work patterns. See Stockmeyer's interpretation of the Rood approach.[195] Rood's skill as a clinician is not refuted. Her rationale for the effectiveness of heavy work patterns reflected the knowledge of the 1950s. Today, the concepts of motor learning more clearly explain why postural holding for periods of time and eccentric lengthening in and out of the shortened range are an effective treatment technique. If repetition within the environmental context leads to motor learning, then the postural systems need to learn coactivation within the shortened range of the postural pattern and need to practice directing the limbs both during closed-chained and open-chained activities.

Feldenkrais. Feldenkrais's concepts[69,70] of sensory awareness through movement place emphasis on relaxation of muscle on stretch and distracting and compressing joints for sensory awareness. Both techniques reflect combined proprioceptive techniques. Taking muscles off stretch slows down general efferent firing and thus overload to the CNS.

Compression and distraction of joints enhance specific input from a body part while simultaneously facilitating input of a lesser intensity from other body segments. This combined proprioceptive approach enhances body schema awareness in a relaxed environment. It also integrates empowerment of the client by using visualization and asking for volitional control.

Manual therapy: specifically Maitland's. "The peripheral and central nervous systems need to be considered as one since they form a continuous tissue tract."[33] Manual therapy or mobilization of joint or soft tissue structures are not specific to orthopedic conditions, nor are neurotreatment principles ineffective on orthopedic patients. Irrespective of the diagnostic reason leading to joint immobility, the functional consequences can be synonymous. With immobility of joints, the peripheral nerve begins to lose its adaptability to change in the length of the nerve bed. This change in elasticity then creates additional problems in connective tissue function, which in turn affects the function of the motor system's control over the musculoskeletal component.[32,33] For this reason alone, discussion of musculoskeletal mobilization needs to be included in this section as a component of classification.

"Pathological processes may interfere with both of these mechanisms: extraneural pathology will affect the nerve/interface relationship and intraneural pathology will affect the intrinsic elasticity of the nervous system."[32] Patients complaining of pain that limits functional movement is the primary reason clients get referred to therapist for musculoskeletal evaluation. Besides subjective and observational evaluation, the physical examination must include tension tests that are used to determine the degree of pain and joint limitation, to differentiate between somatic and radicular symptoms, and to identify adverse neurophysiological changes in the peripheral nervous system.[32] "The increased muscle tone is considered to be a protective mechanism for the inflamed tissue."[65] This increase of tone may be due to a dampening of presynaptic activity of flexor reflex afferent by supraspinal mechanisms. This same mechanism may be triggered with a CNS injury. The difference between the orthopedic and neurological patient may be the trigger to the CNS. In a central lesion the motor generators after injury often are not adequately maintained, which results in hypotonicity. The hypotonicity causes peripheral instability, stretches peripheral tissue, and potentially causes peripheral damage. In both orthopedic and neurological cases, there is peripheral instability, the first due to peripheral damage and the second due to hypotonicity. The CNS's response to the instability may be the same: increase in muscle tone by dampening presynaptic inhibition. A result of a decrease in presynaptic inhibition on incoming afferents would cause an increase in spinal generator activity. With an isolated musculoskeletal problem and an intact CNS, the motor system would have the adaptability and control to modulate the spinal generators and only isolate those components in which an increase in tone might directly affect the problems.

The client with CNS may lose some of the flexibility of the motor system's control over the pattern generators, and thus high tone synergistic patterns may develop.

In either case, the peripheral system needs evaluation and treatment remediation when necessary. Tension tests look for "adverse responses to physical examination of neural tissues. The adverse responses being muscle tone increases as a result of painful provocation of sensitized neural tissue nociceptors, thus serving to prevent further pain."[65] This increase in pain increases tone and leads to limited range of passive movement.[65,127] Painfree range suggests CNS sensitivity to the large highly myelinated alpha fibers. Pain range encompasses the degree of joint motion where the nociceptors play a primary role in CNS attention. It is believed that with the inflamed neural tissue the nociceptors become hypersensitized or more reactive to mechanical or chemical changes in the joint and thus react significantly to movement at the end ranges.[32]

Treatment will be based on the degree of immobility, the pain range, and the degree of pain. Butler[33] not only looks at joint problems but considers many joint problems as having an adverse neural dynamics (tension on the peripheral nervous system). Treatment still incorporates Maitland's grades of passive movement listed in Fig. 6-6.

Butler[32] divides treatment of joint limitations, pain, and thus adverse mechanical tension into three categories:

1. *Selective nervous system mobilization.* Butler believes the therapist needs to mobilize the nervous system rather than stretching it. These techniques may be either gentle (grade 1) or strong (grade IV), through the range (grade II and III), or endrange only (grade IV). Different disorders (irritable verses nonirritable) will require different treatment approaches.

2. *Treatment via interfacing and relating tissues.* When joint immobility is interfaced with muscle and fascia tightness, all components must be treated simultaneously. If the focus of treatment is joint and muscle signs, the constant reassessment of nervous system effect is crucial. This aspect would seem even more crucial in clients with CNS injury and peripheral joint pain.

3. *Indirect treatment.* Indirect treatment includes the use of movement patterns, especially postural based patterns, as part of the treatment itself. When individuals experience nervous system changes, static and dynamic postural patterns often emerge as compensatory reactions to the problem state. Pain posturing, tension, or stiffness due to prolonged positioning, forced postures due to synergy patterns, to name a few; all seem to respond well to indirect treatment with or without passive CNS mobilization. The use of posturally based movement patterns during functional activities also provides for variability and repetition and thus should lead to greater carry-over in motor learning.

Grades of Movement

Grade I   A small amplitude movement performed near the beginning of range.

Grade II   A large amplitude movement carried well into range. Its a movement that occupies any part of the range that is free of pain or resistance.

Grade III   A large amplitude movement that moves up to the limit of range or into resistance.

Grade IV   A small amplitude movement performed near the end of range or slightly into resistance.

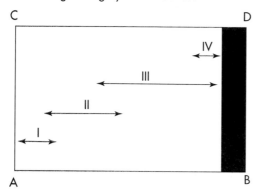

Maitland has also been using the pluses (1) and minuses (2) in his grades of movement for many years now. It enables the therapist to communicate better with other therapists as well as treat the patient with accuracy and skill.

Grade IV――: just nicking resistance

Grade IV―: touching resistance

Grade IV: into resistance about 25%

Grade IV+: into resistance about 50%

Grade IV++: into resistance about 75%

Fig. 6-6. Grades of movement adapted from Maitland's Theory of Joint and Tissue Mobilization. (By: John Sievert, P.T., GDMT.)[184] References: Course Notes Graduate Diploma in Manipulative Therapy. Curtin University of Technology, Perth, WA, 1990. Maitland GD: Peripheral Manipulation, ed 3, Boston, 1991, Butterworth Heinemann Ltd.

Much of manual therapy approaches affect and use the proprioceptive system as a measure to change motor responses. The reader is again reminded that the proprioceptive system affects all systems within the CNS and vice versa. The end effect of all systems interactions will be the behavior observed by the therapist as the client initiates motor strategies in response to functional goals.

Exteroceptive

The somatosensory system is usually subdivided into two distinct systems. One system is phylogenetically older and nonspecific in nature. The other system is phylogenetically newer and specific in function.

The concept of the dual quality of the somatosensory system was first suggested by Head.[102] The older sensory system was said to be *protopathic* in that it mediated primitive stimuli for protective responses. The newer sensory system was described as *epicritic* in that it mediated the discriminative aspects of somatic sensibility. The dual systems were further researched and elaborated on by Mountcastle and his associates.[151] Today the systems are described in more anatomical terms as the *spinothalamic* (protopathic) and the *lemniscal* (epicritic) systems, which include both exteroceptive and proprioceptive information.[6]

A fundamental understanding of the anatomy and physiology of the dual sensory systems is important before undertaking therapeutic intervention techniques. A brief explanation is presented here. The lemniscal system consists of pathways that are clearly distinguishable anatomically and neurophysiologically. Afferent signals are projected to two cortical regions of the parietal lobe from the spinal cord and the trigeminal nerve. From the spinal level, afferent impulses travel through the posterior and lateral columns, ascend through the medial lemniscus to the ventrobasal nuclei of the thalamus, and on to specific regions of the cortex. The afferent impulses entering the CNS by way of the trigeminal nerve synapse with nuclei in the medulla and continue through the medial lemniscus, thalamus, and parietal region of the cortex. The fibers of the lemniscal system are large and well myelinated. Therefore signals are transmitted rapidly, with a minimum of three synaptic relays. A striking characteristic of this system is its somatotopic organization. There is an orderly spatial topographical representation of the surface of the skin in the fiber bundles of the dorsal columns and the synaptic organization of the thalamus. This highly developed organization of sensory relays allows the lemniscal system to discriminate among specific proprioceptive and tactile stimuli. This system transmits conscious proprioceptive and kinesthetic information such as touch, pressure, localization, contour, quality, and spatial details of mechanical stimuli. In general the receptors that feed into the lemniscal system are encapsulated, slowly adapting with type I and II (Aα) fibers. Many of these receptors are found in the joints, muscles, and glabrous (nonhairy) surfaces of the skin.[31,223]

The spinothalamic system is less well defined anatomically than the lemniscal system. Different impulses are linked to this system by way of the anterior and lateral spinothalamic tracts or the reticulospinal tracts (anterolateral funiculus). Ascending impulses either terminate in or send collateral connections to the reticular formation. These fibers continue upward to synapse with the nonspecific thalamic nuclei (medial) and then diverge to make connections with practically all regions of the cerebral cortex. Other collaterals of this system project to the regulators of the autonomic nervous system (ANS), limbic system, and brainstem nuclei.[31,121]

Because the spinothalamic system synapses with the

reticular formation and the ANS, it serves more as an energizing or arousal mechanism to potentially harmful stimuli. Therefore this system is involved in perception of pain, light touch, pleasurable sexual sensations, and aversive stimuli and in the production of primitive orientations and protective responses.[26,31,178]

This subdivision into spinothalamic and lemniscal systems can mislead one into thinking that they can be activated separately. Most sensory stimuli will activate both systems simultaneously—for example, light touch. The lemniscal system can carry both exteroceptive and proprioceptive stimuli. However, it is possible to "load" one system more than the other by using selective stimuli in a fast or slow manner.[6]

Poggio and Mountcastle[170] suggest that the lemniscal system can have an inhibiting influence on the spinothalamic system. Ayers[7] and Wilbarger[219] have proposed that "touch defensiveness" constitutes the predominance of the spinothalamic (protective) system over the lemniscal system. Many of the therapeutic techniques used in sensory integrative therapy are designed to activate the lemniscal system and establish a better balance between the two systems. In addition, the facial region receives its sensory innervation from the trigeminal nerve, which can be regarded as a third somatosensory system because it supplies a body surface that is outside of the dermatomal segments supplied by the spinal cord.[151] A soft, low-intensity stimulation to the facial region can elicit a relaxation response, because the soft tissues are also richly innervated by the parasympathetic nervous system.[95,120] Wilbarger[219] postulates that if the protective system becomes hypersensitive, its generalized effect will lead to sympathetic overactivity, avoidance behaviors of all types, inability to handle or dampen extraneous input, and potential attention deficits. By desensitizing the touch system through maintained deep rubbing with a surgical-type scrub brush, she states the system will dampen its firing, and the discriminatory (lemniscal) system can begin to function. This discriminatory system will further override the older system and better homeostasis will follow.

Cutaneous exteroceptive system. Exteroceptors are sensory end organs located in the superficial layers of the skin, the subcutaneous layers, and the external mucous membranes.[191] Some authors include the special sense organs, such as gustatory, olfactory, visual, and auditory, as part of the exteroceptive system. This section describes only the nonencapsulated and encapsulated end organs found in the skin and around hairs.

The skin is the organ of touch. Exteroceptors in the skin are activated by stimuli from outside the body. Therefore the exteroceptors inform the CNS about changes taking place in the external environment. These receptors tend to be especially sensitive to specific kinds of energy, such as pain, temperature, touch, and pressure. Before an exteroceptor will discharge, it must receive the appropriate amount of energy, which is called the adequate stimulus. Exteroceptors

also have different thresholds. When the stimuli are adequate, the neuron reaches its action potential and discharges according to the intensity of the stimulus.[92,191] The duration of discharge depends on the receptor's ability to adapt. Some receptors adapt quickly, and others adapt slowly.

Exteroceptors transmit impulses along fibers of different diameters. Thick fibers are more myelinated and transmit impulses at a faster rate. Thin fibers have little or no myelin and transmit more slowly.[15,167] Exteroceptors innervate certain areas of the skin in an overlapping fashion. The area of skin innervation is called a receptor field. There is much variation in the number of receptors that innervate a given field of skin. Generally, the palmar surface of the hand contains a greater number of receptors with overlapping fields because the hands are used for prehension and touch. The shoulder region, on the contrary, has fewer receptors with less overlap and ability to discriminate stimuli. For example, the fingertips, lips, and tip of the tongue have a greater capacity for fine discrimination of touch stimuli. These areas contain more encapsulated receptors and more afferent neurons, and they transmit along the thicker fibers.[117,225] They also have greater representation on cortical gyri.[121]

Cutaneous system

Free nerve endings. Free or bare nerve endings are phylogenetically the oldest unencapsulated receptors. Free nerve endings transmit principally along thin fibers classified as Aδ (group III) or C fibers (group IV) (see Table 6-1). These fibers have little or no myelination. Free nerve endings are widely distributed throughout the dermis of the skin's connective tissue and in the viscera. Their greatest concentration is found along the midline axis of the body. For example, the area of the skin along either side of the vertebrae (the ramus posterior) has a 5:1 ratio of free nerve endings to other skin receptors.[92]

Free nerve endings transmit pain, temperature, and light touch sensations. Because these receptors are in greater concentration along the midline axis, pain sensitivity is 20 times greater in skin of the abdomen than in the skin of the fingertip. Pain awareness in the cornea has been estimated to be 30 times greater than in the abdomen. In addition, sensitivity to cold stimuli is 10 times greater along the midline than in the extremities. An exception to this midline rule can be found in the mucosal linings and the posterior surface of the tongue.[45,121]

Free nerve endings seem to serve as primitive protective receptors because they are centrally located and alert the organism to potential dangers to vital organs. Most of the impulses derived from free nerve endings travel to the CNS by way of the spinothalamic tracts.

Hair receptors. Hair follicles are quickly adapting receptors that discharge when displaced. Brushing against the natural direction of hairs sends impulses into the spinothalamic tract, which has many collaterals to the reticular-activating system. In general, this causes an excitatory response because the reticular-activating system links to the ANS. Stimulation to hair follicles or skin located on a dermatome at the same segmental level can facilitate the underlying muscle.[64,100] This stimulus activates a cutaneous fusimotor reflex. The reflex sends impulses carried along Aβ (group II) fibers to the interneurons and alpha motor neurons that terminate at the myoneural junction of the skeletal muscle.[64,100] This creates a dermatone-myotone relationship.

Merkel's disks. Merkel's disks can be found in the deepest layer of the epidermis, primarily in glaborous (nonhairy) skin. The greatest number are located in the volar surface of the fingers, lips, and external genitalia. Slowly adapting touch-pressure receptors, they are highly responsive to slow movements across the skin surface and to pressures. They transmit impulses along Aβ fibers (group II) and produce a prolonged discharge. These receptors have also been associated with the sense of tickly and pleasurable touch.[31,44]

Meissner's corpuscles. Meissner's corpuscles are highly developed, encapsulated receptors commonly found in the glaborous skin. The greatest numbers are found in the tip of the tongue, lips, fingertips, nipples of the breasts, and the pads of the feet. These receptors are highly discriminative, providing instantaneous sense of contact and flutter sensation. These receptors are used in two-point discrimination and stereognosis. Histological studies show that these receptors have a close relationship to the skin. In the fingertips they are uniformly arranged in line with the fingerprint patterns. During digital exploration, the neighboring sweat glands secrete and the liquid aids discriminative touch. Highly skilled braille readers are able to perceive 100 words/minute. There is some evidence that elderly individuals have a reduction of sensation resulting from a combination of skin inelasticity and loss of Meissner's corpuscles.[174,175]

Pacinian corpuscles. Pacinian corpuscles are the largest encapsulated and most studied cutaneous receptors. They are located very deep in the dermis of the skin; in viscera, mesenteries, and ligaments; and near blood vessels. Interestingly, they are most plentiful in the soles of the feet, where they seem to exert some influence on posture, position, and ambulation.[175] The pacinian corpuscles adapt very quickly, and they are activated by deep pressure and quick stretch of tissues.[64] In addition, they are responsive to vibration and show maximal discharge when vibrated at 250 to 300 Hz.[128] It has not been demonstrated, however, that the pacinian corpuscles are implicated in the tonic vibration reflex.[177]

A list of treatment techniques using the tactile or exteroceptive system as their primary mode of entry can be found in Table 6-4.

Treatment alternatives

For an overview of exteroceptive techniques, refer to Table 6-4. The function of the exteroceptive system is to inform the nervous system about the surrounding world. The CNS will adapt behavior to coexist and survive within this environment. Although many protective responses are

patterned within the motor system, these **patterned responses** can be changed or modulated according to momentary inherent chemistry, attitude, motivation, alertness, etc. Thus the function of the input system is not reflexive but rather informative and adaptable.

Quick phasic withdrawal. The human organism reacts to painful or noxious stimuli at both conscious and unconscious levels. If the stimulus is brief and of noxious quality, it will elicit a protective reaction of short duration, which is thought to be a spinal-level phasic withdrawal reflex (Fig. 6-7). Simultaneously, afferent impulses ascend to higher centers to evoke prolonged emotional-behavioral responses. Stimuli such as pain, extremes in temperature, rapid movement, light touch, and hair displacement are the most likely to cause this reaction by activating free nerve endings. It would seem that these stimuli are perceived as potentially dangerous, and most of the impulses are transmitted along C fibers and Aδ fibers. Although both sensory systems would be activated, the majority of the impulses would be channeled to the spinothalamic system. As already mentioned, this system communicates directly with the reticular-activating system and nonspecific thalamic nuclei. These structures have diffuse interconnections with all regions of the cerebral cortex, ANS, limbic system, cerebellum, and motor centers in the brainstem.

There are some real therapeutic limitations to using stimuli that "load" the spinothalamic system. A painful stimulus will be excitatory to the nervous system and produce a prolonged reaction after discharge. According to Wall's "gate-control" theory,[72,130,213] all sensory afferent neurons converge and synapse in the dorsal horn in an area called the substantia gelatinosa. Thick well-myelinated fibers—Aα, Bβ, and γ (group I and II)—synapse with cells in the substantia gelatinosa, causing an inhibition of the second-order tract (T) cells. Thus according to the theory, the gate is closed and a limited number of impulses are permitted to ascend to higher centers. The thick fibers carry impulses from receptors in tendons, joint capsules, muscles, and deep-pressure receptors (pacinian corpuscles), whereas the fibers that conduct painful stimuli have less myelination, are thinner, and conduct more impulses than the thick fibers, but at a slower rate. These pain fibers have an inhibitory influence on the cells of the substantial gelatinosa, which in turn decreases the inhibition on the second-order T cells so that the gate is open and painful stimuli are allowed to ascend the spinothalamic tract. This phenomenon may have some positive implications for pain management because the "gate can swing both ways." Curiously, the large fibers outnumber the small fibers.[217] Therefore physical activity, frequent positioning, deep pressure, and proprioceptive and cutaneous stimulation should cause enough impulses to converge on the T cells of the substantia gelatinosa to close the gate and thus block transmission of pain messages to the brain. Recent studies have demonstrated that physical activity (types of physical stress) stimulates the production of endorphins, which in turn

Table 6-4. Exteroceptive input techniques

Receptors	Stimuli	Response
Free nerve endings: C + A fibers	Pain, temperature, touch	Seems to protect and alert, perception of temperatures, protective withdrawal
Hair follicles	Mechanical displacement of hair receptors	Increased tone of muscle below stimulus site
Merkel's disk	Touch: pressure receptors	Touch identification
Meissner's corpuscles	Discriminative touch	Postural tone; two-point discrimination
Pacinian corpuscles	Deep pressure and quick stretch to tissue, vibration	Position sense, postural tone and movement
Ruffini's corpuscles	Touch mechanoreceptor	Touch/spatial discrimination

Suggested treatment procedures using cutaneous stimuli

Quick phasic withdrawal

1. Stimuli
   a. Pain
   b. Cold: one-sweep with ice cube—Rood's quick ice
   c. Light touch: brush (quick stroking), finger, feather
2. Response
   a. Stimulus applied to an extensor surface: elicits a flexor withdrawal
   b. Stimulus applied to flexor surface: may elicit flexor withdrawal or withdrawal from stimulus into extension

Repetitive icing should be used with caution because of rebound effect

Prolonged icing

1. Stimuli
   a. Ice cube
   b. Ice chips and wet towel
   c. Bucket of ice water
   d. Ice pack
   e. Immersion of body part or total body
2. Response: inhibition of muscles below skin areas iced

Neutral warmth

1. Stimulus
   a. Air bag splints
   b. Wrapping entire body or individual body part with towel
   c. Tight clothing such as tights, fitted turtle-neck jerseys
   d. Tepid water or shower
2. Response: inhibition of area under which neutral warmth was applied

Light touch/rapid stroking: to facilitate muscle below stimulus area

Maintained pressure or slow continuous stroking with pressure

- Response: adaptation of many cutaneous receptors to stimulus, thus decreasing exteroceptive input, decreasing reticular activity, and decreasing facilitation of muscles underlying stimulated skin

---

release opiate receptors and act as the body's own morphine[24,134,135,140] (see Chapters 30 and 31).

Stimuli, such as brushing or stroking the skin with a soft brush, generate impulses along both spinothalamic and lemniscal pathways because they both transmit light touch and will elicit a withdrawal at the spinal level. What specific withdrawal pattern occurs depends on a variety of circumstances. If the stimulus is applied to an extensor surface, then a flexor withdrawal will be facilitated. If the stimulus is placed on a flexor surface, one of two responses occurs. First, the client might withdraw from the stimulus, thus going into an extensor pattern. Second, the stimulus may elicit a flexor withdrawal and cause the client to go into a flexor pattern. Which pattern occurs depends on preexisting motor programming bias as a result of positioning and the predispo-

sition of the client's CNS. Both responses would be considered normal. The condition or emotional state of the nervous system will determine the sensitivity of the response, again reinforcing the system's interdependence.

If resistance is immediately applied to the withdrawal pattern, the technique no longer is considered exteroceptive because spindle, joint, and tendon proprioception has been added. By adding such a procedure, the number of adverse effects, such as a rebound phenomenon caused by eliciting only a withdrawal reflex, can be drastically reduced. Quick phasic withdrawal responses are best elicited by applying the stimulus dermatomally to activate specific target muscles (myotomes). For example, a moving light-touch stimulus from midline to lateral along T10 can elicit a quick withdrawal response in the hip flexors.[66] A light-touch

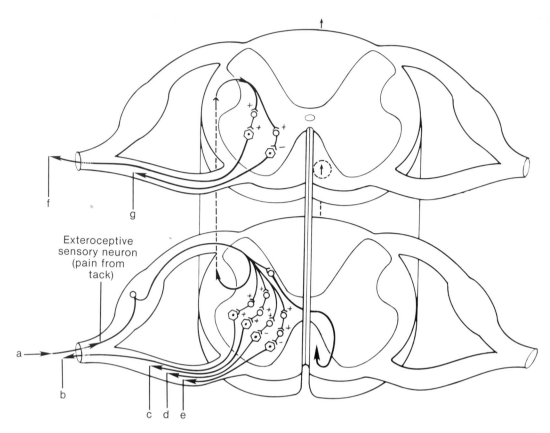

Fig. 6-7. Example of flexor withdrawal multisegmental response. *a,* Exteroceptive sensory neuron triggered by stimulus in skin—will elicit the entire quick phasic with manual/protective response. *b,* Primary flexor muscle to draw distal body part away from stimulus (facilitated). *c,* Flexor muscles in synergy with primary flexor and innervated at same segmental level (facilitated). *d,* Antagonist to primary flexor muscle (inhibited). *e,* Muscle in antagonistic synergy innervated at same segmental level (inhibited). *f,* Muscles in agonistic synergy at different segmental level (facilitated). *g,* Muscles in antagonistic synergy at different segmental level (inhibited). The quick phasic withdrawal visually elicits a flexor withdrawal pattern that facilitates a flexor synergy. This requires activation of flexor and extensor motor neurons at the cord level of the afferent stimulus as well as at other segments. Similarly, the antagonistic synergy is modified at multisegmental levels. Remember, this only illustrates a simplistic spinal neuronetwork.

stimulus along dermatome C6 on the dorsum of the forearm can facilitate the extensor carpi radialis muscle and encourage extension of the wrist. The response occurs because the light touch causes rapid changes in muscle spindle sensitivity through a complex cutaneous fusimotor system reflex.[180,195] Stepping on a tack quickly elicits a strong total flexor withdrawal of the foot and leg (Fig. 6-7). These responses are protective and do not lead to repetition of movement and thus motor learning. For that reason, along with the emotional and autonomic reactions, a phasic withdrawal is not recommended as a treatment approach unless all other possibilities have been eliminated.

Repetitive icing. Cold is another stimulus that the nervous system perceives as potentially dangerous. The use of ice as a stimulus to elicit desired motor patterns is an early technique developed by Rood. An ice cube is rubbed with pressure for 3 to 5 seconds or used in a quick-sweep stimulus over the muscle bellies to be facilitated. Obviously, this method would activate both exterocepters and proprioceptors and cause a brief arousal of the cortex. This method can produce unpredictable results. At the spinal level it would elicit a phasic withdrawal pattern. Yet immediately after the reflex has taken place, the "rebound" phenomenon deactivates the muscle that has been stimulated and lowers the resting potential of the antagonistic muscle.[185] Therefore a second stimulus to the muscle originally stimulated may not elicit a reflex, but because of reciprocal innervation, the antagonistic muscle may effect a rebound movement in the opposite direction. Icing may also cause prolonged reaction after discharge in the connections to the reticular system, limbic system, and ANS. Thus the ANS would be shifted toward the sympathetic end. Too much sympathetic tone causes a desynchronization of the cortex.[86] Although the resting state of the spinal generator may be altered briefly, if the heightened state persists it is most likely due to fear or sympathetic overflow. This state is destabilizing to the system and most likely will not lead to any motor learning. Because of unpredictable response patterns to Rood's repetitive icing, this technique is seldom used.

Ice should not be applied to the facial region above the level of the lips. Again, the spinothalamic system has two afferent pathways: the trigeminal and spinal. The trigeminal nerve innervates three divisions of the facial region: the ophthalmic, maxillary, and mandibular. The trigeminal nerves have a powerful influence on the somatosensory system because they feed directly into the reticular formation. Thus icing around the forehead can set off unwanted behavioral and ANS responses. It is also ill advised to apply ice to the midline of the trunk because the greatest concentration of C fibers are in that region of the body.[43,177]

Ice should not be used behind the ear as it may produce a sudden lowering of blood pressure.[58] The therapist should also avoid using ice in the left shoulder region in patients with a history of heart disease because referred pain secondary to angina pectoris manifests itself in the left shoulder area, indicating the cold stimulus might cause a reflexive constriction of the coronary arteries.[214]

In addition, the primary rami located along the midline of the dorsum of the trunk have sympathetic connections to internal organs. The cold stimulus may alter organ activity and perhaps produce vasoconstriction, causing increased blood pressure and less blood supply to the viscera.[80,159]

Ice can also have beneficial effects if the nervous system's inhibitory mechanisms are in place. For instance, in children with learning disabilities or sensory-motor delays, the application of ice to the palmar surface of the hands will cause arousal at the cortical level because of the increased activity of the reticular activating system. This arousal response presumably produces increased adrenal medullary secretions, resulting in various metabolic changes. Therefore icing should be used selectively. If the patient has an unstable ANS, it should be eliminated as a potential sensory modality.[81]

Prolonged icing. A variety of approaches incorporate prolonged icing techniques. The proprioceptive neuromuscular facilitation approach may be the most common.[124] Inhibition of hypertonicity or pain is the goal for use of any of these methods. With prolonged cold the neurotransmission of impulses, both afferent and efferent, is reduced. Simultaneously, the metabolic rate within the cooled tissue is reduced (see Chapter 31). Caution must be exercised with regard to use of this modality. For effective treatment results, the client (1) should be receptive to the modality, (2) should be able to monitor the cold stimulus—thus sensory deficits should not be present, and (3) should have a stable autonomic system to prevent unnecessary adverse effects of hypothermia.

Ice massage is a form of prolonged ice and is often used to treat somatic pain problems. It is also used over high-toned muscles to dampen striated muscle contractions. Caution must be used when eliminating pain without

correcting the problem causing pain. For example, if instability causes muscle tone and pain, then icing might decrease pain while causing additional joint instability and potential damage. The end result would be an increase, not decrease, in pain.

Neutral warmth. Like icing, this approach alters the state of the motor generators, either directly or indirectly through the motor system. According to Farber,[66] the temperature range is between 35° and 37° C. The length of application depends on the client. A 3- to 4-minute tepid bath may create the same results as a 15-minute total body-wrapping procedure. As with any input procedure, the effects should be incorporated into the therapeutic session to maximize the effect and promote client learning through active movement participation by the client in functional activities.

Maintained stimulus or pressure. Because of the rapid adaptation of many cutaneous receptors, a maintained stimulus will effectively cause inhibition by preventing further stimuli from entering the system. This technique is applied to hypersensitive areas to normalize skin responses. Vibration, used alternately with maintained pressure, can be highly effective. It should be remembered that these combined inputs use different neurophysiological mechanisms. It is often observed that low-frequency maintained vibration is especially effective with learning-disabled children who have hypersensitive tactile systems that prevent them from comfortably exploring their environment. By having them hold and vibrate themselves on the extremities, their hypersensitive system seems to normalize and become receptive to exploring objects. If that exploration is accompanied by additional prolonged pressure, such as digging in a sandbox, the technique seems to be more effective due to the adaptive responses of the nervous system.

Maintained pressure approaches using elastic stockings, gortex clothing, and other means can be incorporated into a client's daily activity without altering life-styles. In this way clients can self-regulate their system, allowing greater variability in adapting to the environment.

Vestibular system

Sensory receptors and physiology. The vestibular apparatus is a mechanoreceptor organ.[31] Functionally, it is involved in the maintenance of head and body equilibrium. Proprioception informs the CNS where the body is in space, and the vestibular system relays the head's position in space. Because the vestibular system is intimately connected with the auditory, visual, proprioceptive, and motor systems, it works cooperatively with a number of other systems to modulate important functions.[53,60] The vestibular system has been credited with influencing muscle tone; maintaining visual gaze, spatial directionality, and head and body orientation; and influencing learning and emotional development.[146,221]

The vestibular apparatus is a membranous structure located in the temporal region of the skull. It is subdivided into the cochlea (which is primarily involved in hearing), the vestibule, and the three semicircular canals. Phylogenetically, the receptors of the vestibular system are similar to the receptors that transduce sound. In both cases the receptors are hair cells; however, the anatomical arrangement and the physiological properties allow the receptors to transduce different sensory modalities. Another commonality between the auditory and the vestibular system is that they share the same cranial nerve root. Yet the connections to brainstem nuclei and other neurological structures are explicitly different.[43,121]

The vestibule (utricle and saccule) is located between the semicircular canals and the cochlea. It is often called the static labyrinth because it elicits tonic reflexes on postural muscles in response to changes in head and body positions and gravitational influences.[121] The vestibule contains two communicating chambers, the sacculus and the utriculus. The hair cells in the sacculus and utriculus are similar: Each chamber contains a thickened patch of sensory hair cells called the macula. The hair cells are arranged in a fixed position so that their hair tufts project up through a gelatinous mass called the *otolithic membrane*. Embedded in this gelatinous substance are small calcium carbonate crystals called *otoliths* (otoconia). This anatomical arrangement allows the hair cells to be highly responsive to changes in head position. As the head is tilted to one side, the force of gravity displaces the otolithic membrane, which causes the cilia of the hair cell to bend. This bending or shearing action causes the hair cell to discharge and transmit afferent impulses to the CNS.[13]

It should be emphasized that the hair cells are tonic receptors. Therefore even in the neutral position, the hair cells are constantly discharging. The bending of the cilia in a single hair cell in one direction will cause an increase in firing, and bending in the opposite direction will cause a slowing of the rate of discharge.[121] The mechanism that allows this to happen is inherent in the cilia of the hair cell. The cilia are arranged in a steplike gradation in length, becoming progressively larger toward the end of the bundle of cilia. At the outer side of the bundle, a conspicuously large cilium called the *kinocilium* serves as a regulator. That is, if the cilia bend toward the kinocilium, the rate of firing increases; if the cilia bend away from the kinocilium, the rate of discharge decreases.[31,121]

The sacculus lies between the utricle and cochlear duct. The majority of the cilia (hair cells) in the saccule are arranged in a side-lying fashion when the head is in the normal upright position. Therefore if the head moves in a vertical plane in linear acceleration and deceleration, the cilia will discharge. Any up-and-down motion, such as bouncing on a trampoline, is an adequate stimulus to the cilia in the saccule. In contrast, the majority of the cilia in the utricle are arranged vertically and the head is in the upright position. Thus linear acceleration and deceleration in the horizontal plane are the adequate stimulus for the cilia in the utricle. One may think of a child in a prone position propelling down an incline on a scooter board. As the child hits the horizontal plane, the head is upright, causing the cilia to deflect and discharge. Quick deceleration, caused by running into a mat on the floor, causes the hair cells to whip forward, deflecting the cilia once again. In most instances, the cilia in both the sacculus and utriculus are sensitive to a variety of stimuli. For example, forward and backward movements will activate cilia in both chambers. In summary, the adequate stimuli for the cilia of the utricle and saccule (vestibule) are the static position of the head in space and linear acceleration and deceleration in horizontal and vertical planes. The greatest tonal changes occur in extensor groups of the postural muscles. In addition, the vestibule (saccule and utricle) contributes to the maintenance of righting reactions and equilibrium responses.

Rood[180] suggested that the side-lying position of the head is useful to diminish unwanted extensor tone caused by poorly integrated tonic labyrinthine information. In this position the symmetrical input of the vestibule receptors on the vestibular nuclei is eliminated, modifying the outflow of the vestibulospinal tract and thus its influence over postural extensors.

The semicircular canals are referred to as the kinetic labyrinth, because they respond to movements of the head. The semicircular canals also exert influences on the limbs and the extraocular muscles of the eyes, as well as assist in equilibrium responses and orientation in space. The semicircular canals are arranged approximately at right angles to one another, one for each axis of rotation. The anterior and posterior canals are sensitive to movement in the sagittal plane. The horizontal canal reacts to rotation around the central body axis.[121,148]

The three membranous semicircular canals are contiguous with the vestibule. The canals are enlarged at the juncture where the canals terminate into the vestibule. This enlargement, called the *ampulla*, contains neuroepithelial receptors similar to the vestibule. These receptors consist of mounds of cilia termed the *crista ampullaris*. The crista are composed of cilia attached firmly to the base of the ampullae. The tufts of cilia project into a dome-shaped gelatinous substance called the *cupula*. The cupula differs from the otolithic membrane in that it does not contain otoliths. Instead it sits on top of the cilia like a hat and is stimulated by the movement of the endolymph in the canal. Therefore any angular (rotatory) acceleration or deceleration of the head will cause the endolymph to circulate through the canals, which in turn displaces the cupula and causes the cilia to fire.[13,121,221]

It should be emphasized that the cupula-endolymph mechanism has not evolved to be responsive to prolonged spinning at constant velocity. Numerous physiological studies[10,29,95] have demonstrated that during the beginning of rotation, the cupula is deflected from its resting position and the cilia discharge at a greater rate. If the rotation is continued, the cupula gradually reassumes its resting position in about 20 seconds and the ciliary firing is reduced. When rotation is stopped, the cupula is again deflected, but in the opposite direction because the endolymph continues to circulate through the canals. This bending of the cilia causes the firing to diminish until the endolymph comes to rest. After about 10 to 30 seconds, the endolymph stops circulating, and the cupula returns to its resting position and resumes its tonic level of discharge.

Based on this information, prolonged spinning is physiologically nonproductive. It should be remembered that the initial acceleration is the force that causes the cupula to be deflected and fire at a greater rate. Also, the semicircular canals are most responsive to short rotational movements as opposed to prolonged rotation.[?] A good formula for semicircular canal stimulation is to spin the subject approximately 10 times in 20 seconds, stop abruptly, wait about 20 seconds, and spin again at the same rate in the opposite direction. It is also beneficial to consider the position of the head while spinning. For example, if the subject is side lying on a large spinning apparatus, the endolymph in both the anterior and posterior canals will circulate, causing a more powerful response.

Spinning is not to be used without proper precautions. In infants and disinhibited patients, it may induce seizures or depress respiration. It is best to allow patients to control the initial rate of spinning or vestibular stimulation so they can accommodate to the stimulus.

Because of its diffuse connections, the vestibular apparatus has a tremendous capacity to alter electrical states within the nervous system. Generally, impulses are dispatched to key centers of the nervous system from the vestibular nuclei located at the pontomedullary junction. For instance, there are extensive interconnections to the 12 cranial nerve nuclei (III, IV, and VI in particular), the cerebellum (flocculomodular lobe), spinal motor generators,

the ANS, motor nuclei in the brainstem, postcentral gyrus of the cerebral cortex, and the reticular formation.[28,31]

To review, the receptors of the vestibule (macula) seem to be concerned with static orientation of the head in space and "directionality." In this context, directionality refers to the ability to move from a beginning point *A* to a designated point *B* without becoming disoriented or veering off in the wrong direction. For example, we rely on the macula for orientation when we are swimming under water. Because the feet are not in contact with the ground and gravitational forces are altered, the proprioceptors in joints and muscles provide little information about position in space. Thus the brain is not receiving its normal proprioceptive input from the legs and postural muscles. In addition, vision is of little assistance because to work properly, the cornea must have air in front of it. Water causes a refractive error, and vision becomes distorted.[93] Consequently, if the vestibular mechanism were not receiving gravitational feedback, the underwater swimmer would become disoriented and unable to determine the direction of the surface.

The semicircular canals detect movements of the head in all planes and are involved in the maintenance of the upright posture. The pathways of the semicircular canals are extremely important for visual gaze, ocular movements, and alignment of head and body. The connections of the semicircular canals and the otoliths work cooperatively with the joint receptors of the neck to accomplish head and neck-righting reaction.[5,75,148]

Treatment alternatives. Because the vestibular system is a unique sensory system, critical for multisensory functioning, it is a viable and powerful input modality for therapeutic intervention. Table 6-5 summarizes the receptor, stimulus, and response patterns of this system and also suggests treatment procedures. Because any static position, as well as any movement pattern, will facilitate the

Table 6-5. Vestibular system

Receptor	Stimulus	Response
Static Vestibule (sacculus, utriculus)	Pressure on hair cells caused by position of head in space (linear movements)	Biasing of lateral and medial vestibular nuclei in response to head position and gravity: Influence of ventral medial division of motor generators
Kinetic Semicircular canals	Pressure on hair follicles caused by change of direction of head in various planes (angular [rotatory] movements)	Tendency of slow movement to dampen muscle tone Tendency of rapid movement to heighten muscle tone Linked to perception of space and directionality Linked to labyrinthine righting especially a vertical head position Linked to balance reactions Linked to extraocular muscles to control visual gaze: VOR

labyrinthine system, vestibular function and dysfunction play a role in all therapeutic activities. To conceptualize vestibular stimulation as spinning or angular acceleration minimizes its therapeutic potential and also negates an entire progression of vestibular treatment techniques.[66,103,106,107] Horizontal, vertical, and forward-backward movement occurs very early in development and should be considered one viable treatment modality. These movements seem to precede side-to-side and diagonal movements, followed by linear acceleration and ending with rotatory movements. All of these movements can be done with assistance or by the client independently in all developmental patterns. *It is important to remember that the rate of vestibular stimulation determines the effects. A constant, slow rocking tends to dampen the motor system, whereas a fast spin or linear movement tends to heighten both alertness and the motor responses.* Again the vestibular mechanism is only one of many that influences the motor system. Thus the systems interaction must be constantly reassessed.

General vestibular treatment techniques. As already indicated, slow, repetitive rocking patterns, irrespective of plane or direction, generally cause inhibition of the total body responses. Yet any stimulus has the potential of causing undesired responses, such as increased tone. When this occurs, the procedure should be stopped and reanalyzed to determine the reason for the observed or palpated response. For example, assume a client, whether a child with cerebral palsy, an adolescent with head trauma, or an adult with anoxia, exhibits signs of severe generalized extensor spasticity in supine position. To dampen the general motor response, the therapist decides to use a slow, gentle rocking procedure in supine and discovers the spasticity has increased. Obviously the procedure did not elicit the desired response and alternative treatment is selected, but the reason for increased spasticity needs to be addressed.

It is possible that the static positioning of the vestibular system is causing the release of the original tone and that by increasing vestibular input the tone also increases. It may also be that the facilitory input did indeed cause inhibition, but the movement itself caused fear and anxiety, thus increasing preexisting tone and overriding the inhibitory technique. Instead of selecting an entirely new treatment approach, a therapist could use the same procedure in a different spatial plane, such as side lying, prone, or sitting. Each position affects the static position of the vestibular system differently and may differentially affect the excessive extensor tone observed in the client. The vertical sitting position adds flexion to the system, which has the potential of further dampening extensor tone. This additional inhibition may be necessary to determine whether the slow rocking pattern will be effective with this client. It would seem obvious that if a vestibular procedure were ineffective in modifying the preexisting extensor tone, then using a powerful procedure, such as spinning, is inappropriate. Selection of treatment techniques should be determined

according to client needs and disability. Clients with either an acoustic tumor that perforates into the brainstem or with generalized inflammatory disorders may be hypersensitive to vestibular stimulation while other clients, such as a child with a learning disability, may be in need of massive input through this system. See Heiniger and Randolph[103] and Farber[66,67] for in-depth analysis of various specific vestibular treatment procedures commonly used in the clinic. A general summary of the treatment suggestions is summarized in the accompanying box.

Treatment suggestions*

General body responses leading to relaxation

1. Slow rocking
2. Slow anterior-posterior: horizontal or vertical movement (chair, hassock, mesh net, swing, ball bolster, carriage)
3. Rocking bed or chair
4. Slow linear movements, such as in a carriage, stroller, wheelchair, or wagon
5. Therapeutic and/or gymnastic ball

Techniques to heighten postural extensors

1. Rapid anterior-posterior or angular acceleration
   a. Scooter board: pulled or projected down inclines
   b. Prone over ball: rapid acceleration forward
   c. Platform or mesh net: prone
   d. Slides
2. Rapid anterior-posterior motion in prone, weight-bearing patterns such as on elbows or extended elbows while rocking and crawling
3. Weight-shifting in kneeling, ½ kneel or standing

Facilitory techniques influencing whole body responses

1. Movement patterns in specific sequences
   a. Rolling patterns
   b. On elbows, extended elbows, and crawling: side by side, linear and angular motion
2. Spinning
   a. Mesh net
   b. Sit and spin toy
   c. Office chair on universal joint
3. Any motor program that uses acceleration and deceleration of head
   a. Sitting and reaching
   b. Walking
   c. Running
   d. Moving from sit to stand

Combined facilitory and inhibitory technique: inverted tonic labyrinthine

1. Semi-inverted in-sitting
2. Squatting to stand
3. Total inverted vertical position

*Remember all of these treatment suggestions involve other input mechanisms and all aspects of the motor system and its components.

General body responses leading to relaxation. Any technique performed in a slow, continuous, even pattern will cause a generalized dampening of the motor output.[115] During handling techniques, these procedures can be performed with the client in bed, on a mat while horizontal, sitting at bedside or in a chair, or standing. The movement can be done passively by the therapist or actively by the client. Carry-over into motor learning will best be accomplished when the client performs the movement actively, without therapeutic assistance. In a clinical or school setting, a client who is extremely anxious, hyperactive, and hypertonic may initiate slow rocking to decrease tone or feel less anxious or hyperactive. The reduction of clinical signs allows the client to sit with less effort and to be more attentive to the environment, thus promoting the ability to learn and adapt.

It is the type of movement, not the technique, that is critical. The concept of slow, continuous patterns is used in Brunnstrom's rocking patterns[30] in early sitting, in proprioceptive neuromuscular facilitation mat programs and in gymnastic ball exercise programs; the use of these patterns can be observed in every clinic. Although the therapist may be unaware of why Mr. Smith gets so relaxed when slowly rocked from side to side in sitting, this procedure elicits an appropriate response. The nurse taking Mr. Smith for a slow wheelchair ride around the hospital grounds may do the same thing. Once the relaxation or inhibition has occurred, the groundwork for a therapeutic environment has been created to promote further learning, such as activity of daily living (ADL) skills. The technique in and of itself will relax the individual but not create change or learning.

Motor learning will occur as the motor system adapts and modifies its responses to the existing environment and functional goals. As the client begins to succeed, repetition and variance in practice is critical. Changes in environments, such as rate of movement, angle of trajectory, support surfaces, all can place greater demands on vestibular processing and the motor system's control over balance. By using the vestibular system to dampen the generalized heightened motor generators, the control needed to modulate motor patterns during activities should be less or easier to achieve. This allows the motor programmers to practice with success. Success may be accompanied by error and thus error correction, but it still allows the motor system to determine available and usable pattern alternatives. As the client practices, changes in task demands must accompany that practice to provide variance in motor selection.[181,222]

Pelvic mobilization techniques in sitting often use relaxation from slow rocking to release the fixed pelvis. This release allows for joint mobility and thus creates the potential for pelvic movement performed passively by the therapist, with the assistance of the therapist, or actively by the client. This technique often combines vestibular with proprioceptive techniques, such as rotation and elongation of muscle groups, which physiologically modify existing fixed tonal response through motor mechanisms or systems

interactions. Simultaneously, slow, rhythmic rocking, especially on diagonals, is used to incorporate all planes of motion and thus all vestibular receptor sites to get maximal dampening effect, whether direct via vestibulospinal or indirect via cerebellum or through another motor system. The same pelvic mobility can be achieved by placing the patient (child or adult) over a large ball. The ball must be large enough for the patient to be semiprone while arms are abducted and externally rotated and legs relaxed (either draped over the ball or in the therapist's arms). Again, this position allows for maintained or prolonged stretch to tight muscles both in the extremities and trunk while doing slow, rhythmical rocking over the ball. The pelvis often releases and the patient can be rolled off the large ball to standing on a relaxed pelvis, preliminary to gait activities.

Techniques to heighten postural extensors. Any technique that uses rapid anterior-posterior or angular acceleration of the head and body while the client is prone will facilitate a postural extensor response. Scooter boards down inclines, rapid acceleration forward over a ball or bolster, going down slides prone, or using a platform or mesh net to propel someone will all facilitate a similar vestibular response of righting of the head with postural overflow down into shoulder girdle, trunk, hips, and lower extremities. Rapid movements while on elbows, on extended elbows, and in a crawling position can also facilitate a similar response. Depending on the intensity of the stimulus, the response will vary. In addition, the client's emotional level during introduction to various types of stimuli may cause differences in tonal patterns. Clinical experience has shown that facilitory vestibular stimulation promotes verbal responses and affects oral motor mechanisms. Children with speech delays will speak out spontaneously and respond verbally.

Because facilitatory vestibular stimulation biases the sympathetic branch of the ANS, drooling diminishes and a generalized arousal response occurs at the cortical level. Therefore the appropriate time to teach adaptive rehabilitative techniques is after vestibular stimulation.[75]

Facilitory techniques influencing whole body responses. One primary reason movement facilitates motor responses is that vestibular influences over motor tracts regulate tone and behavioral mechanisms. Thus rolling patterns, a rocking pattern on elbows, and extended elbows either while prone, sitting, kneeling, or standing using an elevated table—especially in fast side-to-side, linear, and angular motions—tend to elicit total-body responses. Tactile and proprioceptive inputs also assist in the regulation of the body's responses to movement.[6,67]

The vestibular system, when facilitated with fast, irregular, or angular-movement, such as spinning, not only induces tonal responses but also causes massive reticular activity and overflow into higher centers. Thus increased attention and alertness are often the outcome. The tracts going from the spinal cord, brainstem, and higher subcortical structure must be sufficiently intact to permit the desired responses from this type of input. If a lesion in the brainstem blocks higher-center communication with the vestibular apparatus, then massive input may cause a large increase in abnormal tone. The therapist needs to closely monitor any distress or ANS anomalies.

Total body relaxation followed by selective postural facilitation. The use of the inverted position in therapy has become increasingly more popular in recent years. The labyrinthine influences on posture were first studied by de Kleijn[55] and Magnus[132] in the 1920s. In a series of short papers Magnus described some studies performed with decerebrate cats, which entailed progressively positioning the cat until its head was in an inverted position. Magnus discovered that the inverted position activated the cilia of the vestibular system, which in turn promoted "extension maximum." Tokizane (cited by Payton and others[165]) replicated Magnus' and de Kleijn's work with human subjects. Tokizane used a tilt-table apparatus and electromyographic readings to gather data. Although there was a discrepancy in the angles used by the researchers, the net results were the same. Total inversion (angle of 0 degrees) produced maximal extensor tone, and the normal upright position elicited maximal flexor tonicity.[165] There seems to be much confusion in the literature about the clinical effects of inversion. Kottke[125] reports the static labyrinthine reflex is maximal when the head is tilted back in the semireclining position at an angle of 60 degrees above the horizontal. Conversely, minimal stimulation occurs when the head is prone and down 60 degrees below the horizontal position. Stejskal[194] studied the effects of the tonic labyrinthine position in spastic patients. This study failed to show labyrinthine reflexes in subjects with hypertonia.

The explanation for this incongruity seems to be one of interpretation. Any time a subject is put on a tilt table or even a scooter board, the weight bearing of the body on the surface must cause firing of the underlying exteroceptors, as well as potential fear.[59] As the body shifts and presses onto the underlying surface, stretch reflexes associated with posture must contribute some bias to muscle tone.[223] In addition, if the subject is flexing or extending the head, the proprioceptors of the neck (tonic neck reflex) could also alter the muscle tone of the limbs.[178]

Another factor that contributes to tonal changes in the extremities is the cervicoocular reflex.[9,10] Reflex eye movements to center the eyes as the body or neck rotates also exert influences on the muscles of the limbs. Since all the influences brought about by gravity and postural mechanisms in a clinical situation cannot be controlled, the inverted position does not elicit a purely tonic labyrinthine reflex (TLR). Instead, there appears to be an interplay of cutaneous receptors, proprioceptors, and tonal changes in the labyrinthine system.[164]

Several highly recognized therapists have reported using the inverted position as a therapeutic modality.[66,103,195] Generally, the inverted position produces three major changes. First, because of the gravitational forces on

circulation, the carotid sinus sends messages to the medulla and cardiac centers that ultimately lower heart rate, respiration, and resting blood pressure through peripheral dilation. This position may be contraindicated for certain patients with a history of cardiovascular disease, glaucoma, or completed stroke. Clients with unstable intercranial pressure, for example, those with traumatic head injuries, coma, tumor, or postinflammatory disorders, and many children with congenital spinal cord lesion would also be at high risk for further injury if the inverted position were used. However, this position has been used with some success for adult patients with hypertension. In any case, scrupulous recording of blood pressure and other ANS effects should be taken before, during, and after positioning.

Another benefit of the inverted position is generalized relaxation. Farber[66] recommends its use as an inhibitory technique. Because the carotid sinus stimulates the parasympathetic system, the trophotropic system is influenced and muscle tonicity is reduced. This has been found to be beneficial to patients with upper motor neuron lesions and also to children who exhibit hyperkinetic behavior. Heininger and Randolph[103] report that severe spasticity in the upper extremities is noticeably reduced.

The third benefit of the inverted position is an increased tonicity of certain extensor muscles. This phenomenon is not purely a function of the labyrinth; it is also a result of activation of the exteroceptors being stimulated by the body's contact with the positioning apparatus.[164] Therapists have capitalized on this reaction to activate specific extensor muscles of the neck, trunk, and limb girdles.[125,178,194]

The inverted position can be achieved in several ways. A child can be lowered over a ball or bolster into the inverted position. When the client is placed in a squat pattern, the head can effectively be lowered below the level of the heart. This position is more often used with children. Adults are usually seated and tilted forward until the head is in an inverted, semivertical position.

Because the inverted position decreases hypertonicity and hyperactivity and facilitates normal postural extensor patterns, the responses to the technique should be incorporated into activities. For example, if the position of total inversion over a ball is used, then postural extension of the head, trunk, and shoulder girdles and hips should be facilitated next. Additional facilitation techniques, such as vibration or tapping, could help summate the response. Resistance to the pattern in a functional or play activity would be the ultimate goal. If the inverted position is used in a squat pattern, then squatting to standing against resistance would probably be a primary goal. This can be accomplished by the therapist positioning her or his body behind and over the child—not only to direct the child initially into the inverted position but also to resist the child coming to stand. If the inverted position is used in sitting, activities of the neck, trunk, and upper extremities would be the major focus following the initial responses.

As the inverted position elicits both labyrinthine and ANS responses, this technique needs to be cross-referenced within the classification schema. Because of its ANS influence, close monitoring is important for all clients placed in an inverted position. As with all labyrinthine treatment techniques, this approach, considered a normal, inherent human response, is used outside the therapeutic setting. For example, standing on one's head in a yoga exercise causes the same physiological state as that observed in the clinic. In many respects the yoga stance is done for the same reasons: decreasing hypertonicity (generally caused by tension), relaxation, and increasing postural tone and altered states of consciousness. Clients can certainly be taught to control their own ANS activity and hypertonicity by placing their hands between their legs when they need a generalized dampening effect on motor generators.

Summary of the vestibular system. This section has described procedures that use the vestibular system as a primary input modality to alter the client's CNS. If the client's vestibular system itself is dysfunctional, it has the potential of altering the functional state of the motor system.

Hypovestibular problem: peripheral vestibular imbalance. A variety of clinical symptoms are associated with unilateral and bilateral vestibular dysfunction. Unilateral problems present as vertigo, nausea, dizziness, and postural instability, whereas bilateral problems include those mentioned before along with blurred vision, oscillopsia, and gait ataxia.[111,112] When clinical symptoms persist vestibular therapy seems to be an effective treatment approach but must be patient specific and based on whether the function of the vestibular system is reduced or absent.[89,111]

In cases of total vestibular loss, treatment approaches will either teach the client a substitution approach using proprioception and vision, or a combination approach using both substitution and adaptation in clients with reduced vestibular function. A variety of researchers[89,111,112,190] have shown therapeutic intervention to be the most effective treatment for most clients. The specifics of the adaptive treatment approach include, but are not exclusive to, head movements in many directions and various frequencies, working through nausea and/or vertigo with head movements to allow for adaptation and resolution of error signals, discouraging fixation on targets real or imaginary to eliminate voluntary control of vestibular-ocular reflex (VOR), extraocular movements (self-selected speeds), static or quiet stance (eyes open and closed), various gait width with emphasis on decreasing width, marching in place, and active neck range of motion in all directions. When using a substitution approach, visual and somatosensory systems become the focus of treatment. Exercises that encourage compensation for the VOR include active eye-hand movements as the eyes move from one preselected target to another, looking at imaginary targets in front of the client, while holding on a target visually, keeping the head in alignment while twisting the trunk back and forth and sideways. Exercises that encourage substitution of visual and proprioceptive cues to improve postural stability by performing various quiet standing and ambulatory activities include standing with feet close together and with hands on a wall and slowly decreasing time needed in upper body support; repeating this exercise with the head in a different spatial position, with eyes closed; and then beginning to walk and then decreasing the base of support, turning the head to both sides, and finally turning around while walking.[89,106,107,111,190]

Normal vestibular input with central vestibular processing deficits. Horak and others and Shumway-Cook[189] found that upon further testing, some children and adults who demonstrated clinical vestibular impairment did not have true vestibular deficits but did demonstrate impaired postural reactions under all conditions of sensory conflict between visual, vestibular, and somatosensory systems. They concluded that these patients had a central processing disorder and recommended treatment that dealt with the total sensory motor systems. Approaches such as sensory integrative theory,[143] Feldenkrais,[224] or neurodevelopmental therapy (NDT)[143] might be possible options. The critical link or recommendation would be to integrate all treatment activities into normal activities that the client is self-motivated to practice randomly.

Autonomic nervous system

The ANS has become a focus of clinical interest.[103] Traditionally, the ANS regulates, adjusts, and coordinates visceral activities. Many aspects of emotional behavior and primitive drives are controlled by the ANS.[81,158,159] Maintaining homeostasis within the body's internal environment is critical because it strongly influences the CNS response to the external world. The intricate interconnections between the ANS and CNS have led clinicians to discover viable treatment approaches that depend on both systems.[66,103] Input to the spinal cord, brainstem, cerebellum, thalamus, limbic system, and cerebrum has the potential of influencing both the somatic and visceral systems. Many tract systems, such as the reticulospinal tract, are common to both systems.[121] The importance of these interconnections seems obvious. If the external world is threatening the system, then both somatic and visceral systems need to modify responses to optimally protect the organism. For example, if your visual system identified an angry bear ready to attack you as you walk through the forest, both autonomic and somatic responses are needed. Your somatic system needs to ready your neuromuscular system for immediate action. Your autonomic system needs to ready your heart and respiration for increased rate to provide oxygen and nourishment to muscles for increased metabolism. Your emotional system needs arousal to attend to and deal efficiently with the crisis. All systems must react simultaneously and at appropriate intensities to protect the organism from imminent danger. If any system malfunctions and creates too little or too much output, imbalance and inefficiency results. This decreases your flexibility and ability to solve the problem and remove yourself from the dangerous environment[214] (see Chapter 5).

The input and processing systems, as well as the ANS itself, are often impaired in clients with brain damage. This can create ANS responses that are not always appropriate to the situation. Understanding the intricate balance of sympathetic and parasympathetic responses of the ANS and how these behaviors affect functional output are important to conceptualizing the client's total needs. All systems of the person who perceives imminent danger, whether real or imaginary, will change; the clinician will observe these altered responses to the environment, for example, in a gait session or an ADL task. Anxiety level, emotional responses, increased blood pressure, heart rate, or respiration, hypertonicity, and hyperactivity are but a few of the signs a therapist might use to identify an ANS response. These signs should alert and orient the clinician to the causes of the change. Slight alterations in the external environment are often sufficient to produce homeostasis. For example, if a kneeling client feels about to fall forward, it is important to check the patient's perception, even if the therapist believes it to be inaccurate. If the perception is wrong, then the clinician needs to help the client relearn perception of vertical. If the perception is correct, the client's response was appropriate and provided important internal feedback. Even more important, the therapist has respected and responded to the opinion and judgment of the client. This helps begin and kindle trust and mutual respect, important clinical tools for modifying the client's ANS responses to new situations.[42,81]

The ability to differentiate tone created by emotional responses versus tone resulting from CNS damage is a critical aspect of the evaluation process. Emotional tone can be reduced when stress, anxiety, and fear of the unknown have been reduced. This is true for all individuals. The client with brain damage is no exception. Seven treatment modalities that normally produce a parasympathetic response are:

1. Slow, continuous stroking for 3 to 5 minutes over the paravertebral area of the spine
2. Inversion, eliciting carotid sinus reflex and tonic labyrinthine response
3. Slow, smooth, passive and active assistive movement within pain-free range (Maitland's grade II movements)[134]
4. Maintained deep pressure on the abdomen, palms, soles of the feet, peroneal area, and skin rostral to the top lip
5. Deep breathing exercises
6. Progressive muscle relaxation
7. Cranial sacral manipulation[207]

When pressure is applied to both the anterior and posterior surfaces of the body, measurable reductions can be recorded in pulse rate, metabolic activity, oxygen consumption, and muscle tone.[197,199]

These pressure techniques are identified as an intricate part of the many identifiable approaches such as therapeutic touch,[176,214] Feldenkrais,[69,70,119,224] Maitland,[134] rolfing, and myofacial release.[11,14,138,200,201] Although not verbally identified, other techniques (such as NDT,[23,24] Rood,[67,103,195] Brunnstrom,[30] and proprioceptive neuromuscular facilitation[196]) certainly place an important emphasis on the response of the patient to the therapist's touch.

Treatment alternatives

Slow stroking. Slow stroking over the paravertebral areas along the spine from the cervical through lumbar components will cause inhibition. The technique is performed while the client is in the prone position. The therapist begins by stroking the cervical paravertebral region in the direction of the thoracic area, using a slow, continuous motion with one hand. Usually a lubricant is applied to the skin, and the index and middle fingers are used to stroke both sides of the spinal column simultaneously. Once the first hand is approaching the end of the lumbar section, the second hand should begin a downward stroking at the cervical region. This maintains at least one point of contact with the client's skin at all times during the procedure. The technique is applied for 3 to 5 minutes—and no longer—because of the potential for massive inhibition or rebound of the autonomic responses.[66,115] It is also recommended that at the end of the range of the last stroking pattern, the therapist maintain pressure for a few seconds to alert both the somatic and visceral systems that the procedure has concluded. Eastern medicine recognizes the importance of the ANS in total body regulation to a greater extent than western medicine. The concepts of meridians and acupressure/acupuncture points are all intricately intertwined with the ANS. For that reason, a technique such as slow stroking would potentially interact with meridians and does extend over the row of acupoints referred to as *shu* points and relates to visceral reflexes connecting smooth muscle and specific organ systems. It is believed that this continuous slow downward pressure modulates the sympathetic outflow, causing a shift to a parasympathetic reaction or relaxation. Whether the result of the pressure on the sympathetic chain, some energy pressure over meridian points, a pleasant sensation, or something unknown, slow stroking does elicit relaxation and calming.[67,103] Clients with large amounts of body hair or hair whorls are poor candidates for this procedure because of the irritating effect of stroking against the growth patterns and the sensitivity of hair follicles.

Inverted tonic labyrinthine therapy. See the section on vestibular procedures.

Slow, smooth, passive movement within pain-free range. Increasing ROM in painful joints is a dilemma frequently encountered by therapists caring for clients with neurological damage. We have found that by having the client communicate the first perception of pain and then move the limb in a slow, smooth motion toward the pain range, a variety of behaviors occur. First, the client generally gestures or verbalizes that pain is present 10 to 15 degrees before it may, in reality, exist. We believe this occurs because on previous occasions, the therapist has responded to the client statement of pain by saying, "Let's just go a little farther." That additional range is usually 10 to 15 degrees. We have found that if we stop impinging on the stated pain range, go back into a pain-free area, and approach again—possibly with a slight variation in the rotatory direction—the client relinquishes the safety range and a true picture of pain range is obtained. The second finding is that if the motion toward the pain range is slow, smooth, and continuous, very frequently much of the range that was initially painful becomes pain free. The hypothesis is that slow, continuous motion is critical feedback for the ANS to handle imminent discomfort. The slow pattern provides the ANS time to release endorphins, thus modifying the perception of pain and allowing for increased motion. If the therapist stabilizes the painful joint and prevents the possibility of that joint going into the pain range, rapid, oscillating movements can often be obtained within the pain-free range. This maintains joint mobility and often, as an end result, increases the pain-free range. This technique is not unique to the treatment of clients with neurological problems; it is often used as a manual therapy procedure.[72,137,140]

Manual therapy philosophy[134,204] will describe the pain and joint changes occurring at the joint level. As the fields of orthopedics and neurology merge into one system,[33] with the brain acting as an organ, controlling the entire system and its components, the question of whether the pain reduction is centrally or peripherally triggered may be an insignificant question. It is probably both.

Maintained pressure. Farber[66] discusses a variety of techniques that elicit a reduction of tone or hyperactivity. Pressure to the palm of the hand or sole of the foot, to the tip of the upper lip, and to the abdomen all seem to produce this effect. The pressure need not be forceful, but it should be firm and maintained. It is hypothesized that some, if not all, of these responses are parasympathetic.[87]

Progressive muscle relaxation. Progressive muscle relaxation is practiced both during meditation and during treatment approaches such as Feldenkrais.[118,119,224] These methods of relaxation tend to trigger parasympathetic reactions, which in turn slow down heart rate and blood pressure and triggers slow deep breathing. With so many clients with neurological injury suffering ventilatory insufficiency, it is important in some way to emphasize oxygen exchange due to the metabolic demands of exercise.

Cranial sacral manipulation. Summarizing the complexity of cranial sacral theory is not within the scope of this book. The reader is referred to references to gain a global understanding of the treatment interactions and the ANS's response to cranial therapy.[12,207]

Olfactory system: smell

The sense of smell is the least understood of all the senses. Because of the inaccessibility of the olfactory receptors, to date little research has been conducted. Unfortunately, there are more theories than facts about how we sense odors.[120]

Olfaction or the sense of smell is a chemical process. Receptors for smell are located in the olfactory epithelium in the roof of the nasal cavity between the median septum and the superior turbinate bone. The olfactory epithelium has a yellowish-brown color and contains three types of cells: the receptor cells, supporting cells, and basal cells. Interspersed among the epithelial cells are minute ducts from Bowman's gland, which secrete mucous substances onto the cells and aid in dissolving odorous materials.

The olfactory receptor cells are bipolar sensory neurons. Each cell has a single crownlike dendrite projecting to the surface of the epithelium. The distal end of this dendrite contains 10 to 20 cilia. These cilia are actually fine hairlike nerve endings. Aside from a thin layer of mucus, these nerve endings are virtually uncovered, making them the most exposed in the body.[121] Although the olfactory epithelium occupies an area only about the size of a dime, it is estimated to contain 100 million receptor cells.[31] These have an equal number of fibers but converge on principal neurons at a ratio of 1000:1.[44]

How the receptor cells transduce odors into meaningful perception of smell is not well understood. One theory, called the stereochemical theory, suggests that primary odors have specific molecular shapes. The molecular shapes of the odors are thought to correspond to molecular configurations of specific receptors. Thus certain receptors will accept a molecule the way a given lock accepts a particular shape of key.[45] There has been some support for this theory because action potential studies have shown that different odors do selectively activate some receptors and not others.[188] Other theories suggest that odorous molecules simply alter the sodium permeability of the receptor membrane and cause an inactivation of enzymes, thus changing its chemical reactions and electrical states.

Several attempts have been made to classify types of odors. In 1895, odors were grouped into nine classes, each of which contained two or more subdivisions.[226] Current findings indicate that humans can distinguish between 2000 and 4000 different odors. What is more confusing is that individual perception of the same odor will vary considerably; what is nauseating to one may be fragrant to another.[66,162]

Receptors for smell adapt rather quickly to a constant stimulus. Physiological studies indicate that olfactory receptors adapt as much as 50% in the first few seconds of stimulation.[36,172] The strength of the odor has to change by approximately 30% before the receptors are reactivated. There is also some evidence that part of the adaption takes place in the CNS.

The impulses arising in the olfactory mucosa pass along axons that pierce the cribriform plate of the ethmoid bone to enter the cranial cavity. In the cranial cavity the axons synapse on primary neurons (mitral and tufted cells) in the olfactory bulb. The axons of the olfactory bulb make up the olfactory tract (cranial nerve I) and cranial nerve V. This band of fibers courses posteriorly and fans out at the olfactory trigone. Some of the fibers terminate in the trigone, and other fibers form three diverging striae; the lateral, medial, and intermediate. The lateral olfactory stria projects to the temporal lobe of the cortex (uncus, hippocampus). The fibers proceed rostrally to the prefrontal cortex. The medial stria projects to nuclei located in the septal area of the brain below the corpus callosum. The intermediate stria terminates in the anterior perforated substance. The medial and intermediate striae are not well developed in humans.[36,121]

There are also a number of secondary association fibers that course to important subcortical nuclei. For example, impulses are transmitted to the autonomic nuclei of the hypothalamus. Although this connection is not well understood, it has been demonstrated in mammals to be associated with reproduction.[149,150] It has also been demonstrated that olfaction is not mediated exclusively by the olfactory nerve. The nasal region also derives sensory innervation from branches of the trigeminal nerve. Experimental evidence shows that the trigeminal fibers respond to burn smells and also make a general contribution to the sense of smell. With some severe head injuries the cribriform plate and the olfactory epithelium are ruptured. Although the sense of smell is severely compromised, some odor sensation may be preserved via the fibers of the trigeminal nerve.[98,121]

One of the most remarkable characteristics of the olfactory system is that some impulses travel from the receptors via alternative routes and synapses to the temporal lobe without passing through the thalamus. All other major sensory systems pass through a relay in the thalamus en route to the cortex.

The primary olfactory cortex (temporal lobe) projects efferent impulses to cortical and subcortical structures. Output to the thalamus, hypothalamus, and limbic system is believed to influence behavior and emotion. Pleasant odors, such as vanilla or perfume, can evoke strong moods. Unpleasant odors can facilitate primitive protective reflexes, such as sneezing and choking. Sharp-smelling substances like ammonia can elicit a reflex interruption of breathing.[146]

As a result of arousal, protective reflexes, and mood changes caused by odors, the use of smell as a treatment modality has been implemented especially during feeding procedures. Odors such as vanilla and banana have been used to facilitate sucking and licking motions.[193] Ammonia and vinegar have been used clinically to elicit withdrawal patterns and increase arousal in semicomatose patients.[116] When using odors as a stimulant, the therapist must be aware of all behavior changes occurring within the client. Arousal, level of consciousness, tonal patterns, reflex behavior, and emotional levels—all can be affected by odor. Because of limited research in this area, caution must be exercised to avoid indiscriminate use of the olfactory system. Odors such as body odor, perfumes, hair spray, and urine can affect client's behavior even though the smell was not intended as

a therapeutic procedure. Some clients, especially those with head traumas and inflammatory disorders of the CNS, often seem to be hypersensitive to smell. In these cases the therapist needs to be aware of the external olfactory environment surrounding the client and to make sure those odors that are present facilitate or at least do not hinder desired response patterns.[63]

Many clinical questions arise regarding smell as a therapeutic modality. If the choice of odors is pleasant versus noxious, a pleasant odor will theoretically be perceived in a way that should be enjoyable, relaxing, and thus potentially tone reducing. On the other hand, noxious odors should have a sympathetic reaction and, although alertive, may also create a fight/flight internal reaction that, if repeated frequently, could cause an adverse response to the client's perception of the world. This has the potential of having a profound effect on his or her feelings toward the therapist and the therapeutic environment. The effect may not be observable until the client reaches a level of consciousness or motor skill in which he or she has some ability to react.

Gustatory sense: taste

The sense of taste is a chemical sense, involving not only the receptors of the tongue, but also olfaction and tactile receptors. Therefore the term *taste* encompasses not only gustatory sensations derived from food, but the smell, temperature, and texture of the material to be ingested.[40]

Taste receptors are found in the tongue, soft palate, and the beginning of the throat. The receptors for taste are complicated end organs of the neuroepithelium commonly called taste buds. Most of the taste buds, which are located on the tongue, are distributed in definite patterns. Taste buds are surrounded by raised structures called papillae. These papillae are visible on the surface of the tongue and give it a roughened appearance. The papillae vary in shape and form, and each papilla is surrounded by a small depression or moat. Taste buds can be found on the crest of the papilla or more commonly in the depressions. The papillae are distributed in three different locations. On the base of the tongue are seven to twelve circumvallate papillae arranged in a V configuration. Scattered over the entire dorsal surface are small papillae called the *fungiform*. A third type, called *foliate papillae,* are closely packed along the sides of the tongue.[110] They are well developed in children but less numerous in adults.[31]

Each taste bud is made up of approximately 50 receptor cells. Each bud contains supporting cells, basal cells, and receptor cells. The receptor cells have hairlike projections (microvilli) passing into the pore opening. These microvilli increase the surface area and probably help to trap molecules flowing through the moat surrounding the papillae.[44]

The physiology of taste is rather complicated. Because it is a chemical sense, only substances that dissolve in water or saliva can be tasted. Once the water-soluble substances are bathed in fluid, they can diffuse through the taste pore and come in contact with microvilli of the receptor cells. Although the mechanism is not well understood, the contact appears to evoke generator potentials followed by action potentials in the nerve terminals.[67,160,168]

Four primary taste sensations have been identified: salty, sour, bitter, and sweet. These primary tastes are believed to blend together in various combinations to form additional tastes, similar to the way mixing the colors yellow and blue produces green. Histologically, the taste buds appear to be the same, yet they tend to be selective to specific stimuli. Action-potential studies have shown that any one taste bud will respond to all four primary tastes.[96] However, the quantitative responses differ considerably, allowing some buds to respond more vigorously to bitter and some to sour, sweet, or salty stimuli. It is also commonly known that regions of the human tongue vary in sensitivity to the four primary tastes. The base of the tongue best detects bitter, the sides sour, and the tip is sensitive to sweet substances. The ability of taste buds to discriminate changes in concentration of a substance is relatively crude; a 30% change in concentration is needed before a difference in taste intensity is detected.[160]

The number of taste buds on the front, sides, and back of the tongue varies from 500 to 1200.[44] Taste buds have a tremendous capacity to reproduce. The average life span of a taste bud is 7 to 10 days. Each cluster of taste buds (approximately 20) contains mature and young cells; the mature lie toward the center of the cluster.[85]

Afferent transmission of impulses from taste receptors may travel to the CNS by three cranial nerves. Taste sensations from the base of the tongue are served by the glossopharyngeal nerve (cranial nerve IX); the sides and the tip are served by the vagus nerve (cranial nerve X) and the facial nerve (cranial nerve VII). The pharyngeal surface of the tongue is innervated by the laryngeal branch of the vagal nerve (cranial nerve X). Taste buds begin to degenerate during the fifth decade of life, contributing to diminished taste sensation in the elderly.[44,45]

Taste sensation adapts rapidly. Action-potential studies have shown that when first stimulated, taste buds fire a burst of impulses and only partially adapt. As with the olfactory system, the additional adaption is suspected to come from the CNS.[121,150]

Afferent taste impulses transmitted from the tongue and pharyngeal region pass through branches of the appropriate cranial nerves (facial, glossopharyngeal, and vagal) to the solitarius tract in the brainstem. The fibers of the first-order neurons terminate in portions of the nucleus solitarius. The second-order neurons send a number of collaterals to reticular nuclei before crossing to the opposite side of the brainstem and coursing to the ventral posteromedial nucleus of the thalamus. Before reaching the thalamus, other collaterals project to nuclei associated with reflex activity. The third-order neuron transmits signals to the somatesthetic region of the parietal lobe.[31,76,121]

Gustatory input is generally used as part of feeding and prefeeding activities. As already mentioned, the oral region is sensitive not only to taste, but also to pressure, texture, and temperature. For that reason feeding would be classified as a multisensory technique that uses gustatory input as one of its entry modalities. Specific input modalities are based on the combined taste, texture, temperature, and affective response pattern. That is, a banana and an apple both may be sweet, yet the textures vary greatly. When mashed, both fruits may have a puddinglike texture, yet the client's emotional response may differ. Disliking the taste of banana but enjoying apple may cause startling differences in the client's response to various sensations. Although feeding and other complex treatment procedures are discussed in more detail under the classification of combined sensory systems, the importance of the clinician's sensitivity to the client's response patterns within each sensory modality cannot be overemphasized.[67]

Auditory system

The auditory system is fundamental to survival and also to human communication. Together with vision, the auditory system enables human beings to perceive events in the external world that takes place at a distance from the body as well as to localize in space the exact position of the sound.[31]

The auditory nerve shares a common cranial nerve (VIII) with the vestibular system, thus creating a close anatomical and physiological relationship between these two senses.[76,144] Thus individuals with hearing loss may show simultaneous vestibular imbalances. Approximately 10% of adults suffer to some extent from hearing loss. Therapists need to discuss with clients whether they have difficulty hearing specific tones or frequencies. Similarly, clients with auditory figure-ground problems will have difficulty hearing in noisy environments, and compensatory types of communication may need to be used.

The anatomy and physiology of the ear are described only briefly here—with greater emphasis placed on the characteristics of the auditory receptors.

The organ of hearing consists of three components: the external, middle, and internal ear. The ear receives sound waves that are radiated from some source in the external environment. Sound waves are directed by the external ear, travel through the auditory meatus, then strike the tympanic membrane (eardrum) and cause it to vibrate. These vibrations move a series of three small articulating bones (malleus, incus, and stapes) that extend from the tympanic membrane to the inner ear. The chain of three bones is attached to two muscles, the tensor tympani and stapedius. These minute muscles serve as a protective mechanism (tympanic reflex) during excessive stimulation. Strong sound waves elicit contraction of the tensor tympani muscle, causing increased tension on the tympanic membrane.[31,121]

The ossicles serve as a mechanical receptor that converts

sound waves to fluid motion in the cochlea. The fluid motion causes pressure waves that stimulate receptor cells, and the stimulus is once again converted to an electrical-chemical impulse.[40,121]

The organ of hearing is located in the cochlea, which is a fluid-filled tube resembling a small shell that spirals around itself two and a half times. The space within the bony canal of the cochlea is divided into three compartments by the vestibular and basilar membranes. The upper compartment is called the scala vestibuli. The scala vestibuli ends at the oval window and receives pistonlike action from the stapes to produce pressure waves in the perilymph. The lower compartment, the scala tympani, ends at the round window. The round window serves as a dampening mechanism for the pressure waves. The scala vestibuli and scala tympani connect at the apex of the spiral, and both contain perilymph. The third compartment, the cochlear duct (scala media), is bordered by the vestibular and basilar membranes. Lying on the basilar membrane of the cochlear duct is a complex structure consisting of numerous receptor cells. This is the organ of Corti, the sensory mechanism for hearing. The organ of Corti consists of cilia, groups of supporting cells, and fibers from bipolar neurons derived from the spiral ganglion. The receptor cells are cilia similar to the receptors of the vestibular system—with an estimated 23,000 cilia on the basilar membrane of each cochlea.[40,121]

The receptor cells of the organ of Corti have some specific characteristics. First of all, they do not have axons. Actually, they transmit directly to the dendrites of the bipolar cells in the spiral ganglion. The inner cilia may have only one dendrite attached, whereas the outer cilia receive synaptic input from many bipolar ganglion cells.

The arrangement of the cilia and the tectorial membrane is such that a movement of the basilar membrane causes the cilia to bend against the tectorial membrane. Therefore when sound strikes the ear, vibrations are passed from the tympanic membrane to the ossicles and converted to hydrodynamic waves in the cochlea. The basilar membrane vibrates up and down in response to the frequency of the sounds. The mechanical bending or shearing of the cilia releases chemical transmitter substances at their basal pool. This constitutes the adequate stimulus, and action potentials in the bipolar cells cause neuronal transmission.[121]

The auditory pathway to the CNS is very diffuse. Impulses pass from ciliary receptors along nerve fibers of the spiral ganglion to synapse on neurons in the dorsal and ventral cochlear nuclei in the upper region of the medulla. The second-order neurons project mainly to the opposite side of the brainstem and terminate in the superior olivary nucleus. However, some of the second-order neurons do not cross and ascend to the superior olivary nucleus on the same side. Other collaterals pass directly to the reticular-activating system. There are also important connections to the cerebellum, particularly in the event of a sudden noise.[31,121]

The majority of the impulses reaching the superior olivary nucleus ascend by way of the lateral lemniscus, which continues to the inferior colliculus. The next group of neurons continues to ascend and synapse in the medial geniculate nucleus, a sensory nucleus of the thalamus. From this juncture impulses fan out along the auditory radiation to reach the auditory cortex at the superior temporal gyrus, or area 41. At this very small area of the cortex, a sound is "heard," but more specific recognition requires connections with additional auditory associative centers.[44,121]

The inferior olivary nuclei regulated by descending and feedback pathways from the auditory system send projections to the superior olivary complex. Efferent neurons leaving the lateral olivary nucleus are projected ipsilateral via the cochlear nerve to both the inner and outer hair cells of the cochlea. The efferents are important to auditory sensitivity and selective tuning of the cochlea. With this efferent control over the auditory afferents, the cortex has a way of focusing in on certain sounds while ignoring others.[31] This may be the mechanism for auditory figure-ground or selective hearing.

Treatment alternatives. Because of the complexity of the auditory system, a potentially large number of input modalities exists. Although some of them might not be considered traditional therapeutic tools, they are nonetheless techniques that affect the CNS. Some treatment alternatives focus on:

Quality of voice (pitch and tone)
Quantity of voice (level and intensity)
Affect of voice (emotional overtones)
Extraneous noise (sound)
Auditory biofeedback
Language

Levels, volume, and affect of voice. The therapist's voice can be considered one of the most powerful therapeutic tools.[57] Even, constant sound has the ability to cause adaptation of the auditory system and thus inhibition of auditory sensitivity.[34] Similarly, intermittent, changing, or random auditory input can cause an increase in auditory sensitivity.[82] Because of auditory system connections, an increase or decrease in initial input or auditory sensitivity has the potential of drastically affecting many other areas of the CNS.[61] The connections to the cerebellum could affect the regulation of muscle tone. The collaterals projecting into the reticular formation could affect arousal, alertness, and attention, in addition to muscular tone. The importance of voice level has been acknowledged by colleagues for decades with respect to encouraging clients to achieve optimal output or maximal effort. The use of voice levels is a critical aspect of the entire PNF approach.[81,196] Yet the volume or intensity of a therapist's voice is only one aspect of this important clinical tool. Through clinical observation, we have observed that clients respond differently to various pitches. The response patterns and specific range of comfortable pitch seem to be client dependent. The concept that each individual may have a range within the musical scale or even a specific note that is optimal for his or her biorhythm function has been posed by one composer-musician.[27] This concept needs research verification but may prove to relate to one of those innate talents some therapists have that distinguish them as gifted therapists.

The emotional inflections used by the clinician certainly have the potential of altering client response. For example, assume the therapist asks Tim, a child with cerebral palsy, to walk. The specific response from the child may vary if the clinician's voice expresses anger, frustration, encouragement, disgust, understanding, or empathy. Knowing which emotional tone best coincides with a client's need at a particular moment may come with experience or sensitivity to others' unique needs.

Extraneous noise. The varying level of sound or extraneous noise in a clinical setting can at times be overwhelming. Dropping of foot pedals, messages over loud speakers, conversations, typewriters, telephones, moans, a jackham mer outside the clinic, water filling in a tank, a drip in a faucet, whirlpool agitators, a burn patient screaming, a child crying—all are encountered in the clinical environment, and all could be occurring simultaneously. A therapist, whose CNS is intact, usually can inhibit or screen out most of the irrelevant sound. A client with CNS damage may not have the ability to filter his or her sensitivity to all these intermittent noise sensations. The protective arousal responses these sounds might produce in a client could certainly elevate tone, block attention to the task, heighten irritability, and generally destroy client progress during a therapy session. Awareness of the noisy environment and the client's response to it is important not only to treatment modalities; it is also critical to the problem-solving process.

Decreasing auditory distracters or sudden noises can drastically improve the client's ability to attend to a task and/or succeed at the desired movement.[91] The therapist is reminded that if the environment has been externally adapted for a client to procedurally practice successfully the goal, then independence in that functional skill has not been achieved. Reintroduction of the noises of the external world must be incorporated into the client's repertoire of responses so that the individual can feel competent in dealing with any auditory environment the world might present.

Music as an adjunct to therapy has been suggested as a viable way to help clients develop timing and rhythm to a movement sequence (see Chapter 21 for a discussion of basal ganglia disorders). Consistent sound waves and tempos, such as soft music, allow the patient to develop a neuronal modal or an engram for the stimulus. The use of background music during therapy sessions enables the patient to make an association to the sounds, producing an autonomically induced-relaxation response to a particular musical composition.[46]

Music is used for encouraging not only motor function, but also memory[173] and socialization.[161,171] Rhythmic sound perceived as an enjoyable sensation certainly has the effect of creating motor patterns in response to that rhythm. Individuals, young and old, will tap their fingers or feet to a beat. If the beat has words people will often sing along recalling from memory the appropriate words. The movement, memory, and willingness to interact are all critical aspects of the therapeutic environment.[1] Having clients dance with a significant other twice a day to music they have enjoyed in the past encourages both the physical function and the social bonding so important for quality of life.[3] Music affects heart rate, blood pressure, and respiration. It has even been suggested that easy listening music may bolster the immune system.[42,78,192]

Auditory biofeedback. Biofeedback as a total therapeutic modality is discussed under the treatment section in Chapter 30. Auditory biofeedback is generally thought of as a procedure in which sound is used to inform the client of specific muscle activity. The level or pitch may change in relation to strength of muscle contraction or specific muscle group activity. Yet auditory biofeedback also encompasses feedback as simple as a foot slap that communicates that a client's foot is on the floor or verbal praise after a successful therapeutic session. The importance of the auditory feedback system as a regulatory mechanism between internal and external homeostasis cannot be overlooked. However, the clinician should not assume that this system is intact and can automatically be used as a normal feedback mechanism for clients with CNS damage.[1,94]

Language. Although most therapists thoroughly appreciate the complexity of the language system as a whole, they have little if any in-depth background to help them understand the components or the sequences leading to the development of language.[35] Thus many therapists are extremely frustrated when confronted with clients who show perceptual or cognitive deficits involving the auditory processing system. The reader is referred to Chapter 26 to better understand the development of the language system and alternative treatment methods appropriate for use with clients having difficulty within this area.

Therapists easily identify language comprehension difficulties with adults who have first language differences and with young children due to their age and lack of language experience. Nevertheless, many clients have language processing dysfunction that lead to communication difficulties, both in reception and appropriate expression. The elderly often can understand a conversation in a quiet room, but have difficulty in rooms that are noisy.[61] The environment within which communication occurs can drastically affect both reception and the ability to express back to the world inner feelings and thoughts.[42] Creating an environment conducive to that exchange will dramatically affect the motivation and drive of a patient within the therapeutic setting.[78]

Visual system

Vision is considered the most important and relied-on sense. The eye is also the most complex of all the sense organs in our body. Its uniqueness is attributed to the biochemical or biophysical mechanism used to transduce a light stimulus to a neurological action potential. Rather than review the anatomy of the eye in great detail, this discussion will focus on tracking a light stimulus through the eye and describing some of the salient processes that occur en route to visual perception.

The stimulus for vision is light. Light is electromagnetic energy that travels outward in waves at a rate of 186,000 miles per second. Light entering the eye first passes through the cornea and then through a clear, viscous fluid called the aqueous humor. The next structure light passes through is an opening in the iris known as the pupil. The amount of light allowed through is regulated by the diameter of the pupil. Next, the light passes through the lens and vitreous humor (a gelatinous material) and reaches the retina, where light energy is transformed into neuronal-electrical impulses.[31,121,158]

The retina lines a major portion of the inside of the eye. It is composed of three distinct layers of cells: the photoreceptor layer, the bipolar cell layer, and the ganglion cells. Light must first travel through the ganglion and bipolar cells to reach the sensory photoreceptors.

There are two types of photoreceptors: the rods and cones. The rods, which number about 120 million, are reactive to light intensity, that is, shades of gray. Unable to distinguish different colors, rods are said to provide "night vision." The cones (about 6 million) are responsible for color vision and require more light energy to become activated. The rods and cones are fairly evenly distributed throughout the retina. However, a central part of the retina, called the *fovea* (macula lutea), is in direct line with the lens and cornea. Therefore when we fixate on an object, the image of that object is projected upside down and backward on the fovea.[114,121]

The rods and cones are unique sensory receptors. As light enters the eye, it strikes the rod and cone cells and is absorbed by pigments (photopigments) contained in these cells. This stimulus produces a chemical reaction that results in a change in the movement of ions through the cell membranes of the bipolar cells. This ionic movement generates an action potential in the afferent axons of the bipolar cells. Synaptic activity occurs between the bipolar and ganglion cells. The ganglion cell axons project posteriorly and leave the eye in an area called the optic disk. The ganglion axons combine to form the optic nerve.[96,121,182]

The rods and cones require a rich blood supply to maintain their metabolic functions. The major blood supply is derived from the choroid, a layer between the retina and the sclera. The choroid has a pigmented layer that absorbs light not transduced by the rods and cones. In addition, this structure is a storage site for vitamin A, a necessary element for reproduction of the visual pigments used by rods and cones for the absorption of light energy.

The visual pathway begins at the optic foramen. Each optic nerve consists of about 1 million nerve fibers. The combined 2 million nerve fibers of both optic nerves make up about 38% of all sensory and motor fibers entering and leaving the CNS.[121]

The optic nerve contains two types of fibers: large, fast-conducting fibers concerned with visual perception and small, slower-conducting fibers concerned with reflexive activity. The optic nerve fibers originate from nasal and temporal portions of the retina to form the retinogeniculate fibers. These fibers project directly to the optic chiasm just anterior to the pituitary gland. At this juncture a partial crossing of fibers takes place. Fibers originating in the nasal halves of each retina cross at the chiasm. Conversely, the fibers originating in the temporal portion of the retina pass through the chiasm without crossing. The fibers from the temporal side also carry the fibers from the fovea (macula), where visual acuity is sharpest.[114,121]

Once the optic nerve passes through the optic chiasm, it is referred to as the optic tract. The two optic tracts continue uninterrupted to the left and right lateral geniculate bodies of the thalamus and to midbrain centers (superior colliculus and pretectal region). Fibers terminating in the lateral geniculate bodies give rise to the geniculocalcarine tract (optic radiations). These fibers spread out as they go and turn posteriorly to the occipital lobe of the cortex. The principal location of the visual receptive cortex is the area surrounding the calcarine fissure, which encompasses Brodmann's areas 17, 18, and 19. Area 17 is the site where the optic radiations terminate. Functionally, area 17 is said to be associated with conscious but not with interpretive vision; areas 18 and 19 are believed to be involved in associative aspects of visual perception.[114]

The visual system is extremely helpful to physicians and medical personnel for diagnosing disorders of the CNS. The eye provides a window through which a physician can examine the integrity of blood vessels and neurological tissue. Because the system extends through so much of the subcortical and cortical regions of the brain, many disorders manifest themselves in the visual system. Aside from the more obvious visual-field problems, nervous system disorders can interrupt visual reflexes and impede eye movements.

Eye movements are subserved at the cortical and subcortical levels. Areas 18 and 19 of the occipital lobe produce a reflexive visual pursuit in response to visual stimuli. Voluntary eye movements elicited on command derive from neurons in the frontal lobe of the cortex (area 8). Protective reflexes, such as blinking and quick localization of eyes, head, and neck toward a startling stimulus, are mediated by the retinotectal system (superior colliculus). Reflex eye movements activated by rotation of the head are mediated at the brainstem level by the vestibular system. The size of the pupil and lens is reflexly controlled by light stimulus. Pretectal areas, such as the Edinger-Westphal nucleus of cranial nerve III, act on the sphincter muscle of the iris and the ciliary muscle. Psychosocial research has demonstrated that pupils dilate and constrict in response to emotional feelings elicited by a visual stimulus.[45] Objects that are pleasing to the eye cause the pupil to dilate, whereas repugnant visual stimuli constrict the pupil. The higher-level cortical association pathways are very complex, and our understanding of them continues to grow.[121]

Child development studies suggest that the efficiency with which an infant uses its eyes is a strong indicator of verbal ability and performance on intelligence tests.[25] The therapist should reinforce eye pursuits by pointing out objects in the environment and by encouraging the hand to follow the eye toward the object. According to Stejskal,[194] as the eyes turn toward an object, the head has a natural tendency to turn, and when the neck rotates, a volley of neuromuscular events takes place that better enables the upper extremities to perform a task such as reaching. Program generators are much more than a pure reflex action and thus manifest motor response with great adaptability and variability within the environment.

Because of the complexity of the visual system, treatment procedures can vary from simple to extremely complex. Simple treatment alternatives, such as hues or types of lighting, are often overlooked by therapists, yet they have the potential of altering patient response. Complex treatment procedures, such as those discussed in Chapter 27, are also often ignored by therapists because of lack of understanding of and frustration with the visual system. Although we are not suggesting that all therapists become experts in visual processing and training, clinicians should become more aware of this input system, its potency as a treatment modality, and, when damaged, its devastating effect on normal response patterns.

Treatment alternatives. To help the therapist obtain a better understanding of treatment alternatives, a variety of categories (each encompassing a spectrum of treatment considerations) follows.

1. Colors (such as room, clothes, objects)
   a. Hues: brightness usually alerts the CNS and increases tone, whereas dark colors decrease muscle tone[67]
   b. Colors and shades of color: for example, pinks versus blues
2. Types of lighting: fluorescent, incandescent, or sunlight
3. Degree of visual complexity within environment
   a. Isolated room, blank walls with one floor mat
   b. Busy clinic with a table mat in the center of the room
4. Cognitive-perceptual sequential treatment methods— for example, figure and ground, depth, visual object

permanency, visual position in space, spatial relationships
5. Treatment approaches to compensate for deficits in other sensory systems
6. Internal visualization

Because light is an adequate stimulus for vision, any light, no matter the degree of complexity, has the potential to affect a client's CNS. That input not only reaches the optic cortex for sight recognition and processing, but also projects to the cerebellum via the tectocerebellar tract, and affects the reticular-activating and limbic systems via the interneuronal pathway. It even has influence over cervical spinal generators via the tectospinal tract.[31,71] Thus as long as light is entering a client's CNS, that stimuli has the potential of altering response patterns either directly—via the tectospinal system or the corticospinal system via occipitofrontal radiations—or indirectly through the influence of the ANS and limbic system on muscle tone resulting from emotional levels.[56]

The five categories of visual-system treatment alternatives should not be considered fixed, all-inclusive, or without overlap. The first three categories (color, lighting, and visual complexity) are common everyday visual stimuli. Combined, they make up the visual world.

Colors. By varying the colors or by changing hues, tones, or the type of lighting and degree of complexity of the combined visual stimuli, the treatment modality and the way the CNS processes change.[90,202,211] Because the visual system tends to adapt to sustained, repetitive, even patterns, any input falling under those parameters should elicit visual adaptation.[85,121,172] This response will lead to decreased firing of sensory afferent fibers and have an overall effect of decreasing CNS excitation. A clinician would expect to see or palpate a decrease in muscle tone, a calming of the client's affective mood, and a generalized inhibitory response. Cool colors, a darkened room, monotone color schemes—all seem to have an inhibitory effect.

In contrast, intermittent visual stimuli, bright colors, bright lights, and a random color scheme seem to alert the CNS and have a generalized facilitatory effect.[47] Research in the area of criminology is producing evidence to suggest that specific shades of colors can produce either a sedating response (such as certain pinks) or general arousal (certain blues).[157] Although a tremendous amount of research is required to substantiate these results if the clinician is to apply them with confidence, research is beginning to show that specific shades of colors and hues may drastically affect a client's general response to the world and specific response to a therapy session.[209] Within the next few years, many facts regarding the reaction of the CNS to specific visual stimuli may be uncovered, and the clinician will be responsible for integrating this new information into the present categorization scheme.[179] In Holland at the Institute de Hartenbuer, playrooms have been designed in different colors.[77] Except for color all rooms are exactly the same and originate from a central hub or core.[77] Children are allowed to select which room they wish to play or be treated in. Children seem to pick the color room that most suits their moods, alertness and creates an environment in which they can learn.[77]

Lighting. Two types of lighting are found in a clinical environment. Fluorescent or luminescent lighting comes by definition from a nonthermal cold source. This type of lighting is generally emitted by a high-frequency pulse. Umphred[205] has found that many individuals within a normal population complain that this high-frequency flutter is irritating and causes distraction. For this reason, it is recommended that each clinician observe clients' responses to various types of lighting to determine whether fluorescent visual stimuli cause undesirable output. This is especially true with clients who already have an irritated CNS, such as with inflammatory disorders or head trauma. The clinician should also remember that clients frequently lie supine and look directly at overhead lighting, while the therapist looking at the client is unaware of that particular visual stimulus.

Incandescent lights by definition come from hot sources and emit a constant light without a frequency. The brightness of this type of lighting has the potential of altering CNS response. The visual system quickly responds to bright lights with pupil constriction. Following prolonged exposure to a bright environment, the visual system adapts and becomes progressively less sensitive to it.[85,121] Similarly, when exposed to darkness, the retina becomes more sensitive to small amounts of light. Because of the response of the visual system to incandescent lighting, it is recommended that a therapist monitor the brightness of the lighting, especially preceding any type of visual-perceptual training or visually directed movement.

Although the sun is a natural source of light, it is not generally the primary source in a clinical setting. The sun can effectively be used as indirect lighting, thus eliminating the problems produced by artificial lighting. Sunlight is also more acceptable psychologically. Some clinics have designed the buildings to allow for maximum use of natural light.[75]

Visual complexity. The visual system is the primary spatial sense for monitoring moving and stationary objects in space.[105] An infant continually refines the ability to discriminate objects in external space until capable of identifying specific objects amid a complex visual array.[172] When brain damage occurs, the ability to identify objects, localize them in space, pick them out from other things, and adapt to their presence may be drastically diminished.[7] Because of the distractibility of many clients, reducing the visual stimuli within their external space can help them cope with the stimuli to which they are trying to pay attention. Using rooms that have been stripped of such stimuli as furniture and pictures can reduce not only distractibility but also hyperactivity and emotional tone. If this method of reduction of stimuli is used, the clinician must remember that this

procedure has a sequential component. The client must once again adapt to extraneous visual stimuli. Thus as the client's coping mechanisms improve, the therapist needs to monitor and change the visual environment. The therapist can monitor the amount of input according to the response patterns of the client but in time needs to have the client function in everyday environments and practice adaptation.

Cognitive-perceptual sequencing with the visual system. This large category is the focus of many professionals' entire career. In sighted individuals the visual system is important in integrating many areas of perceptual development, such as body schemes, body image, position in space, and spatial relationships.[7] Vision as a processing system is so highly developed and interrelated with other sensory systems that, when intact, it can be used to help integrate other systems.[104] Simultaneously, if the visual system is neurologically damaged, it can cause problems in processing of other systems.

For example, assume a child is asked to walk a balance beam while fixating on a target. The child is observed falling off the beam. On initial assessment vestibular-proprioceptive involvement would be primarily suspected. On further testing the therapist might discover that the child, while looking at the target, switches the lead eye in conjunction with the ipsilateral leg. As the child switches from right to left eye, the target will seem to move. Knowing the wall is stationary, the child will assume the movement is caused by body sway, will counter the force, and will fall off the beam. The problem is a lack of bilateral integration of the visual system versus other sensory modalities. The visual system deficit is overriding normal proprioceptive-vestibular input in order to avoid CNS confusion. Unfortunately, the client is attending to a deficit system and negating intact ones. This visual conflict would be overriding normal processing of intact systems.

This same problem of the visual system overriding other inputs is often seen when clients are trying to relearn the concept of verticality. Clients with hemiplegia who demonstrate a "pusher" syndrome illustrate this conflict. Because the intact visual system can often be used to help reintegrate other sensory systems, the reverse should also occur. Teaching clients to attend to vestibular-proprioceptive cues while vision is occluded or visual stimuli tremendously reduced will help them orient to intact systems. Once the orientation is reestablished, visual input will often be perceived in a more normal fashion.

Familiarity with the visual-perceptual system and its interrelationships with all aspects of the therapeutic environment is crucial if the clinician is to have a thorough concept of the client's problem. (See Chapter 27 for specific information regarding visual deficits and treatment alternatives.)

Compensatory treatment alternatives. The visual system can be used effectively as a compensatory input system if the sensory component of the tactile, proprioceptive, or vestibular system has been lost or severely damaged. The procedure of using vision in a compensatory manner should not be attempted until the clinician is convinced the primary systems will not regain needed input for normal processing. Although vision can direct and control many aspects of a movement, it is not extremely efficient and seems to take a tremendous amount of cortical concentration and effort.[205,206] Vision was meant to lead and direct movement sequences.[105,194] If used to modify each aspect of a movement, it cannot warn or inform the CNS about what to expect when advancing to the next movement sequence. Thus using vision to compensate eliminates one problem but also takes the visual system away from its normal function. For example, assume a hemiplegic man is taught to use vision to tell him the placement of his cane and feet, thus decreasing his need to attend to proprioceptive cues. When advancing to ambulatory skills such as crossing the street, the client may be caught in a dilemma. As he is crossing the street, if he attends to the truck coming rapidly down the road, he will not know where his cane or foot are and thus become anxious and possibly fall. If, on the other hand, he attends to his foot and cane, he will not know if the truck is going to hit him. That may increase emotional tone and make it difficult to move. If normal sensory mechanisms could be reintegrated, this client would have freedom to respond flexibly to the situation. Thus caution should be exercised to avoid automatic use of this high-level system to compensate for what seem to be depressed or deficit systems.

Visual input should be used to check or correct error if other systems are not available. Movement should be programmed on a feedforward mode unless change is indicated. Vision often recognizes the need for that change. If a client is taught a motor strategy in which vision is used as feedback to direct each component of the pattern, the pattern itself will generally be inefficient and disorganized and will lack the automatic nature of feedforward procedural motor plans. If the client is too anxious to practice the procedure physically without overusing vision, then visual mental practice can be introduced.

Internal visual processing. The use of visualizing some aspect of bodily function has been and continues to be used in many forms of therapy.[26] It has been shown that individuals can modulate their immune responses through visualization.[192] Smith and others[192] showed that individuals could dictate through their thoughts and visualization various control over what was thought to be mindless internal processes. Athletic trainers have used mental imaging with athletes for years to reinforce the motor pattern needs to be programmed during an event. These concepts have been used therapeutically but usually when the client is resting or totally relaxed.[69,70,224]

Today, these concepts can be integrated during active treatment in a variety of ways. Before a client begins to initiate a plan of movement the therapist could ask the client to close his or her eyes and imagine the movement and what

it felt like in that functional activity before the CNS injury. In this way, the patient is using prior memory and visualization to access the motor systems and hopefully initiate better motor plans. Similarly, if during a movement plan the state of the motor generators builds to such a level that the client is becoming dysfunctional, the therapist can stop the movement, ask the client to visualize a calm quiet place, and then continue with the movement pattern when the tone is reduced or extraneous patterns cease.

Another way to use the visual system to access the processing strategies of the client is to observe his or her eye gaze. Neurolinguistic theory postulates that the eyes gaze in the direction of brain processing.[8,120,145] Fig. 6-8 illustrates the eye gaze direction along with the suggested processing activity. For example, a client who needs to access and processes motor plans via frontal lobe will look down. A client who needs to visually construct an idea of something new will look up and to the right. Various cortical lobes and hemispheres serve specific global processing functions. There are many ways to apply and interpret this theory. By observing the patient's eye gaze, the therapist can determine if processing is conducted in what would be believed to be the appropriate areas. Even more clinically relevant is observing where the eyes are gazing before and during successful functional activities. It may be that the area once used in processing is no longer available to do the function. If gaze to the right and down always leads to motor success, then the therapist can empower the patient to look down and right before dressing or transferring. Similarly if a patient always looks down at the feet during ambulation, the reason may not be "to look at the feet," but instead may be accessing the motor cortex to gain better motor function. By asking the client to visualize the movement before and during the activity, the head often comes to a posturally correct position as the eyes gaze upward toward the occipital lobe. If the client is asked to walk while visualizing the movement, again the

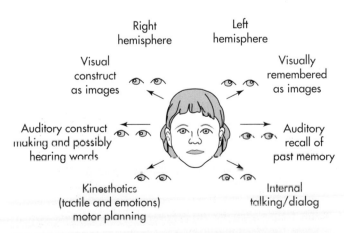

Fig. 6-8. Eye gaze: correlation with lobe and hemispheric processing based on right handed individuals. (Adapted from: handout from New Learning Pathways: Denver, 1988. Illustrations by Ben Burton.)

therapist may find a more upright, posturally efficient pattern. Once the program is set and practice scheduling begun, the patient may no longer need to look down and into the frontal lobe. Thus in this case, the client not only learned the procedure but also avoided practicing and learning a posturally incorrect ambulation strategy.

CLASSIFICATION OF MULTISENSORY TREATMENT TECHNIQUES

Although all techniques have the potential of being multisensory, the specific mode of entry may focus on one sensory system, as already described, or it may target two or more input modalities. Table 6-6 categorizes a variety of treatment techniques that are clearly multisensory. Since new methods of treatment are discovered daily, this table is not all inclusive, but it allows the clinician to identify familiar techniques and their multisensory input channels. The therapist, analyzing how the summated effect of the combined input influences client performance, gains direction in anticipating treatment outcomes in terms of the problem-solving process. Because the potential combinations of multisensory classification are enormous, only a few examples of combinations are included in the text to illustrate the process a clinician might use when classifying a new technique.

As mentioned in Chapter 1, many therapeutic techniques used to assist client learning are contrived and need to be eliminated from the therapeutic environment to achieve true independence in functional activity. The clinical decision regarding which technique should be dropped first must be based on client need. Yet a simple rule a therapist might follow would be to choose the least natural technique. That technique would be the most artificial or contrived. For example, a therapist might teach a client to assist with elbow flexion during a feeding pattern by (1) vibrating the biceps, (2) quick tapping the biceps, or (3) quick stretching the biceps a little beyond midrange using gravity. The first option would be the least natural and obviously the least socially acceptable at a dinner party. The third option is the most natural and closest to the real environment the client will need to function within. Remember, these contrived techniques are used to assist clients who cannot perform the motor strategy or functional activity without assistance or who need assistance in learning to modulate motor control for greater functional adaptability and independence.

Combined approaches

Proprioceptive: tactile integration

Sweep tapping. Many isolated techniques, such as sweep tapping[67] or rolling,[30] would be considered primarily proprioceptive-tactile in sensory origin. During *sweep tapping* the clinician first uses a light-touch sweep pattern over the back of the fingers of one of his or her hands. This stimulus is applied quickly over the dermatome area, innervating the muscles the client is to contract. Second, the therapist applies some quick tapping over the muscle belly of the hypotonic muscle. The first technique is tactile and believed to stimulate the reflex mechanism within the cord to heighten motor generators and increase the potential for muscle contraction. The second aspect, tapping, is a proprioceptive stimulus used to facilitate afferent activity within the muscle spindle, thus further enhancing the client's potential for muscle contraction. At the same time the client will be asked to voluntarily move to activate the entire motor system.

Rolling of the hand. Before Brunnstrom's rolling pattern is implemented, the client's upper extremity is placed above 90 degrees to elicit a Souques's sign, which decreases abnormal excessive tone in the arm, wrist, and hand.[30] This phenomenon may well be a proprioceptive reaction of joints and muscle. The rolling technique consists of two alternating stimulus patterns. The wrist and fingers are placed on extensor stretch. The ulnar side of the volar component of the hand is the stimulus target. A light-touch sweeping pattern is applied to the hypothenar aspect, which has the potential of eliciting an automatic opening of the hand beginning with the fifth digit.[30] Immediately after the light touch, a quick stretch is applied to the wrist and finger extensors. These two techniques are applied quickly and repeatedly, thus giving the visual impression that the therapist is rolling his or her hand over the ulnar aspect of the dorsum of the client's hand. In reality, tactile and proprioceptive stimuli are being effectively combined to facilitate the extensor motor neurons leading to the wrist and fingers. Because the tone is felt in the client's extensors and thus induces relaxation of the spastic flexors, the therapist can easily open the client's hand. As the client obtains volitional control, some resistance can be added by the therapist to further facilitate wrist and finger extension. A hemiplegic client can also be taught to use this combined approach to open the affected hand and give it increased range. This technique is a noninvasive, relaxing approach to opening the hand stuck in wrist and finger hypertonicity. The technique itself seems to trigger spinal generator patterns that dampen the existing neuron network. It does not teach the patient anything unless that individual begins to assist or take over control of the extensor pattern. This usually occurs first by the therapist feeling the flexors relax when the patient is trying to extend the wrist and fingers even if no active extension is palpated. Encouraging the patient at this time that he or she is thinking correctly is very important to motivate continued practice.

Withdrawal with resistance. A therapist could combine the technique of eliciting a *withdrawal* with *resistance* to the withdrawal pattern. This can be an effective way to release spastic tone, especially in the lower extremities. The withdrawal can be elicited by a thumbnail, a sharp instrument, a piece of ice, or any adequate light-touch stimulus to the sole of the foot. As soon as the flexor withdrawal is initiated, the therapist must resist the entire pattern. Once the resistance is applied, the input neuron network changes and the flexor pattern is maintained through proprioceptive input. The one difficulty with this technique is the application of resistance. The withdrawal pattern directly affects alpha motor neurons innervating those muscles responding in the flexor pattern and simultaneously suppresses alpha motor neurons going to the antagonistic muscles. If the antagonistic muscles are spastic, then initially the spasticity is suppressed. Because of the pattern itself, as soon as the flexor response begins, a high-intensity quick stretch has been applied to the extensor muscles. If resistance is not applied to the flexors to maintain inhibition over the antagonistic muscles, the extensors will respond to the stretch. The client will very quickly return to the predisposed spastic pattern and may even exhibit an increase of abnormal tone. This extensor response is a complex reaction within the spinal generators. The therapist should instruct the patient to assist with the flexor pattern to recruit other components of the motor system in order to enhance the system's modulation over the spinal generators.

Modification of a hypersensitive touch system. Another example of a proprioceptive-tactile treatment technique is modification of a hypersensitive touch system through a touch-bombardment approach. The goal of this approach is to bombard the tactile system with continuous input to elicit light-touch sensory **adaptation** or desensitization. Deep pressure is applied simultaneously to facilitate proprioceptive input and conscious awareness. Proprioceptive discrimination and tactile-pressure sensitivity are thought to be critical for high-level tactile discrimination and stereognosis. A hypersensitive light-touch system elicits a protective, altering, withdrawal pattern that prevents development of this discriminatory system and the integrated use of these systems in higher thought. This method of treatment can be implemented by having an individual dig in sand or rice. The continuous pressure forces adaptation of the touch system, and the resistance and deep pressure enhance the proprioceptive-discriminatory touch system by a very complex adaptation process that most likely affects all areas involved in light and discriminatory touch, as well as the complex interaction of all motor system components.

Pool therapy can be used effectively for the same purpose with the added advantage of neutral warmth. Any client perceiving touch as noxious, dangerous, and even life threatening will not greatly benefit from any therapeutic session in which touch is a component part. Touch includes contacts such as touching the floor with a foot, reaching out and touching the parallel bar railings, and touching the mat. The client may not respond with verbal clues such as "Don't touch me" or "When I touch the floor it hurts" but will often respond with increased tone, emotional or attitude changes, and avoidance responses. Nevertheless, this treatment approach has application in many areas of intervention with clients having neurological deficits. As an adjunct to this method, a clinician should cautiously apply light touch when in contact with the client. Deep pressure or a firm hold should

elicit a more desirable response for the client even if the light-touch system is functional.[87,199] The use of gortex material for clothing can greatly enhance the client's ability to tolerate the external world where light-touch encounters cannot be avoided.

The therapist may also consider systematic desensitization as strategy to integrate the touch system. By allowing patients to apply the stimuli to themselves, they can grade the amount that they can tolerate. In this respect they are empowered to control their own environment. They can practice adaptation in many situations. When the environment seems overwhelming, they have learned techniques to dampen the input both from within their own systems and by controlling the external world. For example, the therapist may place a box containing objects of different textures before the patient and encourage exploration and active participation to learn which textures are acceptable or offensive. A gradual exposure to the offensive stimuli will raise the threshold of the mechanoreceptors in the skin. There are also the benefits to the patient being in control of the stimulus and having awareness of the treatment objective. In addition, vibratory stimuli through a folded towel provide proprioceptive input to desensitize the touch system.[7,87,212] Desensitizing the touch system from a need to protectively withdraw is an important process within the CNS if normal stereognosis is to develop.

Orthokinetic cuff. The use of an *orthokinetic cuff* is another example of a proprioceptive-tactile treatment approach. The concept of orthokinetics is credited to Julius Fuchs,[19] an orthopedic surgeon who was dissatisfied with "common static devices" for the correction of fracture dislocations and scoliosis.[16] The term *orthokinetics* is derived from Greek; roughly translated it means "righting of motion." Having observed the problems of prolonged immobilization, Fuchs wanted to design a dynamic device that used tactile and proprioceptive stimulation.

Today, the orthokinetic cuff is made from rubber-reinforced elastic bandage material. Half of the bandlike cuff is designed to be elastic and to stretch; this is called the *active field.* The other half of the cuff is sewn in a criss-cross fashion to reduce its stretch; this is referred to as the *inactive field.* The active field of the cuff is worn over the muscle belly to be activated, and the inactive field is placed over the antagonistic muscle. The client wears the cuff during therapeutic exercise or in some cases throughout activities of daily living.

Orthokinetic orthoses have been reported to remediate both dyskinesia and pain.[9,153-156] Whelan[218] conducted a study on the use of orthokinetics on the upper extremity of the adult hemiplegic patient. She reported significant results in the reduction of spasticity and an increase in active range of motion. Blashy and Fuchs[19] reported successful results with 81 of 100 clients over a 4-year period.

The neurophysiological rationale for the orthokinetic cuff has not been fully established. Nevertheless, some important

Table 6-6. Combined input sensory systems: treatment modalities

Technique	Proprioceptive: joint, tendon, spindle	Exteroceptive	Vestibular	Gustatory	Olfactory	Auditory	Visual	ANS	Inherent response Labeled	Inherent response Not labeled
Sweep tapping[66]	X	X							Automatic extension of hand	
Brunnstrom's rolling (hand)[30]	X	X								?
Raimiste's sign[30]	X	X								
Stretch pressure[66]	X	X								
Digging in sand, etc.	X	X					?			
Gentle shaking[66]	X	X	X							
Prone activities over ball[35,66]	X	X	X				X		Automatic righting of head (tectospinal/ vestibulospinal)	
Sitting activities on ball[35]	X	?	X				X	X	OLR and equilibrium (all systems)	
Mat activities	X	X	X			?	?			
Resistive exercises										
1. Resistive rolling	X	X	X			If verbal command	If visual leads			Rotatory integration
2. Resistive patterns: PNF[124,196]	X	X	Depends on pattern			X	X			
3. Resistive gait	X	?	Depends on pattern			If verbal command	X			
4. Isokinetics	X	Some					X			
5. Wall pulleys	X		X (if done in body rotation)				X (if guided toward target)			
6. Rowing[30]	X	?	X			If verbal command	X			Body rotation
Feeding[35,66,152]										
1. Maintained pressure: walking to back of tongue	X	X		?	?					
2. Resistive sucking										
a. Straw	X	X		?	?					
b. Popsicle	X	X		X	X				X	
3. Use of textures										
a. Peanut butter	X	X		X	X				X	
b. Apple sauce	X	X		X	X					
4. Maintained pressure to top lip	X	X						X	Automatic closing of mouth	

									Comments
Inverted TLR [66,103]	X	X			X		X		
Touch bombardment [66]	X	X			X	X	?	X	Decreased hypersensitive tactile system and thus withdrawal pattern stereognosis
1. Tactile discrimination in sand, etc.									
2. Pool therapy	X	X						X	
Joint compression more than body weight [13-195]	X	X			X				
Throwing and catching									
1. Balloon	?	X			X	X	?	?	? (withdrawal to light touch)
2. Heavy ball	X	?			?	X		Result of light touch	
Variance in movement									
1. Quick action directed by vision	X				X	X			
2. Postural activities in front of mirror	X				?	X			
3. Therapist using voice command to assist client with movement	X			X	X				
High-level movement									
1. Walking balance beam	X	X		?	X	?	X		Labyrinthine righting and equilibrium; possible OLR
2. Trampoline activities	X	X			X	If visually directed			
3. Running, jumping, skipping	X	X			X	If visually directed	X		OLR and equilibrium

variables have been identified. First, it appears that the best results are obtained when the cuff is worn on the extremities. It would appear that the postural muscles do not lend themselves to orthokinetics because of their more postural function. Sensory receptors within extremity musculature tend to adapt, whereas receptors found in postural muscles do not readily adapt.[64] Second, the cuff should fit snugly— not enough to impede circulation but enough to apply circumferential pressure. Obviously, this cutaneous stimulation should activate the exteroceptors of the skin and afferent neurons of the muscle spindle. Thus the active field of the cuff would provide touch pressure and a pinching stimulus. In theory, the active field elicits action potentials in both the exteroceptors and proprioceptors resulting in an increased modulatory effect on motor generators and leading to ultimate motor neuron activity. The inactive field would appear to provide sustained deep pressure, which produces a dampening response. The research to date confirms the need for combining active and inactive kinetic fields for the cuff to be effective. However, which field provides the strongest influence on the nervous system has not yet been verified;[37,87,154] and whether the motor system will be able to internally self-regulate will depend on its plasticity and degree of damage.

Another important component of orthokinetics is the use of therapeutic exercise. Incorporating active resistive exercises using the shoulder wheel, pulley apparatus, machinery, weights, the stationary bicycle, etc., should provide sustained resistance to promote motor learning and long-term motor adaptability.[19,191]

The last and most obvious variable is the placement of the cuff. For patients with spasticity, the active (elastic) field should be placed over the weaker muscle in need of facilitation, whereas the inactive (inhibitory) portion should cover the hypertonic muscles.[156]

The concept of orthokinetics has given rise to dynamic splinting devices for upper-extremity hypertonicity. Several dynamic orthokinetic splints and slings have been developed in recent years, and they appear to be more successful than previous attempts at static splinting. Most of the devices are based on variations of the principles derived from orthokinetics. (For a more thorough discussion of the concepts of orthokinetics and the therapeutic application of orthotics, see Chapter 32.) Tapping procedures used in peripheral orthopedic muscle imbalances and pain have the same potential for patients with neurological problems. This adaptation would be a modification of both splinting and slings.

Proprioceptive, tactile, and gustatory input. The complexity of combined proprioceptive-tactile input becomes enhanced by adding another sensory input, such as taste. Implementations of one of a variety of feeding techniques clearly identifies the complexity of the total input system. When taste is used, smell cannot be eliminated as a potential input, nor can vision if the client visually addresses the food. The following explanation of feeding techniques is included to encourage the reader to analyze the sensory input, processing, and motor response patterns necessary to accomplish this ADL task. The complexity of the interaction of all the various systems within the CNS is mind boggling; but if the motor response is functional, effortless, and acceptable to the client and the environment, then the adaptation should be encouraged.

Several feeding techniques have been developed by Knickerbocker,[123] Mueller,[152] Farber,[67] Rood,[180] and Huss.[115] These techniques are not easily mastered or understood through reading alone. Competency in feeding techniques is best achieved from empirical experience under the guidance of a skilled instructor. The following techniques are eclectic, and they have been adapted for basic understanding.

Oral motor facilitation. The facial and oral region plays an important role in survival. Facial stimulation can elicit the rooting reaction. Oral stimulation facilitates reflexive behaviors, such as sucking and swallowing. Deeper stimulation to the midline of the tongue causes a gag reflex. These reactions and reflexes are normal patterns for the neonate. When these reactions/reflexes are depressed or hyperactive, therapeutic intervention is a necessity. Oral facilitation is an important treatment modality for infants and children with CNS dysfunction. Therapeutic intervention during the early stages of myelination can be crucial to the development of more normalized feeding and speech patterns.

Similarly, adults suffering neurological impairment often have difficulty with oral motor integration. Problems with swallowing, tongue control, hypersensitive and desensitive areas within the oral cavity, and problems with mouth closure and chewing are frequently observed in adults with CNS damage.

Before describing basic feeding techniques, some significant neurology should be highlighted. The innervation of the facial and oral musculature is complex. Therefore only the salient information pertaining to feeding is described here.

Facial sensation is conveyed by the trigeminal cranial (V) nerve. The fibers of the trigeminal nerve are among the earliest to become myelinated. This nerve contains both sensory and motor components. The sensory root of the trigeminal nerve contains two types of fibers: exteroceptive and proprioceptive. The exteroceptive fibers originate from cutaneous receptors of the face and head and enter the trigeminal ganglion through three branches: ophthalmic, maxillary, and mandibular.[31,121] The ophthalmic and maxillary are purely sensory fibers; the mandibular division contains sensory and motor fibers. As the fibers from the three divisions come together in the trigeminal ganglion, they enter the brainstem at the level of the pons and terminate in one of two nuclei. Some fibers descend, becoming the spinal trigeminal tract, and send collaterals to the trigeminal nucleus. These descending fibers convey pain and temperature sensation and participate in a variety of preprogrammed motor behaviors that, without adequate modulation from the cerebellum and cortical structures, will present as stereo-typical responses.[44] Other fibers ascend and terminate in the principal sensory nucleus. These fibers subserve two-point discrimination, pressure, and touch. Cutaneous innervation of the occipital region of the scalp and the dorsum of the upper neck is supplied by spinal roots C2 and C3.[220]

Proprioceptive fibers rise from deep structures, such as the muscles of mastication, temporomandibular joint (TMJ), and ligaments and fascia of facial expression. The proprioceptive fibers have their cell bodies in the mesencephalic nucleus of the trigeminal nerve in the caudal portion of the mesencephalon. This represents the only example of first-order neuron cell bodies located within the brain. The pathways from the mesencephalic nucleus are not well understood, but the nucleus is believed to have projections to the cerebellum, motor nuclei of the brainstem, reticular formation, and the thalamus.[62,98]

The motor branch of the trigeminal nerve controls the muscles of mastication. These muscles include the masseter, temporalis, and medial and lateral pterygoids. The integrity of the mastication muscles is evaluated by having the client move the mandible from side to side or bite down on a tongue depressor.[67]

The process of chewing is a complicated motion requiring movement in all four directions. This movement is permitted by the TMJ. The TMJ and its supporting ligaments provide proprioceptive feedback concerning jaw position and force of bite. The alignment of this joint is very critical. Slight malocclusion has been associated with chronic pain and headaches. Other branches of the motor root control the tensor tympani, tensor veli palatini, mylohyoid, and the anterior belly of the digastric muscle.[66]

The muscles of facial expression are innervated by the facial nerve. Sensory branches provide proprioception from muscles of facial expression, exteroception from the external ear, and taste sensation from the anterior two-thirds of the tongue. The facial nerve also has a motor component to the stylohyoid and digastric muscles, stapedius muscle of the ear, and various secretory glands of the eyes and mouth. Certain muscles of the soft palate and tongue are innervated by branches of the trigeminal, facial, hypoglossal, glossopharyngeal, and vagal nerves.

The tongue is a versatile organ with tremendous mobility. It plays a role in taste sensation, mastication, swallowing, and speech articulation. The tongue is also a discrete tactile receptor. The most precise two-point discrimination in the body is found on the tip of the tongue. The tongue also contains muscle spindles. Tongue proprioception and movement are controlled by the hypoglossal nerve (cranial nerve XII).[97,121]

Feeding therapy is preceded by observation and assessment. With a pediatric client, the therapist should observe breathing patterns while the client is feeding to determine if the child can breathe through the nose while sucking on a nipple. In addition, the child's lips should form a tight seal around the nipple. Formal assessments should include functional assessments, developmental milestones, and behavioral manifestations. Medical charts and results from neurological examinations should be consulted for baseline data.

Postural mechanisms can influence feeding and speech patterns in clients with neurological dysfunction.[178,195] A client with a strong extensor pattern may have to be placed in the side-lying, flexed position to inhibit the forces of the TLR pattern. The ideal pattern for feeding is the flexed position, which promotes sucking and oral activity. Basic reflexes such as rooting, sucking, swallowing, and bite and gag reactions should be elicited and graded in children and evaluated in adults.

As already indicated, the facial region and the mouth have an extraordinary arrangement of sensory innervation. Therefore oral techniques must be used with utmost care. Anyone who has visited the dentist can attest to the feeling of invasiveness when foreign objects are placed in the mouth. With this in mind, the therapist should begin each treatment session by moving the autonomic continuum toward the parasympathetic end. Activation of the parasympathetic system should lower blood pressure, decrease heart rate, and, more important, increase the activity of the gastrointestinal system. Neutral warmth, the inverted position, and slow vestibular stimulation should help to promote parasympathetic "loading." Another approach that is applicable to feeding techniques is the application of sustained and firm pressure to the upper lip. An effective inhibitory device is a pacifier with a plastic shield that applies firm pressure on the lips. Perhaps this is why a pacifier is a "pacifier." Adults can acquire resistive sucking patterns with a straw and plastic shield and achieve the same results.

Sometimes children or adults are not cooperative and will not open their mouths. Rather than pry the mouth open, the jaw is pushed closed and held firmly for a few seconds. On releasing the pressure, the jaw reflexively relaxes. The receptors in the TMJ and tooth sockets may be involved in the production of this response.

The facial and trigeminal nerves work in concert to augment reflexes in the muscles of mastication. A common problem seen in neurologically impaired infants and adults with head trauma is the "hyperactive tongue," which is often accompanied by a hyperactive gag reflex. To alleviate this problem, the receptors have to be systematically desensitized. The technique, called *tongue walking,* has met with clinical success.[66,103] It entails using an instrument such as a swizzle stick or tongue depressor to apply firm pressure to the midline of the tongue. The pressure is first applied near the tip of the tongue and progressively "walked back" in small steps. As the instrument reaches the back of the tongue, the stimulus sets off an automatic swallow response. The instrument is withdrawn the instant the swallow is triggered. This technique is repeated anywhere from 5 to 30 times a session, depending on individual responses.

Another technique, which might be called *deep stroking*

is used to either elicit or desensitize the gag reflex. Again, an instrument such as a swizzle stick is used to apply a light stroking stimulus to the posterior arc of the mouth. The instrument should lightly stretch the lateral walls of the palatoglossal arch of the uvula. Normally, the palatoglossus muscle elevates the tongue and narrows the fauces (opening between the mouth and the oral pharynx). Just behind the palatoglossal arch lies another called the palatopharyngeal arch. Normally, this structure elevates the pharynx, closes off the nasopharynx, and aids in swallowing. Touch pressure to either arc incites the gag reflex. This touch pressure should be carefully calibrated. A hyperactive gag reflex may be best diminished by prolonged pressure to the arcs, whereas light, continuous stroking may be more facilitory in activating a hypoactive gag reflex. A child or adult who has been fed by tube for extended periods of time will often have both hypersensitive reactions in various parts of the oral cavity and hyposensitive areas in other locations. This needs to be assessed in order to formulate a complete picture of the client's difficulties.

The use of vibration over the muscles of mastication appears to be physiologically valid. Muscle spindles have been identified in the temporal and masseter muscles.[48] Selected use of vibration on the muscles of mastication enhances jaw stability and retraction. To facilitate protraction the mandible is manually pushed in.[67,101]

To promote swallowing, some therapists use manual finger vibration in downward strokes along the laryngopharyngeal muscles and follow up with stretch pressure. Ice is beneficial as a quick stimulus to the ventral portion of the neck or the sternal notch. In addition, chewing ice chips provides a thermal stimulus to the oral cavity and a proprioceptive stimulus to the jaw and teeth; it also increases salivation for swallowing.

Certain foods can be used to stimulate salivation. The sight of a dill pickle stimulates salivation in certain individuals. Ingestion of milk tends to thicken saliva, whereas warm beef broth thins saliva. Sweet flavors are universally accepted, and secretion increases with taste concentrations that are watered down. Concentrations of the same flavor should be increased by 30% so that difference in taste intensity is detected.

The therapist can quickly realize that feeding as a proprioceptive, tactile, and gustatory input modality is extremely complex and often incorporates other sensory systems. Breaking down the specific approaches into finite techniques helps the clinician categorize each component and then reassemble them into a whole. The job of dividing and reassembling the parts becomes more and more difficult as the number of input systems enlarges.[214]

Proprioceptive and vestibular input. Proprioceptive and vestibular input is one of the most frequently combined techniques used by therapists. In fact, client success in almost all therapeutic tasks depends on the coordinated input of these two sensory modalities.

Head and body movements in space. If the head is moving in space and gravity has not been eliminated from the environment, vestibular and proprioceptive receptors will be firing to inform the CNS whether it should continue its feedforward pattern or adapt the plan because the environment no longer matches the programmed movement. Depending on the direction of the head motion and the way gravity is affecting joints, tendons, and muscle, the specific bodily response will vary according to the degree of flexibility within the motor system. Bed mobility, transfers, mat activities, and gait all incorporate these two modalities. Although all these functional movements can be performed without these feedback mechanisms, the CNS can not adapt effectively to changing environments without input from these systems. For that reason alone a thorough assessment of the integrity of both systems and the effect of their combined input seems critical if any ADL activity is to be used as a treatment goal.

The use of a large ball or a gymnastic exercise ball can be classified under the category of proprioceptive-vestibular input. Many activities can be initiated over a ball. When a child or adult is prone on a ball, righting of the head can often be elicited by quickly projecting the child forward while the therapist exerts control through the feet, knees, or hips. As the head begins to come up, approximation of neck can be added. Vibration of the paravertebral muscles might also assist. Rocking forward or bouncing the client who is weight bearing on elbows or extended elbows would facilitate postural weight-bearing patterns via the two identified sensory input systems. Having a client sitting on a gymnastic ball doing almost any exercise will require vestibular and proprioceptive feedback to make appropriate adaptive responses. The combination seems to play a delicate role in maintenance of normal righting and equilibrium response so important in functional independence.

A trampoline, equilibrium board, or a similar apparatus has the potential of channeling a large amount of vestibular-proprioceptive input into the client's CNS. In fact, a trampoline is so powerful it can often overstimulate the client and cause excitation or arousal in the CNS.

The trampoline and balance boards are generally used to increase equilibrium reactions, orient the client to position in space and to verticality, and increase postural tone. A client with poor equilibrium, poor postural tone, or inadequate position in space and verticality perception may be justifiably fearful of these two apparatuses because of the rate, intensity, and skill necessary to accomplish the task. Because fear creates tone and that tone may be in conflict with the motor response from the client, caution must be exercised with either modality. Refer to Chapter 28 for further discussion of the interactions of sensory systems and balance.

Gentle shaking. A specific technique of gentle shaking can be listed under a combined vestibular, muscle spindle, and tendon category. This technique is performed while the client is in a supine position and the head ventroflexed in midline. The head is flexed 35 to 40 degrees to reduce the influence of the otolithes and unnecessary extensor tone via lateral vestibulospinal tract. This flexed position should be maintained throughout the procedure. The therapist places one hand under the client's occiput and the other on the forehead. Light compression is applied to the cervical vertebrae. This technique activates the deep-joint receptors (C1 to C3) and muscle spindles in the neck along with the vestibular mechanism, which in turn connects with the cerebellum and motor nuclei with the brainstem. If the technique is performed slowly and continuously in a rhythmical motion, total body inhibition will occur. If the pattern is irregular and fast, facilitation of the spinal motor generators will be observed.

Any one of these techniques can be implemented as a viable treatment approach in considering vestibular-proprioceptive stimuli. The selection of an approach or a method will depend on client preference, client response, the clinician's application skills, and the need for therapeutic assistance.

Modalities: auditory, visual, vestibular, tactile, and proprioceptive

Most, if not all, therapeutic activities activate five sensory modalities: auditory, visual, vestibular, tactile, and proprioceptive. Auditory and visual input are used as the therapist talks to the client and demonstrates the various movement or response patterns to be accomplished during an activity. As the client moves, vestibular, tactile, and proprioceptive receptors are firing. Thus the complexity of any activity with respect to analysis of primary input systems is enormous. Even a sendentary activity like card playing requires a certain amount of proprioception for postural background adaptations, tactile input from supporting body parts and limbs, and visual input for perception and cognition.

The tactile and proprioceptive sensory information is usually filtered by the reticular formation so the cortex can be "sensitive" to the stimuli. At the same time, visual input is formulating higher-order perceptions of the images projected on the retina. The turning of the head, postural control, and quick ocular pursuits bring in the vestibular mechanism.

Thus when considering the categorization of techniques—such as a PNF slow reversal,[124] a Brunnstrom marking time,[30] marking time with music,[3,46] Feldenkrais' sensory awareness through movement,[69,70] neurodevelopmental therapies,[23,37] Rood's mobility on stability,[180,195] or any mat or ADL activity—the therapist must observe the sensory system being bombarded during the activity. At the same time, if the therapist has determined which sensory systems are intact, which are suppressed, and which seem to be registering faulty data, then altering duration and intensity of stimuli through any one system and the combined input through all modalities creates tremendous flexibility in the clinical learning environment. Highly gifted therapists seem

to know instinctively which input systems to use. Simultaneously, they sense the quantity and duration of combined input that best meets the needs of the client. They also seem to know when to release external control and encourage the client to use normal inherent monitoring systems to adapt to changing environments. The key to carry-over will be the client's empowerment over his or her motor control system and the degree of practice, self-monitoring, and adaptation available to the client. By analyzing and categorizing input as well as patients' responses, many therapists may develop skills that were initially considered out of reach.

INNATE CNS PROGRAMMING

The responses of peripheral and central nervous systems (PNS and CNS) to various external stimuli determine the individuality of an organism and its survival potential in the environment. As organisms become more and more complex, the types of external stimuli as well as the internal mechanisms designed to deal with that input also increase in complexity. As the CNS develops structurally and functionally, inherent control over and responses to certain common environmental stimuli seem to be manifested. Different areas of the motor system play different roles in the regulation of motor output. No area is dominant over another. Each area is interdependent on both the input from the environment and the intrinsic mechanisms and function of the nervous system.

As mentioned before, the PNS is intricately linked to the CNS and vice versa. Damage to one could potentially alter the neuropathways, their function, and ultimately behavior anywhere along the dynamic loops. Nevertheless, although researchers today emphasize the dynamic interactions of all components (II STEP and APTA conference), clinicians have observed for decades different motor problems when different areas of the brain are damaged. Thus when discussing clients with neurological damage, it seems paramount to identify inherent synergy patterns available to humans, especially if those patterns become stereotypical and limit the client's ability to adapt to a changing environment.*

The author does not recommend or discredit the use of any stereotypical or patterned response as a treatment procedure. She is only acknowledging their presence and stressing the importance of knowing how these motor programs affect client responses. Without this knowledge, therapists working with either children or adults with CNS dysfunction limit their understanding of the normal CNS, normal motor control mechanism and its components, and the interactive effect of all systems on the end product: a motor response to a behavioral goal.

Overview of patterned responses

For decades it was generally thought that patterned responses were hard-wired and that if a lesion occurred responses were released from control and were exhibited as

* References 39, 52, 73, 74, 103, 110, and 141.

a reflex or stereotypical behavior.[49] This structure was fixed in a hierarchical design where the spinal system was the lowest level and the cortex the master controller. Relearning was also thought to be based on development and developmental sequencing.

Clinicians have observed for years the inconsistencies in this hierarchical/developmental model through clients' behavior. For example, a client might demonstrate equilibrium patterns thought to be cortical while still presenting extensor reflex patterns thought to be spinal or lower brainstem. The same client may be able to ambulate but not roll over. These inconsistencies become explainable with the adoption of a systems model. The reader is referred to Chapters 2, 3, and 4 for an in-depth analysis of motor development, the use of motor control and learning theories, and evaluation procedures used to differentiate the components of motor control. This chapter focuses on classification of alternative methods that activate or assist in activating neuronetworks to help the client produce desired responses.

To conceptualize a systems model, the reader must replace the hypothesis of a stimulus-response based concept of reflexes to a theory of neuronetworks that may be more or less receptive to environmental influences. That sensitivity is modulated by a large number of interconnecting systems throughout the CNS, as well as the internal molecular sensitivity of the neurons themselves. Specific patterns seem to be organized or programmed at various levels or areas within the CNS. These synergies or patterned responses are thought to limit the degrees of freedom available to programming centers such as the basal ganglia and cerebellum[53,122] and enable more control over the entire body. Having soft-wired preprogrammed patterned responses allows organizing systems to activate entire sequences of plans as well as modify any components within the total plan. Modification and adaptation then become the goal or function of the motor system in response to both internal and external goal-directed activities. The specific location of soft-wired programs is open to controversy as is the complexity of programming at any level within the CNS. The following discussion identifies motor patterns observed in humans and possible levels of their programming organization.

Recognizing that these neuronetworks exist with or without external environment influences would suggest that patterns can and will present themselves without an identified stimulus. In the past when an external influence was not correlated with an identifiable stereotypical motor pattern, it was referred to as a synergy. When a stimulus was identifiable, the entire loop was called a reflex. Reflexes and preprogrammed soft-wired neuronetworks such as walking are interactive or superimposed on one another to form the background combinations for more complex program interactions. This superimposed network may encompass spinal and supraspinal coactivity, which makes it very difficult to specify a level of processing. The exact control mechanisms

that regulate the specific pattern may again be a shared responsibility throughout the nervous system, thus providing the plasticity observed when disease, trauma, or environmental circumstances force adaptation of existing plans.

One way to conceptualize this complex neuronetwork is to picture a telephone system linking your home to any other home in any city in any country on earth. If the relay between a friend in New York and you in California develops static, the system may self-correct, relay through another area, or even traject through a nonwired mechanism such as a satellite. The options are infinite but priorities for efficiency, and adaptability exist both within the telephone network and the brain. If the wires to your home are cut the phone will not ring. If your peripheral nerve is cut or the alpha motor neuron damaged, the muscle will not contract. If the relay centers at one end of your block are short circuiting and not working properly, then your phone and those of your neighbors may still function, but not in a fluid or specific manner. That is, someone may be calling your neighbor but both your phone and your neighbor's phone might ring. Spinal involvement can create a similar problem. The muscles are innervated, the input from the environment accurate, but the neuronetwork faulty. Regulation or modulation may be less efficient or controlled, but the system will use all available resources to try to respond to internal and external environmental requirements. This rule seems consistent throughout the nervous system, and the degree of plasticity is tremendous.[57]

When specific patterned responses are observed, the reader must always hold simultaneously the interaction of all other motor programming options. In this way the therapist can easily conceptualize the variations within one response and the reason why, under different environmental and internal constraints, the motor response pattern may show great variations within the same general plan. Similarly, the expected motor response may not be observable even though it would seem appropriate and anticipated. The clinician must remember that the more complex the action (e.g., rolling versus dressing versus playing hockey), the greater the need for integration and coordination over pattern generators. Similarly, the more complex the desired action (especially in new learning), the greater the potential for needed perceptual/cognitive and affective interactions, as well as the greater the potential for gratification and also for failure.

Certain patterned responses or neuronetworks might be considered more simplistic or protective in function. These patterns were once thought to be hard-wired spinal reflexes. It is now known that these reflexes, as well as very complex pattern generators, exist at the spinal level and that their responses effect brainstem, cerebellar, and cortical actions. These centers simultaneously affect the specifics of the spinal neuronetwork responses. With clients who have low functional control over the spinal or brainstem motor networks, identification of existing patterns, optional patterns as response to environmental demands, and obligatory patterns not within the control of the client's intentional repertoire of patterns becomes a critical evaluative component before goal setting or treatment planning.

Spinal neuronetwork. The spinal neuronetwork seems to have many preprogrammed complex interconnections that may be intrinsically activated through program generators, modulated from within and by ventral-medial and lateral motor generator systems within the brainstem, as well as by cerebellar and cortical neuromechanisms.[31,121] It is through these mechanisms therapists try to alter existing states of spinal generators. Ultimately, the therapist is activating systems within the CNS that normally modulate spinal level activity and will self-correct to achieve internal homeostasis and control. Some of the identified patterns thought to be spinal regulated are listed in Table 6-7. The specific input system that has the greatest external affect on the spinal modulation of these patterns is also listed. The therapist must always monitor the client's general CNS response to any input. If for example, the therapist uses some stretch and it makes the client angry, the postural extensor response will be anticipated from the stretch but will be due in reality to the limbic neurochemical response to anger. What the therapist is trying to teach and what the patient is learning may be very different and will not lead to the modulatory control the therapist hopes the patient will achieve. Fig. 6-9 illustrates what might be occurring with a reciprocal multisegmental organizational neuronetwork of the crossed-extension pattern. This figure is used to show some of the complexity of the spinal pattern generators. Realizing that the interneural connections may number in the hundreds of

thousands at the spinal level and hundreds of times that when supraspinal loops are considered, helps the learner to realize why control of systems must be accomplished in patterns, not in individual connections to motor neurons.

The specific reaction of the motor generators depends on the preexisting state of the motor pools when the input (either from the peripheral afferent or the supraspinal mechanism) arrives at the synaptic junctions. Peripheral stretch to a muscle as stated in previous sections will heighten agonist and agonistic pattern generators and reciprocally dampen the antagonistic synergies. The tendon organ will have the opposite effect. With movement or postural holding there is tension and stretch from the peripheral system; thus both input systems will send information supraspinally while helping to modulate spinal motor generators. The automatic grasp pattern and the automatic extension of the hand have this same reciprocal relationship. These patterns have intralimb reciprocal relationship. The flexor withdrawal and the crossed-extension, although reciprocal, illustrate a between-limb synergy that can be modulated into a crude walking pattern even within the spinal generators. The galant modulates lateral flexion, automatic extension of the trunk helps modulate postural extension, and touch to the abdominals heightens the resting level of the trunk flexors. These three patterns together demonstrate a crude total pattern neuronetwork over the motor function of the trunk. The addition of multisupraspinal control centers gives flexibility and variability over these patterns and with specific neuromodulation could recombine existing patterns to modulate new patterns of motor behavior.

Recognizing specific patterns and how those patterns and other might affect functional movement or positional patterns has clinical significance. A child with spastic cerebral palsy, for instance, shows extension and "scissoring" when the pads of the feet are stimulated. Sometimes the extension pattern is so strong that the child will arch backwards. Sustained positions that oppose pathological patterns are believed to elicit autogenic inhibition. Contraction-relaxation techniques also work on the autogenic inhibition principle.[124]

Just as afferent input can be used to alter tone and elicit movement, it can also become an obstacle when the therapist tries to coordinate complex movement patterns. A persistent grasp pattern is a common occurrence in children and adults with CNS insult. This dominant grasp is often reinforced by the client's own fingers and frequently prevents functional use of the hand. If a withdrawal pattern is elicited every time a client is touched, the client not only will be unable to explore the environment through the tactile-proprioceptive systems but also will experience arousal by the influence of the cutaneous system over the reticular activating system. Severe agitation could likely be a behavioral outcome from such a persistent reflex.

As with any treatment procedure, a clinician should determine whether the technique will help the client obtain

Table 6-7. Spinal level reflexes

Pattern generators (listed as)	Input system modulated by
Myotatic/or stretch reflex	Proprioceptive: muscle spindle
Reverse myotatic reflex	Proprioceptive: TO
Withdrawal	Any noxious exteroceptive stimuli
Extensor trust	Exteroceptive: light touch
Crossed extension	Exteroceptive to 1 side with control at response
Stepping and premature walking	Exteroceptive and proprioceptive to foot
Grasp reflex	Exteroceptive or proprioceptive to palm
Automatic extension of wrist and fingers	Exteroceptive or proprioceptive to hypothenar and extensor surface
Galant or incurvation of the trunk	Exteroceptive to trunk
Automatic trunk extension	Proprioceptive: joints and spindle: pressure through hips

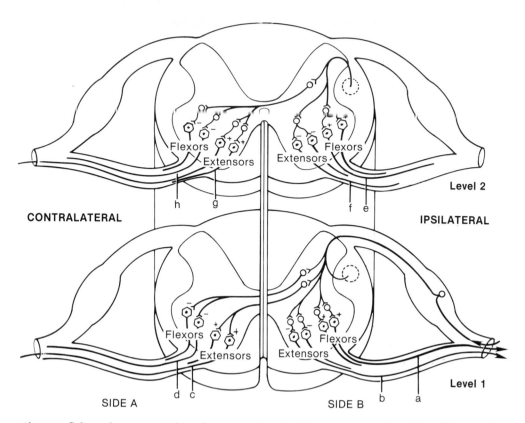

Fig. 6-9. Schematic representation of a neuronetwork of the cross-extension reflex. The stimulus enters at level one and elicits motor responses on both the ipsilateral and contralateral sides at the segmental level it entered and at other levels within the spinal cord. The specific response includes: *(a)* ipsilateral facilitation of flexor motor neurons at the same segmental level (level 1) going back to the leg; *(b)* ipsilateral inhibition of extensor motor neurons at the same segmental level going back to the stimulated extremity (level 1); *(c)* contralateral facilitation of extensor motor neurons at the same segmental level going to the other leg (level 1); *(d)* contralateral inhibition of flexor motor neurons at the same segmental level going to the other leg (level 1); *(e)* facilitation of ipsilateral flexor motor neurons located at other segmental levels but innervating the ipsilateral leg (level 2); *(f)* inhibition of ipsilateral extensor motor neurons located at other segmental levels (level 2); *(g)* facilitation of contralateral extensor motor neurons at other segmental levels (level 3); and *(h)* inhibition of contralateral flexor motor neurons at other segmental levels (level 2).

a higher level of function. As in the case of spinal patterns that in and among themselves may be adequate for movement (see Chapters 3 and 9), lack of a controlling or regulatory system will prevent acquisition of functional skills. Thus eliciting a withdrawal over and over again to get ankle eversion does not teach the client anything and will be effective only if it is incorporated into a higher-level activity. For example, initial use of withdrawal to elicit eversion followed immediately by resistance incorporates a spinal response with higher-order systems modulation. As soon as the resistance is applied, the neuronetwork response pattern has changed.

The clinician must learn to recognize not only specific patterns but what combinations of responses of pattern generators would look like. If the reader overlayed Figs. 6-5, 6-7 and 6-9, a combined reaction to multiinput would be observed. The neuronetwork complexity of multiple input can be overwhelming, even at a spinal level. Thus a therapist

must always be observant of the specific behavioral response and the moment-to-moment changes in behavior during a treatment session, even if the specific neuronetwork is not understood.

Brainstem neuronetwork. The lower brainstem includes the upper spinal cord, the medulla, the pons, and their substructures, especially (for our purposes) the facilitory portion of the reticular formation, and some vestibular nuclei.[121]

Patterns mediated at this level via a large variety of motor nuclei alter motor generators at the spinal level and thus potentially alter muscle tone throughout the body (Table 6-8). The major motor influence via the ventral medial brainstem motor generators is directed toward the postural and antigravity muscles. The principal afferents, which have some modulatory effect over these spinal and brainstem nuclei, are the joint and muscle proprioceptors of the neck (C1 to C3) and the otoliths and cristae of the labyrinth.

Table 6-8. Pattern-generators originating within upper cervical and lower brainstem areas

Patterns	Afferent influence
Tonic labyrinthine reflexes (TLR)	Static position of labyrinth
Tonic neck reflexes Symmetrical (STNR) Asymmetrical (ATNR)	Neck proprioceptors
Positive supporting reacton	Proprioceptors of hands and feet
Tonic lumbar reflex (? location in CNS)	Lumbar proprioceptors
Associated reactions	Proprioceptors and exteroceptors
Shifting reaction	Proprioceptors and labyrinth
Landau	Proprioceptors and labyrinth

Table 6-9. Reactions at the pons, midbrain, diencephalon level

Reaction	Stimulus
Neck righting	Rotation neck proprioceptors
Body on head righting	Rotation neck proprioceptors
Body on body righting	Rotation trunk proprioceptors
Body on body on head righting	Rotation trunk and neck proprioceptors
Labyrinthine righting	Gravity influence of labyrinth Vestibular and proprioceptors
Moro reflex	Neck proprioceptors
Emotional tone	ANS response to any arousal stimuli

The slow adaptation and thus repetitive firing rate of these afferents contribute to a tonic enhancement on specific motor nuclei, which have the potential of activating specific spinal generators. They in turn can trigger prolonged static positioning of body parts. Clear descriptions of these reflexes and their effect on tonal patterns in clients with CNS dysfunction can be found in a variety of references.[20,73,74,88,166] In a normally developing CNS the combined interactions of all these soft-wired programs may lay the foundation for integration of reaching, visual fixation, balance between flexors and extensors, turning of the head and body, bringing limbs to midline and across, and a myriad of other critical components leading to higher-level positioning and movement.[67]

Controversy exists as to whether these brainstem patterns or synergies should be encouraged or discouraged as treatment procedures. Proponents of their use emphasize the importance of these behaviors in the development of normal response patterns.[30] Opponents stress the difficulty clients encounter when obligated to assume the pattern once the stimulus is present.[20] Both groups are analyzing a similar system. It may be that both are viewing only half of the whole. Neither group wants a client severely limited in volitional motor control. Nor would either group teach the client to use the stereotypical patterns that limit functional movement. Thus the first group teaches the client to use these patterns to modify and control antagonistic function, which creates a more flexible dynamic interaction of muscle groups and encourages functional control in movement. The second group never teaches the clients to use these patterns. These clinicians use these patterns only when the client is effectively controlling these patterns in functional goal-directed activities. Although the language sounds contradictory, clinical observation of both therapist behavior and client response would lead many observers to think clinicians in both groups were performing the same procedures.

The clinician needs to observe whether the specific patterned response is (1) triggered by afferent input, (2) triggered by volitional intent, or (3) activated by brainstem nuclei without environmental input or cortical intent. In the third case, the entire cerebellar synergistic system needs to be evaluated to determine which portion might be modulating the observable behavior. Differentiating these motor components will help to set appropriate goals and treatment procedures.

Another group of patterned responses may be programmed within the middle to upper brainstem (pons, midbrain) and diencephalon (thalamus and hypothalamus).[121] When these patterns (Table 6-9) are generated, the overall effect on the spinal motor pool seems to keep the body and head in symmetrical alignment, the head oriented to vertical and regulate postural adjustments. The complexity of these programs incorporate both flexion and extension as well as rotatory interactions during automatic or volitional initiation of these responses. The tectospinal tracts are thought to play a key role in regulation over the head and neck reactions for orientation of the head in space.[148] That orientation can be triggered by vestibular, visual, or auditory stimuli or volitionally by the client.[31,148] The body reactions also incorporate flexion, extension, and rotation, which suggests modulation via both the lateral and ventral medial systems originating from within the brainstem[121] and terminating on the neuronetwork within the spinal system. Remember: The spinal system has tremendous influence over the brainstem; thus the term *modulation* rather than *control* is more accurate.

Traditionally, the principal reactions or patterns generated from the upper brainstem are termed *righting* or *displacement reactions*.[125] These reactions are used (1) in a contrived manner where the therapist guides or handles a patient who is unable to volitionally elicit the responses, (2) in a contrived manner in which the therapist guides the client who volitionally assists, or (3) in a functional, independent manner where the client initiates and practices the activity independently.

Many available treatment alternatives incorporate the two general functions of righting reactions: rotation within the body axis to realign body parts and righting of the head to face vertical.

The first function, keeping the body in alignment, incorporates rotation with either flexion or extension. Rotation within the trunk axis or between the head and trunk elicits a variety of innate reactions: righting of neck, body on head, body on body, and body on body on head. Clinicians, regardless of their orientation, have discovered that rotation within the client's body axis causes dampening of excessive tone in the trunk, shoulders, hips, and often into the extremities. The specific release of tone depends on positioning of the client, direction of the rotatory pattern, and client's individuality. Brunnstrom's rowing technique in sitting position incorporates a large amount of trunk rotation.[30] This rowing maneuver releases trunk, shoulder, hip, and often upper-extremity excessive tone. Simultaneously, by actively moving the head in space, optic labyrinthine righting of the head (OLR) brings the head to face vertical. This tends to elicit a postural pattern in the neck, upper trunk, and shoulder girdle. PNF activities always incorporate rotation as a key element to facilitate normal patterns of movement.[124] Bobath and neurodevelopmental therapists using handling techniques to elicit righting reaction stress rotation as a critical element in eliciting normal coordinated movement.[22] The greatest carry-over or learning should occur when the client actively or volitionally initiates a procedure and controls the movement patterns within a variety of functional activities and environmental contexts.[51,222]

The importance of rotation as a treatment technique does not stop with movement within the trunk axis. Forearm rotation, usually into supination against hypertonic pronators, will often elicit opening of the hand and release of elbow and wrist flexors. Often, shoulder flexion, internal rotation, and adduction are also reduced in tone.[21]

When a client becomes hypertonic in shoulder or hip internal rotation, external rotation seems to be a key to releasing entire hypertonic patterns within the respective limb. Why the proprioceptive stimuli of rotation, which obviously stimulate spindle afferent fibers, joints, and tendons, has such a potent effect on abnormal excessive tone is not known. Yet clinical evidence through observation certainly reinforces rotation as a powerful therapeutic tool. Whether these reactions are modulated within the spinal, brainstem, or cerebellar system is not as critical to the clinician as to the researcher. More important to the clinician is whether the client regains control over functional movement patterns as procedural programs.

The second function of righting reactions is to orient the head to be upright and vertical—in prone OLR by extending the neck to orient the head to vertical and in supine OLR by facilitating flexors. With the client in a sitting position, the head should right to vertical no matter the plane or diagonal the body is tilted toward. In addition to the use of scooter boards, bolster platforms, and horizontal acceleration while

the client is prone over a ball, techniques that automatically facilitate righting of the head to face vertical include (1) the second phase of the inverted tonic labyrinthine technique that elicits postural extension and righting of the head and (2) tipping off vertical while sitting. Vertical patterns may be easier initially because less strength is needed to hold the head against gravity.

These righting reactions often produce complex movement patterns. The specific stimulus, degree of rotation, or angle of the head off vertical determines the individual client's response. As the specific stimulus has a large degree of variance, so does the specific response. Therapists must be keen observers with respect to both the specific afferent input and the client's specific motor programming response in order to flexibly use righting reactions as a treatment modality.

Cerebellum. The cerebellum is a primary motor programmer within the motor system. It might be considered the primary modulator over the synergistic system acting unconsciously yet regulating both voluntary and automatic motor activity.[121,148] Generally, the cerebellum and its connections are the regulators of muscle tone. Within certain parameters the cerebellum monitors the range, rate, force, and direction of voluntary movement. It serves to correct errors in movement by reaffirming for the cortex the current length and tension of skeletal muscles.

Cerebellar lesions affect the ipsilateral side of the body. Affected individuals may fatigue easily and exhibit ataxia, dysmetria, dysdiadochokinesia, asynergia, and intention tremor. The flocculonodular lobe of the cerebellum works intimately with the vestibular nuclei to orchestrate certain equilibrium reactions and directional orientation.[60,121]

As the cerebellum modulates tone for posture and volitional movement, it relies on input from proprioceptive and vestibular mechanisms as well as higher-center regulatory mechanisms. Loss of higher-center feedback or peripheral input drastically affects the functional capacity of the cerebellum. (See Chapter 23 for specific treatment techniques that focus on cerebellar involvement.) Classification of treatment modalities with respect to cerebellar integration can be divided into two areas. The first identifies the sensory input system and the second focuses on the rate, direction, and intensity of the stimuli. For example, assume resistance is the proprioceptive input. The intensity or amount of resistance would determine the rate of movement. By increasing the resistance and decreasing the rate, the cerebellum has more time to adjust and set appropriate base tone. Thus in a cerebellar categorization scheme, input needs to be cross-referenced with rate, intensity, and duration. In the example cited, optimal facilitation would correlate with a high degree of resistance. The gradient would sequence from maximal to minimal resistance in terms of the range of optimal to minimal facilitation.

Another proprioceptive input would be joint traction and approximation. Assume the two techniques are implemented with a weighted ankle cuff and a weighted waist belt, respectively. Both techniques would increase the joint input and heighten cerebellar function. Because of the added weight, both procedures would slow down the movement or rate component and thus give additional time for the cerebellum to regulate tone. Yet traction correlates with movement; approximation promotes joint coactivation. Traction sends conflicting input to the cerebellum when coactivation or slowing of movement is desired. The weight slows down and controls the movement, but the traction enhances it. On the other hand, approximation with resistance summates consistent afferent information and should drive the system toward a more desirable response; it encourages coactivation to further control the movement. If the problem has already been identified as a rate deficit in which movement patterns occur too rapidly, then approximation rather than traction would be a preferred treatment. The specific technique for approximating—whether manual or with equipment such as a dental dam—would be the choice of the therapist. Refer to Chapter 23 for additional information on the cerebellum's function in motor control.

Cortex and basal ganglia. The circuitry interconnecting the cortex, cerebellum, and basal ganglia has generated voluminous research (refer to Chapters 3 and 21 for more information on basal ganglia). There are complex relay loops between the basal ganglia and cortical structures. The motor circuit linking basal ganglia and frontal lobe follows a loop from the supplementary motor to putamen, globus pallidus, thalamus, and back to premotor cortex.[31,121] This motor circuit uses direct and indirect circuitries within the basal ganglia, and its effect will be to modulate frontal lobe activity over brainstem and spinal program generators, as well as to communicate with the cerebellum.[121] Many other loop systems within the basal ganglia deal more directly with cognitive and eye function and emotional control over movement.[31,121]

With regard to motor function, the basal ganglia have been credited with refining displacement reactions, mediating rhythmical automatic movement patterns and associated movements, and regulating postural tone in antigravity muscles.[121]

Lesions to the basal ganglia result in disturbances in muscle tone and involuntary movements. Clients exhibit resting tremors, hemiballismus, athetosis or choreo-type movements (hyperkinesia or hypokinesia).[31,129]

The cerebral cortex maintains an "advice and consent" relationship with the basal ganglia and cerebellum. The three structures interact cooperatively to complement and modulate voluntary movement (see Chapter 3). The added dimension of the motor cortex enables the individual to isolate movement to one muscle or group of muscles during performance of a task. When fast and skillful movements are required, the primary motor cortex may direct the distal function, but the basal ganglia and cerebellum play the primary role in orchestrating the entire plan.[44]

The cortex is intimately involved in learned skill. The term *praxis* or motor planning has a sensory planning component, which depends on input from the periphery to make accurate decisions. Once the plan is learned, that same feedback may not be as critical but will still be used to compare feedforward plans with existing environmental restrictions and demands (See Chapter 11 for addition information on sensory and motor praxis.)

Equilibrium or balance reactions were once thought to be under the total control the cerebral cortex.[215] Today the complexity of balance is much better understood.[60] Refer to Chapter 28 for an in-depth discussion of balance and balance problems. In order for the CNS to respond with the finite sensitivity needed for normal equilibrium, integration of spinal, brainstem, cerebellar, and basal ganglia areas are needed. If a client is dominated by abnormal tone or movement responses, then distortions in or lack of normal equilibrium reactions would be expected. Thus before establishing the goal of normal balance, a therapist needs to identify the client's CNS potential for integration. Because of the complexity of balance reactions, almost every combination of synergistic muscle action can be elicited. It has been observed that once balance responses can be facilitated, the client's freedom in all planes of space and thus control over functional activities are vastly improved. That improvement seems to simultaneously lead to client confidence and an ANS response that relaxes the individual and decreases the undesired emotional tone (refer to Chapters 5 and 14 for additional information).

Cortical function with intact or adequately functioning systems within the basal ganglia, cerebellum, brainstem, and spinal mechanisms is certainly the ultimate goal for all clients. The specific relationships and functional use of the various areas will depend on each client and on the therapist's ability to help the client reintegrate. The specific methods used will obviously vary from client to client and therapist to therapist. Flexibility and willingness to let the client teach the clinician which procedures best matches that individual's CNS are probably the most important therapeutic tools available. Unfortunately, this tool cannot be categorized within a specific scheme because it falls within all sensory systems, is critical at all levels within the CNS of both the client and the therapist, and is based on the client's neuroplasticity.[57,147]

Summary

The importance of understanding the various patterns and synergistic responses programmed within the CNS is obvious. Their interactions affect the ultimate outcome of motor responses. It was once thought that the CNS was totally hierarchical and needed to be learned or retaught using a type of building block design. Today, research has shown that a variety of systems affect motor control (see Chapters 2, 3 and 5). Each system can be approached as an inroad to the CNS. New theories and treatment approaches will be added to the clinical model as creative and visually astute colleagues challenge their clinical expertise and allow patients to show them alternative treatment techniques. Each therapist must be open to new advances while being analytical and cautious if those techniques are presented without any scientific or behavioral research or rationale.

HOLISTIC TREATMENT TECHNIQUES BASED ON MULTISENSORY INPUT

As already mentioned in this chapter and in Chapter 1, a variety of accepted treatment methodologies exist.* Each approach focuses on multisensory input introduced to the client in controlled and identified sequences. These sequences are based on the inherent nature of synergistic patterns[5,158] and the patterns observed in humans[5,22,187] and lower-order animals[68] or a combination of the two.[124,195] Each method focuses on the total client, the specific clinical problems, and alternative treatment approaches available within each established framework. Certain methods have traditionally emphasized specific neurological disabilities. Cerebral palsy in children[14,22,163,195] and hemiplegia in adults[21,30,38,141] are the two most frequently identified. In the last decade substantial clinical attention has been paid to children with learning difficulties.[6,75] Yet the concepts and treatment procedures specific to all the techniques have been applied to almost every neurological disability seen in the clinical setting. This expansion of the use of each method seems to be a natural evolution because of the structure and function of the CNS and commonalities in clinical signs manifested by brain insult.

Nevertheless, dogmatism still persists with respect to territorial boundaries identified by clinicians using specific methods. The question remains as to whether these boundaries are clearly delineated or superficially established. It seems there are many more commonalities than differences among approaches. For example, in the case of a hemiplegic client with a hypertonic upper-extremity pattern of shoulder adduction, internal rotation, elbow flexion, and forearm pronation with wrist and finger flexion, Brunnstrom would identify that pattern as the stronger of her two upper-extremity synergies.[30] Michels, although using an explanation similar to Brunnstrom's to describe the pattern, would elaborate and incorporate additional upper-extremity synergies.[141] Bobath would assert that the client was stuck in a mass-movement pattern resulting from abnormal postural reflex activity.[21] Although the conceptualization of the problem certainly determines treatment protocols, the pattern all three clinicians would work toward is shoulder abduction, external rotation, elbow extension, forearm supination, and wrist and finger extension. Motor control theorists would also work on the same pattern although they would try to encourage the initiation of the pattern during a

functional movement leading to a specific goal.[49] Another clinician might describe the pattern as a reflex-inhibiting position. One description might identify the weakest components of the various synergies, whereas still another might identify the extreme stretch and rotatory element that reciprocally inhibits the spastic pattern. How a clinician sequences treatment from the original hypertonic pattern to the goal pattern will again vary. Push-pull patterns in supine, side lying, and rolling; propping patterns in sitting; or weight-bearing patterns in prone, over a ball or bolster, or in partially kneeling—all have the potential of eliciting the functional pattern and modifying the hypertonic pattern. It may be true that one method is better than others. That truth, however, stems not from the method itself but rather the preferential CNS biases of the client and the variability of application skills among clinicians themselves.

No matter the treatment methodology selected by a clinician, all techniques focus on the active learning process of the client. *The client is never a passive participant,* even if the level of consciousness is considered vegetative. With a multiinput approach that requires a motor response, whether an increase or a reduction of tone, movement, or postural holding, the client's CNS is being asked to process and respond at multisegmental levels to the external world. That response need not be at a cortical level, but it must be present. In time, it is hoped that the client's internal drive system begins to self-regulate and orchestrate **modulation** over this very **adaptable** and dynamic motor system.

Because of overlapping of treatment methodologies and the infiltration of therapeutic management into all avenues of neurological dysfunction, various multisensory models have developed over the last few years.* Although these models have attempted to integrate existing techniques, in reality they may have created a new set of holistic treatment approaches. The ultimate goal is to develop one all-encompassing methodology that allows the clinician the freedom to use any method that is appropriate for the needs and individual learning styles of the client as well as tapping the unique individual differences of the clinician. Although that approach does not yet exist, its development is a challenge to future therapists.

CLINICAL EXAMPLE: HOW TO USE A CLASSIFICATION SCHEME
Clinical problem: lack of head control

There is a potential for lack of head control after any severe injury to the CNS. For that reason it is a common clinical problem. Further, because of the importance of head and neck control, virtually all functional activities are affected by its absence.

Before discussing a classification schema, the clinical problem must be analyzed and identification made of those

---

* References 5, 14, 22, 30, 38, 39, 45, 53, 75, 77, 79, 84, 124, 134, 141, 142, 176, 184, 187, 189, 195, and 196.

*References 39, 67, 75, 88, 97, and 103.

sensory and inherent systems to be facilitated. In considering the specific problem of lack of head control, let us assume that Timothy, a 16-year-old with a closed head injury, suffered a lesion within his CNS 3 months ago. He has the following signs regarding head control.

1. Mild extensor hypertonicity is present in supine, and Timothy is unable to flex and rotate his head off the mat.
2. In prone, extensor hypertonicity is absent, and hypotonicity prevails. The client is able to briefly bob his head off the mat in a hyperextension pattern. Mild tonal shifts occur to either side when the head is turned and when it is symmetrically flexed or extended.
3. Timothy is unable to roll or perform any functional activity in the horizontal plane.
4. When placed in long sitting, he is unable to hold the position or sit with flexed hips and extended knees. His head remains in total flexion with his chin on his chest.
5. When sitting over a table mat, he is unable to hold his position. General hypotonicity prevails, although slightly more flexion is palpable. His head remains flexed. When asked to pick up his head, he extends into a hyperextension pattern followed by extensor relaxation into flexion. He is unable to hold the head in a vertical position.
6. Timothy does not mind being touched and responds well to handling techniques.

From the analysis of these clinical signs, the following clinical interpretations are presented.

1. In horizontal Timothy has persistence of a TLR. In this client this pattern is extensor dominant. While he is supine, extension prevails. While he is prone, extension is inhibited, although flexion tone is not dominant. Because of the persistence of hyperactivity among the extensor motor generators, the ability to initiate rolling using a neck-righting pattern is prevented. Presence of mild ATNR to both sides and an STNR has been noted. Due to his instability and low tone, Timothy seems to be using these stereotypical patterns volitionally to assist in gaining some control over his motor patterns. In prone Timothy has the ability to move into a neck extension or OLR pattern but is unable to hold. Thus movement and range are present, but postural holding is missing.
2. As a result of ventroflexion of the head in sitting, the vestibular apparatus is placed in a similar position to that when prone. In a like manner, the total patterns remain fairly consistent. The increase in flexor tone may result from the positioning of hip and knee flexion and kyphosis of the back. The inability to flex the hips with knee extension suggests that total tonal patterns or synergies prevail. The client is unable to break out

of those dominant patterns. Dominant OLR is not present.
3. Timothy, when asked, carries out the command to the best of his motor ability. This suggests the presence of some intact verbal processing, which is translated into appropriate motor acts. Similarly, when asked to pick up his head, he does just that, suggesting some perceptual integrity of body image, body schema, and position in space. Knowing where his head is in space and where to reposition it also suggests that some proprioceptive-vestibular input and processing are occurring.
4. Timothy's enjoyment of being moved in space with handling techniques again suggests proprioceptive-vestibular integrity. Similarly, his tactile systems seem to be functioning in a discriminatory manner and modifying negative responses of withdrawal and arousal. Specific tactile perception would need a great deal of further testing.

Treatment sequence: development of head control.

Now that the clinical problem has been analyzed and the goal of development of head control set, a treatment sequence or protocol must be established. Timothy lacks head control in all planes and in all patterns of movement. Thus flexors and extensors must be facilitated to develop a dynamic coactivation or postural holding pattern of the neck. The categorization scheme can now be of some assistance. The therapist can ask, "Are there any inherent mechanisms that enhance flexors or extensors in a holding pattern?" OLR should elicit the desired response. Similarly, the clinician can ask, "Are there any inherent processes that would prevent righting of the head to face vertical OLR?" The TLR would block or modify the facilitation of OLR. Knowing the TLR is most dominant in horizontal and least dominant (if at all affected) in vertical is of clinical significance. It is also important to know that the OLR is most frequently tested in a vertical position and seems most active in that position. Awareness that the client is sensitive to total patterns (e.g., flexion facilitates flexion or extension facilitates extension) gives additional treatment clues.

After all this information is assimilated, the following treatment protocol could be established.

1. To enhance neck flexors, the client will be placed in a totally flexed position in vertical with the head positioned in neutral. The client will be rocked backward toward supine, allowing gravity to quick stretch the flexors (Fig. 6-10, A). As soon as the neck flexors are stretched, the head should be tapped forward, back to vertical but not beyond. This avoids hyperextension, extreme stretch to the proprioceptors, and the horizontal supine position of the labyrinths— all of which dampen the flexors and facilitate the extensors. The quick stretch and position should

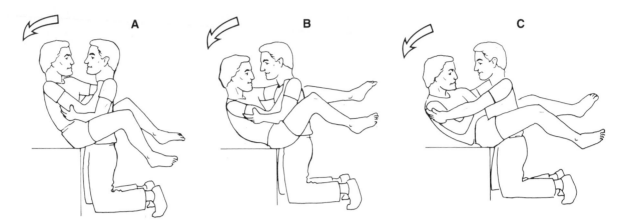

Fig. 6-10. Development of flexor aspect of head control. **A,** Vertical position: head midline and midrange (total body flexion) to optimally facilitate neck flexors. **B,** Facilitating symmetrical neck flexion, using position, gravity, and flexor positions. **C,** Facilitating flexion and rotation to develop pattern necessary for neck righting pattern.

optimally facilitate OLR, which should activate the neck flexors. The total flexion of the body similarly facilitates the neck flexors. Once the neck flexors respond, Timothy can be rocked farther and farther backward while maintaining the head in vertical or ventroflexion (Fig. 6-10, *B*). Once Timothy can be rocked from vertical to horizontal and back to vertical while maintaining good flexor control, his CNS has demonstrated inherent control and modification over the stereotypical patterns, such as the TLR in supine with respect to its influence over the neck musculature. This rocking maneuver can be done on diagonals to practice flexion and rotation (Fig. 6-10, *C*), the key to eliciting a neck-righting, rolling pattern from supine to prone. The total flexed pattern can also be altered by adding more and more extension of the extremities. This decreases the external facilitation to the flexors and demands that Timothy's CNS take more and more control (internal regulation). Additional treatment procedures can be extracted from a variety of sensory categories. To add additional proprioceptive input, any one of those listed techniques might be used. The rotation and speed of the rocking pattern affect the vestibular mechanism.

a. Auditory and visual stimuli can be used effectively. If the therapist takes a position slightly below the client's horizontal eye level, the client (to look at the therapist) will need to look down and flex his head, thus encouraging the desired pattern. Any type of visual or auditory stimulus that directs the client into the desired pattern would be appropriate.

b. The therapist must remember that neck flexion was the goal. Rotation was added to incorporate and set the stage for inherent programming. Since the extensor component still needs integration, total head control has not been attained.

2. To facilitate neck extension a procedure similar to the one for flexion can be established. A vertical position, thus eliminating the influence of the TLR, would again be the starting position of choice. With extension facilitating extension, the client should be placed in as much extension as possible without eliciting excessive extensor tone. Both an inverted tonic labyrinthine position and a kneeling position would be viable spatial patterns to facilitate OLR of the head with focus on postural extensors. The vestibular system sensory category can be checked to identify the treatment procedure for use with an inverted TLR.

a. The kneeling position places the client in a vertical position with hip and trunk extension. Kneeling rather than standing is used because of the influence of the positive supporting reaction in standing and the massive facilitation of total extension. Kneeling avoids the total extension while maintaining a predominant extensor pattern. As a result of the gravitational pull of body weight through the joints, approximation to facilitate postural extension is constantly maintained. The upper extremities can be placed in shoulder abduction and external rotation, which tends to inhibit abnormal upper extremity flexor tone and facilitate postural tone into the shoulder. This extensor tone has the potential through associated spinal reactions to facilitate neck and trunk extension. The arms can be placed in this position over a bolster or ball or by the therapist handling the client from the rear (Fig. 6-11, *A*). The head should begin again in a neutral position. The client is rocked forward (Fig. 6-11, *B*) to facilitate OLR of the head and to elicit a quick stretch to the extensor. If the head begins to fall forward, the therapist can tap the client's forehead immediately following the quick stretch. This

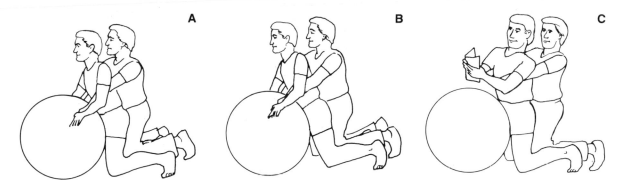

Fig. 6-11. Development of extensor aspect of head control. **A,** Vertical position: head midline with long extensor in midrange and postural extensors in shortened range; body in postural weight-bearing pattern. **B,** Facilitating symmetrical extension of head, trunk, and hips while inhibiting abnormal upper extremity tone. **C,** Facilitating head and trunk extension and rotation to encourage neck righting pattern; client reaches for an object, which is then placed on the opposite side.

tapping action is the reverse tap procedure described under the muscle spindle proprioceptive category. The tapping is done to passively move the head back to vertical. A variety of additional procedures can easily be combined to summate facilitation to the extensors. Tapping, vibration, and approximation through the head to shoulders are only a few of the proprioceptive modalities. All would be facilitory. A variety of auditory and visual stimuli could be used to orient the client to a position in space and thus righting of the head. Techniques listed under the exteroceptive and vestibular systems could also be part of the treatment protocol.

b. The therapist would want to sequence the client toward prone while the head remained in a vertical postural holding pattern. As the therapist rocks the client toward prone again, a rotatory component should be added (Fig. 6-11, *C*). The client will extend and rotate to counterbalance the movement, thus incorporating the neck-righting pattern of extension and rotation necessary when rolling from prone to supine. Resistance to neck extension with or without rotation is an important element in regaining normal functional control.

c. If the client is alert and has some functional use of the arms or legs, this rocking pattern in kneeling can be done as a functional activity. The therapist tells the client that he is going to reach toward an object with one upper extremity. The therapist can guide the client in the reaching pattern in a forward, sideward, or cross-midline direction. While reaching, the client can be rocked forward to elicit OLR. By incorporating an activity into the treatment of head control, the client not only is entertained but also attends to the task rather than to keeping his head up. In this way automatic head control is facilitated, and often

postural patterns follow. In a partial kneeling pattern the client can be sequenced to on-elbow over a bolster or ball or on a chair. These activities should be sequenced from vertical to prone to ensure both total integration of the TLR prone and optimal integration of OLR, as well as letting the client experience control of various motor strategies in many different environmental contexts.

Once the client can maintain good flexor, extensor, and rotational components of head control, the activity should, if possible, be practiced with eyes closed. If the client can still maintain head control, labyrinthine righting would be adequate for any functional activity. If the client loses head control, then additional labyrinthine facilitation would be indicated. If a client uses only vision to right the head, then any time vision is needed to lead or direct another activity, head control might be lost. Because symmetrical vestibular simulation plays a key role in activating the neck muscles to hold the head in vertical, it also is a key element leading to the perception of vertical and all the directional activities sequencing out of the concept of verticality.

• • •

Head control is a complex motor response. A therapist can facilitate inherent mechanisms to assist a client in regaining function. Simultaneously, multitudinous external input techniques classified under the various sensory modalities and combined modalities can be used to give the client additional information. Awareness of one technique and the ability to categorize it appropriately allow easy identification and implementation of many additional approaches. The therapist always needs to remember that the client must practice the behavior (head control) in a variety of spatial positions during various functional activities. This practice must be functional and no longer contrived

SUMMARY

There are treatment techniques that are universally applied from the very young to the aged. The CNS is in a constant state of development throughout life. The brain is unique to each individual: It has idiosyncracies, but it also has an enormous number of predictable responses. Because these factors affect the success or failure of a client-clinician interaction, a classification scheme is only one of the many ways therapists can increase their repertoire while developing more clinical expertise. Both seem to be important factors in the growth and longevity of our professions. It is hoped this chapter will be useful for your practice.

REFERENCES

1. Aitkin LM: The auditory system. In Bjorklund A, Hokfeld T, and Swanson LW, editors: *Handbook of chemical neuroanatomy, vol 7: Integrated systems of the CNS Part II,* New York, 1989, Elsevier.
2. Alexander FM: *The use of the self,* Palo Alto, Calif, 1985, Centerline Press.
3. Allensworth A: A practical guide to the use of music with geriatrics, *Aging to Perfections,* 16(1):9, 1993.
4. Andrew BL and and Dodt E: The deployment of sensory nerve endings at the knee joint in a cat, *Acta Physiol Scand* 28:287-296, 1953.
5. Ayers AJ: *Sensory integration and learning disabilities,* Los Angeles, 1972, Western Psychological Services.
6. Ayers AJ: *The development of sensory integrative theory and practice,* Dubuque, Iowa, 1974, Kendall/Hunt Publishing Co.
7. Ayers AJ: *Sensory integration and the child,* Los Angeles, 1979, Western Psychological Services.
8. Bandler R and Grindler J: *The structure of magic,* Palo Alto, Calif, 1975, Science and Behavior Books.
9. Barnes GR: Head-eye coordination in normals and in patients with vestibular disorders, Proceedings of the Barany Society, Uppsala, Sweden. In *Adv Otorhinolaryngol* (Basel) 25:15, 1978.
10. Barnes GR and Forbat LN: Cervical and vestibular afferent control of oculomotor response in man, *Acta Otolaryngol* (Stockh) 88:79-87, 1979.
11. Barnes JF: The body is a self-correcting mechanism, *Phys Ther Forum* 6:8-10, 1987.
12. Barnes JF: *Myofascial release,* ed 3, Paoli, Pa, 1990, Rehabilitation Service.
13. Barr ML and Kiernan JA, editors: *The human nervous system: an anatomical viewpoint,* ed 6, Philadelphia, 1990, JB Lippincott.
14. Bertoti DB: Effect of therapeutic horseback riding on posture in children with cerebral palsy, *Phys Ther Forum* 68(10):1505-1512, 1988.
15. Bessou P and others: Dynamic properties of mechanoreceptors with unmyelinated (C) fibers, *J Neurophysiol* 34:116-131, 1971.
16. Bessou P and LaPorte Y: Responses from primary and secondary endings of the same neuromuscular spindle of the tenesmus muscle of the cat. In Barker D, editor: *Symposium of muscle receptors,* Hong Kong, 1962, Hong Kong University Press.
17. Bishop B: Vibration stimulation. I. Neurophysiology of motor responses evoked by vibratory stimulation, *Phys Ther* 54:1273-1281, 1974.
18. Bishop B: Vibratory stimulation. II. Vibratory stimulation as an evaluation tool, *Phys Ther* 55:29-33, 1975.
19. Blashy MRM and Fuchs R: Orthokinetics: a new receptor facilitation method, *Am J Ther* 8:5, 1959.
20. Bobath B: *Abnormal postural reflex activity caused by brain lesion,* London, 1978, William Heineman Medical Books, Ltd.
21. Bobath B: *Adult hemiplegia: evaluation and treatment,* ed 2, London, 1978, William Heinemann Medical Books, Ltd.
22. Bobath K and Bobath B: Cerebral palsy. In Pearson PH and Williams CE, editors: *Physical therapy services in developmental disabilities,* Springfield, Ill, 1972, Charles C Thomas.
23. Bobath B: *Abnormal postural reflex activity caused by brain lesions,* ed 3, Frederick, Md, 1985, Aspen Publications.
24. Booker J: Pain: it's all in your patient's head (or is it?), *Nursing* 82:47-51, 1982.
25. Borenstein M and Sigman M: Infant intelligence quotient predictable by gaze, *Child Dev* 57:251-274, 1987.
26. Brecker LR: Imagery and ROM Combine to Create, *Adv Phys Ther* 5(2):18-19, 1994.
27. Brewer S: Personal correspondence with composer, pianist, and theoritician in use of sound in harmony with body rhythms, Aug 1983.
28. Brodal A and Pompliano V: *Basic aspects of central vestibular mechanisms,* Amsterdam, 1972, Elsevier/North Holland Biomedical Press.
29. Brookhart JM, Mori S, and Reynolds PJ: Postural reactions to two directions of displacement in dogs, *Am J Physiol* 218:719, 1970.
30. Brunnstrom S: Movement therapy in hemiplegia, ed 2, 1992 Philadelphia, Pa, 1970, JB Lippincott.
31. Burt AM: *Textbook of neuroanatomy,* Philadelphia, Pa, 1993, WB Saunders.
32. Butler DS: Adverse mechanical tension in the nervous system: a model for assessment and treatment, *Aust J Physiother* 35(4):227-238, 1989.
33. Butler DS: *Mobilization of the nervous system.* New York, 1991, Churchill Livingstone.
34. Butler RA: The cumulative effects of differential stimulus repetition rates on the auditory evoked response in man, *Electroencephalogr Clin Neurophysiol* 35:337-345, 1973.
35. Buttram B and Brown G: *Developmental physical management for the multi-disabled child,* Tuscaloosa, 1977, University of Alabama Press.
36. Cain WS, editor: *Odors, evaluation utilization and control, Ann NY Acad Sci* 2371:439, 1974.
37. Campbell S: *Clinics in physical therapy,* ed 2, vol 5, New York, 1992, Churchill-Livingstone.
38. Carr JH and Sheperd RB: *A motor relearning for stroke,* Frederick, Md, 1987, Aspen Publishers.
39. Carr JH and Sheperd RB: *Movement science-foundations for physical therapy in rehabilitation,* Frederick, Md, 1987, Aspen Publishers.
40. Case J: *Sensory mechanisms: current concepts in biology,* New York, 1966, Macmillan.
41. Cauna N: The effects of aging on the receptor organs of the human dermis. In Montagna W, editor: *Advances in biology of skin,* vol 6, Aging, New York, 1965, Pergamon Press.
42. Cherney L: Aging and communication. In Lewis C, editor: *Aging: the health care challenge,* Philadelphia, 1989, FA Davis.
43. Clark R: *Clinical neuroanatomy and neurophysiology,* ed 5, Philadelphia, 1975, FA Davis Co.
44. Cohen H, editor: *Neuroscience rehabilitation,* Philadelphia, 1993, JB Lippincott.
45. Colavita F: *Sensory changes in the elderly,* Springfield, Ill, 1978, Charles C Thomas.
46. Cook J: The therapeutic use of music: a literature review, *Nurs Forum* 20(3):252-256, 1981.
47. Cooper BA, Letts L and Rigby P: Exploring the use of color cueing on an assistive device in the home: six case studies, *Phys Occup Ther Geriatr* 11(4):47, 1993.
48. Cooper S: Muscle spindles in the intrinsic muscles of the human tongue, *J Physiol* 122:193, 1953.
49. Craik R: Abnormalities of motor behavior. In Lister MJ, editor: *Contemporary management of motor control problems,* Norman, Okla, 1991, Foundation for Physical Therapy.
50. Craik R: Spasticity revisited. In *APTA Combined Section Meetings,* New Orleans, Louisiana: unpublished.
51. Craik RL: Recovery processes: maximizing function. In Lister MJ,

editor: *Contemporary management of motor control problems,* Norman, Okla, 1991, Foundation for Physical Therapy.

52. Crosby EC, Humphrey F, and Laver EW: *Correlative anatomy of the nervous system,* New York, 1962, Macmillan.

53. Crutchfield CA and Barnes MR, editors: *Motor control and motor learning in rehabilitation,* ed 2, Atlanta, 1993, Stokesville Publications Co.

54. de Groot J: *Correlative neuroanatomy,* ed 21, San Mateo, Calif, 1991, Lange Medical Publications.

55. de Kleijn A and Magnus R: *Korperstellung (body posture),* Berlin, 1924, Julius Springer.

56. Debenham G: The healing art, *Canad Med Assoc J* 149(12):1994, 1993.

57. Dobkin B: Neuroplasticity: key to recovery after CNS injury, *West J Med* 159:56-60, 1993.

58. Downie RA: *Cash's textbook of neurology for physiotherapists,* Philadelphia, 1986, JB Lippincott.

59. Duensing F and Schaefer KP: The activity of various neurons of the reticular formation of the unfettered rabbit during head turning and vestibular stimulation, *Arch Psychiatr Nervenkr* 201:97-122, 1960. (Ger).

60. Duncan PW, editor: *Balance proceedings of the APTA Forum,* Alexandria, Va, 1989, APTA.

61. Dwyer B: Detecting hearing loss and improving communication in elderly persons, *Focus Geriatr Care Rehabil* 1(16):3-4, 1987.

62. Ekelund LG: Exercise, including weightlessness, *Annu Rev Physiol* 31:85-116, 1969.

63. Eklund G and Hagbarth KE: Normal variability of tonic vibration reflexes in man, *Exp Neurol* 16:80-92, 1966.

64. Eldred E: Peripheral receptors: their excitation and relation to reflex patterns, *Am J Phys Med* 46(1):69-72, 1967.

65. Elvey RL: Physical evaluation and treatment of neural tissues in disorders of the neuromusculoskeletal system: neural and brachial plexus tension. Course handout. San Jose, Calif, Northeast Seminars, unpublished.

66. Farber S: *Sensorimotor evaluation and treatment procedures,* ed 2, Indianapolis, 1974, Indiana University—Purdue University at Indianapolis Medical Center.

67. Farber S: A multisensory approach to neurorehabilitation. In Farber S, editor: *Neurorehabilitation: a multisensory approach,* Philadelphia, 1982, WB Saunders.

68. Fay T: The neurophysical aspects of therapy in cerebral palsy. In Payton OP, Hirt S, and Newton RA: Neurophysiologic approach to therapeutic exercise, Philadelphia, 1978, FA Davis.

69. Feldenkrais M: *Awareness through movement,* New York, 1977, Harper & Row.

70. Feldenkrais M: *The elusive obvious,* Cupertino, Calif, 1981, Meta Publication.

71. Felton DL and Felton SY: A regional and systemic overview of functional neuroanatomy. In Farber SA, editor: *Neurorehabilitation: a multisensory approach,* Philadelphia, 1982, WB Saunders.

72. Fields HL: *Pain,* New York, 1987, McGraw-Hill.

73. Fiorentino MR: *Normal and abnormal development: the influence of primitive reflexes on motor development,* Springfield, Ill, 1972, Charles C Thomas.

74. Fiorentino MR: *A basis for sensorimotor development—normal and abnormal,* Springfield, Ill, 1981, Charles C Thomas.

75. Fisher AG, Murray EA, and Bundy AC: *Sensory integration; theory & practice,* Philadelphia, 1991, FA Davis.

76. Fitzgerald MJT: *Neuroanatomy: basic and clinical,* ed 2, Philadelphia, 1992, WB Saunders.

77. Flynn J: "Snoezelen" Hartenberg, Ede, Holland, 1986, unpublished description of Institute de Hartenberg.

78. Frank A, Maurer P, and Shepherd I: Light and sound environment; a survey of neonatal intensive care units, *Phys Occup Ther Pediatr* 11(2):27-45, 1991.

79. Freeman G: Hippotherapy/therapeutic horseback riding, *Clin Man Phys Ther* 4(3):20-25, 1984.

80. Galambos R: Suppression of auditory nerve activity by stimulation of efferent fibers to cochlea, *J Neurophysiol* 19:424-437, 1956.

81. Gandhavadi B and others: Autonomic pain: features and methods of assessment, *Pain* 71(1):85-90, 1982.

82. Gardner E: *Fundamentals of neurology,* Philadelphia, 1975, WB Saunders.

83. Garliner D: *Myofunctional therapy,* Philadelphia, 1976, WB Saunders.

84. Gelb M: *Body learning—an introduction to the Alexander technique,* London, 1981, Auburn Press.

85. Geldard FA: *The human senses,* ed 2, New York, 1972, John Wiley & Sons.

86. Gelhorn E: *Principles of autonomic-somatic integration: physiological basis and psychological and clinical implications,* Minneapolis, 1967, University of Minnesota Press.

87. Gerhart KD and others: Inhibitory receptive fields of primitive spinothalamic tract cells, *J Neurophysiol* 46:1309-1325, 1981.

88. Gilfoyle EM, Grady AP, and Moore JC: *Children adapt,* Thorofare, NJ, 1981, Charles B Slack.

89. Gill-Body KM and others: Physical therapy management of peripheral vestibular dysfunction: two clinical case reports, *Phys Ther* 74:130-142, 1994.

90. Gimbel T: *Healing through colour,* Suffron Halden, England, 1980, CW Daniel.

91. Gladsone VS: Hearing loss in the elderly, *Am J Phys Occup Ther Geriatr* 2:5-20, 1992.

92. Granit R: *Receptors and sensory perception,* New Haven, Conn, 1962, Yale University Press.

93. Green JH: *Basic clinical physiology,* Oxford, 1973, Oxford University Press.

94. Greenberg JH and others: Metabolic mapping of functional activity in human subjects with the flourodeoxglucose technique, *Science* 212:678-680, 1981.

95. Groen JJ: Vestibular stimulation and its effects from the point of view of theoretical physics, *Neurology* 21:380, 1961.

96. Groër MW and Shekleton ME: *Basic pathophysiology,* ed 2, St Louis, 1983, Mosby.

97. Grollman S: *The human body—its structure and physiology,* ed 2, New York, 1970, Macmillan.

98. Guyton A: *Basic neuroscience: anatomy and physiology,* Philadelphia, 1991, WB Saunders.

99. Hagbarth KE and Eklund G: Tonic vibration reflexes in spasticity, *Brain Res* 2:201-203, 1966.

100. Hagbarth KE and Vallbo AB: Single unit recordings from muscle nerves in human subjects, *Acta Physiol Scand* 76:321-334, 1969.

101. Hagbarth KE and Wohlfart G: The number of muscle in cat in relation to the composition of the muscle nerves, *Acta Anat* 15:85, 1952.

102. Head H: *Studies in neurology,* vol 2, Oxford, 1920, Oxford University Press.

103. Heiniger MC and Randolph SL: *Neurophysiological concepts in human behavior,* St Louis, 1981, Mosby.

104. Heinsen A: *Visual motor development,* Palo Alto, Calif, 1973, Learning Opportunities: Stanford Professional Center.

105. Henderson A: Body schema and the visual guidance of movement. In Henderson A and Coryell J: *The body senses and perceptual deficit,* Boston, 1973, Boston University Press.

106. Herdman SJ: Assessment and treatment of balance disorders in the vestibular-deficient patient. In Duncan PW, editor: *Balance,* Alexandria, Va, 1990, APTA.

107. Herdman SJ: Exercise strategies in vestibular disorders, *Ear Nose Throat* 68:961-964, 1990.

108. Herdman SJ: Treatment of benign positional vertigo, *Phys Ther* 70(3):381-388, 1990.

109. Hochreiter N and others: Effect of vibration on tactile sensitivity, *Phys Ther* 63:934-937, 1983.

110. Hodgson ES: Taste receptors, *Sci Am* 204(5):135, 1961.
111. Horak FB and others: Effects of vestibular rehabilitation on dizziness and imbalance, *Otolaryngol Head Neck Surg* 106:175-180, 1992.
112. Horak FB and others: Vestibular function and motor proficiency in children with impaired hearing, or with learning disability and motor impairment, *Dev Med Child Neurol* 30:64-79, 1988.
113. Houk J and Hennemou E: Responses of Golgi tendon organs, J Neurophysiol 30:466-489, 1967.
114. Hubel D and Weisel T: *Brain mechanisms of vision,* Sci Am 241(3):130-162, 1979.
115. Huss J: *Sensorimotor treatment approaches in occupational therapy,* Philadelphia, 1971, JB Lippincott Co.
116. Huss J: Workshop, San Jose State University, Neurophysiological approaches to treatment, Unpublished class notes, 1980.
117. Iggo A: A *single unit analysis of cutaneous receptor with C afferent fibers,* CIBA foundation groups, Springfield, Ill, 1967, Charles C Thomas, Publisher.
118. Jackson O: The Feldenkrais method: a personalized learning model. In Lister MJ, editor: *Contemporary management of motor control problems,* Norman, Okla, 1991, Foundation for Physical Therapy.
119. Jackson O: *Therapeutic considerations for the elderly,* vol 14, Clinics in physical therapy, New York, 1987, Churchill Livingstone.
120. Jacob S and Francone C: *Structure and function in man,* ed 3, Philadelphia, 1974, WB Saunders.
121. Kandel ER, Schwartz JH, and Jessell TM: *Principles of neural science,* ed 3, New York, 1991, Elsevier Medical Science Publishing Co.
121a. Gould JA: *Orthopaedic and Sports Physical Therapy,* St. Louis, 1990, Mosby.
122. Keshner EA: How theoretical framework biases evaluation and treatment. In Lister MJ, editor: *Contemporary management of motor problems,* Norman, Okla, 1991, Foundation for Physical Therapy.
123. Knickerbocker H: *A holistic approach to the treatment of learning disorders,* Thorofare, NJ, 1980, Charles B Slack.
124. Knott M and Voss DE: *Proprioceptive neuromuscular facilitation,* New York, 1968, Harper & Row.
125. Kottke F: The neurophysiology of motor function. In Kottke F, Stillwell K, and Lehmann J, editors: *Handbook of physical medicine and rehabilitation,* ed 3, Philadelphia, 1982, WB Saunders.
126. Knowles R: Through neurolinguistic programming, *Am J Nurs,* 83:1010, 1983.
127. Kornberg C and McCarthy T: The effect of neural stretching techniques on sympathetic outflow to the lower limbs, *J Orthop Sports Phys Ther* 16(6):269-274, 1992.
128. LaMotte RH and Mountcastle VB: Capacities of humans and monkeys to discriminate vibratory stimuli of different frequency and amplitude: a correlation between neural events and psychological measurements, *J Neurophysiol* 38:539-559, 1975.
129. Levitt S: *Treatment of cerebral palsy and motor delay,* Oxford, 1977, Blackwell Scientific Publications.
130. Lim RK: Pain, *Annu Rev Physiol* 32:269, 1970.
131. Loeb GE and Hoffer JA: Muscle spindle function. In Taylor A and Prochazka A, editors: *Muscle receptors in movement control,* 1981, MacMillan.
132. Magnus R: Cameron prize lectures on some results of studies in physiology and posture, *Lancet* 2:531-536, 1926.
133. Maisden DC, Meadows JC, and Hodgson HJ: Observations on the reflex response to muscle vibration in man and its voluntary control, *Brain* 42:829-846, 1969.
134. Maitland GD: *Peripheral manipulation,* ed 3, Boston, 1992, Butterworths.
135. Marx J: Analgesia: how the body inhibits pain perception, *Science* 195:471-473, 1977.
136. McCloskey DI: Kinesthetic sensibility, *Physiol Rev* 58(4):763-813, 1978.
137. McCormack GL: Pain management: a role for occupational therapists, *Am J Occup Ther* 43:4, 1988.
138. Melzack R: Myofascial trigger points: relations to acupuncture and mechanisms of pain, *Arch Phys Med Rehabil* 62:47-50, 1981.
139. Melzack R, Stillwell DM, and Fox EJ: Trigger points and acupuncture points for pain: correlations and implication, *Pain* 1:3-23, 1977.
140. Melzack R, Konrad KW, and Dubrobsky B: Prolonged changes in the nervous system activity produced by somatic and reticular stimulation, *Exp Neurol* 25:416-428, 1969.
141. Michels E: Motor behavior in hemiplegia, *Phys Ther* 45:759-767, 1965.
142. Mills M and Cohen BB: *Developmental movement therapy,* Amherst, Mass, 1979, The School for Body/Mind Centering.
143. Montgomery PC: Neurodevelopmental treatment and sensory integrative theory. In Lister MJ, editor: *Contemporary management of motor control problems,* Norman, Okla, 1991, Foundation for Physical Therapy.
144. Moore JC: Cranial nerves and their importance in current rehabilitation techniques. In Henderson A and Coryell J, editors: *The body senses and perceptual deficit,* Boston, 1973, Boston University Press.
145. Moore JC: The Golgi tendon organ and the muscle spindle, *Am J Occup Ther* 28(7):415-420, 1974.
146. Moore JC: The limbic system, Class notes from Bay Area Sensory Symposium, San Francisco, Calif, Feb 1980.
147. Moore JC: Recovery potentials following CNS lesions: a brief historical perspective in relation to modern research data on neuroplasticity, *Am J Occup Ther* 40(7):459-462, 1987.
148. Moore JC and Umphred DA: *The vestibular-visual-cervical triad: foundations for balance, posture, position sense and movement and treatment implications,* San Francisco, 1993.
149. Moulton DG and Beidler LM: Structure and function in the peripheral olfactory system, *Physiol Rev* 47:1, 1967.
150. Moulton DG, Turk A, and Johnston JW, editors: *Methods in olfactory research,* London, 1975, Academic Press.
151. Mountcastle VB, editor: Sensory receptor and neural encoding: introduction to sensory processes. In *Medical physiology,* vol 2, ed 14, St Louis, 1979, Mosby.
152. Mueller HA: Facilitating feeding and prespeech. In Pearson PH and Williams CE, editors: *Physical therapy services in the developmental disabilities,* Springfield, Ill, 1972, Charles C Thomas.
153. Neeman RL: Burn injury rehabilitation—hand dyskinesia and finger pain-treatment by orthokinetic orthoses, *J Burn Care Rehabil* 6:495-500, 1985.
154. Neeman RL and Numan M: Treatment of dyskinesia and pain by orthokineted orthoses in geriatric practice, *Occup Ther Forum* 2(15):19-21, 1986.
155. Neeman RL and Numan M: Treatment of pain by orthokinetic orthosis (cuffs), *Occup Ther Forum* 2(1): 18-19, 1986, (northeast edition) and *Occup Ther Forum* 2(2):18-19, 1986.
156. Neeman RL, Numan HJ, and Numan M: A single-subject study of clinical utility and social validity of orthokinetics treatment for upper extremity dyskinesia in a subject with spastic quadriplegia, unpublished manuscript, 1986.
157. Ninth National Conference on Juvenile Justice: Open forum discussion, Atlanta, Ga, March 1982.
158. Noback CR, Strominger NL, and Demarest RJ: *The human nervous system: introduction and review,* ed 4, Philadelphia, 1991, Lea & Febiger.
159. Normell LA: The cutaneous thermoregulatory vasomotor response in health subjects and paraplegic men, *Scand J Clin Invest* 4(33):133-138, 1974.
160. Oakley B and Benjamin RM: Neurological mechanisms of taste, *Physiol Rev* 46:173, 1966.
161. Olderog Millard KA and Smith JM: The influence of group singing on the behavior of Alzheimer's disease patients, *J Music Ther* 26(2):58-70, 1989.
162. Ottoson D: Experiments and concepts in olfactory physiology, *Progr Brain Res* 23:83-138, 1967.

163. Page D: Neuromuscular reflex therapy as an approach to patient care, *Am J Phys Med* 46(1):816-837, 1967.
164. Parker DE: The vestibular apparatus, *Sci Am* 243(11):118-130, 1980.
165. Payton OP, Hirt S, and Newton RA: *Scientific bases for neurophysiologic approaches to therapeutic exercise: an anthology*, Philadelphia, 1978, FA Davis.
166. Peiper A: *Cerebral function in infancy and childhood*, New York, 1963, Consultants Bureau.
167. Pertovaara A: Modification of human pain threshold by specific tactile receptors, *Acta Physiol Scand* 107(4):339-341, 1979.
168. Pfaffman C: Taste, its sensory and motivating properties, *Am Sci* 52:187-206, 1964.
169. Phelps ME, Kuhl DE, and Mazziotta JC: Metabolic mapping of the brain's response to visual stimulation: studies in humans, *Science* 211.1445-1448, 1981.
170. Poggio GF and Mountcastle VB: A study of the functional contributions of the lemniscal and spinothalamic systems to somatic sensibility, *Bull Johns Hopkins Hosp* 106:266-316, 1960.
171. Pollack NJ and Namazi KH: The effect of music participation on the social behavior of Alzheimer's disease patients, *J Music Ther* 29(1):54-67, 1992.
172. Pribram KH: *Languages of the brain: experimental paradoxes and principles in neuropsychology*, Englewood Cliffs, NJ, 1971, Prentice-Hall.
173. Prickett CA and Moore RS: The use of music to aid in the memory of Alzheimer's patients, *J Music Ther* 28(2):101-110, 1991.
174. Quillian TA: Neuro-cutaneous relationships in fingerprint skin. In Kornhuber H, editor: *The somatosensory system*, Sachs, Germany, 1975, Thiene Publisher.
175. Quillian TA and Ridley A: The receptors community in the fingertip, *J Physiol* 216:15-17, 1971.
176. Quinn JF: Building a body of knowledge-research on therapeutic touch, 1974-1986, *J Holistic Nurs* 6(1):37-45, 1988.
177. Reith E and Breidenback B: *Textbook of anatomy and physiology*, ed 2, New York, 1978, McGraw-Hill.
178. Roberts TDM: *Neurophysiology of postural mechanisms*, New York, 1967, Plenum.
179. Roitman DM: Age associated perceptual changes and the physical environment: perspectives on environmental adaptation, *Isr J Occup Ther* 2(1):14-27, 1993.
180. Rood M: The use of sensory receptors to activate, facilitate and inhibit motor response, autonomic and somatic in developmental sequence. In Scattely C, editor: *Approaches to treatment of patients with neuromuscular dysfunction*, Third International Congress, World Federation of Occupational Therapists, Dubuque, Iowa, 1962, William Brown Group.
181. Schmidt RA: Motor learning principles for physical therapy. In Lister MJ, editor: *Contemporary management of motor control problems*, Norman, Okla, Foundation for Physical Therapy.
182. Schraidt R: *Fundamentals of sensory physiology*, Berlin, 1978, Springer-Verlag.
183. Scholz J and Campbell S: Muscle spindles and the regulation of movement, *Phys Ther* 60(11):1416-1424, 1981.
184. Seivert J: Manual Therapy: Maitland's concepts, 1993.
185. Selbach H: The principle of relaxation occillation as a special instance of the law of initial value in cybernetic functions, *Ann NY Acad Sci* 98:1221-1228, 1962.
186. Serizawa K: *TsuboL—vital points for oriental therapy*, Tokyo, 1976, Japan Publishing.
187. Seufert-Jeffer U and Jeffer EK: An introduction to the VOJTA Method, *Clin Man Phys Ther* 2(4):26-29, 1982.
188. Shepard GM: Synaptic organization of the mammalian olfactory bulb, *Physiol Rev* 52:864-917, 1972.
189. Shumway-Cook A: Equilibrium deficits in children. In Woolcott MH and Shumway-Cook A, editors: *Development of posture and gait*

across the lifespan, Columbia, SC, 1989, University of South Carolina.
190. Shumway-Cook A and Horak FB: Rehabilitation strategies for patients with vestibular deficits, *Neurol Clin* 8:441-457, 1990.
191. Sinclair D: *Cutaneous sensation,* London, 1967, Oxford University Press.
192. Smith GR and others: Psychological modulation of the human immune response to varicela zoster, *Arch Intern Med* 145:2110-2112, 1985.
193. Steiner JE: Innate discriminative human facial expressions to taste and smell stimulations, *Ann NY Acad Sci* 237:229-233, 1974.
194. Stejskal L: Postural reflexes in man, *Am J Phys Med* 58(1):1-24, 1979.
195. Stockmeyer SA: An interpretation of the approach of Rood to the treatment of neuromuscular dysfunction, *Am J Phys Med* 46:900-961, 1967.
196. Sullivan PE, Markos PD, and Minor MA: *An integrated approach to therapeutic exercise,* Reston, Va, 1982, The Reston Publishing Co.
197. Takagi K and Kobagasi S: Skin pressure reflex, *Acta Med Biol* 4:;31-37, 1956.
198. Talbot WH and others: The sense of flutter-vibration: companion of the human capacity with response patterns of mechanoreceptive afferents, *J Neurophysiol* 31:301-334, 1968.
199. Tappan FM: *Healing massage techniques; holistic, classic and emerging methods,* ed 2, Norwalk, Conn, 1988, Appelton & Lange.
200. Taylor TC: Myofascial release techniques, *Phys Ther Forum* 5(23):2-4, 1986.
201. Travell J: *Myofascial pain and dysfunction,* Baltimore, 1983, Williams & Wilkins.
202. Treisman A and Gormican S: Feature analysis in early vision: evidence from search asymmetries, *Psychol Rev* 95:15-48, 1988.
203. Tuttle R and McClearly J: Mesenteric baroreceptors, *Am J Physiol* 229(6):1514-1519, 1975.
204. Twomey LT and Taylor JR: *Physical therapy of the low back,* ed 2, New York, 1994, Churchill Livingstone.
205. Umphred DA: Clinical observations, 1967 to 1994.
206. Umphred DA: Integrated approach to treatment of the pediatric neurologic patient. In Campbell SK: *Clinics in physical therapy: pediatric neurologic disorders,* New York, 1984, Churchill Livingstone.
207. Upledger J: *Craniosacral therapy,* ed 5, Seattle, 1986, Eastman Press.
208. Urbscheit N: Reflexes evoked by group II afferent fibers from the muscle spindle, *Phys Ther* 59:1083-1087, 1979.
209. Valdez P: *Emotion responses to color,* Doctoral dissertation, UCLA, 1993.
210. Vallbo AB and others: Somatosensory, proprioceptive, and sympathetic activity in human peripheral nerves, *Physiol Rev* 59(4):919-951, 1979.
211. Van Houten R and Rolider A: The use of color mediation techniques to teach number identification and single digit multiplication problems to children with learning disability, *Educ Treat Child* 13(3):216, 1990.
212. Verrillo R: Change in vibrotactile thresholds as a function of age, *Sens Processes* 3:49-59, 1979.
213. Wall P: The gate control theory of pain mechanisms, *Brain* 101:1, March 1978.
214. Weiss SJ: Psychophysiologic effects of caregiver touch on incidence of cardiac dysrhythmia, *Heart Lung* 15(5):495-502, 1986.
215. Weisz S: Studies in equilibrium reaction. In Payton OD and others: *Neurophysiologic approaches to therapeutic exercise,* Philadelphia, 1978, FA Davis.
216. Wells K: *Kinesiology,* ed 4, Philadelphia, 1967, WB Saunders.
217. West A: Understanding endorphins: our natural pain relief system, *Nursing* 7:50-53, 1981.
218. Whelan JK: Effect of orthokinetics on upper extremity function of the adult hemiplegic patient, *Am J Occup Ther* 18(4):141-143, 1964.
219. Wilburger P: Advanced course for treatment of sensory defensiveness

In *Symposium on intervention for persons with mild to severe dysfunction,* Minneapolis, Minn.: unpublished.

220. Willis WD and Grossman RG: *Medical neurobiology,* ed 3, St Louis, 1981, Mosby.

221. Wilson V and Peterson B: The role of the vestibular system in posture and movement. In Mountcastle VB, editor: *Medical physiology,* vol 2, ed 14, St Louis, 1980, Mosby.

222. Winstein CJ: Designing practice for motor learning: clinical implications. In Lister MJ, editor: *Contemporary management of motor control problems,* Norman, Okla, 1991, APTA.

223. Young RR: The clinical significance of exteroceptive reflexes. In Desurdet JE, editor: *New developments in electromyography and clinical neurophysiology,* vol 3, Basel, 1973, Karger.

224. Zemack-Bersin D, Zemach-Bersin K, and Resse M: *Relaxercise: the easy new way to health and fitness,* New York, 1990, Harper & Row.

225. Zotterman Y: *Sensory functions of the skin in primates,* Oxford, 1976, Pergamon Press.

226. Zwaardemaker H: *Physiology of smell,* London, 1895, Collier Macmillan.

CHAPTER 7

Psychosocial Aspects of Adaptation and Adjustment During Various Phases of Neurological Disability

Gordon U. Burton

KEY TERMS

adjustment	family network
adaptation	bonding
loss and grief	sexuality
coping	sensuality
support systems	problem solving
cognitive age	

LEARNING OBJECTIVES

After reading this chapter the student/therapist will:

1. Describe adaptation and adjustment as a flexible and flowing process, not as static stages.
2. Describe elements of the grief process that deal with age, cognition, and developmental level.
3. Respect aspects of sensuality and sexuality in treatment and consider them when treating the client.
4. Integrate the family of the client and the client's styles of coping into therapeutic treatment strategies to be used in the clinic.
5. Integrate the elements of problem solving, loss, cognitive functioning, coping, sensuality, as well as significant others' coping and learning styles into the treatment process to encourage adaptation.

OVERVIEW

Psychological **adjustment** appears to be elusive because it is a fluid process: all people are constantly changing. This is especially true for people who have recently become physically disabled. They do not reach a certain state of adjustment and stay there, but progress through a series of **adaptations**. Therapists commonly see clients in a crisis state[41] and therefore identify their adjustment pattern from this frame of reference. How well the client adjusts to crisis, however, does not necessarily indicate how well the individual will adjust to all aspects of the disability or the rate of progress from one adaptation to another.[5,17,91,128] Disabilities are a massive insult to a person's self-perception.[9,15,19,100] A month, or even a year, after the injury may not be long enough to put the disability into perspective.[9,17,42,76,78]

For most people progressing from the shock of injury to the acceptance of, and later adaptation to, disability is a process fraught with psychologic ups and downs. Several authors have discussed the possible stages of adjustment and grieving.[102,106,128] The research of Kübler-Ross[81] into death and dying also has application to this topic of adjustment to disability. She discusses the concept of **loss and grief** in relation to life; loss of function may induce just as profound a reaction. Peretz[103] discusses the grieving process in relationship to loss of role function as well as loss of body function. These losses must be grieved for before the client can benefit from therapy or adjust to a changed life-style and body. Therapists must be aware that the client can and must deal with the death of certain functional abilities.

The concept of stages of adjustment has been questioned,[41] and a call for more empirical research into adaptation and adjustment has been made.[22,77] Several studies have given some attention to this concept, but much more work is needed.*

The components of successful psychological adjustment to a physical disability are varied. To bring a client to a level of function that is of the highest quality possible for that individual, therapists must look holistically at the psychosocial aspects and at the adjustment processes involved, evaluate each component, and integrate the processes into the therapeutic milieu to promote growth in all areas. There is more to evaluation and treatment than just the physical component; the mind and body have interrelated influences, and both must be understood, evaluated, and treated individually and as a whole.†

This chapter explores the processes of adjustment and adaptation, as well as the influences of culture and societal values as they affect the physically disabled person. The importance of loss as a psychological component will be examined as it relates to the body, sexuality, the personality, and the family. Age will also be discussed as a factor in adjustment to disability. The importance of focusing on the strengths of the client, the family, and the support system, rather than on the weaknesses of the disability will also be explored.

This overview is designed to help therapists think of the client as a whole person, not as a diagnosis to be handled in some prescribed way. As fellow human beings, therapist and client are in the rehabilitation process together.

* References 21, 42, 76, 87, 91, 105, and 128.
† References 5, 10, 13, 17, 25, 33, 42, 46, 50, 60, and 67.

Adjustment using the stage concept

Sequence process. Each person has his or her own **coping** style and each should be allowed to be unique. Kerr[70] describes five stages of adjustment:

1. Shock: "This really isn't happening to me."
2. Expectancy for recovery: "I will be well soon."
3. Mourning: "There is no hope."
4. Defense:
   a. "I will live with this obstacle and beat it." (healthy attitude)
   b. "I am adjusted, but you fail to see it." (neurotic attitude)
5. Adjustment: "It is part of me now, but it is not necessarily a 'bad' thing."

In light of current research, it is important for the therapist to realize that these are not lockstep stages and are to be thought of as concepts to help with the understanding of common reactions of all individuals.[87]

Shock. The client in shock does not recognize that anything is actually wrong. He or she may totally refuse to accept the diagnosis. The client may even laugh at the concern expressed by others. This stage is altered when the person has an opportunity to test reality and finds that the physical condition is actually limiting performance. If this stage continues, it may signify either a lack of mental health or an inability to cognitively realize the situation.

Expectancy for recovery. The client in this stage is aware that he or she is "ill" but also believes that recovery will be quick and complete. The person may look for a "miracle cure" and may make future plans that require total return of function. Total recovery is the only goal, even if it takes a great deal of time and effort to achieve. Key signs of this stage are resentment of loss of function and the feeling that the whole body is necessary to do anything worthwhile. The staff can stimulate a change from this stage by giving clear statements to the client that the damage is permanent, by transferring the person home or to the rehabilitation unit, or by discontinuing therapy. Any one of these occurrences can help make the client realize the permanence of the disability.

Mourning. During the stage of mourning the individual feels all is lost; that he or she will never achieve anything in life. Suicide is often considered. The person may feel that characteristics of the personality (such as courage or fight) have also been lost and must be mourned as well. Thus motivation to continue therapy, to work on improving, may be absent. The prospect of total recovery can no longer be held, but, at the same time, there appears to be no other acceptable alternative. This feeling of despair may be expressed as hostility, and, as a result, therapists may view the individual as a "problem patient." It is possible for a client to remain at this stage with feelings of inadequacy, dependency, and hostility. However, it is also possible for therapeutic intervention to facilitate movement to the next stage by creating situations in which the client may feel that "normal" aspirations and goals can be achieved. In this circumstance, "normal" would not include such low-level activities as dressing or walking—activities that were taken for granted before the injury—but would include doing the work he or she was trained to do. These activities would also include playing with or caring for a child or family. This would be seen as self-actualization by Maslow.[88]

Defense. The defense stage has two components. The first represents a healthy attitude in which the client actually starts coping with the disability. The client can take pride in his or her accomplishments, work to improve independence, and become as normal as possible. The person is still very much aware that barriers to normal functioning exist and is bothered by this fact, but also realizes that some of the barriers can be circumvented. This healthy defensive stage can be undermined and possibly destroyed by well-meaning family, friends, and therapists who encourage the individual to see only the positive aspects and who do not allow the client to examine feelings about the restrictions and barriers of the condition. Conditions that lead to the final stage of adjustment may either be the client realizing that the whole body is not needed to actualize his or her life goals or that needs behind the goals can be actualized in other ways. A therapist should watch for opportunities to facilitate this transition.

The negative alternative during the defensive stage is the neurotic defensive reaction. This is typified by the client refusing to recognize that even a partial barrier exists to meeting normal goals. The client may try to convince everyone that he or she has adjusted.

Adjustment. In the final stage, adjustment, the person sees the disability as neither an asset nor a liability but as an aspect of the person, much like a large nose or big feet. The disability is not something to be overcome, apologized for, or defended against. Kerr[70] refers to two aspects or goals of this stage. The first goal is for the person to feel at peace with his or her god: the client does not feel that he or she is being punished or tested. The second goal is for the client to feel that he or she is an adequate person—not a second-class citizen. Kerr[71] believes that "It is essential that the paths to those more 'abstract goals' be structured if the person is to make a genuine adjustment." She also believes that it is the health professional's job to offer that structure.

Acceptance or adjustment is at least as hard to achieve and maintain in life for the disabled person as happiness and harmony are for the able-bodied person. Adjustment connotes putting the disability into perspective, seeing it as one of the many characteristics of that person. It does not mean negating the existence of or focusing on the condition. Successful adjustment may be defined as an ongoing process in which the person adapts to the environment in a satisfying and efficient manner. This is true for all human beings, able-bodied or disabled. There are always obstacles to overcome in attempting the goal of a happy and successful life.[15,22,69]

People and circumstances change. Maintaining a balanced state of adjustment is not easy, especially for the disabled person. I recall a woman who had achieved a stable state of acceptance of her quadraplegic condition. She called in a panic because, as she saw it, she "wasn't adjusted anymore." She had moved into a college dormitory and wanted to go out for a friendly game of football with her new friends, but suddenly saw how disabled she was. She had grown up in a hospital and had never had to face this situation. After discussing this, she was able to put things into perspective and was able to talk over her feelings of isolation with her friends, who, without hesitation, altered the game to include her. Keeping a balanced perspective is hard in a world that changes constantly.

White[132] states that without some performance, there can be no affecting the environment and thus, no sense of self-satisfaction. Fine[36] and King[74] point out that without satisfaction from affecting the environment, reinforcement is insufficient to carry on the behavior and the behavior will be extinguished. Thus satisfaction and performance must be linked. If the patient has not adjusted to his or her new body, however, little satisfaction can be gained from such everyday activities as walking, eating, or rolling over in bed.[106] To define adjustment on a purely performance basis is to run the risk of creating a "mechanical person" who might be physically rehabilitated, but, once discharged, may find that he lacks satisfaction, incentive, and purpose. The psychological state of adjustment is what makes self-satisfaction possible.

Adaptive process. The therapist can use the concept of the adaptive process to organize therapy sessions that promote the adjustment process as well as attain physical goals. In so doing, the therapist will be promoting and teaching performance and working toward the eventual achievement, client satisfaction.

King[74] describes four characteristics of the adaptive process. They can be worked on singly or simultaneously, and they can be thought of as the means to reach the goal of Kerr's[71] final stage of adjustment. These characteristics are: active response, incorporation of the environment, response organized subcortically, and self-reinforcing adaptation.

Active response. In general, therapy encourages an active response by the client against the environment. The client is expected to produce action to improve. Interaction with environmental factors can be seen even if there is little functional ability, as in the case of a high-level quadraplegic client whose main avenue of interaction is verbal but whose influence can change the environment.

Incorporation of the environment. Another characteristic of the adaptive process is use of the environment to stimulate adaptive responses. An example of this would be setting up a graded walking program that takes the client from a smooth surface, to a rug, and eventually to grassy and rocky terrain. The adaptive process would be enhanced if at the time of discharge the client was not only able but also confident of his or her ability to walk over the lawn to reach the house from the surrounding perimeter.

Response organized unconsciously. King[74] believes that an unconsciously organized response is achieved most effectively by directing the client's conscious attention to a task or an object while allowing the subconscious centers to integrate the response. The example in the previous paragraph can be used to illustrate this characteristic. The client's objective (conscious mind) may be set on getting across a lawn to get into her or his house, but the therapist's goal would be to stimulate automatic equilibrium reactions at a subconscious level. Unconscious adaptive responses generalize to other situations more easily than cognitively taught "splinter skill" reactions. As soon as the client cortically attends to equilibrium, the automatic postural changes are, by definition, lost. That is, if the task is procedural, attention needs to be placed on something else while the client practices the activity.

Self-reinforcing adaptation. Each successful adaptation stimulates the next more complex step. It is essential for the client to succeed because this success stimulates progression to the next more complex "task." It should be remembered that the "task" is adjustment and that the activity only facilitates adaptation or adjustment. Thus the therapist does not need to feel disheartened if the client learns to get into and out of his or her house but does not want to start mountain climbing: The goal of the adaptive process is adjustment in as near a normal pattern as possible for that client.

Combining knowledge of Kerr's stages of adjustment, as outlined previously, with the adaptive process gives the therapist a reality-based, evaluative treatment framework. The stage of adjustment can be assessed, and the adaptive process characteristics can be drawn on in treatment to facilitate progression toward psychological acceptance of the disability as well as to promote physical improvement.

For example, if a person is in the mourning stage of adjustment, the therapist, knowing that the defense stage usually follows (p. 181), can encourage and support the client's entrance into this next stage by adapting a situation that meets the goal of the defense stage—beating the obstacles of disability. The adaptive process may also be used to structure the therapeutic activities that facilitate an active response to overcome the disability, using the environment to organize the response subcortically in such a way that it is self-reinforcing. For example, the client might want to call his or her spouse, and the therapist may be working cortically on increasing upper-extremity strength and wheelchair mobility. The client could be told that the only accessible phone is up a steep ramp and that the client must push him or herself up there to use the phone in privacy. The therapist might also add that it always seems that obstacles are in the way of the disabled and that the client must explore methods to deal with these problems. As the client accomplishes the task, not only will the objectives of

strength and wheelchair mobility be realized, but the client may start thinking that he or she may be able to beat the effects of the disability, thus moving the client from the mourning stage to the defense stage. No single experience will cause this to happen, but if therapy is designed to encourage adjustment and adaption, the client will tend to progress faster and with less trauma.

Awareness of psychological adjustment in the clinic

The problem for the therapist in treating a person with a disability is to see the disability in perspective: to see the whole person in the client's own world and in the context of society and a given time. After this difficult task is achieved, the therapist must develop a program that will appropriately stimulate the client and all significant others around the client to pursue the highest-quality life possible. The successful and skilled therapist evaluates the client's physical capabilities but does not stop there. At some level, assessment of the more subtle psychological aspects of the client's ability to function is needed. This includes the client's family network (**support system**) and its ability to adjust to the imminent change in life-style.

The rest of this section will introduce the reader to some of the psychological change components that may be assessed. The last section will attempt to demonstrate possible ways that these components can be taken into account as an aspect of therapy.

Societal and cultural influences. From an early age, people in our society are exposed to misconceptions regarding the disabled person.[9,15,61] Some of these misguided perceptions are that the physically disabled person is also retarded, not employable, dependent, helpless, asexual, unlovable, and miserable. If a first- or second-grade child is asked how a retarded person walks, the common response is the demonstration of a hemiplegic gait and posture with one arm going into a flexion synergy. This child has already learned not only the "role" of the physically disabled but will have also incorporated other misconceptions about how a disabled person acts. If these misconceptions were held before injury, then it is only reasonable for the newly disabled person to be inclined to fulfill these perceived role expectations.[15,61] Thus the client may undergo a radical change in the perceived self (how the person sees him or herself) as a result of the "new" role expectations. Even worse, the family members and medical personnel may hold the same expectations of the disabled person and thus reinforce the helpless, dependent role.[51,52,59]

If in the therapeutic environment, however, the client and family have their misconceptions challenged constantly, they may start reformulating their concept of the role of the disabled person. As this process progresses, therapists and other staff can help make the expectations of the disabled person more realistic. Therapists can schedule their clients at times when they will be exposed to people making realistic adjustments to their disabilities. Use of successfully rehabilitated individuals as staff members (role models) can help to dispel the misconception that disabled people are not employable.[86]

This process of adaptation to a new disability can be considered as a cultural change from a majority status (able-bodied) to a minority status (disabled). Part of the adaptation process can be considered as an acculturation process, and the therapist can help facilitate this process.[15,18] The cultural background of the individual also contributes to the perception of disability and to the acceptance of the disabled person. Trombly[127] states that perception and expression of pain, physical attractiveness, valuing of body parts, as well as acceptability of types of disabilities can be culturally influenced. One's ethnic background can also affect intensity of feelings toward specific handicaps, trust of staff,[127] and acceptance of therapeutic modalities.[10,126]

The successful therapist will be sensitive to the cultural values of the client and will attempt to present therapy to the client in the most acceptable way. For example, in the Mexican culture it is not polite to just start to work with a client; rapport must first be established. Sharing of food may provide the vehicle to accomplish rapport. Thus the therapist might schedule the first visit with a Mexican client during a coffee break. The therapist must remember that the dysfunctional client may be the one who can least be expected to adjust to the therapist and that the therapist may need to adjust to the client, especially in the early stages of therapy.

Gaining trust is one of the crucial links in any meaningful therapeutic situation.[80] Trust will create an environment that facilitates communication, productive learning, and exchange of information.[95] Trust is important in all cultures and will be fostered by the therapist who is sensitive to the needs of the client. This sensitivity is necessary with every client, but will be manifested in many different ways, depending on the background and needs of the individual in therapy. A client of one culture may feel that looking another person in the eyes is offensive, whereas in another culture refusal to look into someone's eyes is a sign of weakness or lack of honesty (shifty-eyed).[58] Thus although it is impossible to know every culture or subculture with which the therapist may come into contact, the therapist must attempt to be sensitive to the background of the client. Even if the therapist knows the cultural norms, not every person follows the cultural patterns, and thus every client needs to be treated as an individual in the therapeutic relationship. It should be the therapist's job to be sensitive to the subtle nonverbal and verbal cues that indicate the level of trust in the relationship.

Trust is often established in the therapeutic relationship through physical activities. The act of asking a client to transfer from the chair to the bed can either build trust or destroy the potential relationship. If the client trusts the therapist just enough to follow instructions to transfer but then falls in the process, it may take quite some time to

reestablish the same level of trust, assuming that it can ever be reestablished. This trusting relationship is so complex and involves such a variety of levels that the therapist should be as aware of attending to the client's security in the relationship as to the physical safety of the client in the clinic.[80] If the client believes that the therapist is not trustworthy in the relationship, then it may follow that the therapist is not to be trusted when it comes to physical manipulation of a disabled body. If the client does not know how to use the damaged body and thus cannot trust the body, then lacking trust in the therapist will only compound the stress of the situation.[80] (Refer to Chapter 5 for more information on some of the neurological components of this interaction.)

The client's culture may be alien to the therapist, even though they may be from the same geographical region. A client's problems of poverty, unemployment, and a lack of educational opportunities[60] can all result in the therapist and client feeling that therapy will be unsuccessful, even before the first session has begun. Such preconceived concepts held by both parties may not be warranted and must be examined.

Cultural and religious values may also result in the client feeling that he or she must pay for past sins by being disabled and that the disability will be overcome after atonement for these sins. Such a client may not be inclined to participate in or enjoy therapy. The successful therapist does not assault the client's basic cultural or religious values, but may recognize them in the therapy sessions. If the therapist feels that the culturally defined problems are impeding the therapeutic process, the therapist may offer the client opportunities to reexamine these cultural "truths" and may help the client redefine the way the disability and therapy is seen. Religious counseling could be recommended by the therapist, and follow-up support in the clinic may be given to the client to view therapy not as undoing what "God has done," but as a way of proving religious strength. Note that reworking a person's cultural/religious (cognitive) structure is a very sensitive area, and it should be handled with care and respect and with the use of other professionals (social workers and religious and psychological counselors) if needed.

The hospital staff can be encouraged to establish groups in which commonly held values of clients can be examined and possibly challenged.[15,69] Such groups can lead the client to a better understanding of priorities and may help the person see the relevance of therapy and the need to continue the adjustment process. This can also prepare the client to better accept the need for support groups after discharge. The therapist may be able to use information from such group sessions to adjust the way therapy sessions are presented and structured to make therapy more relevant to the client's values and needs. Value groups or exercises[112,120] can be another means used by the therapist for evaluation and understanding of the client.

Values, roles, and body parts may all be grieved for by the client. This is especially true during the mourning stage of adjustment. The following section will look at ways of grieving and will explore some possible losses the therapist may not be alert to.[30,44,52,59,69,97]

Examination of loss. Reaction to loss has been examined by Peretz.[103] Nine types of bereavement states were described. They are as follows:

1. Normal grief
2. Anticipatory grief
3. Absent, delayed, and inhibited grief
4. Chronic grief
5. Depression
6. Hypochondriasis
7. Development of psychophysiological reactions
8. Acting out
9. Neurotic and psychotic states

The individual with normal grief alternates from shock and incomprehension to bewilderment and weeping, which may give way to guilt feelings, irrational anger, and even depressive symptoms. Progress can be judged by a gradual return to the client's level of functioning before the loss. The person with anticipatory grief is grieving for a loss that has not yet taken place. This may be grieving for loss of function or role even before the loss is documented. The client with absent, delayed, and inhibited grief may postpone grief until the crisis is past; or he or she may hide grief, not expressing it and not getting the necessary support. These individuals have been noted to experience "anniversary reactions" (reexperiencing loss at some later date such as the "anniversary" of the accident or diagnosis of the disability). With chronic grief the patient is in a state of persistent mourning, and no change in life-style or environment will be tolerated. Sadness, tension, and gloom characterize the individual in the emotional state of depression. The client may feel sorry for himself or herself and may be rendered nonfunctional. Psychotherapy or chemotherapy may be necessary. The patient with hypochondriasis may express anxiety regarding a physical concern (other than the disability) to avoid dealing with the disability. Usually there is no physical cause for the anxiety expressed, but the symptoms may exist. With development of psychophysiological reactions, depression or loss may be expressed through somatic symptom formation, such as a decreased immune defense system, colitis, hypertension, duodenal ulcers, and other illnesses. These illnesses may become so severe as to cause the person's death. Further research and documentation are needed in this area. Acting out is an attempt to avoid the pain of loss by turning attention to something else. This can be done through involvement in acceptable activities, such as work, or unacceptable activities, such as drug use (abuse). Neurotic and psychotic states may take numerous forms depending on the psychological predisposition of the person.

Knowledge of the types of bereavement as described by Peretz[103] can be used by the therapist to better understand the client's reactions to loss and will allow the therapist the possibility of adjusting the treatment approach to the client's type of bereavement.[81] This knowledge of the grief process can be applied to clients who have terminal illnesses in an attempt to increase the client's quality of life.

Cognitive age and loss. The **cognitive age** of the person experiencing the loss is another aspect that therapists sometimes fail to consider. Harper and Bhattarai[61] and Krause and Crewe[78] have pointed out that the age of the person dealing with loss affects his reaction. It seems likely that this concept may be generalized to further understand loss of function.[5,45,61,114]

The child under 5 years of age views loss as a temporary, reversible phenomenon. From age 5 to 9 years, the average child views death or loss as final but remote. The child thinks of the dead person as someone who went away on a long trip or as someone who will not be around anymore. It is not until the person is older than the age of 9 that the child perceives loss as permanent. Dunton[35] cites the following case history:

A typical family with three children ages 11, 9, and 4½ years suffered the sudden loss of a beloved pet dog. When informed of the sad event the 11-year-old responded at first by saying nothing. Slowly the tears welled up in his eyes and he began to cry softly. When he regained his composure he said, "It's such a horrible thing—it's all over." The 9-year-old listened quietly to the news and said, "He has gone a long way. We'll have to get another one." The 4½-year-old looked puzzled and said repeatedly, "What happened? Why are you crying? Let's go get him!"

As a result of brain damage or shock, cognitive levels in the adult may regress after injury, much as reflex development may regress. The client may be functioning at a low cognitive level and may not be capable of understanding the permanence of the loss suffered. Disabled parents and spouses will have to deal with their children's reactions to the parent's loss in a manner appropriate to the cognitive level of each child.[36,37,45,61,62,69] Values clarification groups can be used to help the family deal with adjustment to loss.[112,120] The very act of being aware of cognitive levels of dealing with loss may help family members and therapists accept how the others are dealing (or not dealing) with the loss.[19,22,36,37]

Preschool-aged children often believe that the disability is a punishment and that they must have done something very wrong to deserve such a punishment.[113] It is thus important to stress that a disability is not a punishment and that accidents and disabilities happen to good people. In this way the therapist dispels the next logical concept—that therapy is further punishment and that the client needs to be punished.

Loss and the family. In this chapter, the client's support system is referred to as the family. The family may be composed of spouses, parents, children, lovers (especially in gay and lesbian relationships), friends, employers, or interested others—church groups, civic organizations, or individuals. The people in the support system may go through the same stages of reaction and adjustment to loss that the client does.[17,36,41,61]

Family needs. The family will, at least temporarily, experience the loss of a loved member from the normal routine. During the acute stage the family may not have concrete answers to basic questions regarding the extent of injury, the length of time before the injured person will be back in the family unit, or possibly whether the person will live.

During this phase, the **family network** will be in a state of crisis.[17,62] New roles will have to be assumed by the family members, and the "experts" will not even tell them for how long these roles must be endured. If children are involved, they will probably demand more attention to reassure themselves that they will remain loved. Depending on the child's age, the child will have differing capabilities in understanding the loss (see the section on examination of loss). Each member of the family may react differently to bereavement, and each may be at a different stage of adjustment to the disability (see the section on adjustment). One member may be in shock and deny the disability, while another member is in mourning and verbalizes a lack of hope. The family crisis that is caused by a severe injury cannot be overstated.[17,36,61,92,111]

Role changes in the family may be dramatic.[37,52,59,69,92] Members who have never driven may need to learn how; one who has never balanced a checkbook may now be responsible for managing the family budget; and those who have never been assertive may have to deal forcefully with insurance companies and the medical establishment.[17,37,110]

The family may feel resentment toward the injured member. This attitude may seem justified to them as they see the person lying in bed all day while the family members must take over new responsibilities in addition to their old ones. The medical staff may not always understand the stress that family members are under and may react to the resentment expressed either verbally or nonverbally with a protective stance toward the client. Siding with the "hurt" client may alienate the family from the medical staff and may also drive a permanent wedge between family members.

Parental bonding and the disabled child. The parent **bonding** process is complicated and is still being studied.[25,75] This process (attachment) may start well before the baby is even conceived.[75] The parents often think about having a child and plan and fantasize about future interactions with the child. After conception the planning and fantasizing increase. During the pregnancy the fetus is accepted as an individual by the mother[75] and father, and after the birth of the child the attachment process is greatly intensified. The "sensitive period" is the first few minutes to hours after the birth. During this time the parents should have close physical contact with the child to strongly establish the attachment that will later grow deeper.[75,133] There is an almost symbiotic relationship between mother and child at this time. Infant and mother behaviors complement each other (e.g.,

nursing stimulates uterine contraction). It is important at this point for the child to respond to the parents in some way so that there is an interaction. In the early stages of bonding, seeing, touching, caring for, and interacting with the child allow for the bonding process. When this process is disturbed for any reason, such as congenital malformations or hospital procedures for high-risk infants, problems may occur later. The occurrence of battered child syndrome and failure to thrive has been noted to be higher than the norm when the child is born prematurely or when there is poor (or lack of) bonding at an early age.[75] Klaus and Kennell[75] have recommended elements that increase the chances of parental bonding: (1) special needs during pregnancy and birth dealt with to support the parents; (2) parent preparation, education, and support; (3) need for a companion at labor and especially at birth; and (4) enhancing attachment—privacy and contact with the child and each other.

When the parents are told that their child is going to be malformed or disabled, it is a massive shock to the family. The parents must start a process of grieving. The dream of a "normal" child must be given up, and the parents must go through the loss or "death" of the child they expected before they can accept the new child. Parents often feel guilty. Shellabarger and Thompson[118] state that parents feel the deformed child was their failure.[41] Fathers are the most distressed about the child initially. The disabled child will always have a strong impact on the family, sometimes a catastrophic one.[5,17,41,118]

Parents must be encouraged to express their emotions, and they must be taught how to deal with the issues at hand. Techniques for accomplishing these goals are discussed in later sections.[118,125,133]

The child dealing with loss. If a parent is injured, the young child may experience an overwhelming sense of loss. Child care may be a problem, especially if the primary caregiver is injured. The child will probably feel deserted by the injured parent and may demand the attention of the remaining parent. This will increase the strain on all family members.[37,123]

If the child is the client, his or her life will have undergone a radical change: every aspect of the child's world will have altered. Loved objects and people will help to restore the child's feeling of security. It is of major importance to explain to the child in very simple terms what is going on and to allow the child the opportunity to express feelings both verbally and nonverbally (perhaps using play as the medium of communication).

The hospital setting is threatening to all people, but children are especially susceptible to loss of autonomy, feelings of isolation, and loss of independence. Bentovim and Nelson (Chapter 9) have stated that the severity of the disability is not as important a variable in the emotional development of the child as are the attitudes of parents and family.[3,17,61] Parents must attempt to be aware of the child's inability to understand the permanence (or transience) of the loss of function.[5,45] They will also need to help the child feel secure by bringing in familiar and cherished objects. A schedule should be established and kept to promote consistency. Play should be encouraged, especially that which allows the child to vent feelings and deal with the new environment. Any procedures or therapies should be presented in a relaxed way (fun, if possible), so that the child has time to think and to feel as comfortable as possible about the change.[19] The parents may often need to be reminded to pay attention to the nondisabled children in the family during this acute stage.

The adolescent dealing with loss. The adolescent is subject to all of the feelings and fears that other clients express. Adolescents are in a struggle to obtain autonomy and independence, and they often feel ambivalent about these feelings. When an adolescent is suddenly injured and has to cope with being disabled, it can be a massive assault on the individual's development.[22,48]

The adolescent appears to react differently from other age groups to the knowledge of his or her own terminal illness. The adolescent often feels that he or she has gone through a very painful process (initiation) that will soon lead to the "joys and rights" of adulthood. Unlike persons in older age groups who might feel that they can look back and gain solace from the past,[122] the adolescent feels that he or she will have what Solnit and Green[122] term "death before fulfillment" and thus may react by feeling cheated by life. This same pattern may occur with the disabled adolescent. The therapist must be acutely aware of these feelings so that therapy may be presented in the most effective manner for the client to find challenge and fulfillment in life.

Family maturation. The family also has a maturational aspect. If the injured person is a child and if the family is young with dependent children at home, the adjustment may not be the problem that it would be for a family whose children are older. In the latter case, parents have begun to experience freedom and independence, and they may find adjusting to a return to a restricted life-style, difficult, or even intolerable. They may have the feeling that they have already "put in their time" and should now be free. If the disability interrupts the child's developmental process, future conflict may arise because the parents will eventually want retirement, relaxation, and freedom. Parents may feel guilty about and try to repress this normal response.

The reverse may also be true. The parents may be feeling that the children have left them ("empty nest syndrome"), and they may be too willing to welcome a "dependent" family member back into the home. This may lead to excessive dependence or anger toward the parents on the part of the client. All of these factors must be taken into consideration by the therapist when therapy is presented to the client and family.

The therapist can develop a greater understanding of the client and family by being aware of the normal human developmental patterns as discussed by Sheehy[117] and Lewis.[84] These patterns identify some of the major hurdles that must be overcome in the client's life.

Coping with transition. In the acute stage of a family member's injury, the family must be helped to deal with the crisis at hand. During this phase, the family must first be allowed to cope with the emotional impact of what is happening with a loved one. Second, the family should be helped to see the situation as a challenge that, if overcome, will facilitate growth. Third, adaptation within the family unit must occur to overcome the situation. Brammer and Abrego[16] have developed a list of basic coping skills that they have broken into five levels. In the first level the person becomes aware of and mobilizes skills in perceiving and responding to transition and attempts to handle the situation. In the second level the person mobilizes the skills for assessing, developing, and using external support systems. In level three the person can possess, develop, and use internal support systems (develop positive self-regard and use the situation to grow). The person in level four must find ways to reduce emotional and physiological distress (relaxation, control stimulation, and verbal expression of feelings). In level five the person must plan and implement change (analyze discrepancies, plan new options, and successfully implement the plan). Using this model, the therapist and family can evaluate the coping skill-level of the family. The therapist and staff can then help promote movement toward the next level of coping with the transition. These levels are also broken into specific skills and subskills so that the therapist can grade them further.

One of the more damaging aspects of hospitalization to all involved is that the hospital staff focuses on the disability rather than on the individual's strengths.[47,73] Centering on the disability can lead to a situation where client, family, and staff see only the disability and not the potential ability of the client.

Decentering from the disability will be examined further in this chapter. If the family relationship was positive before the insult and if the client is cognitively intact, then the focus should be directed toward the relationship's strengths as well as toward the client's and family's individual strengths.[109] In the initial acute stage of adjustment, crisis intervention may help the family use its strengths and at the same time deal with the situation at hand.

To adequately deal with the crisis, the family should:

1. Be helped to focus on the crisis caused by the disability
   a. Identify the situation to stimulate problem solving
   b. Identify and deal with doubts of adequacy, guilt, and self-blame
   c. Identify and deal with grief work
   d. Identify and deal with anticipatory worry
2. Be offered basic information and education regarding the crisis situation

3. Be helped to create a bridge to resources in the hospital and in the community for support, as well as to see their own family resources
4. Be helped to remember how they have dealt successfully with crises in the past and to implement some of the same strategies in the present situation

Working with the family as a unit during crisis will help strengthen the family and facilitate more positive attitudes toward the client, thus improving the client's attitudes or feelings toward the injury and hospitalization.[59,69,76] Encouraging family-unit functioning in this situation will decrease the amount of regression displayed by the client. If the family is encouraged to function without the client, however, more damage than good may be done.[22,41]

Awareness of sexual issues

Sexuality is usually one of the last areas to be assessed, but it is one area mentioned as of great importance to family members and the client. Sexuality involves more than just the sex act; it incorporates characteristics such as sexual attraction, sexual identification, sexual confidence, and sexual validation.* It is a predictor of adjustment to disability, of success in vocational training, and of marital satisfaction when the woman is disabled.[119] Sexuality **(sensuality)** is representative of how the person is dealing with her or his world. If the person feels inadequate as a sexual, sensual, and lovable human being, there is little chance that he or she will also feel motivated to pursue other avenues of life.[108,119] This area of function must be assessed with great sensitivity to the individual's feelings.[27,82,108]

The framework for assessing sexuality differs with the therapist. Some therapists see sexuality as an activity of daily living and incorporate it into this evaluation. Others feel the client needs information about body mechanics to perform the sex act; thus positioning and reflex inhibiting patterns are assessed. Still others have found it a motivating force when range-of-motion and muscle control are worked on. A further discussion of these concerns will follow in the section on adult sexuality.

Development of sensuality (sexuality). Even before birth, the sense of touch[95] and the ability to distinguish pleasurable and unpleasurable tactile sensations begin to develop. Pleasurable feelings are comforting, and attempts are made to prolong them; for example, a baby cries when nursing is stopped. If satisfaction is not derived from this interaction on a regular basis, a feeling of anxiety may develop and the child may withdraw from interaction with others and distrust may develop.[95] If pleasure in interaction with others is obtained in the first 3 years, the ability to maintain the warmth of being close and being nourished is translated into trust (that all needs will be satisfied by the

*References 14, 28, 29, 31, 55, 57, 107, 110, 119, and 134.

caretaker) and lovability (bonding). It is here that a sense of intimacy is initiated.[28,79,95,121] Ego and sensuality are refined as the child develops the ability to stimulate and satisfy itself. By the age of 5, the ability to explore the world by using the hands and mouth, as well as other parts of the body, allows the person to develop communication, self-gratification, and a feeling of competence.[121,132]

This feeling of competence is derived from the effective use of the body to make itself feel good and to accomplish tasks. By the age of 8, body parts and body processes are usually named and the child perceives the body as good. At this time intimacy between the self and another person is further refined, as are roles. During puberty body changes and sexual tension are heightened.[53,95] Self-acceptance is based on the person's perception of how effectively he or she has accomplished the previous tasks.

The preceding is an oversimplification of the first 20 years of life, but the role of sensuality and sensation cannot be overemphasized. This is especially true for those professionals who constantly interact with clients in a physical manner. The intervention the therapist provides when the client is, or feels he or she is, in a dependent state can have direct impact on how the client may perceive himself or herself in the future.

Pediatric sensuality. The child needs to learn to enjoy his or her body. The therapist should help the client to distinguish between therapeutic touch and "fun" sensual touch, such as tickling or cuddling. It is important for clients to distinguish between the two so that they do not "turn their bodies off" to touch. For example, a woman with cerebral palsy stated during an interview that therapy was either painful or so clinical that she disassociated herself from sensations in her body during therapy. Later in life this became a problem when she was married. She stated that it took 7 years of marriage before she could enjoy the sensations of being touched by her husband. She also stated that it was a revolutionary concept for her that a vibrator could be used to give pleasure!

The therapy session should also help the client develop a sense of personal ownership of the body.[4,29,80,95] This aspect is often neglected when working with children.[4,53,121] The therapist often does not ask permission to touch a client, thus suggesting that the client lacks the right to control being touched by others. The last thing the therapist would desire to communicate, especially to a child, is that any person has the right to handle and touch the client's body. Child molestation is just beginning to be recognized as a problem in this country, with possibly one third of the female and male population being victimized.[4] It is hard to think of a more likely victim than a person who has (unintentionally) been taught that he or she does not have the right to say NO to being touched, and who cannot physically resist unwanted advances and in some cases cannot even communicate that abuse has taken place. The effects of this can be seen in adults. When one client was asked why tone increased in her lower extremities when she was touched, her response was "I was sexually abused by my father in the name of therapy, and therapy and sexual abuse are synonymous at this point." No wonder she had been resistant to reentering therapy!

One way of helping clients "own" their bodies (besides asking permission to touch) is by naming body parts and body processes using correct terminology (as opposed to baby talk), thus making it possible for the client to communicate and relate appropriately.[4,40,95,121] This can be accomplished as the need arises, or it can be encouraged through the use of anatomically correct puzzles or dolls during therapy sessions.

One goal of therapy may be to develop the concept that the body (in the case of persons with the congenital disabilities) or the "new body" (in the case of those with acquired disabilities) is acceptable and good,[53,80] thus giving the client a more positive attitude toward his or her body and toward therapy. This attitude can be encouraged by pointing out a particularly positive aspect of the client's body and mentioning this regularly. The feature could be the hair, eyes, or a smile; but it should be an aspect of the client that can be seen and commented on by others as well. Commenting on how well the body feels when it is relaxed or how good the sun feels on the body helps the client recognize that the body can be a positive source of pleasure.

Another message that can affect the client in later life is the concept that the disabled are asexual and will never have sexual needs or partners.[79,110] Although it may not be appropriate to deal directly with the concept in therapy with a child, the therapist might mention that he or she knows of a person with disabilities, such as the client's disability, who is married or who has children. In this way the therapist communicates that there is a possibility that the "normal" sex roles of the child may be fulfilled in the future. Without this possibility being presented, the child may think that there is no chance that all the movies, books, and television programs that deal with normal adult interactions apply to the disabled, a belief that leads to poor socialization and further alienation.[28,79,110]

Adult sexuality. Adaptive devices can be a detriment to one's perceived sexuality. It can be hard to see oneself as sexy with an indwelling catheter or braces, but by discussing this topic the client can get some ideas as how to handle difficult situations when they arise.[28,63,79,98,110] Discussing positioning to reduce pain and spasticity or to enable the client to more comfortably engage in sexual relations will help the client deal with problems before they reveal themselves.* Because sexual hygiene may be considered as an activity of daily living, it may fall within the domain of therapy.

The client may feel that his or her sexual identity is threatened by a newly acquired disability and may try to

---

* References 14, 24, 79, 80, 95, 98, and 110.

---

assert his or her sexuality through jokes, flirting, or even passes toward the therapist. In these cases it is important for the therapist to realize that what is often being looked for is the confirmation that the client is still a sexual and sensual human being; thus the therapist's response is very important.[14,55,90,110,124] If the therapist rejects or even ridicules the client, it may be a very long time before the client can even think of attempting such a confirmation of personal attractiveness. The client may feel that because the therapist rejects the client and the therapist is familiar with the disabled, there is little chance anyone who is not familiar with the disabled could accept the client as lovable.[56] The therapist should not be surprised by such advances and should deal with the situation in a professional manner. The therapist should also realize that approximately 10% of the population is homosexual and be prepared for advances from clients of the same sex. The therapist may need to remember that therapy is not the time to attempt to change the client's sexual orientation nor is it time to be offended, but instead to be as professional in dealing with this client as with any other. All of the therapist's interactions should be directed toward creating an environment that will promote a stronger and more well-adjusted client.[110]

The therapist's response to sexual advances must be tempered with an understanding of the possible cause for the behavior. The client may be cognitively involved and may not even be aware of the inappropriateness of some forms of sexual behavior, or the client may be trying to control others through acting out behaviors. The client may have been sexually aggressive even before the injury. *At no time should the therapist allow himself or herself to be sexually harrassed.* If the therapist feels harrassed, the therapist must take control of the situation and find a way to stop the client's behavior. This is usually achieved be confronting the issue. Not dealing with inappropriate behavior will allow it to continue and may be detrimental to the client and the medical staff.[90,124]

Nowinski and Ayers[99] found that sexuality was of great concern to most people with physical disabilities. As Bogle and Shaul stated, it is difficult to see oneself as lovable and huggable when surrounded by hard, cold, and usually unsightly braces.[12,28,63,98,110] The therapist can assist the client in moving through the stages of self-awareness to the reinstatement of self-appreciation that precede positive feelings that he or she is still sensual, sexual, and huggable. This process can be done through everyday interaction; it may entail encouraging the family to embrace the client and may even call for the therapist to role model these behaviors at times.[33] The therapist may provide reading materials to the client and family directly by reviewing and answering questions or indirectly by having such books as *Enabling Romance,*[79] *Reproductive Issues for Persons with Physical Disabilities,*[63] *Sexuality and the Person with Traumatic Brain Injury: A Guide for Families,*[56] *Who Cares?,*[32] *Sexuality and Physical Disability,*[20] *Sexual Options for*

Paraplegics and Quadriplegics,[96] or the Hite Report on female[65] and male sexuality[66] available. In this way, the individual and significant others are made aware of possible options for the expression of intimacy and of the fact that this part of life is not over.

Because the therapist is in a situation of one-to-one treatment involving touching, moving, and handling the client's body, he or she may frequently be a natural person from whom the individual may seek information. If this natural curiosity does not appear to be forthcoming, however, the therapist can give the client an opening. For example, during an evaluation of motor skills, the person may be asked if there are any problems in such areas as sexual positioning. The topic need not be pursued any further by the therapist, but when the client is ready to deal with the subject area, he or she will probably remember that the therapist brought it up and may be a person to approach when dealing with these issues.[50]

Other ways of presenting sexual information are to have literature available on the client's ward so that those who are interested may pursue the topic in private, to have a group discussion (interested clients, clients and significant others, or whatever group the client and therapist might choose to assemble), or to have literature in the department waiting room.

It is important for the therapist to be aware of some of the aspects of sexuality that may or may not be affected by a disability. Fertility is seldom affected in women.[130] Men, on the other hand, may experience dysfunction of the penis and testicles and/or fertility.* Devices may be used and adapted to allow for sexual gratification of the client (masturbation) or significant others. Safe sex is even more of a problem for clients who may be inclined to get infections,[56,79] especially in or around the genitals, because this may provide an avenue for transmission of disease. Sensation should be checked and sexual activities modified (or the client should be alerted to the problem) to avoid breakdowns or medical complications. Positioning modifications may be needed to allow for better energy conservation, joint protection, motor control, maintenance of muscle and skin integrity, and pleasure. Clients may have questions regarding modifications that may be needed for the use of birth control devices or contraindications regarding the use of such devices.† Complications may arise due to pregnancy that may affect function and mobility of the client. Delivery may present some unique situations that may also need to be dealt with. After delivery the disabled parent may require modifications to the wheelchair or consultations may be needed to achieve an optimal level of function in the parenting role. All of these possibilities point to the fact that sexual issues must be dealt with throughout the treatment of all individuals with disabilities.[63,79,101,130] The therapist may approach these needs or

aspects of function while taking a client's sex history.* Clients have repeatedly called for more attention to be paid to sexual concerns.† This is *not* sex counseling or therapy, and the therapist should not try to deal with deep psychosexual issues. The therapist should be informed and should provide information that relates to the therapist's areas of expertise, especially as other medical personnel may not have the knowledge to correctly analyze the components of some of these activities.[57,63,79]

• • •

All of the clinical problem areas that need assessment and evaluation and that have been mentioned previously are examined in relation to treatment planning in the clinical setting in the following sections.

TREATMENT VARIABLES IN RELATION TO THERAPY

This section examines issues the therapist and staff should know to create a therapeutic environment that will facilitate psychological adjustment and independence of the disabled client. The physical and the attitudinal environment of the treatment facility plays a major role in the way the client views the services that are rendered.

Recall a time before you became a member of the medical community. Think about how awe-inspiring the people in white coats were, how strange the smells of the hospitals were, how busy it all seemed, and how puzzling the secret medical language was. It all seemed overwhelming then, and it still is to newcomers, especially newly admitted patients and their families. The hospital usually appears impersonal,[64] sterile, monotonous, and confusing; and all status accumulated outside the hospital means little inside.

The therapist needs to take the setting into account when dealing with the client. The environment can be altered in a variety of ways. Therapy staff could wear street clothes, decorate the department or hospital with posters and lively colors, and allow clients to bring some personal items into the hospital.

The nature of the therapy process can often lead the therapist to see only the disability and not the person, as occurs for example when a client is referred to by his or her disability, rather than by name. This stereotyping of disability can lead the therapist to concentrate on the lack of ability rather than on the strengths of the client. The real danger is that the client and family will also start to focus on the disability of the client and feel that their family relationship is now permanently altered. The accuracy of this perception may have to be evaluated as part of the adjustment process. The wife of a man with paraplegia said with a sudden burst of insight, "I didn't marry him for his

---

* References 2, 3, 29, 63, 79, and 104.
† References 1, 14, 29, 55, 56, 63, 79, 83, 98, and 130.

*References 2, 27, 29, 82, 108, and 110.
†References 2, 14, 57, 63, 79, 83, and 110.

legs—this doesn't change that much." Very often so much attention is directed toward the disability that tunnel vision develops. One way to try to get a better perspective is to look at the bigger picture. Ask some questions such as:

1. Who will marry this person and why?
2. What are his or her good points?
3. What will this person do for a living?
4. What will this person do for enjoyment?
5. How will this person bring others enjoyment?

After the therapist is aware of the strengths of the client, they may be capitalized on in therapy to help the client realize personal strengths and build confidence. Clients often reported that they were not complimented in therapy and especially that they never received feedback that their bodies' were desirable[12] or that they were doing things correctly.[23,56,63,108] A logical thought by the client is "if the therapist cannot see anything desirable about me, and the therapist deals with the disabled all the time, then there must not be anything good about me." Positive, sincere comments to client and family can add a motivational factor to treatment that may have been missing.[23,76]

The last and possibly the most important aspect in creating an environment that will foster growth and adjustment in the client is a staff that is well-adjusted and aware of their own personal needs. Just as coping skills are necessary for the client, the staff, too, must be capable of coping with the stresses of the emotional and physical pain of the client and the client's family. The therapist must also deal with his or her own personal reactions to the sometimes devastating situations others are in.[39,76] Exposure to such situations often elicits introspection on the part of the staff that can result in emotional turmoil for staff members and for their own personal relationships. This emotional energy needs to be directed in a productive way so that the energy does not turn into chaos within the staff and a destructive force on the client.

To decrease the possibly distractive nature of this emotional energy, the staff should be made aware of their own coping styles, and they should be allowed to vent their reactions to particularly distressing client loads in a positive, supportive group. Group meetings can be used to handle some of the inevitable tension, especially if there is a respected member who is skilled in group work. This is not a psychotherapy session but rather an opportunity to test reality and remove tension before it is incorrectly directed toward fellow staff members. These sessions can make use of the four elements of crisis intervention mentioned in the previous section, as well as information from Combs and others.[30,76,93] Other times that this stress reduction can be achieved are in supervision or during coffee breaks, as long as the sessions are productive.

The staff can use these sessions to better understand their reactions to stress and to explore their coping styles.[26,39,52,76,93] Ideally this knowledge of coping styles and stress reduction will decrease staff burnout as well as aid the staff to help clients and their families deal with stress more successfully.[22,26,39,93]

The need to have a staff that is supportive is of paramount importance, because the attitude of rehabilitation personnel has emerged as one of the chief motivating factors in rehabilitation.[41,69,72] Rogers and Figone[107] developed several suggestions that the therapist could benefit from when trying to create a supportive environment:

1. It is helpful to use the same staff member to develop the relationship and to provide continuity of care.
2. Concerned silence is most appreciated, although pushing is sometimes necessary.
3. Staff members should anticipate the need to repeat information graciously.
4. Cumbersome and hard to repair adaptive equipment should not be used after discharge.
5. Give clients responsibility so that they feel they have some control over therapy.
   a. The client should be allowed to pick his or her own advocate from the team.
   b. The client should be given a choice of activities (e.g., which exercise comes first).
   c. Professionals should avoid placing the client in an inferior status. In time the client starts thinking this way (feeling like a second-class citizen).
6. Psychological support was attributed to noncounseling personnel—personal matters were better discussed with staff members with whom the client had developed a relationship.[17,76,110]
7. Willingness to allow the client to try and fail was more helpful than controlling the client.

CONCEPTUALIZATION OF ASSESSMENT AND TREATMENT
Assessment

The one component that weaves through all of Rogers and Figone's[107] seven points is the need for the therapist to be involved with the client in a therapeutic relationship, that is, to know where the client is "coming from." To know where the client is "coming from" is to be aware of and sensitive to the person's total psychosocial frame of reference.[17,76]

The therapist who knows his or her own beliefs, reference points, and prejudices can evaluate whether an assessment result or treatment sequence reflects the client's needs and values or those of the therapist. In the first half of this chapter, several assessments were discussed that could be summarized into the following three major components:

1. Preinjury
   a. Values and prejudices (value systems, culture, and prejudgments) of the client and family members before the injury

b. Developmental stage of the client and family members

c. Cognitive level of the client and family members

d. Ability of the client and family members to handle crisis

2. Components to be evaluated leading to adjustment

a. Loss and grief process for the client and family members

b. Adjustment process for the client and family members

c. Transitional stages for the client and family members

d. Role changes for the client and family members

e. Age-cognitive level of client and family members[5,17,22,76]

f. Sexual adjustment for the client and spouse

3. Techniques used to elicit adjustment and independence

a. Crisis intervention strategies

b. Letting client and family take control

c. Expression of emotion—both verbally and nonverbally

d. Problem solving

e. Role playing

f. Praise

g. Education

h. Support groups

Once an assessment has been made of the client and family member's stages of psychological adjustment, the client's occupational history and roles, as well as of their preinjury attitudes and beliefs, a treatment protocol can be established. This protocol will need to incorporate steps toward stage change and possibly attitudinal change. Because these changes require learning on the part of the client and family, an environment that optimally facilitates these changes must be established.[44,59,105]

Therapy can be seen as a form of education in which the client and the client's family are taught how the client should use his or her body. The education process is not limited to the physical aspects of therapy, however. The client is also taught how to look at and think about the body and the disability. If the staff is nonverbally telling the client and the family that the client is not capable of making decisions and of being independent, it follows that the client may indeed feel dependent and incapable of making decisions. Giles[52] and others[*] stated that there was an inverse relationship between independence and distress. Distress causes further anxiety and decreases the learning potential of the client. There are ways, however, for the therapist to encourage independence on the part of the client and his family.

Treatment

Problem-solving process—independence. The family unit, including the client, should be encouraged to take active control over as much of the client's care and decision making as possible. This can be done in every phase of the rehabilitation process. A family conference with the rehabilitation staff should actively involve the client and family in all stages of planning and treatment up to and including discharge. The family (including the client) should be briefed ahead of time to prepare questions that they want answered or problems that need to be addressed. Rogers and Figone[107] report that conferences with family members that excluded the client engendered suspicion[17,32,97]; therefore, if the client is capable, the client may educate the family in regard to what is happening in the hospital and in rehabilitation. Conversely, family involvement facilitates and shortens the rehabilitation process and reintegration into the community.[*] The family can also be educated regarding the side effects and interactions of medication with publications like the *Physician's Desk Reference*.[6] Later in the rehabilitation process the client and family can be encouraged to arrange transportation services, find and evaluate housing, and supervise attendant care. All of these activities allow the client and the family to be more in control of the environment and, thus, to feel independent.

In the context of one-to-one therapy, client responsibility and independence can be fostered by giving choices. Making decisions about the order of treatment activities (such as in which direction to roll first) can give the individual a sense of self-worth that can continue to grow. This should lead the client and family toward believing that they are strong, with rights that need to be met. Moving out of the role of the victim, the client begins to exercise responsibility and to take action, such as applying for extended health benefits or getting a second consultation when an important medical decision needs to be made. If the client and family start to realize that they do not have to be a casualty of the medical establishment and if they find ways to control the medical establishment,[8,17,43,97,129] they are better able to discard the role of victim.

In some centers, such as the Occupational Therapy clinic at San Jose State University, the client is even taught the art of self-defense to make sure that the client never has to fall into the victim (dependent) role. It should be noted, however, that this knowledge on the part of the client and family can be used in ways that the therapist may not always agree with. At such times it may help to adopt a philosophical attitude toward the situation and to view it as a positive direction for the client in terms of moving from victim to advocate in the rehabilitation process.

The steps of crisis intervention, which were mentioned in

---

*References 7, 52, 83, 87, 97, and 110.

*References 5, 10, 97, 115, 116, and 119.

the previous section, can be used to help the family understand and analyze their needs in the crisis situation. Once the family has discovered that they are in crisis, they will then be able to create strategies that they can use to overcome present and future problems.

Problem solving is another element the therapist may use to help the client and family gain independence and control.* Rather than having the client routinely learn how to accomplish a specific task, the client or family should be encouraged to think through the process, from the problem, to the solution, and to accomplishment of the task. To achieve this activity analysis, the client would have to know the basic principles behind the activity[107] and may then be responsible for educating the family. An example of this would be a transfer from the wheelchair to the toilet. If the therapist simply has the client memorize the steps in the task, the client or family members will not necessarily be able to generalize this procedure to a transfer to the car. If the client learns the principles of proper body mechanics, work simplification, and movement, the client or family member may be able to generalize this information to almost any situation and to solve problems later when the therapist is unavailable.[7] Rogers and Figone[107] have noted that even though the client and family may fail at times during these trials, the therapist should let them be as independent and responsible as possible: let them try it their way, even if they fail the first time.

Pictures or slides of a restaurant, movie theatre, or public building can be used to facilitate discussion and problem solving by the family unit when analyzing potential architectural barriers in the environment. Thus, in the future, when the family is presented with a problem or a barrier, they will have the resources to overcome it rather than be devastated by it.

Role playing in combination with support groups can also be used to defuse potentially painful situations and operate independently. While still in the safe environment of the rehabilitation setting, simulations of incidents can be created for the family and client to practice problem solving with supervision. They can be asked what they would do when a stranger (possibly a child) approaches the client and asks why he is in a wheelchair or is disabled or what they would do when a waiter asks the family member to order for the disabled client. All of these situations are potentially devastating for all involved; however, if role playing and support groups are used in advance to help all members of the family (client included) to satisfactorily handle and feel in control of the situation, the family will not be as likely to be traumatized by a similar occurrence. The result is that the family will not be as inclined to be overwhelmed by social situations and will be able to socialize in a much freer, more gratifying way.[127]

Throughout the therapeutic process the client and the family need to be praised frequently, and credit needs to be given for the gains made by the client and family members. Granted, the therapist may have engineered the gains, but the family and client are the ones who need the reinforcement. Through gratifying experiences the family will unite to overcome the disability. They need to know that they can survive in the world without having the medical staff constantly there to solve the family's problems. In short, they need the strategies and resources that will allow them to be independent outside the medical model.

Yet another way to encourage independence can be applied to working with parents of disabled children.[38] The parents should be educated about normal and abnormal growth and development, including physical, cognitive, and emotional growth, so that the family can maintain some perspective and objectivity about their child's various levels.[5,9,61,69,121] The parents can then better understand the needs of the disabled and nondisabled children in the family. Armed with this knowledge, the parents and children will not be frustrated with unreal expectations or unreal demands. Education of the parents could take place at local colleges, the hospital, or even in a parent's group.

Support systems. Groups are often used to increase motivation, provide support, increase social skills, instill hope, and help the client and family realize that they are not the only ones who have a disabled family member. This will help the client and family establish a more accurate set of perceptions about the disabled individual and allow for greater independence of the client and family.[17,69,77] Problem solving can be encouraged and value systems can be clarified. Client and/or family support groups can be used to relieve pressure that might otherwise be vented in therapy. Livneh and Antonak[87] found that in a chronic-care ward family involvement helped the client and the family improve their status. Schwartzberg[116] and Schulz[115] and others[8,41,43,44] have reported great success in the use of support groups with individuals who had brain damage. Support groups can also be used to educate the client about the client's disability to increase independence.* Wade[131] found that independent physical functioning and knowledge about one's condition were exceedingly important in moving through the phases of the rehabilitation process. A guide to facilitating support groups has been published by Boreing and Adler,[13] and it has been found to be useful, especially by lay people establishing such groups.[69,94,115,116,131]

Establishment of self-worth and accurate body image. Self-worth is composed of many aspects, such as body image, sexuality, and the ability to help others and to affect the environment. The body image of a client is a composite of past and present experiences and of the individual's perception of those experiences. Because body image is based on experience, it is a constantly changing concept. An adult's body image is substantially different from that which he or she held as a child and will no doubt change again as the aging process continues. A newly disabled person is suddenly exposed to a radically new body, and it is that individual's job to assess the body's sensations and capabilities and develop a new body image. Because the therapist is at least partially responsible for creating the environmental experiences from which the client learns about this new body, he or she should be aware of the concept. In the case of an acute injury, the client has a new body from which to learn. The therapist can promote positive feelings as he or she instructs the client how to use this new body and to accept its changes.*

Because in "normal" life we slowly observe changes in our bodies, such as finding one gray hair today and watching it take years for our hair to turn totally white, we have the luxury of slowly adapting to the "new me." This usually does not happen quite so slowly and "naturally" with a disability. This sudden loss of function creates a void that only new experiences and new role models can fill.

The loss of use of body parts can cause a person to perceive the body as an "enemy" that needs to be forced to work or to compensate for its disability. In all cases the body is the reason for the disability and the cause of all problems. The need for appliances can create a sense of alienation and lack of perceived "lovability" resulting from the "hardness of the hardware." People tend to avoid hugging someone who is in a wheelchair or who has braces around the body, because of the physical barrier and because of the person's perceived fragility;[95] the disabled person is certainly not perceived as soft and cuddly.[15,20,79,95] Both the perception that they are not lovable and their labored movements can sap the energy of the disabled for social interaction. To accept the appliances and the dysfunctional body in a way that also allows the disabled person to feel sexy and sensual is surely a major challenge.

In the case of a chronically disabled person, the therapist is attempting to teach the client how to change the previously accepted body image to one that would allow and encourage more normal function. In short, the therapist has two roles. One role is to take away the disabled body image of the chronically disabled person, such as the person with cerebral palsy or Parkinson's disease. The second is the opposite sequence, that is, to teach a functional disabled body image to a newly disabled person. The techniques may be the same, but in both cases the client will have to undergo a great amount of change. The chronically ill person has based his or her life on the concept that the reason for not accomplishing many things was the disability. If the therapist can change the client's ability level, the individual must now change self-expectations. The newly disabled person must now also change expectations; however, he or she has little concept of what is realistic to expect of this new body. At this point, role models can be used to help shape the client's

expectations. If the client does not adjust to this new body and change his or her body image and self-expectations, life will be impoverished for that individual. Pedretti[102] states that the client with low self-esteem often devalues his or her whole life in all respects, not just in the area of dysfunction.[10,63,79,98,105]

One way the client can start exploring this new body is by exploring it for sensation and performance. The male client with a spinal cord injury may touch the whole body to see how it reacts.[28] For example, is there a way to get the legs to move using reflexes? What, if anything, stimulates an erection? Can positioning the legs in a certain way aid in rolling or make spasms decrease? Such exploration will start the client on the road to an informed evaluation of his abilities.

The therapist's role is to promote expansion of the client's realistic perceptions of body functioning. Exercises can be developed that encourage bodily exploration by the individual and, if appropriate, the significant other. Functioning and building an appropriate body image will be more difficult if intimate knowledge of the new body is not as complete as before injury.[14] Books on body massage or exercises, similar to those found in *Your Child's Sensory World*,[85] can be used to establish such programs. The successes the client experiences in the clinical setting coupled with the client's familiarity with his or her new body will result in a more accurate body image and will contribute to the client's feelings of self-worth.

As mentioned earlier in this chapter, sexuality and sensuality have an enormous impact on how the person feels about his or her adequacy and self-worth.[28,98,123] Societal members often evaluate each other on appearance and sensuality (or sexual attractiveness) and may avoid those who are perceived to have deficits.[12,79] Sensuality and sexuality are some of the major ways that humans express their intimate beings, and in Western society, the expression of the physical intimacy is closely associated with love. Thus a client who feels incapable of expressing sensuality or sexuality may see himself or herself as incapable of loving and being loved. Because love and acceptance are primary driving forces in a human's life,[89] the inability to perceive the self as capable of loving would be devastating.

The last aspect of self-worth to be mentioned here is often overlooked in the health fields: it is the need that people have to help others.[49] People often discover that they are valuable through the act of giving. Self-worth is increased by seeing others enjoy and benefit from the individual's presence or offering. Situations in which the client's worth can be appreciated by others may be needed. Unless the client can contribute to others, the client is in a relatively dependent role, with everyone else giving to him or her without the opportunity of giving back. Achieving independence and then reaching out to others, with therapeutic assistance if necessary, facilitates the individual's more rapid reintegration into society. The therapist should take every opportunity to allow the client to express self-worth to others through helping.

The adult client with brain damage. The adult client with brain damage and the needs of the family will be specifically, yet briefly, examined here because brain damage affects the cognitive and emotional system of the client. When a person receives brain injury and is hospitalized, emotional support for the family (client included) is the primary need to be met initially. Pearson[101] feels that it is not the function of the support but the emotional tone of the support that is most important. The therapist should attempt to convey warmth and a caring attitude, especially during the family's initial contacts. Typical complaints about the acute period involve impersonal hospital routines and lack of definite information about the patient's status.[63,69,98] Unfortunately, definite information is usually not available at the earliest stages.

Later, the family must deal with the physical changes in the client's body; what may be even more injurious to the family is the psychological, cognitive, and social changes in the client.* People with cerebral vascular accidents have been found to be more clinically depressed than orthopedic patients. The libido[11,68] and emotional systems are also affected.[56,63,98] It has further been shown that persons who survive a cerebrovascular accident and who have a full return of function do not return to normal life because of a lack of social and emotional skills.[10,42,84] Families of cerebrovascular accident victims have also reported that social reintegration is the most difficult phase of rehabilitation. Lack of socially appropriate behaviors has been one of the most troublesome complaints of people who deal with the person with chronic brain injury.[56] Therapists may be able to help alter this syndrome by encouraging appropriate behavior and by structuring therapy situations to reteach the client interaction skills. A technique called structured learning therapy[34,54,56] has been used with schizophrenics, and although this approach has not been used by enough clinics to judge its effectiveness completely, it appears to be a promising approach.

Better follow-up care needs to be implemented when dealing with the adult with brain damage.[17,21,41,69] It may not be possible for the client and family to constantly come to the clinic for support and follow-up, but telephone conversations can be scheduled on a periodic basis, or the exchange of letters or audiotapes can also be used. With the increased availability of video recorders, the day may come when a follow-up may be performed on videotapes sent by clients living in rural areas. Support groups are being used increasingly to facilitate client and family adjustment and accommodation to disability, as well as reentry into the community.†

---

* References 5, 11, 15, 17, 41, and 42.
† References 8, 10, 15, 21, 41, 44, 69, 76, 94, 97, 115, and 116.

SUMMARY
Clinical example: putting evaluations and techniques into practice

Joan, a married 30-year-old woman, has suffered a T2 spinal cord injury. She has worked as a computer programmer for the past 8 years, except for a short maternity leave when she gave birth to her daughter, who is now 6 years old. Joan was always very active physically and often stated that she felt sorry for her physically disabled neighbor because the neighbor could not hike, be active, or enjoy the outdoors. Joan's husband, age 33, is attempting to visit Joan regularly and care for their daughter, a role that is new for him.

The therapist has assessed several things regarding Joan's developmental stage, adjustment stage, social/cultural influences, and family adjustment reactions. The two adult family members are probably in Sheehy's[12] "catch-30" stage, in which the person reevaluates his or her life and relationships. Joan already "knows" that the physically disabled cannot enjoy a physically active life and is also feeling that everything she has worked for in her career is lost. She appears to be in the mourning stage of adjustment. Her daughter and husband are having to adjust to radical role changes. Cognitively, Joan's young daughter is not going to understand the permanence of the disability and may be inclined to act out as the result of the turmoil. The husband will have to be assessed to determine his stage of adjustment to her disability.

The therapist has determined that Joan's transfers need further work but would like to use the adaptive process to stimulate adjustment. The therapist has devised a treatment session to meet the goals of promoting the defense stage of adjustment, decreasing her prejudice against the disabled, encouraging problem solving, increasing her feelings of self-worth, proving to her that she can take care of her daughter through interacting with children, as well as having her decenter her focus from her disability to her ability. The therapist has contacted the recreational therapist (RT) (who is a paraplegic) to plan a collaborative session at the park across the street from the hospital. Because the RT works in the pediatrics ward, it is determined that the children with spina bifida should come and play tag transferring from log to log in the playground.

The stage is now set. Joan will be asked to help supervise the children. The adaptive process will be used to teach Joan how to transfer using the environment. The transfer will be organized subcortically because she will be attending cortically to the children's needs and to the game itself. Joan will be actively affecting her personal environment, and if everything goes well, the act of helping the children will increase her self-worth and will also be self-reinforcing. Within this treatment session, the therapist has used the RT as a role model to change Joan's prejudice against the disabled being active in the outdoors as well as to show Joan that she can still be a parent even though she is disabled. The therapist may also increase Joan's knowledge of how to interact with children from a wheelchair by giving a few hints and then having Joan transfer up a set of stairs to reach one of the children.

If we want to carry this fantasy further, the therapist could introduce Joan to a child who is interested in computers and who needs help with a programming problem (Joan's computer background will be used, which will increase Joan's feelings of self-worth and help her focus on her abilities rather than her disabilities). On the way back to the ward, the therapist and Joan may discuss how the family is dealing with the crisis they are in and help her realize how the family has made it through other crises in the past and how those previously successful strategies could be used in this situation. Support groups may be mentioned as resources. The session may end with Joan planning the next therapy session and thus starting to take control of her life.

REFERENCES

1. Aloni R and others: Noninvasive treatment for erectile dysfunction in the neurogenically disabled population, *J Sex Marital Ther* 18(3):243, 1992.
2. Aloni R and others: Sexual function in male patients after stroke: a follow-up study, *Sexuality and Disability* 11(2):121-128, 1993.
3. Andersson KE: Pharmacology of erection: agents which initiate and terminate erection, *Sexuality and Disability* 12(1):53-72, 1994.
4. Andrews AB and Veronen LJ: Sexual assault and people with disabilities, *J Soc Work Hum Sexuality* 8(2):137-159, 1993.
5. Asarnow RF, Satz P, and Light R: Behavior problems and adaptive functioning in children with mild and severe closed head injury, *J Pediatr Psychol* 16(5):543-555, 1991.
6. Baker EJ: *Physicians desk reference,* ed 48 Oradell NJ, 1994, Medical Economics Books.
7. Baker LL: Problem solving techniques in adjustment services, *Vocational Evaluation and Work Adjustment Bulletin* 25(3):75-76, 1992.
8. Balcazar FE and others: Empowering people with physical disabilities through advocacy skills training, *Am J Community Psychol* 18(2):281-296, 1990.
9. Baxter C: Investigating stigma as stress in social interactions of parents, *J Ment Defic Res* 33(6):446-455, 1989.
10. Belgrave FZ: Psychosocial prediction of adjustment to disability in African Americans, *J Rehabil* 57:37-40, 1991.
11. Berrol S: Issues of sexuality in head injured adults in sexuality and physical disability. In Bullard DG and Knight DE, editors: *Sexuality and physical disability,* St Louis, 1981, Mosby.
12. Bogle JE and Shaul SL: Body image and the woman with a disability. In Bullard DG and Knight DE, editors: Sexuality and physical disability, St Louis, 1981, Mosby.
13. Boreing ML and Adler LM: *Facilitating support groups: an instructional guide—Educational Monograph No 3,* San Francisco, 1982, Dept of Psychiatry, Pacific Medical Center.
14. Boyle PS: Training in sexuality and disability: preparing social workers to provide services to individuals with disabilities, *J Soc Work Hum Sexuality* 8(2):45-62, 1993.
15. Braithwaite DO: From majority to minority: an analysis of cultural change from ablebodied to disabled, *Int J Intercultural Relations* 1990. 14:465-483, 1990.
16. Brammer LM and Abrego PJ: Intervention strategies for coping with transitions, *Counsel Psychol* 9(2):19, 1981.
17. Brooks DN: The head-injured family, *J Clin Exp Neuropsychol,* 13:155-188, 1991.
18. Brown SE: Creating a disability mythology, *Int J Rehabil Res* 15(3):227-233, 1991.
19. Bukowski WM and Hoza B: Popularity and friendship: issues in theory, measurement, and outcomes. In Berndt T and Ladd G, editors: *Contributions of peer relationships of children's development,* New York, 1989, Wiley.
20. Bullard DG and Knight DE: *Sexuality and physical disability,* St Louis, 1981, Mosby.
21. Burton L and Volpe B: Sex differences in the emotional status of traumatically brain-injured patients, *J Neurol Rehabil* 2:151-157, 1993.
22. Cairns D and Baker J: Adjustment to spinal cord injury: a review of coping styles contributing to the process, *J Rehabil* 59(4):30-33, 1993.
23. Capell B and Capell J: Being parents of children who are disabled. In Bullard DG and Knight DE: *Sexuality and physical disability,* St Louis, 1981, Mosby.
24. Charlifue SW and others: Sexual issues of women with spinal cord injuries, *Paraplegia* 30(3):192-199, 1992.
25. Coffman S: Parent and infant attachment: review of nursing research 1981-1990, *Pediatr Nurse* 18(4):421-425, 1992.
26. Cohen MZ and Sarter B: Love and work: oncology nurses' view of the meaning of their work, *Oncology Nursing Form* 19(10):1481-1486, 1992.
27. Cole IM: Gathering a sex history from a physically disabled adult, *Sexuality and Disability* 9(1):29-37, 1991.
28. Cole SS and Cole TM: Sexuality, disability, and reproductive issues for persons with disabilities. In Haseltine FP, Cole SS, Gray DB, editors: *Reproductive issues for persons with physical disabilities,* Baltimore, 1993, Paul Brookes.
29. Cole SS and Cole TM: Sexuality, disability, and reproductive issues through the life span, *Sexuality and Disability* 11(3):189-205, 1993.
30. Combs AW and others: *Helping relationships,* Boston, 1971, Allyn & Bacon, Inc.
31. Corbett KS, Klein S, and Bregante JL: The role of sexuality and sex equity in the education of disabled women, *Peabody J Educ* 64(4):198-211, 1987.
32. Cornelius DA and others: *Who cares?,* Baltimore, 1982, University Park Press.
33. Daniels SM: Critical issues in sexuality and disability. In Bullard DG and Knight SE editors: *Sexuality and physical disability,* St Louis, 1981, Mosby.
34. Davis RE: Family of physically disabled children: family reactions and deductive reasoning, *NY State J Med* 75:1039, 1975.
35. Dunton HD: The child's concept of death. In Schoenberg B and others: *Loss and grief: psychological management in medical practice,* New York, 1970, Columbia University Press.
36. Fine SB: Resilience and human adaptability: who rise above adversity? 1990 Eleanor Clark Slagle Lecture. *Am J Occup Ther,* 45:493-503, 1991.
37. Fine S: Interaction between psychosocial variables and cognitive function. In Royeen CB, editor: *American Occupational Therapy Association self-study series on cognitive rehabilitation,* Rockville, MD, 1993, American Occupational Therapy Association.
38. Finnie NR: *Handling the young cerebral palsied child at home,* ed 2, New York, 1974, EP Dutton, Inc.
39. Fisher M: Can grief be turned into growth? Staff grief in palliative care, *Prof Nurse* 7(3):178-182, 1991.
40. Fitz-Gerald M and Fitz-Gerald DR: Involvement in sex education, *Volta-Review* 89(5):96-110, 1987.
41. Flagg Williams JB: Perspectives on working with parents of handicapped children, *Psychol Schools* 28:238-246, 1991.
42. Fleming JM and Maas F: Prognosis of rehabilitation outcome in head injury using the disability rating scale, *Arch Phys Med Rehabil* 75(2):159-162, 1994.
43. French S: Researching disability: the way forward, *Disability Rehabilitation,* 1992. 14(4): p. 183-186.

44. Fuhrer MJ and others: Depressive symptomatology in persons with spinal cord injury who reside in the community, *Arch Phys Med* 74(3):255-260, 1993.

45. Furman RA: The child's reaction to death in the family. In Schoenberg B and others: *Loss and grief,* New York, 1970, Columbia University Press.

46. (GAP), Group for the Advancement of Psychiatry, *Caring for people with physical improvements: the journey back.* Washington, DC, 1993, American Psychiatric Press.

47. Gage M: The appraisal model of coping: an assessment and intervention model for occupational therapy, *Am J Occup Ther* 46:353-362, 1992.

48. Gardner B: *Ways of copying: adolescents with spinal cord injury compared with able-bodied adolescents,* San Jose, Calif, 1993, San Jose State University.

49. Geis HJ: The problem of personal worth in the physically disabled patient, *Rehabil Lit* 33(2):34, 1972.

50. Gender AR: An overview of the nurse's role in dealing with sexuality, *Sexuality and Disability* 10(2):71-70, 1992.

51. Gething L: Judgements by health professionals of personal characteristics of people with visible physical disability, *Soc Sci Med* 34(7):809-815, 1992.

52. Giles GM: Illness behavior after severe brain injury: two case studies, *Am J Occup Ther* 48(3):247-255, 1994.

53. Goldberg RT: Toward an understanding of the rehabilitation of the disabled adolescent, *Rehabil Lit* 42(3-4):66, 1981.

54. Goldstein AP and others: *Skill training for community living,* New York, 1976, Pergamon Press Inc.

55. Goldstein H and Runyon C: An occupational therapy education module to increase sensitivity about geriatric sexuality, *Phys Occup Ther Geriatr* 11(2):57, 1993.

56. Griffith ER and Lemberg S: *Sexuality and the person with traumatic brain injury: a guide for families,* Philadelphia, 1993, FA Davis.

57. Grossenbacher NL: The trauma of spinal cord injury on the adolescent, *Occup Ther Health Care* 2(3):79-90, 1985.

58. Hall ET: *The hidden dimension,* Garden City, NJ, 1966, Doubleday Anchor Books.

59. Hallett JD and others: Role change after traumatic brain injury in adults, *Am J Occup Ther* 48(3):241-246, 1994.

60. Hammond DC: Cross-cultural rehabilitation. In Stubbins J, editor: *Social and psychological aspects of disability,* Baltimore, 1977, University Park Press.

61. Harper DC and Bhattarai PK: Children's attitudes toward disabilities in Nepal, *Dev Med Child Neurol,* 31(35):1989.

62. Harvey RM: The relationship of values to adjustment in illness: a model for nursing practice, *J Adv Nurs* 17(4):467-472, 1992.

63. Haseltine FP, Cole SS, and Gray DB: *Reproductive issues for persons with physical disabilities,* Baltimore, 1993, Paul H Brookes.

64. Heiskill LE and Pasnau RD: Psychological reaction to hospitalization and illness in the emergency dept, *Emerg Med Clin North Am* 9(1):207-218, 1991.

65. Hite S: *The Hite report on female sexuality,* New York, 1976, Dell Publishing.

66. Hite S: *The Hite report on male sexuality,* New York, 1981, Random House.

67. Humphry R, Gonzalez S, and Taylor E: Family involvement in practice: issues and attitudes, *Am J Occup Ther* 47:587-593, 1993.

68. Kaitz S: Strategies to prevent caregiver fatigue, *Headlines* May/June: 18-19, 1993.

69. Kasowski JC: Family recovery: an insider's view, *Am J Occup Ther* 48(3):257-258, 1994.

70. Kerr N: Understanding the process of adjustment to disability, *J Rehabil* 27(6):16, 1961.

71. Kerr N: Understanding the process of adjustment to disability. In Stubbins J, editor: *Social and psychological aspects of disability,* Baltimore, 1977, University Park Press.

72. Kerr N: Staff expectations for disabled persons. In Stubbins J, editor: *Social and psychological aspects of disability,* Baltimore, 1977, University Park Press.

73. Kettl P and others: Female sexuality after spinal cord injury, *Sexuality and Disability* 9(4):287-295, 1991.

74. King LJ: Toward a science of adaptive responses, *Am J Occup Ther* 32(7):429, 1978.

75. Klaus MH and Kennell JH: *Maternal-infant bonding,* ed 2, St Louis, 1982, Mosby.

76. Koscuilek JF, McCublin MA, and McCublin HI: A theoretical framework for family adaptation to head injury, *J Rehabil* 59(3):1993.

77. Krause JS and Crewe NM: Long-term prediction of self-reported problems following spinal cord injury, *Paraplegia* 28:186-202, 1990.

78. Krause JS and Crewe NM: Chronological age, time since injury, and time of measurement: effect on adjustment after spinal cord injury, *Arch Phys Med Rehabil* 72:91-100, 1991.

79. Kroll K and Klein EL: *Enabling romance.* New York, 1992, Harmony Books.

80. Krueger DW: *Rehabilitation psychology,* Rockville, Md, 1984, Aspen Systems Corp.

81. Kübler-Ross E: *On death and dying,* New York, 1969, Macmillan.

82. Lefebvre KA: Sexual assessment planning, *J Head Trauma Rehabil* 5(2):25-30, 1991.

83. Lemon MA: Sexual counseling and spinal cord injury, *Sexuality and Disability* 11(1):73-97, 1993.

84. Lewis SC: *The mature years,* Thorofare, NJ, 1979, Charles B Slack.

85. Liepmann L: *Your child's sensory world,* New York, 1973, Dial Press.

86. Livneh H: A unified approach to existing models of adaption to disability, *J Appl Rehabil Counsel* 17(2):6, 1986.

87. Livneh H and Antonak RF: Reactions to disability: an empirical investigation of their nature and structure, *J Appl Rehabil Couns* 21(4):13-20, 1990.

88. Maslow A: *Motivation and personality,* ed 2, New York, 1970, Harper & Row.

89. Maze JR: The complementarity of object-relations and instinct theory, *Int J Psychoanalysis,* 74(3):459-470, 1993.

90. McComas J and others: Experiences of students and practicing physical therapists with inappropriate patient sexual behavior, *Phys Ther* 73(11):762-769, 1993.

91. McCubbin MA and McCubbin HI: Family stress theory and assessment: the resiliency model of family stress, adjustment, and adaptation. In McCubbin HI and Thompson AI, editors. *Family assessment inventories for research and practice,* Madison, 1991, University of Wisconsin-Madison.

92. McKinley W, Brooks D, and Bond M: Post-concussional symptoms, financial compensation, and outcome of severe blunt head injury, *J Neurol Neurosurg Psychiatry* 46:1084-1091, 1983.

93. McLaughlin AM and Erdman J: Rehabilitation staff stress as it relates to patient acuity and diagnosis, *Brain Inj* 6(1):59-64, 1992.

94. Miller L: When the best help is self-help, or everything you always wanted to know about brain injury support groups, *Cogn Rehabil* 10(6):14-17, 1992.

95. Mims FH and Swenson M: *Sexuality: a nursing perspective,* New York, 1980, McGraw-Hill.

96. Mooney TO and others: *Sexual options for paraplegics and quadriplegics,* Boston, 1975, Little, Brown.

97. Nadig PW: Vacuum constriction devices in patients with neurogenic impotence, *Sexuality and Disability* 12(1):99-106, 1994.

98. Neistadt ME and Freda M: *Choices: a guide to sex counseling with physically disabled adults,* Malabar, Fla., 1987, Krieger.

99. Nowinski JK and Ayers T: Sexuality and major medical conditions. In Bullard DG and Knight SE, editors: *Sexuality and physical disability,* St Louis, 1981, Mosby.

100. Parker JG and Asher SR: Peer relations and later personal adjustment: are low accepted children at risk? *Psychol Bull* 102:357-389, 1987.

101. Pearson R: Support: exploration of a basic dimension of informal help and counseling, *Personnel Guidance J* 61(2):83, 1982.
102. Pedretti LW: *Occupational therapy: practice skills for physical dysfunction,* ed 4, St Louis, 1995, Mosby.
103. Peretz D: Reaction to loss. In Schoenberg B and others, editors: *Loss and grief,* New York, 1970, Columbia University Press.
104. Resources FRI: *Resources for people with disabilities and chronic conditions,* ed 2, Lexington, Resources for Rehabilitation, 1993.
105. Revenson TA and Felton BJ: Disability and coping as predictors of psychological adjustment to rheumatoid arthritis, *J Consult Clin Psychol* 57(3):344-348, 1989.
106. Rodrigue RR: Psychological crises of the ill and handicapped, *Emotional First Aid* 2(1):44, 1985.
107. Rogers JD and Figone JJ: Psychosocial parameters in treating the person with quadriplegia, *Am J Occup Ther* 33(7):432, 1979.
108. Romeo AJ, Wanlass R, and Arenas S: A profile of psychosexual functioning in males following spinal cord injury, *Sexuality and Disability* 11(4):269-276, 1993.
109. Rose MH: The concepts of coping and vulnerability as applied to children with chronic conditions, *Issues Compr Pediatr Nurs* 7(4-5):177, 1984.
110. Sandowski C: Responding to the sexual concerns of persons with disabilities, *J Soc Work Hum Sexual* 8(2):29-43, 1993.
111. Santoro J and Spiers M: Social cognitive factors in brain injury-associated personality change, *Brain Inj* 8(3):256-276, 1994.
112. Satir V: *Peoplemaking,* Palo Alto, 1972, Science & Behavior Books.
113. Schalen W and others: Psychosocial outcome 5-8 years after severe traumatic brain lesions and the impact of rehabilitation services, *Brain Inj* 8(1):49-64, 1994.
114. Schoenberg B and others: *Loss and grief,* New York, 1970, Columbia University Press.
115. Schulz CH: Helping factors in a peer-developed support group for persons with a head injury Part 2 survivor interview perspective, *Am J Occup Ther* 48(4):305-309, 1994.
116. Schwartzberg SL: Helping factors in a peer-developed support group for persons with a head injury Part 1 participant observer perspective, *Am J Occup Ther* 48(4):297-304, 1994.
117. Sheehy G: *Passages,* New York, 1976, EP Dutton.
118. Shellabarger SG and Thompson TL: The clinical times: meeting parental communication needs throughout the NICU experience, *Neonatal Netw* 12(2):39-45, 1993.
119. Sigler G and Mackelprang RW: Cognitive impairments: psychosocial and sexual implications and strategies for social work intervention, *J Soc Work Hum Sexual* 8(2):89-106, 1993.
120. Simon SB and others: *Values clarification,* New York, 1972, Hart Publishing Co.
121. Smith M: Pediatric sexuality: promoting normal sexual development in children, *Nurse Practitioner* 18(8):37-44, 1993.
122. Solnit AJ and Green M: The pediatric management of the dying child. In Solnit A and Provence S, editors: *Modern perspectives in child development,* New York, 1963, International Universities Press.
123. Spanbock P: Children and siblings of head injury survivors: a need to be understood, *J Cogn Rehabil* 10(4):8-9, 1992.
124. Stockard S: Caring for the sexually aggressive patient: you don't have to blush and bear it, *Nursing* 21(11):72-73, 1991.
125. Tedder TL: Using the Brazelton Neonatal Assessment Scale to facilitate the parent-infant relationship in a primary care setting, *Nurse Practioner* 16(3):26-36, 1991.
126. Tharp RG: Cultural diversity and treatment of children, *J Consult Clin Psychol* 59(6):799-812, 1991.
127. Trombly CA: *Occupational therapy for physical dysfunction,* ed 2, Baltimore, 1989, Williams & Wilkins.
128. Vander Kolk CJ: Client credibility and coping styles, *Rehabil Psychol* 36(1):51-62, 1991.
129. Vickery DM and Fries JF: *Take care of yourself: a consumers guide to medical care,* Reading, Mass, 1976, Addison-Wesley.
130. Verduyn WH: Spinal cord injured women, pregnancy, and delivery, *Sexuality and Disability* 11(3):29-43, 1993.
131. Wade OT: Is stroke rehabilitation worthwhile? *Curr Opin Neurol Neurosurg* 6(1):78-82, 1993.
132. White W: The urge towards competence, *Am J Occup Ther* 26:(6)271, 1971.
133. Yellott G: Promoting parent-infant bonding, *Prof Nurs* 6(9):519-520, 1991.
134. Zani B: Male and female patterns in the discovery of sexuality during adolescence, *J Adolesc* 14:163-178, 1991.

APPENDIX A   *SUPPORT GROUPS THAT MAY ASSIST THE THERAPIST AND CLIENT*

Administration on Developmental Disabilities
U.S. Department of Health and Human Services
330 C Street, SW
Washington, DC 20201
(202) 245-2890

American Coalition for Citizens with Disabilities
1346 Connecticut Avenue NW
Washington, DC 20036

American Genetic Association
P.O. Box 39
Buckeytown, MD 21717
(301) 695-9292

American Heart Association
7320 Greenville Avenue
Dallas, TX 75231

Arthritis Foundation
3400 Peachtree Road NE, Suite 1106
Atlanta, GA 30326

Association for Persons with Severe Handicaps (TASH)
7010 Roosevelt Way, NE
Seattle, WA 98115
(206) 523-8446

Beach Center on Families and Disability
c/o Life Span Institute
University of Kansas
3111 Haworth Hall
Lawrence, KS 66045
(913) 864-7600   FAX (913) 864-7605

Center for Independent Living
2539 Telegraph Avenue
Berkeley, CA 96704
(415) 841-4776

Closer Look
National Information Center for the Handicapped
Box 1492
Washington, DC 20013

Coalition on Sexuality and Disability
132 East Twenty-third Street
New York, NY 10010
(212) 242-3900

Council for Exceptional Children
1920 Association Drive
Reston, VA 22091-1589
(703) 620-3660

Disabled American Veterans
National Headquarters
P.O. Box 14301
Cincinnati, OH 45250-0301
(606) 441-7300

Epilepsy Foundation of America
1828 L Street NW, Suite 406
Washington, DC 20036.

Federation for Children with Special Needs
95 Berkeley Street, Suite 104
Boston, MA 02116
(617) 482-2915

Information Center for Individuals with Disabilities
20 Park Plaza, Room 330
Boston, MA 02116

Interdisciplinary Special Interest Group on Head Injury of
  American Congress of Rehabilitation Medicine
5700 Old Orchard Road
Skokie, IL 60077
(708) 966-0095

National Association for Retarded Citizens
2709 Avenue E East
Arlington, TX 76011

National Center for Youth with Disabilities
Adolescent Health Program
University of Minnesota
P.O. Box 721-UMHC
Harvard Street at East River Road
Minneapolis, MN 55455
1-800-333-NCYD or
(612) 626-2825

National Association of the Physically Handicapped, Inc.
76 Elm Street
London, OH 43140

National Committee to Prevent Child Abuse (NCPCA)
332 S. Michigan Avenue, Suite 1600
Chicago, IL 60604
(312) 663-3520 TDD (312) 663-3540
(800) 835-2671

National Council on Disability
800 Independence Avenue, SW, Suite 814
Washington, DC 20591
(202) 267-3846   (202) 267-3232 (TT)
FAX (202) 453-4240

National Council on Independent Living (NCIL)
Troy Atrium
4th Street and Broadway
Troy, NY 12180
(518) 274-1979   (518) 274-0701 (TT)
FAX (518) 274-7944

The National Head Injury Foundation, Inc.
1140 Connecticut Avenue, N.W.
Suite 812
Washington, DC 20036
(202) 296-6443

National Rehabilitation Information Center
8455 Colesville Road, Suite 935
Silver Spring, MD 20910-3319
1-800-346-2742

Office for Handicapped Individuals
U.S. Department of Health and Human Services
200 Independence Avenue, SW
Washington, DC 20201
(202) 245-6568

President's Committee on Employment of People with
  Disabilities
P.O. Box 17413
Washington, DC 20041
(703) 471-5761

Sex Information and Education Council of the
 United States
84 Fifth Avenue, Suite 407
New York, NY 10011

Sexuality and Disability Training Center
University of Michigan Medical Center
Department of Physical Medicine and Rehabilitation
1500 E. Medical Center Drive
Ann Arbor, MI 48109
(313) 936-7067

Stroke Clubs of America
805 Twelfth Street
Galveston, TX 77550
(409) 762-1022

The Task Force on Sexuality and Disability of
 the American
Congress of Rehabilitation Medicine
5700 Old Orchard Road
Skokie, IL 60077
(708) 966-0095

Well Spouse Foundation
P.O. Box 28876
San Diego, CA 92198-0876
(619) 673-9043   In NY, (914) 357-8513
FAX (914) 368-4336

PART TWO

Management of Clinical Problems

CHAPTER 8

Neonatal Care and Follow-up for Infants at Neuromotor Risk

Jane K. Sweeney and Marcia W. Swanson

KEY TERMS

NICU environment	high-risk clinical signs
neonatal neuropathology	neuromotor intervention
subspecialization training	parent instruction
physiological and	
musculoskeletal risks	

LEARNING OBJECTIVES

After reading this chapter the student/therapist will:

1. Identify the physiological and structural vulnerabilities of preterm infants that predispose them to stress during neonatal therapy procedures.
2. Outline supervised clinical practicum components and pediatric clinical experiences to prepare for entry into NICU practice.
3. Describe how the grief process may affect behavior and caregiving performance of parents of high-risk neonates.
4. Differentiate the neuromotor risk signs in infants with emerging neuropathology from the clinical signs in infants with transient movement dysfunction.
5. Identify instruments for neuromotor assessment of high-risk infants in NICUs and in follow-up clinics and compare psychometric features of the tests.

In the last three decades, specialized neonatal intensive care units (NICUs) and technological advances have contributed to a dramatic decline in neonatal mortality, particularly among low-birthweight (LBW, birthweight <2500 grams) infants. Between 1960 and 1983 the survival rate in the United States increased from 1% to 46% for neonates between 500 and 1000 grams and from 42% to 85% for neonates between 1000 and 1500 grams.[74] There is evidence, however, that the improved survival of very small infants may be associated with an increased prevalence of neurodevelopmental abnormality, including cerebral palsy.[78,103] An estimated fivefold to sixfold increase in cerebral palsy has been reported among very-low-birthweight (VLBW, birthweight <1500 grams) infants with the rise continuing through the last decade.[114,175] Neonates requiring intensive care also continue to be at high risk for other forms of neurological impairment and developmental disability. Although new diagnostic techniques, such as cranial ultrasonography, provide more accurate documentation of brain injury during the neonatal period, prediction of subsequent developmental outcome is still not possible. Consequently, careful developmental assessment is required during medical follow-up in the outpatient phase. Pediatric therapists serve these increasing numbers of surviving neonates at developmental risk by: (1) offering valuable adjunctive diagnostic support in neurological and developmental assessment, (2) facilitating expedient interdisciplinary developmental case management for infants and parents, and (3) reinforcing the preventive aspects of health care by providing early intervention and long-term developmental monitoring.

This chapter focuses on at-risk infants and their parents during the clinical management phases of inpatient neonatal intensive care and outpatient monitoring. A theoretical framework for neonatal practice and an overview of neonatal neuropathology related to movement disorders are presented. In-depth discussion in the neonatal section includes indications for referral based on risk, neurological assessment instruments, high-risk profiles in the neonatal period, treatment planning, and therapy strategies in the NICU. In the infant follow-up section, discussion is focused on a service delivery model, neuromotor assessment, high-risk neuromotor markers in the first year of life, and selected intervention strategies.

THEORETICAL FRAMEWORK

Concepts of pathokinesiology, neonatal behavioral organization, and crisis intervention provide a theoretical framework for neonatal therapy practice. In this section are three models to provide a theoretical structure for practitioners designing and implementing neuromotor and neurobehavioral programs for at-risk infants and their parents.

Pathokinesiology model

Pathokinesiology, the science of abnormal human movement, has been described by Hislop[102] as the unique clinical science of physical therapy. Applied to the neonatal population, a pathokinesiology model provides the practitioner with a framework for systematically analyzing the components of an infant's movement dysfunction from the cellular to the community level. Not limited to anatomical and physiological analyses, a pathokinesiological perspective also involves a hierarchy of biobehavioral components that influence the effects of neuromotor deficits on the person, family, and community.

A pathokinesiology hierarchy of spastic diplegia is illustrated in Fig. 8-1. The spastic diplegia hierarchy is adapted from Hislop's model and describes the category of cerebral palsy closely associated with a preterm birth. This paradigm presents a holistic biobehavioral framework for understanding the multiple components of a neonatal movement disorder.

Synactive model of infant behavior

The synactive model of infant behavioral organization is a major theoretical framework for establishing physiological stability as the foundation for the organization of motor, behavioral state, and attention/interactive behaviors in neonates. Als and others[3-6] described a "synactive" process of four subsystems interacting together as the neonate responds to the stresses of the extrauterine environment. They theorized that the basic subsystem of physiological organization must first be stabilized for the other subsystems to emerge and allow the infant to maintain behavioral state control and then interact positively with the environment (Fig. 8-2).

To evaluate infant behavior within the subsystems of function addressed in the synactive model, Als and others[5] developed the Assessment of Preterm Infant Behavior. With the development of this assessment instrument, a fifth subsystem of behavioral organization, self-regulation, was added to the synactive model. The self-regulation subsystem consists of physiological, motor, and behavioral state strategies used by the neonate to maintain balance within and between the subsystems.[130] For example, many preterm infants appear to regulate overstimulating environmental conditions with a behavioral state strategy of withdrawing into a drowsy or light sleep state, thereby shutting out sensory input. The withdrawal strategy is used more frequently than crying because it requires less energy and less physiological drain to immature, inefficient organ systems.

Fetters[80] placed the synactive model within a pathokinesiology hierarchy to demonstrate the effect of a therapeutic intervention on an infant's multiple subsystems (Fig. 8-3). She explained that although a neonatal therapy intervention is offered to the infant at the level of the *person*, outcome is measured at the *systems* level where many subsystems may be affected. For example, the motor outcome from neonatal therapy procedures is frequently influenced by "synaction," or simultaneous effects, of an infant's physiological stability and behavioral state. Physiological state and behavioral state are therefore potential confounding variables during research on motor behavior in neonatal subjects. Neonatal therapists may find this combined pathokinesiology and synactive framework helpful in conceptualizing and assessing changes in infants' multiple subsystems from therapy procedures. In particular, Fetter's model illustrates the cardiopulmonary instability or risk during neuromotor assessment or intervention.

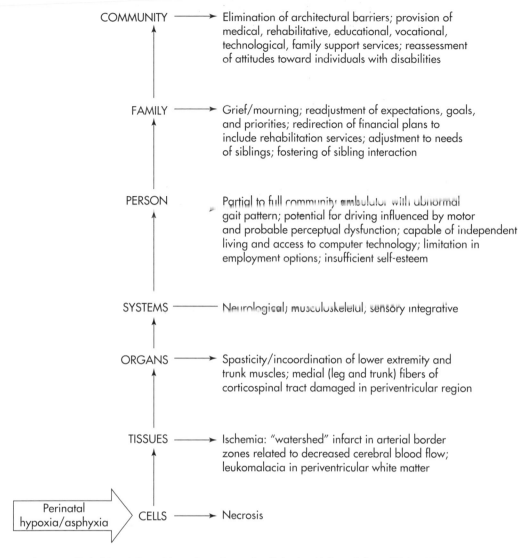

COMMUNITY ⟶ Elimination of architectural barriers; provision of medical, rehabilitative, educational, vocational, technological, family support services; reassessment of attitudes toward individuals with disabilities

FAMILY ⟶ Grief/mourning; readjustment of expectations, goals, and priorities; redirection of financial plans to include rehabilitation services; adjustment to needs of siblings; fostering of sibling interaction

PERSON ⟶ Partial to full community ambulator with abnormal gait pattern; potential for driving influenced by motor and probable perceptual dysfunction; capable of independent living and access to computer technology; limitation in employment options; insufficient self-esteem

SYSTEMS ⟶ Neurological, musculoskeletal, sensory integrative

ORGANS ⟶ Spasticity/incoordination of lower extremity and trunk muscles; medial (leg and trunk) fibers of corticospinal tract damaged in periventricular region

TISSUES ⟶ Ischemia: "watershed" infarct in arterial border zones related to decreased cerebral blood flow; leukomalacia in periventricular white matter

Perinatal hypoxia/asphyxia ⟶ CELLS ⟶ Necrosis

Fig. 8-1. Pathokinesiology hierarchy of spastic diplegia. (Adapted from Hislop HJ: The not-so-impossible dream, *Phys Ther* 55:1060, 1975.)

Hope-empowerment model

A major component of the intervention process in neonatal therapy is the interpersonal helping relationship with the family. A hope-empowerment framework (Fig. 8-4) may guide neonatal practitioners in building the therapeutic partnership with parents, facilitating adaptive coping, and empowering them to participate in caregiving, problem solving, and advocacy. The birth or diagnosis of an at-risk or disabled infant may create both developmental and situational crises for the parents and the family system. The *developmental* crisis involves adapting to changing roles in the transition to parenthood and in expanding the family system. Although not occurring unexpectedly, this developmental transition for the parents brings life-style changes that may be stressful and cause conflict.[191]

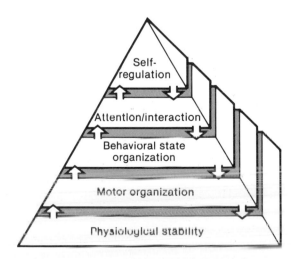

Fig. 8-2. Pyramid of synactive theory of infant behavioral organization with physiological stability at the foundation.

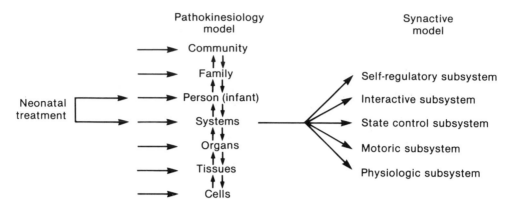

Fig. 8-3. Combined pathokinesiology and synactive models. (Adapted from Fetters L: Sensorimotor management of the high-risk neonate. *Phys Occup Ther Pediatr* 6(3/4):217, 1986.)

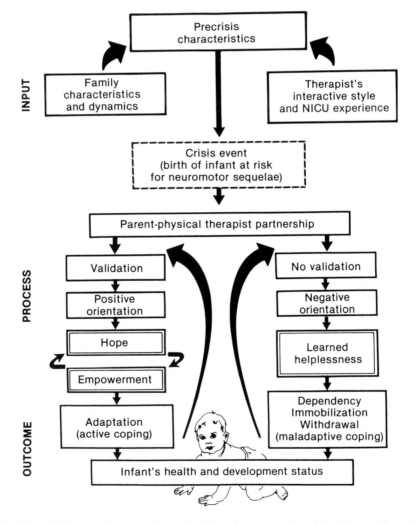

Fig. 8-4. Hope-empowerment versus learned helplessness processes of the therapeutic partnership between parents and neonatal therapist.

A *situational* crisis occurs from unexpected external events presenting a sudden, overwhelming threat or loss for which previous coping strategies are either not applicable or are immobilized.[49,140] The unfamiliar, high-tech, often chaotic **NICU environment** creates many situational stresses that challenge parenting efforts and destabilize the family system. The language of the nursery is unfamiliar and intimidating. The sights of fragile, sick infants surrounded by medical equipment, and the sounds of monitor alarms are frightening. The high frequency of seemingly uncomfortable but required medical procedures for the infant are of financial and humanistic concern to parents. No previous experiences in everyday life have prepared parents for this unnatural, emergency-oriented environment.

The quality and orientation of the helping relationship in neonatal therapy affect the coping style of parents as they try to adapt to developmental and situational crises (Fig. 8-4). Although parents and neonatal therapists come into the partnership with established interactive styles and varying life and professional experiences, the initial contacts during assessment and program planning set the stage for either a positive or negative orientation to the relationship.

Despite many uncertainties about the clinical course, prognosis, and quality of social support, a positive orientation is activated by validation or acknowledgment of parents' feelings and experiences. Validation then becomes a catalyst to a hope-empowerment process in which many crisis events, negative feelings, and insecurities are acknowledged in a positive, supportive, nonjudgmental context where decision-making power is shared.[158] In contrast, a negative orientation may be facilitated inadvertently by information overloading without exploration and validation of parents' feelings, experiences, and learning styles. This may lead to magnified uncertainty, fear, and powerlessness with the perception of excessive complexity in the proposed neuromotor intervention.

In a hope-empowerment framework, parent participation in neuromotor intervention allows sharing of power and responsibility and promotes continuous, mutual setting and revision of goals with reality grounding. Adaptive power can be generated by helping parents stabilize and focus energy and plans and by encouraging active participation in intervention and advocacy activities.[158] Exploring external power sources (Parents of Prematures or Parent-to-Parent support groups) early in the therapeutic relationship may help parents with focusing and mobilizing.[144]

Hope and empowerment are interactive processes. They are influenced by existential philosophy: the hope to adapt to what is, and the hope to later find peace of mind, regardless of the infant's outcome. In describing the effect of a prematurely born infant on the parenting process, Mercer[140] related that "hope seems to be a motivational, emotional component that gives parents energy to cope, to continue to work, and to strive for the best outcome for a child." She viewed the destruction of hope as contributing to the

physical and emotional withdrawal observed frequently in parents who attempt to protect themselves from additional pain and disappointment and then have difficulty reattaching to the infant.

In a hope-empowerment context, parent teaching activities are carefully selected to program the parents and infants for success and pleasurable interaction. Integration and generalization of neonatal therapy into routine caregiving are priorities so that carry-over to the home environment occurs with less disruption to family life-styles.

Conversely, if the parents' learning styles, goals, priorities, values, time constraints, energy levels, and emotional availability are not considered in the design of the developmental program, they are programmed for failure, destruction of self-esteem, powerlessness, immobilization, and dependency. Hopeless outlook, noncompliance, information overload, or negative interaction (power struggles) between infant and parent may be markers of an ineffective teaching style by the neonatal therapist, which can contribute to a learned helplessness outcome.[1]

New events in the infant's health or developmental status may create new crises and destabilize the coping processes.[57] In long-term follow-up many opportunities occur within the partnership to validate new fears and chronic uncertainties within a hopeful, positively oriented helping relationship. The alleviation of hopelessness is a critical helping task in health care. This model provides a caring framework for sharing with parents the gifts of hope and power.

NEUROPATHOLOGY OF MOVEMENT DISORDERS

The pathogenesis of selected, major nonprogressive neurological deficits of hypertonicity, ataxia, and athetosis can be traced to hypoxic and/or ischemic insults. Four lesions have been associated with hypoxic-ischemic brain injury and are linked to the major categories of cerebral palsy.[55,101,237-239] The related **neonatal neuropathology** and neurological sequelae from these lesions are outlined in Table 8-1.

Selective neuronal necrosis

Selective neuronal necrosis is the random, widespread necrosis of neurons from a hypoxic-ischemic event in any of the following sites: the cerebellum (Purkinje cells, dentate nuclei), the deep layers of cerebral cortex including the hippocampus and brainstem (pons, medulla, oculomotor, troclear neurons), and the diencephalon (thalamus, hypothalamus, lateral geniculate body). Hypoxemia can result in an encephalopathy manifested by coma, hypotonia/proximal weakness of the upper extremities in full-term infants or of the lower extremities in preterm infants, seizures, and tremulous movement in a predictable pattern during the first 72 hours after birth. The neurological sequelae associated with selective neuronal necrosis are related to the sites of necrosis and may include spastic hemiplegia, spastic quad-

Table 8-1. Neuropathology of cerebral palsy

Event	Lesion	Category(ies) of CP
Ischemia	Periventricular leukomalacia	Spastic diplegia Spastic quadriplegia Spastic hemiplegia
Hypoxia	Selective neuronal necrosis of the cortex	Spastic quadriplegia Spastic hemiplegia
Ischemia	Parasaggital cerebral lesion	Spastic quadriplegia Spastic hemiplegia
Increased perfusion	Intraventricular hemorrhage	Spastic diplegia Spastic quadriplegia Spastic hemiplegia
Hypoxia	Selective neuronal necrosis of the cerebellum	Ataxia
Brief, total asphyxia	Status marmoratus (hypermyelination in basal ganglia)	Athetoid

riplegia, ataxia, deafness, seizures, or mental retardation. Only 20% to 30% of infants with both hypoxic-ischemic encephalopathy and seizures in the newborn period were neurologically intact at follow-up.[237] Computed tomography (CT) of the brain reveals moderate to marked cerebral atrophy.[105]

Status marmoratus

Status marmoratus refers to basal ganglia lesions in *full-term* infants resulting from acute, brief, total asphyxia. These lesions include neuronal loss and an overgrowth of myelin that causes a unique marbled appearance in the putamen, caudate, and thalamus. The primary neurological deficit associated with status marmoratus is choreoathetosis. This frequently appears in neonates as hypotonia until approximately 10 to 12 months of age, when athetoid cerebral palsy can be confirmed. Normal findings are usually present on the CT scan.[105]

Parasagittal cerebral injury

Parasagittal cerebral injury is the result of incompletely developed autoregulation of cerebral blood flow and the subsequent vulnerability of the brain of the newborn to fluctuations in blood pressure. Parasaggital injury is an ischemic insult in *full-term* infants resulting from generalized reduction in cerebral blood flow associated with intrauterine asphyxia and hypotension. Labeled the "watershed infarct," these lesions imitate a field irrigation system where the most distant section of the field may not get irrigated if the water force is suddenly reduced. The vulnerable "last field" in parasagittal injury is a result of a fall in pressure in the border zones between the "last fields" of the anterior, middle, or posterior cerebral arteries. This fall in blood pressure frequently occurs in a symmetrical distribution with cortical involvement of parietal, temporal, or occipital lobes. The neurological sequelae may include proximal weakness in the shoulder girdle more than in the pelvic girdle musculature during the neonatal period,

perceptual dysfunction (particularly visual-motor), or mental retardation. Spastic hemiparesis or spastic quadriparesis may be present, depending on the topography of involvement of the motor cortex. CT scan data reveal cerebral atrophy from these lesions.[105]

Periventricular leukomalacia

Periventricular leukomalacia (PVL) refers to necrosis in the periventricular white matter of the brain, seen on cranial ultrasound as echodense areas. If it is severe, the elimination of the necrotic tissue over time can lead to the formation of cavities or cysts, which appear as echolucencies on ultrasound. In other infants, areas of increased echogeneity can persist for 2 to 4 weeks without evidence of cyst formation. Periventricular echodensity observed in preterm infants is believed to reflect injury to brain cells during the time of myelination.[129] It is hypothesized that the white matter damage results from a hypoxic-ischemic insult due to disturbances of cerebral blood flow.[79,129] PVL may be in the form of a single large echodense area of multiple small bilateral foci of echodensity. Fig. 8-5 illustrates the vulnerability of the medial corticospinal tract fibers from the motor cortex passing through the periventricular region.

The association between the areas of periventricular echodensities observed on cranial ultrasound and neurodevelopmental outcome depends primarily on the site and extent of the lesions. Transient echodensities that resolve within 2 to 4 weeks appear to be of no prognostic significance when the developmental outcome of affected infants is studied. Conversely, infants with large cystic lesions, usually seen in the frontal-parietal or frontal-parietal-occipital areas of the brain, are at high risk for major neurodevelopmental disability.[64,185,189] Lesions in the parietal area have been associated with cerebral palsy, either spastic diplegia (Fig. 8-6) or quadriplegia, depending on whether the lesions are bilateral or unilateral and the extent of any associated ventriculomegaly.[79,189] Fortunately, less than 10% of VLBW infants demonstrate large (> 1 to 2 cm) cysts.[21,43,89]

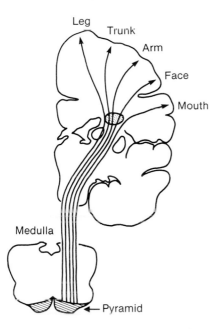

Fig. 8-5. Schematic diagram of corticospinal tract fibers that extend from the motor cortex through the periventricular region into the pyramid of the medulla.

Persistent echodense areas without apparent cysts, observed in 10% to 20% of VLBW infants, have more variable outcome. Small lesions confined to the frontal area usually are associated with a good prognosis for normal outcome, whereas persistent echogenicity in the parietal area, even without cyst formation, has been associated with cerebral palsy.[21,77,89] It is hypothesized that persistent areas of increased echogenicity may reflect permanent microscopic changes. These changes may not be visible as cysts on ultrasound, but may result in later neurological deficits including developmental delay, mental retardation, or minor neuromotor abnormalities.[79,89]

Intraventricular hemorrhage

In addition to the ischemic lesion of PVL, the incidence of *intraventricular hemorrhage* (IVH) associated with preceding perinatal asphyxia is high in the premature population. Papile and others[167] report that close to 50% of the infants with birth weights less than 1500 g (3 lb 5 oz) showed intraventricular changes on CT scan. The thin-walled vasculature in the premature brain is fragile and poorly supported by the gelatinous subependymal germinal matrix in the periventricular region. This anatomical vulnerability and the impaired vascular autoregulation make the premature infant more susceptible to IVH if cerebral blood pressure is increased (as in resuscitation for asphyxia).[124,166,184,234,244]

The relationship between IVH and developmental outcome has been investigated closely since the beginning of routine cranial ultrasound procedures for low-birthweight infants. Attempts to compare the results of different studies

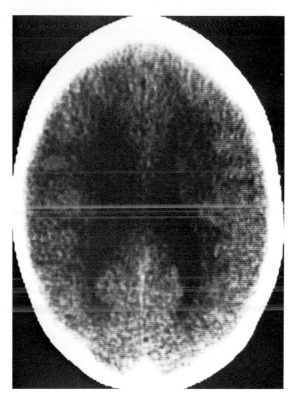

Fig. 8-6. CT findings of dilated ventricles from a child with spastic diplegia category of cerebral palsy.

Table 8-2. Grades of intraventricular hemorrhage

Grade	Extent of hemorrhage
I	Hemorrhage confined to germinal matrix (no ventricular bleed)
II	IVH without ventricular distension
III	IVH with ventricular dilation
IV	IVH extending into brain parenchyma (hydrocephalus present)

Modified from Papile L and others: Relationship of cerebral intraventricular hemorrhage and early childhood neurologic handicaps, *J Pediatr* 103(2):273, 1983.

have been complicated by the absence of a standard grading scale for these bleeds. The grading scale commonly used is a four-level scale (Table 8-2).

When IVH in low-birthweight infants is correlated with developmental outcome, the risk of major neurological handicap for infants with grades I and II bleeds is relatively low: often the degree of risk is not significantly different from that of infants with no IVH[145,168] (see Table 8-3). Infants with grade III have a significantly increased risk of major neurological impairment.

An infant with an identified grade IV IVH can be considered at high risk for developing the neurological sequelae of hydrocephalus, mental retardation, deafness,

Table 8-3. Neurodevelopmental outcome of LBW infants relative to IVH*

Grade of hemorrhage	LBW infants with major handicap
No hemorrhage	0-14%
Grade I	7%-20%
Grade II	10%-30%
Grade III	25%-40%
Grade IV	45%-80%

*References 21, 51, 132, 145, 168, and 211.

seizure disorder, hemiplegia, or quadriplegia. Fig. 8-7 illustrates ventriculomegaly and hydrocephalus as a result of grade IV IVH.

Because an intraventricular hemorrhage often is associated with periventricular echodensities and ventricular dilation, efforts to attribute neurodevelopmental abnormality to a specific type of lesion can be misleading. For example, the incidence of one or more major handicaps for infants with grade IV bleeds was reported to be as high as 100%.[51,145] However, this percentage has not been confirmed by a more recent investigation in which infants with PVL were excluded from the study in order to evaluate the impact of the hemorrhage alone.[211]

CLINICAL MANAGEMENT: NEONATAL PERIOD

Pediatric therapists with precepted subspecialty training in neonatology and infant therapy can expand neonatal medicine efforts by creating clinical protocols designed to optimize the development and interaction of at-risk neonates and parents. The therapeutic partnership between parents and neonatal therapists during developmental intervention in the NICU sets the stage for competency in caregiving and compliance with follow-up in the outpatient period. General aims of NICU clinical management of infants at risk for neurological dysfunction, developmental delay, or musculoskeletal complications are to (1) promote normal movement experiences, (2) reduce active reinforcement of abnormal movement patterns and positions, (3) decrease congenital musculoskeletal deformity and acquired joint-muscle contractures, (4) foster infant-parent attachment and interaction, (5) modify sensory stimulation in the infant's NICU environment to promote behavioral organization and physiological stability, (6) provide consultation or direct intervention for neonatal feeding dysfunction and oral-motor deficits, and (7) enhance parents' caregiving skills (feeding, dressing, bathing, positioning of infant for sleep, interaction/play, and transportation).

Educational requirements for therapists

Assessment and treatment of neonates are advanced-level, not entry-level, clinical competencies. Neonatology is a subspecialty within the specialty areas of pediatric physical

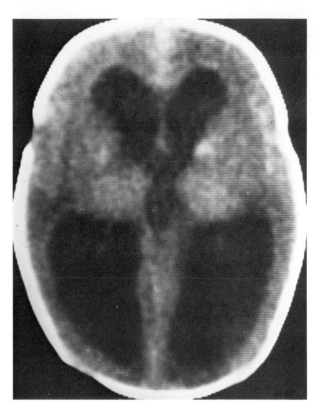

Fig. 8-7. CT findings of ventriculomegaly and hydrocephalus in an infant with a grade IV intraventricular hemorrhage.

therapy and pediatric occupational therapy. Campbell[47] advises that the development of a neonatal therapy program "requires specialized knowledge and skills in neonatal medicine, assessment of development in early infancy, early intervention, parent education, and interdisciplinary interaction in the specialized setting of the intensive care nursery." She further describes the need for studying fetal development, neonatal physiology and pathophysiology, common neonatal medical conditions, nature and management of energy costs in preterm and at-risk full-term infants, parent-infant attachment and interaction, and the ecology of the NICU.

No amount of literature review, self-study, or experience with other pediatric populations can substitute for **subspecialization training** with a preceptor in an NICU. The potential for causing harm to medically fragile infants during well-intentioned intervention is enormous.[172] The ongoing clinical decisions made by neonatal therapists in evaluating and managing **physiological and musculoskeletal risks** while handling small (2 or 3 lb), medically fragile infants in the NICU should not be a trial-and-error experience at the infants' expense. Therapists with adult-oriented training and even those with general pediatric training (excluding neonatal) are not qualified for neonatal practice without a supervised clinical practicum (usually

Table 8-4. Prenatal, perinatal, and postnatal risk factors for neuromotor abnormalities

Study	Birth weight	Outcome age	Risk factors	
			High risk	Low risk
Pape (1978)	≤1000 g	2 years	Birth weight Acidemia ICH† Seizures	Asphyxia IRDS* Apnea Mechanical ventilation
Nelson and Ellenberg (1979)	All	7 years	Birth weight Microcephaly Low Apgar score: 5 and 10 minutes Seizures	Low Apgar score: 1 minute
Knobloch (1982)	≤1500 g	40 weeks	Birth weight Gestational age Low Apgar score: 5 minutes Seizures ICH† IRDS*	SGA‡ Head size
Bennett (1982)	≤2000 g	2 years	Birth weight Gestational age	IRDS*
Kraybill (1984)	≤1000 g	12-34 months	Mechanical ventilation	Birth weight Gestational age Low Apgar score SGA‡ Head size
Stanley and English (1986)	≤2000 g	6 years	Asphyxia score Low Apgar score: 1 minute	Birth weight Gestational age Low Apgar score: 5 minutes
Bull (1988)	≤1500 g	12-30 months	Mechanical ventilation BPD§ Meningitis	Birth weight Gestational age Low Apgar score

*IRDS; Idiopathic respiratory distress syndrome.
†ICH; Intracranial hemorrhage.
‡SGA; Small for gestational age.
§BPD; Bronchopulmonary dysplasia.

3 months). Position papers on advanced level competencies for the physical therapist in the NICU[201] are available from the section on Pediatrics-American Physical Therapy Association. The American Occupational Therapy Association has a similar position paper on knowledge and skills for neonatal practice.

A gradual, systematic entry to neonatal practice is advised. This may be approached by building clinical experience with full-term infants and medically fragile older children and their parents. The experience may include managing caseloads of hospitalized children on physiological monitoring equipment and supplemental oxygen or ventilators. Participating in discharge planning and in outpatient follow up of high risk neonates are other options for providing exposure to assessment, intervention, and family issues when the infants and parents are more stable. This clinical experience and a precepted practicum in the nursery offer the best preparation for appropriate, accountable, scientific, and ethical practice in neonatal therapy.[228]

Indications for referral

Research efforts in recent years have been directed toward determining which LBW infants will have a less-than-optimal outcome. One approach to this task has been the designation of risk factors: prenatal, perinatal, or neonatal conditions that are associated with infants considered to have a statistically higher chance of developing a neuromotor abnormality. The studies in Table 8-4 represent different approaches to medical management at varying time periods and geographical sites. The risk criteria vary because of the absence of uniform definition and grading of conditions, differences in sample selection and follow up procedures, and the absence of standard measures for neurodevelopmental outcome. Changes in obstetrical and neonatal procedures are occurring so rapidly that the findings from reported studies may not be completely relevant to developmental outcome from current practice.

Tjossem's categories[229] of biological, established, and social risk provide a logical framework for listing diagnoses and behavioral observations for neonatal therapy referral. A formal protocol for referral and clinical management validates the therapist as an integral part of the NICU team.[245] An overview of developmental risk categories and risk factors for neonatal therapy referral is listed in the box to assist clinicians in developing a referral mechanism for a clinical protocol based on risk categories.

Biological risk. Biological risk refers to developmental risk created by maturational or medically related complications in the prenatal, perinatal, or neonatal periods.[229] Biological risks may include fetoplacental abnormalities;

Developmental risk indicators for neonatal therapy referral

Biological risk

Birth weight of 1500 g or less
Gestational age of 32 weeks or less
Small for gestational age (less than 10th percentile for weight)
Ventilator requirement for 36 hours or more
Intracranial hemorrhage: grades III or IV
Muscle tone abnormalities (hypotonia, hypertonia, asymmetry of tone/movement)
Recurrent neonatal seizures (3 or more)
Feeding dysfunction
Symptomatic TORCH infections (toxoplasmosis, rubella, cytomegalovirus, herpes virus type II, syphilis)
Meningitis
Asphyxia with Apgar score less than 4 at 5 minutes

Established risk

Hydrocephalus
Microcephaly
Chromosomal abnormalities
Musculoskeletal abnormalities (congenitally dislocated hips, limb deficiencies, arthrogryposis, joint contractures, congenital torticollis)
Multiple births greater than twins
Brachial plexus injuries (Erb's palsy, Klumpke's paralysis)
Myelodysplasia
Congenital myopathies and myotonic dystrophy
Inborn errors of metabolism
HIV infection

Environmental/social risk

High–social risk (single parent, parental age less than 17 years, poor quality infant-parent attachment)
Maternal drug or alcohol abuse
Behavioral state abnormalities (lethargy, excessive irritability, behavioral state lability)

---

labor/delivery complications; and teratogenic, iatrogenic, or physiological factors.

Birth weight is a strong predictor of outcome.[20,117,153] In general, the lower the birth weight, the greater the risk of a suboptimal neurodevelopmental outcome. This finding, however, is not universal.[122,247] In some populations of VLBW infants (1000 to 1500 g) or extremely LBW infants (less than 1000 g), the prevalence of cerebral palsy has been less than expected.[214] In one long-term follow-up study, birth weight was more predictive of the need for special education than for cerebral palsy.[235] Infants who are small for gestational age are at increased risk for cerebral palsy in some studies, whereas in others only the incidence of minor neurodevelopmental abnormalities is greater.[235]

Low Apgar scores, a measure of neonatal asphyxia, are a commonly used risk indicator.[24,85] Because Apgar scores also reflect the relative maturity and neurological integrity of the infant, low scores in preterm infants are not considered as reliable as those for full-term neonates.

Although the presence and severity of respiratory disease did not appear to be predictors of neurodevelopmental outcome in early studies,[20,165] recent comparisons of developmental status between ventilated and nonventilated infants revealed that up to 80% of ventilated infants had developmental abnormalities.[122,190] In other follow-up studies, infants with chronic lung disease or bronchopulmonary disease (BPD) had a higher incidence of cerebral palsy and other neurodevelopmental abnormalities than preterm infants with BPD.[210,235,236] In infants requiring ventilatory assistance, a relationship between duration of ventilatory assistance and outcome has been observed. Increased neurological impairment was associated with prolonged ventilatory assistance[40]; however, this association was not observed in a subsequent study.[132]

Established risk. Established risk is the risk for neurodevelopmental deficits associated with a diagnosis easily established in the neonatal period. Included in this category are congenital malformations, chromosomal abnormalities, central nervous system (CNS) disorders, and metabolic diseases with known developmental sequelae.

Environmental/social risk. Environmental/social risk involves developmental risk related to competency in parenting roles and factors in family dynamics.[124,203] Such risk may be heightened by prolonged hospitalization of infants with suboptimal levels of stimulation and interaction (overstimulation or deprivation) in the intensive care nursery environment, inadequate infant-parent bonding, insufficient educational preparation of parents for caretaking roles, meager financial resources, and limited or absent family support to assist in taking care of and nurturing the infant in the home environment.

• • •

It is common for high-risk neonates to have a combination of risk factors from more than one major category.

In-depth study of perinatal and neonatal medicine and related obstetrical, neonatal nursing, and neonatal therapy literature* is recommended before the development of a neonatal therapy protocol and participation as a member of the special care nursery team.

Neonatal neurological assessment

Multiple neonatal neurological, and neurobehavioral examinations have been developed to assess the integrity of the nervous system, to calculate gestational age, and to describe newborn behavior.[7,131,186,187,193] Five frequently used instruments include the Clinical Assessment of Gestational Age,[71] the Neurological Examination of the Full-term Infant,[177] the Brazelton Neonatal Behavioral Assessment Scale,[36] the Neurological Assessment of the Preterm and Full-term Newborn Infant,[70] and the Assessment of Preterm Infant Behavior.[5] These instruments were selected to familiarize clinicians with a range of neurological and behavioral assessments used in current practice for management of both preterm and full-term infants. Most of these assessment instruments offer *quality* data on motor performance and interactional behavior that are essential for the development of individualized treatment plans.

Clinical Assessment of Gestational Age in the Newborn Infant.[71] The Clinical Assessment of Gestational Age in the Newborn Infant[71] was developed by Dubowitz and others from a total of 167 preterm and full-term infants (28 to 42 weeks gestation) tested within 5 days of birth. It focuses on criteria for calculation of gestational age from a composite of 10 neurological and 11 external features (see Appendix A).

This test rates criteria on a four-point scale; it is commonly administered by nurses or physicians in the newborn nursery. The accuracy (95% confidence limit) of the gestational age score is determined within a variation of ±2 weeks on any single assessment. This measurement error can be decreased to approximately ±1.4 weeks when two separate assessments are performed. From the analyses of multiple assessments on 70 of the 167 infants, the age score was equally reliable in the first 24 hours of age as during the next 4 days of life. The behavioral state(s) of the infant during the assessment is not considered a significant variable in the examination.

Calculation of gestational age is an important adjunct to all other neonatal assessment tools: It guides practitioners in interpreting neurological and behavioral findings relative to the expected performance of newborn infants at various gestational ages. Additional guidelines on gestational differences in neurological, physical, and neuromuscular maturation can be found in the work of Saint-Anne Dargassies,[193] Lubchenco,[131] Carter and Campbell,[50] Amiel-Tison.[7,9,10]

Neurological Examination of the Full-term Infant.[177] The Neurological Examination of the Full-term Infant[177] was designed by Prechtl to identify abnormal neurological signs in the newborn period. The examination was developed from an investigation of more than 1350 newborns and was standardized on infants born at the gestational age of 38 to 42 weeks. If used on premature infants who have reached an age of 38 to 42 weeks of gestation, lower resistance to passive movements (lower tone) may be expected. Delay of testing until a minimum of 3 days of age is advised to maximize the stability of behavioral states and neuromotor responses for improved reliability and validity of results.

The pattern of examination includes an observation period and an examination period. A 10-minute screening examination is offered to determine if the full 30-minute assessment of posture, tone, reflexes, and spontaneous movement is required. Although specific requirements for examiner training are not addressed, Prechtl offers a flow diagram (Fig. 8-8) to assist clinicians with organizing the neurological examination process. Significant findings from the examination are summarized in the following categories: (1) the quality of posture, spontaneous movement, and muscle tone (consistency and resistance to passive movement), (2) presence of involuntary or pathological movements (clonus, tremor, athetoid postures or movements), (3) behavioral state changes and quality of cry, and (4) threshold/intensity of responses to stimulation.

From combinations of these findings, Prechtl identifies four clinical syndromes. The *hemisyndrome* identifies infants with three asymmetrical findings during assessment of movement, tone, posture, or reflexes. The *hyperexcitable syndrome* refers to a behavioral profile that may include instability of behavioral states, prolonged crying, presence of tremor and hypertonus, increased deep tendon reflexes, and hyperkinesis. The *apathetic syndrome,* a frequent precursor of the hemisyndrome, is manifested by hypotonia and a very high threshold for response to stimulation. The *comatose syndrome* is characterized by minimal or absent arousal to pain or other sensory stimuli and by the frequent presence of abnormal respiratory patterns. The presence of these syndromes in newborn infants strongly justifies the need for comprehensive interdisciplinary follow-up to manage potential developmental sequelae. Due to the transient pattern of neurological signs and rapid changes in the developing nervous system, Prechtl advises repeated examinations to monitor neurological status.

Neonatal Behavioral Assessment Scale (NBAS).* To document individual behavioral and motoric differences in full-term infants, Brazelton and others developed a neonatal behavior scale to assess neuromotor responses within a behavioral state context. The 30 to 45 minute

* References 12, 13, 19, 47, 48, 80, 82, 93, 99, 115, 120, 131, 169, 212, 217.

* References 2, 36, 156, 196, 216.

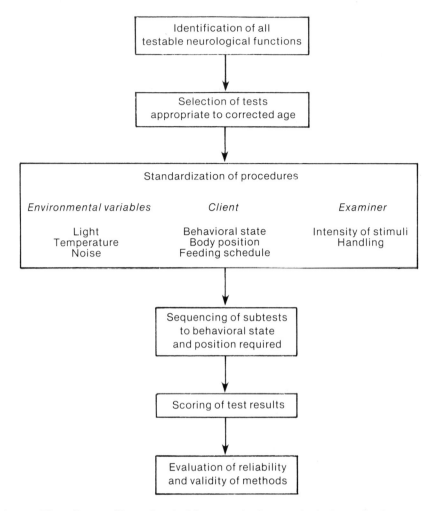

Fig. 8-8. Flow diagram illustrating decision steps in the neurological examination process.

examination consists of observing, eliciting, and scoring 28 biobehavioral items on a 9-point scale and 18 reflex items on a 4-point scale. The reflex items are derived from the neurological examination protocol of Prechtl and Beintema.[178]

The scale was designed to assess newborn behavior on healthy 3-day-old full-term (40-week gestation) white infants whose mothers had minimal sedative medication during an uncomplicated labor and delivery. Use of this examination with preterm infants requires modification of the examination procedure to the environmental constraints of an intensive care nursery and interpretation of findings relative to the gestational age and medical condition of the infant. For preterm infants approaching term (minimum of 36 weeks of gestation), nine supplementary behavioral items are offered. Many of these items were developed by Als and others[5] for use with preterm and physiologically stressed infants.

Although the mean scores are related to the expected behavior of 3-day-old full-term infants, the NBAS is considered an appropriate assessment tool from 37 weeks of gestation until 44 weeks of gestation. Extended use of this

scale for older infants was reported by Provost,[179,180] who described the methods and results from administering the scale with the Kansas Supplements (five additional items on a 9-point scale) to 11 normal, full-term infants during the first 4 months of life.

The NBAS outlines 6 behavioral state categories: deep sleep, light sleep, drowsiness/semidozing, quiet alert, active alert, and crying. Behavioral state prerequisites are provided for each biobehavioral and reflex item to reduce the state-related variables in testing. During the assessment the examiner systematically maneuvers the infant from the sleep states to crying and back to the alert states to evaluate physiological, organizational, motoric, and interactive capabilities during stimulation and physical handling. The scoring is based on the infant's *best* performance with flexibility allowed in the order of testing, repetition of items encouraged, and scheduling of the assessment midway between feedings to give the infant every advantage to demonstrate the best possible responses.

Four dimensions of newborn behavior are analyzed in the Brazelton Scale: interactive ability, motor behavior, behavioral state organization, and physiological organization. Interactive ability describes the infant's response to visual and auditory stimuli (Fig. 8-9), consolability from the crying state with intervention by the examiner, and ability to maintain alertness and respond to social/environmental stimuli.

Motor behavior refers to the ability to modulate muscle tone and motor control for the performance of integrated motor skills, such as the hand-to-mouth maneuver, pull-to-sit maneuver, and defensive reaction (i.e., removal of cloth from face). In the assessment of behavioral state organization, the infant's ability to organize behavioral states when stimulated and the ability to shut out irritating environmental stimuli when sleeping are analyzed. Physiological organization is analyzed by observing the infant's ability to manage physiological stress (changes of skin color, frequency of tremulous movement in the chin and extremities, number of startle reactions during the assessment).

Performance profiles of worrisome or deficient interactive-motoric and organizational behavior are identified by clusters of behavior associated with potential developmental risk.[2,3,127,216] The cluster systems are highly useful for clinical interpretation and for data analysis aspects of clinical research.[246]

The Brazelton Scale has proved to be more sensitive to the detection of mild neurological dysfunction in the newborn period than classical neurological examinations that omit the behavioral dimensions. In predicting neurological outcome at the age of 7 years in 53 high-risk neonates, the Brazelton Scale results provided a lower incidence of inaccuracy (a lower false-positive rate) in the prediction of neuropathology than a standard neurological examination.[230]

Definite strengths of the NBAS are the well-defined indicators of autonomic stress, the analysis of the coping ability of high-risk infants to external stimuli and handling, and the quality of infant-examiner interaction. These features generate specific findings to assist therapists in grading the intensity of assessment and treatment within each infant's physiological and behavioral tolerance and in guiding the development of parent teaching strategies to address the individual behavioral styles of infants.

Participation of the parent in the newborn assessment may yield long-term, positive effects in infant-parent interaction and later cognitive and fine motor development. Widmayer and Field[243] reported significantly better face-to-face interaction and fine motor/adaptive skills at 4 months of age and higher mental development scores at 12 months of age when teenage mothers of preterm (mean gestational age at birth: 35.1 weeks) infants were given Brazelton Scale demonstrations. These demonstrations were scheduled when the premature infants had reached an age equivalence of 37 weeks' gestation.

Nugent[157] developed parent teaching guidelines for using the Brazelton Scale as an intervention for infants and their families. Published by the March of Dimes, the guidelines

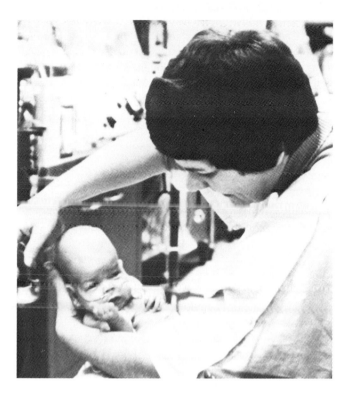

Fig. 8-9. Assessment of auditory orientation to the bell during neonatal assessment using the Brazelton Neonatal Behavioral Assessment Scale.

offer strategies for interpreting each item according to its adaptive and developmental significance, descriptions of the expected developmental course of the behavior (item) over several months, and recommendations for caregiving according to the infant's response to the item.

Four films are available for examiner training.[38] In addition, the administration and scoring of the NBAS on 15 to 25 infants are recommended to establish reliable testing and interpretation skills. Certification for use of the Brazelton Scales in research is coordinated through The Children's Hospital, Boston, Mass.[37] Wilhelm[246] recommends NBAS training for clinicians beginning to develop competence in examining at-risk infants. She explains that it provides a system for developing basic handling skills with full-term, healthy infants without concerns of stressing medically fragile preterm infants during the training period. Learning the Brazelton Scale before the Assessment of Preterm Infant Behavior provides familiarity with similar testing and scoring procedures for preterm infants.[246]

Neurological Assessment of the Preterm and Full-term Newborn Infant.[70] The Neurological Assessment of the Preterm and Full-term Newborn Infant[70] is a streamlined neurological and neurobehavioral assessment designed by Dubowitz and Dubowitz to provide a systematic, quickly administered (10 to 15 minute) examination applicable to *both* premature and full-term infants. A distinct advantage of this tool is the minimal training or experience required by the examiner.

The test includes multiple neurobehavioral components of the Brazelton NBAS: The six behavioral state categories and nine neurobehavioral items are scored on a condensed five-point grading scale and sequenced according to the intensity of response. These neurobehavioral items, selected to reflect higher neurological functioning than the brainstem level reflex responses, consist of the following: (1) habituation to light and sound while sleeping, (2) auditory and visual orientation responses (Fig. 8-10), (3) quality and duration of alertness, (4) defensive reaction to a cloth over the face, (5) peak of excitement—the infant's overall responsiveness and variability of behavioral states during the examination, (6) irritability—the frequency of crying to aversive stimuli during reflex testing and handling throughout the examination, and (7) consolability—the ability after crying to reach a calm state independently or with intervention by the examiner. The appearance of the eyes (sunset sign, strabismus, nystagmus) and the quality of the cry are included in the neurobehavioral category because they also require the awake state for testing.

The 15 items that assess movement and tone and the six reflex items evolved from clinical trials on 50 full-term infants using the Clinical Assessment of Gestational Age by

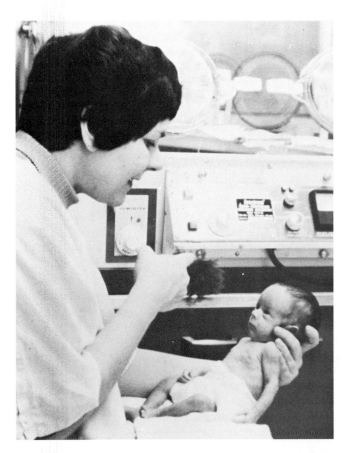

Fig. 8-10. Evaluation of visual orientation responses (i.e., visual fixation and horizontal tracking) during the Dubowitz Neurological Assessment.

Dubowitz and others,[71] the Neurological Examination of the Newborn by Parmelee and others,[170] the Neurological Examination of the Full-term Newborn Infant by Prechtl,[177] and the abnormal inventory protocol described by Saint-Anne Dargassies.[193] The present format was then used during a 2-year period on over 500 infants of varying gestational ages. The authors did not present reliability data in the manual but described modification of the protocol during their clinical trial phase that promoted objectivity in scoring and a high interrater reliability among examiners, regardless of experience level.

The examination protocol is outlined and illustrated on a 2-page form with space allowed for comments. The illustrated form is constructed to accommodate both baseline and repeat assessments, and it can be effectively combined with an additional narrative impression and treatment goals/plan for neonatal therapy programs. Because a total or summary score is avoided in this examination and because emphasis is given instead to patterns of responses, selected parts of the protocol are appropriate for the assessment of premature or acutely ill infants on ventilators, in isolettes, or attached to monitoring or infusion equipment. It is recommended that the scheduling of examinations occur two thirds of the way between feedings.

Dubowitz and Dubowitz[70,72] do not yet have long-term follow-up data beyond 1 year with this examination. Instead they present and discuss seven case histories, describe experiences using the tool in the evaluation of infants with intraventricular hemorrhage, and report outcome data at 12 months of age. The abnormal neonatal clinical signs that correlated with long-term neurological sequelae were persistent asymmetry, decreased lower extremity movement, and increased tone. Infants with IVH had significantly higher incidence of abnormally tight popliteal angles, reduced mobility, decreased visual fixing and following, and roving eye movements.

Dubowitz and others[73] reassessed 116 infants (27 to 34 weeks of gestation) at 1 year of age. Of 62 infants assessed as neurologically normal in the newborn period, 91% were also normal at 1 year of age. Of 39 infants assessed as neurologically abnormal in the newborn period, 35% were found to be normal at 1 year of age. According to Wilhelm,[246] the predictive value of a negative test with this instrument was 92%, but the predictive value of a positive test was only 64%.

Clinicians interested in using the Neurological Assessment for Preterm and Full-term Infants in clinical studies may assign numerical values to the range of descriptive criteria within the items under each major examination category. This technique was used by Morgan and others[146] in efforts to quantitate neonatal neurological status for data analysis.

Interpretations of evaluative findings from the Neurological Assessment for Preterm and Full-term Newborn Infants for neonatal therapy practice are described comprehensively in a case study format by Heriza[99] and Campbell.[48] Dubowitz[69] discussed the clinical significance of neurological variations in infants and offered decision guidelines to clinicians on when to worry, reassure, and intervene with developmental referrals.

Assessment of Preterm Infant Behavior.[5] Als and others[3,5,6] designed the Assessment of Preterm Infant Behavior (APIB) to structure a comprehensive observation of a preterm infant's autonomic, adaptive, and interactive responses to graded handling and environmental stimuli. As described previously in the theoretical framework section, this assessment is derived from synactive theory and is focused on assessing the organization and balance of the infant's physiological, motor, behavioral state, attention/ interaction, and self-regulation subsystems. The APIB follows similar testing sequences and scoring as the NBAS with increased complexity and expansion for premature infants.

Administration and scoring of the Assessment of Preterm Infant Behavior totals 2 to 3 hours per infant, depending on examiner experience. Although the APIB is an instrument of choice for the clinical researcher, it may not be practical (time efficient) for many neonatal clinicians with heavy caseloads.

Extensive training and reliability certification are required to safely administer and accurately score and interpret the test for clinical practice or research. The training is available in Boston and Tucson.[3]

Neonatal Individualized Developmental Care and Assessment Program.[3] Als and others[3,6] developed the Neonatal Individualized Developmental Care and Assessment Program (NIDCAP) to document the effects of the caregiving environment on the neurobehavioral stability of newborn infants. This naturalistic observation protocol includes continuous observation and documentation at 2-minute intervals of an infant's behavioral state and autonomic, motor, and attention signals with simultaneous recording of vital signs and oxygen saturation. This documentation occurs before, during, and after routine caregiving procedures. A narrative description of the infant's responses to the stress of handling by the primary nurse and to auditory and visual stimuli in the NICU environment is provided for developing care plans. Options are described in the care plans for reducing aversive environmental stimuli and adapting physical handling procedures. This clinical tool allows neonatal therapists to determine the infant's readiness for assessment and intervention by observing the baseline tolerance of the infant to routine nursing care before superimposing neonatal therapy procedures.[6] Examiner training in the NIDCAP may be coordinated through the National Training Center at the Children's Hospital, Boston, Mass, for regional training in North Carolina, Oklahoma, Colorado, Arizona, and California.[221]

Summary. It is essential that practitioners be aware of the normative and validation data and of the predictive

characteristics of the test(s) administered to allow appropriate interpretation of the results. Specific clinical training with a preceptor is essential to accurately administer, score, and interpret neonatal assessment instruments; to establish interrater reliability; and to plan treatment based on the evaluative findings. Even low-risk, healthy preterm infants are vulnerable to becoming physiologically and behaviorally destabilized during neurological assessment procedures.[236] This risk is reduced with precepted clinical training in the NICU.

Testing variables. Neuromuscular findings and interactional behavior in the newborn period may be influenced by several variables. Increased reliability in examination results and in clinical impressions may occur when these variables are recognized.[12,55,88] *Medication* may produce side effects of low muscle tone, drowsiness, and lethargy. Such medications include anticonvulsants, sedatives for diagnostic procedures (CT scan, electroencephalography, electromyography), and medication for postsurgical pain management. *Intermittent subtle seizures* may produce changes in muscle tension and in the level of responsiveness. These may be mild, ongoing seizures that are manifested in the neonate by lip smacking or sucking, staring or horizontal gaze, apnea, bradycardia, or stiffening of the extremities more frequently than clonic movement. *Fatigue* from medical/nursing procedures can result in decreased tolerance to handling, decreased interaction, and magnified muscle tone abnormalities. Fatigue may also result when neurodevelopmental assessment is scheduled immediately after laboratory (hematologic) procedures, suctioning, ultrasonography, or respiratory (chest percussion) therapy. *Metabolic/physiological factors* such as tremulous movement in the extremities may be linked to conditions of metabolic imbalance (hypomagnesemia, hypocalcemia, hypoglycemia); low muscle tone may be associated with hyperbilirubinemia, hypoglycemia, hypoxemia, and hypothermia. *Racial factors* produce unique differences in infant temperament among racial groups. Freedman[84] described the calm temperament of Chinese, Polynesian, and Navaho Indian newborns as clearly different from the comparatively more sensitive, irritable temperament of white or Japanese infants. Similarly in clinical practice, normal muscle tone variations among racial groups are common. Tone variations may involve decreased consistency to palpation in Asian babies and increased muscular firmness in black infants as compared to white infants. The normal variations in palpable muscle tension in the extremities among racial groups have not yet been validated by quantitative measurement.

Treatment planning

Level of stimulation. The issue of safe and therapeutic levels of sensorimotor intervention must be addressed in the design of developmental intervention programs for infants who have been unstable medically. The concept of "infant stimulation," which was introduced by early childhood educators to describe *general* developmental stimulation programs for healthy infants, is highly inappropriate in an approach based on concepts of pathokinesiology and infant behavioral organization.

For intervention to be therapeutic in a special care nursery setting, the amount and type of stimulation must be individually graded to each infant's physiological tolerance, movement patterns, unique temperament, and level of responsivity. Rather than needing more stimulation, many infants, especially those with hypertonus or those with tremulous, disorganized movement, have difficulty adapting to the routine levels of noise, light, position changes, and handling in the nursery environment. General stimulation can quickly magnify abnormal muscle tone and movement, increase behavioral state lability and irritability, and stress fragile physiological homeostasis when it is not individualized to the specific motor and interactive needs and responses of preterm or chronically ill infants. Implementation of careful physiological monitoring and graded handling techniques are essential to prevent compromise in patient safety and to facilitate development. Infant *modulation,* rather than stimulation, is the aim of intervention.

Physiological and musculoskeletal risk management. Many maturation-related anatomical and physiological factors predispose preterm infants to pulmonary dysfunction (Table 8-5). For this reason many at-risk neonates will require the use of a wide range of respiratory equipment and physiological monitors (Table 8-6). Pediatric therapists preparing to work in the NICU and those involved with designing risk management plans are referred to Crane's analysis[58,60] of neonatal cardiopulmonary management for therapists.

In this new subspecialty of pediatric practice, neonatal therapists are responsible for the prevention of physiological jeopardy in high-risk infants during developmental intervention in special care units. Before assessment, discussion with the supervising neonatologist is advised regarding specific precautions and the safe range of vital signs for each infant. Medical update and identification of new precautions by the nursing staff before each intervention session are recommended because new events in the last few hours may not be recorded or fully analyzed at the time therapy is scheduled. It is essential that the nurse be invited to maintain ongoing surveillance of the infant's medical stability during neonatal therapy activities in case physiological complications occur. If medical complications develop during or after therapy, immediate, comprehensive codocumentation of the incident with the supervising nurse and discussion with the neonatology staff are essential to analyze the events, outline related clinical teaching issues, and minimize legal jeopardy.

Areas of particular concern during neonatal therapy activities include the following: potential incidence of fracture, dislocation, or joint effusion during the management of limited joint motion; skin breakdown or vascular compromise during splinting or taping to reduce deformity; apnea or bradycardia during movement therapy with potential deterioration to respiratory arrest; aspiration during feeding assessment or emesis with oral-motor therapy; hypothermia from prolonged handling of the infant away from the neutral thermal environment of the Isolette or overhead radiant warmer; and propagation of infection from inadequate compliance with infection control procedures in the nursery. Signs of overstimulation may include labored breathing with chest retractions, grunting, nostril flaring, color changes (skin mottling to red or cyanotic appearance), frequent startles, irritability or drowsiness, sneezing, gaze aversion, bowel movement, and hiccoughs.[3,130] Signals of overstimulation expressed through infants' motor systems are finger splay (extension and abduction posturing), arm salute (shoulder flexion with elbow extension), and trunk arching away from stimulation.[3]

Even a baseline neurological assessment, usually presumed to be a benign clinical procedure, may be destabilizing to the newborn's cardiovascular and behavioral

Table 8-5. Factors contributing to pulmonary dysfunction in preterm neonates*

Anatomical	Physiological
Capillary beds not well developed before 26 weeks of gestation	Increased pulmonary vascular resistance leading to right-to-left shunting
Type II alveolar cells and surfactant production not mature until 35 weeks of gestation	
Elastic properties of lung not well developed	Decreased lung compliance
Lung "space" decreased by relative size of the heart and abdominal distention	
Type I, high-oxidative fibers compose only 10% to 20% of diaphragm muscle	Diaphragmatic fatigue; respiratory failure
Highly vascular subependymal germinal matrix not resorbed until 35 weeks of gestation, increasing infant's vulnerability for hemorrhage	Decreased or absent cough and gag reflexes; apnea
Lack of fatty insulation and high surface area/body-weight ratio	Hypothermia and increased oxygen consumption

*From Crane L: In Irwin S and Tecklin JS, editors: *Cardiopulmonary physical therapy,* St Louis, 1985, Mosby.

organization systems. The physiological and behavioral tolerance of low-risk preterm and full-term neonates to evaluative handling by a neonatal physical therapist was studied in 72 newborn subjects.[226] During and after administration of the Neurological Assessment of the Preterm and Full-term Newborn Infant, preterm subjects (30 to 35 weeks of gestation) had significantly higher heart rate; greater increase in blood pressure; decreased peripheral oxygenation inferred from mottled skin color; and higher frequencies of finger splay, arm salute, hiccups, and yawns than full-term subjects. Neonatal practitioners must examine the safety of even a neurological assessment and weigh the risks and anticipated benefit of the procedure given the expected physiological and behavioral changes in low-risk, medically stable neonates.

High-risk profiles. Three general high-risk profiles are observed from a pathokinesiological perspective. These profiles identify movement abnormalities, related temperament/behavioral characteristics, and interactional styles associated with motor status.

Table 8-6. Equipment commonly encountered in the NICU

Equipment	Description
Radiant warmer	Unit composed of mattress on an adjustable table top covered by a radiant heat source controlled manually and by servocontrol mode. Unit has adjustable side panels. *Advantage:* provides open space for tubes and equipment and easier access to the infant. *Disadvantage:* open bed may lead to convective heat loss and insensible fluid loss.
Self-contained incubator (isolette)	Enclosed unit of transparent material providing a heated and humidified environment with a servo system of temperature monitoring. Access to infant through side portholes or opening side of unit. *Advantage:* less convective heat and insensible water loss. *Disadvantage:* infection control; more difficult to get to infant; not practical for a very acutely ill neonate.
Thermal shield	Plexiglass dome placed over the trunk and legs of an infant in an Isolette to reduce radiant heat loss.
Oxygen hood	Plexiglass hood that fits over the infant's head; provides environment for controlled oxygen and humidification delivery.
Mechanical ventilator: Pressure ventilator	Delivers positive-pressure ventilation; pressure-limited with volume delivered dependent on the stiffness of the lung.
Volume ventilator	Delivers positive-pressure ventilation; volume-limited delivering same tidal volume with each breath.
Negative-pressure ventilator	Ventilator that creates a relative negative pressure around the thorax and abdomen thereby assisting ventilation without endotracheal tube. NOTE: Difficult to use in infants weighing less than 1500 g.
Nasal and nasopharyngeal prongs	Simple system for providing continuous positive airway pressure (CPAP) consisting of nasal prongs of varying lengths and adaptor to pressure-source tubing.
Resuscitation bag	Usually a self-inflating bag with a reservoir (so high concentrations of oxygen may be delivered at a rapid rate) attached to an oxygen flowmeter and a pressure manometer.
ECG, heart rate, respiratory rate, and blood pressure monitor (cardiorespirograph)	Usually one unit will display one or more vital signs on oscilloscope and digital display. High and low limits may be set, and alarm sounds when limits exceeded.
Transcutaneous oxygen (Tc Po$_2$) monitor	Noninvasive method of monitoring partial pressure of oxygen from arterialized capillaries through the skin. The electrode is heated, placed on an area of thin epidermis (usually abdomen or thorax). The monitor has capability of providing both a digital display and a continuous recording of TcPo$_2$ values.
Intravenous infusion pump	Used to pump intravenous fluids, intralipids, and transpyloric feedings at an ongoing rate. Pump has alarm system and capacity to monitor volume delivered, obstruction of flow, and other parameters.
Neonatal vital signs monitor	Measures mean blood pressure and mean heart rate from plastic blood pressure cuff; values are digitally displayed on monitor.
Pulse oximeter	Measures peripheral oxygen saturation and pulse from a light sensor secured to the infant's skin; values are digitally displayed on the monitor; some models have continuous recording of values on strip charts.

*Modified from Crane L: In Irwin S and Tecklin JS, editors: *Cardiopulmonary physical therapy*, St Louis, 1985, Mosby.

The first high-risk profile involves the irritable *hypertonic* infant. These infants classically have a low tolerance level to handling and are frequently in a state of overstimulation from routine nursing care, laboratory procedures, and the presence of respiratory and infusion equipment. They express discomfort when given quick changes in position by the caregivers and when placed in any position for a prolonged time. Predominant extension patterns of posture and movement are associated with this category of infants. Quality of movement may appear tremulous or disorganized with poor midline orientation and limited antigravity movement into flexion as a result of the imbalance of increased proximal extensor tone. Visual tracking and feeding may be difficult because of extension posturing or the presence of distracting, disorganized upper extremity movement. In addition, increased tone with related decreased mobility in oral musculature may complicate feeding behavior. Hypertonic infants frequently demonstrate poor self-quieting abilities and may require consistent intervention by caregivers to tolerate movement and position changes. These temperament characteristics and the signs of neurological impairment discussed earlier place infants at considerable risk for child abuse or neglect as the stress and fatigue levels of parents rise and as coping strategies wear thin during the demanding care required by irritable, hypertonic infants.[112]

Conversely, the lethargic *hypotonic* infant excessively accommodates to the stimulation of the nursery environment and can be difficult to arouse to the awake states even for feeding. The crying state is reached infrequently, even with vigorous stimulation. The cry is characteristically weak, with low volume and short duration, related to hypotonic trunk, intercostal, and neck accessory musculature and decreased respiratory capacity. These infants are exceedingly comfortable in any position, and when held they easily mold themselves to the arms of the caregiver. Depression of normal neonatal movement patterns is common. To compensate for low muscle tone when in the supine position, some preterm infants appear to push into extension against the surface of the mattress in search of stability. Although potentially successful in generating a temporary increase in neck and trunk tone, the extension posturing from stabilizing or "fixing" against a surface in supine lying interferes with midline and antigravity movement of the extremities. Such infants respond dramatically to containment positioning in side-lying and prone. Drowsy behavior limits these infants' spontaneous approach to the environment and decreases their accessibility to selected interaction by caregivers. Feeding behavior is commonly marked by fatigue, difficulty remaining awake, weak sucking, incoordination/inadequate rhythm in the suck-swallow process, and supplementation of caloric intake by gavage (oral or nasogastric tube) feeding. The risk for sensory deprivation and failure to thrive is high for hypotonic infants because they infrequently seek interaction, place few if any demands on caregivers, and remain somnolent.

The third high-risk profile is the disorganized infant with fluctuating tone and movement, who is easily overstimulated with routine handling but remains relatively passive when left alone. Disorganized infants usually respond well to swaddling or to containment when handled. When calm, these infants frequently demonstrate high quality social interaction and efficient feeding with coordinated suck-swallow sequence. When distracted and overstimulated, however, these infants appear hypertonic and irritable. Caregiving for intermittently hypertonic, disorganized, irritable infants can be frustrating for parents unskilled in reading the infant's cues, in implementing consolability and containment strategies, and in pacing during feeding.

While these profiles address the extremes in sensorimotor and interactional behavior, they suggest a need for identifying different tolerance levels of handling neonates with abnormal tone and movement, even though long-term developmental goals may be similar. Few neonates will demonstrate all behaviors described in the high-risk profile, but outpatient surveillance of neonates with worrisome or mildly abnormal motor and interactive behavior is advised to monitor the course of those behaviors and the developing styles of parenting.

Timing. The timing of developmental assessment and treatment for infants with high-risk histories or diagnoses is based on the medical stability of the infant and, in some centers, gestational age. All therapy activities need to be synchronized with the intensive care nursery schedule so that nursing care and medical procedures are not interrupted.

Neonatal therapists should not interrupt infants in a quiet, deep sleep state, but instead wait about 15 minutes until the infant cycles into a light, active sleep or semi-awake state. Higher transcutaneous oxygen saturation has been correlated with quiet rather than with active sleep in newborn infants. Preterm infants reportedly have a higher percentage of active sleep periods in contrast with the higher percentage of quiet sleep observed in full-term infants.[91] Allowing the preterm infant to maintain, rather than interrupting, a deep, quiet sleep is a therapeutic strategy for enhancing physiological stability.

Timing of parent teaching sessions is most effective when readiness to participate in the care of the infant is expressed. Some parents need time and support to work through the acute grief process related to the birth of an imperfect child before participation in developmental activities is accepted. Other parents find the neonatal therapy program to be a way of helping in the care of their child that assists them through the mourning process.

Treatment strategies

This section addresses components of treatment designed to enhance movement, minimize contractures and deformity, promote feeding behaviors appropriate to corrected age, develop social interaction behaviors, and foster attachment to primary caregivers. The areas of developmental intervention presented include management approaches to body positioning, extremity taping, graded sensorimotor intervention, neonatal hydrotherapy, oral-motor/feeding therapy, and parent teaching. In managing an intensive care nursery caseload, the constant physiological monitoring, modifying of techniques to adapt to the constraints of varying amounts of medical equipment, scheduling of intervention to coincide with visits of the parents and peak responsiveness of the infants, and ongoing coordination and reassessment of goals, plans, and follow-up recommendations with the nursery staff create many interesting challenges and demand a high degree of adaptability and creativity from the clinician. Willingness to change a preestablished assessment plan, treatment strategy, or therapy schedule to meet the immediate needs of the infant, parents, or nursery staff is paramount.

Positioning. A diligently administered positioning program can greatly assist infants on mechanical ventilators, under oxyhoods, or in Isolettes to simulate the flexed, midline postures of the normal full-term newborn swaddled in a bassinet. Preterm infants characteristically demonstrate low postural tone with the amount of hypotonia varying with gestational age. Infants born prematurely do not have the neurological maturity or the prolonged positional advantage of the intrauterine environment to assist in the development of flexion. They are instead placed unexpectedly against gravity and presented with a dual challenge of compensating for maturation-related hypotonia and adapting to ventilatory and infusion equipment that frequently reinforces extension of the neck, trunk, and extremities.

The imbalance of excessive extension can occur quickly in preterm infants from repeated efforts to gain postural stability or containment in the nonfluid extrauterine environment by leaning into or "fixing" against a firm surface, usually the mattress. Fixing by the neonate is demonstrated initially as neck hyperextension in supine or side-lying

positions and appears to block further development of mobility and cocontraction in the neck region. As described by Bly[27] and Quinton,[181] the neck hyperextension posturing may herald the development of a host of related abnormal postural and mobility patterns to compensate for inadequate proximal stability. From neck hyperextension, abnormal postural fixing for stability can classically lead to sequential blocking in the shoulder, pelvis, and hip regions. In many preterm neonates, the active postural fixing to compensate for hypotonia contributes to a commonly observed postural profile associated with prematurity and the extension-producing forces of gravity. The components of this high-risk postural profile follow:

1. Hyperextended neck
2. Elevated shoulders with adducted scapulae
3. Decreased midline arm movement (hand-to-mouth)
4. Excessively extended trunk
5. Immobile pelvis (anterior tilt)
6. Infrequent antigravity movement of legs
7. Weight bearing on toes (supported standing)

The use of blanket or cloth diaper rolls or customized foam inserts in a neonatal positioning program can modify the increasing imbalance of extension in preterm or chronically ill infants and can promote movement and postural stability from positions of flexion. Postural principles to incorporate into a positioning program include elongation of neck extensor musculature for chin tucking, trunk flexion, shoulder protraction to encourage engagement of hands at midline, posterior pelvic tilt, and symmetrical flexion of the legs. After the infant is facilitated into a flexed position in the side-lying position, posterior rolls behind the head, trunk, and thighs provide a surface against which the infant can posturally stabilize while a flexed midline position is maintained (Fig. 8-11). An additional anterior roll between

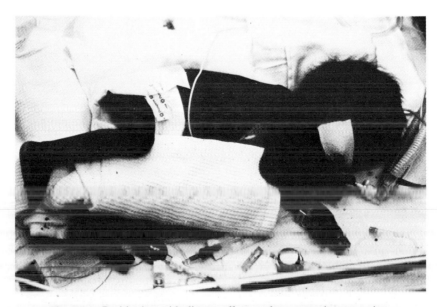

Fig. 8-11. Positioning with diaper rolls to reduce extension posturing.

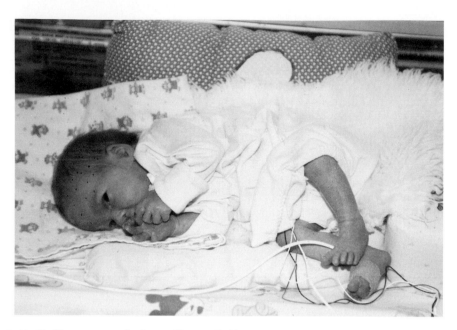

Fig. 8-12. Pacifier promotes flexion and long roll allows anterior and posterior containment of flexed sidelying position.

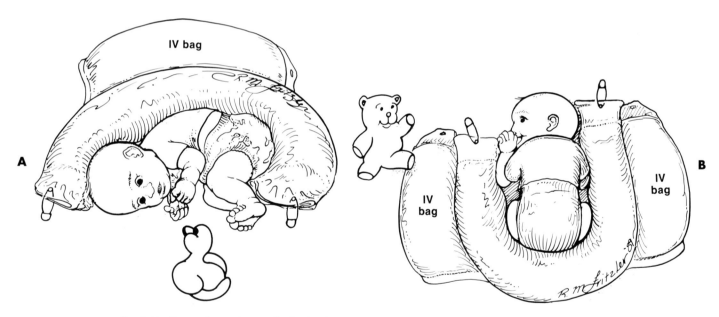

Fig. 8-13. Postural containment in flexion by body stabilization from a long-blanket roll reinforced by a sand or intravenous fluid bag.

the extremities and the use of a pacifier may promote further midline stabilization in flexion (Fig. 8-12). Small neonates can be maintained in a flexed symmetrical position with a long blanket roll pinned to the mattress at each end. Larger neonates may need additional stabilization from a water bag, sand bag, or dextrose IV bag against the blanket roll (Fig. 8-13). Cloth buntings with circumferential body straps and a foot roll (Fig. 8-14) provide positioning support and containment of extremity movement.

Endotracheal tube placement frequently contributes to the neck hyperextension posture in infants who require mechanical ventilation (Fig. 8-15). This iatrogenic component can be avoided by repositioning the endotracheal tube to allow enough mobility for the slightly tucked chin and flexed trunk postures. For neurologically impaired infants with severe pulmonary disease necessitating prolonged ventilatory support, inattention to the alignment of the neck and shoulders can lead to the development of a contracture in the neck

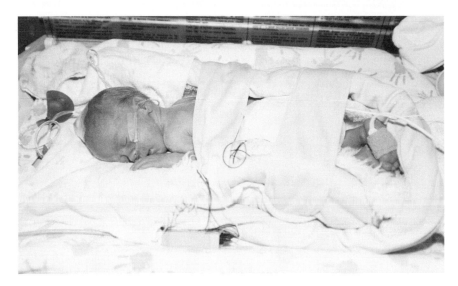

Fig. 8-14. Use of cloth bunting with circumferential straps, interior foot roll, lateral rolls and sheepskin to promote body containment in prone flexion.

extensor muscles (Fig. 8-16) and occlusion of the airway.

Since flexion is enhanced in the prone position by the influence of the tonic labyrinthine reflex, the incorporation of prone positioning is strongly advocated even for infants on ventilators (Fig. 8-17). In fact, infants in the prone position have shown increased oxygenation[136,240] and less crying[38] than in those in the supine position. Placing infants on a sheepskin surface (Fig. 8-14) offers increased tactile input and has been correlated with increased weight gain in VLBW infants compared with a matched group of infants on standard cotton sheets.[204]

Water mattresses are a highly effective adjunct to a nursery positioning program. They provide a soft, intermittently oscillating surface that is not conducive to postural fixing. Other recognized advantages of waterbeds include increased vestibular and proprioceptive stimulation, decreased apnea, reduced head flattening, and improved skin condition.[53,119,135] When the infant is moved from intensive care to intermediate care, transition from a waterbed to a standard mattress is recommended to allow time for adaption to the type of mattress likely to be used at home.

Extremity taping. The presence of perinatal elasticity encourages early management of congenital musculoskeletal deformities in the neonatal period (birth to 28 days of age). A temporary ligamentous laxity is presumed to be present in the neonate because of transplacental transfer of relaxin and estrogen from the mother. In addition to the influence of maternal hormones, the rapid growth of the neonate can foster correction of malalignment if the deforming forces are managed expediently. This peak period of hyperelasticity offers pediatric therapists with advanced orthopedic expertise many opportunities to manage congenital joint deformities.[98]

Intermittent taping of foot deformities (Fig. 8-18) has

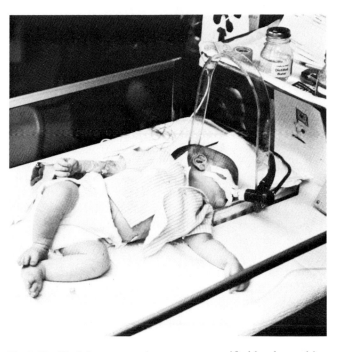

Fig. 8-15. Neck hyperextension posture magnified by the position of the endotracheal tube.

been more adaptable to the nursery setting than either casts or splints and is clearly more effective in gaining mobility than range of motion exercises. Access to the heel for drawing blood, inspection of skin and vascular status, and placement of intravenous lines can be accomplished with the tape in place or by temporary removal of the tape as needed. Therapists without a sound knowledge of arthrokinematic principles and techniques should not attempt the taping procedure, because it involves articulation of the joint(s) into

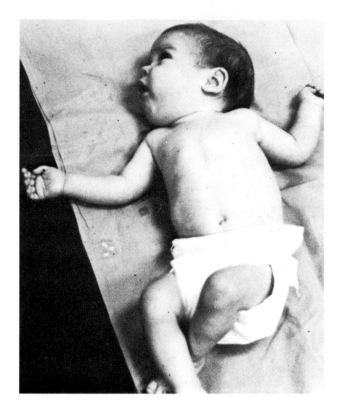

Fig. 8-16. Clinical presentation of contracture in neck extensor muscles related to hyperextension posture during prolonged mechanical ventilation.

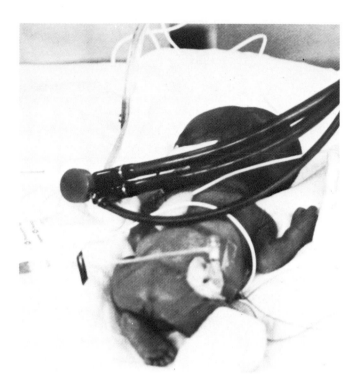

Fig. 8-17. Flexion posture enhanced in the prone position by the influence of the tonic labyrinthine reflex.

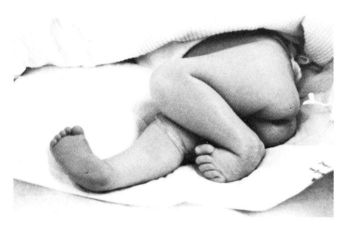

Fig. 8-18. Infant with lumbar meningomyelocoele demonstrating marked varus foot deformities before taping.

a corrected position before taping. Other components of the taping process include application of an external skin protection solution under the tape, application of an adhesive removal solution when removing the tape, observance of skin condition and vascular tolerance, development of a taping schedule beginning with 1-hour and increasing by 1-hour intervals as tolerated, and clinical teaching with selected neonatal nurses for continuation of the taping if needed on night shifts and weekends. Infants with congenital foot deformities required shorter periods of casting in the outpatient period after taping of the extremity (Fig. 8-19) is implemented during the inpatient phase. In 12 years of experience by the author (JKS), using silk or knitted tape to reduce deformity in neonates, neither skin nor vascular complications have occurred, even in infants with absent lower extremity sensation resulting from meningomyelocele.

The availability of thin self-adherent foam or cotton material now allows taping on a bandage layer, rather than on the infant's skin (Fig. 8-20). Although this method creates a definite advantage in skin protection, it may cover the calcaneal region for blood drawing and compromise alignment if the bandage layer loosens after the tape is applied.

Infants with wrist drop from radial nerve compression related to intravenous line infiltration also benefit from the use of taping (Fig. 8-21). The wrist is supported in a

functional position of slight extension. As muscle function returns, the taping is used intermittently to reduce fatigue and overstretching of the emerging, but still weak, wrist extensor musculature.

Sensorimotor intervention. The use of the sensory modalities of tactile, vestibular, proprioceptive, visual, and auditory stimuli to facilitate infant development has been reported* and reviewed[81,208] by many authors. Regardless of

---

* References 54, 118, 123, 150, 183, 197, 241, and 242.

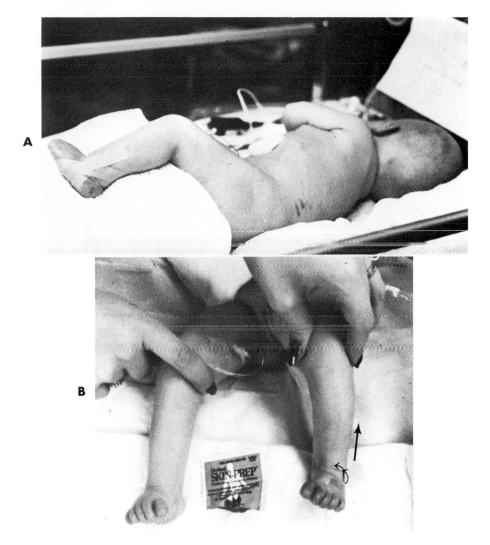

Fig. 8-19. Significant correction in alignment of varus foot deformities in neonate with a lumbar meningomyelocoele. A, Lateral stirrup with open heel taping procedure. B, Moderate correction.

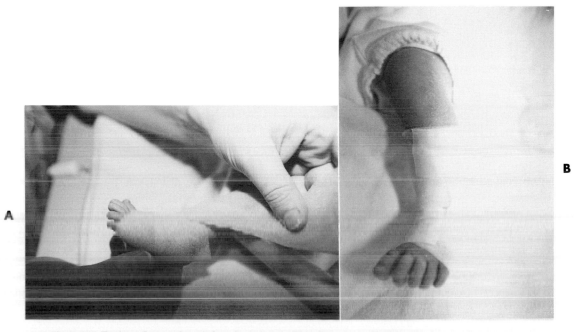

Fig. 8-20. Taping of varus foot deformity using A, Thin foam layer. B, Silk tape in lateral stirrup over foam layer.

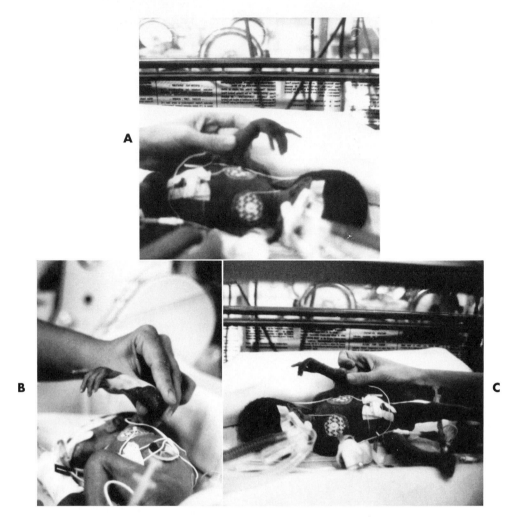

Fig. 8-21. Management of wrist drop in medically fragile neonate. **A,** Wrist drop before taping. **B,** Taping procedure. **C,** One week after taping.

the sensory modalities or neurophysiological treatment approaches selected for neonatal therapy, attention to sensory overload and related physiological consequences should guide the type, intensity, duration, and frequency of intervention.

Primary aims of sensorimotor intervention are to assist the newborn to achieve maximum interaction with parents and caregivers and to facilitate the experience of normal postural and movement patterns. For lethargic, hypotonic infants, intervention may focus on arousal to the alert states and facilitation of cocontraction in the hypotonic proximal (neck, trunk) musculature. Conversely, movement therapy for irritable, hyperexcitable, hypertonic infants may be directed toward calming the infant to the quiet, alert state and inhibiting proximal hypertonus. Attainment of the quiet, alert behavioral state and temporary normalization of postural tone enhance opportunities for visual and auditory interaction and for normal movement experiences. These normal, early movement experiences include hand-to-mouth movement, shoulder protraction/retraction, anterior/posterior pel-

vic tilt, free movement of the extremities against gravity, and momentary holding of the head and midline.[48,63]

Preparation of the neonate for the development of righting reactions may include early-movement experiences in weight shifting and facilitation of postural alignment in the side-lying position for trunk elongation on the weight-bearing side and lateral trunk flexion on the unweighted side.[27]

Behavioral state and movement abnormalities can be clinically influenced by swaddling and graded vestibular stimulation. Swaddling the infant in a blanket with flexed, midline extremity position appears to promote flexor tone, increase hand-to-mouth awareness, and inhibit jittery or disorganized movement. Slow, rhythmical vestibular stimulation (lateral or vertical rocking of the swaddled infant in the face-to-face position with caregiver) usually elicits a calming response in irritable infants. Slightly quicker, more abrupt rocking movement without swaddling often generates an alerting response in drowsy infants. When used by parents during visits to the nursery, these techniques help to elicit quiet, alert behavior and maximal infant-parent interaction. Application of neonatal therapy techniques must be contingent on both the infant's readiness for interaction and need for a recovery break in interaction because of sensory overload.

Incorporation of sensorimotor activities into routine nursing care in the neonatal intensive care unit greatly increases developmental opportunities for the neonate during prolonged hospitalization.[241] While feeding the infant in an Isolette, the nurse may facilitate head lifting and momentary maintenance of the head in midline during the "burping process" in supported sitting (Fig. 8-22). Techniques for inhibiting of trunk and lower extremity hypertonus may be added during diaper changes. Visual and auditory stimulation may be integrated into nearly all parts of child care (Fig. 8-23), or they may be specifically reinforced as appropriate (i.e., visual stimulation: human face, mobile, brightly colored toy, a picture with geometrical pattern; auditory stimulation: human voice, rattle, music box, radio). Easily overstimulated preterm infants may not tolerate multimodal sensory stimulation, but may instead respond to a single sensory stimulus.[25]

Implementation of a positioning program, oral-motor therapy, and reinforcement of developmental activities with parents can all be managed expertly by the neonatal nursing staff when ongoing clinical teaching and intermittent supervision by a pediatric therapist occurs.

A semiinverted supine flexion position (Fig. 8-24) with preterm neonates should be used with caution to facilitate elongation of neck extensor muscles and decrease the neck hyperextension posture. This position may compromise breathing from positional compression of the chest and from potential airway occlusion associated with maximal flexion of the neck. The use of a pulse oximeter during therapeutic handling activities is recommended for objective measurement of physiological tolerance. Although the peripheral oxygen saturation values from monitors may be intermittently unreliable because of motion artifacts from either the infant's spontaneous movement or the therapist's handling of the infant, reliable readings of oxygen saturation may be taken approximately 1 minute after the infant's body is not moved.

Neonatal hydrotherapy. Modified for use in an intensive care nursery setting, the traditional physical therapy modality of hydrotherapy has been implemented as an adjunct to individual developmental intervention for high-risk neonates. Neonatal hydrotherapy was conceptualized in 1980 at Madigan Army Medical Center in Tacoma, Washington.[224]

Indications for referral of medically stable infants to the hydrotherapy component of the developmental intervention program include the following: (1) muscle tone abnormalities (hypertonus or hypotonus) affecting the quality and quantity of spontaneous movement and contributing to the imbalance of extension in posture and movement (Fig. 8-25);

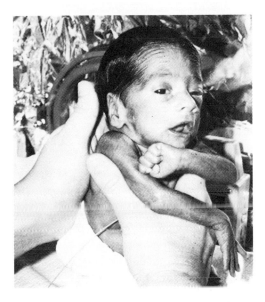

Fig. 8-22. Facilitation of head lifting by a neonatal nurse while "burping" the infant after feeding.

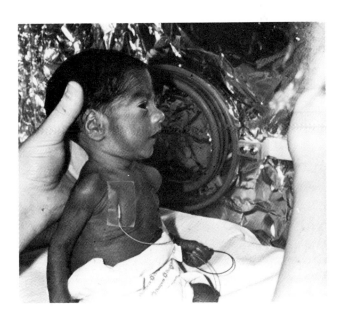

Fig. 8-23. Facilitation of visual following by a neonatal nurse during a change of the infant's position in the isolette.

(2) limitation of motion in the extremities related to muscular or connective tissue factors; and (3) behavioral state abnormalities of marked irritability during graded neuromotor handling or, conversely, excessive drowsiness during "handling" that prevents social interaction with caregivers and contributes to depression of normal movement patterns and tone.

Infants are considered medically stable for aquatic intervention when ventilatory equipment and intravenous lines are discontinued and when resolution of temperature

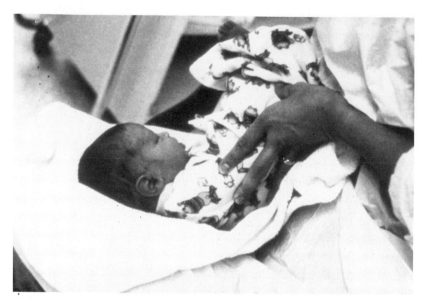

Fig. 8-24. Potential respiratory compromise to the infant from neck extensor muscle elongation in excessively flexed position while in supine position.

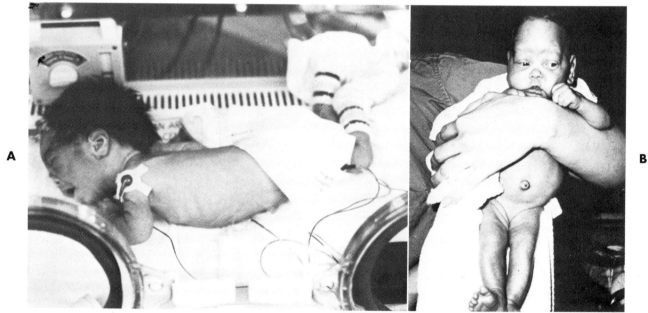

Fig. 8-25. Neonates demonstrating opisthotonic trunk posture, **A,** and marked lower extremity hypertonus, **B,** before hydrotherapy.

instability and apnea/bradycardia are demonstrated. A standard plastic bassinet is used with preparation of the water temperature at 37.2° to 38.3° C (99° to 101° F). Use of an overhead radiant heater decreases temperature loss in the undressed infant, thereby maximizing thermoregulation.

After receiving medical clearance and individualized criteria for the maximum acceptable limits of heart rate,

blood pressure, and color changes during hydrotherapy from the neonatal staff, the baseline heart rate and blood pressure values are recorded and pretreatment posture and behavioral states are observed. The undressed infant is then moved into a semiflexed, supine position, with the blood pressure cuff on one thigh, before being lifted into the water. After a short period for behavioral adaptation to the fluid environment, a second caregiver (i.e., nurse or parent) is recruited to stabilize the infant's head and shoulder girdle region while the pediatric therapist provides support at the pelvis.

The neuromuscular techniques consistent with neurodevelopmental treatment[29-31,128,133] involve midline positioning of the head, proximal hand placement of the therapist and second caregiver, and slow, graded tone-normalizing movement (incorporating flexion and rotation) of the trunk, followed by progression distally to the pelvic girdle region and finally to the shoulder girdle and neck regions. After gentle elongation of cervical and trunk extensor musculature and facilitated dissociated movement at shoulder or pelvic girdle, most infants will demonstrate active extremity movement in the water. The improved range and smoothness of spontaneous extremity movement is facilitated by the buoyancy and resistive properties of the water. Movement experiences in the supine, side-lying, and prone positions are offered as tolerated. If the movement therapy becomes too stressful, with resultant agitation or crying by the infant, the movement is immediately stopped, and the infant is either consoled or, if unconsolable, removed from the water and swaddled. Compromise in hemodynamic stability (increased heart rate, increased blood pressure, decreased respiratory rate) and a decrease in arterial oxygen tension during crying have been well documented in newborn infants recovering from respiratory distress syndrome.[65] Careful monitoring of behavioral tolerance to hydrotherapy (with avoidance of crying) is considered critical for reducing physiological risk with hydrotherapy.

Multiple therapeutic benefits are obtained from selective use of 10- to 15-minute aquatic intervention sessions. Improvement of abnormal muscle tone and facilitation of semiflexed posture are obtained with less time and effort by the therapist and with higher behavioral tolerance by the infant than when a similar movement therapy approach is used without the medium of water (Fig. 8-26). Muscle tone changes are frequently maintained for 2 to 3 hours when aquatic intervention is followed by flexed, midline body positioning in the side-lying position on a water mattress. Enhancement of visual and auditory orientation responses (i.e., visual fixing and tracking, auditory alerting, and localization to human voices), prolonged high-quality alertness, and longer periods of social interaction with caregivers are demonstrated during and after hydrotherapy sessions. Significant improvement in feeding behavior can occur when hydrotherapy is scheduled for 1 hour before feeding to prepare the infant for complete arousal and for flexed, midline postural changes conducive to optimal feeding. If the potential side effects of fatigue and temperature loss during hydrotherapy are not carefully monitored, exhaustion of the infant and a deterioration in feeding abilities may result with a requirement for gavage feeding. Mild flexion contractures of knees and elbows and dynamic hip adduction contractures (Fig. 8-27) can be safely and quickly eliminated by gentle muscle/joint mobilization and elonga-

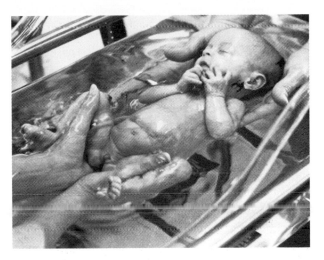

Fig. 8-26. Facilitation of flexed posture and hand-to-mouth movement with calm, behavioral response in infant previously irritable with handling.

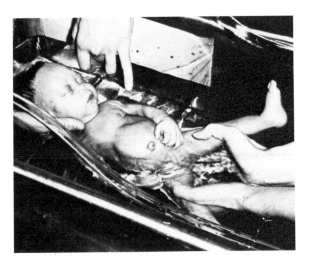

Fig. 8-27. Aquatic intervention for contracture control and inhibition of hypertonus.

tion techniques in warm water as opposed to the traditional range-of-motion and stretching techniques frequently prescribed for adult orthopedic clients.

Therapeutic bathing techniques are incorporated into the parent teaching program to foster early parent participation in child care and in specific developmental activities during the inpatient period to prepare for carry-over into the home environment at hospital discharge. This early pleasurable involvement of parent and child in hydrotherapy and bathing may provide a strong base for future participation in aquatics as a family leisure sports activity and, if needed, as an adjunct to an outpatient developmental therapy program.

When oriented to treatment goals and trained in specific hydrotherapy techniques for individual infants, the nursing staff can effectively carry on the hydrotherapy program established by the pediatric therapist. This release of the pediatric therapist's role to the neonatal nurse allows additional use of hydrotherapy on evening and night shifts and continued teaching and supervision of parents during evening and weekend visits (Fig. 8-28).

An additional advantage of neonatal hydrotherapy is cost effectiveness. The use of equipment readily available in the newborn nursery and the short time period (10 to 15 minutes) required for therapeutic bathing in the nursing care plan and in the parent participation program in the nursery combine to make aquatic intervention cost effective for equipment, time management, and personnel resources.

Although many clinical benefits may be obtained by judicious use of hydrotherapy in the newborn nursery, pilot study data obtained on physiological changes in high-risk infants during hydrotherapy clearly indicate a physiological risk.[224] This risk (increased blood pressure and heart rate) must be carefully evaluated relative to each infant's general medical stability and individual heart rate and blood pressure patterns before hydrotherapy can be included safely in an inpatient neonatal therapy program. In collaboration with the neonatology and nursing staff, preestablished criteria for general medical stability and the maximal limits during hydrotherapy for blood pressure, heart rate, and acceptable color changes are essential requirements for risk management. Physiological monitoring of mean blood pressure and heart rate by a neonatal vital signs monitor (i.e., DYNAMAPP Model 847 by Critikon, Inc., Tampa, Florida) during aquatic intervention is recommended. The blood pressure cuff is a pneumatically driven device that is not electronically connected to the infant and can be safely immersed in water. Since hypothermia is a recognized risk with hydrotherapy, body temperature should be measured routinely before and after the hydrotherapy session using a

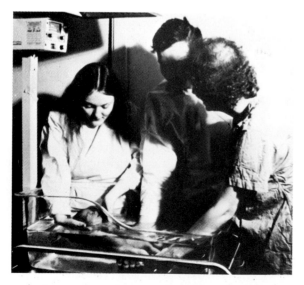

Fig. 8-28. Parents being trained in hydrotherapy techniques for later therapeutic bathing at home.

thermometer with a digital display. A risk-benefit analysis of the potential physiological risk to each infant and the expected therapeutic benefits is strongly advised before hydrotherapy techniques are incorporated into a neonatal therapy program.

Oral-motor therapy. Feeding difficulties are common among infants with neurological immaturity, abnormal muscle tone, depressed oral reflexes, or prolonged use of an endotracheal tube for mechanical ventilation. Because behavioral state affects the quality of feeding behavior, feeding performance may be improved significantly by specific arousal or calming procedures before feeding. Other variables influencing feeding may include decreased tongue mobility, presence of tongue thrusting, decreased lip seal on nipple, nasal regurgitation, tactile hypersensitivity in the mouth, irregular respiratory patterns, insufficient proximal stability from hypotonic neck and trunk musculature, or hypertonic posturing of the neck and trunk in extension.[148,149]

Two instruments for assessing oral-motor and feeding behaviors in the nursery are the Neonatal Oral-Motor Assessment Scale (NOMAS)[35] and the Nursing Child Assessment Feeding (NCAF) Scale.[15] The NOMAS is used to evaluate the following oral-motor components during sucking: rate, rhythmicity, jaw excursion, tongue configuration, and tongue movement (timing, direction, and range). Tongue and jaw components are analyzed during nutritive and nonnutritive sucking activity. Cut-off scores were derived from a pilot study[35] with the instrument: a combined score of 43 to 47 indicated "some oral-motor disorganization"; a score of 42 or less indicated oral-motor dysfunction. Reliability and validity studies are not available on this instrument.

The NCAF Scale is used to analyze parent-infant feeding interaction. It provides a method for evaluating the responsiveness of parents to infant cues, signs of distress, and social interaction opportunities during the feeding process. In concurrent validity studies, NCAF scores were positively correlated with the Home Observation for Measurement of the Environment Inventory at 8 months (r = .72) and at 12 months (r = .79).[15]

Management strategies during feeding may include semiflexed positioning with the chin slightly tucked and with elevated shoulder posture inhibited by elongation of the upper trapezius muscles through use of downward traction on the anterolateral shoulder region bilaterally (Fig. 8-29). Techniques of tactile facilitation of the facial muscles, tactile stimulation of specific intraoral structures, use of a pacifier during gavage feedings, manual stabilization of the jaw and thickening of formula are frequent components of oral-motor therapy programs.[93,147-149,248]

For some infants, oral intake by bottle may be improved by using a "premie nipple," which contains a larger hole and is more easily compressed than standard newborn nipples. Wolf and Glass[248] advise evaluating the flow rate of liquid

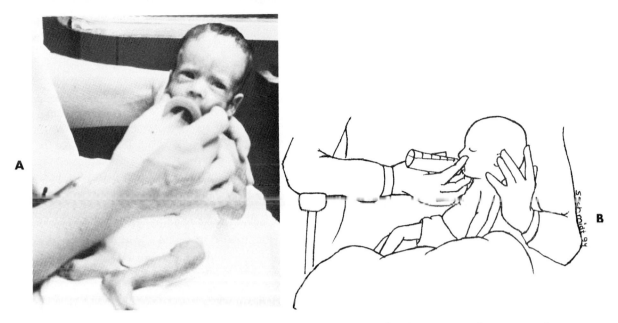

Fig. 8-29. A semiflexed feeding position with **A,** Elongation of neck extensor and upper trapezius muscles and occasional facilitation of buccinator muscles. **B,** Firm pressure of therapist's third finger applied upward toward the mandible for jaw control.

from various types of nipples and analyzing the effect of nipple size, shape, and consistency on an infant's sucking proficiency. Feeding infants in the side-lying position may improve tongue position, particularly if marked tongue retraction is present (Fig. 8-30).

The increasing popularity of breast-feeding has encouraged the development of breast-feeding aids (e.g., "Lact-Aid," Division of J.J. Avery, Inc., Denver). These devices allow supplementation of oral intake during breast-feeding through a small tube that goes to the mouth from a presterilized bag containing infant formula. The feeding performance of infants with severe cleft palate deformities is frequently improved by a dental obturator. This custom-fabricated prosthesis is inserted before feeding to cover the defect in the palate. The timing of movement therapy or neonatal hydrotherapy 1 hour before feeding may significantly improve performance by preparation of total body muscle tone, facilitation of oral musculature, and enhancement of alertness.

Expected outcomes of oral-motor treatment supported by clinical research include: (1) increased number of nutritive sucks after perioral stimulation,[126] (2) increased volume of fluid ingested during nipple feedings,[231] (3) decreased number of gavage feedings and earlier bottle feeding,[120] (4) accelerated weight gain,[139] and (5) earlier hospital discharge.[139] Measel[139] found that use of a pacifier during tube feedings allowed a discharge 4 days earlier in experimental subjects (n = 29) compared with controls (n = 30). With the cost of NICU care at approximately $1300 per day, a discharge 4 days earlier for infants with alterations in feeding may represent a cost saving of $6200 per infant.

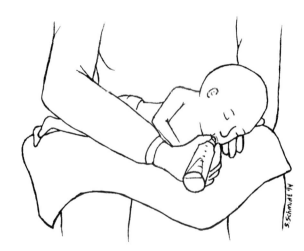

Fig. 8-30. Feeding in sidelying position for infants with marked tongue retraction.

Monitoring the infant's physiological tolerance to oral-motor evaluation and intervention is crucial. Heart rate values may be monitored from the cardiorespirograph or the DYNAMAPP neonatal vital signs monitor. Tissue oxygen saturation is routinely followed from a pulse oximeter. Color changes and behavioral signs of stress should also be observed. Regurgitation with aspiration of milk or formula into the lungs may occur during oral-motor assessment or feeding therapy; complications of pneumonia, cardiopulmonary arrest, and associated asphyxia may also develop after aspiration. Significant physiological risk to the infant and medicolegal risk to the therapist are inherent in oral-motor treatment of medically fragile neonates.

Parent-infant interaction and perceived competency in parenting may be negatively affected by feeding experiences in the NICU. Success during feeding activities has been identified as an important variable in developing a positive parent-infant relationship.[32] Parents of infants with feeding problems describe higher stress than parents of infants who "eat well."[197] Because alteration in feeding caused by oral-motor dysfunction has been reported as an early functional deficit in infants at high risk for later neuromotor sequelae,[203] early support to parents coping with a challenging feeding situation sets the stage for attitudes about and compliance with later developmental follow-up.

Parent support

Grief process. Strong, continuous support is essential to help parents through perhaps the most frightening crisis in their adult lives—the potential death or disability of their infant.[111,125] It is not uncommon for parents to initially establish emotional and physical distance from the infant as they cope with the knowledge that the infant may die. During this time of anticipatory grief, peer-group support by other parents of prematurely born children can be of immeasurable value. Actively listening to the parents' feelings and concerns and providing support, without judgment, through their episodes of detachment and anger are critical. Although long-range plans include parent participation in all aspects of the developmental program, the timing and amount of initial teaching must be individualized to the levels of stress and acute grief present.

When an infant dies, the neonatal therapist begins the important work of closure. This work includes attending memorial or funeral services to support the family and initiating a personal closure process. Neonatal therapists are advised to find a senior nurse mentor to guide them through the closure process of identifying and dealing with frustrations and other feelings regarding the infant and family. Finding meaning and value to the *process* of caregiving rather than solely to functional *outcomes* is an important task in the work of closure and in preventing professional burnout.

Parent teaching. Components of the parent teaching process may include: (1) discussion of the program goals, purposes, and services in the NICU; (2) orientation to the follow-up plan after discharge; (3) guidelines for recognizing and understanding the infant's temperament, stress cues, and ability to interact with the environment; and (4) specific instructions on selected developmental activities and handling techniques. When used in conjunction with verbal instructions and demonstrations, a packet of written guidelines and pictures that are individualized to the infant's needs can improve parents' overall skills and understanding of the program. General handling guidelines for parents of preterm infants are available for purchase (Appendix B).

Occasionally, when geographical distance prevents participation by parents in the inpatient phase of the developmental program, the developmental guidelines may be mailed and later reviewed during outpatient follow-up. During times of separation, telephone contact with parents is imperative to foster attachment to the infant, to explain the purpose and content of the home developmental intervention program, and to discuss the critical need for follow-up. Parents need this ongoing dialogue to make the infant seem real to them and to allow ventilation of their fears and concerns during the separation.

The teaching strategies are most effective when adapted to the learning style of the parents. This may involve more demonstrations and an increased opportunity for supervised practice for some parents, particularly those with reading difficulties that limit use of a written instructional packet.

In the inpatient period, the quality of infant-parent attachment and the comfort level and proficiency of participation in routine care and developmental therapy set the stage for later parenting styles. Helping parents find and appreciate a positive aspect of the newborn infant's neuromotor or other developmental behavior gives them a spark of hope from which emotional energy can be generated to help them through the marathon of the NICU experience. Empowering parents early in their parenting experience with the infant is crucial. *In the life of the child, the effects of parent empowerment will last far longer than neonatal movement therapy and positioning.*

CLINICAL MANAGEMENT: OUTPATIENT FOLLOW-UP PERIOD
General purposes of follow-up period

Regular follow-up of the at-risk neonate after discharge from the NICU is a critical component of the total management of high-risk infants. The purpose of this follow-up is threefold:

1. To monitor and manage ongoing medical problems, such as respiratory complications and feeding difficulties
2. To provide support and instruction to parents in the care and nurturance of at-risk infants
3. To assess the neurodevelopmental progress of infants so that abnormalities may be identified and treated

Issues of assessment, intervention, and developmental profiles of the high-risk infant following discharge from the NICU are discussed in this section.

Medical management. The routine medical care of LBW infants after discharge may be provided by a pediatrician, family practitioner, or health clinic. The infant with medical or sensorimotor complications is often cared for later by a number of additional medical specialists, including neurologists, ophthalmologists, cardiac or pulmonary specialists, nutritionists and gastrointestinal specialists, public health nurses, as well as physical and occupational therapists and infant educators. Communication among these specialists may be minimal, particularly when they are located at different sites. The parent or caregiver may be confronted with conflicting opinions, demands, and expectations of the family and their infant. The follow-up clinic can play a valuable role in this situation by designating one professional as case manager to assist the parents in coordinating services, to verify that all needs of the infant are being met, to set realistic and compatible goals, and to help set priorities.

Family support. The stress that a vulnerable, premature or at-risk infant brings to a family is well documented. Anxiety, grief, anger, and depression are common reactions of parents of premature infants.[106,125] The primary caregivers of high-risk infants are required to become knowledgeable about complex medical terminology and equipment. At discharge they often become responsible for the administration of complicated feeding procedures requiring measurement and recording of intake and output, multiple medications of varying dosages and protocol, and cardiopulmonary procedures and equipment. Frequently, families must cope with a tremendous financial obligation and manage different billing agencies and funding sources.

The LBW infant is often irritable, hypersensitive to stimulation, less responsive to the affective interactions of his parents, and more irregular in sleeping and feeding schedules than the full-term infant.[8,63] The demands that such an infant places on the parents can have a long-term negative impact on the parent-infant relationship and the infant's social and affective development.[14,18,61] Regular follow-up by trained professionals who are knowledgeable about the developmental patterns and specific needs of the LBW infant is essential.

Assessment of neurodevelopmental status. Because LBW infants are at increased risk for neurodevelopmental disorders, close follow-up is necessary during the first 6 to 8 years of life. The prevalence of cerebral palsy is significantly greater in LBW infants than in full-term infants, and the frequency of handicap increases with decreasing birthweight levels (Table 8-7).[24,78,153,164,192] Cerebral palsy is one of several major neurological conditions that are observed sequelae of prematurity; others include mental retardation, hydrocephalus, sensorineural hearing loss, visual impairment, and seizure disorder. When examined as a group, these major handicapping conditions occur with increased prevalence in LBW infants, and again the frequency increases in the LBW groups[78,192] (Table 8-8).

The frequency of so-called minor neurodevelopmental and neurobehavioral abnormalities, observed in long-term follow-up of LBW infants, is also increased.* Problems in visuomotor skills, language comprehension, reading and math skills, static balance, coordination, as well as muscle

Table 8-7. Incidence of cerebral palsy relative to birthweight[24,78,153,164,192]	
Infant birth weight (g)	Rate of cerebral palsy (per 1000 live births)
All birth weights	2.2-2.3
>2500	1.1-1.3
1501-2500	8.5
<1500	60-120
<1000	120-150

Table 8.8. Incidence of major neurodevelopmental handicaps in low-birthweight infants[78,192]	
Infant birthweight (g)	Neurodevelopmental handicap
1500-2500	10%
1000-1500	20-25%
<1000	20-25%

tone abnormalities and behavior disorders, such as attention deficits and impulsivity, occur at greater frequency among children born prematurely. Outcome studies indicate that by school-age approximately one-half of LBW infants will have educational and learning deficits as compared with a reported rate of 24% in the general population.[42,74,154]

Overall, it is estimated that approximately 10% to 30% of LBW infants will have major neurological handicaps, and up to 40% will have "minor" neurological handicaps. A primary objective of developmental follow-up of at-risk infants is the early identification of neurodevelopmental abnormalities so that therapeutic intervention can be initiated. LBW infants who participate in a follow-up clinic have demonstrated advanced performance on cognitive measures and receive more intervention services relative to nonmonitored infants.[210]

The benefits of early therapy have not been substantiated consistently by scientific research, although results of some studies indicate positive change.* However, early recognition of the presence of a developmental disorder is important for directing resources toward family support and/or school management. A developmentally delayed infant may evoke negative maternal responses of anxiety, frustration, and withdrawal even before a medical diagnosis is made.[143] Early recognition by professionals of a developmental problem enables them to assist the parents during this time of adjustment and to help maintain positive, affectionate interaction. A "minor" neurodevelopmental abnormality is not at all minor in the life of that child or his family.

High-risk infant follow-up model

The neurodevelopmental progress of the at-risk infant requires careful monitoring with systematic evaluation at intervals in the first year of life. An organizational model of a high-risk infant follow-up clinic is shown in Fig. 8-31. It is based on the format of the Neonatal Intensive Care Unit (NICU) Follow-up Clinic of the Child Development and Mental Retardation Center established at the University of Washington in Seattle, Washington.

Before discharge from the NICU, very-high-risk infants (infants with seizures, cystic PVL, grade IV bleeding, and obvious neurological abnormalities) are distinguished from infants at relatively low risk. The *high-risk infant* receives therapeutic intervention as described in the previous neonatal section. The infant who is not showing indications of abnormality is closely monitored, but usually without specific intervention. Instead, the role of the therapist with the lower risk infant is primarily to provide guidance to the nurses and parents regarding positioning and developmental intervention.

At discharge, the high-risk or abnormal infant is referred to an ongoing therapy program in the community. It is recommended that the therapy services be provided in the home to minimize the stress to the infant and the family,

although this objective cannot always be accommodated. Infants who do not require therapy are referred to the follow-up clinic for developmental follow-up and to their community pediatrician for medical management.

Age correction. Premature infants are scheduled for evaluation in the follow-up clinic according to their *corrected age* (age adjusted for weeks of prematurity). The issue of whether to adjust according to the gestational age of the infant when assessing psychomotor development is an ongoing question.[137,142,162,207] In several studies the authors have demonstrated that if uncorrected ages are used, the *normal* premature infant will have a lower developmental quotient and delayed acquisition of milestones relative to full-term peers.[142,162] If ages are adjusted for prematurity, the performance of the premature infants is comparable to that of full-term infants at 1 year. In assessment done before 1 year of age, however, adjustment for prematurity tends to result in overcorrection, particularly in infants less than 33 weeks of gestation at birth. Consequently, abnormal infants have had developmental quotients in the normal range of standard tests when age was adjusted for prematurity.

In a follow-up program, the decision of whether to correct for prematurity depends on the following factors: (1) testing instruments used, with attention to the competencies evalu-

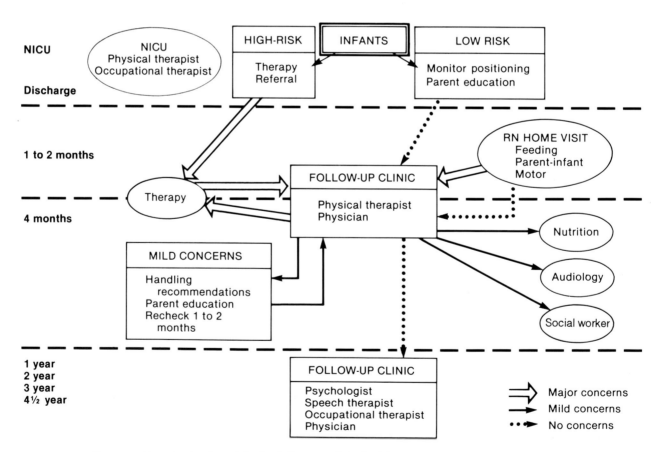

Fig. 8-31. Organizational model of a follow-up clinic for high-risk infants. Infants are evaluated through the interdisciplinary clinic from the time of discharge from the NICU. When problems are identified referral is made to appropriate specialist.

ated by the tool and the number of premature infants in the normative sample and (2) the purpose of the assessment. If the objective is to detect infants who may be neurologically impaired, it is recommended that using uncorrected ages provides a more sensitive index of abnormality. If the purpose of the assessment is to document developmental progress of the at-risk infant relative to a normal population, using corrected age appears to be the more appropriate approach.

In the High-Risk Infant Clinic at the University of Washington, all premature infants are evaluated to age 8 years using the child's corrected age. Developmental quotients in the normal range, however, do not preclude concerns or referral to intervention services when neuromotor or behavioral abnormality is observed.

Follow-up clinic evaluation schedule. The schedule of routine appointments for all infants in the follow-up clinic is shown in Table 8-9. Although the first *routine* appointment is at 4 months (corrected age), infants may be seen earlier at the recommendation of the hospital discharge team, physical therapist, community pediatrician, public health nurse, or parent. The examinations typically performed by each specialist are listed in Table 8-9.

Home visit. At 4 to 6 weeks after discharge from the hospital, a pediatric nurse practitioner makes a home visit when geographically and logistically possible. In addition to providing support and assistance to the family in home management, the nurse practitioner evaluates the infant's feeding and nutritional status, the parent-infant interaction, the infant's social and cognitive development, and the infant's motor development. If there are concerns regarding neuromotor status, the infant is referred to the follow-up clinic for an early comprehensive assessment by the physical therapist.

Four-month evaluation. Four months of age has been determined to be an optimal time for the initial follow-up evaluation for the following reasons:

1. Examinations of older infants are better predictors than neonatal examinations. The neonatal period and the first 2 to 3 months of life are characterized by variability in infant behavior as well as instability of tone, reflex activity, and functional skills.[3] Predictive studies that have examined the results of sequential examinations have demonstrated that neonatal examinations are less accurate in their ability to predict neurodevelopmental outcome than examinations performed on older infants.[76,179,181]

2. Four months is a critical time in the developmental maturation of infants. In the normal infant, muscle tone tends to be stable,[182] reflexes have minimal influence, balance reactions are emerging, and infants develop functional skills with an orientation to the midline (Fig. 8-32). At this time, when medical

Table 8-9. High-risk infant clinic: scheduled evaluations

Corrected age of child	Examiners*	Standard tests administered
4 months	Physical therapist	Movement Assessment of Infants
		Bayley Scales of Infant Development (BSID)
	Pediatrician*	
1 year	Pediatrician	Denver Developmental Screening Test (DDST)
		Neurological examination
	Psychologist	BSID
	Audiologist	
	Physical therapist*	
2 years	Pediatrician	Neurological examination
		DDST
	Psychologist	BSID
	Physical therapist*	
3 years	Pediatrician	DDST
		Neurological examination
	Psychologist	Stanford-Binet
		Peabody Picture Vocabulary Test
	Physical therapist*	
	Speech/Audiologist*	
4½ years	Pediatrician	DDST
		Neurological examination
	Psychologist	Wechsler Preschool and Primary Scale of Intelligence (WPPSI)
	Occupational therapist	Peabody Developmental Motor Scales
		Miller Assessment of Pre-School
	Physical therapist*	
	Speech/Audiologist*	
6 years	Pediatrician	DDST
		Neurological examination
8 years	Psychologist	Wechsler Intelligence Scale for Children—Revised (WISC-R) or WPPSI
		Peabody Individual Achievement Test (PIAT)
	Physical therapist*	
	Speech/Audiologist*	

*Consultant examiner.

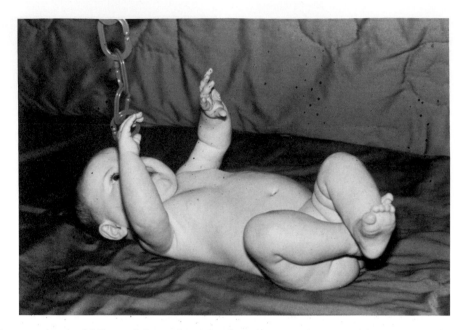

Fig. 8-32. A normal full-term infant at 4 months of age demonstrating symmetrical alignment of trunk and extremities, functional movement against gravity, and no influence of the tonic labyrinthine reflex.

concerns about the high-risk infant are resolving, parents often begin to form questions about developmental expectations. Although for most infants it is not possible to make definitive statements about long-term prognosis at 4 months of age, a systematic evaluation at this age provides an important baseline for comparative assessment of developmental progress in subsequent evaluations.

3. When the initial follow-up evaluations occur at later ages, such as 6 or 9 months, the potential impact of the follow-up clinic in family support is diminished. Many adjustment crises and management problems occur before this time. Although neuromotor abnormality is usually more obvious and therefore more readily detected at later examinations,[221] equivocal findings are still common.[9,188] By delaying the time of assessment until the time when neuromotor abnormalities are conclusive, intervention for the infant and the family is also delayed.

• • •

At the 4-month evaluation the therapist assumes the role of case manager. Because infants at this age express their capabilities and consequently their neurological integrity through their movements, the therapist, as a specialist in movement, is the most highly skilled professional in observing and interpreting the motor activity of the infant. By using both the Movement Assessment of Infants (Appendix C) and the Bayley Scales of Infant Assessment, the therapist can examine the infant's neuromotor and developmental status. The developmental pediatrician pro-

vides medical consultation at the request of the therapist when health, neurological, or developmental concerns are noted during the examination. The infant is referred to a specialist for further investigation if problems are noted in nutrition, vision, hearing, or musculoskeletal alignment. Because of the increasing number of infants born to single mothers, low-income families, and women who used drugs and alcohol during their pregnancy, a social worker has become an important member of the follow-up clinic team. This professional evaluates the family's home and living status, identifies indicators of environmental risk, and assists the caregiver in accessing necessary financial and personal resources.

If the infant demonstrates normal neuromotor and developmental progress at the 4-month evaluation, the next scheduled evaluation is at 1 year (corrected age). The parents or caregivers are informed of their infant's level of function, given recommendations according to their child's performance, and advised regarding appropriate expectations for their child in the next months. They are encouraged to call the therapist if questions arise in the interim period. If the therapist notes an area of minor concern, a telephone interview can be made with appropriate questions to the parents.

If the infant demonstrates definite abnormality or significant delay or shows strong indications of neurological impairment, the child is referred to an appropriate intervention program. This could consist of physical therapy for the infant who demonstrates only motor impairment or a developmental program for the infant who is delayed in multiple areas.

At 4 months many infants demonstrate immaturity or mild neuromotor abnormality. The parents are given handling and positioning recommendations and are shown activities to facilitate developmental progress. The infant is scheduled for a reexamination at an appropriate interval relative to the level of concern, often 6 to 8 weeks. At that time, the infant is reassessed and may be referred for therapy if the concerns persist, reexamined in 2 months to confirm continuing improvement, or scheduled to return for the 1-year evaluation.

One-year evaluation. Beginning at 1 year, the follow-up evaluations become increasingly multidisciplinary as the infant becomes a more complex individual. The clinic schedule is designed to allow for maximum assessment of various areas of competency while not exhausting the infant and family. Because the infant has been followed by the physical therapist throughout the first year of life, formal motor evaluation is not scheduled. Motor skills are assessed by the psychologist and the pediatrician using the Bayley Scales. The physical therapist is available to provide consultation when delay or deviance is noted. The protocol for the 2- and 3-year evaluations is similar in format to the 1-year evaluation.

Four-and-one-half year evaluation. A scheduled evaluation at 4½ years provides an opportunity to inform families of their child's developmental status as they are making decisions regarding school entry. In addition to assessment by the psychologist, speech pathologist, and pediatrician, the occupational therapist evaluates the child's motor development with particular attention to balance, coordination, and fine motor and perceptual motor dysfunction. The objective is to identify potential learning disorders before school placement and to minimize their effect on school performance.

Neuromotor assessment of the high-risk infant

Assessment tools. In addition to the tools designed to assess the neonate, several systematic assessments of the infant have been developed. Based on content and emphasis, these instruments can be viewed in two broad categories: developmental/behavioral and neurological. The Bayley Scales of Infant Development and the Denver Developmental Screening Test are well-known developmental tests, whereas Amiel-Tison's Neurological Evaluation of the Infant is an assessment tool for the full-term and premature infant during the first year of life. The examination of Milani-Comparetti and the Movement Assessment of Infants are neuromotor examinations that include neurological components, such as the evaluation of reflexes, as well as assessment of some developmental functions.

The choice of instrument for a particular clinical situation will depend on the emphasis and focus of the clinic and the disciplines involved in its organization. Neurological findings tend to be more stable in the young infant and are less subject to the influence of the infant's affective state and the environment. Individual neurological signs can be transient, however, and may not be indicative of overall neurological competency, particularly in infants with identified lesions. Over time, neurological integrity is demonstrated best by the achievement of developmental skills. The results of a major collaborative follow-up study indicate that neurological abnormalities are predictive of later cerebral palsy only when they are associated with failure to perform one or more developmental milestones.[76]

A brief review of the infant assessments commonly used in follow-up clinics is presented below.

Neurologic Evaluation of the Newborn and Infant.[9] The Neurologic Evaluation of the Newborn and the Infant[9] was developed by Amiel-Tison for the assessment of the neuromotor behavior of infants in the first 12 months of life. It was designed to be administered monthly, and its primary purpose is to detect neurological abnormalities or deviations.

The test includes examination of the skull, evaluation of muscle tone and primary reflexes, and observation of posture and movement. The assessment of passive muscle tone is based in part on methods described by Andre-Thomas.[11] Important factors include *extensibility,* in which the range of movement is expressed in terms of an angle or specific anatomical sign, and *passivity,* or flapping of the distal segments of the limbs. Active tone is assessed by observing the infant's motor responses to specific physical manipulation by the examiner. Control of the neck flexors and extensor musculature is emphasized as well as the traction response. Developmental milestones and functional skills are not assessed.

The infant's responses are recorded on a grid that provides a record of the infant's performance on successive tests throughout the year. Visual and written descriptions on the score sheet indicate how to score a particular response. Scores considered to be abnormal for a given item at a designated age are shaded on the record sheet. The individual scores do not yield a summary score. The examiner is given descriptive guidelines for formulating a clinical impression based on one examination and on the pattern of development on repeated evaluations.

The Neurologic Evaluation has a standardized procedure, but normative data is not provided. Interrater reliability is available only for the passive tone items. Reported percentage of agreement ranges from 50% to 90%. Test-retest reliability is not given, and specific validity data have not been reported. The results of longitudinal studies of the outcome of infants evaluated with this instrument indicate that the abnormalities detected on early examinations frequently resolve. In a follow-up study of 168 LBW infants, 41% had abnormal examinations when examined at term age, with the principal findings including abnormalities of tone, hyperreflexia, and deviant eye movements. On follow-up examination at 12 months, only 13% of these infants had major neurodevelopmental disorders and another 20% infants had minor neurological abnormalities.[218]

Bayley Scales of Infant Development (BSID-II).[17] The Bayley Scales of Infant Development[17] is a standardized assessment of mental and motor abilities of infants and children between the ages of 2 months and 3½ years. The test is divided into two primary areas: The mental scale includes test items rating performance in the areas of problem solving, memory, visual perception, learning, and verbal communication; the motor scale evaluates gross and fine motor skills. For the infant younger than 12 months of age, successful performance on the mental scale requires competency in visual following and fine motor manipulation. The mental test becomes more heavily weighted toward language items at the older-age intervals. The motor scale is predominantly an assessment of gross motor milestones, with fine motor and visuoperceptual skills included. The BSID-II also provides a behavior rating scale that evaluates the child's behavior during the testing session.

The Bayley Scales were first published in 1969 in a format used extensively in clinical and research settings throughout the United States. The BSID-II, a revised, updated version of the Bayley, was published in 1993. The goals of the revision process included updating the normative data, expanding the upper age level of the test from 30 to 42 months, and adding more relevant test items and materials. The revised test was standardized on 1700 young children representing a distribution of race, gender, geographical regions, and level of parent education as an indicator of socioeconomic status. In addition, approximately 370 children with various clinical diagnoses, including autism, Down syndrome, developmental delay, preterm birth, and prenatal drug exposure were tested with the BSID-II. Test scores from these children were not included in the normative data and are intended to provide a "baseline of performance" for children with these diagnoses.

Administration procedures and grading criteria are clearly described in the manual. Items are scored on the basis of presence or absence of response. The raw scores are converted to standard scores, the Mental Developmental Index (MDI) and the Psychomotor Developmental Index (PDI), both of which have a mean of 100 and a standard deviation variation of ± 15. The authors note that the BSID-II scores are comparably lower than the scores from the original Bayley, with the Mental Scale 12 points lower on average and the Motor Scale 10 points lower. A "moderate" level of correlation was demonstrated between the original Bayley and the BSID-II: 0.62 for the Mental Scale and 0.63 for the Motor Scale.

Test-retest reliability was evaluated for the BSID-II using a sample of 175 children ages 1, 12, 24, and 36 months. The "stability coefficients" for ages 1 and 12 months were r = .83 for the Mental Scale and r = .77 for the Motor Scale. Inter-rater reliability, determined with a sample of 51 children, was 0.96 for the Mental Scale and 0.75 for the Motor Scale.[17]

Concurrent validity of the BSID-II was evaluated by comparing the BSID-II results with a number of assessment tools, including tests of language, cognitive, and intellectual function. The correlations between the Mental Scale and subscales of language and cognitive tests ranged from 0.57 to 0.99 indicating moderate to high positive correlations. The strongest correlation with the Motor Scale was obtained with the Motor subscale of the McCarthy Scales of Children's Abilities (r = .59).[17] No predictive validity was given for the BSID-II. Numerous studies have evaluated the relationship between performance on the original Bayley Scales in infancy and later outcome. Although the Bayley Mental Scale appeared to predict later cognitive development more accurately than the motor scale, the neurological status of a child at 7 years of age was predicted more efficiently by the motor scale.[22] The Bayley Motor PDI reportedly identified cerebral palsy in 3-month-old infants with a sensitivity of 89%,[45] but this was not confirmed by subsequent studies with 4-month-old infants.[96,159,222,223]

Milani-Comparetti Developmental Examination.[141] The Milani-Comparetti Developmental Examination[141] was an early attempt to evaluate neurological and developmental components of infant movement within one screening examination. The stated objective of this test is to selectively include items that reflect the "correlation between functional motor achievement and the underlying reflex structure."[141, p. 285] It assesses gross motor skills between birth and 24 months and the underlying postural reactions that support these skills: righting reactions, tilting reactions, and parachute reactions. Five primitive reflexes—the palmar and plantar grasp reflexes, asymmetrical and symmetrical tonic neck reflexes, and Moro reflex—are included. Muscle tone is not assessed. The test reportedly can be administered in 3 to 10 minutes. This includes minimal time for observation of spontaneous movement, because the test primarily involves physical maneuvers applied to the infant.

In the original description of the examination, descriptive notes are provided for selected items with guidelines for administration and recognition of the desired reaction. Responses are graded only by presence or absence. Observations are recorded on a chart organized as a developmental grid extending from birth to 24 months, and items are arranged according to the time of "usual appearance" along the horizontal axis. Reflexes and reactions related to specific motor function are aligned along the vertical axis. The underlying assumption is that "a particular reaction must be present in order that a particular item of motor behavior can occur."[141, p. 295]

The Milani-Comparetti in its original form is not quantified and does not yield a numerical score. Subsequent modifications of the test have included numerical scoring systems with a total score achieved by summation.[77,210] Reliability was calculated for a revised version of the test. Interrater reliability was in the 90% to 93% range for mean percentage of agreement, whereas test-retest reliability was 93% for percent of agreement.[220] With a modified Milani-Comparetti scored on a 5-point scale, the test reportedly distinguished normal and abnormal infants at 6 months.[77] In subsequent studies the Milani-Comparetti administered at 3 months of age was not predictive of later neurodevelopmental outcome.[159] It was noted that the test did identify infants with severe cerebral palsy and that predictive validity was better at 6 months, although still not adequate for a screening tool. For additional information refer to Chapter 15, Fig. 15-9.

Movement Assessment of Infants.[52] The Movement Assessment of Infants (MAI) was developed by Chandler and others[52] specifically for use in a high-risk infant follow-up clinic. It is a systematic examination of muscle tone, primitive reflexes, automatic reactions of balance and equilibrium, and volitional gross and fine motor skills.

In the manual the authors recommended that the MAI be considered for the following purposes: (1) to identify motor dysfunction in infants up to 12 months of age, (2) to establish the basis for an early intervention program, (3) to monitor the effects of physical therapy on infants or children whose motor behavior is at or below 1 year of age, (4) to assist in data collection and clinical research on motor development through the use of a standard system of movement assessment, and (5) to teach skilled observation of movement and motor development through evaluation of normal and handicapped children.[52]

The 45-minute test period allows time for scoring, parent counseling, and rest/feeding breaks for the infant. A flexible order of testing is allowed, but grouping of items by infant position (supine, prone, sitting, vertical suspension, standing, prone suspension) is advised to minimize fatigue and stress.

The categories of primitive reflexes (14 items), automatic reactions (16 items), and volitional movement (25 items) are graded on a 4-point scale; muscle tone (10 items) is rated on a 6-point scale. The manual provides full descriptions of the examination and scoring procedures.

The assessment provides a profile of motor behavior for 4- and 8-month-old infants, and a risk score indicating deviant or abnormal neuromotor function can be computed (Appendixes C and D). A 6-month-old profile is currently being developed. Early data reported in the manual indicate that total-risk scores greater than 7 were suggestive of neuromotor delay or abnormality. The authors recommended a higher cut-off point, however, because of scoring revisions made at the time of publication of the manual. Recent MAI data collected with full-term and premature infants suggest that total risk scores of 10 or above indicate increased risk for neuromotor abnormality.[92,202,222,223] Norms have not yet been established, although the performance of small samples of full-term and premature infants on the MAI at 4 and 8 months of age has been recorded.

Early studies of interrater reliability based on percent of agreement reported a 90% level,[52] whereas a later study indicated a 72% interrater reliability and a 76% test-retest reliability.[95] A recent investigation of interrater and test-retest reliability with high-risk infants reported reliabilities (intraclass correlation coefficient) of 0.91 and 0.79, respectively.[34] Concurrent validity between the MAI and the Bayley Motor Scale has been reported as −0.63.[95] The predictive validity has been examined in relation to later performance on the Bayley Scales as well as neurodevelopmental outcome. The correlation between the MAI at 4 and 8 months of age and the mental and motor scales of the Bayley at 1 and 2 years of age is highly significant.[95,221] The MAI at 4 months of age is a more discriminating predictor of later outcome than several other tools, including the Milani-Comparetti and the Prechtl Neurological Examination.[159] The MAI was also more accurate in discriminating abnormality than the Bayley Motor Scale at 4 and 8 months of age.[221]

Chandler Movement Assessment of Infants Screening Test. The Chandler Movement Assessment of Infants Screening Test is a 15-minute screening tool for health professionals in primary care (pediatricians, family practice physicians, and nurse practitioners), designed to identify infants needing referral for definitive neurological and developmental assessment. The test retains the basic categories of the Movement Assessment of Infants, but it is limited to selected items considered predictive of movement disorders. Publication will occur after the collection of normative data has been completed.

Alberta Infant Motor Scale (AIMS).[176] This assessment scale was designed to evaluate gross motor function in infants from birth to independent walking, or 0 to 18 months. The instrument was developed recently and has not yet had widespread clinical use. The stated purposes of the AIMS are (1) to identify infants who are delayed or deviant in their motor development and (2) to evaluate motor maturation over time. The AIMS is described as an "observational assessment" that requires minimal handling of the infant by the examiner. The test includes 58 items, organized by the infant's position, to evaluate three aspects of motor performance: weight-bearing, posture, and antigravity movements. The normative sample consisted of 2200 infants born in Alberta, Canada; racial diversity, if any, in this population was not discussed.[176]

Test-retest and inter-rater reliabilities, established on normally developing infants, ranged from 0.95 to 0.98 depending on the age of the child. The AIMS originally had high agreement with the Bayley Scales and Peabody Scales ($r = 0.93$ and $r = 0.98$, respectively, at the 4- to 8-month age range). An evaluation of concurrent validity between the AIMS and the MAI at 4 and 8 months demonstrated "good" agreement ($r = 0.70$ and $r = 0.84$). When infants with abnormal motor development and "at-risk" development

Table 8-10. Prediction accuracy of an infant test

| Evaluation (at specified age) | Outcome (at specified age) | |
	Normal	Abnormal
No-risk	Correct nonreferrals*	Under-referrals (false negatives)
Risk	Over-referrals (false positives)	Correct referrals†

Adapted from Stangler SR and others: *Screening growth and development of preschool children,* New York, 1980, McGraw-Hill Book Co.

$$*Specificity = \frac{Correct\ nonreferrals}{Total\ normal} \times 100 = \text{Percentage of normal cases classified normal}$$

$$†Sensitivity = \frac{Correct\ referrals}{Total\ abnormal} \times 100 = \text{Percentage of abnormal cases identified}$$

Table 8-11. Predictive validity of infant assessment tools

Assessment	Outcome age	Sensitivity (%)	Specificity (%)
Neonatal examinations			
Amiel-Tison (modified) (Stewart, 1988)	1 year	80	67
Dubowitz (Dubowitz, 1984)	1 year	83	67
Paine (Nelson and Ellenberg, 1979)	7 years	57	88
Prechtl (Bierman-van Eendenburg, 1981, 1984)	18 months	87	54
4-month examinations			
Bayley Motor Scale (Swanson, 1992)	18 months	16	97
MAI (Swanson, 1992)	18 months	83	78
Paine (Ellenberg and Nelson, 1981)	7 years	64	89
8-month examinations			
Bayley Motor Scale (Swanson, 1992)	18 months	77	88
MAI (Swanson, 1992)	18 months	96	65
Motor Scale (Swanson, 1992)	18 months	16	97
MAI (Swanson, 1992)	18 months	83	78
Paine (Ellenberg and Nelson, 1981)	7 years	64	89
8-month examinations			
Bayley Motor Scale (Swanson, 1992)	18 months	77	88
MAI (Swanson, 1992)	18 months	96	65

were examined by "blind" examiners, the AIMS accurately identified 89% of the abnormal infants and categorized 30% of the at-risk infants as "abnormal" or "suspicious."[176]

• • •

Infant neuromotor assessment using an objective, standard instrument serves the following two major functions in a follow-up clinic:

1. It documents the infant's current neuromotor status relative to developmental norms and to the infant's previous examinations to determine progress, rate of change, and degree of delay, if any.
2. It identifies neuromotor abnormality indicative of a movement disorder, so that therapeutic intervention can be initiated. Early identification is not simply a task of recognizing signs of neuromotor deviation or CNS injury. The challenge is to distinguish among those infants with abnormal clinical signs the relatively few who will have an abnormal motor outcome. The goal of infant assessment is to predict the neurodevelopmental outcome of the child on the basis of a clinical examination of the infant.

Predictive value of infant assessment tools. The predictive accuracy of a test is stated in terms of sensitivity and specificity and positive and negative predictive values[215] (see Table 8-10). *Sensitivity* is the ability of the test to identify abnormal as abnormal. It is calculated as the percentage of abnormal children who were correctly identified as such when examined as infants. *Specificity* is the ability of the test to identify normal as normal. It is the percentage of normal children who were correctly identified as normal when examined as infants. Table 8-11 shows the sensitivity and specificity of several infant assessment tools.

When neonatal assessments are compared, it is evident that comprehensive instruments, such as the Prechtl,[177] have a good sensitivity. Low specificity indicates a high rate of "false positives": infants who were considered high risk on the basis of the infant examination, but were *normal* at the time of the outcome evaluation. Less comprehensive examinations, such as the Paine assessment,[161] had better specificity but lower sensitivity. This indicates a lesser ability to identify as *abnormal* infants who will later develop cerebral palsy.

The improved predictive ability of examination at 4 months compared with a neonatal examination is demonstrated by the higher sensitivity of the Paine evaluation at this age. The Movement Assessment of Infants, a comprehensive and detailed evaluation, demonstrated good sensitivity (83%) at 4-month examination and increased to 96% at 8 months. However, specificity declined between 4- and 8-month testing.[221] In contrast, the sensitivity of the Bayley Motor Scale is low at 4 months and increases at 8 months.

A modest decline in specificity was observed in the Bayley Motor Scale between 4 and 8 months.[95,221]

• • •

The positive predictive value of a test indicates the proportion of infants initially classified as abnormal or deviant who are determined to be abnormal at a subsequent time. The negative predictive value relates to the outcome of infants categorized as normal on early examination. The positive predictive values for the MAI at 4 and 8 months were 59% and 52%, respectively, indicating that just over one half of the infants identified as "at risk" by the MAI did have an abnormal outcome. A positive predictive value derived for the Bayley Motor Scale performed on the same infants, based on scores <84 (−1 S.D.) as indicative of risk status, yield positive predictive values of 57% and 63% at 4 and 8 months. Negative predictive values for the MAI were 85% and 91% at 4 and 8 months, while a negative prediction for the Bayley was 70% and 82%. These results indicate that for both tests a negative, or normal, rating for an infant is a more stable prediction of outcome than a positive or abnormal rating.

Prediction of neuromotor outcome is difficult in LBW infants because of several complicating factors.

Impact of medical status on test performance. LBW infants often exhibit delay and neurological instability because of their medical status, not central nervous system dysfunction. This can occur at the following two levels:

1. Temporary depression or deviation in posture and movement because of weakness, shock, or medication. Abnormalities tend to diminish as the infant's condition stabilizes.
2. Prolonged retardation and neurological changes because of chronic disease, such as bronchopulmonary dysplasia. Infants with chronic lung disease typically exhibit low muscle tone, delayed gross motor function, and immature balance reactions (Fig. 8-33). Delay is evident as long as their pulmonary capacity is compromised, but developmental progress accelerates when the respiratory condition resolves.

Influence of in utero exposure to drugs and other substances. Infants who have been prenatally exposed to drugs, such as marijuana, cocaine, heroin, and methadone, may exhibit deviations in their neuromotor behavior, which complicate neurodevelopmental assessment during the first months of life. Neonatal abstinence syndrome, exhibited by infants exposed to heroin and methadone, typically is characterized by irritability, tremulousness, and inconsolability. This condition is treated during the neonatal period; following treatment, the abnormal signs usually resolve. In some infants exposed to heroin, hypertonicity has persisted for 6 months before resolution.[200]

Since 1985 when "crack" cocaine became available, a significant number of infants, including both full-term and LBW infants, have been prenatally exposed to cocaine. Reliable scientific documentation of the effects of in utero cocaine exposure on the neurobehavioral outcome of the neonate and infant is still preliminary and qualified by the methodological complications involved in the required research. Reports suggest that prenatal cocaine exposure may contribute to tremulousness, irritability, increased muscle tone, hypotonia, abnormal reflexes, and motor impairment in the neonatal period. These findings are not consistently observed and when present, often do not persist beyond 2 to 4 months of age. If seen in a LBW infant, however, these clinical findings could be perceived as early signs of cerebral palsy or other major neuromotor abnormalities. Further research may clarify the specific neonatal

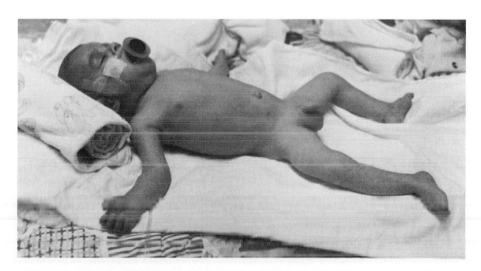

Fig. 8-33. A premature infant with chronic lung disease at 4 months of age with characteristic hypotonic posture and minimal movement against gravity.

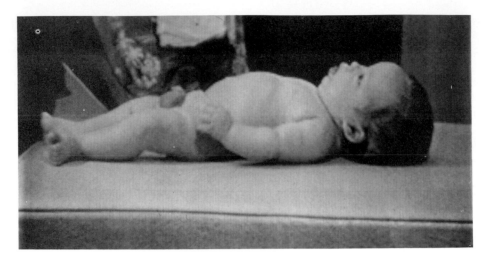

Fig. 8-34. A healthy premature infant at 4 months of age demonstrating shoulder retraction, neck hyperextension, and limited antigravity movement into flexion.

and long-term effects of prenatal exposure to cocaine and other substances. Currently, it is important for therapists working with infants to be aware of the past history of drug exposure because of the potential impact on clinical assessment of neuromotor behavior in the first months of life. Schneider and others[200] provided detailed analyses of the effects of prenatal drug exposure on the developing infant and implications for pediatric therapists working with drug-exposed infants.

Differences between premature and full-term infant neuromotor behavior. Premature infants demonstrate deviation from full-term infants in neuromotor function even when they have not experienced chronic illness and do not have neurological impairment. These variations may reflect predominant positioning during hospitalization, other extrauterine influences, or neurological immaturity.

When compared with full-term infants, healthy premature infants demonstrate variations in their passive and active muscle tone. They initially show greater joint mobility, but may exhibit areas of increased tone, particularly in the hips and ankles, from 2 to 4 months of age.[77,195] Their movements reflect a tendency towards extension posturing, with shoulder retraction, and less antigravity movements in supine[85,232] (Fig. 8-34). Primitive reflexes, such as the asymmetrical tonic neck reflex, the Moro, and the positive support reflex, which are often less pronounced in the young premature infant, tend to persist longer in LBW infants, even when assessed at corrected age.[134]

Balance reactions, including head righting, are immature in the healthy premature infant when compared with full-term infants of comparable age (Fig. 8-35, *A* and *B*). Gross and fine motor skills, especially activities requiring flexion control such as bringing hands to midline and feet to hands, are also less mature.

For most premature infants, these early variations in

movement and posture eventually resolve. In the first months of life, however, they influence both the infant's performance on a neuromotor evaluation and the examiner's clinical impression.

Transient dystonia. Up to 60% of all LBW infants, as well as a number of full-term infants, exhibit abnormal neurological signs that resolve without evidence of major neurological sequelae.[67,90,193] This phenomenon is referred to as "transient dystonia." The abnormalities reportedly are observed in the first 4 months of life, they are most evident between 4 and 8 months, and they are resolved by 1 year of age (Fig. 8-36). The clinical characteristics of transient dystonia that have been most frequently described are given in Table 8-12.

Manifestation of these findings on examination presents a challenge to the examiner. Similar clinical signs are indicative of developing cerebral palsy. It is usually not possible to distinguish the early signs of cerebral palsy from transient neurological signs on one examination. Moreover, long-term follow-up has revealed that even infants whose abnormalities are transient are at increased risk for minor neurodevelopmental abnormalities. Infants who demonstrate abnormal neurological findings in the first year, although developmentally normal at 1-year evaluations, have a higher rate of mental, motor, and behavioral deficits in preschool and schoolage assessments.[10,67]

It is evident that even transient abnormal neuromotor signs in the first year should not be considered as clinically insignificant. They may indicate a child who is at risk for neuromotor problems other than cerebral palsy that may not be functionally evident until school age. In addition, the abnormal behaviors of the infant, although transient, may interfere with the parent-infant bonding process. The infant who is arching instead of cuddling, the infant with poor head control and consequently diminished eye contact with his

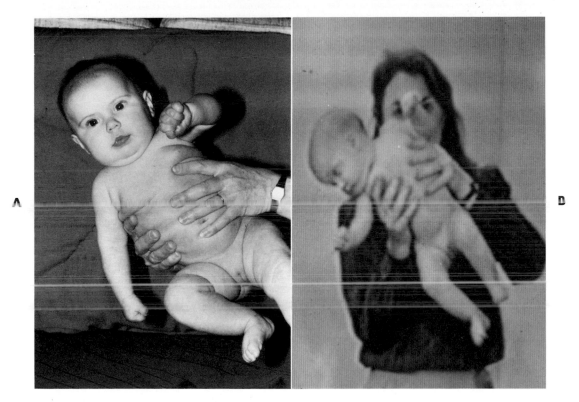

Fig. 8-35. A, A normal full-term infant at 4 months of age demonstrating lateral head righting. When tipped to the side she is able to maintain her head in midline. **B,** A healthy premature infant at 4 months of age demonstrating immature lateral head righting. When tipped to the side the head is not maintained in midline and falls to the side.

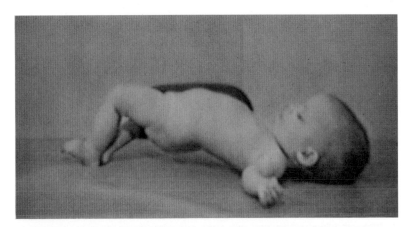

Fig. 8-36. A premature infant at 4 months of age demonstrating excessive arching and extension posturing in supine position, but developmental outcome was normal at 1 year.

parents, or the infant who is irritable and less engaging threatens the quality of the affective and social environment. This may have a serious, detrimental impact on the child's outcome with residual consequences long after the neurological signs have resolved.

High-risk clinical signs. Numerous attempts have been made to identify specific **high-risk clinical signs** that are early manifestations of cerebral palsy. Historically, these were based on subjective qualitative impressions of experienced clinicians.[28,100,180] These observations were a major contribution to the effort to develop methods for early diagnosis of cerebral palsy. However, there were no standard criteria for the observed findings, no control for personal bias and interpretation, and, in general, no evidence that the observations were significantly related to outcome.

Recent data from follow-up studies based on objective

measures have been examined to determine which individual clinical findings are most predictive of abnormal outcome. Conclusions are inconsistent, which may reflect the variability of infants as well as the lack of standard criteria for clinical variables and outcome measures. Results from these studies are summarized in Table 8-13.

Neonatal period. During the neonatal period, the clinical signs reported to be indicative of later cerebral palsy include jerky or abnormal movements and abnormal cry. The tone abnormality most frequently associated with later cerebral palsy is truncal hypotonia with head lag when pulled to sit.[193] However, this finding is not specific to cerebral palsy, because it is also a characteristic of many infants with normal

Table 8-13. High-risk clinical signs indicative of neuromotor abnormality in infants

Neonatal period	4 Months of age	6 Months of age
Abnormal tone	Hypertonicity Lower extremities (hips/knees) Extensibility Neck extensor Hypotonia	Hypertonicity: Upper extremities (flexion) Lower extremities (ankles)
Tremulousness	Tremulousness	
Ankle clonus	Persistent reflexes: Asymmetrical tonic neck Tonic labyrinthine	Persistent asymmetrical tonic neck reflex
		Delayed postural reactions: Head righting Parachute
Abnormal or absent cry Jerky movements Abnormal eye movements	Delayed motor skills: Head control Sit with support Support in prone Open hands Hands to midline Visual following	Delayed motor skills: Rolling Sitting Reach Grasp

Table 18-12. Clinical characteristics of dystonia and abnormality of movements in premature infants that often are transient and resolve spontaneously

Neonatal period	4 Months of age	6 to 8 Months of age
Neck extensor hypertonia	Hypertonicity: Extensor posturing Scissoring	Hypertonia of lower extremities
Hypotonia	Truncal hypotonia	Hypotonia
Irritability	Persistent reflexes: ATNR Positive support	Delayed postural reactions
Lethargy	Head lag	Delayed sitting

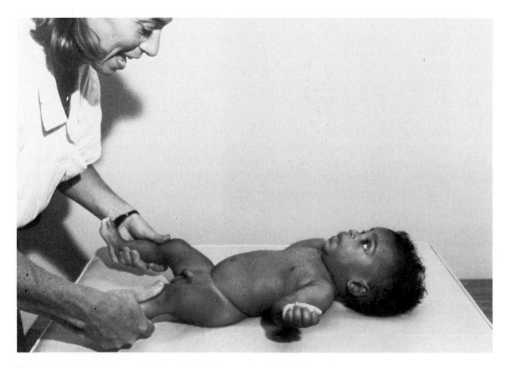

Fig. 8-37. Infant diagnosed with cerebral palsy at 5 months of age; limited hip abduction when passive mobility is examined.

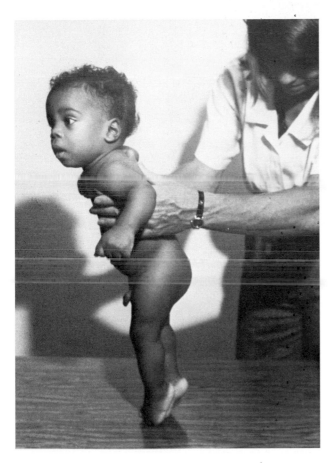

Fig. 8-38. Infant diagnosed with cerebral palsy at 5 months of age; persistence of the positive support reflex.

outcome.[77] Although hypotonia and head lag are frequently observed in young premature infants, in *most* infants these conditions resolve as they mature.

Four months. By 3 to 4 months of age, the abnormal tone often associated with later cerebral palsy is hypertonicity, observed primarily in the lower extremities but usually not in the ankles at this age. Hypertonicity of the extremities in combination with truncal hypotonia is a particularly high-risk sign. The increased tone is detected by the "angles" method of passive assessment of tone used by the Amiel-Tison and Dubowitz examinations and the "extensibility" item of the MAI (Fig. 8-37). Neck extensor hypertonicity is highly predictive of cerebral palsy.[8] Although it was the single most predictive item in one study, however, the majority of infants (60%) who exhibited this clinical sign did not subsequently develop cerebral palsy.[76]

Persistent reflexes at 4 months have been equivocal. Reflexes and neurological signs such as the ATNR and tremulousness have been correlated with cerebral palsy in some studies[76,188,193] but not in others[44,97] (Fig. 8-38). Of the four sections of the MAI, "primitive reflexes" was the least predictive of later outcome.[95]

In contrast, the "volitional movement" section of the MAI was the most predictive at 4 months.[95] This finding is supported by other studies in which delayed developmental milestones were significant predictors of later cerebral palsy[44,76] (Figs. 8-39 and 8-40). Asymmetry of tone and movement is often considered to be an early indication of neurological dysfunction, but this has not been documented.[76,97] It has been commonly observed in premature infants, but its presence does not correlate with later cerebral

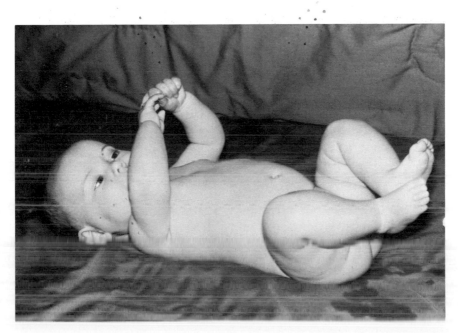

Fig. 8-39. A normal full-term infant at 4 months of age demonstrating ability to bring hands to midline and elevate legs with flexion and abduction of hips, dorsiflexion of ankles.

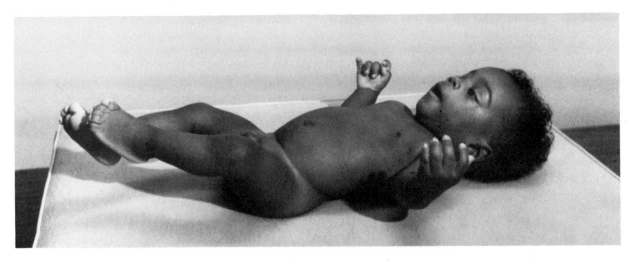

Fig. 8-40. Infant diagnosed with cerebral palsy at 5 months of age; inability to bring hands to midline because of shoulder retraction, extension and adduction of hips with limited movement into flexion, plantar flexion of ankles.

palsy. Fisting of the hands at this age is a significant finding.[97,193]

Six months. Because of the prevalence of transient neurological abnormalities in the LBW infant, 6 months is a less-than-optimal time for prediction of neurodevelopmental outcome on the basis of clinical observation.[10,188] Tone abnormalities most consistently associated with later cerebral palsy include hypertonicity of the upper and lower extremities. The increased tone in the lower extremities can be detected by examination of passive tone and in vertical suspension of the infant, which produces extension posturing of the legs. The upper extremity tone is commonly indicated by shoulder retraction and increased flexor tone.

Interpretation of infant assessment. A review of follow-up studies examining early identification of cerebral palsy indicates that the long-term predictive value of infant assessment, although limited, is of clinical importance. Although it is not possible to predict with certainty the outcome of a specific child, systematic, objective assessment does allow clinicians to make a reasonably accurate statement about a child's degree of risk. This information is important for appropriate medical and family management.

Interpretation of an infant assessment should reflect the following conclusions:

1. Risk is increased with specific abnormal neurological signs, but the majority of infants with any abnormal sign develop normally.
2. A normal neonatal or infant assessment is more predictive than an abnormal examination.
3. Multiple factors are more significantly related to outcome than single factors, indicating the need for a comprehensive evaluation.
4. Periodic examinations over time are the most useful method of determining the developmental outcome of an individual infant.

Neuromotor Intervention

Levels of intervention. Therapeutic intervention for the high-risk infant after discharge from the NICU occurs at multiple levels. Type and intensity of intervention depend on (1) the needs of the infant and family, (2) the structure and organization of the follow-up clinic, and (3) the availability of therapy resources in a particular clinical and geographical setting.

Assessment as intervention. The clinical assessment of an infant by a therapist (or another professional such as a physician or pediatric nurse) is a unique opportunity for intervention on behalf of the infant and his family. For the full potential of this interaction to be realized, parents or caregivers must be informed and involved participants, not passive observers. The focus of the intervention process during an assessment is parent support with two primary components: (1) parent education and (2) positive reinforcement for parenting skills.

Parent education involves demonstrating to the parents of an at-risk infant their child's unique capabilities, strengths, and ability to respond to and influence the environment. They learn about their infant's levels and types of responses to stimuli: what causes the child to pay attention and what elicits stress reactions. Parent education includes describing for parents typical temperamental and developmental patterns of the LBW or medically fragile infant that may differ from expectations based on observations and published descriptions of healthy full-term infants.

Parents of at-risk infants need to be informed about the appropriate level of function for their child and the sequence and pace of development so that they can be realistic in their expectations and interpretation of their infant's progress. This anticipatory guidance enables parents to prepare for and reinforce learning opportunities.

Opportunities to provide *positive reinforcement* to parents need to be emphasized. It is particularly important when working with an infant who may respond inconsistently to the caregiver's affective cues that parents be given positive feedback for their investment of emotion and energy in their child. They should be reassured that they are providing beneficial parenting and that the infant's behavioral responses reflect neurobehavioral immaturity or instability rather than "personality" or negative affective feelings toward the caregiver.

Intervention as instruction in home management. A critical mode of intervention is the process of **parent instruction** in specific techniques for home management. This often occurs at the conclusion of a clinical assessment. The recommendations are based on knowledge of the individual infant's medical and neurological history, current health status, and assessment of neurodevelopmental progress. The objective may be to maximize a healthy child's growth potential or to promote developmental progress in an infant who demonstrates delay or neuromotor abnormality.

In either case it is crucial that the parent or caregiver has a clear understanding of the purpose of the activity, what it is intended to facilitate or counteract, the underlying neurodevelopmental process that this activity will support, and the desired response on the part of the infant. This enables the parent to participate more creatively in the process of intervention by adapting and modifying the recommendation according to the individual temperament of the infant (and parent).

Although handling recommendations are specific to the individual child, some intervention activities are appropriate for many preterm infants. These include the following:

1. *Activities to counteract shoulder retraction.* Fifty percent of LBW infants reportedly demonstrate shoulder retraction.[86] This predominant posture inhibits the infant's ability to move against gravity while supine and results in delayed upper extremity function and rolling. To overcome this retraction, play activities and carrying techniques that bring shoulders forward and hands to midline are demonstrated to parents of premature infants.

2. *Reaching.* Most premature infants are delayed in their reaching skills, decreasing their opportunity to interact with their environment. Although activities to counteract shoulder retraction will promote reaching, it is essential that the infants also be provided with opportunities for practice. Many infants are ready to develop this skill at 3 to 4 months of age, but have only a visually stimulating mobile suspended *beyond their reach* in the crib. Parents are advised to hang toys within the child's reach in the crib, playpen, or other suitable place. Objects that are suspended, rather than handed to or placed in front of the infant, are ideal for the development of directed reach and grasp and shoulder stability (Fig. 8-41).

3. *Centering and symmetrical orientation.* Midline positioning of head with symmetrical alignment of trunk

and extremities is encouraged to counteract the residual effects of asymmetrical positioning during hospitalization. Midline orientation will also promote even development of tone and function in the right and left sides of the body. Asymmetry that is not caused by neurological dysfunction tends to resolve when positioning and environmental influences are modified.

4. *Prone positioning.* Active play time in the prone position is beneficial for the development of neck and back postural control and shoulder stability in weight-bearing, and to counteract the extension posturing of the supine position. However, parents of vulnerable premature infants are often hesitant to place their infants in the prone position. LBW infants, particularly those who have relatively large heads and are very visually attentive, often demonstrate a low tolerance for prone positioning.

Parents are advised to gradually increase the infant's time in the prone position according to the infant's tolerance. When positioned on the floor in front of the infant, visually stimulating toys and objects, including mirrors and the faces of caregivers and siblings, increase acceptance of the prone position. A roll or wedge can facilitate positioning in prone, particularly for the infant with low muscle tone. The infant who is apprehensive or stressed when prone often accepts this position on the parent's chest, where reassuring eye contact can be maintained.

1. *Head balance.* Balance activities to develop head control are frequently recommended. Tilting responses are generally achieved most effectively with the infant in the parent's lap. During parent instruction, emphasis is placed on the importance of (a) adequate trunk support; (b) movement through small ranges; (c) slow, graded motion; (d) the desired head-righting response; and (e) indications of stress or fatigue.

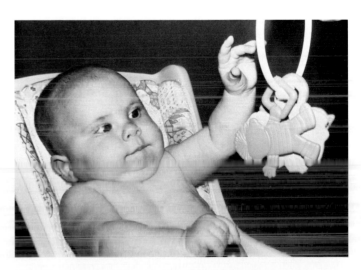

Fig. 8-41. Toys suspended directly in front of infant to encourage symmetrical reaching and midline orientation of head.

2. *Restricted use of infant jumper and walker.* For infants with increased lower extremity tone or tendency toward toe-standing, the infant walkers and jumpers are not recommended because they tend to increase stiffness and extension posturing of the legs. However, these forms of infant equipment are often highly enjoyable for infants and may provide the parent of a very irritable infant with valuable moments of respite within a stressed household. Therefore it is important to assist the parents in finding alternative methods of positioning and amusement for the infant while recommending that time in the walker or jumper be minimized. Caregivers are often reluctant to discard the walker, believing that it promotes early ambulation and is beneficial for infants. Informing them of the hazards of infant walkers and of studies showing that their use may delay the onset of independent ambulation encourages their cooperation.[107,109,110]

Intervention as ongoing therapy. Referral to a regular program of therapeutic intervention is usually made after at least two assessments and a trial period of interim home activities. Criteria for referral include the following:

1. Persistent or progressive indications of abnormal tone
2. Developmental delay in volitional skills or postural reactions
3. Increasing asymmetry or disparity between right and left sides of the body, especially if accompanied by tone differential
4. Loss of joint mobility
5. Feeding difficulties

A decision regarding therapy referral would be influenced by consideration of relevant factors including the following:

1. The infant's medical status
2. Parental concerns
3. Home environment
4. Availability of therapy services relative to geographical, financial, and personnel factors

Effectiveness of early therapy for infants. The effectiveness of therapy for high-risk or neurologically abnormal infants is currently being investigated and discussed.[16,100,138,163,206,208] Numerous studies address this question with inconclusive and, at times, conflicting results. The clinical therapist involved in the treatment of infants needs to critically analyze these studies with respect to the validity of their research methodology and their clinical relevance. Specific questions to be addressed include the following:

1. The sample of infants receiving therapy: Are they "at risk" or neurologically abnormal?
2. The frequency of therapy: Is it an accurate representation of the standard of practice?
3. The duration and timing of therapy: Is it appropriate to critical periods of development?

4. The therapy techniques used: Are they specifically described?
5. The quality and amount of parent participation: Is it realistic?
6. Assessment of results: Are the outcome measures of the study appropriate relative to the goals of therapy?

A review of early intervention studies that demonstrated measurable positive change as a result of an infant intervention program suggests several characteristics critical to effective intervention.[138,163,182,206]

1. *High degree of parent involvement.* For the therapist this implies that the parent or caregiver must be a participant in the therapy session as well as the therapy program at home. This requires that the activities and techniques to be carried out by the parents are comprehensible and manageable by them.
2. *Comprehensive program of developmental intervention.* Motor skills cannot be addressed in isolation from other aspects of an infant's development. To improve quality of life, not just quality of movement, the therapist must explore a broad perspective of infant learning and incorporate a transdisciplinary approach.
3. *Well-defined curriculum of sequential activities.* Physical therapy for infants traditionally is accomplished through a flexible and variable selection of therapy activities rather than structured curriculum. However, a defined program of learning objectives and activities enables the therapist and parents (as well as daycare workers and others participating in the infant's care) to have a clear and consistent understanding of the current therapeutic activities, the goals of the program, and the steps involved in achieving those goals.

Design of an individualized therapy program. The therapy program for a specific infant should incorporate the

Table 8-14. Efficacy and feasibility of physical therapy intervention for at-risk infants

Realistic goals of physical therapy	Potential goals of physical therapy not yet documented	Goals that are not in domain of physical therapy
Home management of disability (feeding, handling)	Change abnormal motor patterns	Cure cerebral palsy
Equipment design for position and function	Prevent physical deformities	Release contractures
Parent support and guidance	Reduce impact of minor neurodevelopmental abnormalities by early therapy	Diagnose abnormal neurological conditions
Document motor development in at-risk infants	Predict outcome of at-risk infants	

CASE 1   **High-risk Infant 1**

The infant was born prematurely at 29 weeks of gestation with a birthweight of 940 g. Her neonatal course was complicated by idiopathic respiratory distress syndrome (IRDS), which was treated with surfactant.

She was first evaluated in the high-risk infant follow-up clinic at 4 months corrected age (6½ months chronological age). Bayley Scale scores at that time were a Mental Scale score (MDI) of 94 and a Motor Scale score (PDI) of 82. On the Movement Assessment of Infants, this infant had a total risk score of 7. She had mildly increased muscle tone in her lower extremities, which was evident in slight resistance to passive manipulation. She demonstrated persistent primitive reflexes including an asymmetric tonic neck reflex, a Moro reflex, and influence of the tonic labyrinthine reflex in supine. Head balance was immature, but emerging righting reactions were noted. When observed in supine her posture was extended, but she was beginning to bring her hands to midline. In prone, she had started to push up on elbows but posture was immature. Her parents were given recommendations for handling to include carrying position with shoulders forward to inhibit retraction, frequent play in the prone position, and increased opportunities for reaching in supine.

The infant returned at 8 months corrected age. Bayley Scale scores at this time were MDI of 101 and PDI of 81. The MAI total risk score was 9. Increased muscle tone observed previously was no longer evident. Muscle tone of the trunk was mildly hypotonic, and greater-than-normal joint mobility was noted at the hips. She demonstrated antigravity movements of the extremities in all positions. Primitive reflexes were all integrated. Balance reactions were present but immature in some areas including head righting into flexion and protective extension reactions. In volitional skills, the infant is now sitting independently for up to 30 seconds, can roll from supine to prone, and can pivot on her stomach. She can pick up a block with either hand and transfer objects. Immaturity is seen in her sitting balance, her inability to move out of sitting, and her failure to progress forward on the floor. She attempted to pick up a pellet but was unable to do so. Her parents were advised to maximize play time on the floor and provide her with tiny edible bits of food to practice fine dexterity.

When seen at 12 months corrected age, the infant had Bayley Scale MDI of 108 and PDI of 94. Although not yet not walking independently, she was cruising with good weight shift and balance. She creeped reciprocally on hands and knees and pulled to stand. She picked up a pellet with an inferior pincer grasp. No deviations of muscle tone or reflex development were observed during examination by the developmental pediatrician. The infant was developing normally and will return for follow-up at 2 years of age. Her parents were advised to call if she is not walking within 2 months or if they have any concerns regarding her pattern of independent walking.

In the management of this child who demonstrated abnormal signs, the primary responsibilities of the pediatric therapist were on-going assessment and parent guidance and teaching. Although there were initial concerns about this infant because of mild tone and reflex abnormalities, it would have been inappropriate to diagnose her with a particular condition. When followed over time, the abnormalities resolved and proved to be transient. This child would continue to be followed in the high-risk infant clinic because she remains at risk for neurodevelopmental problems, which may not become evident until school age.

---

preceding recommendations into a treatment plan that is individualized for the infant and the environment. Progress is monitored by systematic, quantified assessment performed at regular intervals. Effectiveness is determined relative to the rate of progress and the specified goals for each infant.

The long-range goals of an intervention program for a neurodevelopmentally impaired infant must be realistic and stated in terms of clear, measurable objectives. When defining goals, it is important for therapists to make distinctions among (1) objectives that are generally accepted as achievable by therapists, (2) those believed but not yet conclusively demonstrated to be accomplishable by therapeutic intervention, and (3) changes that are not within the domain or capability of physical therapy. Examples of objectives in these categories are provided in Table 8-14.

For example, physical therapy cannot "cure" cerebral palsy (i.e., it cannot heal areas of infarcted brain tissue). LBW infants who demonstrate neurological abnormalities, receive a course of physical therapy intervention, and subsequently do not exhibit residual signs of abnormality demonstrate a clinical course typical of transient dystonia, in which the abnormalities resolve even without therapy. To imply that the therapy "cured" the cerebral palsy could be a misrepresentation and a disservice to families, funding agencies, and the profession. Nevertheless, the value of the support and guidance provided by the therapist to the family during this critical time of intervention should not be underestimated.

Therapists are currently attempting to demonstrate and document their ability to change motor patterns and to improve motor function in neurologically impaired infants. While this effort is in progress, it is necessary to emphasize the unique professional skills and services that are indisputably provided, such as home management, equipment design, and functional training. Other aspects of intervention, such as the relationship between early therapy for "suspect" infants and later minor neurodevelopmental abnormalities, require further investigation.

SUMMARY

This chapter on the NICU management and follow-up of at-risk neonates and infants presented three theoretical

CASE 2 ▼ High-risk Infant 2

The infant was born prematurely at 29 weeks of gestation with a birthweight of 1200 g. The neonatal course was complicated by IRDS and persistent apnea and bradycardia. Cranial ultrasound revealed a large left subependymal hemorrhage with ventriculomegaly and left periventricular leukolmalacia.

She was first seen in the high-risk infant follow-up clinic at 4 months corrected age (6 months 17 days chronological age). The parents stated that they had no concerns regarding their daughter's development, but had observed that she tended to use her left hand more than her right. On the Bayley Scales the infant received a Mental Scale score (MDI) of 102 and a Motor Scale score (PDI) of 102. On the Movement Assessment of Infants the infant received a total risk score of 14. Muscle tone was normal at rest but increased when she was active or agitated. Tone in the lower extremities was increased and restricted passive mobility in the hip abductor and gastrocsoleus muscles bilaterally. In supine she had a stiff, extended posture and brought her hands to midline only once during the examination. In prone she was able to push up and elevate her head while kicking actively. In the prone suspended position she showed good postural elevation, but movements were stiff. Persistent primitive reflexes included the tonic labyrinthine reflex in supine, asymmetrical tonic neck reflex, neonatal positive support reflex, and bilateral ankle clonus. Plantar grasp with persistent toe curling was observed on the right. Righting and equilibrium reactions were emerging. She showed a mature Landau with full extension in prone suspension, which is atypical for her age. In volitional movement, mild asymmetry was evident, as she had difficulty bringing her right arm forward in prone and brought her left arm to midline frequently. Her kicking pattern in supine was low, with a strong extensor pattern often observed on the right side. She was not yet reaching out for objects, and hands were frequently fisted, particularly on the right. Parents were advised in handling skills to reduce shoulder retraction and extension posturing and to facilitate more symmetry in movements and posture. They were advised to return in 6 months.

When seen again at 6 months corrected age the MDI was 94, PDI was 86 and the MAI total risk score was 13. The infant had made the following developmental progress: (1) rolling from supine to prone (over the left side only), (2) beginning sitting balance, and (3) reaching out and grasping objects. She showed a preference for and greater skill and dexterity with her left hand. Occasional fisting was still observed on the right

hand. She transfered objects only from right to left. Muscle tone continued to be increased in the lower extremities with restricted passive mobility of the gastrocsoleus muscles bilaterally. Toe clawing was observed on the right with minimal spontaneous dorsiflexion. Primitive reflexes were integrated except for persistent neonatal positive support and asymmetrical tonic neck reflex to the right. Automatic reactions were more improving, but balance responses were asymmetrical in equilibrium reactions and protective extension reactions delayed on the right. Although the developmental progress was encouraging, the persistent asymmetry remained a major concern. The infant was referred to a local therapy program with regular therapy in the home at least once a week.

The infant was seen in follow-up clinic at 12 months corrected age (14½ months chronological age). On the Bayley Scales, the MDI was 95 and the PDI was 82. She now creeped reciprocally on hands and knees. When she pulled to stand she consistently brought the left foot up first. She cruised at furniture with a tendency to stand on toes on the right. She was able to reach out for objects with either hand. She picked up cubes with either hand but showed partial palmar grasp on the right. She picked up a pellet with an inferior pincer grasp on the left but scooped it into the palm of the right hand. Muscle tone continued to be mildly increased in the lower extremities with tight heelcords, particularly on the right. She sat independently, but her back was not straight. When moving in and out of sitting she used partial rotation over the left side only. Language development was considered appropriate for her age. The infant was diagnosed with mild right hemiplegic category of cerebral palsy. She will continue in a therapy program and return for reevaluation at 2 years of age.

In the management of this child, the role of the pediatric therapist was assessment of neurodevelopmental status and referral to therapy when it became evident that the abnormalities of muscle tone were persisting and interfering with her developmental progress. It should be noted that this child's Bayley Motor Scale scores were in the normal range at both the 4- and 8-month examinations. Because the Bayley Scale does not require infants to perform tasks with both hands, a normal score can be obtained using just one side of the body. This child would continue to be followed in the high-risk infant clinic after 2 years of age to provide periodic reassessment and guidance to the family as they confront questions of school placement and program planning for their child.

models for practice, reviewed neonatal neuropathology related to movement disorders, and described expanded professional services for at-risk neonates and infants in a relatively new subspecialty within pediatric practice. Pediatric therapists participating in intensive care nursery and follow-up teams in the care of high-risk neonates and their parents are involved in a subspecialty of clinical practice that requires heightened responsibility for accountability and for precepted clinical training (beyond general pediatric spe-

cialization) in neonatology and infant therapy techniques.

Inherent in this new area of practice is the challenge to design comprehensive neonatal therapy protocols that include standardized evaluation instruments, comprehensive risk-management plans, long-term follow-up strategies, and systematic documentation of outcome. Ongoing analyses of the physiological risk/therapeutic benefit relationship of neuromotor and neurobehavioral treatment for chronically ill and prematurely born infants must guide the NICU intervention process. The quality of collaboration between therapists and neonatal nurses largely determines the success of neonatal therapy implementation during the 24-hour care environment of the nursery.

Pediatric therapists working in nursery settings are encouraged to participate in follow-up clinics for NICU graduates to identify and analyze the development of movement dysfunction and behavioral sequelae that may, in the future, be minimized or prevented with creative neonatal treatment approaches. The important preventive aspect of neonatal treatment must be guided by careful analyses of neurodevelopmental and functional outcomes in the first year of life.

The LBW or medically fragile infant is at increased risk for major and minor neurodevelopmental problems that may be evident in infancy or not until later childhood. Prenatal and perinatal risk factors indicate infants who have a greater likelihood of neurological complications, but the relationship between single factors and outcome is neither direct nor consistent. Abnormal neurological signs in the first year are also not reliably predictive of abnormal outcome. Attempts to identify factors that definitively indicate significant brain injury are complicated by changing NICU technology, management procedures, environmental variables, and the variability among and within individual infants.

In deciding whether and when an infant requires regular therapeutic intervention, consideration must be given to both the observed capacity for LBW infants to "normalize"[195] during the first year as well as the time span that may elapse before definitive evidence of cerebral palsy. The pediatric therapist's long-term clinical management of the at-risk infant is guided by the developmental course of the individual infant over time, including behavioral and cognitive growth as well as neuromotor progress, considered within the context of the priorities and values of the family. For additional information regarding treatment of those neonates who develop the motor impairments of the clinical problem of cerebral palsy, please refer to Chapter 9.

REFERENCES

1. Abramson L and others: Learned helplessness in humans: critique and reformulation, *J Abnorm Psychol* 87:49, 1978.
2. Als H and others: The Brazelton neonatal behavioral assessment scale, *J Abnorm Psychol* 5:215, 1977.
3. Als H: A synactive model of neonatal behavioral organization: framework for the assessment of neurobehavioral development in the premature infant and for support of infants and parents in the neonatal intensive care environment, *Phys Occup Ther Pediatr* 6 (3/4), 3, 1986.
4. Als H and others: Dynamics of the behavioral organization of the premature infant: a theoretical perspective. In Field TM, editor: *Infants born at risk*, pp 173-192, New York, 1979, Spectrum Publications.
5. Als H and others: Toward a research instrument for the assessment of preterm infants' behavior (APIB). In Fitzgerald HE and others:, editors: *Theory and research in behavioral pediatrics*, New York, 1982, Plenum Press.
6. Als H and others: Individualized behavioral and environmental care for the VLBW preterm infant at high risk for bronchopulmonary

7. dysplasia: NICU and developmental outcome, *Pediatrics* 78: 1123, 1986.
7. Amiel-Tison C: Neurological evaluation of the maturity of newborn infants, *Arch Dis Child* 43:89, 1968.
8. Amiel-Tison C and others: Neck extensor hypertonia: a clinical sign of insult to the central nervous system of the newborn, *Early Hum Dev* 1(2):181, 1977.
9. Amiel-Tison C and Grenier A: *Neurologic evaluation of the newborn and the infant*, New York, 1980, Masson Publishing.
10. Amiel-Tison C and Grenier A: *Neurological assessment during the first year of life*, New York, 1986, Oxford University Press.
11. Andre-Thomas and others: *The neurological examination of the infant*, London, 1964, William Heinemann Medical Books Ltd.
12. Avery GB, editor: *Neonatology*, ed 2, Philadelphia, 1981, JB Lippincott.
13. Babson SG and others: *Management of high risk pregnancy and intensive care of the neonate*, ed 3, St Louis, 1975, Mosby.
14. Barnard KE and others: Developmental changes in maternal interactions with term and preterm infants, *Infant Behav Dev* 7:101, 1984.
15. Barnard KE and Eyres SJ: Feeding scale, in *Child Health Assessment* (DHEW Publication No HRA 79-25), Hyattsville, Md: U.S. Department of Health, Education, and Welfare, Health Resources Administration, Bureau of Health Manpower, Division of Nursing.
16. Barrera ME and others: Early home intervention with low-birth-weight infants and their parents, *Child Dev* 57:20, 1986.
17. Bayley N: *Manual for the Bayley scales of infant development*, ed 2, New York, 1993, The Psychological Corp.
18. Beckwith L and others: Caregiver-infant interaction and early cognitive development in preterm infants, *Child Dev* 47:579, 1976.
19. Behrman RE: *Neonatal-perinatal medicine: diseases of the fetus and newborn*, ed 2, St. Louis, 1977, Mosby.
20. Bennett FC and others: Hyaline membrane disease, birth weight, and gestational age, *Am J Dis Child* 136:888, 1982.
21. Bennett FC and others: Periventricular echodensities detected by cranial ultrasonography: usefulness in predicting neurodevelopmental outcome in low-birth-weight, preterm infants. *Pediatrics* 85:400, 1990.
22. Berk RA: The discriminative efficiency of the Bayley scales of infant development, *J Abnorm Child Psych* 0:113, 1979.
23. Bierman-van Eendenburg MEC and others: Predictive value of neonatal neurological examination: a follow-up study at 18 months, *Develop Med Child Neurol* 23:296, 1981.
24. Bhushan V, Paneth N, and Keily JL: Impact of improved survival of very low birth weight infants on recent secular trends in the prevalence of cerebral palsy, *Pediatrics* 91:1094, 1993.
25. Blackburn ST: Fostering behavioral development of high-risk infants, *JOGN Nurs* 12:76, 1983.
26. Blackburn ST: Assessment of risk: perinatal, family, and environmental perspectives, *Phys Occup Ther Pediatr* 6(3/4):105-120, 1986.
27. Bly L: The components of normal movement during the first year of life. In Slayton DS, editor: *Development of movement in infancy*, Chapel Hill, 1981, University of North Carolina Press.
28. Bobath K and Bobath B: The diagnosis of cerebral palsy in infancy, *Arch Dis Child* 31:408, 1956.
29. Bobath B and Bobath K: The neurodevelopmental treatment of cerebral palsy, *Phys Ther* 47:1039, 1967.
30. Bobath B and Bobath K: *The motor development in the different types of cerebral palsy*, London, 1975, William Heinemann Medical Books Ltd.
31. Bobath K and Bobath B: Cerebral palsy. In Pearson PH and Pieber N, editors: *Physical therapy services in the developmental disabilities*, Springfield, Ill, 1972, Charles C Thomas.
32. Bowlby J: The child's tie to his mother: attachment behavior. In *Attachment and loss*, vol I: Attachment, 1969, New York, Basic Books.

33. Brackbill Y and others: Psychophysiologic effects in the neonate of prone versus supine placement, *J Pediatr* 82:82, 1973.

34. Brander R and others: Inter-rater and test-retest reliabilities of the movement assessment of infants, *Pediatr Phys Ther* 5:9, 1993.

35. Braun MA and Palmer MM: A pilot study of oral-motor dysfunction in "at-risk" infants, *Phys Occup Ther Pediatr* 5:13, 1985.

36. Brazelton TB: Neonatal behavioral assessment scale, ed 2, *Clinics in Developmental Medicine*, No 88, Philadelphia, 1984, JB Lippincott Co.

37. Brazelton neonatal behavioral assessment scale certification program: Child Development Unit, Children's Hospital Medical Center, 300 Longwood Avenue, Boston, Mass.

38. Brazelton neonatal behavioral assessment scale training films: Educational Development Corporation, 8 Mifflin Place, Cambridge, Mass.

39. Brothwood M and others:: Mortality, morbidity, growth and development of babies weighing 501-1000 grams and 1001-1500 grams at birth, *Acta Paediatr Scand* 77:10, 1988.

40. Bull MJ, Bryson CQ, and Schreiner RL: Perinatal status and neonatal treatment as predictors of the neurologic integrity and development of very low birth weight infants, *J Perinatol* 5:16, 1988.

41. Burns WJ and others: Developmental assessment of premature infants, *J Dev Behav Pediatr* 3:12, 1982.

42. Calame A and others: Neurodevelopmental outcome and school performance of very—low-birth-weight infants at 8 years of age, *Eur J Pediatr* 145:461, 1986.

43. Calvert SA and others: Periventricular leukomalacia: ultrasonic diagnosis and neurological outcome. *Acta Paediatr Scand* 75:489, 1986.

44. Campbell SK and Wilhelm IJ: Development from birth to 3 years of age of 15 children at high risk for central nervous system dysfunction, *Phys Ther* 65:463, 1985.

45. Campbell SK and others: Evidence for the need to renorm the Bayley scales of infant development based on the performance of a population-based sample of 12-month-old infants, *Top Early Child Spec Ed* 6:2, 1986.

46. Campbell SK: The developing infant: neuromuscular maturation. In Wilson J, editor: *Infants at risk: medical and therapeutic management*, ed 2, Chapel Hill, 1982, University of North Carolina Press.

47. Campbell SK: Organizational and educational considerations in creating an environment to promote optimal development of high-risk neonates, *Phys Occup Ther Pediatr* 6(3/4):191, 1986.

48. Campbell SK: Clinical decision making: management of the neonate with movement dysfunction. In Wolf SL, editor: *Clinical decision making in physical therapy*, Philadelphia, 1985, FA Davis.

49. Caplan G: Patterns of parental response to the crises of premature birth, *Psychiatry* 23:365, 1970.

50. Carter RE and Campbell SK: Early neuromuscular development of the premature infant, *Phys Ther* 55:1332, 1975.

51. Catto-Smith AG and others: Effect of neonatal periventricular haemorrhage on neurodevelopmental outcome, *Arch Dis Child* 60:8, 1985.

52. Chandler LS and others: *Movement assessment of infants: a manual*, Rolling Bay, Wash, 1980, Authors.

53. Clark JE: Waterbeds: therapeutic devices for handicapped children, *Phys Ther* 61:1175, 1981.

54. Clarr DL and others: Vestibular stimulation influence on motor development in infants, *Science* 196:1228, 1977.

55. Coleman M: Congenital brain syndromes. In Coleman M, editor: *Neonatal neurology*, Baltimore, 1981, University Park Press.

56. Coolman RB and others: Neuromotor development of graduates of the neonatal intensive care unit: patterns encountered in the first two years of life, *J Dev Behav Pediatr* 6:327, 1985.

57. Cowan D: Personal communication, School of Nursing, University of Washington, August, 1987.

58. Crane L: Physical therapy for the neonate with respiratory disease. In Irwin S and Tecklin JS, editors: *Cardiopulmonary physical therapy*, St Louis, 1985, Mosby.

59. Crane L: Cardiorespiratory management of the high-risk neonate: implications for developmental therapists, *Phys Occup Ther Pediatr* 6(3/4):255, 1986.

60. Crane L: The neonate and child. In Frownfelter DL, editor: *Chest physical therapy and pulmonary rehabilitation: an interdisciplinary approach*, ed 3, Chicago, 1983, Year Book Medical Publishers.

61. Crnic KA and others: Social interaction and developmental competence of preterm and full-term infants during the first year of life, *Child Dev* 54:1199, 1983.

62. Dancsak M and others: Concurrent validity of two infant motor scales: the Alberta Infant Motor Scale (AIMS) and the Movement Assessment of Infants (MAI), *Dev Med Child Neurol* 35 (Suppl 69):4, 1993.

63. Davis DH and Thoman EB: Behavioral states of premature infants: implications for neural and behavioral development, *Dev Psychobiol* 20:25, 1987.

64. DeVries LS and others: Neurological, electrophysiological and MRI abnormalities in infants with extensive cystic leukomalacia, *Neuropediatrics* 18:61, 1987.

65. Dinwiddle R and others: Cardiopulmonary changes in the crying neonate, *Pediatr Res* 13:900, 1979.

66. Drillien CM: Actiology and outcome in low-birthweight infants, *Dev Med Child Neurol* 14:563, 1972.

67. Drillien CM: Abnormal neurologic signs in the first year of life in low-birthweight infants: possible prognostic significance, *Dev Med Child Neurol* 14:575, 1972.

68. Drillien CM and Drummond MB, editors: *Neurodevelopmental problems in early childhood*, Oxford, England, 1977, Blackwell Medical Publishers.

69. Dubowitz L: Neurologic assessment. In Ballard R, editor: *Pediatric care of the ICN graduate*, Philadelphia, 1988, WB Saunders.

70. Dubowitz L and Dubowitz V: The neurological assessment of the preterm and full-term newborn infant, *Clinics in Developmental Medicine*, No 79, Philadelphia, 1981, JB Lippincott.

71. Dubowitz L and others: Clinical assessment of gestational age in the newborn infant, *J Pediatr* 77:1, 1970.

72. Dubowitz L and others: Neurologic signs in neonatal intraventricular hemorrhage: a correlation with real-time ultrasound, *J Pediatr* 99:127, 1981.

73. Dubowitz L and others: Correlation of neurologic assessment in the preterm newborn infant with outcome at 1 year, *J Pediatr* 105:452, 1984.

74. Eilers BL and others: Classroom performance and social factors of children with birth weights of 1,250 grams or less: follow-up at 5 to 8 years of age, *Pediatrics* 77:203, 1986.

75. Ellenberg JH and Nelson KB: Birth weight and gestational age in children with cerebral palsy or seizure disorders, *Am J Dis Child* 33:1044, 1979.

76. Ellenberg JH and Nelson KB: Early recognition of infants at high risk for cerebral palsy: examination at age four months, *Dev Med Child Neurol* 23:705, 1981.

77. Ellison PH and others: Development of a scoring system for the Milani-Comparetti and Gidoni method of assessing neurologic abnormality in infancy, *Phys Ther* 63:1414, 1983.

78. Escobar GJ, Littenberg B, and Petitti DB: Outcome among surviving very low birthweight infants: a meta-analysis, *Arch Dis Child* 66:204, 1991.

79. Fawer CL, Dievold P, and Calame A: Periventricular leucomalacia and neurodevelopmental outcome in preterm infants, *Arch Dis Child* 62:30, 1987.

80. Fetters L: Sensorimotor management of the high-risk neonate, *Phys Occup Ther Pediatr* 6(3/4):217, 1986.

81. Field T: Supplemental stimulation of preterm neonates, *Early Hum Dev* 4:301, 1980.

82. Fitterman C: Physical therapy in the NICU. In Connolly BH and Montgomery PC, editors: *Therapeutic exercise in developmental disabilities,* Chattanooga, 1987, Chattanooga Corp.

83. Forslund M and Bjerre I: Growth and development in preterm infants during the first 18 months, *Early Hum Dev* 10:201, 1985.

84. Freedman DG: Ethnic differences in babies, *Hum Nature,* p. 36, Jan. 1979.

85. Freeman JM and Nelson KB: Intrapartum asphyxia and cerebral palsy, *Pediatrics* 82:2, 1988.

86. Georgieff MK and Bernbaum JC: Abnormal shoulder girdle muscle tone in premature infants during their first 18 months of life, *Pediatrics* 77:664, 1986.

87. Georgieff MK and others: Abnormal truncal muscle tone as a useful early marker for developmental delay in low birth weight infants, *Pediatrics* 77:659, 1986.

88. Goodman M and others: Effect of early neurodevelopmental therapy in normal and at-risk survivors of neonatal intensive care, *Lancet* II, 1327, 1985.

89. Graham M and others: Prediction of cerebral palsy in very low birth-weight infants: prospective ultrasound study, *Lancet* II, 593, 1987.

90. Hack M and others: The very low birth weight infant: the broader spectrum of morbidity during infancy and early childhood, *J Dev Behav Pediatr* 4:243, 1983.

91. Hansen N and Okken A: Transcutaneous oxygen tension of newborn infants in different behavioral states, *Pediatr Res* 14:911, 1980.

92. Hardy S: Personal communication, Toronto, Ontario, January, 1988.

93. Harris M: Oral-motor management of the high-risk neonate, *Phys Occup Ther Pediatr* 6(3/4):231, 1986.

94. Harris SR and others: Reliability of observational measures of the Movement Assessment of Infants, *Phys Ther* 64:471, 1984.

95. Harris SR and others: Predictive validity of the Movement Assessment of Infants, *J Dev Behav Pediatr* 5:335, 1984.

96. Harris SR: Early detection of cerebral palsy: sensitivity and specificity of two motor assessment tools, *J Perinatol* 7:11, 1987.

97. Harris SR: Early neuromotor predictors of cerebral palsy in low-birthweight infants, *Dev Med Child Neurol* 29:587, 1987.

98. Hensinger RN and Jones ET: *Neonatal orthopedics,* New York, 1981, Grune & Stratton.

99. Heriza C: The neonate with cerebral palsy. In Scully R and Barnes ML, editors: *Physical therapy,* Philadelphia, 1989, JB Lippincott.

100. Herndon WA and others: Effects of neurodevelopmental treatment of movement patterns of children with cerebral palsy, *J Pediatr Orthop* 7:395, 1987.

101. Hill A and Volpe JJ: Seizures, hypoxic-ischemic brain injury, and intraventricular hemorrhage in the newborn, *Ann Neurol* 10:109, 1981.

102. Hislop HJ: The not-so-impossible dream. *Phys Ther* 55:1060, 1975.

103. Hoffman EL and Bennett FC: Birth weight less than 800 grams: changing outcomes and influences of gender and gestation number, *Pediatrics* 86:27, 1990.

104. Illingworth RS: The diagnosis of cerebral palsy in the first year of life, *Dev Med Child Neurol* 8:178, 1966.

105. Ito M: Computed tomography of cerebral palsy: evaluation of brain damage by Volume index of CSF space, *Brain Dev* 4:293, 1979.

106. Jeffcoate JA and others: Disturbance in parent-child relationship following preterm delivery, *Dev Med Child Neurol* 21:344, 1979.

107. Johnson CF and others: Walker-related burns in infants and toddlers, *Pediatr Emerg Care* 6:58, 1991.

108. Kaback MM, editor: Prenatal diagnosis, *Pediatr Ann* 10:13, 1981.

109. Kauffman IB and Ridenour M: Influence of an infant walker on onset and quality of walking pattern of locomotion: an electromyographic investigation, *Percept Mot Skills* 45:1323, 1977.

110. Kavanagh CA and Banco L: The infant walker: a previously unrecognized health hazard, *Am J Dis Child* 136:205, 1982.

111. Kennell JH and Klaus MH: Caring for parents of a premature or sick infant. In Klaus MH and Kennell JH, editors: *Maternal-infant bonding,* 1976, St Louis, Mosby.

112. Kennell J and others: Parent-infant bonding. In Helfer RE and Kempe CH, editors: *Child abuse and neglect,* Cambridge, Mass, 1976, Ballinger.

113. Kitchen WH and others: Collaborative study of very-low-birth-weight infants, *Am J Dis Child,* 137:555, 1983.

114. Kitchen WH and others: Cerebral palsy in very low birthweight infants surviving to 2 years with modern perinatal intensive care, *Am J Perinatol* 4:29, 1987.

115. Klaus MH and Fanaroff AA: *Care of the high-risk neonate,* Philadelphia, 1973, WB Saunders.

116. Klein N and others: Preschool performance of children with normal intelligence who were very-low-birth-weight infants, *Pediatrics* 75:531, 1985.

117. Knobloch H and others: Considerations in evaluating changes in outcome for infants weighing less than 1,501 grams, *Pediatrics* 69:285, 1982.

118. Korner AF and Thoman EB: The relative efficacy of contact and vestibular-proprioceptive stimulation in soothing neonates, *Child Dev* 43:443, 1972.

119. Korner AF and others: Effects of waterbed flotation on premature infants: a pilot study, *Pediatrics* 56:361, 1975.

120. Korones SB: *High risk newborn infants,* ed 3, St Louis, 1981, Mosby.

121. Krabill E: Who is the infant at risk for CNS deficit? In Wilson J, editor: *Infants at risk: medical and therapeutic management,* ed 2, Chapel Hill, 1982, University of North Carolina Press.

122. Kraybill EN: Infants with birth weights less than 1,001 g, *Am J Dis Child* 138:837, 1984.

123. Kukla A, Fry C, and Goldstein FJ: Kinesthetic needs in infancy, *Am J Orthopsychiatry* 30:452, 1960.

124. Lacey DJ and Terplan K: Intraventricular hemorrhage in full-term neonates, *Dev Med Child Neurol* 24:332, 1982.

125. Leander D and Pettett G: Parental response to the birth of a high-risk neonate: dynamics and management, *Phys Occup Ther Pediatr* 6(3/4):205, 1986.

126. Leonard E and others: Nutritive sucking in high risk neonates after perioral stimulation, *Phys Ther* 60:299, 1980.

127. Lester BB: Data analysis and prediction. In Brazelton TB: *Neonatal behavioral assessment scale,* ed 2, Philadelphia, 1984, JB Lippincott.

128. Levine MS and Kliebhan L: Communication between physician and physical and occupational therapists: a neurodevelopmental based prescription, *Pediatrics* 68:208, 1981.

129. Levitron A and Paneth N: White matter damage in preterm newborns—an epidemiologic perspective, *Early Hum Dev* 24:1, 1990.

130. Linton PT: Behavioral development of the premature infant, *Pediatrics* 29:175, 1986.

131. Lubchenco LO: *The high risk infant,* Philadelphia, 1976, WB Saunders Co.

132. Luchi JM, Bennett FC, and Jackson JC: Predictors of neurodevelopmental outcome following bronchopulmonary dysplasia, *Am J Dis Child* 145:813, 1991.

133. Manning J: Facilitation of movement—the Bobath approach, *Physiotherapy* 58:403, 1972.

134. Marquis PJ and others: Retention of primitive reflexes and delayed motor development in very low birth weight infants, *J Dev Behav Pediatr* 5:124, 1984.

135. Marsden DJ: Reduction of head flattening in preterm infants, *Dev Med Child Neurol* 22:507, 1980.

136. Martin RJ and others: Effect of supine and prone positions on arterial oxygen tension in the preterm infant, *Pediatrics* 63:528, 1979.

137. Mattilainen R: The value of correction for age in the assessment of prematurely born children, *Early Hum Dev* 15:257, 1987.

138. Mayo NE: The effect of physical therapy for children with motor delay

and cerebral palsy: a randomized clinical trial, *Am J Phys Med Rehabil* 70:258, 1991.

139. Measel CP: Non-nutritive sucking during tube feedings: effect on clinical course in premature infants, *Obstet Gynecol Neonat Nurs* 8:265, 1979.

140. Mercer RT: *Nursing care for parents at risk,* Thorofare, New Jersey, 1977, Slack Inc.

141. Milani-Comparetti A and Gidoni EA: Routine developmental examination in normal and retarded children, *Dev Med Child Neurol* 9:631, 1967.

142. Miller G and others: Follow-up of preterm infants: is correction of the developmental quotient for prematurity helpful? *Early Hum Dev* 9:137, 1984.

143. Minde K and others: Impact of delayed development in premature infants on mother-infant interaction: a prospective investigation, *J Pediatr* 112:136, 1988.

144. Mitchell JS: *Taking on the world: empowering strategies for parents of children with disabilities,* New York, 1982, Harcourt Brace Jovanovich.

145. Morales WJ: Effect of intraventricular hemorrhage on the one-year mental and neurologic handicaps of the very low birth weight infant, *Obstet Gynecol* 70:111, 1987.

146. Morgan AM and others: Neonatal neurobehavioral examination, *Phys Ther* 68:1352, 1988.

147. Morris SE: Assessment and treatment of children with oral-motor dysfunction. In Wilson JM, editor: *Oral-motor function and dysfunction in children,* Chapel Hill, 1974, University of North Carolina Press.

148. Morris SE: *The normal acquisition of oral feeding skills: implications for assessment and treatment,* New York, 1982, Therapeutic Media Inc.

149. Mueller HA: Facilitating feeding and prespeech. In Pearson PH and Fieber N, editors: *Physical therapy services in the developmental disabilities,* Springfield, Ill, 1972, Charles C Thomas.

150. Neal MV: Vestibular stimulation and developmental behavior of the small premature infant, *Nurs Res Rep* 3:2, 1968.

151. Nelson KB and Ellenberg JH: Neonatal signs as predictors of cerebral palsy, *Pediatrics* 64:225, 1979.

152. Nelson KB and Ellenberg JH: Children who "outgrew" cerebral palsy, *Pediatrics* 69:529, 1982.

153. Nelson KB and Ellenberg JH: Antecedents of cerebral palsy, *N Engl J Med* 315:81, 1986.

154. Nickel RE, Bennett FC and Lamson FN: School performance of children with birth weights of 1,000 g or less, *Am J Dis Child* 136:105, 1982.

155. Noble-Jamieson CM and others: Low birth weight children at school age: neurological, psychological, and pulmonary function, *Semin Perinatol* 6:266, 1982.

156. Nugent JK: The Brazelton neonatal behavioral assessment scale: implications for intervention, *Pediatr Nurs* 42:18, 1981.

157. Nugent JK: *Using the NBAS with infants and their families: guidelines for intervention,* White Plains, New York, 1985, March of Dimes Birth Defects Foundation.

158. O'Neil S: Personal communication, School of Nursing, University of Washington, Seattle, Wash, May, 1986.

159. Paban M and Piper MC: Early predictors of one year neurodevelopmental outcome for "at risk" infants, *Phys Occup Ther Pediatr* 7:17, 1987.

160. Paine RS: Early recognition of neuromotor disability in infants of low birthweight, *Dev Med Child Neurol* 11:455, 1969.

161. Paine RS: Neurologic exam of infants and children, *Pediatr Clin North Am* 0:471, 1960.

162. Palisano RJ and others: Chronological vs. adjusted age in assessing motor development of healthy twelve-month-old premature and full-term infants, *Phys Occup Ther Ped* 5:1, 1985.

163. Palmer FB and others: The effects of physical therapy on cerebral palsy, *N Engl J Med* 318:803, 1988.

164. Paneth N: Etiologic factors in cerebral palsy, *Pediatr Ann* 15:193, 1986.

165. Pape KE and others: The status at two years of low-birth-weight infants born in 1974 with birth weights of less than 1,001 000 gm, *J Pediatr* 92:253, 1978.

166. Pape KE and Wigglesworth JS: Hemorrhage, ischemia and the perinatal brain, In *Clinics in Developmental Medicine,* Nos 69 and 70, Philadelphia, 1979, JB Lippincott.

167. Papile L and others: Incidence and evolution of subependymal and intraventricular hemorrhage: a study of infants with birth weights less than 1,500 gm, *J Pediatr* 92:529, 1978.

168. Papile L and others: Relationship of cerebral intraventricular hemorrhage and early childhood neurologic handicaps, *J Pediatr* 103:273, 1983.

169. Parer JT: Evaluation of the fetus during labor, *Curr Probl Pediatr* 12:1, 1982.

170. Parmelee AH and Michaelis MD: Neurological examination of the newborn. In Hellmuth J, editor: *Exceptional infant,* vol 2, New York, 1971, Brunner/Mazel Inc.

171. Partington MD and others: Head injury and the use of baby walkers: a continuing problem, *Ann Emerg Med* 20:652, 1991.

172. Peabody JL and Lewis K: Consequences of newborn intensive care, In Gottfried AW and Goither JL, editors: *Infant stress under intensive care,* Baltimore, 1985, University Park Press.

173. Piper MC and others: Early physical therapy effects on the high-risk infant: a randomized controlled trial, *Pediatrics* 78:216, 1986.

174. Piper MC and others: Resolution of neurological symptoms in high-risk infants during the first two years of life. *Dev Med Child Neurol* 30:26, 1988.

175. Pharaoh POD and others: Birthweight specific trends in cerebral palsy, *Arch Dis Child* 65:602, 1990.

176. Piper MC and Darrah J: *Motor assessment of the developing infant,* Philadelphia, 1994, WB Saunders.

177. Prechtl H: The neurological examination of the full-term newborn infant, ed 2, *Clinics in Developmental Medicine,* No 63, Philadelphia, 1977, JB Lippincott.

178. Prechtl H and Beintema D: The neurological examination of the newborn infant, *Clinics in Developmental Medicine,* No 12, London, 1964, Heinemann Educational Books Inc.

179. Provost B: Normal development from birth to 4 months: extended use of the NBAS-K, Part I, *Phys Occup Ther Pediatr* 2:39, 1980.

180. Provost B: Normal development from birth to 4 months: extended use of the NBAS-K, Part II, *Phys Occup Ther Pediatr* 1:19, 1981.

181. Quinton M: Personal communication, Neurodevelopmental treatment baby course, Puyallup, Washington, July 1982.

182. Resnick MB and others: Developmental intervention for low birth weight infants: improved early developmental outcome, *Pediatrics* 80:68, 1987.

183. Rice RD: Neurophysiological development in premature infants following stimulation, *Dev Psychol* 13:69, 1977.

184. Robinson RO: Pathogenesis of intraventricular hemorrhage in the low-birthweight infant, *Dev Med Child Neurol* 21:815, 1979.

185. Rogers B and others: Cystic periventricular leukomalacia and type of cerebral palsy, *Dev Med Child Neurol* 35 (Suppl 69):22, 1993.

186. Rosenblith JF: Relations between neonatal behaviors and those at eight months, *Dev Psychol* 10:779, 1974.

187. Rosenblith JF and Anderson-Huntington R: Behavioral examination of the neonate, In Wilson J, editor: *Infants at risk: medical and therapeutic management,* ed 2, Chapel Hill, 1982, University of North Carolina Press.

188. Ross G and others: Perinatal and neurobehavioral predictors of one-year outcome in infants < 1500 grams, *Semin Perinat* 6:317, 1982.

189. Roth SC and others: Relationship between ultrasound appearance of the brain of very preterm infants and neurodevelopmental impairment at eight years, *Dev Med Child Neurol* 35:755, 1993.

190. Rothberg AD: Infants weighing 1,000 grams or less at birth: developmental outcome for ventilated and nonventilated infants, *Pediatrics* 71:599, 1983.

191. Russell C: Transition to parenthood: problems and gratifications, *J Marriage Fam* 36:294, 1974.

192. Saigal S and others: Decreased disability rate among 3-year-old survivors weighing 501 to 1000 grams at birth and born to residents of a geographically defined region from 1981 to 1984 compared with 1977 to 1980, *J Pediatr* 114:839, 1989.

193. Saint-Anne Dargassies S: Neurodevelopmental symptoms during the first year of life, *Dev Med Child Neurol* 14:235, 1972.

194. Saint-Anne Dargassies S: Long-term neurological follow-up study of 286 truly premature infants I: neurological sequelae, *Dev Med Child Neurol* 19:462, 1977.

195. Saint-Anne Dargassies S: Normality and normalization as seen in a long-term neurological follow-up of 286 premature infants, *Neuropadiatrie* 10:226, 1979.

196. Sameroff AI, editor: Organization and stability of newborn behavior: a commentary on the Brazelton neonatal behavioral assessment scale, *Monogr Soc Res Child Dev* No. 5-6, 1978.

197. Scarr-Salapatek S and Williams ML: A stimulation program for low birth weight infants, *Am J Public Health* 62:662, 1972.

198. Scarr-Salapatek S and Williams ML: The effects of early stimulation on low-birth-weight infants, *Child Dev* 44:99, 1973.

199. Scafidi FA and others: Effects of tactile/kinesthetic stimulation on the clinical course and sleep/wake behavior of preterm neonates, *Infant Behav Dev* 9:91, 1986.

200. Schneider JW, Griffith DR and Chasnoff IJ: Infants exposed to cocaine in utero. Implications for developmental assessment and intervention, *Inf Young Child* 2:25, 1989.

201. Scull S and Deitz J: Competencies for the physical therapist in the neonatal intensive care unit (NICU), *Pediatr Phys Ther* 1:11, 1989.

202. Schneider JW, Lee W, and Chasnoff IJ: Field testing of the Movement Assessment of Infants, *Phys Ther* 68:321, 1988.

203. Schertzer AL and Tscharnuter I: *Early diagnosis and therapy in cerebral palsy*, New York, 1982, Marcel Decker.

204. Scott S and others: Weight gain and movement patterns of very low birthweight babies nursed on lambs wool, *Lancet* II, 1014, 1983.

205. Sell EJ and others: Early identification of learning problems in neonatal intensive care graduates, *Am J Dis Child* 139:460, 1985.

206. Shonkoff JP and Hauser-Cram P: Early intervention for disabled infants and their families: a quantitative analysis, *Pediatrics* 80:650, 1987.

207. Siegel LS: Reproductive, perinatal, and environmental variables as predictors of development of preterm (<1501 grams) and fullterm children at 5 years, *Semin Perinatol* 6:274, 1982.

208. Simeonsson RJ, Cooper DH, and Scheiner AP: A review and analysis of the effectiveness of early intervention programs, *Pediatrics* 69:635, 1982.

209. Skidmore MD, Rivers A, and Hack M: Increased risk of cerebral palsy among very low-birthweight infants with chronic lung disease, *Dev Med Child Neurol* 32:325, 1990.

210. Slater MA and others: Neurodevelopment of monitored versus nonmonitored very low birth weight infants: the importance of family influences, *Dev Behav Pediatr* 8:278, 1987.

211. Sostek AM and others: Developmental outcome of preterm infants with intraventricular hemorrhage at one and two years of age, *Child Dev* 58:779, 1987.

212. Spellacy WN, editor: *Management of the high-risk pregnancy*, Baltimore, 1975, University Park Press.

213. Stanley FJ: The changing face of cerebral palsy, *Dev Med Child Neurol* 29:263, 1987.

214. Stanley FJ and English DR: Prevalence of and risk factors for cerebral palsy in a total population cohort of low-birthweight (<2000 g) in infants, *Dev Med Child Neurol* 28:559, 1986.

215. Stangler SR and others: *Screening growth and development of preschool children*, New York, 1980, McGraw-Hill Book Co.

216. Stengel TJ: The neonatal behavioral assessment scale: description, clinical uses, and research implications, *Phys Occup Ther Pediatr* 1:39, 1980.

217. Stevenson RE: *The fetus and newly born infant—influences of the prenatal environment*, St Louis, 1973, Mosby.

218. Stewart A and others: Prediction in very preterm infants of satisfactory neurodevelopmental progress at 12 months, *Dev Med Child Neurol* 30:53, 1988.

219. Stewart AL and others: Probability of neurodevelopmental disorders estimated from ultrasound appearance of brains of very preterm infants, *Dev Med Child Neurol* 29:3, 1987.

220. Stuberg W and others: *The Milani-Comparetti motor development screening test: test manual*, Omaha, Nebraska, 1987, Meyer Children's Rehabilitation Institute.

221. Swanson MW and others: Identification of neuromotor abnormality at 4 and 8 months by the Movement Assessment of Infants, Abstract, *Dev Med Child Neurol* 30:23, 1988.

222. Swanson MW: Neuromotor assessment of low birthweight infants with normal developmental outcome, *Dev Med Child Neurol* 31 (Suppl 59):27, 1989.

223. Swanson MW and others: Identification of neurodevelopmental abnormality at four and eight month by the movement assessment of infants, *Dev Med Child Neurol* 34: 321, 1992.

224. Sweeney JK: Neonatal hydrotherapy: an adjunct to developmental intervention in an intensive care nursery setting, *Phys Occup Ther Pediatr* 3:20, 1983.

225. Sweeney JK: Physiological adaptation of neonates to neurological assessment, *Phys Occup Ther Pediatr* 6:155, 1986.

226. Sweeney JK: Physiological and behavioral effects of neurological assessment in preterm and full-term neonates, abstracted, *Physical Occup Ther Pediatra* 9(3):144, 1989.

227. Sweeney JK: Assessment of the special care nursery environment: effects on the high risk infant. In Wilhelm IJ, editor: *Physical therapy assessment in early infancy*, New York, 1993, Churchill Livingstone.

228. Sweeney JK and Chandler LS: Neonatal physical therapy: medical risks and professional education, *Inf Young Child* 2(3):59, 1990.

229. Tjossem TD: Early intervention: issues and approaches. In Tjossem TD, editor: *Intervention strategies for high risk infants and young children*, Baltimore, 1976, University Park Press.

230. Tronik E and Brazelton TB: Clinical uses of the Brazelton neonatal behavioral assessment scale. In Friedlander BZ, Sterritt GM, Kirk GE, editors: *Exceptional infant*, vol 3, New York, 1975, Brunner/Mazel.

231. Trykowski L and others: Enhancement of nutritive sucking in premature infants, *Phys Occup Ther Pediatr* 1:27, 1982.

232. Valvano J and DeGangi GA: Atypical posture and movement findings in high risk pre-term infants, *Phys Occup Ther Pediatr* 6:71, 1986.

233. vanderLinden D: Ability of the Milani Comparetti developmental examination to predict motor outcome, *Phys Occup Ther Pediatr* 5:27, 1985.

234. Vaucher YE: Understanding intraventricular hemorrhage and white-matter injury in premature infants, *Inf Young Children* 1:31, 1988.

235. Vohr BR and Garcia Coll CT: Neurodevelopmental and school performance of very low-birth-weight infants: a seven year longitudinal study, *Pediatrics* 76:345, 1985.

236. Vohr BR and others: Neurodevelopmental and medical status of low-birthweight survivors of bronchopulmonary dysplasia at 10 to 12 years of age, *Dev Med Child Neurol* 33:690, 1991.

237. Volpe JJ: Perinatal hypoxic-ischemic brain injury, *Pediatr Clin North Am* 23:383, 1976.

238. Volpe JJ: *Neurology of the newborn,* ed 2, Philadelphia, 1987, WB Saunders.
239. Volpe JJ and Koenigsberger R: Neurologic disorders. In Avery GB, editor: *Neonatology,* ed 2, Philadelphia, 1981, JB Lippincott.
240. Wagaman MJ and others: Improved oxygenation and lung compliance with prone positioning of neonates, *J Pediatr* 94:787, 1979.
241. Webb ZW: Developmental care in the neonatal intensive care unit, *Dimens Crit Care Nurs* 1:221, 1983.
242. White JL and Labarba RC: The effects of tactile and kinesthetic stimulation on neonatal development in the premature infant, *Dev Psychobiol* 9:569, 1976.
243. Widmayer SM and Field TM: Effects of Brazelton demonstrations for mothers on the development of preterm infants, *Pediatrics* 67:711, 1981.
244. Wigglesworth JS and Pape KE: An integrated model for haemorrhagic and ischaemic lesions in the newborn brain, *Early Hum Dev* 2:197, 1978.
245. Wilhelm IJ: The neurologically suspect neonate, In Campbell SK, editor: *Pediatric neurologic physical therapy,* New York, 1985, Churchill Livingstone.
246. Wilhelm IJ: The neurobehavioral assessment of the high-risk neonate. In Wilhelm IJ, editor: *Physical therapy assessment in early infancy,* New York, 1993, Churchill Livingstone.
247. Williamson WD and others: Survival of low–birth-weight infants with neonatal intraventricular hemorrhage, *Am J Dis Child* 137:1181, 1983.
248. Wolf LS and Glass RP: *Feeding and swallowing disorders in infancy: assessment and management,* Tucson, 1992, Therapy Skill Builders.

APPENDIX A

Neurological sign	SCORE					
	0	1	2	3	4	5
Posture						
Square window	90°	60°	45°	30°	0°	
Ankle dorsiflexion	90°	75°	45°	20°	0°	
Arm recoil	180°	90°-180°	<90°			
Leg recoil	180°	90°-180°	<90°			
Popliteal angle	180°	160°	130°	110°	90°	<90°
Heel to ear						
Scarf sign						
Head lag						
Ventral suspension						

App. A. Evaluation Form of Clinical Assessment of Gestational Age in the Newborn Infant. (From Dubowitz LMS and others: *J Pediatr* 77;1, 1970.)

Scoring system for external criteria

External sign	Score*				
	0	**1**	**2**	**3**	**4**
Edema	Obvious edema of hands and feet; pitting over tibia	No obvious edema of hands and feet; pitting over tibia	No edema		
Skin texture	Very thin, gelatinous	Thin and smooth	Smooth; medium thickness; rash or superficial peeling	Slight thickening; superficial cracking and peeling especially of hands and feet	Thick and parchment-like; superficial or deep cracking
Skin color	Dark red	Uniformly pink	Pale pink, variable over body	Pale; only pink over ears, lips, palms or soles	
Skin opacity (trunk)	Numerous veins and venules clearly seen, especially over abdomen	Veins and tributaries seen	A few large vessels clearly seen over abdomen	A few large vessels seen indistinctly over abdomen	No blood vessels seen
Lanugo (over back)	No lanugo	Abundant; long and thick over whole back	Hair thinning especially over lower back	Small amount of lanugo and bald areas	At least half of back devoid of lanugo
Plantar creases	No skin creases	Faint red marks over anterior half of sole	Definite red marks over > anterior half; indentations over < anterior third	Indentations over > anterior third	Definite deep indentations over > anterior third
Nipple formation	Nipple barely visible; no areola	Nipple well defined; areola smooth and flat, diameter <0.75 cm	Areola stippled, edge not raised, diameter <0.75 cm	Areola stippled, edge raised, diameter >0.75 cm	
Breast size	No breast tissue palpable	Breast tissue on one or both sides, <0.5 cm diameter	Breast tissue both sides; one or both .05-1.0 cm	Breast tissue both sides; one or both >1 cm	
Ear form	Pinna flat and shapeless, little or no incurving of edge	Incurving of part of edge of pinna	Partial incurving whole of upper pinna	Well-defined incurving whole of upper pinna	
Ear firmness	Pinna soft, easily folded, no recoil	Pinna soft, easily folded, slow recoil	Cartilage to edge of pinna, but soft in places, ready recoil	Pinna firm, cartilage to edge; instant recoil	
Genitals Male	Neither testis in scrotum	At least one testis high in scrotum	At least one testis right down		
Female (with hips half abducted)	Labia majora widely separated, labia minor protruding	Labia majora almost cover labia minora	Labia majora completely cover labia minora		

From Dubowitz LMS and others: *J Pediatr* 77:1, 1970.
*If score differs on two sides take the mean.

APPENDIX B   *PARENT EDUCATION MATERIALS*

Parent's guide: developmental support of low-birthweight infants
Susan Dockendorf Thurber, PT
Lynda Brookshire Armstrong, OTR
Source: Office of Educational Resources
          Texas Children's Hospital
          P.O. Box 20269
          Houston, TX

Handling your young premature baby at home
Joanne Valvano, PT
Rochelle Gevens, MS
Source: R. R. Givens
          P.O. Box 2922
          Alexandria, VA 22301

Guiding your child through preterm development
Tim Healy MS
Source: Tim Healy MS, PRT, Inc.
          Infant and Child Development Specialist
          Orange, CA 92666

Homecoming for babies after intensive care nursery: a guide for parents in supporting their baby's early development
Marci J. Hanson PhD
Kathleen VandenBerg MA
Source: Pro-Ed
          8700 Shoal Creek Blvd
          Austin, TX 78758

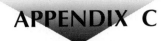

APPENDIX C

Movement Assessment of Infants with 4-Month Profile

Name_____

Case number_____

Examiner_____

Total risk score [____]

Date of examination_____

Birth date_____

Chronological age_____

Gestational age_____

Corrected age_____

Muscle tone

Items 1 to 6, 9, and 10 should be coded by the scale below.
Code items 7 and 8 as explained in the instructions for these items in the manual.

0—Item omitted
1—Hypotonic
2—Greater than hypotonic but less than normal
3—Normal
4—Greater than normal but less than hypertonic
5—Hypertonic
6—Fluctuating, variable

								Distribution variations		Asymmetries		
								Upper	Lower	Left	Right	
1	2		4	5	6	___	1. Consistency	___	___	___	___	1
1	2		4	5	6	___	2. Extensibility	___	___	___	___	2
1	2		4	5	6	___	3. Passivity	___	___	___	___	3
1	2		4	5	6	___	4. Posture in supine	___	___	___	___	4
1	2		4	5	6	___	5. Posture in prone	___	___	___	___	5
1	2		4	5	6	___	6. Posture in prone suspended	___	___	___	___	6
		3	4			___	7. Asymmetry					
		3	4			___	8. Distribution variation					
1	2		4	5	6	___	9. Summary of tone extremities	___	___	___	___	9
1	2		4	5	6	___	10. Summary of tone truck	___	___	___	___	10

[_____]

Primitive reflexes

Items 1 to 12 should be coded by the scale below.
Code items 13 and 14 as explained in the instructions for these items in the manual.

0—Item omitted
1—Integrated or not elicited
2—Incomplete response
3—Complete response
4—Dominant

					Asymmetries		
					Left	Right	
2	3	4	___	1. Tonic labyrinthine reflex in supine	___	___	1
2	3	4	___	2. Tonic labyrinthine reflex in prone	___	___	2
	3	4	___	3. Asymmetrical tonic neck reflex (evoked)	___	___	3
	3	4	___	4. Asymmetrical tonic neck reflex (spontaneous)	___	___	4
	3	4	___	5. Moro	___	___	5
	3	4	___	6. Tremulousness	___	___	6
	3	4	___	7. Palmar grasp	___	___	7
		4	___	8. Plantar grasp	___	___	8
	3	4	___	9. Ankle clonus	___	___	9
	3	4	___	10. Neonatal positive support	___	___	10
	3	4	___	11. Walking reflex	___	___	11
	3	4	___	12. Trunk incurvation (galant)	___	___	12
	3	4	___	13. Asymmetry			
	3	4	___	14. Summary of primitive reflexes			

[_____]

App. C. Scoring sheet for Movement Assessment of Infants with 4-month profile. (From Chandler LS and others: *Movement assessment of infants: a manual.* Rolling Day, Washington, 1980. Copyright © 1980 by Lynette S. Chandler, Mary Skillen Andrews, Marcia W. Swanson.)

Automatic reactions

Items 1 to 14 should be coded by the scale below.
Code items 15 and 16 as explained in the instructions for these items in the manual.

0—Item omitted
1—Complete and consistent response
2—Incomplete or incorrect response
3—Partial response
4—No response

							Asymmetries		
							Left	*Right*	
	3	4	_____	1.	Head righting (lateral)		_____	_____	1
2	3	4	_____	2.	Head righting (extension)		_____	_____	2
	3	4	_____	3.	Head righting (flexion)		_____	_____	3
		4	_____	4.	Landau		_____	_____	4
		4	_____	5.	Rotation in trunk		_____	_____	5
		4	_____	6.	Equilibrium reactions in prone		_____	_____	6
			_____	7.	Equilibrium reactions in sitting				7
			_____	8.	Equilibrium reactions in vertical suspension				8
			_____	9.	Downward parachute		_____		9
			_____	10.	Protective extension (forward)		_____		10
			_____	11.	Protective extension (side)		_____		11
			_____	12.	Protective extension (backward)		_____	_____	12
	3	4	_____	13.	Placing of feet		_____	_____	13
	3	4	_____	14.	Placing of hands		_____	_____	14
	3	4	_____	15.	Asymmetry		_____	_____	15
	3	4	_____	16.	Summary of automatic reactions		_____	_____	16

[   ]

Volitional movement

Items 1 to 23 should be coded by the scale below.
Code items 24 and 25 as explained in the instructions for these items in the manual.

0—Item omitted
1—Complete and consistent response
2—Incomplete or incorrect response
3—Partial response
4—No response

							Asymmetries		
							Left	*Right*	
		4	_____	1.	Hearing		_____	_____	1
	3	4	_____	2.	Visual following		_____	_____	2
	3	4	_____	3.	Peripheral vision		_____	_____	3
		4	_____	4.	Vocalization		_____	_____	4
2	3	4	_____	5.	Head centering		_____	_____	5
	3	4	_____	6.	Head position (anterior/posterior)		_____	_____	6
	3	4	_____	7.	Head balance		_____	_____	7
	3	4	_____	8.	Active weight bearing through shoulders		_____	_____	8
	3	4	_____	9.	Open hands		_____	_____	9
	3	4	_____	10.	Hands to midline		_____	_____	10
			_____	11.	Large grasp		_____	_____	11
			_____	12.	Small grasp		_____	_____	12
			_____	13.	Reaches out		_____	_____	13
			_____	14.	Combines		_____	_____	14
			_____	15.	Transfers		_____	_____	15
		4	_____	16.	Back straight in sitting		_____	_____	16
		4	_____	17.	Active use of hips		_____	_____	17
			_____	18.	Rolling		_____	_____	18
			_____	19.	Prone progression		_____	_____	19
			_____	20.	Sits when placed		_____	_____	20
			_____	21.	Coming to sit		_____	_____	21
			_____	22.	Coming to stand		_____	_____	22
			_____	23.	Walking		_____	_____	23
	3	4	_____	24.	Asymmetry		_____	_____	24
	3	4	_____	25.	Summary of volitional movement		_____	_____	25

[   ]

App. C, cont'd. Scoring sheet for Movement Assessment of infants with 4-month profile.

APPENDIX D

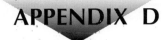

Movement Assessment of Infants with 8-Month Profile

Name_____ Date of examination_____

Case number_____ Birth date_____

Examiner_____ Chronological age_____

Gestational age_____

Total risk score [   ] Corrected age_____

Muscle tone

Items 1 to 6, 9, and 10 should be coded by the scale below.
Code items 7 and 8 as explained in the instructions for these items in the manual.

0—Item omitted
1—Hypotonic
2—Greater than hypotonic but less than normal
3—Normal
4—Greater than normal but less than hypertonic
5—Hypertonic
6—Fluctuating, variable

							Distribution variations		Asymmetries		
							Upper	Lower	Left	Right	
1	2		4	5	6	___	1. Consistency	___	___	___ ___	1
1	2		4	5	6	___	2. Extensibility	___	___	___ ___	2
1	2		4	5	6	___	3. Passivity	___	___	___ ___	3
1	2		4	5	6	___	4. Posture in supine	___	___	___ ___	4
1	2		4	5	6	___	5. Posture in prone	___	___	___ ___	5
1	2		4	5	6	___	6. Posture in prone suspended	___	___	___ ___	6
		3	4			___	7. Asymmetry				
		3	4			___	8. Distribution variation				
1	2		4	5	6	___	9. Summary of tone (extremities)	___	___	___ ___	9
1	2		4	5	6	___	10. Summary of tone (truck)	___	___	___ ___	10

[   ]

Primitive reflexes

Items 1 to 12 should be coded by the scale below.
Code items 13 and 14 as explained in the instructions for these items in the manual.

0—Item omitted
1—Integrated or not elicited
2—Incomplete response
3—Complete response
4—Dominant

					Asymmetries		
					Left	Right	
2	3	4	___	1. Tonic labyrinthine reflex in supine	___	___	1
2	3	4	___	2. Tonic labyrinthine reflex in prone	___	___	2
2	3	4	___	3. Asymmetrical tonic neck reflex (evoked)	___	___	3
2	3	4	___	4. Asymmetrical tonic neck reflex (spontaneous)	___	___	4
2	3	4	___	5. Moro	___	___	5
2	3	4	___	6. Tremulousness	___	___	6
2	3	4	___	7. Palmar grasp	___	___	7
		4	___	8. Plantar grasp	___	___	8
2	3	4	___	9. Ankle clonus	___	___	9
2	3	4	___	10. Neonatal positive support	___	___	10
2	3	4	___	11. Walking reflex			11
2	3	4	___	12. Trunk incurvation (galant)	___	___	12
	3	4	___	13. Asymmetry			
2	3	4	___	14. Summary of primitive reflexes			

[   ]

App. D. Scoring sheet for Movement Assessment of Infants with 8 month profile. (From *Movement assessment of infants*, PO Box 4631, Rolling Bay, Washington, 98361. Copyright © 1980 by Lynette S. Chandler, Mary Skillen Andrews, Marcia W. Swanson.)

Automatic reactions

Items 1 to 14 should be coded by the scale below.
Code items 15 and 16 as explained in the instructions for these items in the manual.

0—Item omitted
1—Complete and consistent response
2—Incomplete or incorrect response
3—Partial response
4—No response

						Asymmetries		
						Left	*Right*	
2	3	4	____	1.	Head righting (lateral)	____	____	1
2	3	4	____	2.	Head righting (extension)	____	____	2
	3	4	____	3.	Head righting (flexion)	____	____	3
	3	4	____	4.	Landau	____	____	4
2	3	4	____	5.	Rotation in trunk	____	____	5
2	3	4	____	6.	Equilibrium reactions in prone	____	____	6
	3	4	____	7.	Equilibrium reactions in sitting	____	____	7
	3	4	____	8.	Equilibrium reactions in vertical suspension	____	____	8
	3	4	____	9.	Downward parachute	____	____	9
2	3	4	____	10.	Protective extension (forward)	____	____	10
2	3	4	____	11.	Protective extension (side)	____	____	11
			____	12.	Protective extension (backward)	____	____	12
2	3	4	____	13.	Placing of feet	____	____	13
2	3	4	____	14.	Placing of hands	____	____	14
	3	4	____	15.	Asymmetry	____	____	15
2	3	4	____	16.	Summary of automatic reactions	____	____	16

☐

Volitional movement

Items 1 to 23 should be coded by the scale below.
Code items 24 and 25 as explained in the instructions for these items in the manual.

0—Item omitted
1—Complete and consistent response
2—Incomplete or incorrect response
3—Partial response
4—No response

						Asymmetries		
						Left	*Right*	
2	3	4	____	1.	Hearing	____	____	1
2	3	4	____	2.	Visual following	____	____	2
2	3	4	____	3.	Peripheral vision	____	____	3
	3	4	____	4.	Vocalization	____	____	4
2	3	4	____	5.	Head centering	____	____	5
2	3	4	____	6.	Head position (anterior/posterior)	____	____	6
2	3	4	____	7.	Head balance	____	____	7
2	3	4	____	8.	Active weight bearing through shoulders	____	____	8
2	3	4	____	9.	Open hands	____	____	9
2	3	4	____	10.	Hands to midline	____	____	10
2	3	4	____	11.	Large grasp	____	____	11
		4	____	12.	Small grasp	____	____	12
2	3	4	____	13.	Reaches out	____	____	13
			____	14.	Combines	____	____	14
2	3	4	____	15.	Transfers	____	____	15
	3	4	____	16.	Back straight in sitting	____	____	16
	3	4	____	17.	Active use of hips	____	____	17
2	3	4	____	18.	Rolling	____	____	18
2	3	4	____	19.	Prone progression	____	____	19
2	3	4	____	20.	Sits when placed	____	____	20
		4	____	21.	Coming to sit	____	____	21
			____	22.	Coming to stand	____	____	22
			____	23.	Walking	____	____	23
	3	4	____	24.	Asymmetry	____	____	24
2	3	4	____	25.	Summary of volitional movement	____	____	25

☐

App. D, cont'd. Scoring sheet for Movement Assessment of infants with 8-month profile.

Cerebral Palsy

Christine A. Nelson

KEY TERMS

cerebral palsy
athetosis
hypotonia
handling

direct verses indirect
  intervention
spastic diplegia
spastic quadriplegia
rhizotomy

LEARNING OBJECTIVES

After reading this chapter the student/therapist will:
1. Identify the parameters of the diagnosis of cerebral palsy including motor, family, and psychosocial components.
2. Analyze the multifaceted aspects of the clinical problem and appreciate a multifaceted approach to evaluation and treatment.
3. Identify treatment approaches and their appropriate match with clinical problems.
4. Recognize the role of the therapist as a guide in helping the child reach his or her optimal level of functional independence within the social, family, and financial limitations of the child's environment.

OVERVIEW
Definitions, parameters, anticipated changes

Cerebral palsy presents a conglomerate of complexities.[2] The diagnosis has historically referred to a lack of oxygen or some related insult to the brain shortly before, during, or shortly after the birth process. The repercussions of that insult to the brain fall into patterns that are not always neatly organized. Earlier categorizations of the types of cerebral palsy have proved inconsistent because a single child may move from one diagnostic category to another during the maturation process. There may be associated perceptual and learning problems, as well as developmental deprivation of movement experience. Record keeping is inaccurate because of the various definitions applied. In one center a child is identified as having cerebral palsy, whereas in another the same child is labeled as having "psychomotor dysfunction" or developmental delay. At times the diagnosis is applied rather carelessly to infants who have sustained gross damage to the entire brain or who have conditions such as primary microcephaly. As we are confronted by new concepts of brain functioning,[15,46,54,62] we may have to completely revise our hypotheses of causation.

The Little Club, named for the physician who first defined the condition of cerebral palsy, described it as "a persistent disorder of movement and posture appearing early in life and due to a developmental nonprogressive disorder of the brain."[44] Dr. Bobath elaborates that "the lesion affects the immature brain and interferes with the maturation of the central nervous system, which has specific consequences in terms of the type of cerebral palsy which develops, its diagnosis, assessment, and treatment."[11]

Another controversy has been the span of time over which the diagnosis may be applied. Vining and others[63] report that their center uses a limit of 3 years of age for applying the diagnosis, whereas the American Association for Cerebral Palsy (AACP) recognizes damage occurring to the central nervous system (CNS) before 5 years. The age limit set is somewhat arbitrary, but it tends to recognize the early plasticity of the immature brain.[32] This also creates some confusion in specific diagnosis, because there is immediately an overlap with traumatic head injuries, brain infections, near-drownings, and episodes that directly affect brain function. The alert therapist, however, will find more similarities than differences in the treatment for the clinical consequences of these events. More complete coverage of these conditions may be found in Chapters 14 and 17.

Milani-Comparetti[45] has presented for consideration a new classification of cerebral palsy based on characteristic fetal movement patterns. Ultrasound now permits professionals to appreciate the wide variability of movements in utero, as well as the movement responses to specific changes in the external environment. Researchers have also identified changes in the rate and type of movement that precedes death of the fetus.

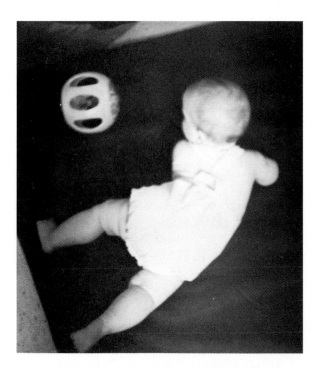

Fig. 9-1. Normal babies accumulate a multitude of experiences as they move smoothly in their environments.

Clinically, therapists have to deal with the visible signs. These observable changes can be evaluated early in a child's development.[9] Therapists are attempting to evaluate the interference of pathological signs and symptoms in comparison to normal or nearly normal responses made by the child. The lack of or distortion of righting reactions against gravity is a strong clue to the presence of a neuromotor disorder.[8] As these righting reactions normally occur early in development, they provide one means of early identification of the infant who is in trouble.[9] Informed individualized home handling can change the outlook for this population. Older children also change significantly with intensive physical treatment that takes into account the tactile, proprioceptive, and vestibular aspects of the condition. It is essential for therapists to realize that they are dealing with a developing human being with emotional needs—an emerging personality within a personal environment. Physical limitations as well as perceptual distortions are to be assessed. Nothing less than a holistic view of the problem will change the life pattern of the client who requests assistance to make change.[37]

The pathological signs observed in cerebral palsy can be related to postural adjustments against gravity with uncoordinated movement of poorly dissociated body parts. The interference with function therefore is greater as normal developmental tasks demand control of the body in an upright alignment. To the naive observer, the increased difficulty may give the erroneous impression that the basic condition is worsening. There is no evidence to suggest that the condition itself worsens, but the will of children directs them to use whatever movement potential they possess to explore their environment and to become acquainted with their own bodies. Vining and others state unequivocally that cerebral palsy "is not a specific disease state with an accepted cause, pathogenesis, pathological picture, clinical presentation, treatment, or prognosis."[63] Bobath[10] has documented the course of development in the presence of various forms of cerebral palsy, but also stresses the uniqueness of each child and that child's particular constellation of pathological and normal responses. It is true that active use of the abnormal patterns of movement tends to reinforce the pathology and consequently block the expression of the more differentiated normal developmental progression[9] (Fig. 9-1).

The osteopathic profession calls our attention to their correlation of constellations of physical characteristics with cranial findings that offer the possibility of relieving specific pressures that impede proper craniosacral rhythms as well as venous and cerebrospinal fluid circulation.[61] Documentation of cranial abnormalities in the newborn has been in the literature for the last 40 years.[1] The infant or young child treated in this way by the cranial osteopathic physician tends to move the head more appropriately and postural tone is modified.[27] General alertness is often affected in a positive way. The intervention is accomplished in a limited number of sessions, and the child generally is better able to retain the changes obtained by the therapist in direct therapeutic handling.

Because early development depends so heavily on motor responses, all areas of development are potentially affected.[46,53,56] There can also be primary physiological limitations. The most common of these is the limited movement of the eyes when head control fails to develop. There is a paucity of eye movement and frequently limitations in the use of the two eyes together. Malnourishment, often compounding the intrauterine conditions, can develop or be continued because of poor sucking patterns and inadequate processing of ingested food. In fact, low birthweight for age is a significant feature of infants who become identified as having cerebral palsy.[30] Poor circulation relates directly to inadequate respiratory patterns and lack of movement. The sensory system is deprived from the beginning and conse-quently fails to mature appropriately. There is no question that cerebral palsy must be considered a sensorimotor dysfunction (Fig. 9-2).

The parents' concern and their feelings of inadequacy in dealing with this atypical infant further compound the developmental frustrations and thus affect personality development. Early therapeutic and educational programming can play a strong role in fostering emotional health for the child and the family. It is essential to support positive developmental responses and to avoid overidentification of inabilities. Parents are caught in the therapist's professional dilemma of symptomatic diagnosis. The very characteristics that constitute the base for the labeling process are those features that change with the application of treatment strategies. This makes documentation of change vital for the continued learning of family and professional alike. Slides, film, or videotape sequences can provide a sample of a

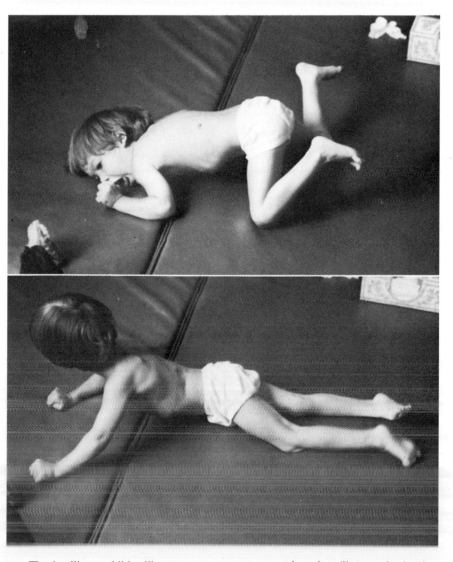

Fig. 9-2. The intelligent child will attempt movement even when the effort results in abnormal patterns.

child's function on a particular date. The therapist gains much from the review of such visual aids and has a base from which change may be evaluated more objectively.

The overwhelmingly positive aspect of cerebral palsy is that its outcome can be positively influenced by informed and specific therapeutic intervention. Changes in population statistics have been clearly documented.[38] Individual cases can also be used as their own control, because the presence of pathology makes certain outcomes predictable with no intervention. Intelligence and motivation also have their role in anticipating potential direction of change, particularly as the child grows older and initiates activity.

Family reactions

No one ever expects to give birth to a disabled child. Parents are looking for normal, healthy responses from their infant and, consequently, allow a wide latitude in their labeling of "normal."[2] In spite of this, most parents identify a problem long before it is acknowledged by professionals. Well-intentioned pediatricians are more fully prepared to cope with the medical needs of the normal child and tend to believe that this child will follow the majority of high-risk infants and "outgrow" the problematic delay. At our present level of knowledge, only the more severely damaged child can be identified at birth, although the traumatized newborn needs evaluation by the skilled professional. Dealing with premature infants and their high risk factors is addressed in detail in Chapter 8.

As the early months pass, suspicions accumulate to the point that they can no longer be ignored. Even when a "problem" is acknowledged, a formal diagnosis may not be applied. Humanistically, this is an advantage to the infant who joins the ranks of the "normal" after a relatively brief period of intensive treatment. A series of visits to specialists may be the next experience of the family. It may be assumed that the parents in most instances make clear observations of developmental difficulties during this period, but in general they do not have the background to relate one finding to another nor the cause to the effect. Because there tends to be a reluctance on the part of professionals to begin intervention without a diagnosis, this period of searching by the family may require extended expenditure of time, energy, and financial investment. This investment without immediate return results in varying levels of frustration. Siblings may be somewhat neglected during this critical search for help. No wonder parents appear suspicious and less than totally cooperative when they first arrive in the new therapeutic environment.

Diagnosis and the time of intervention

In some instances there is an early diagnosis, which offers the possibility for better parental understanding. An early diagnosis, however, may be accompanied by dire predictions as to the limited future of the child. Because these forecasts are presented to the parents in a moment of extreme emotional stress, they tend to make a strong impression. This colors the interaction between parent and infant and severely restricts the expectations of the parents. The therapist needs to be aware of these early experiences and the parents' view of their child when discussing treatment goals. Even early communicative attempts on the part of the child may be rejected as "not possible" and thus not reinforced. Inexperienced therapists should learn from this situation and avoid giving a specific prognosis until they have sufficient clinical experience to be certain of the observations made. It is important to encourage the parents to be alert to responses of the infant and young child and to offer consistent psychosocial stimulation. If the infant has merely spent developmental time resting in bed or sitting passively in the same chair, the therapist may find deprivation compounding the physical and sensory limitations (Fig. 9-3). In actual practice, parents more often need help in seeing the positive responses and specific changes of their child. They need to acknowledge the child as a unique human being.

Although there is reason to supplement the young child's learning environment when definite limitations exist, clinicians must also maintain a strong sense of respect for the child's capacity to compensate. There are numerous examples of persons developing better than normal intelligence in spite of their inability to move or even speak.[54] Therapists can not be expected to have all the answers for how this is accomplished. By keeping a balanced perspective, therapists can offer meaningful help at a moment when the parents are ready to receive it. The child does not exist in a vacuum, nor is treatment the only activity in the life of the family.

The most important contribution of therapists may be their ability to provide practical information based on clinical experience with similar children.[18] It is vital that the guidance offered be appropriate to the family's view of the situation. Once the parents begin to see results from the new positioning and home handling (Fig. 9-4), they find their tension sufficiently reduced and begin to ask questions and regain some of their shaky self-confidence in parenting. A problem that is unknown is always more threatening and "impossible" than one that is understood.

Parents sometimes need specific reminders to avoid focusing all their energy on the disabled child.[66] Siblings often feel as helpless and guilty as the adults in this situation. Their life experience has been altered dramatically. Older children may profit from talking with the therapist directly to understand the movement problems of their sister or brother. It is important to enlist their cooperation in avoiding overstimulation that strengthens abnormal reactions. Some children born into the family after the disabled child may accept the situation without question. However, others may have vague fears that something like that could happen to them. At times, children may find it appealing to have the attention received by the disabled child. Normal siblings may even "wish" to have cerebral palsy themselves in order to receive more attention from parents or to experience the

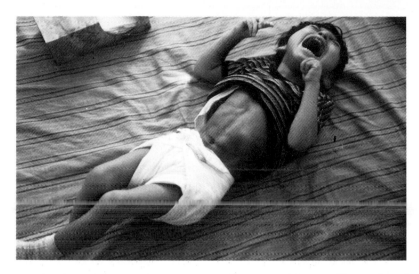

Fig. 9-3. Emotional reactions are also translated into further spasticity (see Chapter 5 on the limbic system).

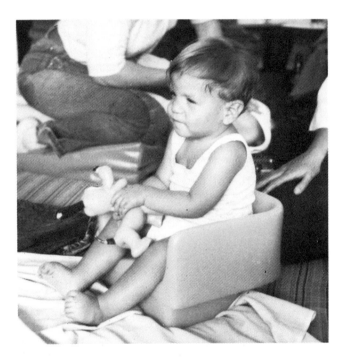

Fig. 9-4. Positioning need not be complicated to achieve a new play opportunity while primitive abduction is inhibited.

relationship that the sibling has with therapists or special teachers.

Cultural and familial value systems bear directly on the interaction of the family with the professional help they seek and receive. Socioeconomic factors and the existence of insurance may determine what assistance the family is able to offer the child. It is always helpful to determine how the family is currently viewing the problem and what they consider to be the major difficulty of the moment. The more therapists take these psychosocial factors into account, the

more effective their influence will be to help the child. (See Chapter 7 on psychosocial adjustment.)

Diagnostic categorization of the characteristics of cerebral palsy

In general, diagnosis of cerebral palsy suggests that the individual in question has some central disorder of posture and movement. In addition, the labeling process often identifies the parts of the body that are primarily involved. Diplegia, hemiplegia, and quadriplegia, respectively, indicate that the lower extremities, one side of the body, or all four extremities are affected.

The clinician must be aware that the categorization of cerebral palsy is based on descriptions of observable characteristics: it is a symptomatic description. Both Dr. Little, who first identified the condition, and Dr. Winthrop Phelps, who differentiated the characteristic types of cerebral palsy, were describing the spontaneous movement attempts away from the resting posture. These characteristic movement patterns were identified as spasticity, athetosis, hypotonicity, and ataxia (Fig. 9-5).

The hypertonus of spasticity prevents a smooth exchange between mobility and stability of the body. Incrementation of postural tone occurs with an increase in the speed of even passive movement. Although diagnostic terms reflect the distribution of excessive postural tone, the entire body must be considered to be involved. Spasticity by nature involves less movement, which makes its distribution easier to identify.

The term **athetosis** refers to a lack of posture. The excessive peripheral movement occurs without central stability. Athetosis may occur with greater involvement in particular extremities, although it most often interferes with postural stability as a whole. Athetoid distribution of postural tone is changeable, particularly during attempted movement.

Hypotonicity is another category of cerebral palsy, but may also mask undiagnosed degenerative conditions (see Chapter 10). A young infant with the picture of **hypotonia** may also be a precursor of athetosis. Often the athetoid movements are not noticed until the infant is attempting antigravity postures, although there may be some disorganization apparent to the careful observer. Tone changes with attempted movement may be present even without the peripheral signs of athetosis.

Ataxia is a cerebellar disorder that is seen more frequently as a sequela of tumor removal (see Chapters 22 and 23) than as a problem occurring from birth. Probably because of changes in delivery practices, it seems to occur with less frequency now than it did when Dr. Phelps categorized the types of cerebral palsy. Ataxic reactions are often noted in the gait of an athetoid individual. However, more specific analysis may reveal compensatory responses to the athetoid tone changes while the body is in motion through space. (See Chapters 3 and 4 on motor control evaluations.) It has also been my clinical experience that a high proportion of these individuals can be assisted more effectively by working with the visual system than with the postural system alone.

There are also individuals who demonstrate athetoid tone changes within a range of hypertonicity or hypertonic distributions of postural tone superimposed on athetotic disorganization. The developing child may move from one predominant postural tone to another. Treatment intervention may reveal finer nuances of difference in the distribution of postural tone as total patterns are inhibited[58] and reflexive reactions are integrated.

These classifications, when accurately applied, give the therapist only a general idea of the treatment problem. Supplementation of this information will occur with a specific analysis of posture and movement, an interview for homecare information, and assessment of treatment responses. The therapist is then ready to establish treatment priorities for the individual child.

Many of the characteristics described in the preceding paragraphs also apply to children who have suffered closed head traumas or brain infections. Further information can be obtained in Chapters 14 and 17. Some of the treatment suggestions that follow may also be applied in such cases. As with cerebral palsy, early positioning and handling may deter many problems later.

EVALUATIVE ANALYSIS OF THE INDIVIDUAL CHILD
Initial observations

Assessment of the individual child begins with careful observation of the interaction between parents and the child, including parental handling of the child that occurs spontaneously (Fig. 9-6).

Much insight can be gained about the relationship

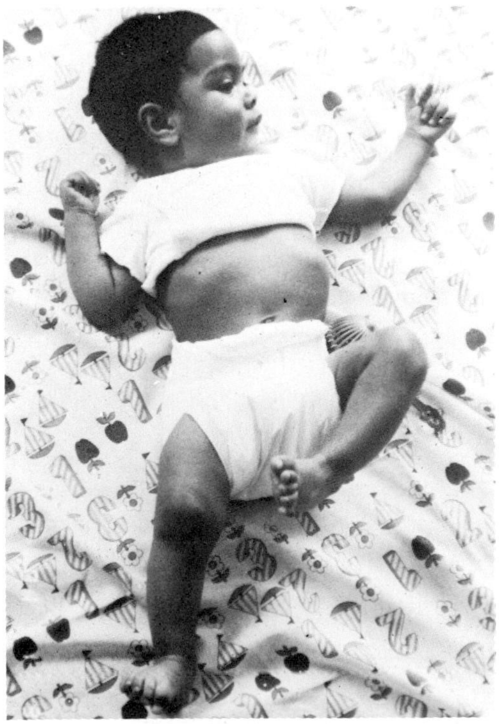

Fig. 9-5. Asymmetry in this immobile 8-month-old infant is a clue to right hemiparesis caused by porencephaly.

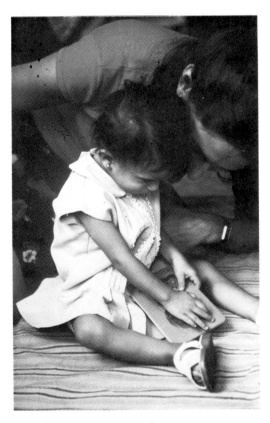

Fig. 9-6. Emotional nurturing by the parent is vital for the child's optimal development.

between parent and child by observing whether the child is overprotected or perhaps thrust toward the therapist immediately. Does the child receive and respond to verbal reassurance from the parent in this new situation? Are excessive bribes offered to the child? Does communication convey the idea of negativity in the therapy situation or an "unfortunate experience that will soon come to an end"? This orientation directly affects the response of the child while working with the therapist.

The therapist working as part of a team will have the advantage of a social worker or psychologist who will work to understand the problems and motivations of the parents. Much of parent behavior toward the disabled child arises from their own uncertainty, fear, concern for the future, disappointment, distress and other reactions to this unforeseeable life experience. The therapist will observe positive changes in parent orientation to the child as the parent is educated as to what can be done to help their child move forward. They will be further assisted by contact with well-adjusted parents of older children so that their bleak or absent image of the future begins to have some hope.

While observing the child, the experienced therapist may extend this initial interaction by eliciting from the parents their view of the problem. By listening carefully, the therapist will also be able to discern the emotional impressions that have surrounded previous experiences with professionals. Sometimes what is not said is more important than what is offered immediately. Listening carefully and clarifying facts are more important than overwhelming the parents with excessive information and suppositions during this early contact. Observation of the response to information will keep the therapist on track in developing a positive relationship with parents that will grow over time.

The next general step is to observe, in as much detail as possible, the spontaneous movement of the child when separated from the parent. Is the child very passive? Does he or she react to the supporting surface? Are there abnormal patterns of movement to reach a toy (Fig. 9-7)? Are clearly normal responses occurring with specific interference by reflexive synergies or total patterns of movement? Does the child rely heavily on visual communication? Do the eyes focus on a presented object? Do they follow hand activity? Does an effort to move result only in an increase of postural tone with abnormal distribution?

This type of observation is valuable, because movement patterns directly reflect the state of the CNS and can generally be obtained while the parent is still handling the child.[13] Once the child is on the mat, one can more easily remove outer clothing to observe movement patterns. Movement responses of the child can gradually be influenced directly by the therapist. Many disabled children associate immediate undressing in a new environment with a doctor's office, and the chance to establish rapport is lost. In some instances it is preferable to have the parent gently remove the child's clothing.

Assessment of the child's status is more likely to be adequate if the therapist follows the child's lead where possible. Notes can later be organized to conform to a specific format. It is often possible to jot down essential information while observing the child moving spontaneously or while the parent is still holding the child. The reactions to the supporting surface will differ in these circumstances. After the session one can dictate the salient information into a tape recorder. Attention should be given to the normal movements of the child as well as to those postures that the child spontaneously attempts to control. It is important to notice the interaction between the two sides of the body. In noting abnormal reactions and compensatory movement patterns, one must also indicate the position of the body with respect to gravity. One tends to compile more pertinent data by learning to cluster observations, relating one to the other. Children are vibrant beings. Choices of position tell us something about their habits and how comfortable they are in this situation. To be the slave of a preformulated sequence destroys the decision-making initiative appropriate to the situation at hand. This is true for the therapist as well as the child.

Each child will differ in ability to separate from his or her parents. Spontaneity of movement, interest in toys, general activity level, and communication skills will also vary from child to child. Responding to the specific needs of the child enables the therapist to set priorities more effectively. If fatigue is likely to be a factor, it is important to evaluate first those reactions that present themselves spontaneously, followed by direct handling to determine near normal responses. Those for which there is a major interference by spasticity or reflexive responses may better be checked at the termination of the assessment. Information regarding favor-

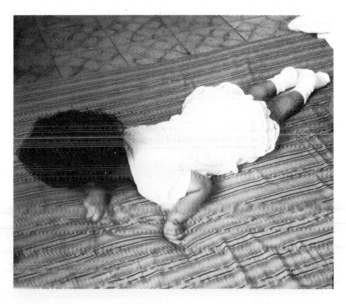

Fig. 9-7. Play experience or exploration for this child is limited to abnormal patterns of movement.

ite sleeping positions and chair supports used can be requested as the session comes to a close.

Reactions to placement in a position

If the child totally avoids certain postures during the spontaneous activity, these are likely to be the more important positions for the therapist to evaluate. Placement of the child in the avoided position will permit the therapist to feel the resistance that prevents successful control by the child. The parent should play an active role in the assessment whenever possible. Continued dialogue with the parent reveals factors such as the frequency of a poor sitting alignment at home or a habitual aversion to the prone position. These contributions by the parent establish the importance of good observation and the need for parent and therapist to work cooperatively.

Following the guide of normal development,[29,43] infants should be able to maintain a posture in which they are placed before they acquire the ability to move into that position alone.[39] The problems presented by cerebral palsy occur primarily as a reaction to the field of gravity in which the child moves.[9] Visual perceptions of spatial relationships motivate and determine movement patterns, but the child must react at a somatic level to the support surface. It is helpful therefore to attempt placement of the infant or child into developmentally/functionally appropriate postures that are not assumed spontaneously (Fig. 9-8). Resistance to placement indicates an increase in postural tone, a structural problem, or an inability to adapt to the constellation of

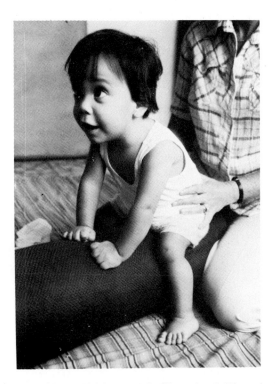

Fig. 9-8. Simple positioning can facilitate head lift and visual contact with the environment.

sensory inputs for that alignment. It is important to keep in mind that a movement that resists control by the therapist will be even less possible for the child. What appears to be a passive posture may in some children hide rapid increases in postural tone when movement is initiated. Such a child has learned to avoid excitation of the unwanted reactions and may fix the body position to avoid the alignment for which he or she is not prepared. Another child may enjoy the sensory experience of accelerated postural tone changes and deliberately set them off.

Abnormal interferences

Abnormal responses that interfere with postural adjustments by the infant or child with cerebral palsy may have been normal at some point in development. Reflexive reactions that are retained beyond the point at which they should have been integrated block the normal differentiation of movement. Postural transitions or movement sequences become distorted and poorly timed if they are initiated at all. In normal development the integration of reflexive reactions follows a sequence that correlates with the acquisition of motor skills.[8] Fiorentino[26] and others[12,29] view these early reflexive reactions as the establishment of efficient patterns of movement that are used even in adult life. These synergistic combinations of movement patterns help to limit degrees of freedom (see Chapter 4) and allow success or function in a desired movement strategy. They may also be viewed as systematic, organized cues that guide the motor responses. Hellebrandt and others[33] predictably elicited the asymmetrical tonic neck reflex (ATNR) in normal college students by placing them in a prone position across a hammock-type support. With the subjects blindfolded and the arms unsupported, voluntary turning of the head to the side was resisted by the examiner. The response obtained in the arm position was the typical ATNR with the face arm extended and the skull arm flexed. Children with cerebral palsy will also vary greatly as to the amount of effort required to activate a stereotypical synergy. The most severely involved individuals almost never move out of the stereotypical patterns, whereas the mildly involved child who runs or reacts emotionally to a situation becomes transiently bound by reflexive reactions. The level at which the reflexive responses interfere with function is most significant. The therapist must also be aware of the reflexive synergies most active in each position of the body (Fig. 9-9, *A* and *B*).

These patterns of movement may be used by the child to accomplish functional skills of daily living, but the patterns are limited in degrees of freedom and thus would be considered abnormal. In such cases reflexive reactions and abnormal distribution of postural tone are reinforced by constant use. Differentiated levels of motor control are prevented from developing, and the child seems to plateau in motor development. At this point parents may seek help to elaborate the necessary sensorimotor base for more sophisticated function. It is more effective to avoid the child's early use of abnormal patterns than to attempt to change established habits superimposed on the use of abnormal synergies.

Motor learning depends on many factors, and there is not yet agreement on the motor development process.[20] By understanding more clearly why abnormal responses become dominant, therapists will become more effective in guiding new motor control.[16] Refer to Chapters 2-4 for additional information.

Primary and compensatory patterns

Compensatory patterns must be taken into account when assessing function. They commonly are mistaken for primary postural reactions, possibly resulting from the distribution of spasticity. One of the most common misunderstandings occurs with the presence of the "toe-walking" response. The distribution of postural tone usually is stronger in flexor patterns, serving to pull the individual down into gravity. In the standing alignment, as the body weight is displaced forward, it is accentuated by hip flexion and the forward position of the center of gravity. With undifferentiated responses of the legs and lack of lateral weight shift, the spastic child counteracts the pull of flexion with a total pattern of extension. The plantar flexion of the foot is only one small component of the total postural picture. This same postural response will be observed in a person with a shift forward of the visual midline.[48]

Careful analysis of the postural adjustments and movement patterns of the cerebral palsied child is crucial to initiating effective therapeutic intervention. The interaction of many factors creates the final picture (Fig. 9-10). Normal reactions to abnormal distribution of tone may distort gait as easily as a lack of adequate trunk extension or marked pelvic immobility. In addition to the physical factors, the sensory aspects of the condition often interfere with the quality of movement. Tactile sensitivity may interfere with foot placement or prevent sustained grasp of a toy or an eating utensil. It is important for the therapist to intervene at the proximal articulation first to determine whether tissue immobility is the interfering factor, which is especially likely in the case of retraction of the upper limbs. Learning experiences associated with firm pressure input to the hands and feet are prevented, and the consequent normal evolution of the sensory system is limited. The therapist may want to simulate normal weight-bearing by the application of firm pressure against the palms of the hands and the soles of the feet. Slight movement of the extremity will facilitate the adaptation. This experience of firm pressure tends to inhibit the withdrawal and prepare for weight-bearing over the limb.

Consideration of foot support is crucial to influence a more normal distribution of postural tone and a better alignment. Heavy controls and limitation of ankle mobility are to be avoided. Detailed attention to the dynamic balance of the foot itself, a stability that permits mobility in gait, brings greater successful adaptation.

The orthotic that seems the most efficient and applicable in the clinical setting was developed by orthotist D. Buethorn[16] working in close coordination with physical therapists N. Hylton and B. Uhri. Various trim lines address the need for more or less ankle stability, but the base always

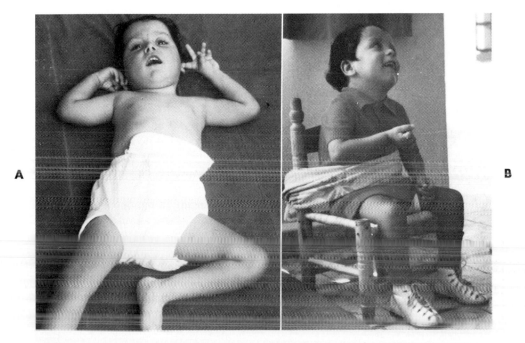

Fig. 9-9. **A,** Strong asymmetry and abnormal tone. **B,** Simple seating can inhibit strong asymmetry and make function a possibility.

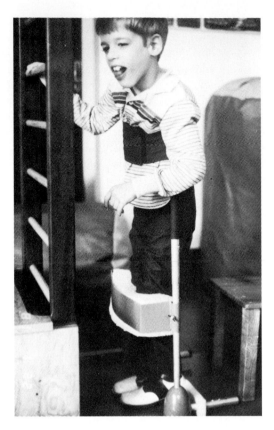

Fig. 9-10. The upright position can help to integrate abnormal postural patterns.

gives full support to the foot. A detailed tracing is made of the individual foot, and a plaster base is gradually formed to support the foot medially and laterally. The metatarsal heads and the heel are lowered into carved recesses. The toes are supported only to the extent that relaxation is achieved. Most often the leg is permitted forward-back mobility over the foot. With the additional security of anatomically correct support for the foot, tone is reduced in the legs, and weight-bearing is aligned to protect foot development. (For additional information on orthotic devices refer to Chapter 32.)

Compensation processes have their positive aspects. The independence finally achieved by the older child reflects his or her intelligence and motivation, as well as the family attitude toward the child and the disability. The most debilitating "handicap" of cerebral palsy may be social or psychological in nature, when the child is not accepted by the family and therefore cannot accept himself or herself.[66] Early treatment not only prevents physical limitations, but also assists the parents in understanding their child and the disability.

The visual system in cerebral palsy

The visual system in its development has many parallels with the postural system.[6] Binocular control and freedom of movement are necessary for the system to function properly. Too often a simple "eye exam" checks acuity at 20 feet on the eye chart or simply checks the health of the eye structure. These tests do not relate to true function of the system.

In the case of a child with cerebral palsy there has been, by definition, a lack of adequate control of the head position, which would allow the eyes to develop sustained focus and orientation to the environment.[51] Without stable control of the neck, it is difficult for the eyes to develop adequate movement. With inadequate alignment of the head in relation to the base of support, the visual system accumulates distortions and inconsistent input, which leads to the formation of an inadequate perceptual base for later learning. Even after improvement in the control of posture and movement, the visual system continues to adapt to the faulty learning, resulting in perceptural confusion and inefficient organization of movement in space. Adequate visual skills develop from the establishment of a sound experiential base formed by the organized input and output of the primary and secondary visual abilities.

Working with children with cerebral palsy and with head trauma clients, Dr. William Padula,[48] behavioral optometrist, has defined a visual midline shift syndrome that can be easily tested. He has demonstrated impressive change in gait patterns by correcting the visual midline orientation to match the body orientation in space. Athetoid children who have plateaued in physical handling are able to reduce their base of support and their extraneous movement while walking after a few weeks of specific vision work. Children who walk on their forefoot or their toes, without having true Achilles contractures, also demonstrate a forward shift in their visual orientation. In many instances gait improves immediately by placing the proper lenses on the individual and is further established by using the lenses during facilitated movement provided in the therapy session. The eyes permit the individual to anticipate movement into space and provide constant feedforward to the system.

In some instances there will be an observable movement of the eyes, further apart or closer together, as the body has the opposite reaction while the child walks.[6] This suggests that the visual system may try to compensate for inadequacies of the postural system, just as the postural system will adjust the head to accommodate the eyes. Understanding the nature of the ongoing interaction between the two systems and attending to the needs of a visuo-postural function will increase the successful evolution of clients with cerebral palsy.[5]

DIRECT TREATMENT OR CASE MANAGEMENT

Simple documentation of observed changes in a child over a series of regular clinic visits is still too common for many children with cerebral palsy. Regular appointments, with periodic assignment of a new piece of apparatus, do not constitute active treatment. Although physical intervention in the form of direct handling of the child is considered a "conservative treatment" by most physicians,[55] there are relatively few children who receive sufficient physical treatment at an early age.[34] Therapists need to demonstrate their unique preparation and describe their interventions in ordinary language so that families understand the importance of specific treatment versus general programs of early "stimulation."

The prognosis for change in cerebral palsy is too often based on records of case management rather than on the effect of direct treatment. Bobath[10] documented more accurately the developmental sequence expected in the presence of spasticity or athetosis. This volume[10] consolidates some observations of older clients that help professionals understand the uninterrupted effects of the cerebral palsy condition. In any institution one can observe the tightly adducted and internally rotated legs, the shoulder retraction with flexion of the arms, and the chronic shortening of the neck so common as the long-term effects of cerebral palsy. The athetoid component provides movement to avoid contractures while creating a need to experience reliable postures for stability.

Responsible surgeons now recognize the improved outcome of their intervention if physical treatment, or a "conservative approach," is applied before and after the surgical procedure.[42] Tendon lengthenings for older children with average intelligence may be preceded by "muscle energy" work, in which the therapist assists the child in activating the desired muscle group. The therapist may then follow the controlled release with isometric activity inside the cast. Early standing in casts is to be highly recommended, as are specific footplates, to reduce potential sensory deprivation and to promote more rapid healing with improved circulation.[6,59,64]

Within the clinical community there is increasing evidence that soft tissue restrictions further limit spontaneous movement in children with cerebral palsy. That these local myofascial restrictions are often found in infants and very young children suggests that they originate early rather than as a gradual result of faulty movement patterns. Because of the tendency of fascial tissue to change in response to any physical trauma or strong biochemical change, some of these responses might be originating with traumatic birth experiences. They can also occur with immobilization or general infectious processes. Applying specific soft tissue treatment techniques to any person with a neuromotor disorder creates the need for immediate follow-up with appropriate motor learning activities. Creating excessive tissue mobility in a given area can also destroy the delicate patterns of coordination that permit function in the person with cerebral palsy.

As myofascial changes are closely related to biochemical changes, much research is needed in nutritional supplementation for young children with cerebral palsy. In many cases there has been poor intrauterine development, possibly complicated by an early birth and consequent immaturity.

Ecological medicine may provide some specific assistance in this area.

There is clear documentation[33,38] of epidemiological or population changes as a result of early intervention while the CNS is in a period of rapid growth and change. It is also important to offer the flexibility that permits short periods of intensive treatment for an individual child. Informed evaluation by developmentally knowledgeable physicians permits optimal use of effective treatment. We have long had evidence that neurological change occurs in small mammals as a result of physical handling and specific environmental experiences.[31] Now evidence for change in the human CNS as a result of therapeutic intervention is accumulating rapidly.[49]

Dr. Josephine Moore has highlighted some important points for therapists in her concept of "forcing" the system and her observations of the significance of the neck structures in developmental sequences.[3] The righting reactions used by both Rood and Bobath are completely dependent on neck functions. Spastic children often have a lack of developmental elongation of the neck, whereas athetoid children lack neck stability as well as postural stability. Moore suggests that our concept of "cephalo-caudal development" should be amended to consider development beginning at the neck and moving in both a "cephalo" and "caudal" direction. This is useful to the therapist who realizes that tone change most often originates with changes in the delicate interrelationship between head and body. Tone itself is developing in a caudocephalic direction, whereas antigravity control follows the cervico-cephalo-cervico-caudal pattern.

In applying Dr. Moore's notion of "forcing" the system, professionals must first gain an understanding of the function of various subsystems as well as the integrative action of the CNS as a whole. Appreciation of the abundance of polysynaptic neurons and polysensory receptors[3] will provide a much more optimistic view of the therapist's role as a "facilitator" of the system. At the same time, therapists have a responsibility to interpret and apply the feedback that they receive from the entire organism. Any stimulus that is of sufficient strength to make a positive change is also capable, under the right circumstances, of making a negative change to influence the quality of "output" in that moment. For example, excessive treatment to obtain extensor responses in the prone position can result in failure of the neck to elongate and inadequate balance of flexor tone to permit normal standing.

Treatment intervention is far from innocuous when responsibly applied. A truly "eclectic" treatment approach comes only after years of experience and a comprehensive understanding of various approaches. The effective therapist will gradually formulate a personal philosophy of treatment, with space for new ideas that arise from treatment feedback or from new knowledge about the CNS. One can never learn "too much" about the intricacies of normal development and its implications. With high quality treatment intervention there will be no doubt about the need for this service as a crucial aspect of case management.

ROLES OF THE THERAPIST
Role of the therapist in direct intervention

Nature of direct treatment for specific problems. The primary role of the therapist is in direct treatment or **handling** of the child with cerebral palsy. This should precede and accompany the making of recommendations to parents, teachers, and others handling the child. As with the initial assessment, many interventions will cause a reaction unique to the particular youngster.[23,52] It is the role of the therapist to ascertain the response of the child with accompanying difficulties in adaptation, to analyze the problems and choose the most effective intervention (Fig. 9-11). It will then be possible for other persons to manage play activities and supervise independent functioning that reinforces treatment goals.[57]

The child who is bound within the limitations of hypertonicity suffers first of all from a paucity of movement. As early attempts to move have resulted in the expression of limited synergistic postural patterns, the child generally loses incentive to attempt movement. The easily observed tightness in the limbs is not the major problem of these children. Looking past the obvious, one sometimes discovers that the stability that should be present in the shoulder structure to support good arm movement or in the pelvis to free the leg is replaced by mobility and low tone. The limb has

then taken on the role of "stabilizer" with the abnormal distribution of excessive tone or hypertonicity as a compensatory reaction due to lack of stabilization. As the trunk tone is normalized, the abnormally high tone in the limbs will be reduced. The compensatory reaction is no longer necessary.

Postures that are associated with an abnormal distribution of postural tone or that express abnormal patterns of movement should be avoided initially. Later in the treatment process the therapist will want to return to these positions to reduce tone in the active posture and gradually to turn over control to the child. One might think here of the child who lies in the supine position with extreme pushing back against the surface. The therapist would initially eliminate the supine position entirely but would incorporate into the treatment plan the activation of normal flexor tone in sitting with variations of pelvic tilt. Only gradually would the child be reintroduced to the independently controlled supine position.

A primary consideration for the spastic child is sufficient mobility of the chest wall and abdominal area to allow for near-normal respiration. Because rotation within the longitudinal axis of the body is frequently of poor quality or completely absent, respiratory patterns remain immature and superficial; differentiated or segmental rolling does not occur. A lack of sitting or antigravity postural control will limit even the physiological shaping of the rib cage itself, because the ribs do not have an opportunity to change their angle at the spine (Fig. 9-2). Initial treatment sessions with an older child must take into account the physiological stress induced by respiratory adaptation and tolerance must be

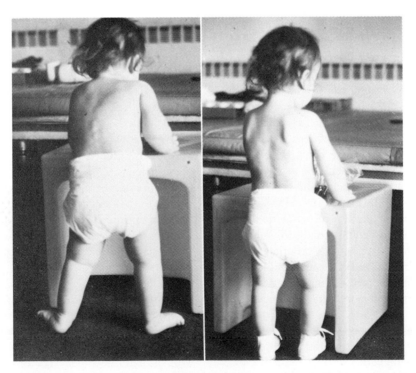

Fig. 9-11. Supportive shoes for the low-tone child unquestionably facilitate more normal trunk reactions and permit use of the hands for play.

increased gradually. The therapist is literally "forcing" an adaptation in the breathing pattern, which will then reinforce postural tone changes in the trunk itself. Normal respiratory adaptation will help to maintain normal trunk tone.

When working to change spasticity or excessive muscle tension, the therapist may find it useful to inhibit unwanted posturing, such as extension, by placing the body in an opposite alignment, such as flexion. While controlling the flexed position, one can deliberately stimulate extension by changing the body position in space or by controlled weight-bearing over the extensor surface. From a flexed body posture maintained by the therapist, the child might protectively extend an arm for support. Once the hand makes contact, the therapist can move the body weight over the limb to further normalize the postural tone while preventing the expression of total extensor patterns. In this way the threshold is gradually altered so that the child begins to tolerate some stimulation without immediately responding with the unwanted posturing—in this case, extension. By orienting more to the disordered learning process in movement control[60] the therapist can elicit new improved responses by manipulating environmental factors.

When there are distinct differences between the two sides of the body, the same control of position might be used in company with lateral weight shifts in standing. For example, the supporting leg may be maintained in extension while the body weight is guided over that side. Frequently, changes near midline are some of the more difficult stimuli for the disorganized system to accept. The shoulders must be assisted to align over the hip of the same side. Thus it may be necessary for the therapist to offer more specific cues for the change and even repeat the experience with a marked pause to allow integration of the new alignment at the sensory-proprioceptive level and time for the CNS to process the information.

While working with CNS disorders, the therapist often uses an intensity of stimulation somewhat beyond the range that is generally considered "normal." However, therapists must take into account that they are addressing a system that is deficient in its ability to perceive and to use the available input. If the microcosm of experience given the child during a treatment session is no more intense than an equal amount of time in his or her everyday living environment, the therapist has failed to utilize this unique opportunity to deliver a meaningful message that developmentally integrates the system.

Reassessment of direct treatment. The therapist actually functions as an extension of the child's CNS, organizing input as to intensity, frequency, and distribution to anticipate a desired response. The child may react positively, negatively, or inadequately to the sensory experience. The therapist immediately is confronted with the need to evaluate the quality of the motor response, much as an intact system monitors its own output and seeks further experience. Has the needed adaptation been achieved? Is the body tolerating

a variety of positions? Does the child adapt to the supporting surface? Is the movement of a limb graded and without unwanted associated reactions in other parts of the body? Is the child now ready to take over more independent control?

The therapist acts on the judgment made regarding the nature of the response obtained. The next "feedback" provided for processing by the child's CNS needs to challenge the system while assuring success and moving toward more normal control. In various ways, depending on the technique found to be most effective, the therapist is interrupting the child's customary abnormal feedback. At times the input of the therapist may only be a slight modification of the child's own response, such as an elongation of a limb as it is being moved. At other times the therapist may introduce a substitute for missed experiences. For example, with firm pressure on the sole of the foot, approximation of the lower extremity gives the system an impression similar to the pushing of a foot against the surface during normal movement within the home environment. This can be considered a component of the sensory experience of normal development (Fig. 9-12). Visual experiences can be altered with prism lenses to cause new postural responses.[48]

Too often professionals consider sensory input to be on a simple graded continuum. The picture is not so elementary.[22] It must be considered as at least a three-dimensional and possibly a four-dimensional phenomenon. Multiple sensory systems are simultaneously activated by most therapeutic input, while a variety of sights and sounds may be available in the immediate environment. Memory, previous learnings, and cognition are often activated by the therapist-child interaction. The therapist must be accustomed to continuous

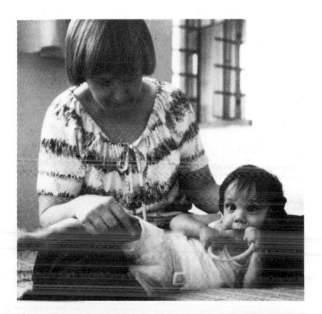

Fig. 9-12. Treatment sessions can consider a child's need for a teething experience while facilitating good postural patterns and tone distribution.

reassessment of the child's experiential needs as compared with the current input provided. The entire CNS is activated by the treatment experience. Input modification is determined by the therapist.

To philosophically explore the developmental meaning attached to the sensory experience of normal movement, therapists must take into account the ability to process contrasting stimuli. While several parts of the body are stable, another is moving. Stability of the proximal body permits a limb to extend forcefully or to be maintained in space. Each new level of differentiation or disassociation of movement increases the complexity of processing by the CNS (Fig. 9-13). Stimuli from within the body and from the environment impinge simultaneously on the CNS. This is easily illustrated with a review of self-feeding. Initially the process of guiding a full spoon into the mouth engages the child's full attention. In time this aspect of the task becomes automatic as the child participates in social exchanges with the family at the same time that he or she manages the physical task of taking the spoon to the mouth.

A solid understanding of normal developmental sequences is essential for the clinician. These insights confirm that earlier, simpler responses of the normal infant are constantly being integrated more completely by the acquisition of new developmental competence. (Elaboration of balance in sitting only occurs with the ability to pull to standing.) How is this knowledge to be applied by the therapist? The implication is that the therapist, functioning to screen input for the child's nervous system, can offer the child the experience of postural activities at a higher level than his or her present function permits. For this reason the assisted self-dressing process is an effective way to introduce and integrate new movement while using established skills. To sit well, the child must practice sitting, moving over the seated surface, coming in and out of sitting, which begins the plans of coming to standing (Fig. 9-14). To walk well, the child may need to run with control by the therapist. This allows practice in change of rate, direction, range, balance, etc. in walking patterns and leads to a new plan of running. At the same time, some of the treatment session is spent filling in gaps that represent missed experiences, such as squatting to play or coming to stand from kneeling or even attending to specific shifts over midline in prone. Preparation of the entire body with the most normal alignment and postural tone is vital to maximize the sensory experience of postural control. Specific techniques can be reviewed thoroughly in Chapter 6.

With the athetoid child, the therapist's role relates primarily to organization and grading of seemingly erratic movement. Initially, therapists provide the postural control that the child has not been able to achieve independently. Through their handling of the child they give stability from which movement can emerge. At a more sophisticated level the therapist grades the movement of limbs by structuring the postural control of the proximal body with special attention to head-trunk relationships. In some instances the therapist may maintain a limb in position to elicit active proximal

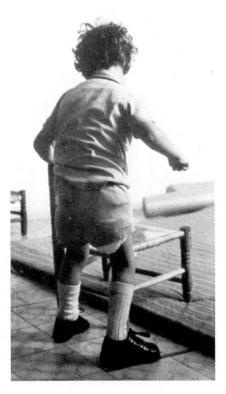

Fig. 9-13. This hemiplegic boy tries to move a chair by orienting only his more active side to the task and bearing weight only briefly on the more affected side.

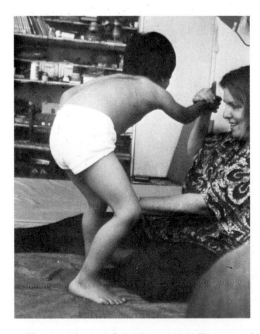

Fig. 9-14. The experience of coming to standing over the more affected side activates diagonal patterns of postural adjustment.

adjustments that are the basis of true postural control. The astute therapist will find that careful analysis of tone changes reveals, in many cases, a predictable pattern. One particular movement will initiate the interfering spasm or series of spasms that interrupt stability. This may be part of a reflexive or synergistic pattern, or it may be an isolated reaction. It is often useful to check for soft tissue restriction in the localized area. In the ambulatory athetoid child it is often the spontaneous depression or elevation of a scapula or the protraction of a shoulder that initiates tone change throughout the body. If this particular initiating action can be effectively inhibited, while righting reactions of the head and trunk are stimulated, the body begins to build a repertoire of responses that does not include the customary interference. With functional use of the upper extremity for support, reach, and grasp, the client shares with the therapist inhibition of the abnormal response. Gradually, the more normal use of the whole upper trunk integrates the interfering response, resulting in improved control for a variety of independently controlled postures. The therapist continues to introduce graded stress during treatment sessions to normalize even further the threshold for the unwanted reaction. Environmental stimuli such as sights, sounds, and social interaction should be considered as stimuli along with positional stress. Visual disorganization is a particularly difficult problem for the athetoid child, and it improves most when balanced activity of the visual and the postural systems have been achieved. Movement control must become procedural if independence is to be accomplished. Thus distracting the child's cognitive attention off the motor act onto the activity will allow for better procedural learning. This concept of graded stress is considered more thoroughly in Chapters 5 and 7.

Direct intervention for the hemiplegic child takes into account the obvious difference in postural tone between one side of the body and the other. However, treatment that addresses itself only to the more affected side of the body has seldom proved effective. The critical therapeutic experience seems to be that of integration of the two sides of the body. Normally, this begins early, with the lateral weight shifts of the infant in a variety of developmental patterns and the same postural organization that permits later reaching for a toy. The hemiplegic child needs assistance to experience those developmental patterns that include rotation within the longitudinal body axis and lateral flexion of the trunk. The therapist will find it profitable to spend time achieving active lateral flexion responses in the trunk. This may be controlled initially in side-lying and coming to sitting before active responses are expected in sitting and in prone. As with other instances of spasticity, one may find that true flexion of the more affected side of the body is fully as difficult for some children as the initial elongation of that side. There tends to be a high incidence of soft tissue restrictions in the shoulder and neck of the affected side. These children also seem to have difficulty in sustaining a posture against the influence

of gravity. This characteristic may contribute to the development of seemingly "hyperactive" behavior. The therapist must also be aware that hyperkinetic responses in one side of the body may compensate for inactivity in the opposite side. One goal of treatment is to approximate these divergent response levels.

The limbs of the hemiplegic child will change in postural tone as the trunk reactions are brought under control. Specific attention must also be given to sensory normalization. The two hands need to sustain the body weight simultaneously, as do the two feet. In effect, the discrepancy between the experiences of the two sides seems to lead the system to reject one of the messages. This can lead to distortions in verticality and is a major interference in bilateral integration. As body weight is shifted to the more normal side, flexor withdrawal patterns of the limbs increase in frequency and strength. The visual system often has a lateral midline shift, which increases the avoidance of weight on the more affected side.[48] One important therapy goal is the achievement of true weight shift in the pelvis during ambulation. Treatment preparation must incorporate a wide variety of more basic developmental alignments in which pelvic weight shift is a factor. The choice of prone, half-kneeling, or a simple weight shift, for example, will depend on the constellation of factors observed by the therapist at the time. Diagonal adaptations are particularly useful in normalizing the system. Dynamic foot supports will facilitate this lateral weight shift when the child is not in treatment. Careful attention must be given to pelvic alignment and mobility, because the more affected side of the pelvis is often rotated back, which causes hip flexion and may easily mislead the therapist during analysis of leg position. Although the more affected hand may not have sensation adequate for skilled activity, it needs to acquire sufficient shoulder mobility to move across the body midline and to assume a relaxed alignment during ambulation. This goal is best reached through a wide variety of weight-bearing postures, from the obvious developmental alignments to horizontal protective responses or walking the hands upward against a wall from the standing position (Fig. 9-15).

The low-tone child is perhaps the greatest challenge for therapist and parent alike. Adequate developmental stimulation is difficult unless positioning can be varied. Placing the child in a more upright alignment, even though it is achieved with complete support initially, seems to aid the incrementation of postural tone. To prepare the low-tone body for function, it is helpful to review areas of the articulations for possible soft tissue restrictions. The neck and shoulder girdle are particularly vulnerable. Strong proprioceptive input, while ensuring accurate postural alignment, is an important part of the treatment session. Direct "tapping," as described by the Bobaths,[11] also assists in maintaining antigravity positions. At all times the therapist must be cautious of high-tone responses only belatedly evident. This spasticity, which can be distributed in the deeper musculature, contrib-

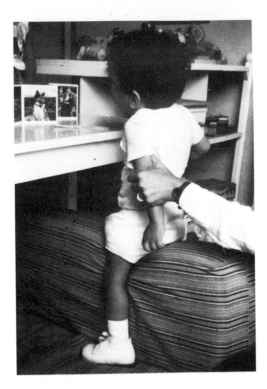

Fig. 9-15. Good upright alignment may be facilitated for brief periods of time to utilize the proprioceptive experience and to inhibit interfering tone changes.

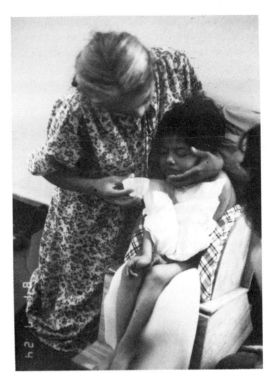

Fig. 9-16. Feeding the child with severe cerebral palsy requires patience and is made easier by an understanding of abnormal reactions and how to avoid them.

utes to fixation rather than differentiated postural control. Similarly, even though the child's motor output may remain low, the sensory and emotional systems may be on overload; thus keen observation by the therapist is critical.

The process of undressing and dressing can be a dynamic part of the treatment program. The diagonal patterns of movement incorporated into the removal of socks and shoes assist in the organization of midline. Weight shifts and changes in stability-mobility distribution occur throughout the dressing process. Concepts of direction and spatial orientation are applied to the relation of body parts and clothing. A bench is useful as it permits the adult to sit behind the beginner. The older child with difficult balance reactions can use the bench in a straddle sit alignment. Aside from the physical and perceptual benefits, this achievement is one that offers the child a feeling of pride and independence. It is also a very practical preparation for the future when it is introduced in keeping with the individual's developmental and emotional needs.

Developing a personal philosophy of treatment. The practicing therapist can never learn too much about the nuances of normal human development.[21] The dynamic interaction of developmental components rises to a new level of significance as the clinician gains awareness of this phenomenon as a reflection of CNS maturation. Increasing knowledge of the functional nature of sensory systems and CNS processing will influence the choice of treatment

techniques (Fig. 9-16). This knowledge will offer more depth and specificity to concepts of posture and movement, as well as a better understanding of the disorders of posture and movement in cerebral palsy. Based on individual experience, each therapist must develop a personal philosophy of treatment to incorporate emerging ideas and new perceptions of the problem of CNS dysfunction. Without this base, it is easy to become "victimized" by each promising treatment idea that presents itself. The therapist, without an internalized treatment goal toward which independent "techniques" are applied, remains ineffective and unconvincing. The therapist in a direct treatment situation must be secure in a concise, personalized visualization of what is to be achieved in the particular session with the individual child.

All of treatment like all of development is potentially a preparation for functional skills. Training in specific skills must begin with a thorough analysis of the whole person who happens to have cerebral palsy. Some have learned self-care along with brothers and sisters. Others have needed therapy guidance for each achievement. Intelligent children with strong motivation may only need some assistance in avoiding use of abnormal reactions, whereas others have poor spatial orientation and minimal motivation to achieve independence.

Adaptations of position and special equipment may be necessary to initiate independent activity. Finnie[25] has given many practical suggestions for new therapists and parents.

Brereton and others[14] have done an excellent job of grading perceptual-motor tasks and suggest alternate presentations that may better suit the individual child. Furth and Wachs[28] have also presented precognitive skill development according to the child's thinking strategy in a useful reference that is organized for the busy therapist.

Active involvement of the family. To be successful active treatment entails active home follow-up in the form of both physical and psychological handling of the child. This allows for variability of practice in different environments, which should promote greater motor learning. Parents who learn to help begin to understand the importance of their participation. This is not easy because parents have suffered in their own self-image when they learned of their child's disability. Although they should not be expected to become therapists per se, close observation of treatment sessions offers insight as to the child's current strengths and weaknesses. Parents can consequently adapt their expectations in keeping with the child's ongoing change. Parenting a child with cerebral palsy is no easy task, and the therapist will do well to develop respect for this demanding role. No one provides more for the cerebral-palsied child than the nurturing parent who guides the child to self-acceptance without destroying initiative.

The therapist must give serious thought to priorities in home recommendations. To be considered are the size of the family, outside employment of mother and father, physical capacity of the child, general health status of the child, and psychological acceptance of the problem within the family. The emotional needs of some parents demand a period of less, rather than more, direct involvement with the child. Other parents must be cautioned that repetition of an activity more times than recommended will not result in faster improvement. Both parent and therapist must appreciate the need for the CNS to have some time to integrate new experiences and to perfect emerging control of postural adjustments. Excessive control of movement patterns by an adult tends to reduce initiation of postural change and decrease motor learning. Health needs for good nutrition and adequate rest must also be considered.

Criteria for equipment recommendations. Equipment recommendations must take into account the physical space in the home and the amount of direct treatment available to the child (Fig. 9-17). Young children, in particular, can often use normal seating with slight adaptations. This is not only more socially acceptable, but also permits changes as required by developmental progress. Portability of supportive seats or standers encourages the family to take the apparatus along for weekend outings. Chair designs should also place children at an age-appropriate level in their environments. This permits a better quality of visual exploration and facilitates social exchange with siblings and visiting peers.

When planning the amount of physical support needed by the child, the therapist will do well to consider varying the

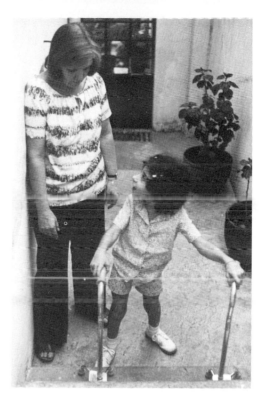

Fig. 9-17. True ability to "walk" must include problem solving for architectural barriers in the child's own environment.

structural control in relation to activity (Fig. 9-18). The child who is merely watching the play of others or a television presentation may successfully control trunk and head balance independently. However, concentration on hand skills or self-feeding may necessitate trunk control assistance by a chair insert to avoid the use of abnormal reactions. As the postural reactions become more integrated and hence more automatic, support should be diminished.

Particularly for the more severely disabled child, equipment should be easily and completely washable. Mothers, using one free hand, should be able to place special seating inserts into wheelchairs or travel chairs. Wheels should suit the family environment. Control straps and seating should be adaptable and allow for future change. The severely limited child needs seating changes at least once every hour during the day. Pleasing color, good quality upholstery, and professional finishing are important not only for the child, but also for the family who is accepting the equipment as part of a personal living environment.

As prices rise and the applicability of insurance changes, cost effectiveness must be considered more carefully by the therapist. Parents are often desperate to do everything possible for their child and tend to be very susceptible to high-powered advertising and reassuring sales personnel. By providing a list of essential equipment features, the therapist will aid the parents in becoming informed consumers. Perusal of several catalogs permits some comparison of

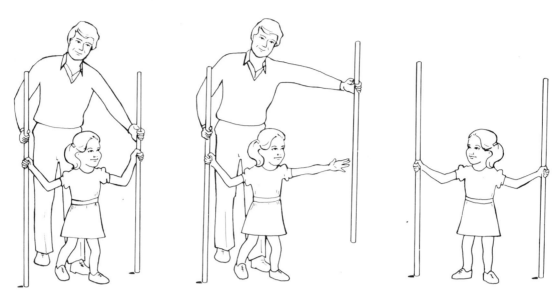

Fig. 9-18. The use of poles was introduced by the Bobaths as a transitional support for increasingly complex postural adjustments in standing.

quality and prices. Periodic review of equipment in use will encourage the family to stay current with the child's needs and pass along items that are no longer used to someone in need. Investment in expensive equipment also has the hidden effect of influencing both parent and therapist to continue its use when its effectiveness as a dynamic supplement to treatment has passed. For this reason more than any other, large investments must be thoroughly researched as to their long-term applicability.

The direct treatment of infants deserves special mention, as there are significant differences between the infant and the older child. Aside from the delicate situation of the new parents, the infant is less likely to have a diagnosis and presents a mixture of normal and abnormal characteristics. It is essential that the clinician has a strong foundation in the nuances of normal developmental movement and early postural control. Direct intervention can be offered as a means of enhancing development and overcoming the effects of a difficult or an early birth. It will be important, however, to secure a diagnosis for the infant who reaches 8 or 9 months of age and continues to need therapy.

Infants with early alterations in motor control should be followed until they are walking independently, even if they no longer need weekly therapy. Infant responses can change very rapidly as the therapist organizes the components of movement control. Soft tissue restrictions should be treated initially to have more success with facilitated movement responses. Careful observation is essential, as all but the severely involved infant will change considerably between visits.

Referral to other professionals is essential in the presence of possible allergies, new neurological signs, visual or auditory alterations, and persistent reflux. There is always the possibility of convulsions, which can occur in infants for a variety of reasons.

Role of the therapist in indirect intervention

For many children with cerebral palsy, active treatment is not available. Geographical isolation, socioeconomic factors, and lack of qualified therapists may interfere with the delivery of direct service. The therapist must then assume the role of teacher, counselor, or consultant. More often the new role emerges as one in which the therapist tries to meet a combination of needs and is frequently frustrated by lack of time, energy, and community resources. The therapist may be a member of a community team that includes a psychologist, a social worker, and a public health nurse. This sometimes creates more of a behavioral than a traditional medical orientation. Therapists can also be primarily responsible to the public school systems, introducing therapeutic positioning to classroom teachers. For these types of situations the clinician will now find videotape a valuable adjunct. The individual child may be filmed with equipment, positions or procedures. Useful topic oriented videotapes are also beginning to be available.

Physical positioning for the child who lacks direct treatment. When the therapist is seeing children who have no access to direct treatment, positioning is of paramount importance. The support must attempt to avoid contractures, scoliosis, and permanent limitations in range of movement. Even the most severely limited child should have a minimum of three positions that can be alternated during the day. In addition, the position selected should be as functional as possible for the individual child. In some cases this may mean encouraging eye contact. For another child, hand use becomes a possibility with proper trunk support.

All supports, whether they be chairs, prone boards, standers, or floor seats, should be checked carefully for their effect. A child may appear to be properly positioned for the first few minutes and then be pulled into excessive flexion or collapse to one side. Positions that appear simple to the therapist may be viewed quite differently by a person who does not have experience with reflexive reactions and postural alignments. It is helpful to have a photo of the client in the chair, with important points of control noted. If the therapist has not seen this particular client over a period of time, careful interview of the family to understand typical behaviors and planning some options in case of problems is advisable.

Mention must be made of the importance of communication for the nonverbal client with cerebral palsy. A simple start may be made with pictures to permit choices in food, clothing, and therapy activities. While computers have their place, the child should have the communication device with him or her at all times. Language development in the young child is enhanced by having this type of alternative while articulation is still difficult. Affordable electronic systems, with a voice recording and portability and growth features are available. Communication can make the difference between passivity and active participation in the environment and can be achieved by coordinating efforts with the speech pathologist.[41] (Refer to Chapter 26 for additional information.)

Consultation for the family and other helpers. If at all possible, some opportunity for in-service exchange should be provided when persons with a variety of professional backgrounds are brought together to accomplish a task. The therapist, along with other specialists, must forfeit some professional jargon in the interest of true communication to benefit the child. One may practice with familiar persons who lack training in therapy. The therapist can try talking this volunteer through the task of positioning a child or feeding the child according to written directions. The therapist should then note the areas of miscommunication and adapt the instructions accordingly.

Therapists should encourage parents, teachers, and others to understand why certain positions are being used. This will make them more conscious of both positive and negative changes that may call for further adaptations. It is safer to overexplain than to leave persons with a partial understanding or outright confusion as to why the positioning may have an effect on the child's development. When feasible, it is helpful to let persons caring for the child assume some of the abnormal postures to personally experience the difficulties that the child experiences.

Communication systems for the more severely disabled child should be evaluated by the therapist to determine which normal patterns may be utilized. Repeated activation of total

patterns of flexion or extension will eventually interfere with trunk control in sitting and may cause a child to regress physically. Use of a simple, normal response will help toward the goal of better function. All activities that are repeated on a daily basis should be examined in light of possible interference by abnormal patterns. For example, secure seating for toileting is fundamental for success in the required physiological control. Self-feeding assistance can be most effectively introduced with abduction at the shoulder and the overhand grasp of the normal toddler. This normal alignment fosters the development of proximal control and facilitates grasp.

The therapist in the schools. Children with mild cerebral palsy may be successfully incorporated in physical education classes as part of the trend to "mainstreaming." Teachers generally appreciate the opportunity to discuss with the therapist specific limitations and those movements that should be encouraged. For better success, the disabled child can be incorporated into a class that follows the guidelines of "movement education," which places much less emphasis on intragroup competition and encourages each child to progress at his or her own rate.

Most teachers who lack experience with disabled persons are understandably reluctant to incorporate a disabled child into their classroom. A meeting with the therapist might be used to help the child demonstrate his or her strengths and physical independence. The child may also be a part of the problem solving necessary for a successful classroom experience. Children may have their own ways of managing the water fountain, the locker door, or personal care needs. This reinforces strengths rather than limitations and arms the child with some positive responses for curious peers.

New directions in the community

As programs that hire therapists move into prevention and early intervention, the therapist is dealing directly with a population that is not familiar with therapy per se nor aware of the need for this intervention. The therapist may discover a need to reorient previously accepted concepts of rehabilitation. Clarification in one's own mind is essential to effective communication with others. In some instances active intervention will precede the labeling process. Philosophically, therapy may become an enhancement of normal development rather than a remedial process.

It is important to keep direct active treatment available for older children, adolescents, and adults who are motivated to change. Now that more effective procedures are available for changing some of the basic neurophysiological characteristics of cerebral palsy, it is possible to obtain change with direct treatment of the older client. Motor learning concepts are better understood [see Chapters 3 and 4] and can be applied after normalizing the tissues that have been unused for so many years. With present program directions, many older clients will not have had the opportunity for direct treatment over time by a qualified therapist.

The movement toward a health orientation as opposed to crisis intervention for illness will also affect services for children and adults with cerebral palsy. This population does not have an illness or active disease process. Many adults with neuromotor disabilities express their preference to participate in the decisions that are made for them regarding their ultimate life-style. Certainly, optimal health for the person with residuals of cerebral palsy has yet to be described.

PSYCHOSOCIAL FACTORS IN CEREBRAL PALSY

We have defined cerebral palsy as a condition existing from the time of birth or infancy. The developing child has no memory of life in a different body. Movement limitations circumscribe the horizon of the child's world unless the family is able to provide compensatory experiences. The development of both intelligence and personality relies heavily on developmental experiences and self-expression.

The child with **spastic diplegia or spastic quadriplegia** may be hesitant in making decisions or reaching out for a new opportunity because the world may seem overwhelming and somewhat threatening. The child may find it easier to withdraw toward social isolation. Parents and professionals can help to avoid these reactions by encouraging independence in thought and in physical tasks. Early choices can be made by the child regarding which clothes to wear or which task to do first. Understanding the child's limitations helps build successes rather than failures. To function in spite of the constraints of spasticity demands considerable effort.

Athetoid children, in contrast, have adapted to failures as a transient part of life. However disorganized their movements, they repeatedly attempt tasks and eventually succeed. Their social interactions reflect this life experience. Most people will sooner or later succumb to the positive smiling approach without assessing the underlying communication offered by the child. These children are difficult for parents to discipline and structure during their early years. Early treatment with concomitant guidance for young parents does ameliorate some of the problems by making more appropriate the developmental expectations for the child.

Intelligent children with low tone demand that the world be brought to them. Mentally limited children may fail to receive sufficient stimulation for optimal development. Whatever the learning potential of the child with cerebral palsy, it is not always evident early. Parents find it difficult to know how to guide a child when they are not certain that an assigned task is understood.

Parental guidance of the disabled child is also influenced by the adults' adaptation to their offspring's problem. They need to have resolved in their own way the emotional impact of the child's disability. Most parents feel inadequate, ignorant, and relatively helpless at being unable to remedy the situation for their child. They need help in feeling good about themselves before they can effectively guide the child toward acceptance of himself or herself as an adequate human being.

The therapist plays an important role in the psychosocial development of children who receive regular treatment. The child may perceive the therapist as a confidant, disciplinarian, counselor, or friend at various stages of development. Some children accept the therapist as a member of their extended family. This is natural considering the extent to which therapists influence clients' own self-awareness through changes in their physical bodies. However, it also places a personal responsibility on the therapist to be cognizant of the ongoing interaction and its effect on the maturational process.

Any evaluation of personality characteristics in a disabled child must take into account the unnatural life-style that is superimposed by the need for therapy, medical appointments, and hospitalization, for example. The child is expected to separate from parents earlier than the average child and usually confronts many more novel situations. There is little time or physical opportunity for free play. Continuous demands are placed on children to prove their intellectual potential in evaluations of various types. Their social interaction is most often monitored by adults, while they assume a dependent role. Nonetheless, these children's social acceptance frequently rests on their skill in interacting with persons in their environments. It is not easy to evaluate the evolution of personality without considering these experiential factors.

MEDICAL INFLUENCES ON TREATMENT

Because the problems of cerebral palsy are so varied, the condition lends itself to diverse interventions, some of which have a longer life than others. The cerebellar implant so popular in the late 1970s offered the possibility of regulating tone by supplementing cerebellar inhibition.[19,21,65] As time goes on the procedure is used less often and patients have difficulty getting repairs or replacement parts for the implant. The procedure that largely replaced the cerebellar implant was the placement of four electrodes in the cervical area to offer more control over postural tone.[35] These had the advantage of being adjustable so that the individual or a family member could make daily choices as to the optimal tone distribution. In some cases early success gave way to disappointment as the system adapted to the inputs.[35] Therapy was always recommended after the procedure, although the nature of the program was left to the family to decide.

In 1908 a **rhizotomy** procedure was developed by Dr. Otfrid Foerster and some success was reported.[40] It remained for Dr. Peacock to apply the procedure more selectively and functionally and to bring it to the United States from South Africa.[50] Based on his experience, he insisted on daily neurodevelopmental (Bobath) treatment for at least 1 year after the surgical intervention. An electrophysiological system is used to determine which posterior nerve rootlets are creating the spasticity in the lower extremities. Ideally, the child cooperates actively in treatment as more normal movement patterns are learned. There is a need to have some trunk function and fairly normal underlying tone.[17,35] The child must also adapt psychologically to the temporary loss of physical control, as the previous ability to walk or move about may be impaired for some months as new patterns of movement are learned. The long-term gains can be impressive[24] although experienced therapists state the need for 1 to 3 years of treatment after surgery because of the child's completely new tone distribution. The foundation for success is accurate selection of the child, an experienced surgeon, and accurate analysis of therapy goals.

The more recent improvement in the rhizotomy procedure has been developed by Lazareff and others[42] who enter two rather than five levels and prefer to work close to the cauda equina, following the technique of Fasano.[24] The children operated with this technique tend to recuperate more rapidly, and children of 6 to 9 years resume walking within weeks. Older clients have a slower process of learning new motor patterns, but the reduction of spasticity frees them for better control. Lazareff prefers to have recommendations from the child's therapist and considers 2 years for CNS maturation plus 2 years of quality therapy as a minimum for consideration of the limited selective posterior rhizotomy (LSPR) as an intervention. Lazareff has also operated more severely involved older youngsters with improvements noted in respiration, postural adaptation, and ease of daily care.

Orthopedic intervention continues to be effective in cerebral palsy when there are tendon contractures or specific structural limitations that are not accompanied by excessive levels of spasticity. In any surgery the outcome is much improved by close coordination between therapist and surgeon. Using early standing postsurgery, dynamic footplates inside the casts, and orthotics to follow cast removal will generally improve outcomes. Bone surgeries to offer better stability are usually planned for the termination of growth. The orthopedist is also able to guide conservative positioning measures to prevent hip problems due to spasticity while direct treatment intervention continues. Children with cerebral palsy differ in the ability to relax completely during sleep. The orthopedist should participate in any plan for immobilization or temporary casting that will be used on a 24-hour schedule.

RECORD KEEPING AND CLINICAL RESEARCH

Data collection is an important task in the treatment of cerebral palsy. Change occurs at variable rates, but it is important to document the cause and effect of change whenever possible. Slides, super 8 film, or videotapes are useful in recording functional comparisons over time. Film lends itself to a formal frame-by-frame analysis. A motor drive unit or "automatic advance" on a 35 mm single lens reflex (SLR) camera also records a sample of movement five or more times per second. Placing the subject against a spaced grid in the same alignment to perform the same movement task allows for measurement of efficiency of movement. These ideas may be applied to documentation of treatment effectiveness or elaborated for a statement regarding similar movement problems.

Matching of groups is an approach doomed to failure or at least to considerable inaccuracy in cerebral palsy because of a wide range of individuality. It is analogous to making a statement regarding the mean in a widely variable population. This does not mean that methods of intervention or treatment are not measurable or that research is not applicable to the problems of cerebral palsy. Once a specific question has been formulated, systematic recordings of appropriate data can be gathered over time to accumulate the number needed for a viable study. There is value in longitudinal reporting of a single case or a small group of individuals who have some characteristics in common.

The way in which therapists are taught to view a problem determines, to a large extent, the potential range of solutions available to them. Cerebral palsy is a complex of inabilities that cluster about the inadequacy of CNS control. For the purpose of productive study, therapists may look critically at qualities of movement, postural adjustments, timing of movements, or changes in range of functional movement. New areas of motor learning, systems, and chaos theories offer the researcher new approaches to the challenge of cerebral palsy and the resultant disorder of posture control and movement learning. Tscharnuter[60] has theorized that environmental factors may have more influence than specific CNS limitations. Therapists are improving a disorder of posture and movement through their treatment. Analysis of the postural components and movement characteristics will help them toward meaningful research more quickly than reliance on the traditional definitions of the condition.

CASE STUDIES

To understand the problems of children with cerebral palsy, it is essential to follow some children over time to capture the evolution of family problems. Functional treatment must change according to the developmental level, chronological age, and neuromotor responses of the child. Intervention must be specific to the presenting problem of the moment while considering the missing aspects of complete motor development. The case study comparison of two boys illustrates the typical lack of clinical correlation between history and manifest characteristics of cerebral palsy.

CASE 1 ▾ L.P.

A young mother was pregnant with her first child. She was middle class, well nourished, and had no identified risk factors. In her seventh month of pregnancy, her older sister died, causing considerable emotional upheaval. The much anticipated baby was born, small for gestational age, at her correct date. It was theorized that there had been inadequate intrauterine nourishment during the first 6 to 7 months. L.P. weighed 3.5 pounds (1587 grams) and was fed initially by nasogastric tube. Her movements were quick and eye movement was very active for a new infant. She was received for therapy at 17 days of age, immediately after hospital discharge.

Initial therapy focus was on the practical task of adequate nutritional intake so that the nasogastric tube could be removed before scarring occurred from repeatedly passing the tube. Swaddling was suggested to calm the baby and assist her organization of body movement. Simple handling was oriented to moving the trunk over midline to let the head follow and assisting the infant to assume age-appropriate antigravity postures.

At 3 years of age L.P. continued to have difficulty with control of her head position in space and was unable to initiate postural change with her head. Her clinical picture was one of low tone with athetoid movement. She could not speak, communicated with looks and a few word approximations and hitched along the floor in a seated position with one hand supporting.

By 5 years of age L.P. was still receiving therapy three times per week and could walk in a hesitating way with her hands held. At this stage she was evaluated by a behavioral optometrist and started vision therapy to prepare her to participate in preschool activities. As a secondary benefit her balance in walking improved markedly. L.P. began walking up and down 27 steps daily in her new home.

Now at 7 years of age L.P. can walk independently on level surfaces. She has physical therapy once a week and vision therapy once a week to maintain her control of posture and movement. Her school performance is adequate to keep her with her age peers and she attends a regular school.

CASE 2 ▾ D.D. and E.D.

D.D. and E.D. were born within 6 months of each other at 6 months, 1 week gestation. Both were first-born infants for their respective mothers. D.D.'s mother was discovered to have a double uterus when she had a miscarriage early in the pregnancy. E.D. suffered malnutrition during his intrauterine development. D.D. started therapy just before he was 5 months old. E.D. began therapy at almost 7 months old.

At 6 years of age D.D. walks alone with very mild athetotic "overflow." He wears corrective lenses that were fit at 2 years of age and returns for follow-up examinations with the behavioral optometrist once a year. Vision therapy was an important adjunct to physical handling as it introduced changes in spatial perception based on specific sessions with prism lenses. At 4 years of age D.D. was discovered to have a mild to moderate hearing loss, and still uses a hearing aid in one ear. He speaks English and Spanish, as do his parents, and he understands the French spoken to him by his grandparents. He functions in a regular school with his age peers and is a well-adapted, active child.

At 6 years of age E.D. presents as a moderately severe diplegic, with some immaturity of hand use and trunk control. He speaks English and Spanish well, although he demonstrates some emotional instability and difficulty in dealing with his disability. He is creative in storytelling and offers to tell original stories for other children in therapy. He is just beginning to walk with a walker within interior environments and with low resistance.

REFERENCES

1. Arbuckle BE: *The selected writings of Beryl E Arbuckle,* Newark, Ohio, 1947, American Academy of Osteopathy.
2. Arnold GG: Problems of the cerebral palsy child and his family, *Va Med Monthly* 103:225-227, 1976.
3. Bach-y-Rita P, editor: *Recovery of function: theoretical considerations for brain injury rehabilitation,* Berne, Switzerland, 1980, Hans Huber, Publishers.
4. Benabib RM: *Vision training for neurologically impaired children,* Albuquerque, NM, 1993, Clinician's View video.
5. Benabib RM and Nelson CA: Efficiency in visual skills and postural control: a dynamic interaction, *J Occup Ther Pract,* 3(1), 1991.
6. Bertoti DB: Effect of short leg casting on ambulation in children with cerebral palsy, *Phys Ther* 66(10):1522-1529, 1986.
7. Bleck E: *Orthopedic management in cerebral palsy,* Philadelphia, 1987, JB Lippincott Co.
8. Bobath B: The very early treatment of cerebral palsy, *Dev Med Child Neurol* 9(4):373-390, 1967.
9. Bobath B: *Abnormal postural reflex activity caused by brain lesions,* London, 1975, William Heinemann Medical Books, Ltd.
10. Bobath B: *Motor development in the different types of cerebral palsy,* New York, 1975, William Heinemann.
11. Bobath K: A neurophysiological basis for the treatment of cerebral palsy, ed 2 of CDM 23, *Clinics in developmental medicine,* no 75, London, 1980, William Heinemann Medical Books, Ltd.
12. Brazelton TB: *Infants and mothers: differences in development,* New York, 1969, Dell Publishing Co, Inc.
13. Brazelton TB: Neonatal behavioral assessment scale. In *Clinics in*

developmental medicine, no 50, London, 1973, William Heinemann Medical Books, Ltd.

14. Brereton B and others: *Cerebral palsy: basic abilities,* Mosman, NSW, Australia, 1975, The Spastic Centre of New South Wales.

15. Brooks VB: *The neural basis of motor control,* New York, 1986, Oxford University Press.

16. Buethorn D: *Dynamic ankle foot orthotics,* (manual and video), Albuquerque, New Mex, 1992, Clinician's View.

17. Cahan LD and others: Electrophysiologic studies in selective dorsal rhizotomy for spasticity in children with cerebral palsy, *Appl Neurophysiol* 50(1-6):459-462, 1987.

18. Conner F and others: *Program guide for infants and toddlers with neuromotor and other developmental disabilities,* New York, 1978, Teacher's College Press.

19. Cooper IS and others: *Correlation of clinical and physiological effects of cerebellar stimulation,* Acta Neurochir (suppl)(Wien), 30:339-344, 1980.

20. Crutchfield CA and Barnes MR: *Motor control and motor learning in rehabilitation,* Atlanta, 1993, Stokesville Publishing Co.

21. Davis R and others: Cerebellar stimulation for spastic cerebral palsy: double-blind quantitative study, *Appl Neurophysiol* 50(1-6):451-452, 1987.

22. Davis R and others: Cerebellar stimulation for cerebral palsy, *J Fla Med Assoc* 63:910-912, Nov 1976.

23. Denhoff E and others: Treatment of spastic cerebral palsied children with sodium dantrolene, *Dev Med Child Neurol* 17(6):736-742, Dec 1975.

24. Fasano VA and others: Long-term results of posterior functional rhizotomy, *Acta Neurochir* (suppl)(Wien), 30:435-439, 1980.

25. Finnie NR: *Handling the young cerebral-palsied child at home,* New York, 1975, EP Dutton, Inc.

26. Fiorentino MR: *A basis for sensorimotor development: normal and abnormal,* Springfield, Ill, 1981, Charles C Thomas, Publisher.

27. Frymann V: Relation of disturbances of craniosacral mechanisms to symptomatology of the newborn: study of 1,250 infants, *J Am Osteopath Assoc* 65:1059-1075, June 1966.

28. Furth H and Wachs H: *Learning goes to school,* New York, 1974, Oxford University Press, Inc.

29. Gilfoyle EM and others: *Children adapt,* Thorofare, NJ, 1981, Slack.

30. Haberfellner H and Müller G: Sequelae of head and neck positions on auditory performance, *Neuropädiatrie* 7(4):373-378, 1976.

31. Hagberg BA: Epidemiology of cerebral palsy: aspects on perinatal prevention in Sweden, Neonatal Neurological Assessment and Outcome Report of the 77th Ross Conference on Pediatric Research, 1980.

32. Held R: Plasticity in sensory-motor systems, *Sci Am* 71-80, 1965.

33. Hellebrandt FA and others: Methods of evoking the tonic neck reflexes in normal human subjects, *Am J Phys Med* 41(90):263-269, 1962.

34. Hochleitner M: Control study of children with cerebral palsy with and without early neurophysiological treatment, *Austrian Med J* 32(18):1091-1097, 1977.

35. Hugenholtz H and others: Cervical spinal cord stimulation for spasticity in cerebral palsy, *Neurosurgery* 22(4):707-714, Apr 1988.

36. Illingworth RS: *The development of the infant and young child: abnormal and normal,* ed 7, Edinburgh, 1980, Churchill Livingstone.

37. Keshner EA: Re-evaluating the theoretical model underlying the neurodevelopmental theory, *Phys Ther* 61(7):1035-1040, July 1981.

38. Knoblock H and Pasamanick B, editors: *Developmental diagnosis,* Hagerstown, Md, 1974, Harper & Row.

39. Köng E: Very early treatment of cerebral palsy, *Dev Med Child Neurol* 8:68-75, 1966.

40. Laitinen LV and others: Selective posterior rhizotomy for treatment of spasticity, *J Neurosurg* 58:895-899, 1983.

41. Langley MB and Lombardino LJ: *Neurodevelopmental strategies for managing communication disorders in children with severe motor dysfunction,* Austin, Tex, 1991, Pro-Ed.

42. Lazareff J and others: Limited selective posterior rhizotomy for the treatment of spasticity secondary to infantile cerebral palsy: a preliminary report, *Neurosurgery* 27(4):535-538, 1990.

43. Leach P: *Babyhood,* New York, 1977, Alfred A Knopf, Inc.

44. MacKeith RC and others: The Little Club memorandum on terminology and classification of cerebral palsy, *Cereb Palsy Bull* 1(27):34-37, 1959.

45. Milani-Comparetti A: Neurophysiologic and clinical implications of studies on fetal motor behavior, *Semin Perinatol* 5(2):183-189, 1981.

46. Montgomery PC and Connolly BH: *Motor control and physical therapy: theoretical framework, practical application,* Hixson, Tenn, 1991, Chattanooga Group, Inc.

47. Niswander KR: The obstetrician, fetal asphyxia, and cerebral palsy, *Am J Obstet Gynecol* 133(4):358-361, 1979.

48. Padula WV: *A behavioral vision approach for persons with physical disabilities,* Santa Ana, Calif, 1988, Optometric Extension Program Foundation.

49. Palmer FB and others: The effects of physical therapy on cerebral palsy: a controlled trial in infants with spastic diplegia, *N Engl J Med* 318(13):803-808, 1988.

50. Peacock WJ and Arens LJ: Selective posterior rhizotomy for the relief of spasticity in cerebral palsy, *S Afr Med J* 62:119-125, 1982.

51. Pearlstone A and Benjamin R: Ocular defects in cerebral palsy, *Eye Ear Nose Throat Mon* 48:87-89, 1969.

52. Pettitt B: Surgery of the lower extremity in cerebral palsy: considerations and approaches, *Arch Phys Med Rehabil* 57:443-447, Sept 1976.

53. Prechtl H: *The neurological examination of the full-term newborn infant,* Philadelphia, 1977, JB Lippincott.

54. Restak RM: *The brain: the last frontier,* New York, 1979, Doubleday.

55. Rosenthal R and others: Levodopa therapy in athetoid cerebral palsy, *Neurology* 22(1):21-24, 1972.

56. Rosenzweig M and others: Brain changes in response to experience, *Sci Am,* Feb 1972.

57. Soboloff HR: Trends in cerebral palsy treatment, *Tex Med* 66(12)82-91, 1970.

58. Sussman M and Cusick B: Preliminary report: the role of short-leg tone-reducing casts as an adjunct to physical therapy of patients with cerebral palsy, *Johns Hopkins Med J* 145(3):112-114, 1979.

59. Tardieu G and Tardieu C: Cerebral palsy: mechanical evaluation and conservative correction of limb joint contractures, *Clin Orthop* 219:63-69, 1987.

60. Tscharnuter I: A new therapy approach to movement organization, PT and OT, *Pediatrics* December, 1993. (scheduled for publication)

61. Upledger JE and Vredevoogd JD: *Craniosacral therapy,* Seattle, 1983, Eastland Press.

62. Van der Knaap MS and others: Myelination as an expression of the functional maturity of the brain, *Dev Med Child Neurol,* 33:849-857.

63. Vining E and others: Cerebral palsy: a pediatric developmentalist's overview, *Am J Dis Child,* 130:643-649, 1976.

64. Watt J and others: A prospective study of inhibitive casting as an adjunct to physiotherapy for cerebral palsied children, *Dev Med Child Neurol* 28(4):480-488, 1986.

65. Whittaker CK: Cerebellar stimulation for cerebral palsy, *J Neurosurg* 52(5):648-653, 1980.

66. Wright BA: *Physical disability—a psychological approach,* New York, 1960, Harper & Row.

ADDITIONAL READINGS

Ames LB and others: The *Gesell Institute's child from one to six: evaluating the behavior of the preschool child,* New York, 1979, Harper & Row.

Aptekar R and others: Light patterns as means of assessing and recording gait. II. Results in children with cerebral palsy, *Dev Med Child Neurol* 18(1):37-40, 1976.

Bach-y-Rita P: *Brain mechanisms in sensory substitution,* New York, 1972, Academic Press.

Barolat G: Dorsal selective rhizotomy through a limited exposure of the cauda equina at L-1, *J Neurosurg* 75:804-807, 1991.

Beintema DJ: A neurological study of newborn infants. In *Clinics in developmental medicine,* no 28, London, 1968, William Heinemann Medical Books, Ltd.

Black R: Visual disorders associated with cerebral palsy, *Br J Ophthalmol* 66(1):46-52, 1982.

Boehme R: *Improving upper body control: an approach to assessment and treatment of tonal dysfunction,* Tucson, Arizona, 1988, Therapy Skill Builders.

Bower TGR: The visual world of infants, *Sci Am* 251(6):349-357, 1966.

Bower TGR: *A primer of infant development,* San Francisco, 1977, WH Freeman.

Briggs DC: *Your child's self-esteem,* ed 2, Garden City, NJ, 1975, Dolphin Books.

Buscaglia L: *The disabled and their parents: a counseling challenge,* Thorofare, NJ, 1975, Slack.

Eccles JC: *The understanding of the brain,* ed 2, New York, 1977, McGraw-Hill Book Co.

Featherstone H: *A difference in the family: life with a disabled child,* New York, 1980, Basic Books.

Feldenkrais M: *Awareness through movement,* New York, 1977, Harper & Row.

Ford E and Englund S: *For the love of children,* Garden City, NY, 1977, Anchor Press.

Gahm NH and others: Chronic cerebellar stimulation for cerebral palsy: a double-blind study, *Neurology (NY)* 31(1):87-90, 1981.

Goffman E: *Stigma: notes on the management of spoiled identity,* Englewood Cliffs, NJ, 1963, Prentice-Hall.

Graham M and others: Prediction of cerebral palsy in very low birthweight infants: prospective ultrasound study, *Lancet* 2(8559):593-595, 1987.

Haeusserman E: *Developmental potential of preschool children,* New York, 1958, Grune & Stratton.

Hannon C: *Parents and mentally handicapped children,* London, 1975, Penguin Books.

Harrell R and others: Can nutritional supplements help mentally retarded children? An exploratory study, *Proc Natl Acad Sci USA,* 78(1):574-578, 1981.

Holt KS: *Developmental paediatrics, postgraduate paediatrics series,* London, 1978, Butterworth & Co.

Hulme JB and others: Effects of adaptive seating devices on the eating and drinking of children with multiple handicaps, *Am J Occup Ther* 41(2):81-89, 1987.

Jones FP: *Body awareness in action: the Alexander technique,* New York, 1976, Schocken Books.

Kane P: *Food makes the difference: a parent's guide to raising a healthy child,* New York, 1985, Simon and Schuster.

Katayama M and Tamas LB: Saccadic eye-movements of children with cerebral palsy, *Dev Med Child Neurol* 29(1):36-39, 1987.

Katz K and others: Seat insert for cerebral-palsied children with total body involvement, *Dev Med Child Neurol* 30(2):222-226, 1988.

Kock J: *Total baby development,* New York, 1976, Wyden Books.

Leboyer F: *Loving hands: the traditional Indian art of baby massage,* New York, 1976, Alfred A Knopf.

Menken C and others: Evaluating the visual-perceptual skills of children with cerebral palsy, *Am J Occup Ther* 41(10):646-651, 1987.

Montagu A: *Touching, the human significance of the skin,* ed 2, New York, 1978, Harper & Row.

Nelson KB and others: Children who "outgrew" cerebral palsy, *Pediatrics* 69(5):529-536, 1982.

Nwaobi OM: Seating orientations and upper extremity function in children with cerebral palsy, *Phys Ther* 67(8):1209-1212, 1987.

Ornstein R and Sobel D: *The healing brain,* New York, 1987, Simon and Schuster.

Pearson P and Ethun-Williams C: *Physical therapy services in the developmental disabilities,* Springfield, Ill, 1972, Charles C Thomas.

Penn RD: Chronic cerebellar stimulation—a review, *Neurosurgery* 10(1):116-121, 1982.

Prechtl Heinz FR: *Continuity of neural functions from prenatal to postnatal life,* Philadelphia, 1984, JB Lippincott.

Restak R: *The brain,* New York, 1984, Bantam Books.

Rolf IP: *Rolfing: the integration of human structures,* New York, 1978, Harper & Row.

Rose S: *The conscious brain, updated edition,* New York, 1976, Vintage Books.

Samples B: *Open mind whole mind: parenting and teaching tomorrow's children today,* Rolling Hills Estates, California, 1987, Jalmar Press.

Scherzer A and Tscharnuter I: *Early diagnosis and therapy in cerebral palsy,* New York, 1982, Marcel Dekker.

Scherzer AL and others: Physical therapy as a determinant of change in the cerebral palsied infant, *Pediatrics* 58:47-52, 1976.

Stockmeyer SA: An interpretation of the approach of Rood to the treatment of neuromuscular dysfunction, *Am J Phys Med* 46, 1977.

Stone LJ and others: *The competent infant, research and commentary,* New York, 1973, Basic Books.

Sweeney JK: *The high-risk neonate: developmental therapy perspectives,* New York, 1986, The Haworth Press.

Szasz S: *The body language of children,* New York, 1978, WW Norton.

Tjossen TD, editor: *Intervention strategies for high-risk infants and children,* Baltimore, 1976, University Park Press.

Touwen B: Neurological development in infancy. In *Clinics in developmental medicine,* no 58, London, 1976, William Heinemann Medical Books, Ltd.

Verny T and Kelly J: *Secret life of the unborn child,* New York, 1981, Delta Books.

Willemson E: *Understanding infancy,* San Francisco, 1979, WH Freeman.

Witkin K: *To move, to learn,* New York, 1977, Schocken Books.

RECOMMENDED READING

Gleick J: *Chaos: making a new science,* New York, 1987, Viking Press.

Thelen E: Developmental origins of motor coordination: leg movements in human infants, *Dev Psychobiol* 18:1-18, 1985.

Thelen E and others: Self-organizing systems and infant motor development, *Dev Rev* 7:39-65, 1987.

Yokochi K and others: Leg movements in the supine position of infants with spastic diplegia, *Dev Med Child Neurol* 33:903-907, 1991.

CHAPTER 10

Genetic Disorders

Gay M. Naganuma, Susan R. Harris, and Wendy L. Tada

KEY TERMS

genetic disorders
developmental physical
  and occupational
  therapist
family priorities

evaluation
functional skills
natural environments

LEARNING OBJECTIVES

After reading this chapter the student/therapist will:

1. Describe the two main types of genetic disorders and
   give examples of each type.
2. Describe the three modes of inheritance for specific
   gene defects.
3. Describe the clinical symptoms and common motor
   problems associated with genetic disorders frequently
   observed in children in developmental therapy
   settings.
4. Explain why it is important to include family
   members in the planning and development of therapy
   programs for children with genetic disorders.
5. Describe and give examples of three types of
   assessment tools and the intended purpose of each.
6. Identify therapy objectives that are outcome-focused,
   rather than focused on a child's deficits.
7. Explain the importance of addressing family priorities
   when designing therapy programs for children with
   genetic disorders.
8. Describe the importance of developing therapy
   programs that focus on functional skills in natural
   environments.
9. Identify three medical treatments that may be used
   for children with genetic disorders to ameliorate the
   effects of the disorder.
10. Explain why it is important for developmental physical
    and occupational therapists to have knowledge of the
    services available through genetic counseling.

Genetic disorders in children frequently result in severe neurological impairments. This chapter discusses disorders of known genetic origin that **developmental physical and occupational therapists** are most likely to encounter in children involved in developmental therapy programs. Minor, isolated anomalies of known genetic origin are addressed only briefly. Types of genetic disorders are dis-

cussed in the first section. Specific examples of each type are presented along with a description of typical clinical characteristics and symptoms, incidence or prevalence estimates, and underlying neuropathology. A summary of typical clinical signs observed in children with genetic disorders concludes the section.

The second section focuses on the physical or occupational therapist's role in the clinical management of children with genetic disorders. Evaluation procedures, treatment goals and objectives, and general treatment principles and strategies are discussed from a family-centered perspective. The final section discusses the medical management of genetic disorders and genetic counseling.

AN OVERVIEW: TYPES OF GENETIC DISORDERS WITH REPRESENTATIVE CLINICAL EXAMPLES

Genetic disorders may be divided into two major categories: chromosomal abnormalities and specific gene defects. Chromosomal abnormalities can be further subdivided into autosomal trisomies, sex chromosome abnormalities, and partial deletion syndromes.[107] Specific gene defects may be transmitted through three different modes of inheritance: autosomal dominant, autosomal recessive, and sex-linked. Fig. 10-1 shows the categories and subcategories of genetic disorders and clinical examples of each.

Chromosomal abnormalities

According to Smith,[107] the defect that produces a chromosomal abnormality is usually one of quantity rather than quality of genetic material. Most chromosomal abnormalities appear as an extra chromosome or as a missing chromosome, with the latter being more lethal than the former. The incidence of chromosomal abnormalities among spontaneously aborted fetuses may be as high as 50% to 60%.[8] About 5:1000 live-born infants have a detectable chromosomal abnormality and in about half of these cases, the chromosomal abnormality is accompanied by congenital anomalies, mental retardation, or phenotypic changes that are manifested later in life.[6] Of the fetuses with abnormal chromosomes that survive to term, about half represent sex chromosomal abnormalities and the other half represent autosomal trisomies.[107]

The autosomal trisomies (trisomies 21, 18, and 13) are discussed first because these chromosomal abnormalities are more apt to include serious neuromotor problems than the sex chromosomal abnormalities. Finally, three deletion syndromes (4p-, 5p-, and 15q-) are described.

Autosomal trisomies

Trisomy 21. Down syndrome is the most common chromosomal cause of moderate to severe mental retardation.[98] It was first identified in 1866 by Dr. Langdon Down who described the syndrome as "mongolism." It was not until 1959 that Lejeune identified the presence of an extra chromosome in the G group as responsible for the syndrome.[67]

Down syndrome occurs in one out of every 800 live births[105] and is equally distributed between the sexes.[119] The presence of an extra twenty-first chromosome (trisomy 21) accounts for 91% of individuals with Down syndrome. The remaining 9% have the mosaic and translocation forms of Down syndrome. The incidence of Down syndrome increases with advanced maternal, and possibly paternal, age.[48] The exact cause of the additional chromosome is unknown.[18]

A list of 10 features characterizing newborns with Down syndrome was published by Hall in 1966.[42] These features included hypotonicity, a poor Moro reflex, joint hyperextensibility, excess skin on the back of the neck, a flat facial profile, slanted palpebral fissures, anomalous auricles, dysplasia of the pelvis, dysplasia of the mid-phalanx of the fifth finger, and simian creases. In his study of 48 newborns with Down syndrome, Hall[42] reported the frequency of these characteristics to vary from 45% to 90% (Fig. 10-2).

In a longitudinal study of 79 infants with Down syndrome from birth to 10 months of age, Cowie[22] reported the universal finding of marked hypotonicity (which appeared to gradually diminish with age) and the persistence of several primitive reflexes, including the palmar and plantar grasp reflexes, the stepping reflex, and the Moro reflex. She also observed a delay in the development of normal postural tone as indicated by the severe head lag evident during elicitation of the traction response and the lack of full antigravity extension noted when the Landau response was tested.

Additional characteristics observed in individuals with Down syndrome include congenital heart disease (occurring in 40% of children with Down syndrome) and musculoskeletal anomalies such as metatarsus prima varus, pes planus, thoracolumbar scoliosis, patellar instability, and an increased risk for atlantoaxial dislocation.[48] It is particularly important for persons working with infants and children with Down syndrome to be aware of this propensity for atlantoaxial dislocation, which has been observed through radiogram in up to 20% of a sample studied.[123] If atlantoaxial instability persists undetected, spinal cord compression with myelopathy may result, leading to leg weakness, decreased walking ability,[89] and increased spasticity or incontinence.[80] Although dislocation is relatively rare, there have been reported cases of quadriplegia.[123]

Other clinical features observed in individuals with Down syndrome include brachycephaly, small stature, epicanthal folds, speckled iris (Brushfield's spots), convergent strabismus, and nystagmus.[32] In addition, craniofacial differences such as a shortened palate and mid-face hypoplasia have been noted. These craniofacial differences together with oral hypotonia, tongue thrusting, and poor lip closure frequently result in feeding difficulties at birth.[80]

Impairments of visual and sensory systems are also common in individuals with Down syndrome. As many as 77% of children with Down syndrome have a refractive error (myopia, hyperopia) or astigmatism. Hearing losses that interfere with language development are reportedly present in 80% of children with Down syndrome. In most cases the hearing loss is conductive; up to 20% are sensorineural or mixed.[80]

Several researchers have explored the neuropathology associated with Down syndrome. The relatively small size of the cerebellum and brainstem has been widely reported.[25,91,101] Researchers have noted that although the overall brain weight of individuals with Down syndrome

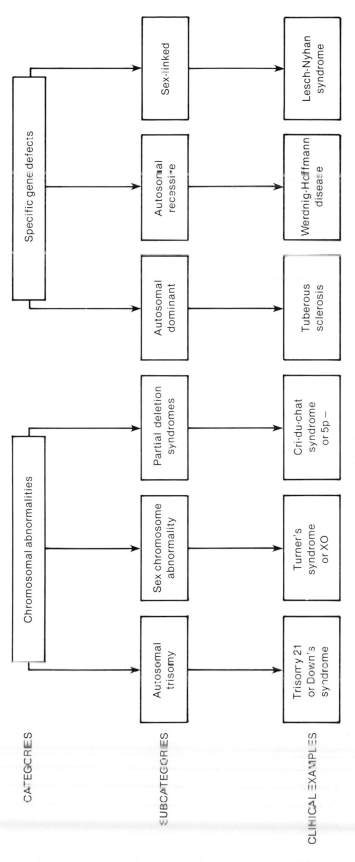

Fig. 10-1. Classification of genetic disorders.

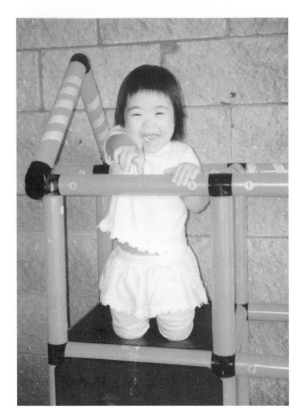

Fig. 10-2. Two-year-old girl with Down syndrome climbing up playground equipment.

averages 76% of the brain weight of normal individuals, the combined brainstem and cerebellum weight averages only 66% of normal.[24]

The reduction in size of the cerebral hemispheres is especially apparent at the frontal poles, causing Cowie[22] to speculate that this particular aspect of the neuropathology may have some bearing on the clinical persistence of the palmar grasp reflex, because a lesion in the frontal lobe of an adult may result in a forced grasp. The brain is abnormally rounded with a relatively narrow anteroposterior diameter and wide lateral diameter (microbrachycephaly) and exhibits reduced convolutions.[92,99]

In addition to these gross neuropathological differences, a number of cytological distinctions characterize the brains of individuals with Down syndrome. Marin-Padilla[74] studied the neuronal organization of the motor cortex of a 19-month-old child with Down syndrome and found various structural abnormalities in the dendritic spines of the pyramidal neurons of the motor cortex. He suggested that these structural differences may underlie the motor incoordination and mental retardation characteristic of individuals with Down syndrome. Loesch-Mdzewska[71] also found neurological abnormalities of the pyramidal system (in addition to reduced brain weight) in his neuropathological study of 123 individuals with Down syndrome aged 3 to 62. Finally, Benda[4] noted a lack of myelinization of the nerve fibers in the precentral areas, frontal lobes, and cerebella of infants with Down syndrome. As McGraw[75] has pointed out, the amount of myelin in the brain reflects the stage of developmental maturation. The delayed myelinization characteristic of newborns and infants with Down syndrome is thought to be a contributing factor to the generalized hypotonicity and persistence of primitive reflexes characteristic of this syndrome.[21]

Trisomy 18. Trisomy 18 is the second most common of the trisomic syndromes to occur in term deliveries, although far less prevalent than Down syndrome (Fig. 10-3). The incidence has been reported as 1:8000 live births, with females affected more often than males (3:1).[105] As with Down syndrome, advanced maternal age is positively correlated with trisomy 18.[32] Only 10% of infants born with trisomy 18 survive past the first year of life. The survival of girls averages 7 months; the survival of boys averages 2 months.

Individuals with trisomy 18, known also as Edwards syndrome, generally have far more serious organic malformations than do those with Down syndrome.[119] Typical malformations include the cardiovascular, gastrointestinal, urogenital, and skeletal systems. At birth, infants with trisomy 18 are of low birthweight and small stature, with long, narrow skulls, low-set ears, flexion deformities of the fingers, and rocker-bottom feet. Muscle tone is initially hypotonic, but becomes hypertonic.[119] Based on our experience in providing developmental physical therapy to two sisters with trisomy 18, the period of hypertonicity in the early years once again gave way to low tone and joint hyperextensibility by preschool and school age.

Common skeletal malformations that may warrant attention from the developmental physical or occupational therapist include scoliosis,[31] limited hip abduction, flexion contractures of the fingers, rocker-bottom feet, and talipes equinovarus.[119] Infants with trisomy 18 may also experience feeding difficulties as a result of a poor suck.[89] Profound mental retardation is another clinical factor that will affect the developmental therapy programs for children with trisomy 18.

Microcephaly, abnormal gyri, cerebellar anomalies, myelomeningoceles, hydrocephaly, and corpus callosum defects have been reported in individuals with trisomy 18. Cytological abnormalities such as heterotopic ganglion cells and abnormal stratification of the cerebellum have also been noted.[119]

Trisomy 13. Trisomy 13 is the least common of the three major autosomal trisomies, with an incidence of 1:20,000 live births.[105] As in the other trisomic syndromes, advanced maternal age is correlated with the incidence of trisomy 13.[19] Fewer than 10% of individuals with trisomy 13 survive past the first year of life.[105]

Described in 1960 by Patau,[91] trisomy 13 is characterized by microcephaly, deafness, anophthalmia or microphthalmia, and cleft lip and palate. As in trisomy 18,

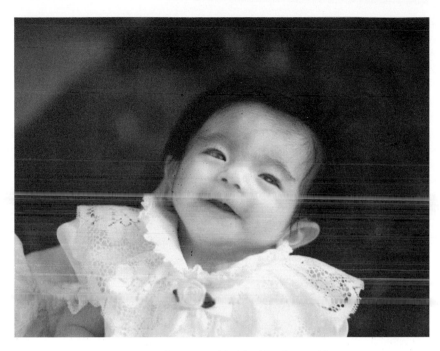

Fig. 10-3. One-year-old girl with trisomy 18.

infants with trisomy 13 frequently have serious cardiovascular and urogenital malformations, and typically have severe to profound mental retardation. Skeletal deformities and anomalies include flexion contractures of the fingers and polydactyly of hands and feet.[105] Rocker-bottom feet also have been reported, although less frequently than in individuals with trisomy 18. Reported central nervous system (CNS) malformations include arrhinencephalies, cerebellar anomalies, defects of the corpus callosum, and hydrocephaly.[120]

Sex chromosome abnormalities. The two most prevalent sex chromosome anomalies are Turner syndrome and Klinefelter syndrome.

Turner syndrome. Turner syndrome is the most common chromosomal anomaly among spontaneous abortions.[13] Known also as gonadal dysgenesis or XO syndrome, Turner syndrome occurs in 1:2500 births.[43] Unlike the autosomal trisomy syndromes, the incidence of Turner syndrome does not increase with advanced maternal age.

The syndrome was first described in 1938 by Turner,[117] who noted three primary characteristics: sexual infantilism, a congenital webbed neck, and cubitus valgus. Other clinical characteristics noted at birth include dorsal edema of hands and feet, hypertelorism, epicanthal folds, ptosis of the upper eyelids, elongated ears,[119] and shortening of all the hand bones.[43] Growth retardation is particularly noticeable after the age of 5 or 6 years, and sexual infantilism, characterized by primary amenorrhea, lack of breast development, and scanty pubic and axillary hair is apparent during the pubertal years. Ovarian development is severely deficient, as is estrogen production.[119]

Congenital heart disease is present in 20% of individuals with Turner syndrome;[20] 33% to 60% of individuals with Turner syndrome have kidney malformations.[43] There are numerous incidences of skeletal anomalies, some of which may be significant enough to require the attention of a pediatric therapist. Included among these are hip dislocation, pes planus and pes equinovarus,[119] dislocated patella,[43] deformity of the medial tibial condyles,[32] and osteoporosis.[53] Decreased lumbar lordosis[43] and idiopathic scoliosis are also common.[31]

Sensory impairments include decreases in gustatory and olfactory sensitivity,[119] deficits in spatial perception and orientation,[78] and moderate hearing losses. (Up to 80% of individuals with Turner syndrome experience chronic otitis media.)[43] Although the average intellect of individuals with Turner syndrome is within normal limits, the incidence of mental retardation is higher than in the general population.[119]

Klinefelter syndrome. The most common type of Klinefelter syndrome, XXY, is usually not clinically apparent until puberty when the testes fail to enlarge and gynecomastia occurs.[32] Eighty percent of males with Klinefelter syndrome possess a karyotype of XXY, 10% are mosaic, and 10% include karyotypes of XXXY, XXYY, and XXXXY.[32] The incidence of Klinefelter syndrome (XXY) is about 1:1000 liveborn males.[89] Advanced maternal age is positively correlated with an increase in births of XXY males.[32]

Most individuals with karyotype XXY have normal intelligence, a somewhat passive personality, and a reduced libido. Nearly all individuals with a nonmosaic karyotype are sterile. Individuals with the karyotypes XXXY and XXXXY tend to display a more severe clinical picture. Individuals with XXXY usually have severe mental retardation, with multiple congenital anomalies, including microcephaly, hypertelorism, strabismus, and cleft palate.[119] Skeletal anomalies include radioulnar synostosis, genu valgum, malformed cervical vertebrae, and pes planus. Parental age does not appear to be a factor in the incidence of the more severe types of Klinefelter syndrome.[32]

Partial deletion syndromes

Wolf-Hirschhorn syndrome (4p-). Wolf-Hirschhorn syndrome appears karyotypically as a partial deletion of the short arm of chromosome 4.[32] It was first described separately by Wolf and others[124] and Hirschhorn and others[52] in 1965. As of 1992, 120 cases of Wolf-Hirschhorn syndrome have been reported.[105] One third of infants born with Wolf-Hirschhorn syndrome die within the first 2 years of life.[32]

Clinically, infants with Wolf-Hirschhorn syndrome present with severe psychomotor and growth retardation, hypotonicity, seizures, and microcephaly. Other congenital characteristics include craniofacial anomalies, ocular malformations, cleft lip or palate, and heart malformations. Skeletal deformities such as scoliosis,[105] dislocated hips, club feet, and proximal radioulnar synostosis may also be present.[32]

Cri-du-chat syndrome (5p-). Cri-du-chat syndrome, also referred to as cat-cry syndrome, results from a partial deletion of the short arm of chromosome 5. The syndrome was first described in 1963 by Lejeune and others.[68] Over 300 cases have been reported, and the incidence of the syndrome is estimated to be 1:20,000 live-births.[105] Although approximately 70% of individuals with cri-du-chat

syndrome are female, there is an unexplained higher prevalence of older males with cri-du-chat.[10] Advanced parental age is not related to this syndrome.

Primary identifying characteristics at birth include a definitive high-pitched cat-like cry, microcephaly, and intrauterine growth retardation.[119] The characteristic cry results from abnormal laryngeal development and disappears in the first few years of life.[89] It should be noted that the characteristic cry is not present in all individuals.

Other features of individuals with this syndrome include hypertelorism, strabismus, "moon face," and low-set ears.[119] Associated musculoskeletal deformities include scoliosis, hip dislocations, clubfeet, and hyperextensibility of fingers and toes. Severe mental retardation and muscular hypotonicity are associated with this syndrome, although cases with hypertonicity have also been noted.[103] Severe respiratory and feeding problems have also been reported[89] (Fig. 10-4).

Prader-Willi syndrome (15q-). Prader-Willi syndrome was initially described by Prader, Lablart, and Willi in 1956.[95] Its incidence is estimated to be 1:10,000 births.[66] Characteristics include obesity, hypogonadism, short stature, hypotonia, dysmorphic facial features, dysfunctional CNS performance,[54] and a compulsive preoccupation with food.

Because Prader-Willi syndrome is characterized by a distinct combination of physical and behavioral features, diagnosis has been based largely on clinical phenotype. Diagnosis by chromosome studies, however, has been reported in 50% to 60% of cases, where a cytogenetic microdeletion is apparent at 15q11-13.[20] The deletion occurs on the paternally derived chromosome.[12]

Most studies of parental chromosomes have been normal, indicating that the deletions are de novo events.[12] Recent

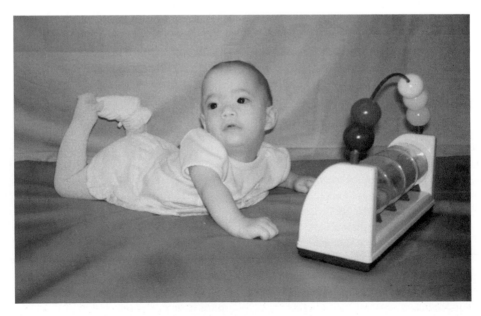

Fig. 10-4. Nine-month-old girl with cri-du-chat syndrome.

literature reviews have documented at least 30 cases of chromosome 15 translocations in Prader-Willi syndrome.[66] Parental studies are important in translocation cases because 20% of cases cited in the literature involved familial rearrangements, which may significantly increase the recurrence risk.[1]

Generalized hypotonia is present at birth and is severe in the majority of cases.[14] Most infants have an expressionless face, flaccid muscles, a weak cry, and little spontaneous movement. Muscle tone generally improves after the first few months of life; however, poor coordination and motor delays persist. Hypotonia often results in a poor suck with early feeding difficulties and slow initial weight gain.[14] At an average age of 2 years, children develop a persistent appetite, and the focus shifts from initial concerns about weight gain to preventing obesity.[72]

The majority of individuals with Prader-Willi syndrome have mild to moderate mental retardation, although some individuals have IQ scores within normal limits.[72] Maladaptive behaviors such as temper tantrums, aggression, self-abuse, and emotional lability have been reported.[114] As a result of extreme obesity, many individuals with Prader-Willi syndrome experience impaired breathing that can produce sleepiness, cyanosis, cor pulmonale, and heart failure.[72] Scoliosis is common but does not appear to be related to obesity.[118]

Specific gene defects

Other genetic disorders commonly seen among children in a developmental therapy setting include those that result from specific gene defects. There are three types of specific gene defects: autosomal dominant, autosomal recessive, and sex-linked. Each of these types of inheritance is discussed separately. Several examples of syndromes or disorders associated with each type are presented. They include those most commonly seen in children attending pediatric therapy programs and those of specific neurological importance to developmental physical or occupational therapists.

Autosomal dominant disorders. Autosomal dominant disorders occur when one parent is affected with the disorder, although spontaneous cases with no family history also have been reported. Each child of a parent with an autosomal dominant trait has a 50:50 chance of inheriting that trait. Many of these are specific isolated anomalies that may occur in otherwise normal individuals[119] such as extra digits or short fingers. Other autosomal dominant disorders include syndromes characterized by profound neurological disability. Three examples of autosomal dominant disorders that can result in serious neurological disabilities are osteogenesis imperfecta, tuberous sclerosis, and neurofibromatosis. Individuals with these disorders may require intervention from a developmental physical or occupational therapist because of the associated musculoskeletal and neuromuscular problems.

Osteogenesis imperfecta. Osteogenesis imperfecta is a spectrum of diseases that results from deficits in collagen synthesis.[89] The four types of osteogenesis imperfecta are characterized by brittle bones, hyperextensible ligaments, blue sclerae, cardiopulmonary abnormalities, discolored and fragile teeth,[73] and hypotonia.[1] Deafness, secondary to otosclerosis, appears in adulthood and is found in 35% of individuals by the third decade of life[60] (Fig. 10-5).

Type I, the mildest form of osteogenesis imperfecta, is characterized by mild-to-moderate bone fragility and joint hyperextensibility. There are no significant deformities and individuals with this type are usually ambulatory. Type II, the most severe form, is lethal before or shortly after birth,[94] Children with type III osteogenesis imperfecta present with severe bone fragility and osteoporosis, often experiencing fractures in utero. An autosomal recessive form of osteogenesis imperfecta, type III, is characterized by progressive skeletal deformity, scoliosis, triangular facies, large skull, normal cognitive ability, short stature, and limited ambulatory ability.[73,94] Type IV osteogenesis imperfecta is characterized by more severe bone fragility and joint hyperextensibility than type I. Bowing of long bones, scoliosis, and short stature are common.[73] Children with type IV osteogenesis imperfecta are often ambulatory but may require splinting or crutches. The overall incidence of osteogenesis imperfecta is 1:20,000 to 30,000, with types I and IV being the most common. Types II and III have an incidence of 1:62,000 and 1:68,000, respectively.[73]

The long bones of the lower extremities are most susceptible to fractures, particularly between the ages of 2 to 3 years and 10 to 15 years,[60] with the frequency of fractures diminishing with age.[89] Intramedullary rods inserted in the tibia or femur may minimize recurrent fractures.[100] Prevention of fractures through careful handling and positioning is

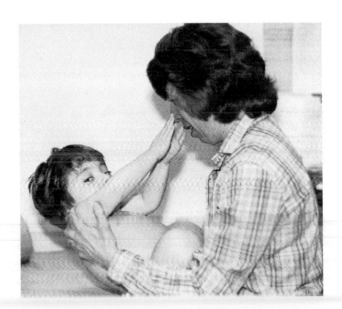

Fig. 10-5. Child with osteogenesis imperfecta during physical therapy session.

the most important goal in working with individuals with osteogenesis imperfecta.[119] Mobility aids and splinting also can be helpful in preventing fractures.[89] We have found the use of pool therapy to be a valuable treatment strategy for children with osteogenesis imperfecta.

Tuberous sclerosis. Tuberous sclerosis is characterized by a triad of symptoms that include seizures, mental retardation, and sebaceous adenomas;[100] however, there is wide variability in expression of the symptoms, with some individuals displaying skin lesions only.[60] Although tuberous sclerosis is inherited through autosomal dominance, 86% of cases occur as spontaneous mutations, with older paternal age a contributing factor. Tuberous sclerosis is a relatively rare condition with a frequency of 1:10,000 births;[121] both sexes are affected equally. Infants are frequently normal in appearance at birth, but 70% of those who go on to show the complete triad of symptoms display seizures during the first year of life.[119]

Hypopigmented macules are often the initial finding. These lesions vary in number and are small and ovoid shaped. Larger lesions, known as leaf spots, may have jagged edges.[89] Sebaceous adenomas first appear between the ages of 4 to 5 years, with early individual brown, yellow, or red lesions of firm consistency in the areas of the nose and upper lips. These isolated lesions may later coalesce to form a characteristic butterfly pattern on the cheeks.[119] Known also as hamartomas or tumorlike nodules of superfluous tissue, the skin lesions are present in 83% of individuals with tuberous sclerosis.[60]

Delayed development is another characteristic during infancy,[23] particularly in the achievement of motor and speech milestones. Mental retardation occurs in 62% of individuals with tuberous sclerosis.[60] Because of the retardation in motor development, as well as associated rigidity or hemiplegia seen in some cases,[119] children with this disorder may be referred to a developmental physical or occupational therapist.

Ultimately, 93% of individuals who are severely affected develop seizures, usually of the myoclonic type in early life, progressing in later life to grand mal seizures. Seizure development is secondary to nodular lesions in the cerebral cortex and white matter.[60] Tumors are also found in the walls of the ventricles. Neurocytological examination reveals a decreased number of neurons and an increased number of glial cells as well as enlarged nerve cells with abnormally shaped cell bodies.[119] Surgical excision of seizure-producing tumors has been successful in some cases.[100]

Other associated anomalies include retinal tumors and hemorrhages, glaucoma, and corneal opacities.[100] Cyst formation in the long bones and in the bones of the fingers and toes contributes to osteoporosis.[119] Cardiac and kidney involvement[89] and catatonic schizophrenia have also been reported.[100]

Neurofibromatosis. Neurofibromatosis is characterized by flat, light brown skin patches, known as café au lait spots, and neurofibromas or connective tissue tumors of the nerve fiber fasciculus.[119] It is a slowly progressive disease, characterized by an increase in the number of tumors with increasing age.[119] The prevalence of neurofibromatosis is 1:3500. Fifty percent of cases are due to new mutations (usually paternal in origin).[20]

Infants usually appear normal at birth, with the initial symptoms of cafe au lait spots first appearing in early childhood.[60] Neurofibromas may be found in either the peripheral or CNS[108] and can lead to secondary disabilities such as optic and acoustic nerve damage,[119] paraplegia, quadriplegia,[100] or hemiparesis.[58] Muscle weakness or incoordination, rather than complete paralysis, may be evident.[89] Neurofibromas may also develop in the kidneys, stomach, or heart.[60] Puberty and pregnancy may exacerbate symptoms of this disorder.[6] Three percent of affected individuals have moderate to severe mental retardation, approximately 30% have learning difficulties, and 3% have seizure disorders.[20] Ultimately, 47% of individuals with neurofibromatosis develop some type of neurological impairment[60] (Fig. 10-6).

Cervical paraspinal neurofibromas may develop in late childhood or early adulthood and are a major cause of chronic disability.[27] Scoliosis occurs in up to 5% of individuals with neurofibromatosis.[20] Severe kyphoscoliotic deformities may lead to spinal cord compression or impaired cardiopulmonary function. Kyphosis usually becomes apparent between ages 6 and 10. Other skeletal deformities include pseudoarthrosis of the tibia and fibula,[119] tibial bowing, craniofacial and vertebral dysplasia,[89] rib fusion, and dislocation of the radius and ulna. Differences in leg

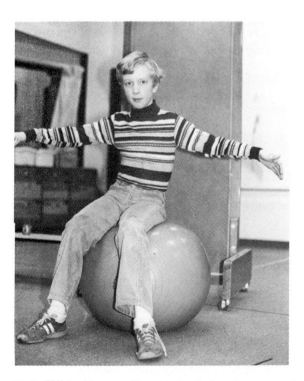

Fig. 10-6. Child with neurofibromatosis during therapy session.

length also have been noted and may contribute to scoliosis.[119]

Autosomal recessive disorders. When parents are unaffected carriers of the trait, they are heterozygous for the abnormal gene, and each of their offspring faces a 25% risk of exhibiting the disorder. When two homozygous affected parents mate, there is a great risk that all children will be similarly affected with the disorder.[119] Consanguinity or marriage between close relatives increases the chance of passing on autosomal recessive traits. Certain types of limb defects, familial microcephaly, and a variety of syndromes such as Laurence-Moon-Biedl and Hurler syndromes are passed on through autosomal recessive genes. Four examples of autosomal recessive disorders that may be of interest to developmental physical or occupational therapists are presented in this section: Hurler syndrome, phenylketonuria, Werdnig-Hoffmann disease, and Kugelberg-Welander disease.

Hurler syndrome (gargoylism, mucopolysaccharidosis I). Hurler syndrome is an inborn error of metabolism that results in abnormal storage of mucopolysaccharides in many different tissues of the body.[1] Although most cases of Hurler syndrome are acquired through autosomal recessive inheritance, some cases have been reported of boys with Hurler syndrome who have acquired the disorder through sex-linked inheritance modes; these cases are usually less severe.[119] The incidence of Hurler syndrome is estimated to be 1:100,000 live births.[89]

Infants born with Hurler syndrome are usually normal in appearance at birth[100] and may be larger in birthweight than their siblings.[119] Symptoms of this progressively deteriorating disease usually appear during the latter half of the first year of life,[107] with the full disease picture apparent by 2 to 3 years.[119] A preponderance of males have been reported to have Hurler syndrome.[1]

Characteristic physical features include a large skull with frontal bossing, heavy eyebrows, edematous eyelids, corneal clouding, a small upturned nose with flat nasal bridge, thick lips, low-set ears, hirsutism, and gargoylelike facial features. Growth retardation results in characteristic dwarfism.[1] Some individuals with the physical characteristics of Hurler syndrome have normal intelligence, but the vast majority have mental retardation.[119]

Spastic paraparesis or paraplegia and ataxia[119] also have been observed in individuals with Hurler syndrome. Commonly reported orthopedic deformities include flexion contractures of the extremities, thoracolumbar kyphosis, genu valgum, pes cavus,[1] hip dislocation, and claw hands secondary to joint deformities.[60] Restriction of neck flexion and extension also may result from hypoplasia of the odontoid process.[89]

Other frequently associated anomalies include deafness, hydrocephaly,[1] an enlarged tongue,[60] hepatosplenomegaly, and delayed dentition with small, pointed teeth.[100] Respiratory involvement results from thickening of the soft tissues in the nasal and pharyngeal area.[89] Progressive mental and physical deterioration leads to early death, usually before adulthood.[1] Death is usually secondary to deposits of mucopolysaccharides in the cardiac valves, myocardium, or coronary arteries.[1]

Gross neuropathological findings include reduced brain size and weight. Cytological findings are distended pyramidal cells, peripherally displaced nuclei, and a decrease in the number of Nissl bodies.[119] Mucopolysaccharide deposits in neurons also have been noted.[1]

Because of the many associated neuromotor and orthopedic problems, infants and children with Hurler syndrome may benefit from developmental therapy services. Delayed motor milestones have been noted in later infancy and early childhood,[119] with severe disabilities occurring with increasing age.[89] Adaptive equipment often is needed and most children with Hurler syndrome become wheelchair users in their later years.[89] We have had experience in providing developmental therapy to a 10-year-old boy with Hurler syndrome who had profound mental retardation, accompanying spastic paraplegia, and severe plantar flexion deformities of the ankles. Because of the ankle deformities, this child was basically a "knee-walker" but occasionally ambulated short distances with weight borne on the dorsum of his feet.

Phenylketonuria. Phenylketonuria (PKU) is one of the more common inborn errors of metabolism. Absence of phenylalanine hydroxylase prevents the conversion of phenylalanine to tyrosine, resulting in an abnormally excessive accumulation of phenylalanine in the blood and other body fluids. If untreated, this metabolic error results in mental and growth retardation, seizures, and pigment deficiency of hair and skin.[104] PKU is most prevalent among individuals of northern European ancestry, with a frequency of 1:10,000 to 15,000 births.[107] It is estimated that 1 of every 50 individuals is heterozygous for PKU.

Children born with PKU are usually normal in appearance, with delayed development becoming apparent toward the end of the first year. Parents usually become concerned with their child's slow development during the preschool years.[104] If untreated, individuals with PKU may go on to develop hypertonicity (75%), hyperactive reflexes (66%), hyperkinesis (50%), or tremors (30%),[64] in addition to mental retardation. IQ levels generally fall between 10 and 50, although there have been reported rare cases of untreated individuals with normal intelligence.[104]

A simple blood plasma analysis, which is mandatory for newborns in many states in the United States, can detect the presence of elevated phenylalanine levels. This test is ideally performed when the infant is at least 72 hours old. If elevated phenylalanine levels are found, the test is repeated along with further diagnostic procedures. Placing the infant on a low phenylalanine diet can prevent the mental retardation and other neurological sequelae characteristic of this disorder.[104] Follow-up management by an interdisciplinary team consisting of a nutritionist, psychologist, and appropriate medical personnel is advised in addition to the special diet.

Werdnig-Hoffmann disease (acute infantile spinal muscular atrophy). Werdnig-Hoffmann disease, or acute infantile spinal muscular atrophy (SMA), is a progressive, degenerative disorder of the anterior horn cells. It is characterized clinically by severe hypotonicity, generalized symmetrical muscle weakness, absent deep-tendon reflexes, and markedly delayed motor development. Intellect, sensation, and sphincter functioning, however, are normal.[49] In one third of individuals with this disorder, onset occurs in utero with a prenatal history of decreased fetal movements during the third trimester. Other neurological signs are observed during early infancy, usually by 6 months of age.[89] Incidence is estimated to be 1:20,000 live births.[88]

Diagnosis may be accomplished through electromyogram (EMG) and muscle biopsy, which reveal neurogenic atrophy.[49] Poor head control, froglike positioning of lower extremities,[56] better use of distal than proximal musculature, and fasciculation and atrophy of the tongue secondary to hypoglossal nucleus involvement[49] are other clinical symptoms. Progressive swallowing problems also have been noted in some cases.[89]

Intercostal muscle weakness leads to diaphragmatic breathing and contributes to the greatly increased susceptibility to pulmonary infection,[49] which usually results in death before the age of 2.[56] A few individuals with Werdnig-Hoffmann disease have survived to adolescence but are unable to stand without support. Neuropathological examination reveals abnormal and decreased numbers of neurons in the spinal cord and medulla as well as demyelinization of anterior roots and peripheral nerves.[56]

Kugelberg Welander disease (intermediate spinal muscular atrophy). Kugelberg Welander disease or intermediate SMA has an age of onset between 3 months and 15 years. Incidence is estimated at 1:24,000 live births.[88] Like the infantile onset form of SMA, Kugelberg Welander disease is characterized by proximal weakness, decreased deep tendon reflexes, and normal intelligence. There is an increased incidence of scoliosis and joint contractures. Chewing and swallowing difficulties are rare. Individuals with this disorder may experience long periods in which the disease appears static, and many survive into adulthood.[89]

We participated in the interdisciplinary evaluation of a 13-month-old girl with Kugelberg Welander disease and found pronounced trunk and proximal muscle weakness and an inability to sit, crawl, or creep. Examination by the neurologist on the team revealed tongue fasciculations and many of the other neurological signs noted earlier. Referral was made to a pediatric physical therapist to provide the parents with positioning techniques and breathing exercises for the infant. A powered wheelchair was prescribed when she was 2 years of age.

Sex-linked inherited disorders. The third mechanism for transmission of specific gene defects is through sex-linked inheritance. Two well-known sex-linked inherited diseases are Duchenne muscular dystrophy (see Chapter 13) and hemophilia. In sex-linked inherited disorders, the abnormal gene is carried on the X chromosome. Female individuals carrying one abnormal gene will not show the trait because of the dominant normal gene on the other X chromosome. Each son born to a carrier mother, however, has a 50:50 chance of inheriting the abnormal gene and thus exhibiting the disorder. Each daughter has a 50:50 chance of becoming a carrier of the trait. Two of these syndromes that result in profound neurological disabilities are discussed in this section: Lowe syndrome and Lesch-Nyhan syndrome.

Lowe syndrome (oculocerebrorenal syndrome). Lowe syndrome is characterized by progressive mental deterioration, renal tubular dysfunction, and cortical cataracts with or without glaucoma.[60] Because of the sex-linked inheritance, all individuals with Lowe syndrome are boys. Clinical symptoms that become apparent during infancy include hypotonicity, joint hyperextensibility, growth retardation and failure to thrive,[98] frontal bossing,[119] and a shrill, piercing cry.[1]

Physical characteristics of individuals with Lowe syndrome include scaphocephaly (long, narrow skull), large low-set ears, pale skin, and blond hair.[1] Neuromuscular findings include diminished or absent deep-tendon reflexes and muscle hypoplasia with fatty infiltration.[60] Neuropathological findings show demyelination and gliosis in the CNS. Moderate to severe mental retardation, hyperactivity, and abnormal electroencephalogram (EEG) findings also are present.[60] Blindness,[119] secondary to the cataracts and glaucoma, and osteoporosis[104] are observed later in life. Death usually results from renal failure.[1]

Lesch-Nyhan syndrome. Another sex-linked disorder that leads to profound neurological deterioration is Lesch-Nyhan syndrome or hereditary choreoathetosis. The primary metabolic symptom that characterizes this disorder is a marked overproduction of uric acid (hyperuricemia),[55] which results in a deficiency of hypoxanthine guanine phosphoribosyltransferase (HGPRT) in the brain, liver,[61] and amniotic cells.[9] First described in 1964 by Lesch and Nyhan,[69] the syndrome has an incidence rate of 1:10,000 males.[20] This disorder is detectable through amniocentesis, and genetic counseling is advisable for parents who have already given birth to an affected son.[9]

Infants appear normal at birth, but begin to self-mutilate at 1 to 2 years of age by biting their lips. The disorder progresses to more severe forms of self-mutilation in which individuals have been known to bite off their finger tips.[55] In spite of the extreme self-mutilation that characterizes this disorder, pain perception appears to be normal.

Motor development is often normal during the first 6 to 8 months of life. Progressive spastic paresis and athetosis, however, become evident during the latter half of the first year of life. Other neuromotor symptoms include chorea, ballismus, tremor, hyperactive deep-tendon reflexes, severe dysarthria, and dysphagia. Bilateral dislocation of hips may occur secondary to the spasticity.[55] An increased incidence of club foot deformity has been noted.[27] Growth retardation is also apparent, as well as moderate to severe mental retardation.[55]

Blood and urine levels of uric acid have been decreased successfully through the administration of allopurinol, with resultant decrease in kidney damage.[27] Death usually occurs before adolescence and is often secondary to uremia from gouty neuropathy or to generalized debilitation.[55]

Other genetic disorders. One other genetic disorder that developmental therapists should be familiar with is Rett syndrome. It is not included under any of the previous categories because its etiology is unknown. The leading hypothesis is that it is an X-linked dominant condition that is lethal in males. Several genetic studies aimed at detecting fragile sites, translocations, and deletions have been performed,[126] with no cytogenetic abnormalities detected on routine chromosomal analysis. Initial reports suggested fragile sites on the Xp22 region, but further studies revealed the incidence to be similar to the normal population.[79] Because no biological marker has been identified for Rett syndrome, clinical symptoms must be used for diagnosis. Some of these symptoms, however, may not be evident until the child is 5 years old; therefore clinical diagnosis before this age is tentative.[38]

Rett syndrome is a pervasive, progressive neurological disorder that occurs exclusively in girls. It is usually sporadic, but occasionally occurs in female siblings and relatives. Over 1000 girls with Rett syndrome have been identified worldwide,[126] with an estimated incidence of 1:15,000 births.[36]

The syndrome is characterized by apparently normal development during the first 6 months of life, with deterioration occurring between 6 to 18 months of age. Virtually all language ability is lost, although some children may produce echolalic sounds and learn simple manual signing. Evidence of minimal receptive language skills may be observed. Previously acquired purposeful hand skills are also lost and replaced by stereotypical hand movements. These nonspecific hand movements have been described as hand wringing, clapping, waving, or mouthing. Almost all individuals with Rett syndrome function in the range of severe to profound mental retardation. Although head circumference is normal at birth, deceleration of rate of head growth occurs between 5 months and 4 years of age.[115]

Onset of walking is usually delayed until about 19 months of age, almost one fourth of girls with Rett syndrome never develop independent ambulation skills.[115] Initially, hypotonia may be evident, but with advancing age, spasticity of the extremities develops.[37] Increased muscle tone is usually observed first in the lower extremities, with continued greater involvement than in the upper extremities. Peripheral vasomotor disturbances and muscle wasting have been noted as associated characteristics.[113]

In a report of 16 patients with Rett syndrome, Hennessey and Haas[50] described musculoskeletal deformities in nearly all patients. Fifteen showed clinical evidence of scoliosis, nine showed heelcord tightening, and hip instability was identified as an area of potential concern. Trevathan and Naidu[115] reported scoliosis in 50% of girls with Rett syndrome after the age of 10 years, many of whom required surgical correction.

Approximately 70% to 80% of individuals with Rett syndrome develop seizures in the first five years of life. Early EEG can be normal before 2 years of age. Cranial CT scans are normal or show mild generalized atrophy. Breathing dysfunction, including wake apnea and intermittent hyperventilation,[115] is also associated with Rett syndrome. Interventions reported in the literature have focused on splinting,[82] behavioral modification techniques to teach self-feeding skills,[93] music therapy, physical therapy, and occupational therapy.[111]

Typical clinical symptoms and common motor problems

Specific examples of genetic disorders in children and their accompanying symptomatology have been presented in the foregoing section. Table 10-1 summarizes the clinical signs common to many of the disorders. Following is a description of those clinical signs and common motor problems that are most relevant for developmental physical or occupational therapists.

Hypertonicity. Children with hypertonus generally display stiff or jerky movements that are limited in variety, speed, and coordination. Movements tend to be limited to the midranges. Total patterns of flexion or extension may dominate with limited ability to selectively move individual joints. Motor development of children with hypertonicity may be further complicated by the retention of primitive reflexes, which can result in stereotyped movements that are dependent on sensory input.

Some children will learn to use these habitual patterns of movement to achieve functional goals and are able to activate the muscle synergies of a reflex without sensory feedback.[7] If a goal of therapy is to facilitate functional movement that is not dominated by persistent reflexes, it is critical to practice new motor patterns to accomplish the functional activity for which that reflex is being used. For example, if a child has learned to activate an asymmetrical tonic neck reflex (ATNR) for reaching, a new method of reaching must be developed if the ATNR is to be inhibited. If a child is unable to learn an alternative method of reaching, however, it may be necessary to allow reflex movements to occur. When using a reflex synergy is the only way a child can perform a task, inhibition for the sake of "normalization" of tone and movement would be detrimental to functional independence.[44]

Differences and similarities observed in children with hypertonicity and hypotonicity are listed in Table 10-2.

Table 10-1. Typical clinical symptoms

Genetic disorder	Hypotonicity	Hypertonicity	Hip Dislocation	Spinal Deformities	Upper Extremity Deformities	Other Deformities	Motor Delays	Cognitive Delays	Cerebellar Dysfunction
Trisomy 21	X			X		X	X	X	X
Trisomy 18	X	X		X	X	X	X	X	
Trisomy 13	X	X			X	X	X	X	
Turner syndrome			X	X	X	X			
Klinefelter syndrome (Type XXY)					X	X			
Wolf-Hirschhorn syndrome (4p-)	X		X	X	X	X	X	X	
Cri-du-chat syndrome (5p-)	X	X	X	X		X	X	X	
Prader-Willi syndrome (15q-)	X			X		X	X	X	
Osteogenesis imperfecta	X			X	X	X	X		
Tuberous sclerosis		X					X	X	
Neurofibromatosis		X		X		X			
Hurler syndrome		X	X	X	X	X	X	X	X
Untreated PKU		X					X	X	X
Werdnig-Hoffmann syndrome	X			X	X	X	X		
Kugelberg-Welander syndrome	X			X		X	X		
Lowe syndrome	X					X	X	X	
Lesch-Nyhan syndrome		X	X			X	X	X	X
Rett syndrome	X	X		X		X	X	X	

Table 10-2. Hypotonicity and hypertonicity: Differences and similarities

	Hypotonicity	Hypertonicity
1. Characteristics	Low tone, floppy, "rag doll"	High tone, spastic, or rigid
2. Distribution	Generalized, symmetrical	Generalized; often asymmetrical
3. Range of motion	Excessive, joint hyperextensibility	Limited to midranges
4. Risk for contractures and deformities	Risk of dislocation (jaw, hip, atlantoaxial joint)	Risks for contractures (flexor), dislocations (hip) and deformities (scoliosis, kyphosis)
5. Deep tendon reflexes	Hypoactive	Hyperactive
6. Integration of primitive reflexes	Hyporeflexive; sometimes delayed integration	Often delayed
7. Achievement of motor milestones	Delayed (amount of delay correlates with severity of hypotonicity)	Delayed (amount of delay correlates with severity of hypertonicity)
8. Influence of body position	Tone remains same	Tone fluctuates with changes in body position
9. Consistency of muscles	Soft, doughy	Hard, rocklike
10. Respiratory problems	Shallow breathing; choking secondary to decreased pharyngeal tone	Decreased thoracic mobility; limited inspiration and expiration
11. Speech problems	Shallow breathing; little sustained phonation	Dysarthria secondary to hypertonicity in oral muscles
12. Feeding problems	Hypoactive gag reflex, open mouth and protruding tongue, incoordination of swallowing	Hyperactive gag reflex, tongue thrust, bite reflex, rooting reflex

Although hypertonicity is often used interchangeably with the term "spasticity" (defined as increased resistance to passive stretch), there is growing recognition that muscles may be hypertonic, but not spastic. One explanation for muscles that are hypertonic, but not spastic, is that such hypertonicity results from an attempt to control excessive movement at a joint.[7] This may be observed during the learning of a new skill in which there is a need to eliminate some of the excessive movement. Such "fixing" keeps the involved joints fairly rigid, thereby "fixing" or "freezing" nonessential movements and resulting in increased muscle tone or stiffness around that joint. As skill increases, a child learns to control the forces of movement and no longer needs to "fix," thereby allowing a greater variety of movements to occur. If skill does not increase, however, a child may "fix" to compensate for his or her lack of active control, thereby exhibiting hypertonus.

Hypotonicity. Whereas movements of the child with high muscle tone are generally limited to the midranges, children with low muscle tone typically display movements in the extremes of the range. Children with hypotonicity tend to lock weight-bearing joints or assume positions that provide a broad base of support to maximize their stability. Although retention of primitive reflexes is less likely to interfere with the development of functional movement patterns, delays in the development of postural reactions are a major concern (Fig. 10-7). As a result of delays in postural development, children with hypotonicity often learn to rely on sources of external support to maintain upright positions.

Limited strength and lack of endurance are often concerns with children who have hypotonicity. Additional concerns that may arise from joint laxity are discussed in the next section.

Hyperextensible joints. Hyperextensible joints are commonly observed in children with low muscle tone, and are noted in many children with genetic disorders. Activities should be modified to avoid undue stress to these joints and the surrounding ligaments, tendons, and fascia. For example, positions that allow knee or elbow joints to lock into extension should be modified so that weight-bearing occurs through more neutral alignment. Varying the placement of toys and support surfaces, providing physical assistance, or using adaptive equipment can help modify weight-bearing forces to achieve more neutral alignment. For example, if hyperextensible ligaments cause excessive pronation in stance, the use of ankle foot orthoses may provide enough support to the structures to allow functional activities in standing. For a child who stands with knee hyperextension, a vertical stander may allow that child to stand and play at a water table with his or her classmates for extended periods with the knees in a more neutral position. Rather than restricting a child's repertoire of upright positions, it is preferable to modify an activity or provide external support to enable a child to participate fully (Fig. 10-8).

Contractures and deformities. Skeletal anomalies and deformities are associated with many genetic disorders. The developmental physical or occupational therapist may work

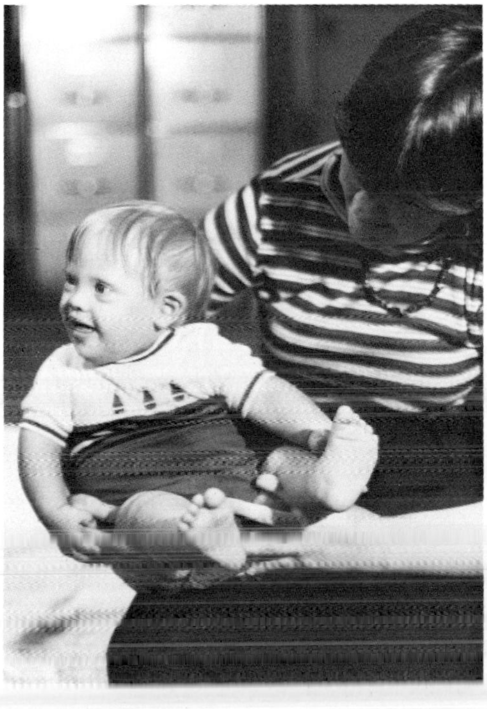

Fig. 10-7. Facilitation of equilibrium reactions in a 10-month-old child with Down syndrome.

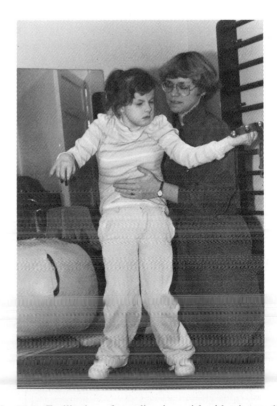

Fig. 10-8. Facilitation of standing in a girl with trisomy 18.

with orthopedists, prosthetists, and orthotists to detect and prevent the progression of a variety of conditions. The therapist should be aware of factors that can contribute to the development of deformities in order to prevent or minimize such problems. For example, the child with hypertonicity is at risk for developing joint contractures because of the limitation of movement around the joint.

Although joint contractures are less likely to occur in a child with hypotonicity, habitual positioning may lead to soft tissue restrictions. For example, children with low muscle tone who adopt a constant position of wide abduction, external rotation, and flexion at the hips ("frog" or "reverse W" position)[113] can develop soft tissue contractures in the hips and knees. Likewise, children whose hips are maintained in a position of adduction, flexion, and internal rotation are at risk for hip subluxation or dislocation.[113] Spinal deformities, such as lumbar lordosis, and thoracic kyphosis and scoliosis, are also common concerns in children with abnormal muscle tone. An imbalance of muscle tone, strength, or immobility may increase the risk of spinal deformity. In general, contractures and deformities are of most concern for children who display a limited variety of postures and movements.

Respiratory problems. Respiratory problems are often observed in children with hypotonicity or hypertonicity, as well as in children whose respiratory functioning is compromised by chest and skeletal deformities. These children may require mobilization techniques, deep breathing, chest expansion exercises, and postural drainage. Some children may find it difficult to tolerate one position for an extended time due to respiratory difficulties. For these children, frequent changes of position and use of adapted positioning devices may be necessary.

Our experience in treating a child with Werdnig-Hoffmann disease necessitated the modification of a prone board as an alternative positioning device. The child was unable to tolerate a completely prone position because of respiratory problems and became easily fatigued when sitting for extended periods, often using her hands to support her head in an upright position. A standard prone board with desk was modified to include an anterior head rest. This adaptation allowed her to rest her neck muscles and free her hands for other activities, and it did not compromise her respiratory status.

FAMILY-CENTERED INTERVENTION FOR CHILDREN WITH GENETIC DISORDERS

This section examines the role of the developmental physical or occupational therapist in providing therapy services for children with genetic disorders. Following a discussion of ways in which therapists can support families of children with genetic disorders, evaluation strategies, goals and objectives, and general treatment principles are discussed. Throughout this section, emphasis is placed on supporting and including family members in all aspects of

therapy and assuring that therapy programs meet the priorities and needs of family members.

Supporting families

Therapists working with children with genetic disorders need to recognize and acknowledge the multitude of tasks that all families work to accomplish. In addition to tasks specifically related to caring for their child with a disability, families must perform functions to address the economic, daily care, recreational, social, and educational/vocational needs of both individual members and the family as a whole.[116] As Turnbull and Turnbull[116] have cautioned, each time professionals intervene with families and children, they can potentially enhance or hinder the family's ability to meet important family functions. For example, intervention that promotes a child's social skills can be an important support to positive family functioning. On the other hand, intervention that focuses on a child's deficits can have a negative impact on how the family perceives that child and the place of the child in the family. For therapists to be supportive of families, they must (1) acknowledge the importance of **family priorities,** (2) respect the family's cultural values, (3) include families as integral team members, and (4) promote and deliver services that build on family and community resources.

Family priorities. Families are the primary agents for promoting the development of their child. It is important, therefore, for developmental physical or occupational therapists and other professionals to acknowledge the values, priorities, and concerns of the families with whom they work. Family resources, support networks, and home/community activities must be considered when planning interventions or suggesting home activities. Such information need not be obtained through a battery of formal assessments.[106] In fact, information about topics such as family roles, life crises, future planning, and stress is more likely to be gathered through informal approaches and open-ended conversations[84] during the course of an ongoing relationship, rather than in the context of a formal "initial intake" session.[106]

Cultural values. Part of understanding a family's values and priorities is understanding their culture. For developmental therapists, it is particularly important to have knowledge about the values of the culture that relate specifically to health care. For example, knowing how persons from a given culture are likely to view disabilities and traditional medicine, and how they seek help from professionals, may minimize the danger of imposing one's values and incorrectly judging as abnormal behaviors that are considered "normal" for a particular culture.[16] In addition, values related to privacy, time, the future, family life, child-rearing, and decision making should be considered.

Family-guided teamwork. It has been recognized for quite some time that no one discipline can meet the diverse and complex needs of children with disabilities and their families. Both Public Law 94-142[97] and 99-457 (and the more recent Public Law 109-112) require professionals to work in teams to plan and provide comprehensive services for all children with disabilities. With the passage of PL 99-457 came the recognition that parents and family members are essential team members who know what is best for their child and family. Therapists and other professionals need to assure that the family's interests, not the professionals', are the foundation for decision making.[70] For this to occur, family members should be involved in goal setting, planning of service delivery, and program evaluation. Family input in each of these areas helps ensure that recommendations for treatment can be incorporated into the family's life-style.

Building on family and community resources. An important aspect of supporting families is providing them with the information and encouragement they need to solve problems and acquire a sense of control over their lives. Families gain competence in solving problems by getting the support that enables them to discover which solutions are best for them, not by getting the "right" solutions from "expert" professionals.[110] Professionals should refrain from providing services that could be provided by someone in the family's own support network. One way that professionals can assist families is by supporting them to seek out the "natural" supports in their own communities. Natural supports include friends, neighbors, and other community members. Because long-term professional services are not available to all families, using these informal sources of assistance can help ensure the availability of adequate resources and support.[26] Facilitating parent-to-parent support networks is another way to strengthen a family's personal support network. A special level of understanding can be shared by people in similar circumstances; families can provide each other with encouragement and support, as well as practical information about topics such as community resources and caregiving.

Supporting and including families in all aspects of therapy should be an important focus of providing developmental therapy services. Taking advantage of the knowledge and expertise of parents is especially important when gathering information about a child's current level of functioning and in developing therapy goals.

Evaluation strategies

Knowledge of a child's diagnosis can aid in the selection of appropriate assessment tools and alert the therapist to any potential medical problems or contraindications associated with the specific syndrome that might affect the **evaluation** procedures. Therapists must be careful, however, not to develop preconceived opinions about a child's capabilities based on how other children with similar diagnoses have performed. It is critical to remember that there is wide behavioral and performance variability among children

within each genetic disorder. For example, wide variability in the achievement of developmental milestones has been reported among children with Down syndrome.[76]

Typically, therapists include in their assessments an evaluation of the neuromuscular status of the child, such as primitive reflexes, automatic reactions, and muscle tone. For children with orthopedic involvement, assessment of muscle strength, joint range of motion, joint play, and soft tissue mobility is also important. In addition to these types of evaluations, an assessment of the child's developmental level and functional ability should be completed. Such assessments can be used to discriminate between typical and delayed development, to identify the constraints interfering with the achievement of functional skills, and to guide the development of treatment goals and strategies. Most developmental assessment tools fall into one of the following categories: (1) discriminitive, (2) predictive, and (3) evaluative measures.[62] Each of these three types of developmental assessment tools yields different types of information. It is important to understand these differences and the intended purpose for each type of assessment to ensure that evaluation tools are used appropriately.

Discriminitive assessments. A discriminitive measure is used to distinguish between individuals with or without a particular feature of interest.[62] Such instruments provide information necessary to document children's eligibility for special services, but rarely provide information useful for planning or evaluating therapy programs.[47] Norm-referenced tests such as the *Bayley Scales of Infant Development* (motor and mental scales),[3] the *Peabody Developmental Motor Scales,*[28] and the *Revised Gesell & Amatruda Developmental & Neurological Examination* (adaptive, gross and fine motor, language, and personal/social development)[63] are examples of norm-referenced tests used with infants and young children to verify developmental delay or assign age levels (Fig. 10-9). Examples of norm-referenced assessments for older children include the *Bruininks-Oseretsky Test of Motor Proficiency*[11] and the *Stott-Moyes-Henderson Test of Motor Impairment.*[112]

It may be possible to detect improved motor performance by administering a developmental test used to discriminate children who have motor delays. Such tests, however, usually cannot detect small increments of improvement, as there are relatively few test items at each age level and developmental gaps between items are often large. In assessing whether intervention has been effective, the use of most discriminitive tools does not examine a child's performance of functional activities in natural environments.[47]

Predictive assessments. Predictive measures are used to classify individuals according to a set of established categories and to verify whether an individual has been classified correctly.[62] Measures designed to predict future performance are often used to detect early signs of motor impairment in infants who are at risk for neuromotor dysfunction.[47] The *Movement Assessment of Infants (MAI)*

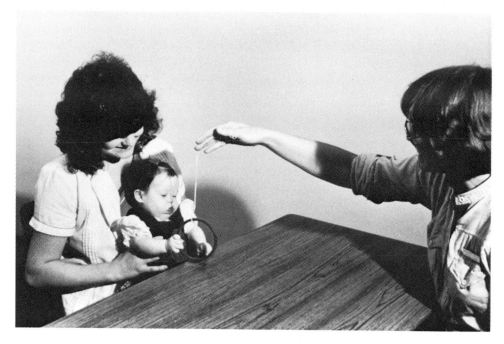

Fig. 10-9. Four-month-old infant with Down syndrome being assessed on the Bayley Scales of Infant Development.

was designed to assess muscle tone, reflex development, automatic reactions, and volitional movement of infants in the first year of life.[15] The ability of the *MAI* to predict later cerebral palsy has been examined.[45]

Evaluative assessments. An evaluative measure is used to document change within an individual over time or change as the result of intervention.[62] The *Hawaii Early Learning Profile (HELP)*[29] is a curriculum-referenced test that provides information about a child's developmental progress relative to a prespecified curriculum sequence. The *HELP* and its accompanying activity guide can be used to plan intervention strategies in the areas of gross motor, fine motor, social, self-help, cognitive, and language skills.

To determine whether a child's ability to perform meaningful skills in everyday environments has improved, a functional assessment should be used. Functional assessments focus on the accomplishment of specific daily activities, rather than the achievement of developmental milestones (Fig. 10-10). Emphasis is placed on the end result in terms of the achievement of a functional task, rather than on the form or quality of the movement. Assistance in the form of people or devices is incorporated into the assessment of progress, with the measurement of progress focusing on the achievement of independence.[41] Qualitative aspects of movement that have important functional implications, such as accuracy, speed, endurance, adaptability, and generalizability, are also considered.

Functional assessments can be used to screen, diagnose, or describe functional deficits and to determine the resources needed to allow the child to function optimally in specific environments (e.g., school, home). Another use of functional

assessments is to evaluate the nature of the problem and the specific task requirements limiting function in order to develop educational plans and teaching strategies.[41] A final use of functional assessments is to examine and monitor changes in functional status. Such assessments can be used for program evaluation and for determining the cost-effectiveness of services or programs.

The *Functional Independence Measure (FIM)* is an example of a functional assessment. The *FIM* assesses the effectiveness of therapy on functional dependence in the areas of self-care, sphincter control, mobility, locomotion, communication, and social cognition.[34] Seven levels of functional dependence ranging from total assistance to complete independence are used to determine an individual's status. An adaptation of the *FIM*[40] places greater emphasis on functional gains as opposed to the level of care. The *WeeFIM*[33] has been developed for use with children through the age of 6 years.

Another example of a functional assessment is the *Tufts Assessment of Motor Performance (TAMP)*. The *TAMP* is a standardized, criterion-referenced tool that has been designed to assess functional motor performance in the areas of mobility, dressing, feeding, and communication.[30] Separate pediatric and adult versions are available.

A final example of a functional assessment is the *Pediatric Evaluation of Disability Inventory (PEDI)*, which focuses on the domains of self-care, mobility, and social cognition. The *PEDI* incorporates three measurement scales: (1) the capability to perform selected functional skills, (2) the level of caregiver assistance that is required, and (3) identification of environmental modifications or equipment

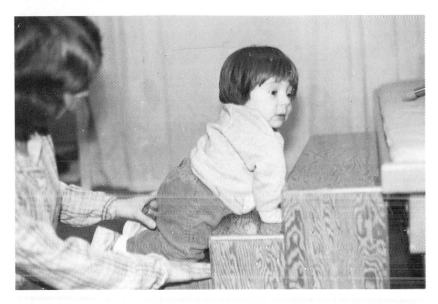

Fig. 10-10. Functional mobility skills in a child with osteogenesis imperfecta.

needed to perform a particular activity.[39] The *PEDI* has been standardized and normed and is intended for use with children whose abilities are in the range of a typical 6-month-old to 7-year-old child.

Family-driven goals and objectives

After a child's strengths and needs are evaluated, therapy goals and objectives can be developed. In the past, this has been the responsibility primarily of professionals. More recently, however, professionals have recognized the value of having families guide the process of establishing intervention goals and objectives. This shift toward collaborative goal-setting has occurred largely as a result of the belief that families should determine their vision of the future for their children, and professionals should act as consultants and resources to assist families in achieving that vision. When parents and therapists jointly determine goals and the means by which to attain them,[2] parents are more likely to commit time and energy to work toward the goals. For children, these goals are developed within the context of individualized service plans.

Individualized service plans. With the enactment of Public Law 94-142 in 1975,[97] physical and occupational therapists working in public school settings were required to establish long-term annual goals and short-term therapy objectives within the framework of each child's Individualized Education Program (IEP). The components of an IEP are as follows:[87]

1. A statement of the child's present levels of educational performance
2. A statement of annual goals, including short-term instructional objectives
3. A statement of the specific special education and related services to be provided to the child

4. The projected dates for initiation of services and the anticipated duration of the service
5. Appropriate objective criteria and evaluation procedures and schedules for determining, at least annually whether short-term instructional objectives are being achieved

Similar requirements are now in effect for infants receiving early intervention services as a result of the enactment of Public Law 99-457 in 1986 and its revision Public Law 102-119 (Individuals with Disabilities Education Act) in 1991. An Individualized Family Service Plan (IFSP) must be written after a multidisciplinary assessment of the strengths and needs of the child is completed. This assessment must include a family-directed assessment of the supports and services necessary to enhance the family's capacity to meet the needs of their child with a disability.[77] The IFSP must contain the following:

1. A statement of the child's present levels of development (cognitive, speech/language, psychosocial, motor, and self-help)
2. A statement of the family's resources, priorities, and concerns related to enhancing the child's development
3. A statement of major outcomes expected to be achieved for the child and family
4. The criteria, procedures, and timelines for determining progress
5. The specific early-intervention services necessary to meet the unique needs of the child and family including the method, frequency, and intensity of service
6. The natural environments in which services shall be provided

7. The projected dates for the initiation of services and expected duration
8. The name of the resource coordinator
9. The procedures for transition from early intervention to the preschool program

Functional objectives. The development of behaviorally written, measurable therapy objectives is crucial for monitoring the effects of intervention in a child with a genetic disorder. Many of the clinical symptoms listed in the descriptions of genetic disorders described earlier in the chapter may be monitored through systematic, periodic, data-keeping procedures. One example is the monitoring of functional hand skills in girls with Rett syndrome. Periodic vital capacity measures for a child with osteogenesis imperfecta or a child with Werdnig-Hoffmann disease could reflect progress toward a goal of maintaining respiratory function.

Typically, therapy objectives focus on a child's deficits. For example, delays in achieving motor milestones are often used to identify gaps in development, and therapy objectives are written and programs established to address these deficits. When the child meets an objective, new deficits are identified and new objectives are developed. A different approach is to begin with the desired outcome and consider what needs to occur to achieve that outcome.

For example, Maile is a 3-year-old girl with Down syndrome. On developmental testing, she displays deficits in single-leg stance stability. A typical developmental therapy objective might be, "Maile will balance on one foot for at least 3 seconds, two out of three trials." In Maile's IFSP meeting, however, her parents expressed the hope that Maile would be able to play safely with her peers at a neighborhood playground—a more functionally relevant goal. The following therapy objectives were developed to address her need to develop single-limb stance stability within the context of the family-identified goal:

1. With standby assistance, Maile will climb up the rungs of a 4-foot high slide and seat herself at the top with feet pointed down the decline of the slide by 6/94.
2. Maile will be able to walk independently across a 25-foot stretch of uneven ground (sand or lawn) without falling by 6/94.

Goal attainment scaling (GAS) is a variation of behavioral objectives that detects small, clinically important changes over time.[90] Similar to behavioral objectives, GAS requires (1) identification of observable goals, (2) the conditions under which performance is measured, (3) the measurable criteria for success, and (4) a time frame for goal achievement. In contrast to behavioral objectives, however, GAS identifies *five* possible outcomes with accompanying score values: two outcomes that surpass the expected level and two outcomes that fall below the expected level. Using five possible levels of attainment, one can determine whether a child has made progress despite not achieving the expected

outcome, or whether progress has exceeded the expected outcome. Following is an example of the use of GAS to assess Maile's first functional objective:

−2 = With physical assistance, Maile will climb up the rungs of a 4-foot high slide by 6/94.
−1 = With physical assistance, Maile will climb up the rungs of a 4-foot high slide and seat herself at the top with feet pointed down the decline of the slide by 6/94.
 0 = With standby assistance, Maile will climb up the rungs of a 4-foot high slide and seat herself at the top with feet pointed down the decline of the slide by 6/94.
+1 = Maile will climb up and seat herself at the top of a 4-foot high slide independently, slide down and stop at the bottom with physical assistance to prevent losing her balance by 6/94.
+2 = Maile will climb up and seat herself at the top of a 4-foot high slide, slide down, and stop at the bottom independently by 6/94.

Rather than focusing on a child's deficits, such "outcome-focused" objectives provide a more positive and supportive context for therapy, and at the same time address the family's needs and priorities. This approach to developing therapy goals and objectives in ways that support positive family functioning is also an important aspect of delivering therapy services to children and their families.

General treatment principles

Several general treatment principles guide the delivery of therapy services to children with genetic disorders. A description of each of these principles is followed by examples illustrating their applicability to particular children.

Focus on functional skills. Many of the classic therapeutic exercise approaches for individuals with neurological disorders are oriented toward making qualitative changes in motor tasks such as normalizing muscle tone or improving gait symmetry. Often, there is little regard for the functional significance of those changes.[46] More recent therapeutic approaches place less emphasis on such qualitative changes, and instead focus on the motor behaviors necessary to acquire **functional skills.** In this approach, environmental adaptations and assistive technology are used to attain functional outcomes such as independence in self-help skills, communication, and mobility[46] (Fig. 10-11).

This shift to a focus on functional skills is consistent with recent task-oriented approaches to neurological rehabilitation. The task-oriented model assumes that control of movement is organized around goal-directed, functional behaviors rather than on muscle or movement patterns.[57] Intervention, therefore, is aimed at teaching motor problem-solving (adaptability to varied contexts), developing effective compensations that are maximally efficient, and providing practice of new motor skills in functional situations.

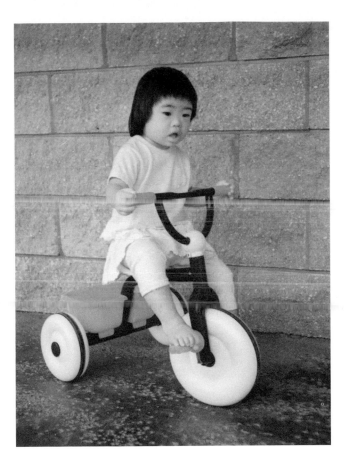

Fig. 10-11. Child with Down syndrome during practice of functional motor skills.

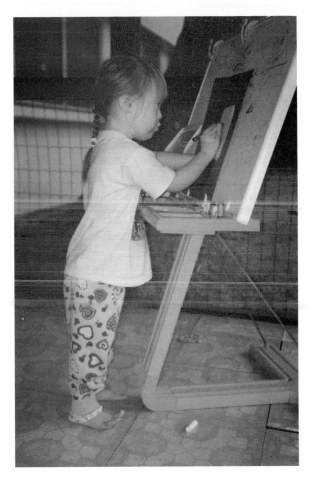

Fig. 10-12. Practice of developmental skills during daily routine at home.

Rather than teaching individuals to perform movement patterns in a controlled therapy setting, this approach focuses on the learning that must take place for an individual to function independent of a therapist's guidance.[51]

Delivery of services in natural environments. Functional skills are most meaningfully taught and practiced within the context where they will be used.[84] The movement toward integrating therapy into classroom settings is one example of providing services in a **natural environment**.[17,109] In an integrated model of service delivery, therapists work in the classroom with teachers, rather than removing students to an isolated therapy room to provide services. Therapists work closely with the teacher to establish common goals for the student and to devise programs that will allow therapeutic activities to be interwoven into a variety of activities throughout the day in a natural manner.

Another example of providing therapy in a natural environment is providing home-based services for infants and young children. Home based programs are "normal" options for very young children because the natural environment for most infants and toddlers is the home— either their own or that of a childcare provider.[84] For children who are medically fragile, it is the preferred option for therapy.[102] For other families, transportation to a center based program

may be difficult because of the expense or length of travel required.

One advantage of working with children in their home environment is that it is often easier to see the whole picture and consider a child's needs within the context of the entire family. Therapists who provide services in the home environment must be especially flexible in the way they offer their services so that they respect the family's daily routines.[59]

Incorporating therapy activities into daily routines. Therapists need to work collaboratively with families to develop activities that incorporate therapeutic activities into the family's daily routine (e.g., during play, dressing, bathing, meals). Rather than practicing narrowly defined tasks in a controlled clinic environment, therapy activities should be interwoven into a variety of activities throughout the day in a natural manner. Practicing skills in the context of daily routines allows the child to learn to adapt to the real life contingencies that arise during a functional task.[51] In addition, activities become more meaningful both to the child and family (Fig. 10-12).

Use of assistive technology devices. As noted previ-

CASE 1 ▼ **Kristy**

Kristy is an 8-month-old girl with cri-du-chat syndrome. She attends an early intervention program weekly and is accompanied by her mother, Nancy, and occasionally a neighbor, Betty, who is very involved with Kristy's care. Kristy has very low muscle tone throughout her trunk and extremities, but is beginning to move against gravity in prone and supine. In her most recent IFSP meeting, Nancy requested that the therapist concentrate on helping Kristy learn to sit independently so that she can play with her hands free. In prone, Kristy relies on her arms for support and as a result, her hands are not readily available for play. Nancy has noticed that Kristy seems to manipulate toys more when in supported sitting than when in prone.

To allow Kristy to sit without adult assistance, a dense, foam insert was added to her highchair to provide additional support. The insert included a pelvic stabilizer, which allowed Kristy to maintain proper postural alignment even during active movement of her upper body. The therapists had several ideas about activities in the home that could assist Kristy to develop independent sitting balance. In talking to Nancy, however, the staff found little time for Nancy to devote to specific therapy activities during the day because of her responsibilities in caring for her four other children. They also learned that her neighbor, Betty, was interested in helping out with Kristy's care and was happy to follow through with the home activities. Plans were made for Betty to accompany Kristy and Nancy to the therapy sessions to learn new activities from Kristy's therapists.

CASE 2 ▼ **Maile**

Maile is a 3-year-old girl with Down syndrome whose therapy goals were discussed in another section of this chapter. As noted previously, her parents' primary concerns regarding Maile's motor skills involve her playground abilities. Therefore, the therapist scheduled Maile's weekly therapy session during the classroom playground time. In this way, the therapist would be able to help Maile improve her strength, endurance, and coordination in the context in which these skills need to be used. Therapy occurring on the playground will provide opportunities for Maile to learn how to assess the demands of the environment and to match them with her abilities. In this natural setting, she will also learn a variety of strategies to adapt to changing conditions. For example, when faced with the task of negotiating the playground slide, Maile will have to learn how to compensate for her low muscle tone and joint laxity so that she can climb up the ladder to sit on the top of the slide. Working on postural stability, single leg stance, and shoulder girdle stabilization in this context will be more motivating than practicing these same skills in an isolated therapy room, and will likely be facilitated by Maile's classmates who can serve as models.

---

ously, an important aspect of providing developmental therapy services is the use of assistive technology devices to maximize a child's functional abilities, level of independence, and inclusion in school and community activities with peers. Examples of assistive technology include mobility devices, augmentative communication devices, and adapted computer keyboards. Assistive technology also includes adaptive devices such as splints, bath chairs, prone standers, and other positioning equipment that can be used to provide optimal body alignment and minimize the risk for contractures/deformities, while encouraging a greater variety of movement patterns. Such devices can be constructed from readily available materials or obtained commercially. The developmental physical or occupational therapist works with the family and other team members to select, construct, and/or order assistive devices, as well as to assist caregivers in the use of the devices.

The above case examples demonstrate how these general treatment principles are applied to particular children receiving developmental therapy services. The case examples also show how the family's priorities and needs are considered and supported in the planning and delivery of services.

MEDICAL MANAGEMENT AND GENETIC COUNSELING

The developmental physical or occupational therapist should have general knowledge of both medical management of children with genetic disorders and genetic counseling for family members. This information allows the therapist to answer the family's general questions and to refer family members to the appropriate persons for more specific information.

Medical management

Few medical therapies have been successful in treating genetic disorders in children, although a number of strategies for ameliorating isolated symptoms have been reported. Of the genetic disorders discussed in this chapter, the only one for which dramatic results have been achieved through early medical management is PKU. With early diagnosis and immediate implementation of a low phenylalanine diet, the infant with PKU can be spared the severe mental retardation and other progressive neurological impairments that have resulted in untreated individuals.[104]

Medical treatment for the other disorders is not curative, but rather palliative or directed at specific associated anomalies. The congenital heart defects present in an estimated 40% to 60% of individuals with Down syndrome can, in most instances, be corrected by cardiac surgery.[80] Orthopedic surgery in the form of insertion of intramedullary rods in the tibia or femur may minimize the recurrence of repeated fractures associated with osteogenesis imperfecta.[100] Surgical correction of scoliosis may be warranted in individuals with neurofibromatosis, Rett syndrome,[115] or Werdnig-Hoffmann disease[65] if the deformity is severe and bracing[83] is not successful. Radiographic screening for atlantoaxial instability in children with Down syndrome can be initiated beginning at age 2 years.[89] If atlantoaxial instability is excessive or results in a neurological deficit, a posterior fusion of the cervical vertebrae is recommended.[89] Surgical removal of obstructive or malignant tumors is advisable in certain cases of neurofibromatosis,[55] as is removal of cerebral nodular growths in individuals with tuberous sclerosis for the control of seizures.[100]

The use of appetite-regulating drugs for individuals with Prader-Willi syndrome has had equivocal results. Surgical interventions such as gastric bypass, small intestinal bypass, and jaw wiring have been attempted for weight control with these individuals but have met with limited success.[72]

Respiratory therapy is an important adjunctive treatment strategy for children with Werdnig-Hoffmann disease[65] and may be implemented as part of the overall developmental therapy program. Specific medical therapies include estrogen therapy to promote feminization in individuals with Turner syndrome and testosterone therapy to enhance masculinity in boys with Klinefelter syndrome.[81] The use of anticonvulsants is an important part of seizure management for individuals with Rett syndrome[115] and tuberous sclerosis.[5] To assist in the management of metabolic acidosis and rickets, which are often present in persons with Lowe syndrome, alkali supplements and vitamin D therapy have been used.[55] Allopurinol has been used for individuals with Lesch-Nyhan syndrome to prevent urological complications, although it has no effect on the progressive neurological symptomatology.[27]

The use of large, potentially toxic, amounts of vitamins and minerals (the orthomolecular hypothesis) has been proposed for children with many different types of developmental disabilities. This approach has been rejected for children with Down syndrome based on results of several investigations. In addition, supplementation of individual metabolites such as 5-hydroxytryptophan or pyridoxine for children with Down syndrome is ineffective.[35] Proponents of cell therapy, which involves intramuscular injection of fetal lamb brain tissue, claim that many of the morphological and developmental characteristics of Down syndrome can be altered. These claims have not been supported by clinical investigations, and opponents of cell therapy warn of the potential risk for serious allergic reactions.[96]

In light of the limited medical treatment strategies available for children with genetic disorders, the developmental physical or occupational therapist must be concerned with maximizing the child's developmental or functional potential within the limitations imposed by the lack of possible cures and the prospect of the shortened life span that characterizes many of these disorders. When deterioration of skills is expected, therapy must be directed at maintaining current functioning levels or at minimizing decline.

Genetic counseling

Of crucial importance in working with children with genetic disorders and their families is a knowledge of genetic counseling. Developmental physical or occupational therapists must have an understanding of the modes of inheritance of the various genetic disorders, as well as information about the services that can be offered through genetic counseling. Although the physician has primary responsibility for informing the parents of a child with a genetic disorder about the availability of genetic counseling, the close professional and personal relationships that therapists often develop with families may prompt family members to seek this type of information from the therapist.

Although we are certainly not advocating that the therapist serve in the role of genetic counselor, it is important that therapists be aware of the availability and location of genetic counseling services so that they may be assured that parents of a child with a genetic disorder have this information. Most major university-affiliated medical centers provide genetic counseling.

Six steps or procedures in genetic counseling have been discussed by Novitski.[86] The first is to make an accurate medical diagnosis of the child's disorder. In the case of a suspected chromosome abnormality, this usually involves conducting a karyotype of the child as well as karyotypes of parents and siblings. Other diagnostic procedures may include a medical examination, muscle biopsy, other laboratory tests, and radiographic examinations. If the disorder is of genetic origin, further procedures should follow.

The next step in genetic counseling is to construct a pedigree or family tree of all known relatives and ancestors of both parents.[86] Pedigree information includes the age and cause of death of ancestors, a history of stillbirths and spontaneous abortions, and a history of appearance of any other genetic defects or unknown causes of mental retardation. The country of origin of ancestors is also important, because certain genetic defects, such as PKU, are far more prevalent in families of a particular ethnic origin. Once the defect has been identified and a pedigree constructed, Novitski[86] advises that further information be obtained from one of the comprehensive resource texts on genetic disorders. Informing family members about the characteristics of the disorder and its natural history may diminish fears of the unknown.[14]

The third procedure in genetic counseling is to estimate the risk of recurrence of the disorder.[86] In specific gene defects, the probability of recurrence is fairly straightforward, with a risk of 25% for autosomal recessive disorders and a 50% risk for each male child in sex-linked disorders. These percentages, however, do not hold true in cases of spontaneous mutations. In cases of chromosomal abnormalities, such as Down syndrome, karyotyping is mandated to determine whether the child has the translocation type of Down syndrome. In that case the risk of recurrence is much greater than with a history of standard trisomy 21 Down syndrome.

Informing parents of the probability of recurrence is the next procedure.[86] Novitski points out the common misunderstanding that if a risk is 1:4 for a child to be affected, as in an autosomal recessive disorder, many parents assume that if they have just given birth to a child with the disorder, the next three children should be normal. It is important to explain that each subsequent child faces a 1:4 risk of inheriting the disorder regardless of how many siblings with the disorder have already been born.

The fifth step in genetic counseling is for the parents to decide on the course of action they will take for future pregnancies once the counselor has presented all available facts to them.[86] Some parents may choose not to have any more children; others may elect to undergo prenatal diagnostic procedures for subsequent pregnancies. These decisions rest entirely with the parents and may be influenced by their individual religious or ethical preferences.

Follow-up counseling and review of the most recent advances in medical genetics are the final steps in the genetic counseling procedure.[86] Genetic counseling can play an important role in opening channels of communication between parents, other family members, and their friends; connecting parents and siblings to support groups; and helping families to address their grief, sadness, or anger.[14] The effect of a child with a disability on the family may modify the parents' earlier decision to have or not to have more children. Recent medical advances may allow a more certain prenatal diagnosis of specific genetic disorders.

The most common prenatal diagnostic procedure is amniocentesis, which is used to detect early genetic disorders in the fetus at 14 to 16 weeks' gestation. This method involves inserting a long, slender needle through the mother's abdominal wall and into the placenta to extract a small amount of amniotic fluid.[122] Laboratory tests of amniotic fluid reveal all types of chromosome abnormalities, as well as a number of specific gene defects, including Tay-Sachs disease and Lesch-Nyhan syndrome, and some disorders of polygenic multifactorial inheritance, such as neural tube defects. Although certain sex-linked disorders are not as yet detectable through laboratory analysis of amniotic cells, it is possible to determine the sex of the fetus and thus elect to abort male offspring who have a 50:50 chance of inheriting the disorder.

Chorionic villi sampling has gained increasing accep-

tance as a prenatal diagnostic procedure because it allows for detection of some genetic disorders as early as 8 to 10 weeks' gestation. Chorionic villi may be used for the same tests as amniotic fluid cells, but this procedure has the advantage of rapid diagnosis because the cells need not be cultured before analysis, thus allowing fetal chromosomal analysis within 24 hours.[20] It is very difficult, however, to detect chromosomal abnormalities involving a loss or gain of small amounts of chromosomal material such as with Prader-Willi syndrome.[125] The biopsy can be performed transcervically under ultrasound guidance between 8 to 12 weeks' gestation. Transabdominal sampling can be performed throughout the pregnancy and may pose a lower risk of infection and allow easier access to the fundal placenta.[27]

Maternal serum alpha-fetoprotein (MSAFP) screening has been used widely in the United States since 1985 to detect prenatally neural tube defects.[78] MSAFP is generally measured at 15 to 16 weeks gestation, and abnormally low levels were first associated with fetal chromosome defects in 1984.[27] One screening program found 7% of women tested with levels below an established risk threshold; an abnormal karyotype was found in 1 out of 90 women who underwent subsequent amniocentesis. Approximately 40% of the abnormalities were trisomy 21, 20% were other trisomies, and the remaining cases involved a variety of different chromosome disorders. In addition to MSAFP screening, two other prenatal diagnostic tests are used to detect trisomy 21. These include tests for elevated maternal serum human chorionic gonadotropin (MShCG) levels and decreased maternal serum unconjugated estriol (MSuE3). Combined use of MSAFP, MShCG, and MSuE3 tests in screening for trisomy 21 decreases false-positive rates and increases detection rates.[78]

SUMMARY

This chapter has addressed several chromosomal abnormalities and specific gene defects that are most apt to appear in children in a typical developmental therapy setting. The inclusion of family members in all aspects of therapy has been stressed along with the need to consider family goals, priorities, and resources in the development and implementation of therapy services. The importance of developing functional goals and delivering services in natural environments has also been emphasized. Readers are encouraged to consult the reference list at the end of this chapter for further information about genetic disorders not described in this chapter (see especially Connor and Ferguson-Smith,[20] Nora and Fraser,[85] Weatherall,[121] and Jones[60]).

REFERENCES

1. Aita JA: *Congenital facial anomalies with neurologic defects,* Springfield, Ill, 1969, Charles C Thomas.
2. Bailey D: Collaborative goal setting with families: resolving differences in values and priorities for services, *Top Early Childhood Special Educ* 7:59, 1987.

3. Bayley N: *Bayley Scales of Infant Development, ed 2,* San Antonio, 1993, Psychological Corporation.

4. Benda CE: *The child with mongolism (congenital acromicria),* New York, 1960, Grune & Stratton.

5. Berg BO: Convulsive disorders. In Bleck EE and Nagel DA, editors: *Physically handicapped children: a medical atlas for teachers,* New York, 1975, Grune & Stratton.

6. Berini RY and Kahn E, editors: *Clinical genetics handbook,* Oradell, NJ, 1968, Medical Economics Books.

7. Bly L: A historical and current view of the basis of NDT, *Pediatr Phys Ther* 3:131, 1991.

8. Boue JG: Chromosomal studies in more than 900 spontaneous abortuses, Teratology Society meeting, 1974.

9. Boyle JA and others: Lesch-Nyhan syndrome: preventive control by prenatal diagnosis, *Science* 169:688, 1970.

10. Breg WR and others: The cri du chat syndrome in adolescents and adults: clinical findings in 13 older patients with partial deletion of the short arms of chromosome no 5 (5p-), *J Pediatr* 77:782, 1970.

11. Bruininks RH: *Bruininks-Oseretsky Test of Motor Proficiency: examiner's manual,* Circle Pines, Minn, 1978, American Guidance Service.

12. Butler MG and others: Clinical and cytotenetic survey of 39 individuals with Prader-Labhart-Willi syndrome, *Am J Med Genet* 23:793, 1986.

13. Carr DH: Chromosome anomalies as a cause of spontaneous abortion, *Am J Obstet Gynecol* 97:283, 1967.

14. Cassidy SB: Management of the problems in infancy: hypotonia, developmental delay, and feeding problems. In Caldwell ME and Taylor RL, editors: *Prader-Willi syndrome: selected research and management issues,* New York, 1988, Springer Verlag.

15. Chandler LS and others: *Movement assessment of infants: a manual,* Rolling Bay, Wash, 1980, Chandler, Andrews & Swanson.

16. Christensen CM: Multicultural competencies in early intervention: training professionals for a pluralistic society, *Infants Young Children* 4:49, 1992.

17. Cole K and others: Comparison of two service delivery models: in class vs. out of class therapy approaches, *Pediatr Phys Ther* 1:49, 1989.

18. Coleman M: Down's syndrome, *Pediatr Ann* 7:90, 1978.

19. Conen PE and Erkman B: Frequency and occurrence of chromosomal syndromes. I. D-trisomy, *Am J Hum Genet* 18:374, 1966.

20. Connor JM and Ferguson-Smith MA: *Essential medical genetics* (4th ed), Boston MA, 1993, Blackwell Scientific Publications.

21. Cowie VA: Neurological aspects of the early development of mongols, *Clin Proc Child Hosp DC* 23:64, 1967.

22. Cowie VA: *A study of the early development of mongols,* Oxford, 1970, Pergamon Press, Ltd.

23. Critchley M and Earl CJC: Tuberose sclerosis and allied conditions, *Brain* 55:311, 1932.

24. Crome L: The pathology of Down's disease. In Hilliard LT and Kirman editors: *Mental deficiency,* ed 2, Boston, MA, 1965, Little, Brown & Co.

25. Crome L and Stern J: *Pathology of mental retardation,* ed 2, Edinburgh, 1972, Churchill Livingstone.

26. Dunst C and others: A family systems assessment and intervention model. In Hanft BE, editor: *Family centered care,* Rockville, MD, 1989, American Occupational Therapy Association, Inc.

27. Emery AEH and Rimoin DL: *Principles and practice of medical genetics* (2nd ed), New York, 1990, Churchill Livingstone.

28. Folio MR and Fewell RR: *Peabody Developmental Motor Scales and Activity Cards,* Allen, TX, 1983, DLM Teaching Resources.

29. Furuno S and others: *Hawaii early learning profile,* Palo Alto, CA, 1979, VORT.

30. Gans BM and others: Description and interobserver reliability of the Tufts Assessment of Motor Performance, *Am J Phys Med Rehab* 67:202, 1988.

31. Goldberg MJ: *The dysmorphic child: an orthopedic perspective,* New York, 1987, Raven Press.

32. Gorlin RJ: Classical chromosome disorders. In Yunis J, editor: *New chromosomal syndromes,* New York, 1977, Academic Press.

33. Granger CR and others: *Guide for the use of the Functional Independence Measure (Wee FIM) of the uniform data set for medical rehabilitation,* Buffalo, NY, 1988, Research Foundation, State University of New York.

34. Granger CV and others: *Guide for the use of the uniform data set for medical rehabilitation,* Buffalo, NY, 1986, Research Foundation, State University of New York.

35. Guralnick MJ and Bennett FC: Early intervention for at-risk and handicapped children: current and future perspectives. In Guralnick MJ and Bennett FC, editors: *Effectiveness of early intervention for at-risk and handicapped children,* Orlando, Fla, 1987, Academic Press.

36. Hagberg B: Rett syndrome: Swedish approach to analysis of prevalence and cause, *Brain Dev* 7:277, 1985.

37. Hagberg B and others: A progressive syndrome of autism, dementia, ataxia and loss of purposeful hand use in girls: Rett syndrome: Report of 35 cases, *Ann Neurol* 14:471, 1983.

38. Hagberg B and others: Rett syndrome, criteria for inclusion and exclusion, *Brain Dev* 7:372, 1985.

39. Haley SM and others: *Pediatric evaluation of disability inventory (PEDI),* Boston, 1989, PEDI Research Group, Department of Rehabilitation Medicine, New England Medical Center Hospitals.

40. Haley SM and others: *Adaptation of the Functional Independence Measure for use with infants and children.* Grant funded by the National Institute of Disability and Rehabilitation Research, US Department of Education, grant no H133G80043, 1988.

41. Haley SM and others: Functional assessment in young children with neurological impairments, *Top Early Childhood Special Educ* 9:106, 1989.

42. Hall D: Mongolism in newborn infants, *Clin Pediatr* 5:90, 1978.

43. Hall JG and Gilchrist DM: Turner syndrome and its variants, *Pediatr Clin North Am* 37:1421, 1990.

44. Harris SR: Early intervention: does developmental therapy make a difference? *Top Early Child Special Educ* 7:20, 1988.

45. Harris SR: Early diagnosis of spastic diplegia, spastic hemiplegia, and quadriplegia, *Am J Dis Child* 143:1356, 1989.

46. Harris SR: Functional abilities in context. In Lister MJ, editor: *Contemporary management of motor control problems: proceedings of the II-Step Conference,* Alexandria, VA, 1991, Foundation for Physical Therapy.

47. Harris SR and McEwen I: Assessing motor skills. In McLean M and others, editors: *Assessing infants and toddlers with special needs,* Columbus, Ohio, (in press), Merrill.

48. Harris SR and Shea AM: Down syndrome. In Campbell SK, editor: *Pediatric neurologic physical therapy,* ed 2, New York, 1991, Churchill Livingstone.

49. Haslam RHA: Neurological disorders. In Smith DW, editor: *Introduction to clinical pediatrics,* ed 2, Philadelphia, 1977, WB Saunders.

50. Hennessey MJ and Haas RH: Orthopedic management of Rett syndrome. In Haas RH, Rapin I, and Moser HW, editors: *J Child Neurol Supplement,* vol 3, 1988.

51. Higgins S: Motor skill acquisition, *Phys Ther* 71:123, 1991.

52. Hirschhorn K and others: Deletion of short arms of chromosome 4-5 in a child with defects of midline fusion, *Humangenitik* 1:479, 1965.

53. Hoffenberg R and Jackson WPU: Gonadal dysgenesis: modern concepts, *Br Med J* 2:1457, 1957.

54. Holm VA: The diagnosis of Prader-Willi syndrome. In Holm VA, Sulzbacher S, and Pipes PL, editors: *Prader-Willi syndrome,* Baltimore, 1981, University Park Press.

55. Holmes LB and others: *Mental retardation: an atlas of diseases with associated physical abnormalities,* New York, 1972, Macmillan.

56. Holvey DN, editor: *The Merck manual of diagnosis and therapy,* Rahway, NJ, 1972, Merck & Co.

57. Horak FB: Assumptions underlying motor control for neurologic rehabilitation. In Lister MJ, editor: *Contemporary management of motor control problems: proceedings of the II-Step Conference,* Alexandria, VA, 1991, Foundation for Physical Therapy.

58. Hudson LH and Cox TR: Brown-Sequard syndrome with bilateral elephantiasis in neurofibromatosis, *JAMA* 161:326, 1956.

59. Johnson BH and others: *Caring for children and families: guidelines for hospitals,* Bethesda, 1992, Association for the Care of Children's Health.

60. Jones KL: *Smith's recognizable patterns of human malformation,* ed 4, Philadelphia, 1988, WB Saunders.

61. Kelley WN: Hypoxanthine-guanine phosphoribosyltransferase deficiency in the Lesch-Nyhan syndrome and gout. *Fed Proc* 27:1047, 1968.

62. Kirshner B and Guyatt GH: A methodological framework for assessing health indices, *J Chron Dis* 38:27, 1985.

63. Knobloch H and others: *Manual of developmental diagnosis: the administration and interpretation of the revised Gesell & Amatruda Developmental and Neurological Examination,* Houston, 1987, Gesell Developmental Materials.

64. Know WE: Phenylketonuria. In Stanbury JB and others, editors: *The metabolic basis of inherited disease,* ed 3, New York, 1972, McGraw-Hill.

65. Koehler J: Spinal muscular atrophy of childhood. In Bleck EE and Nagel DA, editors: *Physically handicapped children: a medical atlas for teachers,* New York, 1975, Grune & Stratton.

66. Ledbetter DH and Cassidy SB: The etiology of Prader-Willi syndrome: clinical implications of the chromosome 15 abnormalities. In Caldwell ME and Taylor RL, editors: *Prader-Willi syndrome: selected research and management issues,* New York, 1988, Springer Verlag.

67. Lejeune J: Le Mongolisme. Premier exemple d'aberration autosomique humane, *Ann Genet* 1:41, 1959.

68. Lejeune J and others: Trois cas de deletion partielle du bras court d'un chromosome 5, *Compt Rend Acad Sci* (Paris) 257:3098, 1963.

69. Lesch M and Nyhan WL: A familial disorder of unric acid metabolism and central nervous system function, *Am J Med* 36:561, 1964.

70. Leviton A and others: The family centered consultation model: practical application for professionals, *Infants Young Children* 4:1, 1992.

71. Loesch-Mdzewska D: Some aspects of neurology of Down's syndrome, *J Ment Defic Res* 12:237, 1968.

72. Luiselli JK and others: Issues in Prader-Willi syndrome: diagnosis, characteristics and management. In Caldwell ME and Taylor RL, editors: *Prader-Willi syndrome: selected research and management issues,* New York, 1988, Springer Verlag.

73. Marini JC: Osteogenesis imperfecta: Comprehensive management, *Adv Pediatr* 35:391, 1988.

74. Marin-Padilla M: Pyramidal cell abnormalities in the motor cortex of a child with Down's syndrome: a Golgi study, *J Comp Neurol* 167:63, 1976.

75. McGraw MB: The neuromuscular maturation of the human infant, New York, 1966, Hafer.

76. Melyn MA and White DT: Mental and developmental milestones of noninstitutionalized Down's syndrome children, *Pediatrics* 52:542, 1973.

77. *Mental Health Law Project: Early intervention advocacy network, new guide to the Part H law and regulations,* July 1992, 1101 15th St. NW, #1212, Washington, DC, 20005.

78. Milunsky A, editor: *Genetic disorders and the fetus,* 3rd ed, Baltimore, 1992, The Johns Hopkins University Press.

79. Moore JW and others: Chromosome studies in 10 patients with the Rett syndrome, *Am J Med Genet* 24:345, 1986.

80. Msall ME and others: Health, developmental and psychosocial aspects of Down syndrome, *Infants Young Children* 4:35, 1991.

81. Myhre SA and others: The effects of testosterone treatment in Klinefelter's syndrome, *J Pediatr* 76:267, 1970.

82. Naganuma GM and Billingsley FF: Effects of handsplints on sterotypic behavior of three girls with Rett syndrome, *Phys Ther* 68:664, 1988.

83. Nagel DA: Temporary orthopedic disabilities in children. In Bleck EE and Nagel DA, editors: *Physically handicapped children: a medical atlas for teachers,* New York, 1975, Grune & Stratton.

84. Noonan MJ and McCormick L: *Early intervention in natural environments,* Pacific Grove, Calif, 1993, Brooks/Cole Publishing Co.

85. Nora JJ and Fraser FL: *Medical genetics: principles and practice,* Philadelphia, 1989, Lea and Febiger.

86. Novitski E: *Human genetics,* New York, 1977, Macmillan.

87. O'Neill DL and Harris SR: Developing goals and objectives for handicapped children, *Phys Ther* 62:295, 1982.

88. Osawa M and Shishikura K: Werdnig-Hoffmann disease and variants, *Handbook Clin Neurol* 15:51, 1991.

89. Oski FA and others: *Principles and practice of pediatrics,* Philadelphia, 1990, JB Lippincott.

90. Palisano RJ: Validity of goal attainment scaling in infants with motor delays, *Phys Ther* 73:651, 1993.

91. Patau K and others: Multiple congenital anomaly caused by an extra chromosome, *Lancet* 1:790, 1960.

92. Penrose LS and Smith GF: *Down's anomaly,* London, 1966, Churchill Livingstone.

93. Piazza CC and others: Teaching self-feeding skills to patients with Rett syndrome, *Dev Med Child Neurol* 35:991, 1993.

94. Plumridge D and others, editors: *The student with a genetic disorder,* Springfield, Ill, 1993, Charles C Thomas.

95. Prader A and others: Ein Syndrom von adipositas, kleinwuchs, kryptochimus and oligophrenie nach myatonieartigem zustand in neugeborenenalter, *Schweiz Med Wochenschr* 86:1260, 1956.

96. Pruess JB and Fewell RR: Cell therapy and the treatment of Down syndrome: a review of research, *Trisomy 21* 1:3, 1985.

97. *Public Law 94-142. Education for all handicapped children act of 1975* (5.6), 94th Congress, 1st Session, 1975.

98. Robinson NM and Robinson HB, editors: *The mentally retarded child: a psychological approach,* New York, 1976, McGraw-Hill.

99. Ross MH and others: Down's syndrome: is there a decreased population of neurons? *Neurology* 37:909, 1984.

100. Rubin A: *Handbook of congenital malformations,* Philadelphia, 1967, WB Saunders.

101. Rubinstein TH: Cranial abnormalities. In Carter CH, editor: *Medical aspects of mental retardation,* ed 2, Springfield, Ill, 1978, Charles C Thomas.

102. Sandall SR: Developmental interventions for biologically at-risk infants at home, *Top Early Childhood Special Educ* 10:1, 1990.

103. Schneegans E and others: Un cas de maladie du cri du chat. D'aael'aaetion partielle du bras court du chromosome 5, *Pediatrie* 21:823, 1966.

104. Scott CR: Inborn enzymatic errors. In Smith DW, editor: *Introduction to clinical pediatrics,* ed 2, Philadelphia, 1977, WB Saunders.

105. Simpson JL and Golbus MS: *Genetics in obstetrics and gynecology,* Philadelphia, 1992, WB Saunders.

106. Slentz RL and Bricker D: Family-guided assessment for IFSP development, *J Early Intervention* 16:11, 1992.

107. Smith DW: Clinical diagnosis and nature of chromosomal abnormalities. In Yunis J, editor: *New chromosomal syndromes.* New York, 1977, Academic Press.

108. Solnit A and Stark M: Mourning and the birth of a defective child. In Menolascino FJ, editor: *Psychiatric aspects of the diagnosis and treatment of mental retardation,* Seattle, 1971, Special Child Publications.

109. Sternat J and others: Occupational and physical therapy services for severely handicapped students: toward a naturalized public school

service delivery model. In Sontag E: *Educational programming for the severely and profoundly handicapped,* Reston, Va, 1977, Council for Exceptional Children.

110. Stewart K: Collaborating with families: reflections on empowerment. In Hanft BE, editor: *Family centered care,* Rockville, Md, 1989, American Occupational Therapy Association.

111. Stewart KB and others: Rett syndrome: a literature review and survey of parents and therapists, *Phys Occup Ther Pediatr* 9:35, 1989.

112. Stott DH and others: *Stott Test of Motor Impairment,* Guelph, Ontario, Canada, 1984, Brook Educational Publishing Limited.

113. Tachdjian MO: *Pediatric orthopedics,* ed 2, Philadelphia, 1990, WB Saunders.

114. Taylor RL: Cognitive and behavioral characteristics. In Caldwell ME and Taylor RL, editors: *Prader-Willi syndrome: selected research and management issues,* New York, 1988, Springer-Verlag.

115. Trevathan E and Naidu S: The clinical recognition and differential diagnosis of Rett syndrome. In Haas RH, Rapin I, and Moser HW, editors: *J Child Neurol Suppl* 3:S6, 1988.

116. Turnbull AP and Turnbull HR: *Families, professionals and exceptionality: a special partnership,* ed 2, Columbus, Ohio, 1990, Merrill.

117. Turner HH: A syndrome of infantilism, congenital webbed neck, and cubitus valgus, *Endocrinology* 23:566, 1938.

118. Wagner CW: Surgical considerations in Prader-Willi syndrome. In Caldwell ML and Taylor RL, editors: *Prader-Willi syndrome: selected research and management issues,* New York, 1988, Springer-Verlag.

119. Warkany J: *Congenital malformations,* Chicago, 1971, Year Book Medical Publishers.

120. Warkany J and others: Congenital malformations in autosomal trisomy syndromes, *Am J Dis Child* 112:502, 1966.

121. Weatherall DJ: *The new genetics and clinical practice,* ed 3, New York, 1991, Oxford University Press.

122. Werch A: Amniocentesis: indications, techniques, and complications, *South Med J* 69:894, 1976.

123. Whaley WI and Gray WD: Atlanto-axial dislocation and Down's syndrome, *Can Med Assoc J* 123:35, 1980.

124. Wolf U and others: Deficiency an den kurzen Armen eines Chromosomes Nr 4, *Humangenitik* 1:397, 1965.

125. Young ID: Genetic counseling. In Liu DTY, editor: *A practical guide to chorion villus sampling,* New York, 1991, Oxford University Press.

126. Zoghbi H: Genetic aspects of Rett syndrome. In Haas RH, Rapin I, and Moser HW, editors: *J Child Neurol Suppl* 3:S76, 1988.

CHAPTER 11

Learning Disabilities

Stacey E. Szklut, Sharon A. Cermak, and Anne Henderson

KEY TERMS

learning disabilities
minimal brain dysfunction
sensory integration
motor deficits
neurodevelopmental treatment (NDT)
motor control
life span disability

LEARNING OBJECTIVES

After reading this chapter the student/therapist will:

1. Become familiar with accepted definitions and terminology used in the field of learning disabilities.
2. Be aware of characteristics that typically identify a child with learning disabilities.
3. Develop an historical perspective of brain dysfunction theories in the field of learning disabilities.
4. Be aware of current thinking in regard to etiologies and research in the field of learning disabilities.
5. Become familiar with members of the specialist team and service provision types for children with learning disabilities.
6. Be aware of the characteristics of the learning-disabled child with motor deficits.
7. Identify areas of evaluation to effectively assess motor deficits in the learning disabled child.
8. Become familiar with theories of etiology and treatment techniques for this population.
9. Understand the lifelong ramifications for the individual with learning disabilities.

AN OVERVIEW OF LEARNING DISABILITIES
Characteristics

Difficulties in learning may manifest themselves in various combinations of impairment in perception, conceptualization, language, memory, and control of attention, impulses, or motor functions.[67,102] The symptomatology of a child with **learning disabilities** is diverse and varied. All of the symptoms are not present in all children, and the symptoms that are present vary in degree of severity from child to child.

The most commonly recognized deficits in learning pertain to academic success. In most instances, attention has been given to deficits in verbal learning, including deficits in the learning of reading, in the acquisition of spoken and written language, and in arithmetic. Deficits in nonverbal learning, however, are equally important, such as disturbances in directional concepts (e.g., right and left, up and down) and body orientation, in the meanings of facial expressions and the behaviors of others, and in music and rhythm.[145,238]

In addition to disorders in the perceptual, conceptual, language, or academic areas, children with learning disabilities often have correlated behavioral disorders that include hyperactivity, lack of attention, and general maladaptive behavior.[3,161] The 10 characteristics most often reported by clinicians of the child with learning disabilities are hyperactivity, perceptual-motor impairment, emotional lability, general coordination deficits, disorders of attention (short attention span, distractibility, perseveration), impulsiveness, disorders of memory and thinking (concept formation and problem solving), specific learning disabilities (reading, arithmetic, writing or spelling), disorders of speech and hearing, and soft neurological signs.[67,206]

Definition. The heterogeneity of the learning-disabled population has made agreement of a single definition difficult. Despite a wide variety of proposed guidelines, the issue of creating a single, standard definition has not been resolved.[151] Within the definitional debate is another dilemma of creating discrete subgroups of disability type. This problem affects not only how diagnosis is determined, but also who receives services and how research studies are interpreted under these varied definitions and subgroups.[143,151,263]

As a variety of disciplines have focused on the child with learning disabilities, each has described the problem according to its own frame of reference. Because numerous names and labels have been given to children who experience difficulties in learning,[3,39,40,102,184] there is a great deal of confusion about terminology in the literature.[234] In general, the terms fall into two broad categories: etiological and behavioral.[3,161] Medical professionals tend to label the disability in terms of cause, and they generally relate it to a deficit in the brain, particularly to cerebral dysfunction. Terms such as *brain-injured*,[273] **minimal brain dysfunction**,[67] and *psychoneurological disorder*[211] imply a neurological cause for the deviation in development.

Educators tend to describe the child's disability in behavioral terms that address the disordered function rather than identify the cause, even though some of the terms may imply a central nervous system (CNS) deficit. These terms include *perceptual handicap, perceptual-motor deficit, visual-motor delay, clumsy child syndrome, reading disability or dyslexia,* and *learning disability.* Educators most often view children with learning disabilities as "children who fail to learn despite an apparently normal capacity for learning."[143] They utilize a discrepancy between the child's potential for learning and academic achievement in one or more of seven areas: oral expression, listening comprehension, written expression, basic reading, reading comprehension, mathematics calculation, and mathematics reasoning as a guide for distinction.[143] Regardless of the terminology, average to high intelligence, adequate hearing and vision, and adequate emotional adjustment together with a deficiency in learning are the salient features that constitute the basis for homogeneity.[145]

The term used in this chapter as a general name for this type of dysfunction is *learning disabilities.* This concept of learning disabilities and its definitions have evolved over time. One of the first formal definitions of learning disabilities was formulated by the National Advisory Committee on Handicapped Children, and incorporated by the United States Office of Education into Public Law 94-142, and is as follows:

Children with specific learning disabilities exhibit a disorder in one or more of the basic psychological processes involved in understanding or using spoken or written language. These may be manifested in disorders of listening, thinking, talking, reading, writing, spelling or arithmetic. They include conditions which have been referred to as perceptual handicaps, brain injury, minimal brain dysfunction, dyslexia, developmental aphasia, etc. They do not include learning problems which are primarily due to visual, hearing, or motor handicaps, to mental retardation, emotional disturbance or to environmental disadvantage (p. 322).[47,235]

This definition of learning disabilities has been challenged, as its applications to various groups of individuals has been unclear. One distinct shortcoming is that it does not specify that learning disabilities are a heterogeneous group of disorders, but rather implies it is a homogeneous condition.[151] It also specifies the word "children," which excludes the persistence of these deficits into adulthood. Although it does recognize that learning disabilities do not include problems in learning due to mental retardation, sensory or motor handicap, emotional disturbance, or cultural disadvantage, it does not identify that a learning disability can occur in conjunction to, or as a consequence of another handicap.[151] The National Joint Committee for Learning Disabilities (NJCLD) attempted to address these concerns through a revised definition in 1981:

Learning disabilities is a generic term that refers to a heterogeneous group of disorders manifested by significant difficulties in the acquisition and use of listening, speaking, reading, writing, reasoning or mathematical abilities. These disorders are intrinsic to the individual and presumed to be due to central nervous system dysfunction. Even though a learning disability may occur concomitantly with other handicapping conditions (e.g., sensory impairment, mental retardation, social and emotional disturbance) or environmental influences, it is not the direct result of those conditions or influences (p. 336).[123]

Due to expanding knowledge of conditions associated with learning problems, and continued definitional debate, Congress created the Interagency Committee on Learning Disabilities (ICLD). Its purpose was to provide a synthesis and overview of present knowledge in the field of learning disabilities.[150] In 1987 this committee suggested a uniform definition based on modifications in the NJCLD definition to include (with changes italicized):

Learning disabilities is a generic term that refers to a heterogeneous group of disorders manifested by significant difficulties in the acquisition and use of listening, speaking, reading, writing, reasoning or mathematical abilities, *or of social skills.* These disorders are intrinsic to the individual and presumed to be due to central nervous system dysfunction. Even though a learning disability may occur concomitantly with other handicapping conditions (e.g., sensory impairment, mental retardation, social and emotional disturbance), *with socioenvironmental influences (e.g., cultural differences, insufficient or inappropriate* instruction, psychogenic differences), *and especially with attention deficit disorder, all of which may cause learning problems, a learning disability* is not the direct result of those conditions or influences (p. 550).[151]

This latest revision is expanded to include deficits in social skills that have been noted in the learning-disabled population. It also addresses the relationship of attention deficit to learning disabilities, indicating that attention deficit may accompany learning disabilities or cause learning *problems*.[151] The interagency committee has suggested that this latest definition be used for epidemiological studies, diagnosis, research, administrative action, and future legislation. The delineation of one accepted definition is essential to consistency in diagnosis, research, and treatment of the learning-disabled population.

Incidence and prevalence. The inconsistencies in the definition of learning disabilities also affect the ability to determine its incidence and prevalence, although both have increased rapidly. Incidence refers to the number of new cases of a disease identified within a given time period; prevalence is the total number of cases in a population at a given time.[153] The estimated prevalence of children with learning disabilities ranges from 1% to 30% of the school population, depending on the criterion used to determine the disability.[3,175,248,299] A more conservative estimate has been made by the National Advisory Committee on Handicapped Children, which estimated children with significant learning disabilities constituted approximately 1% to 3% of the school population.[161] Whichever estimate is used, it is clear that a huge number of children are involved. Incidence of identified cases has grown tremendously, with a 135% gain between 1976 and 1986, whereas the incidence of all other handicapping conditions has increased by only 16%.[150]

Students diagnosed as learning disabled are currently the largest percentage of enrollment in special education programs, ranging from about 25% to 65% of the total handicapped students.[3,150] Most observers agree that learning problems are far more common in boys than in girls. In general, learning disabilities occur from two to five times more frequently in males than in females, although some writers have estimated the ratio as high as 10:1.[145,275]

Subtypes. The search for a single description of learning disabilities has not been successful. Rourke[239] has stated that "the confusion that abounds in the literature dealing with the group of clinical problems known as learning disabilities is, in many ways, a direct reflection of the failure of many scientists and practitioners in this field to acknowledge and address the heterogeneity and diversity extant among the learning disabled population."

The identification of subgroups within learning disabilities is currently a major focus of research.[32] Work continues to specify clusters with discrete symptoms that constitute subgroups and to identify the underlying origin of the disability. There is growing evidence that children with

learning disabilities show different patterns of disorders.* Although similarities can be found in grouping the learning disabled by patterns of academic achievement, the categorization appears to vary with the orientation of the researcher, the types of assessments and observations used, and the age and heterogeneity of the sample.[239,263,275]

In one of the early attempts at classification of subgroups within learning disabilities, Denckla and Rudel[82] determined that approximately 30% of the 190 children she assessed by neurological examination could be classified into three recognizable subgroups. The other 70% exhibited an unclassifiable mixture of signs. Of the 30%, the first subgroup was classified as children having *specific language disability*. These children, who were failing in reading and spelling, showed a pattern of inadequacy on repetition, sequencing, memory, language, motor, and other tasks, all of which required rote functioning. The second group had what was termed a *specific visuospatial disability:* they were children with at least average performance in reading and spelling who were poor in arithmetic, who were seriously inadequate in writing and copying, and who were all socially and/or emotionally maladjusted. The third group manifested a *dyscontrol syndrome* and included children who had poor motor and impulse control, who were behaviorally immature, and who were normal in language and perceptual functioning.

Mattis and others,[187] Boder[44] and others[88] have gone further in attempting to delineate subgroupings within the reading-disabled child, but these subgroupings have not been validated by more current research.[127] Siegal and Ryan[252] demonstrated that the way in which the reading disability was defined and assessed influenced the formation of subtypes. For example, poor reading ability could be assessed through inadequate phonic skills or word recognition, delayed reading comprehension, or slow reading speed.[252] Each of these would have implications for reading performance, yet would require different remediation strategies. This theory stressed the importance of identifying specific functional deficit areas rather than lumping symptoms. Currently, however, reliable categorization of subtypes within the reading disabled population is not possible.[260a]

Nevertheless, more consistent and accepted subtypes may be identified within the learning disabled population. Rourke[239] has identified discrete patterns of academic performance and neuropsychological functioning. Initially, he drew from research on adult patients with brain damage that used the Weschler Adult Intelligence Scale (WAIS) to yield a "verbal IQ" (based primarily on language tasks) and a "performance IQ" (based primarily on visuoperceptual and perceptual motor tasks). Research on adults with brain damage found that patients with left hemisphere

---

* References 11-13, 16, 17, 20, 38, 46, 67, 70, 82, 239, and 250.

dysfunction tended to show a low verbal, high performance WAIS profile and language deficits. Those patients with right hemisphere dysfunction presented the opposite profile of high verbal, low performance on the WAIS, and exhibited predominantly visuoconstructive deficits. Based on patterns of scores on the Weschler Intelligence Scale for Children (WISC), children ages 9 to 14 were placed into similar subgroups.[152,238,241,242,260a] The performance of the high verbal, low performance group was superior for tasks that primarily involved verbal, language, and auditory-perceptual skills. In contrast, the high performance, low verbal was superior on tasks that primarily involved visuoperceptual skills. The investigators suggested that the WISC verbal/performance discrepancy reflected differential integrity of the two cerebral hemispheres in older children with learning disabilities. These same patterns, however, were not identified in the younger children with learning disabilities. Some researchers believe that it is difficult to make inferences about brain dysfunction in children based on behavioral responses, as the relationship between performance on tests often does not correspond to specific types of CNS dysfunction in the same way as in adults.

Rourke and colleagues have continued to explore these subgroups, and have found similar patterns using the Wide Range Achievement Tests (WRAT) to assess patterns of academic performance.[225,260a,272] They identified three distinct patterns of academic achievement. The first group consists of students who have depressed scores in both reading and arithmetic. Subgroup two performs higher on arithmetic relative to reading and spelling, but is still deficient in all areas. The third group exhibits a specific arithmetic deficit, with reading and spelling in the normal range of performance. This latter group also showed delays in psychomotor and tactile-perceptual skills, yet possessed superior verbal skills and auditory-perceptual skills. This group also more often had difficulties in understanding nonverbal cues, as well as having a greater frequency of emotional problems as reported by their parents.[240] This last group of children exhibit many of the same characteristics as the child with motor planning problems referred for occupational and physical therapy services.

Several studies have replicated similar subgroups, with continued emphasis on academic performance. The impact of using more homogeneous subgroups within research is now being explored. Shafir and others[256] performed a study where they substantiated the need for subgroups within research. When looked at as a homogeneous group, learning-disabled children scored more poorly on tests of problem solving and metacognitive strategies than normally achieving children. When the group was separated by reading disability and arithmetic disability, however, the reading-disabled child performed lower on these tasks, but the arithmetic group scored similarly to the normal control. This

has significant implications for future research and remediation.[260a]

It appears that subgrouping within learning disabilities is essential to both assessment and remediation. Review of studies suggests at least three appropriate groups—reading disabled, reading disabled with delays in arithmetic, and arithmetic disabled. In addition another group of children have attentional problems that affect many areas of performance. Personality and socioeconomic dimensions of learning disabilities also are being examined through subtype analysis.[224,232,272]

Various disciplines may continue to identify patterns of strengths and weaknesses in the learning-disabled population. Yet, clinical observations by educators, therapists, and researchers suggest that learning disability is not a unitary syndrome but rather a heterogeneous one.[15,82,94,187] This has resulted in numerous categorization systems. The relationship between these various systems has been explored only minimally; there is no one, agreed-on classification, although for some time it has been recognized that children with learning disabilities need to be classified into subgroups to best plan appropriate treatment interventions.*

Summary. A great deal of attention has been focused on the definition of *learning disabilities,* and many attempts have been made to identify different "types" of learning disabilities. Research has attempted to relate brain mechanisms to the different types of learning disabilities. According to Rourke,[238,239] an important problem is whether and to what extent dysfunction at the level of the cerebral hemispheres causes learning disabilities. Etiological considerations of learning disabilities have contributed to understanding the nature of developmental cerebral dysfunction, and have had practical applications.[238] Several theories about learning disabilities have been proposed. These are discussed in the following sections, with greatest emphasis given to those theories that consider the role of brain function.

Brain dysfunction theories

Numerous hypotheses have been proposed about the causes of learning disabilities. Although some researchers have emphasized emotional and social causes of learning disabilities, the majority of recent research has focused on the role of neurological factors in learning disability. In 1972, Peck and Stackhouse[228] hypothesized that children with reading disabilities were experiencing difficulties as a result of familial conflict. Bannatyne[30] stated that there is a type of dyslexia, termed *primary emotional communicative dyslexia,* that results from a poor communicative (language) relationship between the mother and infant.

Other researchers hypothesize that learning disabilities result from an interaction of organic and nonorganic factors.[192] Keough[156] suggested that hyperactive children may have different conceptual styles than nonhyperactive children. The term *inactive learner* has been used to describe deficiencies in the learning-disabled child's ability to actively problem solve.[278] Other investigators suggested that situational influences play an important role in eliciting maladaptive behavior in children with brain damage, and they have suggested that the behavior is not maladaptive because of the brain damage, but rather that such children are likely to find themselves in situations in which they are continuously frustrated in achieving their hopes and aspirations.[189]

Despite the magnitude and variety of theories proposed to explain learning disabilities, it is clear that no single theory can adequately explain the multifactorial and heterogenous nature of this disability. In general, the cause of learning disabilities is unknown. Diverse causes have received varying degrees of empirical support, but none have been demonstrated to exist for all learning-disabled children.[135,263,293] Frequently studied etiological factors include (1) brain damage or dysfunction from causes such as birth injury, perinatal anoxia, head injury, fetal malnutrition, encephalitis, and lead poisoning; (2) allergies; (3) biochemical abnormalities or metabolic disorders; (4) genetics; (5) maturational lag; and (6) environmental factors, such as neglect and abuse, a disorganized home, and inadequate stimulation.[94,281]

Because learning disabilities are frequently associated with neuropsychological symptoms, such as disorders of speech, spatial orientation, perception, motor coordination, and activity level, and because neuropsychological deficits tend to occur concomitantly, various researchers have attempted to identify aspects of the brain that may be dysfunctional. Several theories will be discussed, but it must be recognized that theories of brain dysfunction are, to some extent, speculative.[169] Many of these theories of the cause of learning disabilities have been based on experimental studies of animals, studies of adults who have received gunshot wounds or other forms of cerebral trauma, or research on epileptics who have undergone brain surgery.

Empirical data of the learning-disabled population gathered at the behavioral level have further refined the thinking about the preceding theories. Tests such as dichotic listening, visual half field, and dichaptic procedures assessed individuals responses to auditory, visual, or tactile input. More recent research includes empirical measures of physiological function such as electroencephalogram (EEG), event-related potentials (ERP), brain electrical activity mapping (BEAM), regional cerebral blood flow (rCBF), and positive emission tomography (PET). Continued research on the behavioral, physiological, and anatomical levels has strengthened the conceptual basis within the field of learning disabilities.[209]

Historical perspective. Data about the profile of an individual with learning disabilities were presented initially through case study analysis. From these early attempts at the classification of functional deficits, many single factor theories evolved. The three most accepted theories were delayed development of cerebral dominance, visuoperceptual deficits, and auditory-perceptual deficits with associated language inefficiencies.[295] Although each of these theories has been criticized as being too simplistic to cover the broad spectrum of learning disabilities, they all have contributed greatly to research and subtyping within the field of learning disabilities. For example, Orton's theory of delayed cerebral dominance was based on his clinical observation of higher incidence of reading problems in children with mixed handedness. He asserted that the left hemisphere did not develop dominance for language processes and, therefore, lead to deficiencies in organizing language information necessary for reading.[218,295] In his reasoning, the term dominance came from the fact that the majority of persons were right handed, and it was known that the left hemisphere governed this right hand preference, and hence was dominant.[209] Although this theory would be refuted by empirical data, it led to at least five different research models including maturational lags in cerebral specialization, left hemisphere impairment, interference of the right hemisphere in the development of the left, lack of hemispheric specialization, and inefficient interhemispheric integration.[295]

Left hemisphere maturational lag or damage. Some researchers proposed that reading problems were a result of a lag in the lateralization of the cerebral hemispheres, particularly the left hemisphere.[250,266,267] These authors also suggested a maturational lag in the differentiation of motor, somatosensory, and language functions that was subserved by the left hemisphere of dyslexic children, which resembled the behavioral patterns of chronologically younger normal children, as opposed to a unique syndrome of disturbance. Geschwind and Galaburda[107] proposed an elaborate model in which the underdevelopment of the left hemisphere is attributed to the effects of testosterone, which selectively inhibits maturation of the left hemisphere.

Recent evidence has suggested that the degree to which the hemispheres will be lateralized is present at birth.[71,209] Results of dichotic listening studies also have been used as a measure of hemispheric lateralization. In these studies subjects respond to different auditory stimuli presented to the right and left ears simultaneously. The information to the right ear goes to the left hemisphere and vice versa. These studies suggest that lateralization is innate, because results in the ear advantage do not strengthen with age.[209] Therefore, the tenability of a maturational lag of this theory has been questioned.

Other researchers found patterns of behavioral deficits in children with dyslexic learning disabilities (including right-left confusion, finger agnosia, calculation difficulty, writing difficulty, visuoconstructive impairment, depressed verbal intelligence, and reading problems) were similar to those of adults who have sustained damage to the left cerebral hemisphere.[106] In addition, dyslexic children, as well as patients with lesions in the left inferior parietal cortex, showed impaired performance in cross-modal tasks, particularly auditory-visual tasks. Some dichotic listening studies supported the theory that children with reading problems had diminished lateralization of language and linguistic auditory function in the left hemisphere.[21,56a,299] Researchers found that poor readers did not show the normal pattern of right visual field (left hemisphere) superiority for word recognition.[117,185,217]

In review, these study results are thought to be affected by the rote nature of the task and are thought to be influenced by deficits in attention, memory, and the use of strategies.[295] They have also been criticized for presenting only the words within the visual field horizontally, and in subsequent studies, where the stimuli was presented vertically, these results were not replicated.[71,295] In fact, the results from the Yeni-Komshian study[298] suggested that poor readers might have difficulty processing information in the right hemisphere or transmitting the information from the right to the left hemisphere. Presently, researchers believe there is little evidence to support the theory that children with learning disabilities have a developmental delay in cerebral lateralization.[295]

Lack of hemispheric specialization. As research findings on brain function have been compiled, evidence mounts that certain functions are specialized within each hemisphere. Semmes[254] hypothesized that the left hemisphere has a more focal, precise organization, with functional units located near each other, which may facilitate the precise coding needed for speech. The right hemisphere is considered to be more diffusely organized, allowing dissimilar information to be synthesized simultaneously. This type of organization would be advantageous for spatial processing and visual perception. The left hemisphere is thought to process information in a sequential, linear fashion, and is more proficient in analyzing details. The right hemisphere processes input in a more holistic manner, grasping the overall organization or the gestalt of a pattern.[209] In regard to function, the left hemisphere is hypothesized to be important for word recognition and reading comprehension, performing mathematical calculations, and processing and producing language. The right hemisphere processes nonverbal stimuli such as environmental sounds and voice intonation, synthesizes mathematical reasoning and judgment, and is able to line up numbers for calculations, as well as other visuospatial functions. In this organization, we can see that although the hemispheres vary in the method of organization of input, they each participate in certain functional outputs such as reading and mathematical calculations. Hence neither hemisphere is thought to be dominant, but rather specialized for types of function. Specialization of function of the cerebral hemispheres is generally considered an optimal neural basis for learning.[17]

Historically, the issue of whether a possible cause for learning disabilities is the failure of one hemisphere to

specialize for language and the other for visuospatial skill has long been controversial. Ayres[13] suggested that in some children with learning disabilities, the two hemispheres do not specialize in their functions and thus develop similar functions, with neither hemisphere being as effective. Levy and others[179] reviewed a number of studies that support the hypothesis that development of language function in both hemispheres is achieved at the expense of the development of visuospatial perceptual-skills. Witelson[296] hypothesized that learning-disabled children have bilateral representation for spatial function rather than representation of spatial function in the right hemisphere as seen in normal children. Specifically, she suggested that the left hemisphere does not exhibit the "normal" focal organization but rather exhibits the right hemisphere type of diffuse organization as described by Semmes.[254] As a result, children with learning disabilities tend to use predominantly spatial, parallel, holistic modes of processing. This leads to poor performance on such linguistic tasks as reading, which demands sequential analysis.

Measures of hemispheric specialization are largely inferential, and definitive statements of function are affected by the focus on dyslexia in research and the heterogeneity of the learning-disabled population. Research does suggest that at least some children with learning disabilities show different patterns of cerebral organization than normal children.[209,295] A strict left-right dichotomy is oversimplified, and does not take into account many aspects of functional brain organization.[209,295] For example, Luria's[183] neuropsychological theory of brain organization proposes three basic functional units within the brain: subcortical, anterior, and posterior. According to this theory, communication between these functional units occurs at many levels, with each of the three units involved with the performance of any behavior. Within this system of organization, the subcortical unit is responsible for maintaining an adequate level of cortical tone and arousal; the posterior portion plays a major role in the reception, analysis, integration and storage of sensory and motor information. The anterior unit holds an executive function in organizing a plan, and is thought to be responsible for future goal-related behavior. This system clearly indicates that the nervous system is highly specialized for function. The use of a left-right dichotomy cannot reflect the complexity of the functioning of the brain.[209,295]

Inadequate interhemispheric communication. The importance of adequate communication between the two sides of the brain, particularly between the cerebral hemispheres, has been emphasized frequently in theories that propose that reading is a process that requires the active participation of both hemispheres and the transfer of information between them.* Gazzaniga[105] suggests that some aspects of minimal brain dysfunction may reflect

* References 55, 105, 231, 287, 289, and 298.

problems in the "shuttling of information between various specialized processing centers in the brain." Myklebust[212] states that the primary deficit of some learning-disabled children is an impairment of the ability of one hemisphere to communicate with the other; this is reflected cognitively by the child's inability to convert verbal learning (left hemisphere) into nonverbal meanings (right hemisphere) and to convert nonverbal learning into verbal meanings. Hardy and others[126] have shown that auditory-to-visual processing is critical to academic achievement.

Support for the hypothesis of impaired interhemispheric communication comes from a tachistoscopic study in which right visual half-field scores (left hemisphere) were at about the same level of accuracy for both poor and good readers while the poor readers showed considerable deficit in their left visual half-field scores.[298] In this study, because the material presented was linguistic in nature and the response mode was verbal, these authors suggested that the poor readers might suffer from some form of processing deficit in the right hemisphere or that the transmission from the right to the left hemisphere was degraded. Gross and others[117] found that students with reading disabilities showed a greater difference between thresholds for left and right hemifield stimuli than normal readers. They suggested that this perceptual asymmetry may reflect inefficient interhemispheric transfer of visual information.

Adequacy of interhemispheric communication has also been assessed using motor tasks. Badian and Wolff[29] examined motor sequencing abilities in boys 8 to 15 years old with reading disabilities, using both single-hand tapping and alternating-hand tapping. The authors found that in the single-hand trials, boys with reading disabilities tapped as well as boys without reading disabilities. However, the boys with the disability showed marked deterioration of performance when tapping with two hands in alternation, resulting primarily from the left hand's performance. The authors suggest that the motor sequencing deficit was the result of inadequate interhemispheric cooperation necessary to coordinate control over the motor actions in the left hand (right hemisphere) and hemispheric specialization for temporal sequencing (left hemisphere).

Sensory integration dysfunction. Ayres[15] originally defined **sensory integration** as the "the ability to organize sensory information for use." She sought to describe the specific relationships between neural functioning, sensorimotor behavior and learning, and identifying subtypes.[95] Ayres[15,17,19,24,28] viewed learning disorders as a reflection of deviation in neural function and hypothesized that certain types of learning disorders may be a result of dysfunction in the ability to organize and interpret sensory information. This dysfunction has been termed *sensory integration dysfunction.* Ayres noted that some children with learning disabilities had indications of subcortical dysfunction.[12,14,16,17,23] She[24] suggested that higher-level perception, language, and cognition depend on the ability of the brainstem/midbrain to organize and integrate sensory processes. Normal development depends on intersensory integration, particularly from the somatosensory and vestibular senses. This processing is considered significant because of the phylogenetically and ontogenetically early development of these systems and because of the many interconnections of the vestibular and tactile system throughout the brain. The functioning of these systems is considered to affect the functioning of the brain as a whole. Impairment in this subcortical processing can result in immature postural reactions, poor eye/motor control, and motor planning problems and can possibly contribute to language and learning disabilities. It is important to note that most of the theories of learning disabilities attribute learning problems to cortical dysfunction, and although sensory integration dysfunction may exist with or contribute to cortical dysfunction, the latter probably causes the actual learning processes.[209] Elaboration of this theory is presented in the treatment section. This theory is especially useful to therapists because it provides an organizing framework for treatment.

Summary. Various researchers have attempted to explain the underlying nature of learning disabilities, and various theories of learning disabilities have been proposed, including psychological and/or social explanations as possible causative factors. The majority of theorists, however, have suggested that learning disabilities are the result of some type of brain dysfunction, with an emphasis placed on anomalous hemispheric specialization. After a review of findings, however, Hiscock and Kinsbourne[135] concluded that "there is very little reason to believe that behavioral skill is in any way correlated with hemispheric specialization." These authors emphasized that "the heterogeneity of learning disabilities militates against a single etiology" and suggested that "the neural basis of learning disorders appears to be brain pathology rather than anomalous brain organization per se." Recently, the emphasis has shifted to looking at differential patterns of cortical activation, which emphasizes the highly complex nature of information processing within the brain. Whatever the cause, learning disabilities do not make up a homogeneous group, and a single theory is not adequate to classify or differentiate these children for assessment and remediation of functional problems.

A multidisciplinary approach to learning disabilities

Service delivery models. Evaluation and treatment of the learning-disabled child are essentially interdisciplinary procedures because the complex cause of learning disabilities results in differing constellations of problems and because remediation is beyond the competency of any individual professional group. Most learning-disabled children are seen by a group of professionals, the make-up of which depends on the purpose, location, philosophical orientation, or available resources of a particular program. The accompanying box lists the different professionals and specialists within professions who might participate in assessment or remediation of learning disabilities. The types of professionals are grouped into the four categories of education, medicine, psychology, and special services; and they have been listed only once although some professions could be categorized more than one way. Indeed, the number of potential professional disciplines is enormous. Although the expertise of a variety of professionals is essential for identifying the strengths and weaknesses of each child with learning disabilities, the method by which service is provided by these specialists has been a matter of debate. In a multidisciplinary approach, separate assessments and isolated programs to remediate weaknesses are used. The weakness here is the lack of consistent communication among specialists. The interdisciplinary approach refers to a team process, where the members assess and treat individually, but share results to plan a more comprehensive treatment program. Communication most often occurs through team meetings, where progress is discussed, and Individual Educational Plans (IEP) are created and revised. The transdisciplinary approach was created to achieve better coordination of therapy services, through the use of one primary therapist who was responsible for providing parental instruction and child programming in all developmental areas. The other team members share their expertise with the primary therapist.[53] This last approach is most often used in early intervention settings, where the overlap of developmental therapy services tends to be greater.

The label of learning disability is given to the child if he or she has a primary problem in academic learning, and the management of learning disabilities most commonly takes place in the school setting. Within this setting the most common form of service delivery is the interdisciplinary team. The goal of the team is to program for success in the educational setting, and a number of educational specialists have emerged to meet programming needs.

In some educational settings, children with learning disabilities are given full-time instruction in a special classroom with a small group of other learning-disabled children. A special education teacher or a learning disability teacher is in charge of the classroom. More commonly, the child is placed in a regular classroom and leaves class for special instruction for some part of the day. The child may go to a resource room, where a special education teacher provides regularly scheduled remedial education for children with a variety of educational handicaps, or the child may receive tutoring from a reading specialist or a private tutor.

With increasing costs of programming for special education and the influences of the education reform bill, a shift in educational models is occurring. Where classrooms and programs were being created to accommodate children with special needs outside the regular classroom, the shift is now toward inclusion into the mainstream. The philosophy of full inclusion asserts that children with disabilities are educated in the same school and classroom they would be if they were not handicapped.[4] Although the Education for All Handicapped Children Act (PL 94-142) was intended to facilitate

---

Types of specialists working with learning disabled children

Education

Classroom teacher
Special educator
Learning disability specialist
Psychoeducational diagnostician
Reading specialist
Early childhood education teacher
Physical educator
Adaptive physical educator

Medicine and nursing

Family physician
Pediatrician
Pediatric neurologist
Psychiatrist
School nurse
Biochemist
Geneticist
Endocrinologist
Nutritionist
Ophthalmologist
Otologist

Psychology

Clinical psychologist
Neuropsychologist
School psychologist
Child psychologist
Counseling psychologist
Guidance counselor

Special services

Occupational therapist
Physical therapist
Speech and language pathologist
Psycholinguist
Audiologist
Optometrist
Social worker
Recreational therapist
Motor therapist
Perceptual-motor trainer
Vocational education specialist

---

the inclusion of children into the "least restrictive environment," in actuality a greater number of special education classrooms were created, and it became the norm that children with special learning needs were placed in special segregated classrooms.[53]

Although there is much support for the model of inclusion, it requires that members of the team work closely together with the regular education teacher to ensure that there is an understanding of the child's special learning needs, as well as a level of comfort with incorporating therapeutic procedures into the regular classroom to facilitate the best learning environment. Within the model of inclusion, therapy services can still be provided through a variety of approaches including direct service, monitoring, and consultation. It is important that the child's services not be provided in isolation from the child's natural environment.[90] This means, that regardless of the choice of service provision, the therapist must, at the very least, observe the child within the classroom and other appropriate environments so that therapies address the functional issues of the child within the educational setting.

Specialists. Because therapists are familiar with the roles of the various medical specialists and of primary care physicians, these specialists will not be described here. School nursing is mentioned, however, because it is a specialty within nursing. The school nurse is usually the key health professional in a school system and is responsible for maintaining information about the child's health history, current health status, medication, home environment, family cooperation, and family problems. The school nurse is the primary liaison between the child and the doctor or health clinic and relays information from the school to medical professionals.

Psychologists have two distinct and often separate roles in the management of learning disorders. The first role is in psychodiagnosis. Psychological testing is essential in the identification of specific learning problems and may be done by clinical psychologists, school psychologists, or clinical neuropsychologists who specialize in diagnosis of learning disorders with an organic base. The second role of psychologists is to provide mental health service. Children with learning disabilities often have problems with self-esteem and peer relationships, resulting from either primary behavior problems or reactions to failure.

A learning-disabled child with a primary behavior problem, such as impulsiveness, disinhibited behavior, or hyperkinetic activity, may receive special treatment for the behavior disorder. A behavior modification specialist may be working with parents and teachers to help the child control his or her behavior. The child may receive psychotherapy from a psychologist or psychiatrist, or family therapy may be provided by a social worker, psychologist, or psychiatrist. These latter interventions are usually provided by public or private mental health clinics. Learning-disabled children with general adjustment problems in peer relationships are often treated within the school setting. School adjustment or guidance counselors offer support and advice on specific academic difficulties, social conflicts, and affective issues. The school psychologist, in addition to the diagnostic role, may offer psychological counseling to students and may help plan strategies for classroom management. Alternatively, the child may be seen outside of the school program by a psychiatrist or psychologist.

Among the professionals listed in the box on p. 319 as providing special services, a number are concerned with motor and perceptual-motor education. The physical therapist is primarily concerned with, although not limited to, the purely motor and postural functions and efficient use of the body. The occupational therapist has similar concerns for the postural basis of movement but stresses fine motor abilities, sensory integration, visual, spatial, and perceptual functions, and activities of daily living. Within the school system, physical educators address gross motor skills and physical fitness. Adaptive physical education teachers generally work with children who have handicaps. Finally optometrists, whose special concern is visual functions, such as visual acuity, visual perception, visual memory, and visual motor learning, may provide perceptual-motor training programs.

In other areas of function, speech and/or language therapists serve children who have problems with stuttering, vocabulary, word finding, articulation, sound sequencing, auditory attention, as well as the comprehension and processing of complex language. Audiologists are concerned with hearing, auditory perception, and auditory training. A related area of language study is psycholinguistics, which combines psychology and linguistics in the study of how language is acquired. This has also been applied to the educational setting.

The liaison between the child's family and the various service organizations may be a social worker. Social workers may also provide family therapy or serve as program coordinators. Finally, recreational therapists or vocational education specialists may be available to provide their special services.

While a single child is rarely seen by all of these professionals, a child with multiple problems may see many specialists. As an example, we describe the program of Paul, a learning-disabled child, in Case 1 on p. 321.

Coordinating multiple interventions. Learning disabilities are complex, multifaceted problems. The varied symptoms have brought the child with learning disabilities to the attention of many disciplines. Over the years, the number of therapeutic disciplines involved in the assessment and therapeutic management of learning disabilities has steadily increased. However, the involvement of so many specialists is both a problem and a benefit. The skill and interest of these disciplines constitute the benefit. However, the view that the more service the better may result in a service delivery overkill, as was the case with Paul. According to Kenny and Burka,[154] because our society values highly trained specialists, it is in jeopardy of expanding itself to the "point of logistic chaos."

Cruickshank and others[72] indicated that one of the major problems confronting the child with learning disabilities was the lack of a true interdisciplinary approach. Each discipline has traditionally been concerned with its own viewpoint of the learning disability field, with the result that research and subsequent remediation of learning problems have been limited in scope. According to Weiner,[292] efforts to educate

---

CASE 1 ▼ **Paul**

Paul, an 8-year-old boy, came to the Sargent College Occupational Therapy Clinic at Boston University because of the severe motor coordination problems that accompanied his learning disability. In addition to Paul's weekly treatment sessions, suggestions were made to his mother for a home program to be accomplished two to three times a week for 15 to 30 minutes each time. Meanwhile, Paul also received other services. Although he was mainstreamed into a regular classroom in accordance with the special education law, he was seen by the resource room teacher on a daily basis and by the adaptive physical education teacher twice a week to meet his specialized needs. Paul's regular teacher told Paul's mother that it was imperative for Paul to read at least one book a night because he needed additional reading practice. A reading tutor came to Paul's house Saturday morning. Paul also had oculomotor problems so he was evaluated by an optometrist who recommended weekly visits plus ocular exercises for one half hour a day. Paul developed secondary emotional problems, partly because he was very bright yet aware of his learning disability and frustrated by it. Thus Paul saw a psychotherapist on a weekly basis. The psychotherapist recommended participation in weekly group sessions, in addition to Paul's individual sessions, to help improve peer relationships. Thus, in all, Paul's "therapists" had developed a 12-hour-a-day program for him and his family. It is no wonder that Paul had difficulty in developing peer relationships—he never had time. Paul's schedule also affected interaction in his own family. His mother felt that her being a "therapist" interfered with her being a mother. She felt unable to carry out the home programs and felt guilty for not doing it.

What became apparent with Paul is that although a number of professionals were involved with him and although each contributed to the evaluation and treatment, the massive input, to some extent, had a detrimental effect on Paul and his family. The potential problems with multiple interventions and the need for coordinated services are discussed in the next section.

---

the child with minimal brain dysfunction have been reminiscent of the fable of the blind man and the elephant. Depending on which part of the elephant was being touched, the elephant was described as "a huge leaf waving in the breeze," "a broad table top," "a short, dangling rope," "a twisting snake," "a wide wall," "a tree trunk," or "a spear." Weiner suggested that similar failures to perceive the whole and to appreciate the behavioral uniqueness of the individual are in part a result of the skewedness and skimpiness of special professional preparation. He emphasized that "the task of educating the child with minimal brain dysfunction requires a repertoire of information, insights, and competencies that draws across arbitrary lines of profession proprietorship" (p. 283).[292]

Kenny and Burka[154] have identified factors that affect the process of achieving effective coordination of intervention services. One problem area is that treatment approaches fall in the skills and domain of a number of disciplines, and the territories often overlap. There is a strong need for each discipline to prove its expertise with the result being the development of territoriality. According to Gaddes,[102] the "proponent of each of these methods (treatment approaches) frequently recommends his or her system with an emotional fervor that reflects a stronger relationship with professional prejudices than with the objective behavior of the child" (p. 376). For reasons of this nature diagnosis of the same child may differ, depending on different professional responsibilities and goals.[34] Kenny and Burka[154] emphasize the need for each discipline to accept fully the skills and competence of other disciplines. Gaddes[102] emphasizes that territoriality is not necessary because none of the procedures by themselves is complete and adequate for dealing with all learning-disabled children or with all the disabilities of one child, and the superiority of any one method over another has generally not been demonstrated for all learning-disabled children. Johnson[144] supports this belief, stating that there is no simple response or treatment program for the learning-disabled population because of the variability and complexity of the problems. In creating a plan that truly encompasses and addresses the issues hindering the child's learning within the academic setting, the team must work together to create relevant and inclusive goals and objectives with the cooperation of the parent. Goals should be functionally based, with team members collaborating to determine appropriate program outcomes for that child.[90]

A final problem that has been identified in achieving effective coordination of intervention services is that no single discipline has trained its students to handle that role.[154] Rather, it seems to be an assumption that all professionals acquire the ability to coordinate services by virtue of learning their own special skills. Kenny and Burka[154] stress the need for a person to act as coordinator for the management and integration of the multiple interventions received by the learning-disabled child. They suggest that leadership be delegated on a functional rather than on a hierarchical basis. By this, they suggest that the coordinator be the team member who could best service the needs of the child.

THE CHILD WITH LEARNING DISABILITIES AND MOTOR DEFICITS
Concept of the clinical problems

Rationale for emphasizing this aspect. Motor deficits are only one aspect of the problems facing the learning-disabled child. This aspect, however, has been selected for the focus of this chapter because physical and occupational therapists working with learning disabled children generally deal with the motor problems. Denckla[81] reported that, across the entire spectrum of developmental disabilities, the most frequent signs leading to medical referral are those related to motor output. Selection of this aspect, however, is not meant to imply that the motor deficits are the paramount problems of the learning-disabled child or that motor deficits should receive priority over other symptoms. It is critical for the therapist who works with the learning-disabled child to be aware of the overall strengths and deficits of the child and of the characteristics of the child's educational program in order to plan optimal intervention strategies.

Terminology. The concept of developmental motor problems is not new. Developmental clumsiness was documented as early as the 1900s, when Collier used the term *congenital maladroitness.*[100] Orton[218] first adopted the term *clumsy* or *developmentally clumsy* to refer to these children. He recognized that disorders in praxis and gnosis resulted in clumsiness in physical performance, which he described as similar to a right-handed person trying to use the left hand, and said that the child seemed to have two left feet. The child with learning disabilities and motor incoordination is most commonly described as being "clumsy"[118-121,133,142,290] in the literature. The term clumsiness has been defined as "a deficit in the acquisition of skills requiring fluent coordinated movement, not explicable by general retardation or demonstrable neurological disease"[122] (p. 375). The term motor *dysfunction* appears to be used interchangeably with *clumsiness.* Other terminology includes *perceptual motor deficits,*[251] *developmental apraxia,*[11,17,24,290] and *sensory integration dysfunction,*[15] all of which generally connote a more specific set of motor coordination problems.

In this chapter the terms *motor dysfunction, deficit, disorder,* or *disturbance* are used as general terms that encompass all disorders that have a motor component. We identify two classes of motor function, which we term *motor coordination* and *visual-motor function.* Motor coordination refers to functions that are more clearly and traditionally defined as motoric and includes gross motor, fine motor, and motor planning (praxic) functions. *Gross motor coordination* is defined as motor behaviors concerned with posture and locomotion, ranging from early developing behaviors to finely tuned *balance.*[137] Fine motor coordination includes motor behavior such as manipulation, discrete finger movements, and eye-hand coordination. *Praxis* and *motor planning* are used only in the specific sense to denote the ability to plan and execute skilled, nonhabitual tasks.[15]

Although visual-motor function is in fact an aspect of motor coordination as we have defined it, it is predominantly used in the literature as a synonym for visuoconstructional abilities and refers to the ability to copy or draw forms or other visual stimuli. Visual-motor functions as thus defined are generally the concern of the special educator or the

occupational therapist and are described and discussed in another chapter of this book. Therefore the emphasis in the discussions of evaluation and treatment is on motor coordination deficits.

Prevalence. The documentation of the prevalence of motor deficits within the learning disabled population is made difficult by the inconsistencies in definition of what constitutes a learning disability, and further how to define the cut-off for inclusion into the subgroup of motor dysfunction. As discussed within the population of learning disabled, children with motor clumsiness do not form a homogeneous group.[132] One problem in definition is that motor competence is not a single entity. The problem may be predominantly in either gross or fine motor skills, but not necessarily both.[122] Other factors influencing prevalence rates include differences in types and methods of testing, reliability of the tests used, and heterogeneity of the test sample.[87,146]

Within the normal population the prevalence rates of motor clumsiness tend to fall between 5% and 15%.[118,146] Johnston and others[146] screened 717 5-year-olds and 757 7-year-olds, and found the prevalence of poorly coordinated children to be 6.5% and 7.2%, respectively. In this study boys outnumbered girls by 2:1. In a sample of 19-year-old boys Keogh[155] found 19% to be physically awkward and clumsy.

Various researchers have attempted to identify the incidence of motor problems in learning-disabled children. A National Collaborative Perinatal Project reported that 75% of the more than 2300 children with positive total "neurologically soft signs" ratings had the symptom of poor coordination.[81] Other frequently noted signs were abnormal reflexes, abnormal gait, mirror movements, and impaired position sense.[81] Tarnopol and Tarnopol[274] reported that about 90% of the children with learning disabilities have motor coordination and visual-motor defects. Clements[67] reported that 98% of children with minimal brain dysfunction showed poor, labored handwriting. In other studies the estimates of motor deficits range for 35% to 60%.[87,173] These figures are greatly affected by the criterion used to determine motor dysfunction. Some of the variables for inclusion/exclusion of any given sample are mixed dominance, choreiform movements, synkinesis, and apraxia.[87]

Descriptions of motor deficits in the learning-disabled child. Although many children with learning disabilities have disorders of motor control, there is no consistent correlation between motor dysfunction and learning disabilities.[182] Because motor functions are the result of complex neurophysiological mechanisms and because the concept of learning disability or minimal brain dysfunction is controversial and not well defined, it is difficult to draw a clear, valid generalization from the study of the relationship between a complex function and a not well-defined concept.[182]

The motor deficits of the learning-disabled child are quite variable, and there does not appear to be any single characteristic pattern.[57] Patterns of movement in children are influenced by age, individual variability, and the environment.[182] For example, research has indicated that younger learning-disabled children show perceptual-motor signs more frequently and in a greater degree of severity than older learning-disabled children.[77,162]

Because there is not a single pattern of motor deficits, two approaches are being used to describe the characteristic motor deficits. This serves to enhance the therapist's awareness of the varied symptomatology and may familiarize the therapist with the focus and type of description that various disciplines provide. The first approach is a descriptive and observational approach and includes the general characteristics of the motor problems. These characteristics are frequently reported by parents and teachers. The second approach, called the neurological approach, focuses primarily on the soft neurological signs. These signs include both motor and nonmotor signs. When evaluating the learning-disabled child, the pediatric neurologist generally looks for soft neurological signs as part of the examination.

Descriptive/observational. Although many developmentally dyspraxic children are not referred for evaluation until they reach school age, many parents report long-standing clumsiness and associated difficulties.[57] Children are described as falling excessively, continuously knocking into things and dropping things, and having more than the usual number of bruises. Although motor milestones such as rolling, sitting, standing, and walking may be within normal or slow to normal limits, there is often a history of relative slowness in self-care skills. The child often appears excessively awkward in daily activities, and there is a history of slowness in dressing, such as buttoning a coat or sweater or tying shoes. Feeding, including handling a spoon, fork, and knife, is often delayed. Play skills, such as learning to ride a tricycle and bicycle, skipping rope, and catching a ball, are often achieved at a later age and seem to take extra effort for the child to perform.

Fine motor coordination problems are also evident. They may be manifested by reluctance to engage in, or incompetence in, small motor tasks such as block building, or constructive manipulatory play such as tinker toys, tracing, and cutting with scissors. Inefficiencies of fine motor performance may manifest themselves educationally in the impairment of the ability to write or draw. Impaired drawing ability is characterized both by poor motor control and spatial disorientation. Handwriting is often labored and spacing problems are evident. Letters are irregular in shape and poorly organized on the page. To compensate for inadequate pencil manipulation, the child may develop a maladaptive grasp that further contributes to making writing prolonged and laborious. Associated articulatory deficits are often present, probably because of the fine motor nature of the demands of articulation.[15,24,61,177]

Although poor motor coordination may be present as difficulty with total body balance, ineptness may be most apparent when complex motor activities are attempted. Physical education class often presents major problems. A 9-year-old boy described his motor problems as follows: "When the gym teacher tells us to do something, I understand exactly what he means. I even know how to do it, I think. But my body never seems to do the job."[178]

Children with motor coordination problems cannot keep up with other children in sports. They often prefer to play more sedentary games, to play alone, or to play with younger children. They are often described as children with whom other children will not play because they are "no fun." These children often get into fights.

A number of characteristics are associated with the motor coordination problems: overactivity or underactivity, a short attention span, spatial disorientation, constructional apraxia, finger agnosia, right-left discrimination problems, low self-esteem, poor peer relationships, and assorted behavior problems.[24,83,255] (See Case 2, page 324.)

Neurological approach/soft neurological signs. Although children with learning disabilities have many symptoms that appear similar to those exhibited by the adult with brain damage, for the most part, they do not demonstrate problems identified by classical neurological examination.[116] Rather, it is felt, they more often demonstrate "soft neurological signs."[233,255,280] These signs suggest minor abnormalities in the function of the CNS.

Studies that have attempted to link soft neurological signs with the diagnosis of learning disabilities and mild motor dysfunction have had varied results. Many studies suggest that a high percentage of children with learning disabilities exhibit certain soft neurological signs. In a study of preschoolers,[166] children that exhibited a greater number of minor neurological indicators had a high likelihood of demonstrating difficulty with tasks of visual perception and gross and fine motor tasks on developmental scales. In general, it appears that a composite of signs is more predictive of dysfunction than single signs. Rie,[233] however, did not find the total number of soft signs predictive of learning disabilities in a study of 80 learning-disabled children. Rather neurological signs requiring complex processes were the most predictive. Peters and others[230] compared learning-disabled boys with a normative sample for the presence of 80 signs and found that 44 of the signs significantly discriminated between the groups.

Research has suggested that soft neurological signs could be more predictive if they were subgrouped, but at present no one sign or discrete group of signs presents a consistent relationship to learning disabilities.[146] Tupper[285] suggests the need for further research in relating specific soft signs to precise behavioral deficits. Rie[233] states, "The phenomenon every clinician has observed for many years, that children who have grave difficulty learning a variety of cognitive tasks, who otherwise appear healthy, are much more likely to show minor motor-sensory dysfunctions than normal ones, should be measurable" (p. 215).

Although a higher proportion of children with learning disabilities manifest soft neurological signs than does a normal control group, neurological involvement is not a

---

CASE 2 ▼   **Paul (continued)**

The following is a mother's description of her child, Paul, who had motor coordination problems and was learning disabled:

"I think when Paul was first born I tried to ignore the problem. Paul is a child who never climbed or ran or drew pictures the way other kids did. But until he went to nursery school, I didn't pay much attention to it. Maybe I didn't want to pay attention to it. Maybe I knew it was there and I didn't want to know about it. I'm not sure. But Paul was always a very verbal child and a very creative and imaginative child. He and I had something special because I used to enjoy that kind of creative imaginative play. We used to have our own world of various fantasies, heroes, and places."

"Paul sat up at about 7 months, he crawled and crept on time. He didn't learn to walk until he was about 15 months old. He walked very cautiously holding on and wouldn't let go of anything. He walked late but he talked early. He said his first clear word, 'cat', at 6 months. He knew what a cat was and could relate to it. My husband and I were so enthusiastic about his sounds. In those days they said that if you stimulated your child and talked to him and got him ready to talk, that this was the important thing, and he could read early. I was very concerned that Paul would be able to talk and have a marvelous vocabulary and read because I had a reading disability and a spelling disability."

"When Paul was 4 years old and in nursery school, at my first conference, the teacher said, 'Look out the window, Mrs. B. See Paul sitting at the bottom. All the other kids are climbing on top of the jungle gym.' And then she showed me some art work. Paul couldn't cut, he couldn't paste, he couldn't do any of it. We could definitely, at the age of 3½ or 4, see his problems. He was very bright but he couldn't cut, paste, or draw, he couldn't climb, he really didn't know how to run. That was where his handicaps were first being noticed, more by other teachers and professionals than by my husband and myself."

"When we had to make the decision as to whether to put Paul into kindergarten or hold him back, we were very frustrated by it because Paul was very very bright and very alert. He has always known everything that was going on in the world."

"Now, the kids Paul knows and the kids who know Paul, know that he can't do motor tasks and they'll come over and play rocket ships with him. But there will come a time, as the kids are getting older, that they won't want to do this."

Paul's mother, who was also learning disabled, described her own disability as follows:

"The hardest course for me was gym. I was unfortunate enough to have the same gym teacher throughout high school. The teacher always used to think I was a lazy kid, that I just never wanted to try to do the exercises. Although I tried, I couldn't do the stunts and tumbling for anything. The other girls would do a somersault and I would still do it like a 4-year-old. I'd just about get over."

"I took dance a couple of times. I never could figure out as a kid why I couldn't point my toes. The teacher would say, "Point your toes" and it never made any sense to me. I always curled my toes up. Only when somebody sat down with me and actually showed me, did I know that that was how you were supposed to point your toes. With other kids, they just did what the teacher did. Nobody had to stop and tell them. I was the klutzy kid. I never could do the nice leaps across the floor. But I would try. After two or three sessions my mother stopped giving me lessons. She was probably embarrassed."

"As a girl, it wasn't as traumatic not being athletic. As I got older, the need for a woman to be athletic tended to decrease, whereas for a boy, the need to be athletic and competitive tends to increase. I foresee this as one of the major problems for Paul."

"Most of my life my friendships with people have always relied on other people. I met most of my friends through other friends because I've gone along to things. I think it goes back to being teased as a child, about the things I couldn't do or the way I looked. If you looked at me, I probably looked like a lot of the learning-disabled kids that you see . . . clothes were not put together properly, shoelaces were untied, my hair was never quite combed properly."

"It was very difficult for me learning how to put on make-up, to use a hairblower. It would take many hours of trying to learn. For a long time, my fingernails were cut very short because I didn't know how to file them. It is still very hard for me to put on eye make-up . . . to look in the mirror and try to figure it out. I still don't feel as though I am completely put together. And I put a lot of effort and energy into looking good."

---

necessary concomitant of learning disabilities.[3,297] Most of the neurological evaluations of learning-disabled children do not attempt to identify a specific site of neurological deficit or to evaluate sensory functions or frank reflexes. Rather, they emphasize the consideration of how the signs may affect a child's functional performance in tasks involving motor skills, spatial understanding, perceptual tasks, and the integration of various modalities for adaptation to demands in the environment. Kinsbourne[159,160] stressed the need to view soft signs from a developmental perspective and stated that "soft signs differed from hard signs in that the child's age is the factor that determines whether the sign represents an abnormality." Accordingly, in a younger child the same sign would be considered normal. Denckla[80] divided soft signs into two groups—developmental and neurological. Developmental signs imply a state of immature neurological function that would be considered normal in a younger normal child. These include awkwardness of motor skills, functional articulatory substitution or distortion, motor overflow and impersistence, persistence in late childhood of extinction to double-tactile stimulation, right-left confusion, and mild oculomotor difficulties. Neurological soft signs, such as reflex asymmetries, are subtle abnormalities that do not occur at any time during normal development and are sufficient but not necessary evidence for brain damage. Tupper[285] has added a third category of signs that results from causes other than neurological damage.

The box on p. 325 lists soft neurological signs frequently used to assess this population. The reader is referred to Tupper,[286] Touwen and Prechtl,[279] and Levine and others[178] for more information on the evaluation of soft neurological signs.

Social and emotional consequences of motor deficits. Poor motor coordination often results in significant social

Common soft neurological signs used in assessment of children with learning disabilities and motor deficits

Minor neurological indicators

Left-right discrimination
Finger agnosia
Visual tracking
Extinction of simultaneous stimuli
Choreiform movement
Tremor
Exaggerated associated movements
Reflex asymmetries

Coordination

Finger-to-nose touching
Sequential thumb-finger touching
Diadochokinesia
Heel to shin
Slow controlled motions

Postural/motor measures

Muscle tone
Schilder's arm extension posture
Standing with eyes closed (Romberg)
Walking a line
Tandem walking (forward and backward)
Hopping/jumping/skipping
Ball throw and catch
Imitation of tongue movements
Pencil/paper tasks
Fine motor tasks (bead stringing, block towering)

Sensory

Graphesthesia
Stereognosis
Localization of touch input

Note: There is considerable variation in assessment measures of soft neurological signs for learning-disabled children, both in what signs are included in assessment and how they are grouped. This chart represents a compilation of possible soft neurological signs.

and emotional consequences. Play, which in the early years is in large part motoric, is essential to psychosocial aspects of development, including self-concept and ego development.[10] As early as 1912, Montessori[204] believed that movement is the basis for personality. In addition, the stimulation that comes from socialization and play is essential to the development of motor behavior.[10] Thus the child with poor play and manipulative skills loses both ways.

Development of gross and fine motor skills and the child's ability to master body movements enhance feelings of self-esteem and confidence. To the extent that the child's perceptual or motor difficulties impede success, self-concept suffers.[91,154,226] Children who are clumsy may be ostracized by their peers. A recent study found that boys with learning

and motor coordination problems demonstrated significantly less effective coping strategies than the normative sample in all domains of functioning.[193] Learning-disabled boys with poor motor coordination were also found to have lower ratings on measures of self-esteem and lower same-sex social relationships and happiness than a matched group of learning-disabled boys with good motor coordination.[257] Shaw and others[257] called this phenomenon 'double developmental jeopardy,' which refers to the double risk factors for poor self-esteem possessed by learning-disabled with motoric impairments. Being unable to compete with peers, having difficulty with the changing demands of cooperative play or feeling self-conscious because of their lack of coordination, learning disabled children often shy away from participation in games. Failure at play and the inability to succeed at school serve to compound the child's feelings of worthlessness, increasing his/her inappropriate responses to the demands of society.[10] Antisocial behavior may occur. Motor performance affects social behavior as exemplified in this statement by a learning-disabled child with motor deficits:

They always pick me last. This morning they were all fighting over which team had to have me. One guy was shouting about it. He said it wasn't fair because his team had me twice last week. Another kid said they would only take me if his team could be spotted four runs. Later, on the bus, they were all making fun of me, calling me a 'fag' and a 'spaz.' There are a few good kids, I mean kids who aren't mean, but they don't want to play with me. I guess it could hurt their reputation (p. 83).[178]

Statements like these highlight the close relationship between motor output, effectiveness, self-image, and social interaction.

Evaluation of motor deficits in the child with learning disabilities

Disciplines involved in evaluation. The disciplines of physical education, adaptive physical education, physical therapy, occupational therapy, and developmental optometry may be involved in the evaluation and training of motor dysfunction in learning-disabled children. Techniques of evaluation have been borrowed as needed among disciplines, and there may be considerable overlap in areas that are assessed both informally and in standardized tests and test batteries. It should be noted that, even though one motor evaluation may resemble another superficially, there are differences between professions in their orientation and rationale for evaluating dysfunction. The unique training of the particular profession influences both the selection of tests and the qualitative aspects of evaluation that come from clinical observation of a child's performance.

Some of the differences in professional orientation and emphasis in evaluation are as follows. Physical educators and adaptive physical educators typically assess skilled tasks necessary for sports-related activities. These include abilities in ball throwing, kicking and catching, jumping, running, and climbing. These professionals are concerned with the child's physical fitness. Physical therapists also evaluate the child's gross motor development and physical fitness, but they assess neuromuscular and neurodevelopmental factors as well. The physical therapy evaluation includes observations of muscle strength and tone, postural refinement, reflex integration including automatic reactions, and sensorimotor functions. Occupational therapists evaluate sensory integrative functions that underlie motor skill development, as well as developmental motor skills. The occupational therapist emphasizes fine motor and visual-perceptual motor realms in assessment and is particularly concerned with the impact of motor deficits on functional abilities. The special attention of the developmental optometrist is on eye movement functions as they relate to visual-perceptual motor skills. The developmental optometrist recognizes the relationship between vision and movement in development and eye-hand coordination.

The areas assessed and the particular tests chosen by a therapist depend on the make up of the professional team serving children in a particular setting and the referral concerns. Careful planning is required in designing an evaluation protocol. Unnecessary duplication of assessment must be avoided; both the child's and the therapist's time are too valuable. Free exchange of information between professionals evaluating motor function is absolutely essential, both of the tests that are used and of the rationale underlying evaluation. The therapist must be aware of information on motor function that is available from other professionals and of information that should be shared with those professionals.

Assessing motor deficits: areas to examine. The learning-disabled child with motor dysfunction can often perform motor tasks with a level of strength, flexibility, speed, and coordination that is virtually normal by the standards of evaluation used by neurologists or by therapists experienced in a population of more severely handicapped children. The child's difficulty with skilled, purposeful manipulative tasks or with finely tuned balance activities may not be readily apparent in the classroom. This appearance of normality, which leads to expectations of age-level motor performance, can create problems and misunderstandings for these children. Therefore identification of subtle motor handicaps is very important.

Areas of testing commonly used in physical therapy, such as muscle strength, range-of-motion, and ambulation; those used in occupational therapy, such as eye-hand coordination and fine motor function; and those used in both professions, such as evaluation of postural control and automatic reactions, are appropriate. It is important, however, to realize that evaluation techniques, for the most part, have been developed for children with moderate-to-severe neurological impairments. To evaluate learning-disabled children, levels of expected performance in these areas may encompass

borderline function. For example, a child might have a normal gait, but lack steadiness standing on one leg, or be unable to tandem walk with the eyes closed. Careful clinical observation becomes of paramount importance, as the deficit in these children is often qualitative rather than quantitative.

To compile a complete picture of the scope and severity of motor deficits in learning-disabled children, the following areas of assessment are important: (1) *postural control and gross motor performance* including muscle tone, strength, functional range of motion, reflex integration, righting, equilibrium and vestibular function, automatic postural reactions, and gross motor skill development; (2) *fine motor and visual motor performance* including proximal and distal movement patterns, eye-hand coordination, handwriting, and fine motor skill development; (3) *motor planning abilities* including ideation, planning, and execution; (4) *sensory integration* including sensory modulation and sensory discrimination; and (5) *physical fitness* including muscular strength, endurance, and flexibility. Each of these interrelated functions is described here as an area of clinical assessment. Because the motor dysfunction of learning-disabled children is subtle, however, a greater reliance on tests with normative data may be necessary, especially for the new therapist or one without experience with neurological disorders. Information on age-appropriate performance is not always available, but sources for provisional information are included when possible. Formal tests and test batteries described in Appendix A provide sources of normative data that can be used as guides for clinical assessment.

Postural control and gross motor performance

Muscle tone and strength. Low muscle tone and poor joint stability have been identified as characteristic of some learning-disabled children.[2,15] Increased tone is not common in children with learning disabilities and may be indicative of minimal cerebral palsy. Learning disabled children with low tone may develop patterns of compensation for low tone called *fixing patterns.* These patterns may include elevated and internally rotated shoulders, internally rotated hips, and pronated feet. To a new observer these patterns may look like slightly increased tone as the child holds himself or herself stiffly for increased stability. Assessment of muscle tone is difficult and subjective, even for experienced testers.[146] It depends on the clinical experiences of the therapist and on a knowledge of normal performance. Judgments of inadequate tone are primarily made through clinical observations. On observation the child may look "floppy," positioning with an open mouth, lordotic back and sagging belly, with knees often positioned close together. Muscle groups may be poorly defined and feel "mushy" or soft on palpation, and joints may be hyperextensible. A common method for assessing muscle tone and proximal joint stability involves placing the child in a quadruped position and observing for inability to maintain the position without locking elbows, winging of the scapula, or lordosis of the trunk. The therapist can determine joint stability by asking the child to "freeze like a statue" and then attempting to move the head sideways and downward, as well as providing intermittent pushes sideways on the trunk looking for ability to remain in the quadruped position. Although manual muscle testing can provide detailed information about the strength of individual muscles, it is not regularly used in the learning disabled population unless there are concerns of a possible degenerative disease. More often strength is assessed by the child's functional ability to move against gravity. Within developmental assessment the therapist is observing range of motion against gravity in skills such as reaching, climbing and throwing, and kicking. The therapist will also frequently have the child attempt to hold positions against gravity to assess strength and endurance.

Integration of primitive postural reflexes. Early reflexes are essential for the development of normal patterns of motor development. Their presence facilitates movement patterns that will later be integrated into purposeful motion.[41] Stereotyped or obligatory responses only occur in pathology and are not expected in the learning-disabled child with motor dysfunction. The residual reactions that might be noted in this population are subtle and most often are seen in stressful nonautomatic tasks. Some learning-disabled children exhibit abnormally persistent asymmetrical tonic neck reflex (ATNR) and symmetrical tonic neck reflex (STNR).[15,207,226,246,262] It is important to note, however, that full integration of these postural reflexes within the normally developing child is not anticipated until 8 or 9 years of age[262,286] or even later.[124,246] Assessment for persistence of primitive reflex patterns with the learning-disabled child should emphasize functional aspects of performance. The lack of full integration of postural reflexes may be observable in the quadruped position,[124,226,227,246] but is more important to view the effect of lack of integration in tasks such as writing at a table or gross motor activities such as ball skills and rope jumping.

To assess for the persistence of the ATNR in the quadruped position, the child assumes the position, the head is passively or actively rotated 90 degrees, and the amount of flexion in the arm on the skull side is measured with a goniometer or scaling devise. Rating scales and age expectations can be found in research studies.[89,226,227,260] Observations of STNR may be seen by passively or actively flexing the neck in this position and looking for elbow flexion or collapse. Residual ATNR also may be observed during the Schilder's Arm Extension Test.[261] In this test the child stands with the arms extended in front of the body at shoulder height with eyes closed. The head is then passively rotated to assess trunk, head, and arm dissociation. Asymmetry in arm flexion on head rotation is normal in 6- to 7-year-olds, but older children should be able to maintain arm position with only slight deviations.

If persistence of these primitive reflexes has an impact on the child's functional performance, it may be seen in the child's inability to sit straight forward at the table for fine

motor or writing tasks. The ATNR influence might be observed by a sideways position at the table with the arm on the face side used in extension. During crawling or climbing games, the younger child might exhibit difficulty maintaining stable arms for success. During ball games the child may have diminished ability to throw with directional control as head movements will influence extension of the face side arm. Another observation of residual ATNR can be seen when the child is asked to pull a rope at midline to propel a swing or scooter board. If the reflex is affecting function the child may lose the bilateral hold on the rope with changes in head position. Although residual reflex involvement may impact performance on the above tasks, many other components are involved in these tasks that will need consideration as well.

Righting, equilibrium and vestibular function. Righting and equilibrium are dynamic reactions essential for the development of upright posture and smooth transitional movements. Righting reactions provide the background for our movements between body positions.[95] Equilibrium reactions are continuous automatic adjustments that maintain the center of gravity over the base of support, and keep the head in an upright position. In simpler terms, righting reactions get us there, and equilibrium reactions keep us there.

Assessment of equilibrium reactions is most often completed on an unsteady surface such as a tilt board or large therapy ball. Equilibrium reactions occur in all developmental positions, and complete assessment will look at reactions in each of these positions. When testing equilibrium, the child's center of gravity is quickly tipped off balance. The equilibrium response is one of flexion of the uphill body side and phasic extension and abduction of the downhill limbs. In daily actions, most of the equilibrium reactions we use are subtle and occur continuously to relatively small changes in the center of gravity.[164] Assessment of righting and equilibrium reactions, therefore, should encompass functional performance in gross and fine motor activities.

The vestibular system plays a role in the mediation and facilitation of equilibrium reactions for the development of balance.[95,258] Automatic righting and equilibrium reactions occur as a response to changes in the center of gravity that facilitate the utricles and semicircular canals of the vestibular system. This stimulation "acts on antigravity extensor muscles so as to elicit compensatory head, trunk, and limb movements, which serve to oppose head perturbations, postural sway, or tilt"[97] (p. 240). Sensory input of proprioception and vision also plays an integral role in balance control.[258] Therefore on assessment of equilibrium and balance, it is important to consider these combined sensory inputs. The therapist tests balance with both eyes open and closed. Traditional tests of vestibular function include (1) the Romberg position—standing with feet together and eyes closed, (2) Mann's position—standing with feet in tandem position (heel to toe) with eyes closed, and (3) standing on one leg with eyes open and eyes closed. The Sensory Integration and Praxis tests[27] includes a 16-item test of standing and walking balance. Refer to Chapter 28, Balance Disorders, for a thorough discussion.

Assessment can include items that involve visual, proprioceptive, and vestibular dissociation such as balancing on an unsteady surface (e.g., dense foam or a tilt board) with and without visual orientation.[258] DeQuiros and Schrager[86] used a changing consistency board to demonstrate vestibular proprioceptive dissociation. The board is a wide walking beam in which irregular lengths of polyurethane foam are alternated with wood to provide an inconsistent walking surface.

Posture and automatic postural reactions. The posture of some learning disabled children is poor.[10,15] The quality of movement is affected both by decreased strength and endurance of the trunk musculature and by diminished automatic reactions to maintain a dynamic upright position. The relationship between posture and muscle tone is also important to consider. A child has " . . . adequate trunk stability when control of the trunk is sufficient to maintain an erect posture, shift weight in all directions, and use rotation within the body axis"[97] (p. 92). These areas are often deficient in the learning-disabled child with motor dysfunction, which affects both gross and fine motor performance.

In gross motor play the child may fatigue quickly and fall often. Other body parts may be used for additional support due to weak postural musculature, such as placing the head on the ground when crawling up an incline, or sticking out the tongue when climbing or pumping a swing. These children may also exhibit lordosis well beyond the age it normally disappears, and recurvatum of the knees is common. In sitting, a child with diminished postural control will fatigue quickly, either leaning on his or her hands for additional support, or moving frequently in and out of the chair. This affects the child's ability to perform fine motor tasks or be available for cognitive learning, as so much effort is spent on sitting up. It is important to observe the effects of fatigue, as both sitting and standing posture may deteriorate over the course of a day. Postural control also is important for the development of fine motor skills because the arms are connected to the trunk, which provides a base of support for distal movements.

Gross motor skills. Learning-disabled children with perceptual-motor or sensory-integrative dysfunction may attain reasonably high degrees of motor skills in specific activities; however, these motor accomplishments remain highly specific to particular movements or to a series of movements and do not generalize to other activities, regardless of their similarities. Whenever variation is required in the motor response, the response breaks down and the motor behavior becomes inaccurate and disorganized. Smyth[264] found that movement time for complex responses was also longer for these children. Thus although the learning-disabled child sits, stands, and walks with

apparent ease, he or she may be awkward or slow in rolling, coming to standing, running, and hopping. The child may be unable to balance on his or her knees or to alternate his or her feet when climbing stairs.

Therefore evaluation of motor skills should include novel motor sequences as well as age appropriate skills. For example, the child can be asked to imitate a hopping sequence or maneuver around a variety of obstacles. Developmentally earlier skills should be assessed as well, and the quality of performance is paramount. It is important to look at the child's ability to make transitions within a position and between positions, as well to observe sequences of motor acts.[200] Learning-disabled children often can perform skill tasks such as skipping, but may do so with increased effort, decreased sequencing and endurance, and a greater amount of associated movements. Gilfoyle and others[108,109] have illustrated qualitative differences in gross motor skills by describing and photographing twins, one of whom was normal while the other demonstrated motor dysfunction. Hughes and Riley[139] have described several gross motor tasks useful in evaluating minor motor dysfunction. Tests of balance, such as those described in the section on vestibular function and in the standardized tests, are important in monitoring achievement as well as in observing exaggerated postural responses. The Test of Motor Proficiency by Bruininks[48] and the Peabody Developmental Motor Scales[99] are examples of standardized assessment of motor skills (see Appendix A).

Fine motor performance

Fine motor skills. It is not uncommon for a child with learning disabilities to be referred for an occupational therapy evaluation because of fine motor concerns. Areas of difficulty typically include awkward manipulation of small objects or avoidance of small manipulatives; diminished grasp and manipulation of tools such as a pencil, spoon, or knife; and delays in activities of daily living requiring dextrous hand use such as buttoning, zippering, and shoe tying. Assessment should include both standardized assessments and structured clinical observations as discussed earlier.

Fine motor movements. Fine motor evaluation should include assessment of proximal control and distal movements, because the control of upper extremity reach and manipulation patterns are thought to be controlled by dual systems.[229] Proximal control is important because movements of the trunk and shoulders have a direct effect on distal function.[73] Trunk control and shoulder stability affect the accuracy and control of reaching patterns and create a stable base from which both hands can be used for bilateral skills.

Distal control includes the fractionated movement patterns that allow the fingers to move independently and with precision and speed.[229] The assessment of distal control involves looking at wrist stability, development of hand arches, and separation of the two sides of the hand, which provide a structural basis for the control of distal movement.[35] In terms of qualitative observations of distal fingertip control, Exner[91] separates manipulative motions into translation, shift, and rotation. Translation involves finger motions to move objects into and out of the palm of the hand. Shift is an alternation of pattern of the thumb and first finger generally used for the final adjustment of an object. Rotation involves turning an object within the hand. The reader is referred to Exner's[91] works for further elaboration of these concepts, and Pehoski[229] for more information on developmental trends.

Although standardized assessments such as The Test of Motor Proficiency by Bruininks,[48] and the Peabody Developmental Motor Scales[99] have fine motor sections, they do not adequately measure manipulative elements as described earlier. Careful clinical observation of movement components during a variety of fine motor tasks is necessary for qualitative analysis. The clinician must have a strong base of reference in normal development for accurate assessment. Soft neurological signs, including diadochokinesis, sequential thumb-to-finger touching, and stererognosis can provide further qualitative information. Several excellent sources provide provisional information on age-appropriate performance.[79,178,279,280,286]

Eye-hand coordination and handwriting. The evaluation of eye-hand coordination is best achieved by using standardized test measures such as the Bruininks-Oseretsky Test of Motor Proficiency,[48] Gubbay's Tests of Motor Proficiency,[118] the Motor Accuracy Test of the Sensory Integration and Praxis Tests,[27] and the Purdue Pegboard Test.[277] Supplemental clinical observations include observations of ball catching and throwing, fine motor tasks such as bead stringing and block towering, and written accuracy tasks such as drawing or coloring within a boundary.

Handwriting requires complex integration of fine motor control, sensory feedback, motor planning, and visual-motor integration.[284] Refinements of accuracy and control have been documented up to the age of 14 in recent studies.[300,301] Although there were developmental trends in the child's finger and hand position during writing, the actual type of grasp on the pencil did not significantly affect the speed and legibility of written work.[301] More important to accuracy is grasp pressure (as measured by the angle of flexion in the index finger) and forearm position.[300] Children who experience difficulties with handwriting most commonly exhibit sloppy work with incorrect letter formations and/or reversals, inconsistent size and heights of letters, variable slant and poor alignment, and irregular spacing between words and letters.[283]

Motor planning. Motor planning involves the ability to carry out a new or unusual motor act, when there is potentially adequate cognitive and motor skill to do so. The child with motor planning deficits has difficulty with performing in, and acting on, the environment.[26] Referral concerns may include clumsiness in performing motor actions, inability to figure out new activities, disorganized approach, poor anticipation of his or her actions, difficulties with peer interactions, and frustration. The child with motor planning problems can often clearly see the differences between his or her performance and other children the same age, which has significant implications for self-esteem. Kephart[157] describes clumsiness, as well as difficulty adapting to changes in external conditions, as being a reflection of a child's inability to plan his or her movements. Children with motor planning deficits often have difficulties in situations characterized by changing demands such as unstructured group play. Transitions also may be difficult because they involve the creation of a new plan, or a change in the program the child is following.

According to Ayres,[26] "Praxis is that neurological process by which cognition directs motor action; motor or action planning is that intermediary process which bridges ideation and motor execution to enable adaptive interaction in the physical world . . . Motor planning is a consciously formulated internal plan of action that occurs before actual motor execution" (p. 23). It involves *ideation* or generating an idea of how one might act in the environment, *planning* or organizing a program of action, and *execution* of the sequences of the motor act.[26]

Standardized assessments of praxis include the tests of Postural Praxis, Sequencing Praxis, Praxis on Verbal Command, Oral Praxis, Constructional Praxis and Design Copy of the Sensory Integration and Praxis Tests[27] (see Appendix A for description of tests). The FirstSTEP by Lucy J Miller is a screening tool for preschoolers that has a section to assess motor planning abilities.[194] Clinical observations can add valuable information about the child's ability to see the potential for action, organize and sequence motor actions for success, and anticipate the outcome of an action. Children with dyspraxia may enter a therapy room filled with equipment and have limited capacity to experiment and play. Other children may move from one activity to the next without truly exploring variations, or completing a task. At times, children with dyspraxia may quickly engage in play with the equipment with little regard for safety. Observations of typically developing children show an incredible amount of variation in play, and spontaneous additions to motor sequences as actions and explorations are successful. These characteristics are important to look for when assessing the child with potential motor planning problems.

Sensory integration. Our system is bombarded with a tremendous amount of sensory information from the world around us and our own bodies. The process of organizing all this information while maintaining our systems at a functional state of arousal is called *sensory modulation*. Deficits in registering and organizing sensory input may be responsible for poor performance noted in motor functioning in learning-disabled children. Sensory information is essential for initiation, execution, and adaptation of motor actions. Consider how difficult it is to speak clearly and chew efficiently after having novocaine at the dentist's office!

Sensory input needs to be efficiently registered for it to be used to learn about or *discriminate* the qualities of objects in the world, as well as the quality of our own body movements within space. Both sensory modulation and sensory discrimination are thought to play integral roles in organized motor behavior.[95]

Kinesthetic perception appears to have a particularly close association with motor performance. Laszlo and Bairstow[172] have developed a Kinaesthetic Sensitivity Test (KST) that measures acuity, perception, and memory. Their initial results on a study of 40 developmentally clumsy children indicated that 73% of the children had deficits in processing kinesthetic input.[171] Hoare and Larkin[125] tested 80 clumsy children using the KST and found that three of the seven kinesthetic measures were deficient. They cautioned labeling children as kinesthetically dysfunctional on the basis of performance on a small number of tasks. Johnston and others[146] found 40% of a sample of 95 children to have abnormal proprioception, and Smyth and Glencross[265] identified slower processing of proprioceptive information in clumsy children. Ayres has repeatedly linked poor tactile, proprioceptive and kinesthetic perception with problems in motor planning.* Other researchers have emphasized the visual and kinesthetic contributions to movement.[133,140,172,215]

Assessment of sensory integration can be best accomplished through the use of the Sensory Integration and Praxis Tests[207] and The Miller Assessment for Preschoolers.[199] Clinical observation of a child's responses to sensory input and ability to organize multiple inputs in the world provide essential additional information in the integration of sensory input.

Physical fitness. The child with motor dysfunction often performs poorly in games and athletic activities and consequently is reluctant to participate. As a result, the level of physical fitness, strength, muscular endurance, flexibility, and cardiorespiratory endurance may be poorly developed. Fitness testing of a group of "clumsy" children in a movement program in Australia indicated that the group performed well below average on a number of fitness tests of aerobic/anaerobic capacity, flexibility, strength, and muscular endurance, even when the tasks were selected to minimize demands on motor coordination.[170] Tests of flexibility indicated that "clumsy" children performed at both ends of the range. Seventy-two percent of the sample scored either below the 25th or above the 75th percentile. One task of the physical therapist is to differentiate between poor physical fitness secondary to low motor activity and problems of low muscle tone, joint limitations, low strength, and endurance that reflect a developmental lag or deviation in motor function. Collaboration among the physical educator, the adaptive physical educator, and the physical therapist is of special importance in these areas. The reader

is referred to Arnheim and Sinclair,[10] and Larkin and Hoare[170] for further discussion of physical fitness and a developmental program for children with problems in motor coordination.

Standardized screening and diagnostic tools for assessment of motor deficits. Several standardized or partially standardized tests of motor function have been used to evaluate children with learning disabilities. The use of a standardized test battery can help to examine the overall developmental status of a child and identify patterns of disability that provide clues to underlying disabilities.[172] A selection of standardized tests is described in Appendix A, which provides an overview of the kinds of tests available for the assessment of motor dysfunction in learning-disabled children and indicates the uses and limitations of the individual tests and test batteries. These tests, as a whole or in part, should be used only by individuals who have knowledge and understanding of the rules of the use and interpretation of standardized tests in general. Furthermore, the use of an individual test requires specific training and/or practice with that test. An examiner should always be thoroughly familiar with all aspects of the administration and scoring procedures of a test and should comply with the requirements for training described in the test manual. Administration and interpretation of some tests (for example, the Sensory Integration and Praxis Tests) require special certification.

In the test descriptions included in the Appendix, comment is generally made on test construction and reliability, but not on validity. Criteria for a satisfactory standardized test should include validation against external criteria. It is difficult to say, however, what external criteria should be selected to validate a motor test because of the fragmentary state of knowledge about patterns of motor deficit and their functional implications. Few of the tests for learning-disabled children reach a desirable level of external validity.[114] In any case, the judicious use of the tests described here must rest on the content validity of the test items. This means that the clinical judgment of the examiner is all important in the selection of tests for an evaluation protocol. The tests must be logical for testing attributes of concern to the therapist, and the interpretation must be made within the overall frame of reference for the evaluation and treatment of children with minimal motor dysfunction.

Setting goals. After assessment the therapist must synthesize areas of strength and weakness and address the functional implications of identified deficits. If deficit areas are clearly affecting the child's functional performance within his or her environment, treatment may be warranted. The treatment process begins with a statement of the child's specific difficulties and with corresponding statements of the type and quality of behavior desired as a result of therapy. In other words, the therapist must set treatment goals to be achieved through remediation.

It is not simple to interpret test data, integrate findings,

---

* References 11, 13, 16, 20, 24, 26, and 27.

identify problem areas, and formulate goals. It may be necessary at times to form initial clinical impressions, which will result in the need for further evaluation to formulate refined goals. This additional assessment may involve formal testing or observation during initial therapy. All therapy is, in a sense, evaluation, and the therapist refines the goals and methods of achieving these goals.

Setting goals for the learning-disabled child with motor problems, as with any child, must be based on consideration of a variety of factors. These include:

1. Referral information, age of the child
2. Medical, developmental, and sensory processing history
3. Parents' and teachers' perception of child's strengths and deficit areas and functional concerns
4. Educational information
   a. Major difficulties experienced in school
   b. How motor problems are interfering with the child's school performance
   c. Current services being received
5. Child's peer relationships, self-esteem, play and leisure activities
6. Therapists' observation/evaluation of the child through informal and formal assessment, both standardized and nonstandardized
7. Functional expectations and abilities at home and school

Goals for the learning-disabled child can be stated in terms of long-term and/or short-term objectives. According to Arnheim and Sinclair,[10] the major long-term objectives in remediation of motor deficits of the clumsy child should be:

effective total body management in a wide variety of activities requiring dynamic balance and agility, object management including manipulation, propulsion and reception, emotional control, ability to socialize effectively, a positive self-concept and a sense of enjoyment in movement.[10]

Short-term objectives should be written to reflect a specific behavior or set of behaviors that is attainable within a predetermined time frame of therapy, usually 6 months to 1 year. Bundy[51] writes that "well written objectives are predictions about how a client will be different, in some meaningful way, as a result of intervention." Behavioral short-term objectives are specific and composed of three parts: (1) The *behavioral statement* is the specifics of what will be accomplished by the child; (2) the *condition statement* provides details regarding how the skill or behavior will be accomplished and; (3) the *performance statement* denotes how the skill or behavior will be measured for success. The most important consideration in compiling goals and objectives is that the objectives chosen are relevant to the child's functional daily performance and are meaningful to all those who are working with the child.

Jonathan was a 6½-year-old referred for occupational therapy evaluation because of concerns by his parents and teacher regarding motor skill development. Assessment revealed several areas of clinical deficit including poor discrimination of his body position and movement in space, diminished postural control and balance reactions, motor planning deficits, delayed eye-hand coordination, qualitative fine motor deficits, and delayed visual-motor integration that affected handwriting. Jonathan's mother reported that he was clumsy and seemed constantly to bump into things. Of greater concern was that Jonathan seemed fearful of activities that his peers found pleasurable such as climbing the jungle gym and coming down the slide at the neighborhood playground. Jonathan tended to play on the outskirts of groups, and when he did attempt to interact he often became frustrated because the children would not play the game by his rules. At home, Jonathan was often frustrated by tasks of daily living such as putting on his coat, snapping his pants, and tying his shoes. His mother reported that Jonathan frequently called himself "stupid" when he could not independently complete self-care skills.

In determining appropriate behavioral objectives for Jonathan it was paramount to look at the areas of functional relevance such as pleasure and safety in gross motor play, peer interactions, and competence and independence in activities of daily living. In discussions with Jonathan and his parents, it became clear that these were common areas of concern for all of us. Jonathan wanted to "not be so stupid that kids won't play with me." His parents wanted him to feel more competent and less frustrated in play, at home, and at school. I felt that through remediation of sensory discrimination and motor deficits Jonathan could develop improved motor competence and planning abilities, which would lead to greater success in peer interactions and improved feelings of self-confidence. From these common desires we created goals and objectives.

One of the general/long-term goals became *to improve Jonathan's gross motor skill development.* Jonathan was interested in learning to ride a bicycle without training wheels, and his parents were hopeful that he could become more confident at the neighborhood playground. It was decided that these were appropriate behavioral objectives that would measure the development of greater control and proficiency in the deficit areas of poor discrimination of his body in space, delayed postural control and balance reactions, and deficient motor planning. The following objectives were written:

1. Jonathan will independently climb the ladder and come down the slide without exhibiting fear, bumping into other children, or falling for 5 minutes.
2. Jonathan will develop the ability to ride his bicycle without training wheels in straight lines and turning corners. (Note: Successfully riding the bicycle becomes the performance measure of behavior in this objective.)

To address *improvement in independence for self-care skills* the following objectives were written:

1. Jonathan will put on his coat independently in correct orientation and successfully zipper it four out of five times.
2. Jonathan will successfully tie his shoes without assistance each day within a timely manner.

To address *greater success in peer interactions* the following were considered appropriate:

1. Jonathan will participate in a structured game for 10 minutes while successfully following the rules.
2. Jonathan will play outside, while interacting with the children in the neighborhood, without conflict for 1 hour at a time.

Although clinically based objectives could have been written to address the same areas, they would be of limited relevance to Jonathan and the people working with him. For example, balance and postural control could be addressed by an objective stating that Jonathan would stand on one foot for 10 seconds, but the functional implications would not have been clear, and Jonathan and his parents would not have had a success measure that was meaningful and measurable to them. Thus it would have negated the effects of working as a cohesive team toward a common goal.

When working as a member of a team within the school, behavioral objectives will have implications for the child's performance in the school environment. In Jonathan's case specific objectives that were meaningful to the classroom situation included ability to sit in the chair to complete written assignments for 15 minutes and increased accuracy of letter formation, size, and spacing on written assignments. The other goal areas related to gross motor, fine motor, and peer interactions also were influential to Jonathan's success at school; but if specific objectives were to be written pertaining to school, our functional outcome measures would have been chosen from tasks within the school environment such as gym class, playground interactions, and classroom expectations.

Under Public Law 94-142 occupational and physical therapy services are considered supportive services, and the need for them should be based on academic relevance for the child.[235] Statements of goals and specific objectives are included in the Individualized Educational Plan that is written as a team process. The parent should be considered an integral part of that team, and objectives should be clear and meaningful to all professionals involved with the child so that there is a common direction of each of the team members. Among the many excellent references on writing goals and objectives and functional outcome measures are Arnheim and Sinclair,[10] Dunn and Campbell,[90] Fisher and others,[95] and LaVesser and Bloomer.[173]

Treatment of the learning-disabled child with motor deficits

What is remediation? In treating the deficits of the learning-disabled child, an important question is, do you try to improve brain function or do you drill the child in the specific perceptual, cognitive, and motor skills? Direct therapy is teaching the child what you want him or her to learn, and indirect therapy is "training the brain."[102]

Indirect therapy techniques are based on the assumption that learning disabilities result from dysfunction of the CNS and that the CNS dysfunction affects one (or more) basic perceptual motor or language processes. Treatment is directed toward the improvement of the underlying abilities. Pioneers in the treatment of learning-disabled children followed this orientation and developed techniques directed toward the improvement of underlying perceptual, perceptual-motor, and psycholinguistic abilities.[3] Direct therapy techniques follow a behaviorist orientation. The presence of CNS dysfunction is not denied, but training in underlying abilities is not considered useful. Treatment approaches emphasize behavior modification, programmed and criterion-referenced instruction, and direct teaching of skills.[3]

The direct technique of teaching the child specific cognitive and academic skills, has been expounded by Sapir,[249] who believes that one should teach to the child's strengths, but at the same time develop methods to help the child deal with interfering deficits. The child should be encouraged to become an active collaborator in diminishing his or her own weaknesses by developing an awareness of the problem and by using his or her conceptual ability to consciously approach his or her perceptual problems and develop compensatory mechanisms. Sapir feels that mobilization of the child's strengths is more effective than training the perceptual skills and hoping for transfer.

Sensory integration procedures are an example of the indirect therapeutic approach. According to Gaddes,[102] this is one of the most articulate and best-developed programs of sensorimotor training for learning-disabled children. The objective of sensory integration procedures is modification of the neurological dysfunction interfering with learning rather than dealing with the specific behavior associated with the dysfunction.[15] This approach emphasizes the role of subcortical functions and structures, including the brainstem, thalamus, and vestibular mechanisms, because they are considered functionally important. The goal of therapy is to improve sensory integration at all levels of the CNS. According to Ayres,[15] "If the brain develops the capacity to perceive, remember and motor plan, the ability can then be applied toward mastery of all academic and other tasks, regardless of the specific content." A sensory integration approach to treating learning disorders differs from many other procedures in that it does not teach specific skills, such as matching visual stimuli, learning to remember the sequence of sounds or movements, or differentiating one sound from another. Rather, the objective is to enhance the brain's ability to learn how to do these things. Ayres emphasizes, however, that sensory integration procedures must be coupled with an educational program to enable optimal integration of sensory and motor functions that subserve language and higher cortical functions.

These descriptions of the approaches of Sapir[249] and Ayres[15] illustrate direct and indirect therapeutic techniques used primarily in the remediation of perceptual and cognitive deficits. The same differentiation occurs in the remediation of motor deficits. The issue then becomes whether one should try to build the underlying foundation abilities or try to develop specific skills. Often the objective of influencing brain function is inherent to the theoretical framework of building foundations. For example, sensory integration theory holds that by increasing integration at all levels of the nervous system, particularly at subcortical levels, the brain also develops better performance. In sensorimotor therapy, as well as in neurodevelopmental therapy (NDT) and proprioceptive neuromuscular facilitation (PNF), techniques are directed toward influencing the CNS through sensory input. These are all indirect approaches in which increased integration of sensation or of basic reflex responses is expected to result in improved specific skills.

One of the concerns of proponents of indirect therapeutic techniques is that teaching a child the specific motor skills that he or she needs in everyday life will result in the development of *splinter skills,* a term used to describe skills that have been learned by the child but that are inefficient because the child did not have the prerequisite sensory integration, postural functions, or movement patterns. For example, in the case of a child with poor balance affecting his or her ability to sit in a chair, having the child attend to his or her balance develops a splinter skill. Research has indicated that this takes much more effort and has a negative influence on the child's ability to concentrate on other learning and skills.[86]

In reality, any compensatory skill could be labeled a splinter skill. For example, walking with crutches could imply insufficient foundation of equilibrium reactions and is an inefficient form of locomotion. However, there is a point in a child's life at which teaching skills, such as crutch walking, is both necessary and appropriate. Therapists should be aware of this need and provide adapted equipment or methods that allow performance of the skill but that prevent the development of maladaptive patterns.

It should be noted that, in some instances, the differences between direct and indirect therapeutic techniques are more theoretical than practical. Both types of techniques may be developmental and the differences between, say, a developmental physical education program and an occupational or physical therapy program are in part a result of the stage of development that is being addressed. Neurodevelopmental

therapy focuses primarily on the development of early motor functions, for example, equilibrium and righting reactions, and physical education historically focuses on higher-level skills, for example, standing balance and ball skills. However, when a developmental motor skills program begins with the early skills, there are fewer differences between direct and indirect therapeutic approaches.

The distinction between these techniques was discussed at length by Ottenbacher,[221] who identified the direct therapeutic approach with an educational model and the indirect therapeutic approach with the medical model. Ottenbacher states that both models are needed and suggests that "The goal of therapists and educators working in the school system should be to create an atmosphere in which models can develop in a synergistic rather than an antagonistic fashion" (p. 84).

In conclusion, both direct and indirect therapeutic techniques of remediation are necessary, because the superiority of any one remedial method has not yet been demonstrated.[102] If we are to deal successfully with all learning-disabled children, we may need to draw on all existing procedures for the management of dysfunction, taking care that proportions of direct and indirect therapy are relevant to the child's age and the severity of his or her disability.[102]

Occupational and physical therapy approaches to treatment. Within treatment there are no delineated formulas or rules for determining the best treatment approach for an individual child. Each child referred for treatment is unique and presents a new challenge to the therapist to set up a plan and achieve functional outcomes. A chosen treatment approach reflects the orientation of the setting the child is referred to, as well as the therapist's beliefs. Selection of treatment methods is tied integrally to the child's presenting problems, and the goals and objectives set up as part of the treatment plan.

The treatment methods presented in the following section are some of the options available to occupational and physical therapists. None is mutually exclusive, and each requires a level of training and practice for competence, as well as experience in how typical development proceeds. Most therapists synthesize information from different treatment techniques and use an eclectic approach to treatment, pulling relevant pieces from a variety of treatment modalities to best meet the needs of each child.

For convenience, occupational and physical therapy approaches to the remediation of motor deficits in children with learning disabilities are classified as sensory integration, neurodevelopmental, motor control, sensorimotor, developmental motor skill, and physical fitness.[10,202] These categories identify emphases in the management of children with minimal motor dysfunction. Sensory integration, as well as neurodevelopmental, motor control, and sensorimotor therapy, relatively speaking, represent the indirect therapeutic approaches, and motor skill training and physical fitness represent a more direct approach.

Sensory integration theory of Ayres. The sensory integration theory was developed and articulated by Ayres,[11,25,27,28] an occupational therapist and psychologist who died in 1988. It includes concepts drawn from neurophysiology, neuropsychology, and development, and was developed to explain the observed relationship between difficulties in organizing sensory input from the body and environment, and deficits in academic and neuromotor "learning" seen in some learning-disabled children with motor clumsiness.[98] Sensory integration theory is based on the premise that higher cortical functions depend on adequate neural organization at subcortical brain levels. The theory postulates that " . . . learning is dependent on the ability of normal individuals to take in sensory information derived from the environment and from movement of their bodies, to process and integrate these sensory inputs within the central nervous system, and to use this sensory information to plan and organize behavior"[98] (p. 4). Ayres[27] used learning in a broad sense to include concept development, adaptive motor responses, and behavioral change.

In her theory Ayres[15] suggested that the child with motor deficits and underlying sensory integration problems could be treated by influencing neurophysiological integration through controlling sensorimotor behavior. She proposed that when provided with appropriate opportunities for enhanced sensory intake, in the context of meaningful activities which encouraged adaptive responses, that CNS processing and integration of sensory inputs could be improved. Improved sensory integration would in turn enhance conceptual and motor learning.[98] Cortical function is thought, in some respects, to depend on brainstem functions, although it is essential to remember that the brain is holistic and integrative in its processing, and both cortical and subcortical processing contribute to sensory integration.[98]

Sensory input is provided in a planned and organized manner, while eliciting adaptive responses enhance the organization of neural structures. "Evincing an adaptive behavior promotes sensory integration, and, in turn, the ability to produce an adaptive behavior reflects sensory integration" (p. 17). The therapist strives to find activities that are self-motivating and tap the child's inner drive, as it is felt that only the child can truly direct the child's body. The therapist works to meld the science of the theory with the art of "playing" with the child. The goal of sensory integration treatment is to elicit responses that reflect better the organization of sensory input, as opposed to improving motor skill for its own sake. It is hoped that skill will generalize for function, and the child will realize his or her potential for action.

For this treatment technique to be appropriate, the motor deficits observed in a child with learning disabilities need to be a result of deficits in processing sensory input.

Ayres[15,16,24] states clearly that sensory integration procedures are designed to remediate sensory integration dysfunction, which accounts for only some aspects of learning disorders. Further research is needed to identify discrete subtypes of children with learning disabilities and sensory integrative dysfunction, who will benefit maximally from this type of treatment.

Although there are general principles for sensory integration treatment, each child's plan must be individualized based on the results of evaluation and responses to sensory input within therapy. It should be mentioned the vestibular-proprioceptive and tactile sensory inputs used in therapy are powerful and must be used with caution. The autonomic and behavioral responses of the child must be carefully monitored. The therapist should be knowledgeable about sensory integration theory and treatment before using these procedures. Monitoring of behavioral responses after the therapy session also is suggested through parent or teacher consultation. Treatment precautions are elaborated in Ayres,[15] and Koomar and Bundy.[164]

Types of sensory integration dysfunction. Through a series of factor analysis studies and cluster analyses, Ayres[11-13,16,20,27] has described certain characteristics that seem to occur together and relate to deficits in processing in certain sensory systems. These types of sensory integration dysfunction are often associated with deficits in tactile and/or vestibular processing. It must be emphasized that these patterns are not absolute. Considerable overlap exists and most children do not fit exclusively into one category. The patterns that have emerged most consistently through factor and cluster analyses include (1) disorders in vestibular-proprioceptive discrimination influencing postural-ocular movements and bilateral integration and sequencing, (2) deficits in somatosensory discrimination resulting in somatodyspraxia, (3) disorders in sensory modulation including tactile defensiveness and gravitational insecurity, (4) deficits in form and space perception including visuomotor and visual construction (visuodyspraxia), and (5) auditory-language problems (praxis on verbal command). (Note: This last category is not thought to be a sensory integration disorder.) The first two categories involve disorders that are most closely associated with motor deficits, and thus are discussed here. Although the motor dysfunction is the sign of a problem, it is the integration of sensory information within the CNS that is being addressed in this treatment technique; the motor output is the means of assessing status and change in sensory integration.

DISORDERS IN VESTIBULAR-PROPRIOCEPTIVE DISCRIMINATION INFLUENCING POSTURAL-OCULAR MOVEMENTS AND BILATERAL INTEGRATION AND SEQUENCING. Children with learning problems often exhibit deficits in vestibular-proprioceptive discrimination that influence the postural and ocular systems. Certain indicators of inadequate vestibular functions have been noted in the learning-disabled child. One of the most frequently used measures of vestibular function is the postrotatory nystagmus response, the back and forth movements of the eyes following rotation. This response is a manifestation of the vestibular ocular reflex and is a normal adaptive response designed to reestablish the original fixation on a visual field.[18] Several studies have linked hyporesponsive (shortened) duration of nystagmus to learning disabilities. DeQuiros[86] and Ayres[18,23] found that more than 50% of the learning-disabled children they each studied had shortened duration of nystagmus. Frank and Levinson[101] found that almost 90% of their learning-disabled children had vestibulocerebellar deficits. Thus a significant percentage of learning-disabled children seem to have a reduced duration of postrotatory nystagmus. Several mechanisms have been suggested to explain this phenomenon.[18]

It should be emphasized that nystagmus is only one manifestation of vestibular functioning. Certain other problems, such as postural and ocular problems, have been associated with vestibular system dysfunction.[205] The vestibular system serves a primary role in the development of postural control and equilibrium. Many learning-disabled children have immature or poorly developed equilibrium and delayed automatic postural reactions. Standing balance is often impaired.[110] Standing balance with the eyes closed may be more impaired than standing balance with eyes open, because when the eyes are closed the child cannot use vision and must rely on vestibular and proprioceptive input.[18,19] The child may also show an inability to assume and maintain the prone extension position (head, trunk, and leg extension against gravity). It has been suggested that this also reflects inadequate vestibular processing.[19,23,52,220] Other indicators of vestibular dysfunction may be inadequate muscle tone and proximal joint stability.[15,75,205,220] Adequate muscle tone enables the body to be readied for movement.[236]

The vestibular system also has been implicated in ocular control. Through its interaction with the oculomotor mechanism, the vestibular system stabilizes the eyes during head and neck movements so that a fixed visual image may be perceived.[15]

A postural and ocular movement disorder is thought to be the basis for bilateral integration and sequencing deficits.[96] Clinically, the deficit is represented by difficulties in coordination of the two body sides, avoidance of crossing the body midline, failure to develop a preferred hand for skill, and possible right-left confusion. Behavioral tasks demonstrating these difficulties may be problems in jumping with both feet together, reciprocal stair climbing, or skipping. The child who tends to avoid crossing the midline may either shift the entire body to avoid crossing the midline or tend to use the right hand on the right body side and the left hand on the left body side. This may interfere with the development of a preferred skilled hand. These children also often have difficulties sequencing and projecting their body movements in space. They are unable to adequately judge, time, and sequence movements of their own bodies in relationship to the environment. This problem can be

observed in difficulties with timing, sequencing and terminating a series of jumps.[96] It may also be assessed in tasks where the child needs to time his or her body in relationship to a moving object, such as catching a ball, or at a harder level, running and kicking a moving ball.

SOMATODYSPRAXIA. Somatodyspraxia refers to the subgroup of children with motor planning delays that are hypothesized to have deficits in somatosensory processing including poor tactile and proprioceptive discrimination.[58] Somatosensory input is important for developing awareness of where the body is in space and body scheme. "If the information that the body receives is not precise the brain has a poor basis on which to build its body scheme"[25] (p. 170). The scheme is developed by sensory awareness initiated by the tactile system, which is a mature sensory system at birth. During early development the child experiences much of the environment through the tactile system and gains a diffuse awareness of his or her own body. The child also discovers the nature of objects through tactile manipulation. Proprioceptive input from the muscles, tendons, joints, and vestibular system work with the tactile system to establish an awareness of his or her body and how it works. "Sensory input from the skin and joints, but especially from the skin, helps to develop in the brain the model or internal scheme of the body's design as a motor instrument"[15] (p. 168). It is suggested that dyspraxic children receive incorrect or inadequate amounts of tactile and proprioceptive input.

According to Ayres,[15] motor planning ability depends strongly on an adequate body scheme and on understanding one's relationship to the environment. "The body scheme which provides the substrate for praxis is a product of intersensory integration" (p. 165). Motor planning depends on the adequate integration of somatosensory, vestibuloproprioceptive, and visual information. As such, disorders in any of these senses may result in poor motor planning ability. Somatodyspraxia represents an impairment in the ability to plan skilled movements that are nonhabitual. Children with dyspraxia can learn specific skills with practice, but they do not have the generalized ability to plan unfamiliar tasks. Gubbay[118-121] refers to the child with developmental dyspraxia as the "clumsy child." Movements are performed with an excessive expenditure of energy and with inaccurate judgment of the required force, tempo, and amplitude.[290] There is an inability to relate the sequence of motions to each other. Ayres[24,26] has suggested that praxis is more than just motor planning. Rather, it involves programming a course of action that includes the ability to organize behaviors and to develop strategies. Children with problems in programming a course of action are often disorganized and have poor work habits—characteristics that frequently accompany developmental dyspraxia.

Manifestations of poor motor planning ability are apparent in many daily tasks. Dressing is often difficult. The child is not able to plan where or how to move his or her limbs to put on clothes. Problems are often demonstrated in constructive manipulatory play, such as tinker toys, cutting, and pasting. Similarly, learning how to use utensils, such as a knife, fork, pencil, or scissors, is difficult. The dyspraxic child often has problems with handwriting. As mentioned previously, dyspraxic children can learn through repetition of a task; however, there is limited generalization of the learned skill to similar tasks.

Critique of sensory integration theory. Sensory integration theory is immensely complex, because it is derived from neurophysiological and psychological knowledge, but it is shaped by ongoing research and therefore is changing and developing. Most critics of sensory integration theory are general in their criticism. Sieben[259] has questioned the theory based on the lack of clinical signs of brainstem malfunction in learning-disabled children and on the lack of clarity in the process by which sensory stimulation is supposed to foster integration in the brainstem. This criticism may result in part from the use of the term *brainstem* as a synonym for subcortical structures. The hypotheses about brain functioning, however, are not directly testable. This criticism of the theory is directed at the lack of support rather than at evidence of contradiction with known facts. Although various individuals have criticized sensory integration because the research has not shown why it works,[9] it is clearly very difficult to substantiate why sensory integration is effective through the research tools and methodologies now available because these aspects are highly theoretical and difficult to observe. According to Tickle,[276] however, it is inappropriate to conclude on the basis of this difficulty that the theory is not correct. Tickle[276] states that the purpose of early research in a field, particularly in a practice field, is to demonstrate whether the given treatment is or is not effective. As the research progresses, researchers start examining factors that influence the effectiveness of therapy. Later they examine why therapy works.

Research on the effects of sensory integration procedures. Many articles have been written on the effectiveness of sensory integration therapy. Within the field of occupational therapy it is the most well-documented treatment procedure. Examination of some of the reviews of sensory integration effectiveness and other related literature* indicates that consistent agreement regarding the effectiveness of sensory integration treatment is lacking. Clinicians who are using sensory integration procedures are convinced that it is effective. There are many testimonials from parents of children who have received occupational therapy using sensory integration procedures. Sensory integration treatment principles are probably the most frequently used in the treatment of learning-disabled children with motor deficits. The knowledge and use of this approach continue to become more widespread, with national and international conferences held on sensory integration theory and treatment.

---

* References 9, 59, 60, 65, 141, 143, 203, 222, and 276.

Nevertheless, the empirical data continue to raise questions about *who, how* and *what* sensory integration procedures affect. Ottenbacher[221] used eight studies for a meta-analysis, which included learning-disabled, mentally retarded, aphasic and at-risk children. A study by Densem and others[84] included subjects who "exhibited a wide array of handicapping conditions, including mild mental retardation, behavioral disturbance, mild cerebral palsy, and epilepsy." Clark and Pierce[66] found 26 effectiveness studies that included four different independent variables including sensory integration procedures, systematically applied vestibular stimulation, multisensory input, and perceptual-motor training. In reviewing effectiveness studies, Cermak and Henderson[59,60] identified at least six different outcome measures including academic measures, language outcomes, motor skills, postrotary nystagmus, self-stimulatory behaviors, and behavioral outcomes. Looking at this incredible variation in the approaches within research studies, it is easy to see that consensus on treatment effectiveness is lacking.

Ottenbacher's meta-analysis of eight studies found that the average child receiving sensory integration performed better on academic measures than three fourths of the control children. He also found a moderate effect size for a motor reflex variable. In summary, Ottenbacher stated that "the meta-analysis of the SI research literature did provide suggestive support for the effects of SI therapy" (p. 319), although the size and the number of research studies that met the criterion for inclusion was quite small. Humphries and others[141] found that subjects treated with a sensory integration approach showed an advantage in motor planning. Depauw[85] reported sensory integration procedures to be more effective than remedial physical education in improving scores on perceptual-motor and fine motor tests.

Two recent studies[141,148] have suggested that sensory integration treatment is not more effective than more traditional skill-based therapies. Part of the difficulty is in how we measure the outcomes of improved sensory integration. Traditional motor tests may not best reflect the changes in organization, adaptability, and planning that children with sensory integration therapy consistently appear to make. Cermak and Henderson[59,60] suggest that "organization, learning rate, attention, affect, exploratory behavior, biological rhythm (sleep-wake cycle), sensory responsivity, play skills, self-esteem, peer interactions and family adjustment" (p. 7) are domains that may change with sensory integration treatment. They also discuss the need for research on short-term effects of sensory integration treatment, which have, for the most part, been unreported in literature.

In reviewing sensory integration research with learning disabilities, Henderson[131] concluded that "the studies . . . provide preliminary evidence of the value of sensory integrative therapy for children with learning disabilities" (p. 45), and that "Certainly they provide sufficient evidence to warrant further investigation of the effects of sensory integrative therapy . . . " (p. 45). In their recent review of sensory integration effectiveness Miller and Kinnealey[203] suggest that future studies need better controls for homogeneous samples, treatment approach, and more clearly defined hypotheses. The complexity of the theory of sensory integration, the individualized approach that treatment warrants, and the lack of good outcome measures create many challenges in designing appropriate and valid research studies.

Neurodevelopmental theory of Bobath. **Neurodevelopmental treatment (NDT)** is a technique that was formulated by the Bobaths[42,43] to enhance the development of gross motor skills, balance, quality of movement, and hand skills in individuals with movement disorders.[244] Its premises and ideas for treatment continue to evolve as the knowledge about neurophysiology expands. NDT is based on the premise that abnormal movement results from deficits in CNS, which is organized with reciprocal connections across many cortical and subcortical structures.[213] Many factors can contribute to abnormal movement patterns including abnormal muscle tone, influence of primitive reflex patterns, delayed development of righting and equilibrium reactions, weakness of specific muscles, inability to counteract the forces of gravity, and deficits in sensory input. It is thought that the learning of movement depends on sensory experiences, and sensory input is essential in initiating and directing movement.[74]

Treatment techniques were designed primarily for use with individuals who had cerebral palsy, with known frank damage within the CNS. It has been applied to various other populations including the at-risk infant population and children with Down syndrome and learning disabilities who demonstrate deficits in motor movement patterns. The framework of NDT is to facilitate normal movement patterns so that the individual does not develop abnormal or compensatory patterns, which lends its use to children with more minimal motor involvement. Of particular relevance to the learning-disabled child with motor deficits is facilitation of improved righting and equilibrium responses, automatic postural adjustments, and balance reactions.

Neurodevelopmental treatment utilizes physical handling techniques directed toward developing the components of movement that underlie functional motor performance. Movement components of neuromotor maturation, postural alignment and stability, mobility skills, weight bearing, weight shifting, and balance are all foundations for smoothly executed movements in space.[244] This is accomplished through a combination of facilitation and inhibition techniques that use sensory input, particularly tactile-proprioceptive cues. Abnormal movement patterns are prevented while normal postural adjustments are guided through key points of control on the body.[74] Proximal stability is promoted for the achievement of distal control.

The ultimate goals of NDT treatment are the normalization of abnormal tonus, facilitation of active adaptive posture and movement, and integration of postural reactions to

encourage the acquisition of functional movement patterns needed for learning and daily living skills.[74] As the theory has grown and evolved the realization of the need to promote better movement within the context of functional task performance has been greatly emphasized.[247] The NDT therapist is working toward using movement patterns as "functional" components of practice tasks (Personal correspondence, Missy Windsor, April 22, 1994). The reader is referred to Chapters 9 and 10 for more extensive reviews of neurodevelopmental theory and treatment.

Research on the effects of neurodevelopmental therapy. Neurodevelopmental therapy is based on principles derived from research in motor development and neurophysiology. The techniques, however, arise from careful and extensive clinical observations. The system of therapy is widely used with children with cerebral palsy, the group for which it was designed, but it has been subjected to little experimental verification. Much of the difficulty with designing effectiveness studies to assess NDT is defining appropriate and measurable outcome measures. Two studies[128a,230a] that used standardized developmental motor tests as a dependent variable did not find significant differences between children treated with NDT treatment techniques and children who were not treated. In her study of infants and toddlers with Down syndrome utilizing NDT treatment techniques Harris[128,128a] also utilized individualized specific objective measures as a dependent variable. According to her findings, 80% of the treatment group reached individualized objectives, compared with only 57% of the control group. Nevertheless, she did find any significant differences on the standardized motor measures. This finding led her to question the appropriateness of these tests in assessing the qualitative motor changes that are anticipated with NDT treatment.

Of the 41 studies initially identified by Royeen and DeGangi[244] for a review of NDT treatment effectiveness, only one quantitative study was performed.[223] In 1986 Ottenbacher and others performed a meta-analysis on the use of NDT procedures in the pediatric population and found that the effect size was small due to the small number of samples, changes in the quality of movement and posture being difficult to measure, and research studies lacking rigorous control. The findings did suggest that clients receiving NDT treatment or some combination of NDT and other related therapy performed better than 62.2% of the subjects not receiving service.

After their review Royeen and DeGangi[244] suggested that the effectiveness studies had methodological problems as manifested in the lack of objective outcome measures, overreliance on subjective clinical observations, and small sample size. Of the 19 studies they reviewed there was also a great deal of variation in the sample populations chosen for studies including adult and pediatric cerebral palsy with varied diagnoses, high-risk infants, and Down syndrome. No studies were found on the use of this technique in the child with learning disabilities and motor deficits. Royeen and

DeGangi[244] suggested that more studies are needed regarding the ability of NDT to answer questions about whether benefits are obtained over time with NDT intervention before the effectiveness of NDT as compared to other therapeutic techniques is studied.

Motor learning and motor control theories. As the understanding of the neurophysiology of the nervous system has increased, therapeutic approaches have been challenged to expand their assumptions and methodologies. Many motor learning and **motor control** theories have been proposed and evolved. The reader is referred to Chapters 3 and 4 for more extensive discussions of these theories. This discussion focuses on those aspects of the theories that are relevant to the treatment of learning-disabled children with motor deficits.

The theoretical models of motor learning and motor control, and their therapeutic uses, have been built on scientific studies in the areas of movement science, including biomechanics, motor control, muscle biology, motor learning, and cognitive psychology.[56] Motor learning refers to the process of acquiring ability to produce skilled movement.[113] The acquisition of skilled movement is thought not only to depend on integration within the nervous system, but also to be influenced by environmental factors and human biomechanics. "A central assumption of the motor control model is that the neural structures that act to control movement must be adapted to constraints imposed by the structure of the musculoskeletal system and by the physical laws governing movement"[115] (p. 25). Due to the influences of environmental factors, task-related intervention is considered essential to the development of motor control. The person with a movement dysfunction needs to learn how to perform the required motor tasks for adequate function in daily life.[56] One of the criticisms of NDT treatment has been the limited carryover of facilitated "normal" movement patterns into functional situations.

Bernstein[37] introduced these concepts with the premise that "purposeful movement is organized to solve motor problems"[247] (p. 523). Motor problems occur from the interaction of the external environment that challenge the neuromuscular system. Bernstein proposed that the human biomechanical system had a huge number of *degrees of freedom* in movement that needed to be controlled. For example, in the upper extremity degrees of freedom occur within each joint, with the shoulder being able to move in three planes of movement, the elbow and wrist one, etc. This creates an incredible complexity and variation of movement patterns to control for a functional activity such as handwriting. Bernstein suggested that individuals reduce the degrees of freedom by creating linkages among muscular activities at various joints. Limitations of degrees of freedom through coordinated kinematic linkages create the basis for motor control or ability to use the body effectively. This has led to the evolution of the more current view that most skilled movements depend on preplanned patterns of neural output to the muscles, called "motor programs."[115]

Motor programs are "command sets" that execute movement without requiring peripheral feedback. This process of motor control is called an *open loop,* or *feedforward system.* A feedback, or closed loop system, depends on the recognition and correction of errors from peripheral feedback such as kinesthesia for performance. If all movement depends on this type of error correction, human behavior would be extremely slow and inefficient.[247] With the open loop (feedforward) system of control, the nervous system utilizes previous motor learning to detect errors in a movement plan before it has been executed, so that the individual can avoid errors in motor performance. Feedforward is the system that lets you know you are going to type an incorrect letter before your finger actually hits the key. The work of Nashner and McCollum[214] indicates that postural control works on a feedforward system. A person makes preparatory postural adjustments before they ever initiate a movement.

Components of these theories of motor control appear particularly relevant to the treatment of a learning-disabled child with motor deficits. Task-oriented behavior has always been a key premise in occupational therapy. When engaged in remediation with the child, progress is seen more rapidly when there is investment in a task-related behavior that is meaningful to the child. For example, eye-hand coordination tasks become more meaningful within the context of a game of hot potato or baseball.

Problems typically seen in this population include clumsiness, difficulty with judging force, timing and amplitude of motions, and deficits in anticipating the results of a motor action. These children often take longer to initiate a motor action and many move in a slow, plodding fashion. Using the concepts of the motor control theories presented here, we can hypothesize that these children are experiencing difficulties with feedforward and feedback systems. Feedforward would be essential to the development of projected action sequences discussed in the earlier section on sensory integration treatment, where the child has difficulty judging and timing movements through space in relationship to another object. Smyth[264] compared normal and clumsy children on a series of simple and complex movements and found that the clumsy group had a longer reaction time and movement time for complex motions. He hypothesized that clumsy children have a deficit in programming the movements; as a result, they need to rely more heavily on feedback for movement control.

Treatment that uses these theories of motor control includes behavioral and biomechanical analyses. Much consideration is given to how the person solves movement problems in the environment.[219] For completion of a successful task-oriented movement, the child must conform to the spatial and temporal demands of the environment.

Visual and verbal cognitive strategies are used to assist the individual in performing the movement more appropriately. At times specific movement components of a task might be practiced, but they are combined in the context of the entire motor task, concentrating on the specific goal or end product of the task. At times the therapist needs to communicate the goal of the task to the child, but independent problem solving is encouraged. It is felt that "active planning, execution, and termination of a movement sequence enable a person to code the movement-related kinesthetic and visual information most effectively"[247] (p. 525).

Critique of motor control theories. Current motor control research involves a multidisciplinary effort, including neurophysiology, anatomy, muscle physiology, biomechanics, and behavioral sciences.[115] Because of the great number and variation of theories presented on motor control, limited consensus has been reached on terminology and definitions, which impedes the ability to adequately test and compare these theories. It also makes it difficult for researchers to understand each other's work and research and limits the ability to search for underlying neural mechanisms of dysfunction.[136]

Sensorimotor therapy. The practice of sensorimotor treatment techniques evolves from the premise that sensorimotor performance requires the child to organize sensory information from the environment for use in executing motor actions.[180] The goal of sensorimotor therapy typically does not evolve around a single, unified theory.[112] More often, the systems of sensorimotor therapy that have been developed for learning-disabled children are a combination of perceptual-motor, neurodevelopmental, motor control, and sensory integration procedures.[93,109,180,202]

In a sensorimotor therapy approach tasks are chosen for their innate sensory and motor components. The child is directed to activities that encourage the use of environmental concepts such as spatial and temporal sequencing within the context of a motor activity. The therapist chooses activities to meet the child's developmental levels and encourage practice of appropriate motor skills. Play interactions are considered important to encourage sensory motor integration within the context of meaningful interactions with persons and objects.[180] For example, the child may propel himself or herself on a scooter board in prone through an "obstacle maze" looking for matching shapes.

The goal of this type of treatment is typically outcome based, with emphasis on the development of age-appropriate perceptual motor and gross motor skills. The approach is developmental, utilizing motor sequences that encourage adaptation and practice of certain skills. Gross motor outcomes of improved muscle strength, postural control, balance, equilibrium, and planning are promoted. For example, the learning-disabled child with motor dysfunction walks and runs, but may demonstrate inadequate postural reactions in lying, sitting, or kneeling positions. Therefore

these positions are encouraged. The child may be having difficulty keeping up with the skilled activities in gym class such as skipping or rope jumping. Components of these activities will be encouraged, with emphasis on sequencing and timing. The therapist may use a heavier jump rope to provide more sensory information.

For further discussion of sensorimotor therapy, the reader is referred to Gilfoyle and Grady,[108,109] Heiniger and Randolph,[129] Knickerbocker,[163] Ayres,[15] and DeQuiros and Schrager.[86] These sources also describe many therapeutic activities for the development of postural functions in learning-disabled children.

Research on sensorimotor therapy. DeGangi and others[76] identify a gap between theoretical thinking about sensorimotor therapy and current research. Studies in this treatment technique are limited. In a comparison study DeGangi and others[76] found that children provided with structured sensorimotor therapy made greater gains in gross motor skills, developmental functions such as self-care, and sensory integrative functions than children who engaged in child-centered activity.

Functionally relevant motor skill training. Sensorimotor therapy includes training in motor skills that are basic, that is, those that develop in preschool and early school years. The skills taught in motor skill training programs are usually of a higher level, and functionally relevant to the child's daily performance. The real difference is in the approach used. Motor skill training involves the learning of skills and subskills sequenced by the ages at which they are accomplished or by steps from less demanding to more demanding skills. Evaluation identifies the point at which a child fails; treatment involves a hierarchy of tasks from gross to fine.[119,120]

Abbie described the motor skills training approach: "One can . . . break down the skills into their simplest forms and give the child opportunities to practice each in as many varied ways as possible so that he does not learn one isolated splinter skill" (p. 200).[1] As an example, Abbie suggested that a child with poor balance in standing practice balance in all positions—kneeling, all fours, sitting, and prone—and on both stable and mobile surfaces. Abbie used multiple approaches, including neurodevelopmental theory, modern dance, and gymnastics.

Knickerbocker[163] has developed a structured approach for developing skills that span a progression from early postural functions to perceptual skills, noting that learning-disabled children are often exposed to learning experiences for which they are not developmentally ready. The development of postural skill is organized around the use of five basic pieces of therapeutic equipment: an indoor climber, a carpeted barrel, a scooter board, inflated equipment, and suspended equipment. Program plans are presented with activities given for three levels of accomplishment. Knickerbocker emphasizes the close relationship between diagnostic assessment and treatment procedures and presents an evaluation system that basically consists of qualitative descriptions of a child's response to the therapeutic equipment. Thus the overall plan provides a graded system that includes an ongoing evaluation of performance.

In general, the recommended approach for motor skill training includes indirect remediation, as well as motor skill development.[129] However, much of the treatment is directed toward the acquisition of basic skills as described by Abbie.[1,2] A basic principle is to provide a great variety of motor activities at the child's developmental motor level to promote motor generalizations. The activities recommended include balance, locomotion, body awareness, and hand-eye coordination. The functional relevance of these skills areas include being able to sit at the desk within the classroom and complete written work, as well as greater success in recess games such as basketball.

A final area of skill that should not be ignored is that of activities of daily living. Clumsy children are frequently delayed in the basic self-care skills of tying shoe laces, using a knife and fork, and blowing their nose, as well as a general inefficiency in dressing for school.[118,120] Inadequacy in self-care is a sensitive area for children whose peers have no such difficulty, and teachers and therapists should be aware of a child's need to learn these basic skills.

Monitoring physical fitness. In addition to the primary deficits in sensorimotor functions, motor skills, and sensory integration functions, a learning-disabled child is at risk for poor posture, body mechanics, and physical fitness. Physical fitness, as defined here, includes strength, endurance, speed, agility, flexibility and cardiorespiratory endurance.

Arnheim and Sinclair[10] pointed out that there is a vicious cycle in the relationship between motor ability and physical fitness. The child with poor motor ability avoids physical activity, and the poor fitness that develops through lack of exercise lessens motor ability.

The physiologically based poor posture and inefficient body use can be exaggerated by a secondary disability. The child's poor self-concept may be reflected in a hunched, withdrawn posture and the avoidance of any physical activity beyond that needed in everyday activities. This latter pattern can also be found in learning-disabled children without a primary motor disability.

The physical therapist should monitor and prevent or correct loss of movement in the joints of the neck and spine and work with the physical educator to ensure that a child receives sufficient exercise to maintain his or her physical fitness. Arnheim and Sinclair[10] presented graded levels of activities for fitness in the four levels of strength and muscular endurance, flexibility, agility and large muscle coordination, and cardiorespiratory endurance. The reader is referred to Arnheim and Sinclair,[10] and Larkin and Hoare[170] for further discussion of physical fitness and a developmental program for children with problems in motor coordination.

Summary. Children with learning disabilities often also present with motor deficits. These deficits may be subtle and difficult to pick up using neurological evaluation or standardized testing. Nevertheless, deficits may have significant impact on the qualitative development of age-appropriate motor skills, which may further affect self-esteem, peer relations, and functional performance at school and home. Whether or not motor deficits affect academic achievement directly is an issue of debate. Motor foundations such as automatic postural control certainly allow more freedom of movement for the child to explore and learn within his or her environment or to sit upright in a chair to participate in academic tasks. Motor deficits may be another manifestation of inefficient cerebral and brainstem processing thought to affect learning. A multitude of factors have to be considered in the development of each individual's capacities. Lerner stated that:

> We cannot conclude that motor development is unimportant or that this aspect of learning should be discarded. Rather, these studies suggest that plans are needed for building the bridge between motor training and academic learning. Efficient motor movement may be a prerequisite but alone it is insufficient[175] (p. 155).

Motor performance is certainly an important aspect of the child's total development. It is important that the motor deficits in children with learning disabilities be assessed by the special education team, with remediation provided by the team members as appropriate for improved functional abilities.

Many theoretical models have been developed in an attempt to explain the qualitative motor deficits observed in the learning-disabled population, as well as to provide constructs in which to develop treatment programs. All have certain relevance to this population and perhaps to each individual child. Many of the approaches share common assumptions, although the rationales for these assumptions and the treatment approaches for remediation may vary markedly. Several theories and treatment approaches have been presented to attempt to give a spectrum of alternatives for use with this population. Each child presents a unique blend of clinical signs and functional deficits, and the therapist is challenged to assess the child appropriately, to identify strengths and weaknesses, and to formulate a treatment program that best addresses both the underlying deficits in foundation skills and the functional weaknesses in daily life tasks. The experienced therapist will combine knowledge from many areas of motor development and remediation to facilitate the best performance in each child.

Organization of occupational and physical therapy services. Traditionally, occupational and physical therapy was provided in clinics that were completely separated from educational services or in special schools or classes for orthopedically or multiply handicapped children. In special schools and classes, the therapists work with teachers but with a philosophy similar to that of a clinic. The service is optimal for interdisciplinary cooperation; teachers and therapists are readily accessible to one another, and the program has the potential for maximizing educational and therapeutic benefits for the child. In such a setting therapists provide direct "hands on" treatment for the child, as well as work with the teacher and the child's parents to facilitate motor functioning in the classroom and at home.

Although in some states occupational and physical therapists have provided services for multiply handicapped children in public schools for many years, therapy for children with minor motor deficits, such as the learning-disabled child, is more recent. During the last 15 years, occupational therapy services for learning-disabled children have become increasingly common; physical therapy for learning disabled children has been even more recently established and is still less common. However, the establishment of the Education for All Handicapped Act (PL 94-142) and the Individuals with Disabilities Education Act (IDEA) is rapidly changing the status of therapy in public school systems. The provision of related services, including occupational and physical therapy as well as special education, is now a mandated part of the educational process. As specialists in the evaluation of motor functions, therapists provide evaluation services for children with all levels of motor dysfunction, and therefore see children not referred for service formerly.

PL 94-142 and recent education reform bills also have changed the location and kinds of services provided to children with special needs. The educational and social disadvantages of segregating handicapped children from their age peers have been cited, and the concept of least restrictive placement has been articulated in the law. "Least restrictive" implies an appropriate education in an environment as close to that of the normal child as possible.

Educational reform is moving more toward a model of full inclusion, where children with handicapping conditions are educated within the context of the regular education classroom. For the learning-disabled child, this includes full mainstreaming into regular classes, with specialists providing direct service, monitoring and consultation within the context of this environment. Meeting the needs of these children requires a change both in occupational and physical therapy evaluation and treatment services and in the methods of delivery of those services.*

Kalish and Presseller[147] have identified five areas of function for the physical or occupational therapist in the educational environment. They include:

1. Screening and evaluating children with a wide variety of functional deficits

2. Program planning based on evaluation results and related to a child's ability to receive maximum benefit from his educational experiences
3. Treatment activities designed to meet program goals
4. Consultation to teachers, other school personnel, and parents around carry-over of services into the classroom and home programming
5. In-service training for individuals and/or group relative to the needs of handicapped children

Because each of these functions is usually required of the public school therapist, the time available for providing direct services to children is limited. Treatment service must be done, in part, through consultation to parents, classroom teachers, and physical educators. The child's motor development needs can sometimes be met, wholly or in part, through the physical education program. The therapist can evaluate the child and suggest therapeutic activities that could be incorporated into an adaptive physical education program.

Kalish and Presseller[147] point out the necessity of integrating therapy into the educational process, first by adapting therapy to reinforce educational goals and then by incorporating therapy into routine classroom activities. The therapist must be flexible and discover alternate methods of reaching therapy goals, such as positioning and using unobtrusive adaptive equipment. The teacher's responsibility for all of the children in his or her classroom must always be kept in mind. Before proposing the incorporation of a therapeutic activity into a classroom, its feasibility must be assured. In some classrooms a teacher's aide might be available for individual attention, but in all instances both the child's time and the teacher's time must be considered in relation to the total program requirements.

In providing direct services, learning-disabled children can often be treated effectively in small groups, and occupational therapy and physical therapy aides are often available. It is important to plan schedules carefully so that the child is not removed from the classroom at times critical to his or her academic education. It must be recognized that what may be considered "optimal therapy" within a medical model may not be possible in an educational model. It is important for therapists to understand that the public schools' principal concern is the educational rather than the medical well-being of the child.

The therapist should become a participant in the educational process.[176] It is essential for the therapist working in the public school to learn about the public school system as a social institution, about the educational philosophies that guide teachers, and about the legislative regulations governing programs for children with special needs, as well as about the legal responsibilities of public school therapists.[208] Within a specific setting the therapist needs to know which model of special education service delivery is being used. The therapist needs to translate medical information for

---

* References 90, 147, 168, 176, 208, and 253.

educational personnel and must write evaluation and progress reports without using medical jargon. In short, the therapist must become a participant in the educational process.[176] Comprehensive discussions of occupational and physical therapy in public school systems are presented in a number of publications.*

BEHAVIORAL AND EMOTIONAL SEQUELAE OF LEARNING DISABILITIES

Although the majority of literature and work in learning disabilities has been addressed to the identification, analysis, and remediation of academic deficits, behavioral and emotional sequelae often accompany a learning disability and may sometimes become of even greater importance than the learning disability itself.[47,69,111,291] Ames[7] stressed that there is no single behavior pattern prevalent in all those who are learning disabled but that there are some commonalities, the most obvious of these being a poor self-image. Although the child with a learning disability may initially be an integral part of the social and educational milieu, because of poor academic progress, disruptive behaviors, and the necessity for special attention from the teacher, guidance counselor, or resource personnel, the learning-disabled child perceives herself or himself and is perceived by others as being "different."[116] A self-defeating cycle may be established: the child experiences learning problems, the school and home environments become increasingly tense, and disruptive behaviors become more pronounced. These responses, in turn, further affect the child's abilities to learn. Lack of success generates more failure until the child anticipates defeat in almost every situation.[299] The learning-disabled child is often discouraged and fearful, attitudes are defensive and negativistic, and motivation may be lost. Self-concept, self-confidence, and peer relationships are often affected.† Research has confirmed that these children tend to be rejected more often and that they are less popular than "normal" peers in regular classrooms.[49,64,178] The child's behavior and impaired learning usually generate a state of perpetual anxiety for the entire family.[7,116]

Life-span learning disabilities

Research with learning-disabled adolescents and adults has indicated that, for the most part, children do not outgrow learning disabilities‡ and that these problems tend to persist in some or all of the following areas: attention and activity, neuromaturation, motor skills, cognition and academic performance, emotional adjustment, and social interactions.

Follow-up studies of hyperactive children indicate that although hyperactivity itself becomes less of a problem as children get older, many other problems exist. Routh and Mesibov[243] found that, of 83 teenagers who had been

hyperactive as children, 58% had failed one or more grades in school, many had low self-esteem, and several had been involved in delinquent behavior. In a 5-year follow-up study of hyperactive children, Weiss and others[293] found that 70% had repeated at least one grade as compared to 15% of matched control subjects. The chief complaints of the children's mothers included distractibility and poor concentration, although the hyperactivity itself had declined. Hoy and others[138] did a 5-year follow-up study of hyperactive children and found that at adolescence, although the activity declined, the hyperactive children still had attentional and stimulus-processing difficulties that affected both their academic and social functioning. Overall, results indicated that childhood hyperactivity seems to be predictive of continued academic failure, poor concentration, impulsivity, low self-esteem, and poor conduct.

Research has also indicated that there are long-term academic effects of learning disabilities during the school years. In looking at whether or not children outgrow learning disabilities, Book[45] tested 472 Utah kindergarten children on standardized tests and assigned each student to one of three categories of presumed risk. Students were retested on academic achievement tests in first through fourth grades. Fewer than 11% of the students assigned to the high-risk group ever performed above the fiftieth percentile. Only 4% in the lowest-risk group ever performed below the twenty-fifth percentile.

Helper[130] reviewed follow-up studies of children with learning disabilities and found that, both emotionally and behaviorally, learning-disabled boys continued to have a much higher frequency of problems than did controls. In addition, persistent deficits in learning skills (e.g., reading achievement) along with deficits in attention and information processing were noted.

Even within the motor domain, there is increasing evidence that children do not outgrow their deficits* despite some arguments to the contrary.[68] In fact, Denckla[81,83] pointed out that although many clumsy children do later master certain motor skills, they fail new age-appropriate ones. The same seems to be true in many domains.

Learning disabilities appear to have a persistent effect on self-concept. Of the adolescent populations with learning disabilities or hyperactivity studied, 40% to 60% have low self-esteem.[269] Depression, thoughts of suicide, and low expectations for the future also seemed to be more prevalent in the learning-disabled adolescent.[190]

The finding that learning disabilities are associated with behavioral problems has resulted, in recent years, in an interest in the relationship between learning disability and juvenile delinquency. A high rate of antisocial behavior in adolescence, "trouble with the law," or "police contact" are frequently found in follow-up studies of children with

---

* References 5, 6, 147, 149, 168, and 282.
† References 32a, 50, 92, 237, 262a, and 294.
‡ References 31, 54, 63, 72, and 181.

*References 63, 134, 174, 181, 255, 268, and 294.

learning disabilities.[54,181] Learning or skill deficiencies are considered an element in a significant number of delinquents.[36] Several studies of delinquent, adolescent boys have shown that 25% to 30% have learning disabilities,[92] and Mauser[188] reported that 50% to 70% of juvenile delinquents in his sample exhibited evidence of learning disabilities. Rubin and Braun[245] found that the major deficits in juvenile delinquents were visual-spatial-orientational and visual-motor coordination deficits. It is recognized that not all children with learning disabilities become juvenile delinquents. Although there is no evidence for a causal link between juvenile delinquency and learning disabilities, there does seem to be a relationship.[167,200] Some clinicians believe that the learning-disabled child is at risk for developing deviant and antisocial behaviors and that educational and psychological trauma occurring in the classroom may be expressed as aberrant social functioning in the community.[299]

Study of the adult with learning disabilities is fairly recent, in part because "learning disabilities" were not diagnostic entities until the 1960s. Many of the current reports on learning disabilities in adulthood are from persons who were diagnosed as learning disabled in their teenage or adult years. Thus they did not receive the early intervention services that learning-disabled children are currently receiving. Moreover, whereas the learning-disabled child of today is recognized as being bright with specific learning disabilities, those persons whose learning disabilities were recognized in their later years may have been considered lazy, unmotivated, or stupid in their formative educational years. Because of the recency of intervention services for learning disabilities, we cannot evaluate the effectiveness of treatment or its effect on long-term disability. For these reasons, it may not be possible to generalize from the learning-disabled adult of today to the learning-disabled adult of the future.

Much of our knowledge about the learning-disabled adult today is largely anecdotal and in the form of case histories. Documentation has clearly been lacking. Few research studies have systematically explored the continued effects of a learning disability in adulthood. In reviewing the current literature in learning disabilities in adulthood, it appears that among adults, as among children, learning disabilities can be expressed throughout the total personality—cognitively, perceptually, and emotionally.[9] Functional difficulties also persist and now are seen in vocational adjustment, work management, and social and family interactions.[62] The same cycle that the person experienced as a child may be repeated as an adult. Chronic anxiety and tension are often present. An example of this is Mrs. B., Paul's mother, who also had a learning disability but was not diagnosed as learning disabled until age 20. Nevertheless, she completed both college and a master's degree in counseling. Although the academic problems were no longer an issue, the learning disability interfered with her home and work performance.

For example, Mrs. B. described her organizational problems and identified a continuous need to make lists in order to function in her job. Mrs. B. said she had to work hard to not look clumsy and that she was fearful that she would trip over things and look foolish. She said that it seemed as though it took a lot more effort for her to learn and accomplish things as compared to her peers. Mrs. B. also discussed how her learning disability interfered with her relationship with her husband and children. Because of her tactile defensiveness, she disliked it when her children would come up from behind and unexpectedly grab her, and she only felt comfortable being touched (hugged, caressed) on her own terms. Thus it is apparent that even as an adult, the learning disability continued to present difficulty.

In the box on p. 344 is a letter from a woman with learning disabilities and sensory integration problems. She describes how her learning disability affects her current functioning and how it affected her when she was a child.

SUMMARY

Meeting the needs of the learning-disabled child offers new challenges in occupational and physical therapy. As a result of the passage of PL 94-142 and IDEA, the treatment of children is moving from the clinical arena to the public school arena. Providing service for any handicapped child requires changes in patterns of service delivery, especially an increase in skills for consultation and in service education. To treat the learning-disabled child with motor dysfunction, a therapist must also develop new skills in evaluation and treatment.

Occupational and physical therapists must assume responsibility for learning-disabled children with motor problems and must make sure that motor problems and their import in the overall development of a child are recognized. It is important for therapists to understand that the principal concern of the public school is the educational rather than the medical well-being of the child. The role of the therapist must be kept in perspective. Occupational and physical therapists are specialists in abnormal motor behavior and can identify problems and possible underlying deficits better than psychologists or teachers. The therapist can help the teacher understand a child's limitations and can offer suggestions that can both facilitate the child's motor performance and reduce the stress of his or her everyday motor activities. Furthermore, it is the therapist who can best explain the child's need for a program to lessen the motor deficit.

On the other hand, the child's motor needs must be assessed in the context of the overall educational and emotional development. The question often is not whether the child would benefit from therapy but which types of remediation are the most essential for the child at a given time in his or her development. Some children with motor incoordination cope quite well as long as their problem is recognized. As Gubbay[13] says, "Bringing the child into

A letter from an adult with a learning disability

I am 26 years old, a professional bassoonist with a master's degree in Music Performance. My name is Wendy. Through Jane, an occupational therapist, I discovered when I was 24 years old that I had learning problems and sensory integration problems.

I invert letters and especially numbers. When people speak English to me, I feel it's a foreign language. There's translation lag time. When learning new things, I either understand intuitively or never. I can't seem to go through step-by-step learning processes.

Physically, I'm extremely sensitive to motion. When I was little, we moved every year. I spent the first 5 years of my life feeling sick. It seems that I feel everything more strongly than most people. I have an extremely low threshold of pain and even pleasure tends to overload me. If I am touched unexpectedly it hurts; it's so jarring. This causes a lot of problems with interpersonal relationships. I can't stand to have people close to me; it produces an adrenalin reaction.

Motor activities are also a problem; my muscles don't seem to remember past motions. Despite the many times I've walked down steps and through doors, I still have to think about how high to lift my foot and about planning my movements. When eating, I have to think about chewing or I bite my tongue or mouth. I don't think other people think about these things. I'm physically inept; I can bump into the same table 10 times running. I'm always bruised, and as a child people constantly labeled me as clumsy. Physical education courses were hell as a child, especially gymnastics, where you are forced to leave the ground and swing or walk on balance beams or uneven bars. I cannot begin to explain the terror or disorientation.

Academically, I was labeled stupid or, more frequently, lazy. I was told that I was not trying. Actually, my I.Q. is very high and my coping mechanisms are very complex. If they only knew how hard I was trying. I was lucky because I taught myself to read at an early age. I would never have learned to read otherwise. Even so, my first grade teacher wouldn't believe that I could read so far past my age. She called me a liar when I said that I had finished each stupid "Dick-Jane" book. I was forced to read each one 50 times before she would give me a new one.

Not all teachers were so insensitive. My fourth grade teacher made every effort to let me go at my own pace, letting me read on a college level and do 2 years of math on my own. Left to my own devices, I can learn and love to do so. My fifth grade teacher forced me to do math the long way with steps. I just know the answer by looking at multiplication or division problems, even algebra problems, but to this day I cannot understand how one does it in steps. If a teacher didn't accept this, I was in for a year of hell. I cried a lot in school, from frustration mostly, and I pretended to be sick a lot.

I never had friends until college. I guess I was too different to be acceptable. I grew up in a very rigid, repressive, religious community which made it especially difficult to be accepted. My differences were labeled evil or, at best, I was ignored. I left high school at age 16 for college, where at least I could structure what I wanted to learn. It's never been easy for me to make friends, although it's better now. Music circles tend to be a bit crazy so I fit in more easily.

My learning disabilities still are problems. My motor and learning problems get in the way of my music, but my coping mechanisms are strong. I deal better with my clumsiness now. Just being diagnosed by Jane has made a big difference. To have things labeled, to be told and realize that it's not my fault, has given me a sense of peace. It's also allowed me to turn from inward depression to outward anger at those who labeled me stupid and clumsy. Just being able to admit anger allows one to let it go.

Other than my testing and subsequent conversations with Jane, I have not received treatment for my problems. I believe that adults with my problems can be helped. I wish programs were available in all areas of the country. At age 26, I feel much better about myself than I did even at age 24. It's a matter of growth and coping with major differences.

The greatest advice I would give to educators and therapists working with problem children is: accept. Accept what they can do well; don't make an issue of what they can't do. We all have our strengths and weaknesses. If a child can't do math, so what! Buy the child a calculator and the child will do a lot better with it than with a label of stupidity following her through life.

focus by the recognition of his problem immediately reduces the pressures to conform" (p. 157). In an environment in which parents, teachers, peers, and the child recognize the nature of the deficit and set reasonable expectations, some children accept their motor disability, and academic skills and alternative forms of recreation assume greater importance.

As this review has indicated, evidence supporting the effectiveness of treatment of motor deficits in learning-disabled children is as yet fragmentary. Learning-disabled children present highly variable patterns of disability that make it difficult to predict or measure response to therapy. Both formal research and careful documentation of clinical outcomes are needed to explore and define the dimensions and significance of motor disorders in learning-disabled children that are relevant to therapy. Only then can we better categorize children, improve the precision of treatment, and validate treatment theory.

REFERENCES

1. Abbie MH: Physical treatment for clumsy children—not enough? *Physiotherapy* 64:198, 1978.
2. Abbie MH and others: The clumsy child: observations in cases referred to the gymnasium of the Adelaide Children's Hospital over a three year period, *Med J Aust* 1:65, 1978.
3. Adelman HS and Taylor L: *An introduction to learning disabilities,* Glenview, Ill, 1986, Scott Foresman & Co.

4. Allen L: Inclusion education: a changing role for occupational therapists, *Occup Ther Forum* 8(32):4-5, 1993.

5. American Occupational Therapy Association: *Occupational therapy in the public school system,* Rockville, Md, 1976, The Association.

6. American Physical Therapy Association Board of Directors: Physical therapy practice in an educational environment. In *American physical therapy house of delegates handbook,* Phoenix, 1980, The Association.

7. Ames TH: Post secondary problems: an optimistic approach. In Weber RE, editor: *Handbook on learning disabilities: a prognosis for the child, the adolescent, the adult,* Englewood Cliffs, NJ, 1974, Prentice-Hall.

8. Anderson CM: The brain-injured adult: an overlooked problem. In Weber RE, editor: *Handbook on learning disabilities: a prognosis for the child, the adolescent, the adult,* Englewood Cliffs, NJ, 1974, Prentice-Hall.

9. Arendt RE, MacLean WE, and Baumeister A: Critique of sensory integration theory and its application in mental retardation, *Am J Ment Defic* 92:401.

10. Arnheim DD and Sinclair WA: *The clumsy child: a program of motor therapy,* St Louis, 1979, Mosby.

11. Ayres AJ: Patterns of perceptual motor dysfunction in children: a factor analytic study, *Percept Mot Skills* 20:335, 1965.

12. Ayres AJ: Deficits in sensory integration in educationally handicapped children, *J Learning Dis* 2:160, 1969.

13. Ayres AJ: Characteristics of types of sensory integrative dysfunction, *Am J Occup Ther* 25:329, 1971.

14. Ayres AJ: Improving academic scores through sensory integration, *J Learning Dis* 5:338, 1972.

15. Ayres AJ: *Sensory integration and learning disorders,* Los Angeles, 1972, Western Psychological Services.

16. Ayres AJ: Types of sensory integrative dysfunction among disabled learners, *Am J Occup Ther* 26:13, 1972.

17. Ayres AJ: Sensorimotor foundations of academic ability. In Cruickshank WM and Hallahan DP, editors: *Perceptual and learning disabilities in children,* vol 2, Research and theory, New York, 1975, Syracuse University Press.

18. Ayres AJ: *Southern California Postrotary Nystagmus Test,* Los Angeles, 1975, Western Psychological Services.

19. Ayres AJ: *Interpreting the Southern California Sensory Integration Tests* Los Angeles, 1976, Western Psychological Services.

20. Ayres AJ: Cluster analyses of measures of sensory integration, *Am J Occup Ther* 31:362, 1977.

21. Ayres AJ: Dichotic listening performance in learning disabled children, *Am J Occup Ther* 31:441, 1977.

22. Ayres AJ: Effects of sensory integrative therapy on the coordination of children with choreoathetoid movements, *Am J Occup Ther* 31:291, 1977.

23. Ayres AJ: Learning disabilities and the vestibular system, *J Learning Dis* 11:18, 1978.

24. Ayres AJ: *Sensory integration and the child,* Los Angeles, 1980, Western Psychological Services.

25. Ayres AJ: *Southern California Sensory Integration Tests Manual,* Revised, Los Angeles, 1980, Western Psychological Services.

26. Ayres AJ: *Developmental dyspraxia and adult onset apraxia,* Torrance, Calif, 1985, Sensory Integration International.

27. Ayres AJ: *The Sensory Integration and Praxis Tests,* Los Angeles 1988, Western Psychological Services.

28. Ayres AJ, Mailloux Z, and Wendler C: Developmental dyspraxia: Is it a unitary function?, *Occup Ther J Res* 7(2):93, 1987.

29. Badian NA and Wolff PH: Manual asymmetries of motor sequencing in boys with reading disabilities, *Cortex* 13:343, 1977.

30. Bannatyne A: *Language, reading and learning disabilities,* Springfield, Ill, 1971, Charles C Thomas.

31. Bax M and MacKeith R: Minimal cerebral dysfunction in the adolescent, *Pediatr Clin North Am* 27:79, 1980.

32. Beale IL and Tippett LJ: Remediation of psychological process deficits in learning disabilities. In Singh NN and Beale IL: *Learning disabilities, nature, theory, and treatment,* New York, 1992, Springer-Verlag.

32a. Beasley DS and others: Learning disabilities: a problem in communication? In Gottlieb MI and others, editors: *Current issues in developmental pediatrics: the learning disabled child,* New York, 1979, Grune & Stratton.

33. Berry KE: *Developmental Test of Visual-Motor Integration,* (VMI) ed 3, Cleveland, 1989, Modern Curriculum Press.

34. Belmont T: Perceptual organization and minimal brain dysfunctions. In Rie RH and Rie ED, editors: *Handbook of minimal brain dysfunctions: a critical view,* New York, 1980, John Wiley & Sons.

35. Benbow M: A neurodevelopmental approach to teaching handwriting. Lecture notes from a workshop presented March 1990.

36. Berman A and Siegal AW: Adaptive and learning skills in juvenile delinquents: a neuropsychological analysis, *J Learning Dis* 9:583, 1976.

37. Bernstein N: *The coordination and regulation of movements,* Elmsford, NY, 1967, Pergamon Press.

38. Birch HG and Walker HA: Perceptual and perceptual-motor dissociation, *Arch Gen Psychiatry* 14:113, 1966.

39. Black PE: *Brain dysfunction in children: etiology, diagnosis and management,* New York, 1981, Raven Press.

40. Black PE: Introduction: changing concepts of "brain damage" and "brain dysfunction." In Black PE, editor: *Brain dysfunction in children: etiology, diagnosis and management,* New York, 1981, Raven Press.

41. Bly L: *The components of normal movement during the first year of life and abnormal motor development,* Oak Park, Ill, 1983, NDT, Inc.

42. Bobath K: The motor deficits in patients with cerebral palsy, *Clinics in Developmental Medicine,* no 23, London, 1966, The National Spastics Society Medical Education and Information Unit in association with William Heinemann Medical Books, Ltd.

43. Bobath KA and Bobath B: Neuro-developmental treatment. In Scrutton D, editor: *Management of the motor disorders in children with cerebral palsy,* ed 2, Philadelphia, 1984, JB Lippincott.

44. Boder E: Developmental dyslexia: a new diagnostic approach based on the identification of three subtypes, *J Sch Health* 40:289, 1970.

45. Book RM: Identification of educationally at-risk children during the kindergarten year: a four-year follow-up study of group test performance, *Psychol Schools* 17:153, 1980.

46. Bortner M and others: Neurological signs and intelligence in brain damaged children, *J Special Educ* 6:325, 1972.

47. Brown JS and Zinkus PW: Screening techniques for early intervention. In Gottlieb MI and others, editors: *Current issues in developmental pediatrics: the learning-disabled child,* New York, 1979, Grune & Stratton.

48. Bruininks RH: *Bruininks-Oseretsky Test of Motor Proficiency,* Minnesota, 1978, American Guidance Service, Inc.

49. Bruininks VL: Actual and perceived peer status of learning disabled students in mainstream programs, *J Special Educ* 12:51, 1978.

50. Bryan TH and Pearl RA: Self concepts and locus of control of learning disabled children, *Education Horizons* 59:91, 1981.

51. Bundy A: A conceptual model of school system practice for occupational and physical therapists. Lecture notes from a conference presented in November 1991.

52. Bundy AC and Fisher AG: The relationship of proximal to distal and other vestibular functions, *Am J Occup Ther* 35:782, 1981.

53. Campbell PH: The integrated programming team: an approach for coordinating professionals of various disciplines in programs for students with severe handicaps, *J Assoc Persons Severe Dis* 12(2):107-116, 1987.

54. Cannon IP and Compton CL: School dysfunction in the adolescent, *Pediatr Clin North Am* 27:79, 1980.

55. Carmon A: The two human hemispheres acting as separate parallel and

sequential processors. In Inbar GF, editor: *Signal analysis and pattern recognition in biomedical engineering,* New York, 1975, John Wiley & Sons.

56. Carr JH and Shepard RB: A motor learning model for rehabilitation. In Carr JH and Shepard RB: *Movement science: foundations for physical therapy in rehabilitation,* Rockville, Md, 1987, Aspen Publications.

56a. Cermak SA and others: The effect of concurrent activity on dichotic listening in boys with learning disabilities, *Am J Occup Ther* 32:493, 1978.

57. Cermak S: Developmental dyspraxia. In Roy E, editor: *Neuropsychological studies of apraxia and related disorders,* New York, 1985, Elsevier Science Publishing Co.

58. Cermak SA: Somatodyspraxia. In Fisher AG, Murray EA, Bundy AC: *Sensory integration: theory and practice,* Philadelphia, 1991, FA Davis.

59. Cermak SA and Henderson A: The effectiveness of sensory integration procedures, Part I *Sensory Integration Q* 17(4):1-5, 1989.

60. Cermak SA and Henderson A: The effectiveness of sensory integration procedures, Part II *Sensory Integration Q* 18(1):1-17, 1990.

61. Cermak S, Ward E, and Ward L: The relationship between articulation disorders and motor coordination in children, *Am J Occup Ther* 40:546, 1986.

62. Cermak SA and Murrary E: The adult with learning disabilities: where do all the children go?, *Work* 2(2):41-47, 1991.

63. Cermak SA and others: The persistence of motor deficits in older students with learning disabilities, *Jpn J Sensory Integration* 2:17-31, 1991.

64. Chapman JW and Boersma FJ: *Affective correlates of learning disabilities,* Lisse, Netherlands, 1980, Sets and Zeitlinger, B.V.

65. Clark FA and Pierce D: Synopsis of pediatric occupational therapy effectiveness: studies on sensory integrative procedures, controlled vestibular stimulation, other sensory stimulation approaches, and perceptual-motor training. Paper presented at the Occupational Therapy for Maternal and Child Health Conference, Santa Monica, Calif, 1986.

66. Clark F and Pierce D: Synopsis of pediatric occupational therapy effectiveness, *Sensory Integration,* 16(2), 1988.

67. Clements SD: Minimal brain dysfunction in children: terminology and identification, *NINDB Monograph* no 3, Washington, DC, 1966, United States Department of Health, Education, and Welfare.

68. Committee on Children with Disabilities: School-aged children with motor disabilities, *Pediatrics* 76(4):648, 1985.

69. Cook LD: The adolescent with a learning disability: a developmental perspective, *Adolescence* 14:697, 1979.

70. Crinella FM: Identification of brain dysfunction syndromes in children through profile analysis: patterns associated with so-called "minimal brain dysfunction," *J Abnorm Psychol* 82:33, 1973.

71. Crowell DH and others: Unilateral cortical activity in newborn infants: an early index of cerebral dominance? *Science* 180:205-208, 1973.

72. Cruickshank WM and others: *Learning disabilities, the struggle from adolescence toward adulthood,* Syracuse, New York, 1980, Syracuse University Press.

73. Danella E and Vogtle L: Neurodevelopmental treatment for the young child with cerebral palsy. In Case-Smith J and Pehoski C: *Development of hand skills in the child,* Rockville, Md, 1992, American Occupational Therapy Association.

74. DeGangi GA: Perspectives on the integration of neurodevelopmental treatment and sensory integrative therapy, *NDTA Newsletter,* 1(4), January 1990.

75. DeGangi GA and others: The measurement of vestibular based dysfunction in pre-school children, *Am J Occup Ther* 34:452, 1980.

76. DeGangi GA and others: A comparison of structured sensorimotor therapy and child-centered activity in the treatment of preschool children with sensorimotor problems, *Am J Occup Ther* 47(9):778-785, 1993.

77. DeHirsch K and others: *Predicting reading failure: a preliminary study,* New York, 1966, Harper & Row.

78. Deloria DJ: Review of Miller Assessment for Preschoolers. In Mitchell, JV Jr, editor: *The ninth mental measurements yearbook,* Lincoln, Neb, 1985, University of Nebraska Press.

79. Denckla MB: Development of motor coordination in normal children, *Dev Med Child Neurol* 16:729, 1974.

80. Denckla MB: MBD and dyslexia: beyond diagnosis by exclusion, *Top Child Neurol* 19:253, 1977.

81. Denckla MB: Developmental dyspraxia: the clumsy child. In Levine MD and Satz P, editors: *Middle childhood development and dysfunction,* Baltimore, 1987, University Park Press.

82. Denckla MB and Rudel R: Rapid Automatized Naming (RAN): dyslexia different from other learning disabilities, *Neuropsychologia* 14:471, 1976.

83. Denckla MB and others: Motor proficiency in dyslexic children with and without attentional disorders, *Arch Neurol* 42:228, 1985.

84. Densem JF and others: Effectiveness of a sensory integrative therapy program for children with perceptual-motor deficits, *J Learning Dis* 22(4):221-229, 1989.

85. Depauw KP: Enhancing the sensory integration of aphasic students, *J Learning Dis* 11:142, 1978.

86. DeQuiros J and Schrager O: *Neurophyschological fundamentals in learning disabilities,* San Rafael, Calif, 1979, Academic Therapy Publications.

87. Deuel RK and Robinson DJ: Developmental motor signs. In Tupper DE: *Soft neurological signs,* New York, 1987, Grune & Stratton.

88. Doehring DG: Reading disability subtypes: interaction of reading and nonreading deficits. In Rourke BP, editor: *Neuropsychology of learning disabilities: essentials of subtype analysis,* New York, 1985, Guilford Press.

89. Dunn W: *A guide to testing clinical observations,* Rockville, Md, 1981, American Occupational Therapy Association.

90. Dunn W and Campbell PH: Designing pediatric service provision. In Dunn W: *Pediatric occupational therapy: facilitating effective service provision.* Thorofare, NJ, 1991, Slack.

91. Exner CE: In-hand manipulation skills. In Case-Smith J and Pehoski C: *Development of hand skills in the child.* Rockville, Md, 1992, American Occupational Therapy Association.

92. Faigel HC: The learning disabled adolescent. In Gottlieb MI and others, editors: *Current issues in developmental pediatrics: the learning disabled child,* New York, 1979, Grune & Stratton.

93. Farber SD: *Neurorehabilitation: a multisensory approach,* Philadelphia, 1982, WB Saunders.

94. Finucci MM: Genetic considerations in dyslexia. In Myklebust HR, editor: *Progress in learning disabilities,* vol 4, New York, 1978, Grune & Stratton.

95. Fisher AG, Murray EA, and Bundy AC: *Sensory integration: theory and practice,* Philadelphia, 1991, FA Davis.

96. Fisher AG: Vestibular-proprioceptive processing. In Fisher AG, Murray EA, Bundy AC: *Sensory integration: theory and practice,* Philadelphia, 1991, FA Davis.

97. Fisher AG and Bundy AC: Vestibular stimulation in the treatment of postural and related disorders. In Payton OD and others, editors: *Manual of physical therapy techniques,* New York, 1989, Churchill Livingstone.

98. Fisher AG and Murray EA: Introduction to sensory integration theory. In Fisher AG, Murray EA, Bundy AC: *Sensory integration: theory and practice.* Philadelphia, 1991, FA Davis.

99. Folio MR and Fewell R: *Peabody Developmental Motor Scales (POMS): revised experimental edition,* Allen, Tex, 1983, DLM Teaching Resources.

100. Ford FR: *Diseases of the nervous system in infancy, childhood and adolescence,* ed 5, Springfield, Ill, 1966, Charles C Thomas.

101. Frank J and Levinson H: Dysmetric dyslexia and dyspraxia, *J Am Acad Child Psychiatry* 12:690, 1973.

102. Gaddes WH: *Learning disabilities and brain function: a neuropsychological approach,* ed 2, New York, 1985, Springer-Verlag.

103. Gardner RA and Broman M: The Purdue Pegboard: normative data on 1334 school children, *J Clin Child Psychol* 1:156, 1979.

104. Gardner MF: *TVMS Test of Visual-Motor Skills,* San Francisco, 1986, Children's Hospital of San Francisco.

105. Gazzaniga MS: Brain theory and minimal brain dysfunction, *Ann NY Acad Sci* 205:89, 1973.

106. Geschwind N: Language and the brain, *Sci Am* 226:76, 1972.

107. Geschwind N and Galaburda A: Cerebral lateralization: biological mechanisms, associations, and pathology: I, II, III, *Arch Neurol* 42:428, 521, 6, 1985.

108. Gilfoyle EM and Grady A: A developmental theory of somatosensory perception. In Henderson A and Coryell J, editors: The body senses and perceptual deficit, *Proceedings of the Occupational Therapy Symposium on Somatosensory Aspects of Perceptual Deficit,* Boston, 1972, Boston University.

109. Gilfoyle EM and others: *Children adapt,* Thorofare, NJ, 1981, Charles B Slack.

110. Gillberg IC: Children with minor neurodevelopmental disorders—III: Neurological and neurodevelopmental problems at age 10, *Dev Med Child Neurol* 27:3, 1985.

111. Goff JR: A neuropsychological approach to the learning disabled child. In Gottlieb MI and others, editors: *Current issues in developmental pediatrics: the learning disabled child,* New York, 1979, Grune & Stratton.

112. Goldman L: Sensory motor activity not necessarily SI, *OT Week* 2(10):8, March 1988.

113. Goodgold-Edwards SA: Clinical application of motor control and motor learning theory, Massachusetts Chapter Physical Therapy Lecture Series, January 1993.

114. Goodwin WL and Driscoll LA; *Handbook for measurement and evaluation in early childhood education,* San Francisco, 1980, Jossey-Bass.

115. Gordon J: Assumptions underlying physical therapy intervention: theoretical and historical perspectives. In Carr JH and Shepard RB: *Movement science: foundations for physical therapy in rehabilitation,* Rockville, Md, 1987, Aspen Publications.

116. Gottlieb MI: The learning-disabled child: controversial issues revisited. In Gottlieb MI and others, editors: *Current issues in developmental pediatrics: the learning disabled child,* New York, 1979, Grune & Stratton.

117. Gross K and others: Duration thresholds for letter identification in left and right visual fields for normal and reading disabled children, *Neuropsychologia* 16:709, 1978.

118. Gubbay SS: *The clumsy child,* New York, 1975, WB Saunders.

119. Gubbay SS: The management of developmental apraxia, *Dev Med Child Neurol* 20:643, 1978.

120. Gubbay SS: The clumsy child. In Rose FC, editor: *Pediatric neurology,* London, 1979, Blackwell Scientific Publications.

121. Gubbay SS and others: Clumsy children: a study of apraxic and agnosic deficits in 21 children, *Brain* 85:295, 1963.

122. Hall DM: Clumsy children, *Br Med J* 296(6619):375-376, 1988.

123. Hammill DD and others: A new definition of learning disabilities, *Learning Dis Q* 4:336, 1981.

124. Hanson C: A study of the presence of the asymmetrical tonic neck reflex in first and second grade children, master's thesis, 1976, Sargent College, Boston University.

125. Hoare D and Larkin D: Kinaesthetic abilities of clumsy children, *Dev Med Child Neurol* 33:671-678, 1991.

126. Hardy M and others: Developmental patterns in elemental reading skills: phoneme-grapheme and grapheme-phoneme correspondences, *J Educ Psychol* 63:433, 1972.

127. Harness BZ, Epstein R, and Gordon HW: Cognitive profile of children referred to a clinic for reading disabilities, *J Learning Dis* 19:426, 1984.

128. Harris SR: Physical therapy and infants with Down's syndrome: the effects of early intervention, *Rehabilitation Literature* 42:339, 1981.

128a. Harris SR: Effects of neurodevelopmental therapy on motor performance of infants with Down's syndrome, *Dev Med Child Neurol* 23:477-483, 1981.

129. Heiniger MC and Randolph SL: *Neurophysiological concepts in human behavior,* St Louis, 1981, Mosby.

130. Helper MJ: Follow-up of children with minimal brain dysfunctions: outcomes and predictors. In Rie HE and Rie ED, editors: *Handbook of minimal brain dysfunctions: a critical view,* New York, 1980, John Wiley & Sons.

131. Henderson A: Research in occupational therapy and physical therapy with children. In Camp BW, editor: *Advances in behavioral pediatrics,* Greenwich, 1981, Jai Press.

132. Henderson SE: The assessment of "clumsy" children: old and new approaches, *J Child Psychol Pschiatry* 28:511-527, 1987.

133. Henderson SE and Hall D: Concomitants of clumsiness in young school children, *Dev Med Child Neurol* 24:448, 1982.

133a. Henderson SE and Sugden D: Movement Assessment Battery for Children (ABC), Kent, England, 1992, Psychological Corporation.

134. Hern A: Neurological signs in learning disabled children: persistence over time, and incidence in adulthood compared to normal learners, doctoral dissertation, Victoria, BC 1984, University of Victoria.

135. Hiscock M and Kinsbourne M: Specialization of the cerebral hemispheres: implications for learning, *J Learning Dis* 20(3):130, 1987.

136. Horak FB: Assumptions underlying motor control for neurologic rehabilitation. In Lister MJ, editor: *Contemporary management of motor problems,* Alexandria, Va, 1991, Foundation for Physical Therapy.

137. Hoskins T and Squires J: Developmental assessment: a test for gross motor and reflex development, *Phys Ther* 53:117, 1973.

138. Hoy E and others: The hyperactive child at adolescence: cognitive, emotional and social functioning, *J Abnorm Child Psychol* 6:311, 1978.

139. Hughes JE and Riley A: Basic gross motor assessment, *Phys Ther* 61:503, 1981.

140. Hulme C and others: Visual, kinaesthetic and cross-modal judgements of length by normal and clumsy children, *Dev Med Child Neurol* 24:461, 1982.

141. Humphries T and others: A comparison of the effectiveness of sensory integrative therapy and perceptual-motor training in treating children with learning disabilities, *Dev Behav Pediatr* 13(1): 31-40, 1992.

142. Illingsworth RS: The clumsy child. In Bax M and MacKeith RM, editors: Minimal cerebral dysfunction, *Clinics in Developmental Medicine,* no 10, London, 1963, The National Spastics Society Medical Education and Information Unit in association with William Heinemann Medical Books, Ltd.

143. Ingersoll BD and Goldstein S: *Attention deficit disorder and learning disabilities, realities, myths and controversial treatments,* New York, 1993, Doubleday.

144. Johnson D: Paper presented at the 85th Convention of the American Psychological Association, Washington, DC, Sept, 1976.

145. Johnson DJ and Myklebust HR: *Learning disabilities: educational practices and principles,* New York, 1967, Grune & Stratton.

146. Johnston O, Short H, and Crawford J: Poorly coordinated children: a survey of 95 cases, *Child Care, Health, and Dev* 13(6): 361, 1987.

147. Kalleh R and Provostler S: Physical and occupational therapy, *J Sch Health* 50:264, 1980.

148. Kaplan BJ and others: Reexamination of sensory integration treatment: a combination of two efficacy studies, *J Learning Dis* 26(5):342-347, 1993.

149. Kauffman NA: Occupational therapy theory, assessment, and treatment in educational settings. In Hopkins HL and Smith HD, editors: *Willard and Spackman's occupational therapy,* ed 5, Philadelphia, 1978, JB Lippincott.

150. Kavale KA and Forness SR: History, definition and diagnosis. In Singh NN and Beale IL: *Learning disabilities, nature, theory,and treatment,* New York, 1992, Springer-Verlag.

151. Kavanagh JF and Truss TJ, editors: *Learning disabilities: proceedings of the national conference,* New York, 1988, York Press.

152. Keim RP: Visual motor training, readiness, and intelligence of kindergarten children, *J Learning Dis* 3:256, 1970.

153. Keogh BK: Learning disabilities: diversity in search of order. In Wang MC, Reynolds MC, and Walberg HJ, editors: *The handbook of special education: research and practice,* vol 2, Oxford, Pergamon Press.

154. Kenny TJ and Burka A: Coordinating multiple interventions. In Rie HE and Rie ED, editors: *Handbook of minimal brain dysfunctions: a critical view,* New York, 1980, John Wiley & Sons.

155. Keogh JF: Incidence and severity of awkwardness among regular school boys and educationally subnormal boys, *Res Q* 39:806-808, 1968.

156. Keough K: A compensatory model for psychoeducational education of children with learning disorders, *J Learning Dis* 4:544, 1971.

157. Kephart NC: Teaching the child with a perceptual-motor handicap. In Bortner M, editor: *Evaluation and education of children with brain damage,* Springfield, Ill , 1968, Charles C Thomas.

158. King-Thomas L and Hacker B: *A therapist's guide to pediatric assessment,* Boston, 1987, Little, Brown.

159. Kinsbourne M: Minimal brain dysfunction as a neurodevelopmental lag, *Ann NY Acad Sci* 205:268, 1973.

160. Kinsbourne M: Editorials: MBD—a fuzz concept misdirects therapeutic efforts, *Postgrad Med* 58:211, 1975.

161. Kirk S: *National Advisory Committee on Handicapped Children: special education for handicapped children, first annual report,* Washington, DC, 1968, United States Department of Health, Education, and Welfare.

162. Klasen E: *The syndrome of specific dyslexia,* Baltimore, 1972, University Park Press.

163. Knickerbocker BM: *A holistic approach to the treatment of learning disorders,* Thorofare, NJ, 1980, Charles B Slack.

164. Koomar JA and Bundy AC: The art and science of creating direct intervention for theory. In Fisher AG, Murray EA, Bundy AC: *Sensory integration: theory and practice,* Philadelphia, 1991, FA Davis.

165. Koppitz EM: *The Bender Gestalt Test for young children,* New York, 1963, Grune & Stratton.

166. Landman GB and others: Minor neurological indicators and developmental function in preschool children, *Dev Behav Pediatr* 7(2):97-101, 1986.

167. Lane BA: The relationship of learning disabilities to juvenile delinquency: current status, *J Learning Dis* 13:20, 1980.

168. Langdon HJ and Langdon LL: *Initiating occupational therapy programs within public school systems: a guide for occupational therapists and public school administrators,* Thorofare, NJ, 1983, Charles B Slack.

169. Lansdell H: Theories of brain mechanisms in minimal brain dysfunctions. In Rie HE and Rie Ed, editors: *Handbook of minimal brain dysfunctions: a critical view,* New York, 1980, John Wiley & Sons.

170. Larkin D and Hoare D: *Out of step,*Nederlands, West Australia, 1991, The Active Life Foundation.

171. Laszlo JI: Child perceptuo-motor development: normal and abnormal development of skilled behavior. In Hauert CA, editor: *Developmental psychology: cognitive, perceptuo-motor, and neuropsychological perspectives,* North Holland, Amsterdam, 1990, Elsevier Science Publishers.

172. Laszlo JI and Bairstow PJ: Kinaesthesis: its measurement, training, and relationship to motor control, *Q J Exp Psychol* 35A:411, 1983.

173. LaVesser P and Bloomer MA: Using functional performance outcomes in a school setting, *OT Week* 4-6, 4(38):7 September 1990.

174. Lebby M: Incidence of mirror and overflow movements in learning disabled and normal young adults, Master's thesis, 1988, Sargent College, Boston University.

175. Lerner J: *Children with learning disorders,* Boston, 1976, Houghton Mifflin Co.

176. Levangie PK: Public school physical therapists, *Phys Ther* 60:774, 1980.

177. Levine M: *Pediatric examination of educational readiness at middle childhood,* Cambridge, Mass, 1985, Educators Publishing Service.

178. Levine MD and others: *A pediatric approach to learning disorders,* New York, 1980, John Wiley & Sons.

179. Levy J and others: Perception of bilateral chimeric figures following hemispheric deconnexion, *Brain* 95:61, 1972.

180. Linquist JE, Mack W, and Parham LD: A synthesis of occupational behavior and sensory integration concepts in theory and practice, part 1, theoretical foundations, *Am J Occup Ther* 36, 365-374, 1982.

181. Losse A and others: Clumsiness in children: do they grow out of it? A 10 year follow-up study, *Dev Med Child Neurol* 33:55-68, 1991.

182. Lucas AR: Muscular control and coordination in minimal brain dysfunctions. In Rie HE and Rie ED, editors: *Handbook of minimal brain dysfunctions: a critical view,* New York, 1980, John Wiley & Sons.

183. Luria AR: *Higher cortical functions in man,* ed 2, New York, 1980, Basic Books.

184. MacKeith RM: Defining the concept of minimal brain damage. In Bax M and MacKeith RM, editors: *Minimal cerebral dysfunction,* London, 1963, The National Spastics Society Medical Education and Information Unit in association with William Heinemann Medical Books.

185. Marcel T and others: Laterality and reading proficiency, *Neuropsychologia* 12:131, 1974.

186. Mathiowetz V and others: The Purdue Pegboard: norms for 14- to 19-year olds, *Am J Occup Ther* 40:174, 1986.

187. Mattis S and others: Dyslexia in children and young adults: three independent neuropsychological syndromes, *Dev Med Child Neurol* 17:150, 1975.

188. Mauser AJ: Learning disabilities and delinquent youth, *Acad Ther* 9:389, 1974.

189. McReynolds LV: Operant conditioning for investigating speech sound discrimination in aphasic children, *J Speech Hear* 9:519, 1966.

190. Mendelson W and others: Hyperactive children as teenagers: a follow-up study, *J Nerv Ment Dis* 153:273, 1971.

191. Michaels WB: Review of Miller Assessment for Preschoolers. In Mitchell JV Jr, editor: *The ninth mental measurements yearbook,* Lincoln, 1985, University of Nebraska Press.

192. Michael-Smith H: Reciprocal factors in the behavior syndrome of the neurologically impaired child. In Hellmuth J, editor: *The special child in century 21,* Seattle, 1964, Special Child Publications.

193. Miller AE: Differences in coping strategies between boys with motor incoordination and learning disabilities and normally developing peers, Masters Thesis Boston University, 1994.

194. Miller LJ: *FirstSTEP (Screening Test for Evaluating Preschoolers),* San Antonio, Texas, 1993, The Psychological Corporation.

195. Miller LJ: *Miller Assessment for Preschoolers,* Littleton, Colorado, 1982, The Foundation for Knowledge in Development.

196. Miller LJ: Longitudinal validity of the Miller Assessment for Preschoolers: study I, *Percep Mot Skills* 65:211, 1987.

197. Miller LJ: Differentiating children with school-related problems after four years using the Miller Assessment for Preschoolers, *Psychol Schools* 25:10, 1988.

198. Miller LJ: Longitudinal validity of the Miller Assessment for Preschoolers: study II, *Percept Mot Skills* 66:811, 1988.

199. Miller LJ: *Miller Assessment for Preschoolers: manual 1988 revision,* San Antonio, Tex 1988, The Psychological Corporation.

200. Miller LJ: *The toddler and infant motor evaluation,* Littleton, Col, 1992, The KID Foundation.

201. Miller LJ and Schouten PGW: Age-related effects on the predictive validity of the Miller Assessment for Preschoolers, *J Psycheducat Assess* 6(2):99, 1988.

202. Miller TG and Goldberg MA: Sensorimotor integration, *Phys Ther* 55:501, 1975.

203. Miller LJ and Kinnealey M: Researching the effectiveness of sensory integration, *Sensory Integration Q* 21(2), 1993.

204. Montessori M: *The Montessori Method: scientific pedagogy as applied to child education in the children's houses* (translated by E George), New York, 1912, FA Stokes.

205. Montgomery P: Assessment of vestibular function in children, *Phys Occup Ther Pediatr* 5:33, 1985.

206. Mordock JB: Behavioral problems of the child with minimal cerebral dysfunction, *Phys Ther* 51:398, 1971.

207. Morrison DC, Hinshaw SP, and Carte E: Signs of neurobehavioral dysfunction in a sample of learning disabled children: stability and concurrent validity, *Percept Mot Skills* 61:863, 1985.

208. Mullins J: New challenges for physical therapy practitioners in educational settings, *Phys Ther* 61:496, 1981.

209. Murray EA: Hemispheric specialization. In Fisher AG, Murray EA, Bundy AC: *Sensory integration: theory and practice,* Philadelphia, 1991, FA Davis.

210. Mutti M and others: *QNST: Quick Neurological Screening Test,* revised edition, Novato, Calif, 1978, Academic Therapy Publications.

211. Myklebust HR: Learning disabilities: definition and overview. In Myklebust HR, editor: *Progress in learning disabilities,* vol 1, New York, 1968, Grune & Stratton.

212. Myklebust HR: Learning disabilities and minimal brain dysfunction in children. In Tower DB, editor: *The nervous system,* vol 3, Human communication and its disorders, New York, 1975, Raven Press.

213. Nash M and Oetter P: A neuroscience based NDT/SI integrated treatment approach in OT. Lecture notes from a conference presented in April 1994.

214. Nashner LM and McCollum G: The organization of human postural movements: a formal basis and experimental synthesis, *Behav Brain Sci* 8:135-172, 1985.

215. O'Brien V, Cermak S, and Murray E: The relationship between visual-perceptual motor abilities and clumsiness in children with and without learning disabilities, *Am J Occup Ther* 42:359, 1988.

216. Obrzut JE: Deficient lateralization in learning disabled children: Developmental lag or abnormal cerebral organization? In Molfese DL and Segalowitz SJ, editors: *Brain lateralization in children: developmental implications,* New York, 1988, Guilford Press.

217. Olson M: Laterality differences in tachistoscopic word recognition in normal and delayed readings in elementary school, *Neuropsychologia* 11:343, 1973.

218. Orton ST: *Reading, writing and speech problems in children,* New York, 1937, WW Norton.

219. Ostronsky KM: Facilitation vs motor control, *Clinical Management American PT Association* 10(3): 34-40, 1990.

220. Ottenbacher K: Identifying vestibular processing dysfunction in learning disabled children, *Am J Occup Ther* 33:317, 1979.

221. Ottenbacher K: Occupational therapy and special education: some issues and concerns related to public law 94-142, *Am J Occup Ther* 36:81, 1982.

222. Ottenbacher K and Short MA: Sensory integrative dysfunction in children: a review of theory and treatment, *Adv Dev Behav Pediatr* 6:267, 1985.

223. Ottenbacher K and others: Qualitative analysis of the effectiveness of pediatric therapy, *Phys Ther* 66:462-468, 1986.

224. Ozols E and Rourke BP: Dimensions of social sensitivity in two types of learning-disabled children. In Rourke BP, editor: *Neuropsychology of learning disabilities: essentials of subtype analysis,* New York, 1985, The Guilford Press.

225. Ozols EJ and Rourke BP: Characteristics of the young learning disabled children classified according to patterns in academic achievement: auditory-perceptual and visual perceptual abilities, *J Clin Child Psychol* 17:44-52, 1988.

226. Parmenter C: The asymmetrical tonic neck reflex in normal first and third grade children, *Am J Occup Ther* 29:463, 1975.

227. Parr C and others: A developmental study of the asymmetrical tonic neck reflex, *Dev Med Child Neurol* 16:329, 1974.

228. Peck BB and Stackhouse T: Reading problems and family dynamics, *J Learning Dis* 6:506, 1973.

229. Pehoski C: Central nervous system control of precision movements of the hand. In Case-Smith J and Pehoski C: *Development of hand skills in the child,* Rockville, Md, 1992, American Occupational Therapy Association.

230. Peters JE, Romine RA, and Dykman RA: A special neurological examination of children with learning disabilities, *Dev Med Child Neurol* 17:63-78, 1975.

230a. Piper MC and others: Early physical therapy effects on the high risk infant: a randomized control trial, *Pediatrics,* 78:216-224, 1986.

231. Pirozzola F and Rayner K: Hemispheric specialization in reading and word recognition, *Brain Lang* 4:248, 1977.

232. Porter JP and Rourke BP: Socioemotional functioning of learning disabled children: a subtypal analysis of personality patterns. In Rourke BP, editor: *Neuropsychology of learning disabilities: essentials of subtype analysis,* New York, 1985, The Guilford Press.

233. Ric ED: Soft signs in learning disabilities. In Tupper DE: *Soft neurological signs,* New York, 1987, Grune & Stratton.

234. Rie HE: Definitional problems. In Ric HE and Rie ED, editors: *Handbook of minimal brain dysfunctions: a critical view,* New York, 1980, John Wiley & Sons.

235. *Public Law 94-142: Education for All Handicapped Children Act,* November 29, 1975, US Congress (Section 5B-4).

236. Roberts TDM: *Neurophysiology of posture mechanisms,* ed 2, Boston, 1978, Butterworth.

237. Rogers H and Saklofske DH: Self-concept, locus of control and performance expectations of learning disabled children, *J Learning Dis* 18:273, 1985.

238. Rourke BP: Brain-behavior relationships in children with learning disabilities: a research program, *Am Psychol* 30:911, 1975.

239. Rourke BP, editor: *Neuropsychology of learning disabilities: essentials of subtype analysis,* New York, 1985, The Guilford Press.

240. Rourke BP: Socioemotional disturbances of learning disabled children, *J Consult Clin Psychol* 58.801-810, 1988.

241. Rourke BP and Telegdy GA: Lateralizing significance of WISC verbal-performance discrepancies for older children with learning disabilities, *Percept Mot Skills* 33:875, 1975.

242. Rourke BP and others: The relationship between WISC verbal-performance discrepancies and selected verbal, auditory-perceptual, visual-perceptual and problem solving abilities in children with learning disabilities, *J Clin Psychol* 27:475, 1971.

243. Routh DK and Mesibov GB: Psychological and environmental intervention: toward social competence. In Rie HE and Rie ED, editors: *Handbook of minimal brain dysfunctions: a critical view,* New York, 1980, John Wiley & Sons.

244. Royeen CB and DeGangi GA: Use of neurodevelopmental treatment as an intervention: annotated listing of studies 1980-1990, *Perceptual Motor Skills* 75: 175-194, 1992.

245. Rubin E and Braun J: Behavioral and learning disabilities associated with cognitive motor dysfunction, *Percept Mot Skills* 26:171, 1968.

246. Rylander P: The ATNR in eight and twelve year old LD and normal boys, master's thesis, 1977, Sargent College, Boston University.

247. Sabari JS: Motor learning concepts applied to activity-based intervention with adults with hemiplegia, *Am J Occup Ther* 45(6):523 529, 1990.

248. Sahler OJ and others: Learning disorders and the hyperactive child; the pediatrician's role. In Smith DH and Hoekelman RA, editors: *Controversies in child health and pediatric practice,* New York, 1981, McGraw-Hill.

249. Sapir SG: Educational intervention. In Rie HE and Rie ED, editors: *Handbook of minimal brain dysfunction: a critical review,* New York, 1980, John Wiley & Sons.

250. Satz P and others: An evaluation of a theory of specific developmental dyslexia, *Child Dev* 42:2009, 1971.

251. Schaffer and others: A study of children with learning disabilities

and sensorimotor problems, *Phys Occup Ther Pediatr* 9(3):101-117, 1989.

252. Siegel LS and Ryan EB: The development of working memory in normally achieving and subtypes of learning disabled children, *Child Dev* 60:973-980, 1989.

253. Sellers JS: Professional cooperation in public school physical therapy, *Phys Ther* 60:1159, 1980.

254. Semmes J: Hemispheric specialization: a possible clue to mechanism, *Neuropsychologia* 6:11, 1968.

255. Shafer S and others: Ten year consistency in neurological test performance of children without focal neurological deficit, *Dev Med Child Neurol* 28:417, 1986.

256. Shafir U, Siegel SL, and Chee M: Learning disability, inferential skills and post-failure reflectivity, *J Learning Dis* 23:506-517, 1990.

257. Shaw L, Levine M, and Belfer M: Developmental double jeopardy: a study of clumsiness and self-esteem in children with learning problems, *J Dev Behav Pediatr* 3:191, 1982.

258. Shumway-Cook A, Horak F, and Black FO: A critical examination of vestibular function in motor impaired learning disabled children, *Int J Pediatr Otorhinolaryngol* 14: 21-30, 1987.

259. Sieben RL: Controversial medical treatment of learning disabilities, *Academ Ther* 13:133, 1977.

260. Sieg K and Shuster JJ: Comparison of three positions for evaluating the asymmetrical tonic neck reflex, *Am J Occup Ther* 33:240, 1979.

260a. Siegel LS and Metsala J: Subtypes of learning disabilities. In Singh NN and Beale IL: *Learning disabilities, nature, theory, and treatment,* New York, 1992, Springer-Verlag.

261. Silver AA and Hagin R: Specific reading disability: delineation of the syndrome and relationship to cerebral dominance, *Comp Psychiatry* 1:126, 1960.

262. Silver S: Psychologic aspects of pediatrics: postural and righting responses in children, *Pediatrics* 41:493, 1952.

262a. Silverman R and Zigmond N: Self-concept in learning disabled adolescents, *J Learning Dis* 16:478, 1983.

263. Singh NN and Beale IL: *Learning disabilities, nature, theory, and treatment,* New York, 1992, Springer-Verlag.

264. Smyth TR: Abnormal clumsiness in children: a defect of motor programming? *Child Care Health Dev* 17:283-294, 1991.

265. Smyth TR and Glencross DJ: Information processing deficits in clumsy children, *Aust J Psychol* 38(1): 13-22, 1986.

266. Sparrow S: Dyslexia and laterality: evidence for a developmental theory, *Semin Psychiatry* 1:270, 1969.

267. Sparrow S and Satz P: Dyslexia, laterality, and neuropsychological development. In Bakker BJ and Satz P, editors: *Specific reading disabilities: advances in theory and method,* Rotterdam, 1970, University of Rotterdam.

268. Spreen O: *Learning disabled children growing up: a follow-up into adulthood,* Victoria, BC, 1983, Department of Psychology, University of Victoria.

269. Stewart MA and others: Hyperactive children as adolescents: how they describe themselves, *Child Psychiatry Hum Dev* 4:3, 1973.

270. Stott DH: A general test of motor impairment for children, *Dev Med Child Neurol* 8:523, 1966.

271. Stott DH and others: *Test of motor impairment,* rev ed, Guelph, Ontario, 1984, Brook Educational Publishing, Ltd.

272. Strang JD and Rourke BP: Adaptive behavior of children who exhibit specific arithmetic disabilities and associated neuropsychological abilities and deficits. In Rourke BP, editor: *Neuropsychology of learning disabilities: essentials of subtype analysis,* New York, 1985, The Guilford Press.

273. Strauss AA and Lehtinen LE: *Psychopathology and education of the brain-injured child,* New York, 1947, Grune & Stratton.

274. Tarnopol L and Tarnopol M: *Brain function and reading disabilities,* Baltimore, 1977, University Park Press.

275. Taylor HG: Learning disabilities. In Mash EJ and Barkley RA, editors: *Treatment of childhood disorders,* New York, 1989, The Guilford Press.

276. Tickle-Degnen L: Perspectives on the status of sensory integration theory, *Am J Occup Ther* 42(7):427, 1988.

277. Tiffin J: *Purdue Pegboard Test,* Lafayette, Ind, 1968, Layfayette Instrument Co.

278. Torgesen JK: The learning disabled child as an inactive learner: educational implications, *Top Learn Learning Dis* 2(1):45-51, 1982.

279. Touwen BCL and Prechtl HFR: *The neurological examination of the child with minor nervous dysfunction,* Philadelphia, 1970, JB Lippincott.

280. Touwen BCL and Sporrel T: Soft signs and MBD, *Dev Med Child Neurol* 21:528, 1979.

281. Towbin A: Neuropathologic factors in minimal brain dysfunction. In Rie HE and Rie ED, editors: *Handbook of minimal brain dysfunctions: a critical view,* New York, 1980, John Wiley & Sons.

282. *Training and management in occupational therapy* (TOTEMS), Rockville, Md, 1980, American Occupational Therapy Association.

283. Tseng MH and Cermak SA: The evaluation of handwriting in children, *Sensory Integration Q* 19(4): 1-6, 1991.

284. Tseng MH and Cermak SA: The influence of ergonomic factors and perceptual-motor abilities on handwriting performance, *Am J Occup Ther* 47(10): 919-926, 1993.

285. Tupper DE: The issues with "soft signs." In Tupper DE: *Soft neurological signs.* New York, 1987, Grune & Stratton.

286. Tupper DE: *Soft neurological signs.* New York, 1987, Grune & Stratton.

287. Vellutino F: *Dyslexia: theory and research,* Cambridge, Mass, 1979, The MIT Press.

288. Vellutino F and others: Reading disability and the perceptual deficit hypothesis, *Cortex* 8:106, 1972.

289. Vellutino F and others: Inter- versus intra-hemispheric learning in dyslexic and normal readers, *Dev Med Child Neurol* 20:71, 1978.

290. Walton JN and others: Clumsy children: a study of developmental apraxia and agnosia, *Brain* 85:603, 1963.

291. Weber RE: *Handbook on learning disabilities,* Englewood Cliffs, NJ, 1974, Prentice-Hall.

292. Weiner BB: Curriculum development for children with brain damage. In Bortner M, editor: *Evaluation and education of children with brain damage,* Springfield, Ill, 1968, Charles C Thomas.

293. Weiss G, MBD: critical diagnostic issues. In Rie HE and Rie ED, editors: *Handbook of minimal brain dysfunctions: a critical view,* New York, 1980, John Wiley & Sons.

294. Whyte L: Characteristics of learning disabilities persisting into adolescence, *Alberta J Educ Research* 30(1):14, 1984.

295. Willis AG, Hooper SR, and Stone BH: Neuropsychological theories of learning disabilities. In Singh NN and Beale IL: *Learning disabilities, nature, theory, and treatment,* New York, 1992, Springer-Verlag.

296. Witelson SF: Developmental dyslexia: two right hemispheres and none left, *Science* 195:309, 1977.

297. Wolff PH, Gunnoe CE, and Cohen C: Associated movement as a measure of developmental age, *Dev Med Child Neurol* 25:417, 1983.

298. Yeni-Komshian GH and others: Cerebral dominance and reading disorders: left visual defect in poor readers, *Neuropsychologia* 13:83, 1975.

299. Zinkus PW: Behavior and emotional sequelae of learning disorders. In Gottlieb MI and others, editors: *Current issues in developmental pediatrics: the learning disabled child,* New York, 1979, Grune & Stratton.

300. Ziviani J: Qualitative changes in dynamic tripod grip between seven and 14 years of age, *Dev Med Child Neurol* 25: 778-782, 1983.

301. Ziviani J and Elkins J: Effect of pencil grip on handwriting speed and legibility, *Educ Rev* 38(3): 247-257, 1986.

APPENDIX A   *SUMMARY OF STANDARDIZED MOTOR TESTS*

1. Bruininks-Oseretsky Test of Motor Proficiency
2. Test of Motor Impairment—Henderson Revision
3. Peabody Developmental Motor Scales
4. Quick Neurological Screening Test
5. Miller Assessment for Preschoolers
6. FirstSTEP
7. Tests for Motor Proficiency of Gubbay
8. Sensory Integration and Praxis Tests
9. Bender Gestalt Test for Young Children
10. Developmental Test of Visual-Motor Integration—3rd revision
11. Test of Visual-Motor Skills
12. Basic Motor Ability Tests—Revised
13. Purdue Pegboard Test

1. Bruininks-Oseretsky Test of Motor Proficiency (1978)[48]

Author: Robert H. Bruininks, PhD
Source: American Guidance Service, Inc.
         Circle Pines, Minn. 55014
Ages: 4½ to 14½ years
Administration: Individual; 45 minutes to 1 hour
Equipment: Test kit needed
Description: The Bruininks-Oseretsky Test of Motor Proficiency is the most recent revision of the Oseretsky Tests of Motor Proficiency first published in Russia in 1923. The Oseretsky Tests were first adapted by Doll in 1946 and then by Sloan in 1955 as the Lincoln-Oseretsky Motor Development Scale. As with the earlier versions, the Bruininks-Oseretsky Test yields an age equivalency score, but standard scores and percentile ranks are also available. The test assesses motor functioning in eight areas, each with standard score information. The areas are:

1. Running speed and agility	Runs 15 yards, picks up blocks, and returns
2. Balance	Eight items ranging in difficulty from standing on one leg to stepping over object on a balance beam
3. Bilateral coordination	Seven items that require use of upper and lower extremities simultaneously or in sequential movement, e.g., tapping feet and fingers and jumping and clapping. Final item requires pencil use with both hands simultaneously
4. Strength	Three items: standing broad jumps, sit-ups, and push-ups
5. Upper-limb coordination	Five items that involve catching and throwing balls and an additional four items assessing precise finger movements
6. Response speed	Requires a quick catch of falling stick
7. Visual motor control	Eight pencil, paper, and scissor items
8. Upper-limb speed and dexterity	Eight items that range from putting pennies in a box to making dots in circles

Construction and reliability: The Bruininks-Oseretsky Test has been carefully standardized on 765 subjects from differing geographical regions and community size. Test-retest reliability coefficients for the subtests ranged from 0.50 to 0.89 and that of the total battery was 0.87 for second graders and 0.86 for sixth graders. With the exception of "response speed," the subtests differentiated significantly between normal and learning-disabled children.

Comment: The Bruininks-Oseretsky Test of Motor Proficiency appears to be one of the better standardized tests of motor performance. A short form, taking 15 to 20 minutes, can be used for screening. In testing children with motor dysfunction, careful attention must be paid to performance on individual items. For example, a child who compensates for poor proprioceptive postural control with vision can score in the normal range on the balance subtest, even though he or she fails the single item of balance with eyes closed. A problem with finger sequencing in the upper limb coordination subtest could be masked by a good ball skills. These kinds of problems could result in not identifying a child's deficit. Another problem with the subtests is that a single item has a disproportionate effect on a child's age equivalence. Nevertheless, this is an excellent test for monitoring the motor development of a dysfunctioning child.

2. Movement Assessment Battery for Children (Movement ABC) (1992)[133a]

Authors: S.E. Henderson and D. Sugden
Source: Psychological Corporation
Ages: 4 to 12 years
Administration: Individual; 20 to 30 minutes
Equipment: Test kit required
Description: The Movement ABC is a revision and expansion of the Test of Motor Impairment (TOMI)-Henderson

Revision. The Movement ABC includes three aspects: *Screening and Evaluation:* The Movement ABC Checklist provides classroom assessment of movement difficulties, screening for at-risk children, and monitoring of treatment programs; *Assessment:* The Movement ABC Test (similar to the TOMI) provides a more comprehensive assessment and includes both normative and qualitative measures of movement competence. The test is divided into four age bands: for children 4-6 years; 7-8 years; 9-10 years; and 11-12 years. *Treatment:* The manual provides guidelines for organizing intervention programs.

The Movement ABC Test includes eight categories, with a single item for each age in each category.

1. Manual dexterity 1	Speed and sureness of movement by each hand
2. Manual dexterity 2	Coordination of two hands for a single task
3. Manual dexterity 3	Hand-eye coordination using the preferred hand
4. Ball skills 1	Ball task emphasizing aiming at a target
5. Ball skills 2	Ball task emphasizing catching a ball
6. Static balance	Balance task
7. Dynamic balance 1	Balance task emphasizing spatial precision
8. Dynamic balance 2	Balance task emphasizing control of momentum

Construction and reliability: Standardization of the Test was done in the U.S. whereas work on the Checklist was based in the United Kingdom. Normative data on the Test were gathered on 1234 children in the U.S. The sample was approximately representative of the general population of children in the U.S. in terms of gender, region, and ethnic origin. Test-retest reliability for consistency of individual item scores with children ages 5, 7, and 9 showed a median percentage of agreement between test and retest from 80% to 90%. Percent agreement for Total Impairment Score ranged from 73% for age 9 to 97% agreement for age 5.

Comment: This revision offers several advantages: (a) the Checklist helps teachers identify children with movement problems; (b) information is provided for a cognitive-motor approach to intervention; (c) the qualitative component of the Test is more clearly defined and incorporated on the record form, and the scoring systems have been refined.

3. Peabody Developmental Motor Scales (PDMS): Revised Experimental Edition (1983)[99]

Authors: M. Rhonda Folio and Rebecca R. Fewell
Source: DLM Teaching Resources
P.O. Box 4000, One DLM Park
Allen, Texas 55002

Ages: Birth to 7 years
Administration: Individual (birth to 3 years) and/or individual or group (4 to 7 years); 40 to 60 minutes (test items may be scored by direct observation or by parent or teacher report)
Description: The Peabody Developmental Motor Scales were designed for use with children who show delay or disability in fine and gross motor skills. Test items are similar to those on other developmental scales but only motor items are included. Items are scored on a 3-point scale, 0 for unsuccessful, 1 for partial, and 2 for successful performance. Age-equivalent, motor quotients, percentile rankings and standard scores are provided. The following skill categories are tested in the gross motor scale (170 test items). These tasks are considered to require precise movements of large muscles of body.

1. Reflexes (12 items)	Includes items such as turning head in response to sound, aligning head on pull to sit, ATNR, protective reaction, and kicking
2. Balance (33 items)	Includes propping, levels of sitting and standing as well as higher-level items such as standing on one foot, beam walking, and walking on tiptoes
3. Non-locomotion (42 items)	Includes items such as head control, rolling, weight bearing as well as higher-level tasks such as jumping and sit ups
4. Locomotion (58 items)	Examples include creeping, cruising, walking, stairs, hopping, tricycle riding, running, and jumping hurdles
5. Receipt and propulsion (25 items)	Catching, throwing, and kicking balls

The fine motor scale has 112 test items considered to require precise movements of small muscles. The following skill categories are included:

1. Grasping (22 items)	Includes reflex grasping and voluntary grasping with the hands and with the fingers as well as crayon grasp
2. Hand use (26 items)	Includes a variety of items ranging from maintaining hands closed to hand preference and including the manipulation of cubes, pegs, and other objects
3. Eye-hand coordination (46 items)	Early items include visual fixation and tracking; later items—form boards, cube building, and copying forms
4. Manual dexterity (18 items)	This category begins with page turning and includes screwing, winding, lacing, and buttons

Construction and reliability: The 617 children making up the normative sample range in age from birth to 83 months, with samples beginning at 2-month intervals and increasing to 1-year intervals in older children. Thus subgroups are small, a majority having 30 or fewer children. Samples were selected to reflect socioeconomic status and rural-urban characteristics. A test-retest reliability of 0.95 for the gross motor scale and of 0.80 for the fine motor scale was reported based on a sample of 38 children. Validity was demonstrated by the significantly lower scores of 104 children with developmental deviations on all but the 0- to 5-month children. Another study of 43 children established a low but significant correlation (0.37) between the PDMS gross motor scale and the Bayley Psychomotor Index and a moderately high correlation (0.78) between the PDMS fine motor scale and the Bayley Mental Scale.

Comment: The PDMS are primarily useful for children with mild to moderate motor deficits, such as a learning-disabled child or a child with developmental delay. The test does not discriminate among children with moderate to severe motor disability, as they fall far below the standard scores given. The standardization sample is small, especially in the age subgroups. The fine motor scale has a high cognitive element as demonstrated by the high correlation with the Bayley Mental Scale. The skill categories are unevenly distributed and have too few items at some age levels to be meaningful. Despite its drawbacks, the PDMS is probably the most valuable motor scale currently available for preschool children.

4. Quick Neurological Screening Test (1978)[210]

Authors: M.A. Mutti, H.M. Sterling, and N.V. Spalding
Source: Academic Therapy Publications
20 Commercial Boulevard,
Novato, Calif. 94947
Ages: 5 years and over
Administration: Individual; 20 minutes
Equipment: None
Description: The Quick Neurological Screening Test (QNST) was developed as a screening device to identify children who have possible learning disabilities. The tasks are adapted from pediatric neurological examinations as well as from developmental assessments. The test is made up of the following fifteen subtests:

1. Hand skill	Writing his or her name and a sentence
2. Figure recognition and production	Naming, then drawing, five geometric forms
3. Palm form recognition	Recognizing numbers written on their palm by examiner with his finger
4. Eye tracking	Following pencil back and forth and up and down
5. Sound patterns	With hands on knees and eyes closed, imitating patterns demonstrated by the examiner
6. Finger to nose	Finger to nose test; includes observation
7. Thumb and finger circle	Forming circle with thumb and each of the fingers; laterality also observed
8. Double simultaneous stimulation of hand and cheek	With eyes closed, child must identify hands and cheeks touched by examiner in various combinations simultaneously
9. Rapid reversing, repetitive hand movements	Observation of diadochokinesis
10. Arm and leg extension	With eyes closed, extending legs, arms, and tongue for 1 to 15 seconds
11. Tandem walk	Walking straight line, heel to toe, forward and backward
12. Stand on one leg	Balancing first on one leg, then on other, 10 seconds each, eyes open, then closed; right-left differentiation observed
13. Skip	Skipping across the room
14. Left-right discrimination	Scored from subtests; 6, 7, and 12
15. Behavior irregularities	General observation for behaviors such as distractibility, perseveration, defensiveness, hyperactivity

The test is scored based on careful observation and requires a subjective evaluation of performance. The manual provides ages at which 75% of neurologically intact children pass each test as well as total scores indicative of probable neurological dysfunction.

Construction and reliability: The QNST has been used in numerous research studies of normal children and of children with suspected learning disabilities. Although the manual reported these studies, the test has not been formally standardized. Reliabilities on the whole test on learning-disabled children of 0.81 and 0.71 are reported, but the data are incomplete. Ages at which 25%, 50%, and 75% of normal children pass each subtest are given based on a compilation of subjects from many studies. Norms for the total test are not given.

Comment: The QNST is a screening device that identifies children with possible neurological dysfunction. It is not and should not be used as a standardized test but rather as an adjunct to clinical observation. It is important to realize that the test is primarily of motor function. It does not include language tests and, therefore, will not identify all children with learning disabilities. The test does screen for possible minimal brain dysfunction or motor deficits.

5. Miller Assessment for Preschoolers (MAP) (1988)[195,199]

Author: Lucy Jane Miller
Source: Psychological Corporation

555 Academic Court,
San Antonio, Texas 78204-0952

Ages: 2 years 9 months to 5 years 8 months

Administration: Individual; 20 to 30 minutes including scoring

Equipment: The MAP Test Kit

Description: The Miller Assessment for Preschoolers was designed to identify children who exhibit mild to moderate developmental delays. The MAP is a developmental assessment intended for use by educational and clinical personnel to identify those children in need of further evaluation and remediation. It can also be used to provide a comprehensive, clinical framework that would be helpful in defining a child's strengths and weaknesses and that would indicate possible avenues of remediation. The test is made up of 27 items and a series of structured observations. The test items are divided into five performance indices:

1. Foundations	Items generally found on standard neurological examinations and sensory integrative and neurodevelopmental tests
2. Coordination	Gross, fine, and oral motor abilities and articulation
3. Verbal	Cognitive language abilities, including memory, sequencing, comprehension, association, following directions, and expression
4. Nonverbal	Cognitive abilities such as visual figure-ground, puzzles, memory, and sequencing
5. Complex tasks	Tasks requiring an interaction of sensory, motor, and cognitive abilities

Construction and reliability: The MAP has been well standardized on a random sample of 1200 preschool children. The sample was stratified by age, race, sex, size of residence, community, and socioeconomic factors. Data were collected nationwide in each of nine US Census Bureau regions. Reported reliabilities are good. In a test-retest on 90 children, 81% of the children's scores remained stable. The coefficient of internal consistency on the total sample was 0.798. Interrater reliability on 40 children was reported as 0.98.

Comment: The MAP was developed by an occupational therapist and provides information that is of particular relevance to therapists. It is carefully standardized and fills a need for early identification of learning and motor deficits in children. Several articles have now been published supporting the validity of this test as a screening instrument.[196-198,201] Reviews of the MAP in the Ninth Mental Measurements Yearbook have described it as "the best available screening test for identifying preschool children with moderate 'preacademic problems'"[78] and "an extremely promising instrument which should find wide use among clinical psychologists, school psychologists, and occupational therapists in assessing mild to moderate learning disabilities in preschool children."[191] A more complete review of this test is provided by King-Thomas and Hacker.[158]

6. FirstSTEP (Screening Test for Evaluating Preschoolers) (1993)[194]

Author: Lucy J. Miller, PhD

Source: The Psychological Corporation
San Antonio, Texas

Ages: 2 years 9 months to 6 years 2 months

Administration: Individual; 15 minutes

Equipment: Test kit needed

Description: The FirstSTEP is a quick screening test for identifying developmental delays in all five areas defined by IDEA (Individuals with Disabilities Education Act) and mandated by PL 99-457: cognition, communication, physical, social/emotional, and adaptive functioning. Twelve subtests assess cognitive, communication and motor domains. An optional Social-Emotional Scale includes 25 items from five areas (task confidence, cooperative mood, temperament and emotionality, uncooperative antisocial behavior, attention communication difficulties) that are scored based on behaviors observed by the examiner during the test session. The Adaptive Behavior Checklist is an optional measure completed by parent interview to assess the child's self-help and adaptive living skills. The Parent/Teacher Scale provides additional information about the child's typical behavior.

Subtest Name	Area Assessed
Cognitive Domain	
Money Game	Quantitative Reasoning

Description: The child is asked a series of questions about coins, regarding quantity, amount, comparisons, size, and numeration. This subtest requires cognitive understanding of simple arithmetic concepts.

What's Missing Game	Picture Completion

Description: The child is asked to identify what is missing from the pictures of common objects or events by naming or pointing. This subtest measures visual figure-ground as well as gestalt closure abilities.

Which Way? Game	Visual Position in Space

Description: The child is asked to look at a stimulus figure that is turned in a specific direction. The child then selects the response figure that matches. This subtest measures visual discrimination and the ability to visually perceive directionality.

Put Together Game	Problem Solving

Description: The child is asked to select the pieces that best fit a certain space. The subtest requires abstract thinking.

Subtest Name	Area Assessed

Language Domain

Listen Game — Auditory Discrimination

Description: This two-part activity requires the child to listen as the examiner names and points to three similar sounding pictures. Then the child chooses the pictures that represent the words. The second part requires the child to discriminate between words that are the same and words that are different. This task taps phoneme discrimination and requires good auditory processing skills.

How Many Can You Say? — Word Retrieval Game

Description: The child's linguistic fluency and word-finding skills are measured by asking the child to count, recall animals, and recite rhyming words.

Finish Up Game — Association

Description: The child is asked to complete a phrase that is initiated by the examiner. The subtest requires the child to demonstrate an understanding of the association between concepts (e.g., big and little).

Copy Me Game — Sentence and Digit Repetition

Description: The child is asked to repeat a series of meaningful verbal stimuli and then a series of numbers. This subtest measures verbal memory, grammatical abilities, and verbal expression skills.

Motor Domain

Drawing Game — Visual-Motor Integration

Description: The child is presented with paper and pencil tasks. This subtest requires the integration of fine motor and visual perceptual abilities.

Things With Strings Game — Fine Motor Planning

Description: The child is asked to perform a series of motor movements with the upper extremities using a wooden cube and a string. These items tap the ability to plan and execute a series of motor actions and measures fine motor planning or praxis.

Statue Game — Balance

Description: The child is asked to assume a series of increasingly more difficult positions that require the child to balance with eyes open and vision occluded. The subtest taps the abilities needed to maintain equilibrium and screens for proprioception, vestibular perception, and/or visual processing difficulties.

Jumping Game — Gross Motor Planning

Description: The child is asked to imitate the examiner through a series of increasingly more difficult tasks that involve jumping in specific patterns. Gross motor and motor planning abilities are measured.

Construction and reliability: The FirstSTEP is norm-referenced and was standardized on 1,433 children. Norms are provided in 6-month intervals for each of seven age groups. Standardization sample closely matches demographic characteristics provided by the US Census Bureau. Scores are reported in standard scores as well as a three-category color coded risk status to indicate whether the child is functioning in the normal or delayed range. The FirstSTEP is a highly reliable instrument. Overall test reliability (Split half) is 0.90, with individual domains ranging from 0.71 to 0.87. Test-retest reliability indicated a high degree of consistency in the classification of a child's performance across two test sessions (90% agreement for composite score; 85% to 93% for individual domain scores). Results also indicated a high level of inter-rater agreement (r = 0.94 on composite scores).

Comment: The FirstSTEP is a new test that shows exceptional promise as a screening instrument. A Spanish version, Primer Paso, will be published in the near future. The FirstSTEP was developed by the occupational therapist who also developed the MAP (The Miller Assessment for Preschoolers), and, like the MAP, the test provides information that is of particular relevance to therapists. Although individual items on the FirstSTEP differ from the MAP, many are derived from the MAP, and the test is based on the same theoretical framework as the MAP.

Initial validity studies of the FirstSTEP appear highly promising and indicate that FirstSTEP has good construct, content, and discriminant validity. The FirstSTEP can effectively identify children with developmental delays. A study of 900 children demonstrated that children with delays perform 1.5 to 2 standard deviations below the mean in all domains.

With regard to the Motor Domain of the FirstSTEP, which taps motor skills, the results of a concurrent validity study suggest that the Motor Domain measures constructs similar to those measured by the Bruininks-Oseretsky Test of Motor Proficiency and support the use of the Motor Domain of the FirstSTEP as an indicator of the child's motor functioning.

7. Tests of Motor Proficiency of Gubbay (1975)[118]

Author: Sasson S. Gubbay

Source: In Gubbay SS: *The Clumsy Child*, Philadelphia, 1975, WB Saunders Co.

Ages: 8 to 12 years

Administration: Individual; 5 minutes

Equipment: Described in book, must be purchased or constructed

Description: Gubbay's Tests of Motor Proficiency make up a quick screening instrument for the identification of developmental dyspraxia. The battery is made up of eight items that best discriminate between clumsy and normal children in a study of 1000 schoolchildren. The test items are:

1. Whistle through pursed lips
2. Skip forward five steps
3. Roll ball with foot around objects
4. Throw tennis ball, clap hands, then catch tennis ball

5. Tie one shoelace with double bow
6. Thread 10 beads
7. Pierce 20 pinholes in graph paper
8. Posting box: fit six shapes in appropriate slots

The first two items are scored pass or fail; the score for the fourth item is the number of claps, and the other items are timed. Percentile values at each age level from 8 to 12 years are reported.

Comment: Gubbay's tests were devised as a rapid screening to be used together with teacher questionnaires to identify clumsy children in a school program. They are valuable if used as intended. One or more of the items could be incorporated into an evaluation protocol using a cutoff based on normative data given. However, this is not a fully standardized test, and further normative data as well as validity and reliability studies are required.

8. The Sensory Integration and Praxis Tests (SIPT) (1989)[27]

Author: A. Jean Ayres
Source: Western Psychological Services
        12031 Wilshire Boulevard
        Los Angeles, Calif. 90025
Ages: 4 years to 8 years 11 months
Administration: Individual; 1½ hours; examiner certification highly recommended
Equipment: SIPT Test Kit
Description: The Sensory Integration and Praxis Tests are a major revision and restandardization of the Southern California Sensory Integration Tests.[25] Four new tests of praxis were added, five tests underwent major revisions, eight tests underwent minor revisions, and four tests were deleted. The tests are designed to identify sensory integration and praxis deficits in children with learning disabilities. There are 17 tests described as follows:

1. Space visualization	Select from two blocks the one that will fit into a form board; it is necessary to mentally manipulate the forms to arrive at the correct choice on the more difficult test items
2. Figure-ground perception	The child selects from six pictures the three that are superimposed or embedded with other forms on the test plates
3. Manual form perception	Part I: a geometric form is held in the hand and the counterpart is selected from a visual display Part II: a geometric form is felt with one hand while its match is selected from several choices with the other hand
4. Kinesthesia	With vision occluded, the child attempts to place his or her finger on a point at which his or her finger had been placed previously by the examiner; a separate recording sheet is provided for each child
5. Finger identification	With hands screened from view, the examiner touches the child's finger, the shield is removed and child then points to the finger touched
6. Graphesthesia	The examiner uses his or her finger to draw a design on the back of the child's hand, without the child looking; the child then reproduces the design
7. Localization of tactile stimuli	With vision occluded, the child touches the spot on his or her hand or arm that was touched by the examiner with a specially designed pen
8. Praxis on verbal command	The examiner verbally describes a series of body movements and the child executes them
9. Design copying	Part I: the child copies a design by connecting dots on a dot grid Part II: the child copies a design without the use of a dot grid; both process and product are scored
10. Constructional praxis	Working with blocks, the child attempts to duplicate two different block structures; in the first structure, the child observes the examiner building the model; the second structure is preassembled
11. Postural praxis	The child imitates unusual body positions demonstrated by the examiner
12. Oral praxis	The child imitates movements of the tongue, lips, and jaw demonstrated by the examiner
13. Sequencing praxis	The child imitates a series of simple arm and hand movements demonstrated by the examiner
14. Bilateral motor coordination	The child imitates a series of bilateral arm and foot movements demonstrated by the examiner
15. Standing and walking balance	The subtest consists of 15 items in which the child assumes various standing and walking postures
16. Motor accuracy	The child traces a printed, curved black line with a red, nylon-tipped pen, first with the preferred hand and then with the nonpreferred hand

17. Postrotary nystagmus

The child is rotated first counterclockwise and then clockwise on a rotation board and the duration of postrotary nystagmus, a vestibulo-ocular reflex, is observed

In addition to these 17 tests, a series of clinical observations aids in interpreting the SIPT. These clinical observations include the following:

1. Eye dominance
2. Eye movements
3. Muscle tone
4. Cocontraction
5. Postural background movements
6. Postural security
7. Equilibrium reactions and protective extension
8. Schilder's arm extension posture
9. Supine flexion
10. Prone extension
11. Asymmetrical tonic neck reflex
12. Hyperactivity, distractibility
13. Tactile defensiveness
14. Ability to perform slow motions
15. Thumb-finger touching
16. Diadochokinesis
17. Tongue-to-lip movements
18. Hopping, jumping, skipping

Construction and Reliability: The construction of the Sensory Integration and Praxis Tests was based on a theoretical model developed from observation of children with learning disabilities and supported by factor analytical and cluster analysis studies. Interpretation follows a clinical model based on patterns of scores rather than a poor score on any one test.

The SIPT was nationally standardized on 1997 children from across the United States and Canada. Sex, geographical location, ethnicity, and type of community are represented in proportion to the 1980 US census.

Test-retest reliability was evaluated in a sample of 41 dysfunctional children and 10 normal dysfunction and ranges from moderate to high. As a group, the praxis tests had the highest reliability's. Inter-rater reliability is excellent, with most correlations between raters at 0.90 or higher.

Comment: The SIPT is computer scored and interpreted, and a full eight-color profile (WPS Chromograph) is provided that summarizes major SIPT testing and statistical results in a clear manner. Initial validity studies of the SIPT indicate a good ability to discriminate between normal and dysfunctional groups and across ages. The SIPT is the most comprehensive assessment of sensory integration and praxis. However, it requires specialized training for administration and interpretation, and the test kit and scoring of protocols are expensive.

9. Bender Gestalt Test for Young Children (1963)[165]

Author: E.M. Koppitz
Source: Grune and Stratton, Inc.
New York, NY
Ages: 5 to 10 years
Administration: Individual; 7 to 15 minutes; special training required
Description: The Bender Gestalt Test for Young Children is an adaptation of the Bender Visual Motor Gestalt Test, which is an individually administered test of performance in copying designs. The test consists of nine designs that are printed on separate cards and presented one at a time to the child. The child is given unlimited time to copy each successive design on a sheet of paper. The developmental scoring system for young children to age 10 was developed by Koppitz.[165] The Bender Gestalt is used by psychologists to assess visual motor functions and possible neuropsychological impairment, and it is also used with the Koppitz scoring system to evaluate perceptual-motor maturity and emotional adjustment. The reproduced design is scored for distortion, rotation, perseveration, method of reproduction, and other factors. The Koppitz scoring system yields an estimate of the child's developmental age.
Construction and reliability: The Bender Gestalt Test is a widely used and heavily researched test of neuropsychological impairment following brain injury in adults. The Koppitz version, standardized for children, makes possible similar diagnoses with children. Test-retest reliability for the Koppitz scoring of the Bender Visual Motor Gestalt test are moderate, ranging from 0.60 to 0.66. Interscorer agreement is 93%.
Comment: The Bender Gestalt Test yields more information about a child's deficit than simpler tests of geometric form reproduction, but it requires special skills for interpretation. Inability to copy geometric forms may occur for several reasons: faulty visual-perceptual discrimination, poor motor ability, or, more likely, problems in the translations of the percept of the form to its reproduction.

10. Developmental Test of Visual-Motor Integration (VMI), 3rd Revision (3R) 1989[33]

Author: K. Berry
Source: Modern Curriculum Press
13900 Prospect Road
Cleveland, Ohio 44136
Ages: 2 years 6 months to 17 years 11 months
Administration: Individual or group; 10 to 15 minutes
Equipment: Protocol booklets (test forms)
Description: The Developmental Test of Visual-Motor Integration tests the ability to copy geometric forms. A booklet is provided with 24 designs in an age-graded

sequence. The child copies each design in a space directly below it. Items are judged pass or fail on criteria given in the manual.

Construction and reliability: The most recent revision of this test includes additional specificity for the scoring of some items. In addition, the range of VMI scores was expanded by weighting the values of the 24 forms according to their developmental difficulty to allow for finer discriminations among individuals, especially at the older ages. The Visual-Motor Integration manual contains information relating to ages at which forms are passed based on Gesell and other researchers as well as age equivalencies, standard scores, percentile equivalents, and T scores based on a sample of 5824 children. This reflects a 1988 sample combined with two previous normative samples. Various studies of reliability and validity are reported in the manual. Studies of test-retest reliability was reported for groups of children of all ages and ranges from 0.63 (7-month interval) to 0.92 (2-week period), with a median of 0.81. There are no reports of reliability at individual ages. Split-half reliability was reported to range from 0.66 to 0.93, and inter-scorer agreement was 0.93.

Comment: The Developmental Test of Visual Motor Integration provides a quick and easy method to assess the development of a child's ability to copy geometric forms. It is useful as an adjunct to other assessments of the learning-disabled child. When the test is presented to the child, he or she is told that the booklet must remain parallel to the edge of the table. This prevents some of the problems of other tests, e.g., the child turning the individual paper on which designs are reproduced. However, the structured format does not allow the assessment of overall organization of copying forms, as can be done when the child copies forms on a blank sheet of paper (e.g., Bender Gestalt Test). Therefore overall organization also should be tested.

11. Test of Visual-Motor Skills (TVMS) (1986)[104]

Author: Morrison F. Gardner
Source: Children's Hospital of San Francisco
Publication Department OPR-110
P.O. Box 3805, San Francisco, Calif. 94119
Ages: 2 to 13 years
Administration: Individual or group; 3 to 6 patients
Equipment: Protocol booklet
Description: The TVMS consists of a series of 26 forms to be copied by the child. Each form is on a separate page of the booklet, which has some forms commonly used in visual-motor tests (lines and circles, for example), but many more forms are unique to this test. Care was taken to avoid forms that resembled language symbols. The forms are scored from 0 to 2. A score of 0 indicates that the child is unable to copy the form with motor accuracy. A score of 2 demonstrates precision in

execution. A score of 1 indicates poor coordination or control. Criteria for scoring at each level are given with examples for each form. Age equivalents and standard scores are provided.

Construction and reliability: The Test of Visual-Motor Skills was administered to 1009 children in the San Francisco Bay area at 11 age levels, from 2 years to 12 years. The number of subjects in each age group ranged from 38 to 132, with about half boys and half girls. Cronbach's coefficient *alpha* was used to determine the internal consistency of the test. These reliability coefficients were lower for the younger children (0.31 at 2 years and 0.69 at 3 years) but otherwise good, ranging from 0.78 to 0.90 for older age groups and reaching 0.97 for the sample as a whole. Test-retest reliability was not reported in the manual, but the author noted the need for research in that area.

Comment: The TVMS is a companion test to the Test of Visual-Perceptual Skills (TVPS), which is a motor-free test of form perception. Using the tests together can determine whether the child's form reproduction reflects incorrect visual perception or whether the problem is in motor execution. The TVMS places greater expectations on motor precision than other visual-motor tests. For example, a line must touch an intersecting line without crossing over it. Therefore it should be used only when motor control and constructive abilities are important.

12. Basic Motor Ability Tests—Revised (BMAT—Revised) (1979)[10]

Authors: D.D. Arnheim and W.A. Sinclair
Source: In D.D. Arnheim and W.A. Sinclair, *The Clumsy Child*, St. Louis, 1979, Mosby.
Ages: 4 to 12 years
Administration: Individual, 15 to 20 minutes; or group, 30 minutes
Equipment: Assembled from description
Description: The Basic Motor Ability Tests—Revised consists of eleven tests:

1. Bead stringing	Bilateral eye-hand coordination and dexterity
2. Target throwing	Eye-hand coordination in throwing
3. Marble transfer	Finger dexterity and speed of arm movement
4. Back and hamstring stretch	Flexibility of back and hamstring muscles
5. Standing long jump	Strength and power in thigh and lower legs
6. Face down to standing	Speed and ability in changing from prone to standing
7. Static balance	One foot standing with eyes open and eyes closed
8. Basketball throw for distance	Arm and shoulder girdle explosive strength

9. Ball striking — Coordination in striking dropped ball with hand
10. Target kicking — Eye-foot coordination
11. Agility run — Ability to rapidly move body and alter direction

Construction and reliability: The data on standardization presented in *The Clumsy Child* are fragmentary. The authors have tested 1563 children and report a test-retest reliability of 0.93, but no additional data are given on breakdown by ages. Normative information for each test is presented in percentiles at each age.

Comment: One or more of the tests can be used individually with normative data providing an indication of expected performance. Use of the test as a whole or in part could be a valuable part of an evaluation program.

13. Purdue Pegboard Test (1948, 1968)[277]

Author: Joseph Tiffin, PhD
Source: Lafayette Instrument Co.
P.O. Box 5728,
Lafayette, Ind. 47903
Ages: 5 years through adult
Administration: Individual; 10 to 15 minutes
Equipment: Pegboard with pins, collars, and washers required
Description: This test of manual dexterity consists of four parts, each described as follows:

1. Right hand — Subject inserts small pegs into holes in pegboard using right hand for a 30-second trial
2. Left hand — Subject inserts pegs into pegboard with left hand for a 30-second trial
3. Both hands — Both hands pick up and insert pegs into board at same time for a 30-second trial
4. Assembly — Using hands cooperatively, subject assembles sequences of pens, collars, and washers for a 60-second trial

Construction and reliability: This test has recently been standardized with 1334 normal schoolchildren, ages 5 to 16, from New Jersey. Means, standard deviations, and percentile scores are presented as a function of age (6-month intervals) and gender. Reliability data on children are not presented in the test manual, although reliability with college students ranged from 0.60 to 0.71. A number of validity studies indicate that learning-disabled subjects perform more poorly than normal controls on this test. Additional normative data are presented in the manual for various age and diagnostic groups.

Comment: This test was originally designed for adults to assist in the selection of employees for manual industrial jobs. It has recently been standardized with school-aged children[103] and adolescents.[186]

Peripheral Neuropathies

Bradley W. Stockert

KEY TERMS

neuropathy	reinnervation
degeneration	diagnosis
neuronal sprouting	treatment
denervation	

LEARNING OBJECTIVES

After reading this chapter the student/therapist will:

1. Classify schemes for traumatic peripheral neuropathies.
2. Understand the pathogenesis and prognosis of traumatic peripheral neuropathies.
3. Understand the status of current knowledge of the degeneration and regeneration phenomena of nerve and muscle.
4. Recognize the typical clinical signs and problems directly caused by traumatic peripheral nerve injury.
5. Recognize the typical clinical problems that develop as secondary complications of traumatic peripheral nerve injury.
6. Understand the evaluation process of clients with traumatic peripheral neuropathies.
7. Understand the treatment procedures for clients with traumatic peripheral neuropathies.

The classification of peripheral **neuropathies** covers a wide range of etiological factors. An anatomical classification has been presented by Schaumberg[37] that describes two overall types: (1) symmetrical generalized neuropathies and (2) focal and multifocal neuropathies. Others have described neuropathies with regard to specific pathology, noting the agent's effect on the peripheral nervous system, but that information appears to be included in Schaumberg's anatomical classification.[37]

Traumatic peripheral neuropathies are classed as focal or multifocal neuropathies in the category of physical injuries, which includes severance, focal crush, compression, stretch or traction, and entrapment.[37] The physical therapy literature has not described peripheral neuropathies with regard to these categories; however, articles describing specific pathological entities have been presented.[32] Some of the specific problems discussed include thoracic outlet syndrome (TOS), specific entrapment syndromes (e.g., suprascapular nerve entrapment), traction injuries (e.g., brachial plexus), and acute compression syndromes (e.g., Saturday night palsy, casting, and splinting). Although the treatment and the signs and symptoms of these syndromes and pathologies have received much attention, less consideration has been afforded the specific pathophysiology of the peripheral nerve injury in traumatic peripheral neuropathies.

This chapter describes traumatic peripheral neuropathies with regard to classification, neuroanatomy, pathogenesis, degeneration, and regeneration phenomena, as well as evaluation and treatment of orthopedic problems relating to traumatic peripheral neuropathies. Although traumatic and degenerative neuropathic problems have many similarities and both have been included, the discussion focuses primarily on peripheral trauma because of its clinical link to orthopedic management.

NEUROANATOMY OF PERIPHERAL NERVOUS SYSTEM

The peripheral nervous system (PNS) may be generally described as that portion of the nervous system outside the central nervous system (CNS), which includes the brain and spinal cord. The major components of the PNS[27,37] include motor neurons, sensory neurons, and autonomic neurons.

Pratt[32] describes three levels in the organization of a peripheral nerve or nerve trunk (Fig. 12-1, A). At the innermost level, the nerve fiber is the conducting component of a neuron or nerve cell. The nerve fiber is surrounded by the endoneurium consisting of connective tissue. The second level is a nerve bundle, the funiculus (fascicle), consisting of several nerve fibers collectively surrounded by the perineurium.[32,37] The third level, the nerve trunk, is formed by one to many funiculi enclosed by another connective tissue layer, the epineurium. Extensions from the epineurium pass into the nerve trunk and connect to the perineurium. The connective tissue is loose and irregular and contains cells, fibers, and ground substance.[31]

Microscopically, a nerve fiber consists of an axon, which may be myelinated or unmyelinated, a Schwann cell and a surrounding basement, or basal, membrane (Fig. 12-1, B). The nerve fiber is separated into segments defined by a single Schwann cell and the myelin sheath produced by that cell (Fig. 12-2, A). Junctions between consecutive Schwann cells are termed nodes of Ranvier. Although the nodes may interrupt the myelin sheath, the basement membrane remains continuous along the length of the axon. The axon forms a continuous tubular structure surrounded by the axolemma. The axon contains axoplasm and a variety of cellular components (e.g., mitochondria, neurofilaments, and neurotubes). Axoplasmic flow to and from the neuronal cell body is termed retrograde and anterograde axoplasmic transport, respectively. This transport process provides for the metabolic needs of the nerves and various end-organ tissues.[27] The substances exchanged through axoplasmic flow between axons and the tissues they innervate are termed trophic factors.[27] The neurotubules and neurofilaments are thought to be connected with the fast component of axoplasmic flow.[2,29,40]

CLASSIFICATION OF TRAUMATIC PERIPHERAL NEUROPATHIES

Seddon's clinical classification of nerve injury[38] is based on mechanical trauma. Neurotmesis ("cutting of the nerve") refers to severance of all essential structures in the neuron, including the axon and endoneurium. A visible disruption may not be apparent in the epineurium. Axonotmesis is a

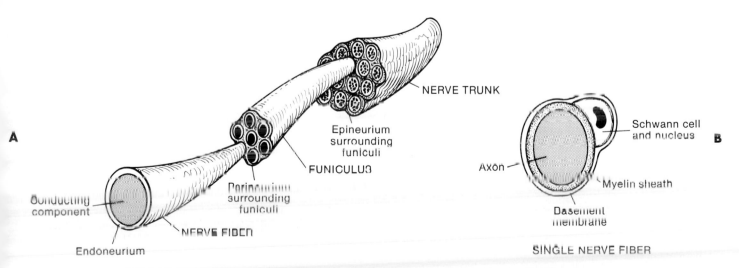

Fig. 12-1. Three levels of organization of a peripheral nerve or nerve trunk. **A,** Nerve trunk and components. **B,** Microscopic structure of nerve fiber.

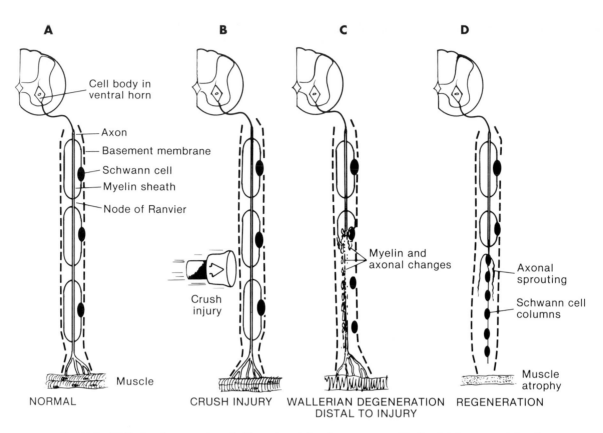

Fig. 12-2. Wallerian degeneration. **A,** Normal peripheral motor nerve. **B,** Crush injury to peripheral nerve. **C,** Wallerian degeneration distal to site of injury. **D,** Regeneration with axonal sprouting guided by Schwann cell columns. (Adapted from Schaumberg HH, Spencer PS, and Thomas PK: *Disorders of peripheral nerves,* Philadelphia, 1983, FA Davis Co.)

lesion to the axon severe enough to cause **degeneration** of the axon distal to the lesion, but with no interruption in the continuity of the endoneurium. Neurapraxia ("nonacting nerve") is an injury to the nerve that causes some degree of paralysis but no peripheral degeneration. This classification is descriptive from the standpoint of morphology, functional loss and recovery, and clinical prognosis.[22]

Schaumberg[37] modified Seddon's classification into an anatomically based scheme. He defined neuropraxia, axonotmesis, and neurotmesis as class I, class II, and class III injuries, respectively (Table 12-1). Class I injuries result in a reversible blockade of nerve conduction that tends to be the result of mild or moderate focal compression. The following two types of class I are described: (1) mild, rapidly reversible blockade resulting from transient ischemia with no anatomical changes and (2) slowly reversible conduction blockade resulting from paranodal demyelination.

Clinically, class I injuries may result in decreased strength, absence of deep tendon reflexes, and a loss of sensation (confined to large diameter fibers); however, there is usually no loss of autonomic nerve function. There is no permanent damage to the axon itself. Recovery is generally spontaneous and occurs within 3 months.[37]

Class II injuries (axonotmesis) result in variable loss of sensory, motor, and sympathetic nerve function.[37] Both myelinated and unmyelinated fibers may be involved. Muscle atrophy may occur and areflexia is consistently found. These lesions generally occur as a result of closed-crush or percussion injuries. The axon is damaged, but the Schwann cell basal lamina remains intact along with the endoneurium. Although Wallerian degeneration occurs distal to the lesion, regeneration is generally effective with a high degree of fidelity because the integrity of the Schwann cell basal lamina and endoneurium is maintained.[37] Recovery is generally slow (several months to more than a year) because the axonal regeneration occurs at the rate of 1 to 8 mm/day, depending on the specific nerve and location of the lesion.[2,40] The prognosis is good, however, because axons can regenerate within the original, uninterrupted connective tissue tubes.[37]

Class III injuries (neurotmesis) are commonly the result of stab wounds, high-velocity projectiles, or nerve traction that disrupts the connective tissue components and completely transects the nerve trunk. Wallerian degeneration occurs distal to the lesion. Regeneration of the damaged nerves may occur, but because of the damage to the

Table 12-1. Classification of acute, traumatic peripheral nerve injury

Anatomical classification	Class I	Class II	Class III
Previous nomenclature	Neurapraxia	Axonotmesis	Neurotmesis
Lesion	Reversible conduction block resulting from ischemia or demyelination	Axonal interruption but basal lamina remains intact	Nerve fiber and basal lamina interruption (complete nerve severance)

Adapted from Schaumberg HH, Spencer PS, and Thomas PK: *Disorders of peripheral nerves,* Philadelphia, 1983, FA Davis.[37]

connective tissue layers and Schwann cell basal lamina, the **neuronal sprouting** will occur with a low fidelity. As a result, the prognosis is poor and proper end-organ function may not be restored. The formation of neuromas is not uncommon.[37]

PATHOGENESIS OF PERIPHERAL NEUROPATHIES

As described previously nerve degeneration is a salient feature of class II and class III traumatic neuropathies. Waller is credited with describing nerve degeneration that occurs distal to the site of injury; this process is called Wallerian degeneration (Fig. 12-2).[2] Primarily, the axon shrinks, fragments, and becomes irregular in shape distal to the lesion. Myelin, if present, breaks down and the associated Schwann cells undergo change. The breakdown of myelin involves chemical alteration of myelin lipids and is accompanied by retraction of the myelin sheath from the axon at the nodes of Ranvier.[2] Axonal fragments and myelin debris are broken down by lysosomal vacuoles in Schwann cells and macrophages that migrate to the area during the early stages of the degenerative process. Loss of axonal proteins within the first 24 hours occurs concomitantly with the axonal and myelin degeneration.[46] These changes are a reflection, in part, of a cessation of normal axonal flow and the disintegration of some cellular organelles. Shortly after the injury, Schwann cells proliferate and then form columns of cells (bands of Bungner) that guide the regenerating axon along the endoneurial tube toward their original target tissue.[40] The entire process of Wallerian degeneration prepares the nerve stump for sprouting and regeneration.[30] Wallerian degeneration and the proliferating Schwann cells may cause the elaboration of neurotrophic factors that promote the regenerative process.[7] Changes occur in the nerve proximal to the site of the injury, including retraction of the axonal stump proximal to the lesion, as well as chromatolysis and other changes in the cell body.[40] These changes are indicative of an attempt by the cell to repair itself. This process is followed either by cell death or by the process of neuronal regeneration. The surviving neurons form axonal sprouts in an attempt to grow from the proximal to the distal stump. The rate of neuronal growth depends on the severity and/or type of injury (i.e., crush versus

severance).[40] Rates of regeneration vary from 1 to 8 mm/day depending, in part, upon the specific nerve and location.[2,40] As regeneration continues distally, axons may become remyelinated and some eventually may reestablish a peripheral connection with an appropriate target tissue.[46]

In muscle, the target tissue of an alpha motoneuron, the effects of denervation are profound. The most obvious change in muscle following denervation is atrophy. Fast (type II) and slow (type I) fibers both undergo a decrease in fiber diameter and show a decrease in the ability to generate force.[24]

In an innervated muscle acetyl choline receptors are found only at the neuromuscular junction.[24] After denervation there is a proliferation of extrajunctional receptors.[24] Lieber[24] suggests that this change may act as a "signal" to promote neuronal sprouting and prepare the muscle for the formation of a new neuromuscular junction and thus **reinnervation.** As the denervated muscle fiber becomes reinnervated, the extrajunctional receptors disappear. Direct electrical stimulation of denervated muscle can prevent the appearance of extrajunctional receptors or diminish their presence once they have appeared.[25] The exact clinical significance of this decrease is unknown.

In the developmental process an extracellular matrix molecule called *neural cell adhesion molecule* (NCAM) is found on the surface of myotubes (primitive muscle fibers) and is speculated to help direct incoming alpha motoneurons to myotubes lacking innervation.[24] Once a myotube becomes innervated and develops into a muscle fiber, the NCAM is no longer found.[24] Denervated muscle fibers have NCAM on the surface of the cell membrane.[36] As the muscle fibers become reinnervated, the NCAM disappears from the surface of the cell membrane.[36] Of particular clinical interest is the effect of electrical stimulation on the denervated muscle. The NCAM "normally" found on the surface of the denervated muscle disappears with electrical stimulation even though the muscle remains denervated.[36] These findings would seem to suggest that electrical stimulation of the denervated muscle might interfere with the reinnervation process. Jansen and others,[18] however, showed that in denervated muscle direct, electrical stimulation did not prevent the reinnervation of the muscle by the original nerve but did prevent the reinnervation by a foreign nerve.

SURGICAL REPAIR OF PERIPHERAL NERVE INJURY

Surgical repair of peripheral nerve injuries has historically been accomplished by either nerve suturing or use of a nerve graft. Although both procedures have been successful, nerve suturing appears to be more effective.[39] End-to-end suturing of peripheral nerves is possible when the transected nerve ends can be closely approximated. If there is a considerable gap between the severed ends of the nerve, a graft may be considered.[28]

Many factors influence the success of a nerve suture procedure. Success or failure depends on the age of the patient, location and/or level of the injury, size of the defect, time between injury and repair, type of nerve, extent of paralysis, and surgical (technical) factors.[9]

Nerve graft procedures have used heterografts, homografts, and autographs as donor material. Autografts seem to provide the best clinical and experimental results.[28] The factors that influence the success of the procedure include graft revascularization, length, caliber, shrinkage, delay in placement, and source of material.[39]

As previously noted, class II and class III nerve injuries cause profound changes to motoneurons and muscle. Some investigators have found that a long period of denervation potentiates the problems associated with denervation.[12,15] Other investigators have shown that suturing a severed nerve after a delay of 20 days[6] or 1 to 2 months[17] resulted in a better long-term outcome.

Most recently Finkelstein[10] showed in rats that more adverse changes in contractile characteristics occurred with increasing periods of denervation. The changes noted included a substantial decrease in the recovery of muscle mass when the denervation period lasted longer than 21 days. Consistent with the loss of muscle mass was a decrease in the absolute force and the force per unit of mass when denervation was greater than 7 days. The results of this study suggest that motoneurons do not lose the capacity to reinnervate a muscle but rather the denervated muscle loses the ability to recover.[10]

TYPICAL CLINICAL SIGNS AND PROBLEMS

Primary and secondary clinical problems resulting from traumatic peripheral nerve injuries are found distal and, to a lesser extent, proximal to the lesion. Although pure motor and pure sensory disturbances are found in some pathological states (e.g., poliomyelitis), the pattern typically seen with trauma is a loss of motor control, sensory loss, and impaired vasomotor control.[45]

Nonneurological injuries directly caused by trauma

Multiple tissue damage is frequently associated with the trauma that results in peripheral nerve damage. Depending on the specific type of trauma (e.g., gun shot, stabbing, traction injury) the damage may take the form of open wound sites, bone fractures, blood vessel damage, muscle tears, edema, internal organ damage, head injury and/or infection. Each of these lesions presents problems and all prolong the period of immobilization, resulting in numerous secondary clinical problems (e.g., vascular stasis, disuse atrophy, and abnormal joint range of motion).

Problems directly caused by peripheral nerve injury

Sensory disturbances. Many sensory disturbances are commonly associated with peripheral nerve injuries. These disturbances can be grossly categorized as either negative phenomena (decreased or loss of a sensation) or positive phenomena (increased sensation or dysesthesia).[4] The exact pattern of the sensory change(s) varies with the specific cause and severity of the injury.

Peripheral nerve injuries typically produce negative phenomena and a decrease in the perception of touch, proprioception, and stereognosis. These sensations are associated with large diameter fibers that are generally more vulnerable to compression than small diameter fibers. Small diameter fibers are associated with temperature and pain sensation.[4] Any absence or decrease in the perception of noxious stimuli diminishes normal protective reactions and may lead to additional problems as a result of neglect.

In addition to the obvious difficulties found with these sensory disturbances, there is the problem of patient neglect associated with an "insensitive" area. The diminished protective reactions and poor hygiene habits commonly found with a neglected area often lead to an increased incidence of repeated trauma and secondary problems (e.g., swelling with dependent positioning of a limb). If the client's CNS also has been damaged as a result of trauma, degeneration, or substance abuse, these problems can become pronounced.

Positive phenomena associated with peripheral nerve injuries include contact dysesthesia, hyperesthesia, burning, and pins-and-needles sensation. An increased perception of pain often is associated with compression applied directly over the injury site, as well as just proximal and distal to the lesion. Hyperalgesia and pins-and-needles sensation are the most common positive phenomena found with peripheral nerve injuries.[4]

Weakness/paralysis of denervated muscle. The specific pattern of weakness and/or paralysis seen with traumatic peripheral nerve injuries is directly related to the site and severity of the nerve injury. Sites that are particularly vulnerable to injury include the peroneal nerve near the proximal fibula, the median nerve at the carpal tunnel, and the radial and ulnar nerves as they respectively pass the radial groove and medial epicondyle on the humerus.[20]

In general, partially denervated muscle shows some degree of weakness, whereas completely denervated muscle becomes flaccid. In both cases, atrophy begins to appear shortly after denervation. Concomitant with partial denervation is the patient's complaint of rapid fatigue and diminished capacity to perform activities of daily living.

Deep tendon reflexes are diminished, or absent, and electromyographic (EMG) readings are abnormal after nerve injury.[3]

After muscle denervation, EMG readings remain electrically silent for 5 to 7 days, at which time fibrillation potentials begin to appear.[3] Frequent fibrillation potentials are characteristic of denervated muscle and are present within 3 weeks after the injury. The EMG pattern after that time depends on the degree of nerve injury and regeneration. The appearance of low amplitude, short duration, polyphasic motor unit potentials is evidence of repair and reinnervation. Motor unit potentials often occur before there is any palpable contraction. As regeneration continues, the fibrillation potentials diminish and the polyphasic motor unit activity increases. Fibrillation potentials typically remain for 2 to 3 years, and sometimes 4 to 5 years in severe injuries.[3]

The force generating ability of partially denervated muscle depends on the number of surviving motoneurons and muscle fibers. The effects of partial denervation in humans and rats were recently studied by Gordon and others.[13] In both models, all of the motor units that survived partial denervation increased in size in proportion to the degree of denervation. From the perspective of force generation, the capacity for the motor units to enlarge through the process of neuronal sprouting (i.e., increase the number of muscle fibers per motoneuron) resulted in the ability to effectively cope with a loss of up to 80% of the motoneurons. The results indicated that the enlarged motor units (1) increased their size by innervating more fibers within their territory rather than expanding their territory and (2) could generate more force per motor unit than a normal motor unit. With a loss of 80% or more of the motoneurons, however, the maximal tetanic force was permanently and significantly reduced.[13] Although neuronal sprouting can compensate, in terms of tetanic strength, for a loss of up to 80% of the motoneurons, other alterations in the neuromuscular unit may develop (e.g., changes in motor control/learning and/or muscular endurance). Some literature on postpoliomyelits suggests that enlarged motor units may carry an increased susceptibility for dysfunction and/or degeneration.

Vasomotor disturbances. In some cases of peripheral nerve injury (e.g., complete transection) the peripheral sympathetic nerve fibers are cut, resulting in a loss in sympathetic control of vasomotor tone and vasodilation.[44] The resultant vasodilation increases the incidence of edema. This situation compounds the problem of swelling in an insensitive limb left in a dependent position.

Changes secondary to traumatic peripheral nerve injury

Soft tissue changes. Connective tissue and muscle changes occur secondary to disuse after paralysis and/or immobilization. Close examination and palpation frequently reveal thickening of tendon sheaths and fibrotic adhesions,

especially in the periarticular areas. These soft tissue changes can decrease the available physiological and accessory range of motion (ROM) at a joint and may ultimately limit a patient's functional recovery after reinnervation.

Joint weakness and instability develop initially from the weakness and/or paralysis of the muscles surrounding the joint. Over time, edema and disuse result in weakness of the joint capsule and ligaments, predisposing the effected joints to hypermobility. In all joints hypermobility increases the probability that degenerative changes will occur. Hypermobility and instability make a joint more susceptible to subluxation, damage to articular surfaces, and further compromise to joint integrity.[44] Additional joint deformities may appear secondary to the unopposed pull of an antagonist or from abnormal biomechanics in weight-bearing joints.

Bony changes. Studies have shown that the changes in bone after nerve section with motor paralysis are similar to the changes in bone following a similar period of immobilizations without nerve section.[1,14,44] The rate of onset and extent of bony changes are more directly related to the degree of disuse than the cause of the neural disturbance. In adults the changes include a decrease in cortical and trabecular thickness, concomitant with an increase in decalcification, porosity, and medullary canal diameter. These changes appear to be only partially reversible following reinnervation and mobilization.[34,44] These alterations in bone structure result in an overall decrease in bone strength and can lead to an increased incidence of fracture, especially in weight-bearing bones.

The pattern is somewhat different in growing bones. Immediately after the injury there is a period of hyperplasia followed by premature cessation of growth.[34,35] This results in a permanent decrease in the length and diameter of the bone, as well as the size of the bony prominences.[44] This childhood injury is one of the causes of leg-length or arm-length discrepancies in adults.

EVALUATION
Patient history

A complete medical history should be taken for each patient. Even when the **diagnosis** is known, the history will give additional valuable information regarding the diagnosis, prognosis, and patient's perceptions of his or her condition. Relevant past medical history, **treatment**, and response should be discussed.

Observation

This portion of the evaluation is used to gain a gross overview of the patient. If the patient walks into the treatment area, the gait pattern should be observed to determine whether further assessment of that activity is necessary. In addition the examiner should observe the patient's general posture, integrity of the skin, and general willingness to move and cooperate. If the patient is seen at bedside, his or her overall appearance should be observed as the examiner enters the room. The therapist should ascertain whether the patient is being treated for any other problems (e.g., vascular compromise, fracture, head injury) that must be considered during the evaluation and treatment process. The patient's willingness to move the affected area and to move in general should be assessed. In addition the patient's overall disposition should be noted and its potential effect on the evaluation and treatment process considered.

Objective examination

A thorough, objective evaluation will help the therapist classify the extent of the peripheral nerve injury. Classification is useful in determining the prognosis, setting realistic goals, and developing an appropriate treatment plan. A good differential diagnosis is especially important in cases of multiple trauma to separate true peripheral nerve injuries from other possible sources of nerve injury (e.g., herniated nucleus pulposus or foramina entrapment).[20] Clients with other confounding problems, such as CNS involvement, must be assessed in their entirety with the peripheral system being one component of the whole.

Nerve conduction test

A thorough evaluation of a patient with a suspected peripheral nerve injury requires equipment and personnel not available in many physical therapy clinics. Nerve conduction velocity should be tested. In a peripheral nerve injury, this test will demonstrate a normal velocity proximal to the lesion, but a decreased velocity or loss of the signal at the injury site and distally. After Wallerian degeneration, regenerated axonal tissue typically demonstrates a conduction velocity equal to only 60% to 80% of the value predicted for normal tissue.[44] (Refer to Chapter 29 for further discussion of electrodiagnosis.)

Electromyography

EMG can demonstrate the presence or absence of normal innervation to a muscle. As denervated muscle becomes reinnervated, the EMG pattern changes in a characteristic fashion that suggests specific stages of recovery have occurred. The time required for nerve regeneration, muscle reinnervation, and normal muscle action potentials to return depends on the severity of the injury and the distance between the muscle and site of injury.[3]

Lester and others[23] made several interesting findings in a study of 22 individuals with a complete transection of the median and/or ulnar nerves at the wrist. The average time between injury and follow-up was 5 years. First, EMG studies demonstrated that reinnervation of the intrinsic muscles occurred in almost every case. Second, the absence of functional use of the intrinsic muscles did not preclude the presence of EMG activity. When the maximum evoked muscle action potential (MEAP) on the effected side was less

than 50% of the MEAP on the unaffected side, there was a consistent lack of clinically detectable intrinsic muscle power. In the muscles that lacked clinically detectable muscle power, however, there was electrical activity, so they were partially reinnervated.[23] Thus a case can be made for the use of electrical stimulation in these patients in an effort to maximize the recovery of intrinsic muscle strength and function. (Refer to Chapters 29 and 30 for additional information.)

Sensory testing

Sensory testing can be performed in any physical therapy facility, and the results can give significant clues about the severity of the injury. Because large-diameter fibers are more vulnerable to injury than small-diameter fibers, the presence or absence of the various sensory modalities gives an indication of the extent of the nerve injury. Touch, proprioception, and stereognosis are senses transmitted along large-diameter fibers, whereas temperature is a sensation transmitted on small-diameter fibers. All of these sensory modalities are readily tested. The Tinel sign is a provocation test used on regenerating nerves to determine the leading edge of the regenerating axon. The test consists of tapping on the end of the regenerating nerve. A positive sign consists of pain or tingling in response to tapping over the distal end of the regenerating axon. The pain or tingling occurs in areas where the nerve has regenerated. No sensation is perceived in those areas still lacking innervation.[26] Although Tinel's sign is commonly used to give an indication of axonal regeneration, in some cases (e.g., class III peripheral nerve injury) the sign can be extremely misleading and unreliable.[44] Sensory testing should be used in cases of multiple trauma to determine whether the loss in sensation follows a true dermatomal pattern or a peripheral nerve distribution. At some point appropriate high level functional testing (e.g., balance and coordination) should be performed to develop a thorough picture of the patient's level of dysfunction and the progress of the rehabilitation program. The patient who develops hypersensitivity should be evaluated carefully and followed for the presence of reflex sympathetic dystrophy.

In the study noted previously of 22 individuals with complete transection of the median and/or ulnar nerves at the wrist, detailed sensory testing was performed.[23] Testing included the assessment of two-point discrimination, ridge discrimination, and the sensations of vibration, light touch, and temperature. All patients except one had some return of "protective sensation." However, the return was not uniform throughout the nerve territory and 10 patients experienced "delays" in the appreciation of the thermal stimuli. In addition, 21 patients had a return of the sensations to light touch and vibration. The degree of sensory recovery was far greater than the recovery of clinically detectable muscle power in the intrinsic muscles but was comparable to the degree of EMG activity detected.[23]

Range of motion testing

ROM testing is essential. Accessory motions (i.e., gliding) and physiological motions need to be assessed for hypomobility as well as hypermobility. All relevant end feels (the sensation perceived by the therapist at the end of a passive ROM) should be assessed. This information is used to help determine prognosis and the need for mobilization, stabilization, and protection of a given area.[8,26]

Manual muscle testing

Thorough manual muscle testing should be performed (1) to determine the pattern (myotome versus peripheral nerve) of any weakness and/or paralysis, (2) to determine whether the nerve injury is unifocal or multifocal, and (3) to assess the completeness and severity of each nerve lesion. Muscle testing provides a baseline to judge the patient's recovery and the effects of treatment. When appropriate, testing should include functional tests to determine a patient's ability to perform activities of daily living. An endurance factor should be included in testing because partially denervated muscle may demonstrate near normal strength but fatigue quickly. These findings should be compared with the EMG report.

Soft tissue palpation

Soft tissue palpation is often an overlooked technique, but it is an important part of the evaluation process. Layer palpation is typically begun superficially and then progresses to deeper tissues. During palpation care must be taken to ensure that the fingers move with the skin. If the fingers slide over the skin, the patient will experience discomfort and skin abrasions. When skin integrity is poor, palpation must be accomplished with precaution to avoid abrasion and tearing of the superficial skin layer. Initially the skin should be inspected for signs of neglect and then palpated to determine temperature and mobility. Palpation progresses to the subcutaneous layers to assess the pulses of relevant blood vessels, the mobility of subcutaneous fascia, and the presence of edematous tissue, especially in dependent, affected limbs. Thorough palpation should include some assessment of skin fat folds, which may mask muscular atrophy. Deep palpation is performed to assess the status of fascial planes, ligaments, tendons, and tendinous sheaths. Careful soft tissue palpation can reveal abnormalities (e.g., adhesions or thickenings) in tissues that may impair joint and/or soft tissue function.[26,42]

TREATMENT PROCEDURES

One of the unfortunate realities of treating peripheral nerve injuries is that physical therapy treatment is directed only at the secondary consequences of the nerve injury. The nerve injury per se is not affected by traditional physical therapy treatment. Our approach eliminates or minimizes these secondary changes while we wait to see how much functional reinnervation will occur. This approach focuses on anticipating changes in an effort to minimize their impact. Patient education is essential to maximize functional return and avoid secondary conditions resulting from sensory neglect.

Weakness/paralysis

In denervated muscle the effectiveness of treatment to prevent atrophy with electrical stimulation remains unproven in humans.[11,41] The classic study by Gutmann and Guttmann[16] in 1942 showed that electrical stimulation was effective in retarding atrophy in denervated muscle of rabbits. Some studies using other animal models have confirmed these results, whereas other studies found no effect.[31,41] No controlled study has proved that electrical stimulation will retard atrophy in denervated muscle in humans, Brown,[5] however, has shown that direct electrical stimulation of denervated muscle prevents terminal sprouting of alpha motoneurons but does not stop the formation of nodal sprouts, which can reinnervate the denervated muscle. As noted previously, electrical stimulation of completely denervated muscle resulted in the disappearance of NCAM.[36] (Remember that NCAM is thought to act as a chemical guide to bring regenerating axons back toward denervated muscle.) The clinical significance of these findings in the overall scheme of reinnervation is unknown at this time. (See the section on pathogenesis for a further discussion of NCAM.)

Successful studies in animal models do suggest some guidelines for the application of electrical stimulation. Treatment should begin as soon as possible after the injury because the rate of atrophy is greatest immediately after the injury and declines exponentially. If the denervation period lasts less than 100 days, however, the recovery will not be significantly modified by the use of electrical stimulation.[41] Because denervated muscle has no "motor point," the current must pass through the bulk of the muscle to cause a contraction. As a result, interrupted galvanic or sinusoidal current alternating at 25 to 60 cycles per second is recommended. Stimulation should be strong enough to produce 15 to 20 strong contractions per session, and the sessions should be repeated three to four times a day.[40] This approach has helped retard atrophy in the denervated muscles of rats[41] and rabbits,[16] but not cats.[31]

In partially denervated muscle the number of alpha motoneurons and the number of innervated muscle fibers determine if any increase in the strength of those fibers will be sufficient to create a clinically significant effect.[41] Rancho Los Amigos Rehabilitation Engineering Center[33] has reported that electrical stimulation has assisted in "carry-over" to voluntary movements in patients with partially denervated muscles. Strengthening exercises for partially denervated muscles generally follow one of two philosophies. Sister Kenny developed a series of exercises that attempts to isolate the effort to the affected muscle. This treatment strategy was originally developed for use on patients with poliomyelitis.

The second approach, proprioceptive neuromuscular facilitation (PNF), consists of therapeutic exercises that use a series of facilitation and synergy patterns in an effort to get muscle strengthening, neuromuscular reeducation, and "overflow" from the stronger muscle groups to the weaker muscle groups.[43] In this system the weaker muscles work with the stronger muscles and not in isolation. For example, consider a patient who has isolated weakness in the tibialis anterior muscle resulting in foot drop. The Sister Kenny approach would involve exercises specifically designed to isolate the effort to that muscle (e.g., resisted dorsiflexion with inversion). In contrast, a therapist using patterns of facilitation and synergy might involve the entire lower extremity in the exercise, using hip flexion, adduction, and lateral rotation with the ankle dorsiflexion and inversion. This pattern would combine the strengthening effort in the affected muscle with the effort in the unaffected muscles. This is an attempt to produce "overflow" from the stronger muscle groups to the affected muscle and adds an element of neuromuscular reeducation. In either case, the results will be limited by the number of motor units and the number of innervated muscle fibers. These exercises do have the additional benefit of assisting in maintenance of ROM and reduction of edema. As has been seen with motor learning and motor control research (Chapters 3 and 4) carry-over into functional patterns become a critical element if motor learning is to occur. Strengthening in isolation, no matter the approach, will be less effective than to practice in functional activities.

Thus the patient should be taught an appropriate home exercise program as soon as possible. Again, if the patient has additional problems, application of either approach must be modified to the needs of the individual.

For example, if the patient is elderly and has cardiopulmonary problems, the response to motor output and overflow would need to be monitored carefully to avoid excessive stress on this and other systems. However, if the patient previously had a cerebrovascular accident that caused a fall with resultant peripheral nerve injury, appropriate modification of the treatment approach would need to be considered. Maximal effort with "overflow" may not be the optimal choice of exercises because of the synergistic patterns often accompanying volitional movement in hemiplegia. Thus any treatment approach needs to be adapted to the individual's needs and based on which functional patterns the patient needs to incorporate into his or her life strategies.

Sensory impairment

Physical therapy treatment of the sensory-impaired area should include extensive patient education about limb neglect. The patient should learn to regularly inspect the affected area in an attempt to reduce further trauma to the area. Monitoring the redevelopment and quality of returning sensations can be helpful in assessing the repair and regeneration of the injured nerve.

Vasomotor disturbances

Though the loss of sympathetic vasomotor control cannot be directly altered, the edema resulting from the loss can be addressed. Primary treatment consists of prevention through patient education about the causes of edema, such as dependent positioning and limb neglect. Reduction of edema can be accomplished through a variety of techniques, including pump massage, compression, and elevation. These techniques are means of assisting venous and lymphatic return from an extremity. For example, someone with swelling around the ankle and foot would benefit from having the distal extremity elevated above the level of the heart whenever possible. Reduction of the edema could be further enhanced with the use of an elastic wrap. This would apply a mild, constant compressive force over the swollen area. Pump massage is a technique that attempts to manually assist venous and lymph return. This technique is done, for example, in the anterior ankle by gently sliding one hand proximally over the swollen area while the other hand guides the foot and ankle into plantarflexion. This combines compression and lengthening of the edematous tissue in an attempt to manually "squeeze" the fluid out of the area. Patients with sensory neglect, whether as a result of peripheral nerve injury or not, will benefit from this type of treatment to eliminate edema associated with decreased muscle function and dependent positioning. This problem is often seen in head trauma. (For further information on vasomotor disturbance, see Chapter 17, inflammatory problems; Chapter 24, CVA; Chapter 25, the elderly.)

Soft tissue changes

Connective tissue and contractile tissue become progressively shorter when not stretched regularly.[21] Normal activities of daily living provide stretching and ROM to the soft tissues and joint structures. With flaccid or weak muscles, however, the ability to perform those activities is diminished, and the potential for developing restrictions and contractures is increased. Again, this is true whether the disuse is a result of peripheral or CNS injury.

The most effective treatment program uses preventive measures, such as ROM exercises. These exercises may initially be performed by the therapist as passive or active-assisted exercises. As soon as possible, however, the patient is taught how to do the appropriate exercises independently. If ROM can be maintained through activities of daily living, then the patient should be encouraged to incorporate these patterns of range into daily procedural tasks.

Basic to any "stretching" exercise is the premise that a

Stage of recovery versus problems to look for and anticipate

Acute Stage Management—What is the patient's current status?

1. Tissue trauma and complications directly related to the original injury
2. Sensory disturbances
   Typically result in a loss of sensation rather than an increase in sensation
   Potential for limb neglect and loss of protective reactions
3. Patterns of weakness/paralysis and what functional groups are affected
   Is there partial or complete denervation of one or more muscle groups?
   Does this affect a weight-bearing or non-weight-bearing extremity?
4. Vasomotor disturbances with the potential for edema
5. Secondary changes in the soft tissues, bones, or articular surfaces

Rehabilitation Stage—How has the patient's status improved?

1. Have the tissue trauma and complications directly related to the original injury resolved with or without further complication?
2. Have the sensory disturbances resolved or continued?
   Is there still a partial or complete loss of proprioception, stereognosis, temperature, and pain?
   Is there still a partial or complete loss of protective reactions and the presence of limb neglect?
3. Is the weakness/paralysis resolving or continuing without change?
   Is there persistent partial or complete denervation?
   How is the extremity being used in activities of daily living?
4. Is there persistent edema?
   Is there persistent limb neglect?
   Does the patient understand the consequences of dependent limb positioning?

5. Are there secondary soft tissue and/or boney/articular changes?
   Are the changes related primarily to denervation, disuse, or both?
   Are weight-bearing joints being adequately protected?
   Are all affected joints and soft tissues being adequately mobilized?

Long-Term Care—What problems appear to be permanent rather than still resolving?

1. Have the tissue trauma and complications directly related to the original injury resolved with or without further complication?
2. Are the sensory disturbances permanent?
   Does this result in a complete or partial loss of sensation?
   Is there a complete or partial loss of protective reactions?
3. What is the long-term pattern of weakness/paralysis?
   Is there partial or complete denervation of one or more functional groups?
   How does this effect the weight-bearing or non-weight-bearing extremity?
4. Is there a potential long-term problem for persistent edema?
   Is there persistent limb neglect?
   Does the patient understand the consequences of dependent limb positioning?
5. What is the potential for permanent soft tissue and bony/articular changes?
   Are the changes related primarily to denervation, disuse, or both?
   Are weight-bearing joints being adequately protected?
   Are all affected joints and soft tissues being adequately mobilized?
6. Is the patient adapting to permanent change and creating an environment that prevents future injury?

slow, prolonged stretch will provide for a more plastic or permanent response than the elastic or temporary response of a ballistic stretch. Special care must be given to protect insensitive structures.

If a restriction to physiological or accessory ROM is found, the cause must be determined. The type of dysfunction normally can be accurately assessed by determining the quality of the end feel in the restricted movement. The quality of the end feel suggests a cause and prognosis as well as an appropriate treatment approach for the restriction. The end-feel may have a bony, hard quality similar to elbow extension. This suggests a poor prognosis when found in an abnormal position, such as less than 20 degrees of elbow extension, or in a joint whose end-feel is not normally bony,

such as extension of the knee. Treatment often will have no beneficial effect in these cases because of the probable presence of a bony block. Tissue stretch is the end-feel often described as being the same feeling perceived with normal hamstring stretching. This end-feel suggests a soft tissue restriction is present. These restrictions should respond to stretching and soft tissue mobilization. A common restriction after immobilization results from adhesions and/or capsular tightness. These dysfunctions give an end-feel similar to the sensation perceived at the end of lateral rotation in the shoulder. The sensation is often described as leathery or capsular. The restriction can usually be successfully treated with soft tissue and joint mobilization techniques.[8,19,26]

For example, following a fracture of the humeral shaft,

which may or may not include trauma to the radial nerve, the shoulder is often immobilized. After this period of immobilization, the glenohumeral joint often lacks abduction and lateral rotation. Other movements may also be affected. Assessment of joint play motion will usually reveal a lack of such accessory movements as inferior glide (needed for normal abduction) and anterior glide (required for lateral rotation) of the humerus. Typically the end-feels of the restricted physiological and accessory motions in this example are leathery. This combination of findings suggests a capsular restriction that should respond well to joint mobilization.

Soft tissue restrictions may be found during the assessment of ROM or through the use of palpation. Many soft tissue dysfunctions respond to stretching programs, but others may require the use of soft tissue mobilization techniques, such as myofascial release. These techniques are particularly effective at removing restrictions in areas where various anatomical structures need to freely slide by one another (e.g., fascial planes between muscles). For example, the trauma that results in peripheral nerve injury quite often causes soft tissue trauma. These lesions frequently produce scar tissue that may abnormally adhere the various soft tissue layers to other superficial or deep structures. As a result, motion may become limited or painful as these adhesions restrict the normal soft tissue movement that should occur. Transverse friction massage and myofascial release techniques are effective at removing soft tissue restrictions and promoting proper collagen fiber alignment. Myofascial release techniques are also effective at helping to restore mobility in soft tissues after prolonged periods of immobilization.[8,42] This immobilization may be the result of external (e.g., casting) or internal forces (e.g., spasticity or rigidity).

Orthotic applications

Peripheral nerve injuries may require the application of an orthotic appliance to protect an extremity, especially the weight-bearing lower extremity. Orthoses can be used to protect bony structures and articular surfaces, as well as muscles, ligaments, and nerves, during periods of rehabilitation. The orthotic appliance assists in preventing deformities and limiting pathological motor patterns that can develop with muscular weakness and aberrant sensory input. (See Chapter 32 for further discussion of orthotics.)

Problem solving process

The box on p. 369 divides clinical problems into acute, rehabilitation, and long-term care. Within each section suggested questions related to each phase have been stated to help the therapist sequence the problem-solving process and recognize how questions change as the problems change.

CASE STUDY PRESENTATIONS: EXAMPLES OF PROBLEMS AND TREATMENT

Two case studies are presented to illustrate general treatment approaches to peripheral neuropathic injuries. Case I describes a patient with a traumatic peripheral neuropathy, concomitant orthopedic problems, and specific intervention. Case II describes a patient with a nontraumatic (alcoholic) peripheral polyneuropathy with orthopedic and neurological implications and outlines a general approach to treatment with relevant references.

CASE 1 ▼   Traumatic Compression Injury

History

J.S. was seen as an outpatient 1 week after he had received a traumatic injury to the right lower extremity. The trauma resulted in a compression injury in the area of the common peroneal nerve, near the head of the fibula. Before coming to physical therapy, a nerve conduction study and EMG were performed. Based on these studies and other findings, the physician described the injury as a unifocal, class I neurapraxia of the common peroneal nerve.

Evaluation

Subjective findings. The patient's chief complaint at the time of our evaluation was weakness and a lack of coordination in the right foot. He reported significant difficulty walking, and he used a cane that a friend has given him. In addition, he reported that the right foot seemed to feel "asleep" or "not there" at times. He had no complaints of pain. Mr. J.S. was an office worker. He had no special outside interest that required specific advanced ambulatory skills.

Observations. When J.S. walked into the treatment area, he used a cane in the left hand. Gait deviations included (1) increased left lateral translation of the trunk and (2) a steppage gait to compensate for a right-foot drop. His posture in standing with the cane was normal. Without the assistive device, his standing posture was unsteady and unsafe. Mr. J.S. demonstrated a willingness to move the entire right lower extremity, but his ankle movements were laborious and accomplished with substitutions. Mild pedal edema was noted on the right. Circumferential measurements of the lower extremities were essentially equal bilaterally, except where swelling was present in the ankle and foot.

Sensory testing. J.S. reported decreased sensation to light touch on the dorsum of the right foot and in the first web space. This pattern corresponds to the cutaneous distribution of the two terminal branches of the common peroneal nerve (i.e., the superficial and deep peroneal nerves). Cutaneous sensation was intact elsewhere.

Proprioceptive awareness was diminished in movements at the talocrural joint (dorsiflexion, plantarflexion), subtalar joint (eversion, inversion), and the phalanges (flexion, extension). Temperature sensation was intact throughout both lower extremities.

Strength and range of motion. Active ROM and manual muscle testing were performed. Strength and ROM were within normal limits in the left foot and bilaterally at the hips and knees. Strength in the distal right lower extremity was diminished. Anterior compartment muscles in the leg (tibialis anterior, extensor hallucis longus, extensor digitorum longus, and peroneus tertius) and lateral compartment muscles (peroneus longus and peroneus brevis) both had 2/5 strength. Toe extensors as a group had less than 3/5 strength. Posterior compartment muscles had normal strength.

Passive ROM tests were equal for all motions bilaterally. The end-feels had the same quality bilaterally with each movement tested.

Palpation. The temperature and the integrity of the skin were within normal limits in the distal right lower extremity as measured by superficial palpation. Pedal pulses were equal bilaterally. Palpation of deeper soft tissues was remarkable for the presence of edema throughout the ankle and dorsum of the foot. Neither significant adhesions nor hypomobility was noted in any of the soft tissues or joint play motions. Skin fat folds of the legs were equal bilaterally, confirming the lack of muscular atrophy suggested by circumferential measurements.

Stage I

Goals. Short-term goals included the following: (1) improving strength from 2/5 to 3/5, (2) decreasing and controlling the swelling, (3) teaching the patient to walk without gait deviations using appropriate assistive devices, and (4) developing a home program to help meet goals 1 through 3. Long-term goals included the following: (1) normalizing strength (5/5) and endurance, (2) elimination of swelling, (3) walking without assistive devices and without deviations, and (4) normal proprioception, balance, and coordination responses.

Treatment. Obvious strength deficits in the anterior and lateral compartments were addressed. We chose to include proprioceptive neuromuscular facilitation (PNF). We used repeated

contractions of the hip patterns combined with knee pivots in an effort to get overflow from the strong proximal musculature to the weaker distal muscle groups. This activity had the additional benefit of (1) assisting venous and lymphatic return from the foot and ankle and (2) providing sensory stimulation to those areas with impaired sensation. Stationary bicycling, with toe clips to hold the right foot safely in position, was done for strengthening, endurance, sensory stimulation, cardiovascular fitness, and to promote a sense of "wellness" in the patient.

Swelling in the right lower extremity was diminished through the combined use of pump massage and elevation. In addition, the edema was affected during the active exercise sessions by the action of the lower-extremity muscles, the muscular pump.

The patient was fitted with a plastic ankle-foot orthosis (AFO). This assistive device was used to help protect the weight-bearing joints and soft tissues in the right lower extremity. These areas are particularly susceptible to trauma during walking when weakness, decreased sensation, and instability are present in the lower extremity.

Home program. The patient's home program was designed to supplement the treatment sessions in the clinic. The home program focused on the same dysfunctions addressed in the clinic—weakness, decreased sensation, swelling, and instability in the distal right lower extremity. Initially, significant amounts of time were used for patient education rather than providing just "direct" treatment of the patient's dysfunctions.

The patient was taught strengthening and ROM exercises. J.S. was shown how to apply manual assistance and manual resistance with his exercises to provide tactile sensation and proprioceptive input. He was instructed to watch the body part move during the exercises while visualizing how normal movement should feel. Exercises focused on toe extension and ankle dorsiflexion, with and without eversion or inversion.

The patient was instructed in the proper use of the AFO and the cane. He was shown how to ambulate without the gait deviations he initially demonstrated. He was encouraged to ambulate as much as possible or until fatigue forced him to ambulate with deviations.

J.S. received extensive instruction on the care of an insensitive limb. He was taught to inspect the area for skin breakdown and swelling on a daily basis. The effects of prolonged dependent positioning and elevation were discussed. The patient was instructed in the use of ICE (*ice, compression, and elevation*) to treat and control the edema.

Stage II

Reevaluation. After approximately 6 weeks of treatment, J.S. had shown significant improvements in the dysfunctions assessed on initial evaluation. His strength had improved from 2/5 to 3+/5 in the affected muscles. Light touch and proprioception were improved but still diminished in the distal

Continued.

CASE 1 ▼ Traumatic Compression Injury—cont'd

right lower extremity. Passive ROM in dorsiflexion and plantarflexion was slightly decreased 5 to 10 degrees on the right. The end-feels of those restricted motions were leathery, suggesting a mild capsular restriction. Swelling was a problem only with prolonged (longer than 3 hours) dependent positioning.

Goals. Short-term goals included (1) improving strength from $^{3+}/_5$ to $^5/_5$, (2) improving endurance with walking, (3) improving proprioception, (4) eliminating the motion restriction at the talocrural joint, and (5) eliminating swelling.

Long-term goals remained the same as stated in Stage I.

Treatment. Weakness ($^{3+}/_5$) was still a problem with the toe extensors and in the anterior and lateral compartment. Strengthening exercises continued using lower-extremity PNF patterns with repeated contractions and knee pivots. Slow reversals and ankle pivots were added to further enhance strengthening and neuromuscular reeducation in the distal components. At this point (strength equal to or greater than $^3/_5$), controlled weight-bearing activities were initiated without the cane and AFO to combine strengthening with functional proprioceptive input. Initially, weight transfers side-to-side and front-to-back provided the focus of our functional activities in a weight-bearing position. PNF gait activities emphasizing the swing phase of gait were utilized to provide additional training in functional patterns in a non-weight-bearing position. Stationary bicycling was continued for the reasons mentioned previously.

Over time, J.S. had developed a mild restriction to plantarflexion and dorsiflexion. The leathery end-feels suggested a capsular restriction that typically responds to joint mobilization procedures. Graded joint play movements were used to produce capsular stretching at the talocrural joint. This approach resolved the motion restrictions within a few treatment sessions. For an explanation of the guidelines, indications, and contraindications to joint mobilization procedures, review the suggested readings of Cyriax,[8] Kaltenborn,[19] and Magee.[26]

Home program. J.S. was instructed to walk without the use of any assistive device when he could do so without any noticeable deviations. With the onset of fatigue and/or deviations in gait, the cane was required. Because swelling was still an intermittent problem, the guidelines regarding dependent positioning and ICE were reviewed. The adverse consequences of swelling, such as diminished balance reactions, were reviewed to emphasize the need to completely control the problem.

J.S. continued with his manually resisted home exercises, but he was encouraged to increase the amount of resistance. Home exercises in weight-bearing positions were added to his home program. He was encouraged to perform weight-shifts and single-leg stances to affect strength and proprioception in functional positions. To improve the safety of these activities, he was encouraged to perform the exercises on nonslippery surfaces, where he could hold onto a stable object for contact assistance (e.g., behind the couch or at the kitchen sink). J.S. was encouraged to begin bicycling as part of his home program.

Stage III

Reevaluation results. At approximately 10 weeks J.S. had shown further significant improvement in the dysfunctions seen on initial evaluation. Swelling was no longer present, even with prolonged sitting. Sensation to light touch was intact and normal throughout. ROM was within normal limits in both lower extremities. Strength had returned to normal ($^5/_5$) in all muscle groups, but endurance was less on the right. He was able to walk short distances (4 blocks) without assistive devices and with no gait deviations. Proprioception, balance, and coordination reactions, however, continued to be mildly decreased on the right.

Goals. Short-term goals included (1) improving endurance in ambulation without assistive devices, (2) maintaining normal ROM in the distal right lower extremity, (3) improving proprioception, balance, and coordination reactions, and (4) discharging the patient with a thorough home program that would allow for continued improvement of his dysfunction. Long-term goals included (1) ambulation without assistive devices, (2) normal endurance, balance, and coordination with ambulation, and (3) no residual dysfunction in the right lower extremity.

Treatment. We continued to work on strength, endurance, and neuromuscular reeducation of the right lower extremity through the use of PNF. Hip patterns were done with full integration and resistance of the distal components. Gait activities included work on the swing and stance phases. To improve diminished coordination and balance reactions, we added high-level functional activities, such as running agility tests and obstacle courses with figure 8s, angular turns, and uneven surfaces.

The patient was encouraged to continue the balance and coordination activities as part of his home program. J.S. was told to continue these activities until he could perform them faultlessly. He was shown how to increase the degree of difficulty in the activities so he could continue to progress independently at home. The patient was encouraged to continue bicycling to improve his endurance and his cardiovascular fitness.

CASE 2 ▼ Nontraumatic Peripheral Neuropathy

History

R.A. is a 60-year-old man with a 40-year history of chronic alcoholism. Diagnosis is progressive, peripheral polyneuropathy, secondary to alcoholism and nutritional (dietary) deficiency and concomitant peripheral vascular compromise.

Evaluation

Findings on evaluation are as follows:
I. Weakness
   A. Bilateral lower extremities
      1. 3/5 posterior compartment muscles
      2. 4/5 anterior compartment muscles
      3. 2+/5 lateral compartment muscles
      4. Generalized weakness intrinsic muscles of both feet
   B. Bilateral upper extremities
      1. 4/5 strength wrist, hand, intrinsics
II. Sensation
   A. Bilateral lower extremities, localized below midcalf
      1. Decreased superficial sensation with moderate impairment of touch, pain, and temperature
      2. Decreased deep sensation with mild impairment of deep pressure, vibration, and position sense (proprioception)
   B. Bilateral upper extremities: wrist and hand
      1. Decreased superficial sensation with mild impairment of touch, pain, and temperature
III. Range of motion
   A. 5 degree flexion contracture at both knees
   B. Dorsiflexion to neutral (passive) bilateral talocrural joints
IV. Gait: mild ataxia with steppage gait (resulting from anterior and lateral compartment muscle weakness) bilateral lower extremities

Patient also has several areas of skin ulceration on dorsum of the right foot, glossiness of the skin around the distal aspect of the leg, ankle, and foot bilaterally. Hyperhidrosis of feet and hands is noted bilaterally. There is also slight and occasional dysphagia and constant hoarseness.

Patient R.A. has relatively classic findings associated with peripheral polyneuropathy secondary to chronic alcoholism. The goal of treatment of the patient with a traumatic peripheral neuropathy may be to return to normal function, depending on the prognosis for regeneration. In this case the peripheral polyneuropathy is a progressive disease and the goal is maintenance.

Suggestions for treatment

Lower-extremity weakness may be addressed by the use of manual active-assisted and/or resisted exercises using linear patterns or proprioceptive neuromuscular facilitation (PNF) techniques. Manual contacts would provide proprioceptive and exteroceptive input and would address sensory deficits as well. PNF techniques, such as repeated contractions or slow reversal, would facilitate strength as well as rhythm and coordination. Upper-extremity weakness might be addressed in the same manner with the inclusion of activities to maintain fine motor skills and coordination.

Sensory deficits may be addressed in several ways. As mentioned previously, manual contacts during exercise may subserve proprioceptive/exteroceptive function. Because this disease is progressive, patient education regarding sensory changes and sequelae (e.g., skin lesions) is critical. Cognitive changes may be a limiting factor in educating the patient. (For further information concerning memory/learning changes, consult Chapter 5 on the Limbic System.)

Ataxia associated with alcoholism may be addressed in relation to cerebellar dysfunction and subsequent changes in coordination of motor function. Consult Chapter 23 on cerebellar dysfunction.

Loss of ROM as a result of weakness and/or contractures may be corrected by either maintaining strength or stretching. Orthotic devices may be helpful but must be used judiciously to prevent skin lesions from pressure. Consult Chapter 28 on orthotics for further information. Dysphagia and hoarseness may be a result of progressive motor weakness. Refer to Chapter 26 regarding speech pathology for further information.

The outcome of alcoholic neuropathy can be good if the disease is not advanced and the drug addiction is stopped. If the alcoholic continues drinking, the peripheral neuropathic outcome will become progressively worse as additional peripheral nerves become involved.

SUMMARY

This chapter focused on the nature and clinical implications of traumatic peripheral neuropathy. Although involving the nervous system directly, the neurological and musculoskeletal effects of trauma to the PNS differ significantly from the effects of trauma to the CNS. In addition, although traumatic peripheral injuries created by an external force are relatively well focused, peripheral neuropathy of a multifocal nature occurring from an internal mechanism (e.g., alcoholic neuropathy) can be quite traumatic as well. Classification of injuries, pathophysiology of degeneration, and regenerative processes were presented. Specific findings on evaluation with guidelines and prescriptions for specific treatment of possible orthopedic problems with reference to peripheral nerve injury were discussed. It is hoped that the information presented, along with case studies, will be valuable to physical therapists and other health professionals in the treatment of traumatic peripheral neuropathies.

ACKNOWLEDGMENT.

The author would like to thank Bill Ogard for his valuable contribution to this chapter.

REFERENCES

1. Allison N and Brooks B: Bone atrophy, *Surg Gynecol Obstet* 33:250, 1921.
2. Allt G: Pathology of the peripheral nerve. In Landon DN, editor: *The peripheral nerve,* London, 1975, Chapman & Hall.
3. Archibald KC: Clinical usefulness of EMG and nerve conduction tests in nerve injury and repair. In Jewitt DL and McCarrol HR Jr, editors: *Nerve repair and regeneration: its clinical and experimental basis,* St Louis, 1980, Mosby.
4. Bradley WG: *Disorders of peripheral nerves,* London, 1974, Blackwell Scientific Publishing.
5. Brown MC: Sprouting of motor nerves in adult muscles: a recapitulation of ontogeny, *Trends Neurosci* 7:10, 1984.
6. Brunetti O and others: Role of the interval between axotomy and nerve suture on the success of muscle reinnervation: an experimental study in the rabbit, *Exp Neurol* 90:308, 1985.
7. Bunge RP: Some observations on the role of the Schwann cell in peripheral nerve regeneration. In Jewitt DL and McCarrol HR, Jr, editors: *Nerve repair and regeneration: its clinical and experimental basis,* St Louis, 1980, Mosby.
8. Cyriax J: *Textbook of orthopedic medicine,* ed 8, London, 1982, Bailliere Tindall.
9. Doyle JR: Factors affecting clinical results of nerve suture. In Jewitt DL and McCarrol HR Jr, editors: *Nerve repair and regeneration: its clinical and experimental basis,* St Louis, 1980, Mosby.
10. Finkelstein DI and others: Recovery of muscle after different periods of denervation and treatments, *Muscle Nerve* 16:769, 1993.
11. Forester R: *Clayton's electrotherapy,* ed 8, London, 1981, Bailliere Tindall.
12. Gordon T and Stein RB: Time course and extent of recovery in reinnervated motor units of cats triceps surae muscles, *J Physiol* 323:307, 1982.
13. Gordon T and others: Recovery potential of muscle after partial denervation: a comparison between rats and humans, *Brain Res Bull* 30:477, 1993.
14. Grey EG and Carr GL: An experimental study of factors responsible for noninfectious bone atrophy, *Bull John Hopkins Hosp* 26:381, 1915.
15. Gutmann E: Effect of delay of innervation on recovery of muscle after nerve lesions, *J Neurophysiol* 11:279, 1948.
16. Gutmann E and Guttmann L: Effects of electrotherapy on denervated muscle in rabbits, *Lancet* 1:169, 1942.
17. Holmes W and Young JZ: Nerve regeneration after immediate and delayed suture, *J Anat* 77:63, 1943.
18. Jansen JKS and others: Hyperinnervation of skeletal muscle fibers: dependence on muscle activity, *Science* 181:599, 1973.
19. Kaltenborn F: *Mobilization of the extremity joints: examination and basic treatment techniques,* Oslo, 1980, Olof Norlis Bokhandel.
20. Kopell HP and Thompson WAL: *Peripheral entrapment neuropathies,* Baltimore, 1963, Williams & Wilkins.
21. Kottke FV: The rationale for prolonged stretching for correction of shortening of connective tissue, *Arch Phys Med Rehabil* 47:345, 1966.
22. Landon DN and Hall S: The myelinated nerve fiber. In Landon DN, editor: *The peripheral nerve,* 1975, Chapman & Hall.
23. Lester RL and others: Intrinsic reinnervation—myth or reality? *J Hand Surg* 18B:454, 1993.
24. Lieber RL: *Skeletal muscle structure and function: implications for rehabilitation and sports medicine,* Baltimore, 1993, Williams & Wilkins.
25. Lomo T and Rosenthal J: Control of ACh sensitivity by muscle activity in the rat, *J Physiol* 221:493, 1972.
26. Magee D: *Orthopedic physical assessment,* ed 2, Philadelphia, 1992, WB Saunders.
27. Mather LH: *The peripheral nervous system: structure, function and clinical correlations,* Reading, 1985, Addison-Wesley.
28. Miyamoto Y and others: Nerve grafting and nerve regeneration. In Sobue I, editor: *Peripheral neuropathy,* Oxford, 1983, Excerpta Medica.
29. Pleasure D: Axoplasmic transport. In Sumner AJ, editor: *The physiology of peripheral nerve disease,* Philadelphia, 1980, WB Saunders.
30. Politis MJ: The role of distal nerve stumps in guiding regenerating fibers. In Sobue I, editor: *Peripheral neuropathy,* Oxford, 1983, Excerpta Medica.
31. Pollock LV: Electrotherapy in experimentally induced lesions of peripheral nerves, *Arch Phys Med Rehabil* 32:377, 1951.
32. Pratt NE: Neurovascular entrapment in the regions of the shoulder and posterior triangle of the neck, *Phys Ther* 66:12, 1986.
33. Rancho Los Amigos Rehabilitation Engineering Center: *Annual report of progress to the rehabilitation services administration,* Washington, DC, 1979, US Department of Health, Education and Welfare.
34. Ring PA: Paralytic bone lengthening following poliomyelitis, *Lancet* 2:551, 1958.
35. Ring PA: The influence of the nervous system upon the growth of bones, *J Bone Joint Surg* 43B:121, 1961.
36. Sanes JR and Covault J: Axon guidance during reinnervation of skeletal muscle, *Trends Neurosci* 8:523, 1985.
37. Schaumberg HH, Spencer PS, and Thomas PK: *Disorders of peripheral nerves,* Philadelphia, 1983, FA Davis.
38. Seddon HJ: Three types of nerve injury, *Brain* 66:237, 1943.
39. Seddon HJ: *Surgical disorders of the peripheral nerves,* New York, 1972, Churchill Livingstone.
40. Seltzer ME: Regeneration of peripheral nerve. In Sumner AJ, editor: *The physiology of peripheral nerve disease,* Philadelphia, 1980, WB Saunders.
41. Stillwell GK: Rehabilitation procedures. In Dyck PJ, editor: *Peripheral neuropathy,* ed 2, Philadelphia, 1984, WB Saunders.
42. Stoddard A: *Manual of osteopathic techniques,* ed 3, London, 1980, Hutchinson & Company.
43. Sullivan P: *An integrated approach to therapeutic exercise,* Reston, 1982, Reston Publishing.
44. Sunderlund S: *Nerves and nerve injuries,* ed 2, Baltimore, 1978, Williams & Wilkins.
45. Trueba JL and others: Problems concerning the diagnosis, clinical course and prognosis of localized neuropathies. In Refsum SA and others, editors: *International conference on peripheral neuropathies,* Oxford, 1982, Excerpta Medica.
46. Weller RO and Cervos-Navarro J: *Pathology of peripheral nerves,* Woburn, 1977, Butterworths.
47. Wolf SL: *Electrotherapy: clinics in physical therapy,* New York, 1981, Churchill Livingstone.

CHAPTER 13

Neuromuscular Diseases

Ann Hallum

KEY TERMS

amyotrophic lateral
  sclerosis (ALS)
disuse atrophy
polyradiculoneuropathy

Guillain-Barré
  syndrome (GBS)
overwork damage
Duchenne muscular
  dystrophy (DMD)

LEARNING OBJECTIVES

After reviewing this chapter the student/therapist will:

1. Describe the basic pathology and medical treatment of amyotrophic lateral sclerosis, Guillain-Barré syndrome and Duchenne muscular dystrophy.
2. Describe the current goals and treatment program for each condition.
3. Describe the "safe" exercise windows related to disuse atrophy and exercise (overwork) damage.
4. Be able to apply treatment concepts discussed in this chapter to other neuromuscular diseases.

This chapter traces the connections between the central nervous system (CNS) and muscle tissue using three disorders, amyotrophic lateral sclerosis (ALS), which affects upper and lower motor neurons; Guillain-Barré syndrome (GBS), which affects the peripheral nervous system, and Duchenne muscular dystrophy (DMD), with affects the muscle. The upper motor neurons that are affected in ALS originate in the motor cortex of the brain (Betz cells). These upper motor neuron axons descend via the corticobulbar and corticospinal tracts to synapse with lower motor neurons (primary motor neurons) in the brainstem and spinal cord (anterior horn cells). From the lower motor neuron, the axon runs within the peripheral nerve, which includes motor and sensory fibers, to synapse with the muscle fibers innervated by that nerve. Depending on the site of the pathology, neuromuscular diseases can be classified as neurogenic or myopathic. ALS and GBS are neurogenic disorders; DMD is a primary myopathy (Fig. 13-1.)

AMYOTROPHIC LATERAL SCLEROSIS
Background information

Amyotrophic lateral sclerosis (ALS), commonly known in the United States as "Lou Gehrig's disease," is a degenerative disease affecting both the upper and lower motor neurons. Massive loss of anterior horn cells of the spinal cord and the motor cranial nerve nuclei in the lower brainstem results in muscle atrophy and weakness (amyotrophic). Demyelination and gliosis of the corticospinal

Neuromuscular diseases

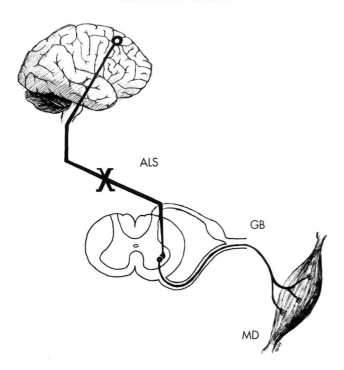

Fig. 13-1. Primary sites of pathology of amyotrophic lateral sclerosis, Guillain Barré syndrome and Duchenne muscular dystrophy.

tracts and corticobulbar tracts caused by degeneration of the Betz cells in the motor cortex result in upper motor neuron symptoms (lateral sclerosis). Diagnosis of ALS depends primarily on the identification of a constellation of motor system changes. Little is known about the early changes occuring in the motor neurons; however, histologically, there is extensive neuronal loss with astrocytic gliosis. Some neurons seem to remain intact, whereas others show nonspecific cytoplasmic and nuclear shrinkage associated with the accumulation of lipofuscin.[4,13]

The etiology of ALS is unknown; however, numerous theories have been proposed. Because of its similarity to poliomyelitis virus, which attacks the anterior horn cells, a viral origin for ALS has been proposed, but has not been identified. Toxic theories related to increased lead and aluminum levels and abnormalities in concentration in calcium and magnesium levels also have been suggested. Other theories suggest that ALS may be related to an accelerated form of normal aging, the loss of androgen receptors in motor neurons, a lack of neurotrophic hormone, abnormal DNA in motor neuron, or problems with thyrotropin-releasing hormone. More recently, excitotoxicity (decreased levels of glutamate in ALS spinal cord with increase in intracellular calcium) and autoimmunity (antibody to calcium channels leading to motoneuron destruction) have been implicated.[4]

ALS is the most common form of motor neuron disease,

with an incidence of approximately 1 to 2 per 100,000. Mean age of onset is 57 years,[1] with two thirds of patients being between 50 and 70 years at time of onset. Men are affected 1.5 to 2 times more frequently than women.[4] Ninety percent to 95% of cases are classified as sporadic, with approximately 5% to 10% of cases classified as having a familial relationship. ALS occurs about as often as muscular dystrophy and is three times more common than myasthenia gravis.[1]

Clinical presentation

No laboratory test is available to confirm a diagnosis of ALS, although creatine phosphokinase levels are elevated in about 70% of patients. Instead the diagnosis must be made based on recognition of a clinical pattern or syndrome. The earliest and first symptom of ALS in 90% of patients is weakness occurring in any striated muscle or group of muscles. The weakness spreads over time to include musculature throughout the body. The onset of ALS is incidious. Most patients are not aware of the changes or have accommodated to the changes until they have difficulty with a functional activity, such as tying shoes or climbing stairs. Physical examination usually demonstrates more widespread weakness and atrophy than reported by the patient.[1,4,18] By the time most patients complain of weakness, they have lost approximately 80% of their motor neurons in the areas of weakness. This demonstrates the plasticity of the nervous system and its drive to adapt to meet functional goals. Succeeding symptoms of weakness in other muscle(s) depend on the continued loss of motor neurons to the 20% threshold needed for perception of weakness.[3,34]

Another common presenting complaint is cramping and muscle twitching within specific muscles or muscle groups that accompanies weakness. Electrophysiological studies confirm presence of widespread lower motor neuron disease without peripheral neuropathy or polyradiculopathy. The typical electromyographic (EMG) study shows spontaneous fibrillations and fasciculations with giant or large unit spikes on voluntary activity. Nerve conduction velocities are usually within normal limits.[4]

Although the atrophy and weakness component of ALS is most obvious, 80% or more of patients show clinical evidence of pyramidal tract dysfunction (i.e., hyperreflexia, spasticity, and Babinsky and Hoffman reflexes).[18] Although in some cases, the upper motor neuron signs may be absent clinically, Chou[6] has shown on autopsy that significant involvement may be present despite the lack of clinical evidence.

The pattern of ALS onset is highly varied, with several patterns identified by primary area of onset. Lower extremity onset is slightly more common than upper extremity onset, which is more common than bulbar onset. Some patients show initial symptoms in distal musculature of upper and lower extremities. A significant diagnostic feature of the pattern of disease is the asymmetry of the weakness and the sparing of some muscle fibers even in highly atrophied muscles. For example, a patient may present with weakness of the right intrinsics and shoulder musculature or weakness of the left anterior tibial muscles. Cranial nerve nuclei deficits, heralded by tongue fasciculations and weakness, facial and palatal weakness, and swallowing difficulties, may be noted; but oculomotor nuclei are almost always spared as are bowel and bladder function.[4] Despite the pattern of onset, however, the eventual course of the illness is similar in most patients with an unremitting spread of weakness to other muscle groups leading to total paralysis of spinal muscula-ture and muscles innervated by the cranial nerves. Death is usually related to respiratory failure.[28] Cognitive functions are not affected, but most patients and their families must undergo considerable psychological adjustments related to the disease.

A consistent diagnostic criterion for ALS has been the absence of sensory involvement. Mulder and Kurland,[18] however, have reported that 20% of their patients show signs of sensory dysfunction. Several investigators have shown possible dysfunction in somatosensory evoked potentials transmitted in the posterior columns.[18,35] In addition to the possible sensory deficits, subclinical abnormalities of the autonomic nervous system (ANS), both sympathetic and parasympathetic, have also been identified in a sample of 74 patients using a quantitative sudomotor axon reflex test (sweat testing) and parasympathetic vascular reflex testing of heart rate change during Valsalva and deep breathing. Thirty-eight percent of patients showed symptoms of autonomic dysfunction. The authors suggested that the problems appear to be associated with atrophy and bulbar changes and that patients with ANS dysfunction seemed to have a faster rate of progression.[7]

In a multisite study of 167 patients with ALS, subjects were followed for 2 years on a monthly basis with 42 strength and functional assessments. Data confirmed find-ings of other studies that showed a more rapid loss of strength in the upper extremities than the lower extremities. There was no difference between men or women in the rate of progression. In contrast to other studies, results indicated that older patients did not show a faster rate of deterioration, although they did enter the study in a weaker, more debilitated state which may be related to their apparent shorter disease course.[28] In an ongoing study using monthly questionnaires, direct patient interviews, record reviews, physician interviews, and family member interviews, Brooks and others[3] followed 702 patients with ALS. Their findings suggest that spread of neuronal degeneration occurred more quickly to adjacent areas than to noncontiguous areas. The spread to adjacent areas was more rapid at the brainstem, cervical, and lumbar regions. Limb involvement after bulbar onset was more aggressive in men than in women.[3]

Several studies have focused on developing methods to assess the natural history of the progression of ALS so that medical and supportive treatment planning and interventions

can be instituted. Hillel and others[12] have developed an Amyotrophic Lateral Sclerosis Severity Scale for rapid functional assessment of disease stage. Their 10-point ordinal scale allows the clinician to score patients in four categories of function: speech, swallowing, lower extremity, and upper extremity (see accompanying box).[12] (Note: A four-point scale of severity is currently being used in ALS clinical drug traits.) See Brooks and others[3] and Pradas and others[25] for information on natural history of ALS and its importance in the design of clinical treatment trials.

Prognosis

In almost all cases, ALS progresses relentlessly and leads to death from respiratory failure. The rate of progression seems to be consistent within each patient but varies considerably between patients. Patients with an initial onset of bulbar (dysarthria, dysphagia) and respiratory weakness (dyspnea) tend to have a more rapid progression to death than patients whose weakness begins in the distal extremi-ties.[28] Caroscio[4] reported that in a study of 397 patients with ALS, the median survival time was 4.08 years after onset of symptoms with a shortening of median survival time with increasing age at onset.[4] A small number of patients have lived for 15 to 20 years after onset. Although time of onset is determined primarily by the patients' recognition of the disease onset, autopsies of patients who have died from respiratory failure soon after diagnosis have shown evidence of more widespread disease in the skeletal musculature even though there was no clinical evidence of skeletal muscle involvement.[18]

Medical management

There is no known cure for ALS and to date there is no definitive treatment. Because of the apparent hopelessness of the diagnosis, many physicians, especially those not asso-ciated with major medical centers having neuromuscular disease units, do not refer patients with ALS for services. In a survey of ALS patients, 90% stated that their referring neurologists made no referrals or follow-up appointments. Most patients had been told to expect death within 1 to 3 years, although evidence shows that the median life span is approximately 4 years. Some physicians are concerned that providing aggressive treatment will only increase or prolong the patient's distress.[15] Other physicians, however, feel that withholding care and symptom relief seriously impairs the patient's quality of life. The fact is supportive medical and therapy interventions are available.

Muscle spasms. Some patients experience muscle cramps and spasms related to the upper motor neuron changes. Although most spasms can be relieved with stretching or increased movement, some patients require medications such as quinine or baclofen to relieve symptoms (see Chapter 33). Because many patients have compromised respiratory function, the physician must take great care when prescribing the medication and dosage. Patients should be

Amyotrophic lateral sclerosis severity scale: lower extremity, upper extremity, speech, swallowing

Lower extremities (walking)

	Normal	
10	Normal ambulation	Patient denies any weakness or fatigue; examination detects no abnormality.
9	Fatigue suspected	Patient suspects weakness or fatigue in lower extremities during exertion.
	Early ambulation difficulties	
8	Difficulty with uneven terrain	Difficulty and fatigue when walking long distances, climbing stairs, and walking over uneven ground (even thick carpet).
7	Observed changes in gait	Noticeable change in gait; pulls on railings when climbing stairs; may use leg brace.
	Walks with assistance	
6	Walks with mechanical device	Needs or uses cane, walker, or assistant to walk; probably uses wheelchair away from home.
5	Walks with mechanical device and assistant	Does not attempt to walk without attendant; ambulation limited to less than 50 ft; avoids stairs.
	Functional movement only	
4	Able to support	At best, can shuffle a few steps with the help of an attendant for transfers.
3	Purposeful leg movements	Unable to take steps, but can position legs to assist attendant in transfers; moves legs purposely to maintain mobility in bed.
	No purposeful leg movement	
2	Minimal movement	Minimal movement of one or both legs; cannot reposition legs independently.
1	Paralysis	Flaccid paralysis; cannot move lower extremities (except, perhaps, to close inspection).

Upper extremities (dressing and hygiene)

	Normal function	
10	Normal function	Patient denies any weakness or unusual fatigue of upper extremities, examination demonstrates no abnormality.
9	Suspected fatigue	Patient suspects fatigue in upper extremities during exertion; cannot sustain work for as long as normal; atrophy not evident on examination.
	Independent and complete self-care	
8	Slow self-care	Dressing and hygiene performed more slowly than usual.
7	Effortful self-care performance	Requires significantly more time (usually double or more) and effort to accomplish self-care; weakness is apparent on examination.
	Intermittent assistance	
6	Mostly independent	Handles most aspects of dressing and hygiene alone; adapts by resting, modifying (electric razor) or avoiding some tasks; requires assistance for fine motor tasks, e.g., buttons, tie.
5	Partial independence independent	Handles some aspects of dressing and hygiene alone; however, routinely requires assistance for many tasks such as make-up, combing, shaving.
	Needs attendant for self-care	
4	Attendant assists patient	Attendant must be present for dressing and hygiene; patient performs the majority of each task with the assistance of the attendant.
3	Patient assists attendant	The attendant directs the patient for almost all tasks; the patient moves in a purposeful manner to assist the attendant; does not initiate self-care.
	Total dependence	
2	Minimal movement	Minimal movement of one or both arms; cannot reposition arms.
1	Paralysis	Flaccid paralysis; unable to move upper extremities (except, perhaps to close inspection).

Amyotrophic lateral sclerosis severity scale: lower extremity, upper extremity, speech, swallowing—cont'd

Speech

Normal Speech Processes

10 Normal speech — Patient denies any difficulty speaking; examination demonstrates no abnormality.

9 Nominal speech abnormalities — Only the patient or spouse notices speech has changed, maintains normal rate and volume.

Detectable speech disturbance

8 Perceived speech changes — Speech changes are noted by others, especially during fatigue or stress; rate of speech remains essentially normal.

7 Obvious speech abnormalities — Speech is consistently impaired, affected are rate, articulation, and resonance, remains easily understood.

Intelligible with repeating

6 Repeats message on occasion — Rate is much slower, repeats specific words in adverse listening situation; does not limit complexity or length of messages.

5 Frequent repeating required — Speech is slow and labored; extensive repetition or a 'translator' is commonly used, patient probably limits the complexity or length or messages.

Speech combined with nonvocal communication

4 Speech plus nonverbal communication — Speech is used in response to questions; intelligibility problems *need* to be resolved by writing or a spokesman.

3 Limits speech to one word responses — Vocalizes one word responses beyond yes/no; otherwise writes or uses a spokesman; initiates communication nonvocally.

Loss of useful speech

2 Vocalizes for emotional expression — Uses vocal inflection to express emotion, affirmation, and negation.

1 Nonvocal — Vocalization is effortful, limited in duration, and rarely attempted; may vocalize for crying or pain.

X Tracheostomy

Swallowing

Normal eating habits

10 Normal swallowing — Patient denies any difficulty chewing or swallowing; examination demonstrates no abnormality.

9 Nominal abnormality — Only patient notices slight indicators such as food lodging in the recesses of the mouth or sticking in the throat.

Early eating problems

8 Minor swallowing problems — Complains of some swallowing difficulties; maintains essentially a regular diet; isolated choking episodes.

7 Prolonged times/smaller bite size — Meal time has significantly increased and smaller bite sizes are necessary; must concentrate on swallowing thin liquids.

Dietary consistency changes

6 Soft diet — Diet is limited primarily to soft foods; requires some special meal preparation.

5 Liquefied diet — Oral intake adequate; nutrition limited primarily to liquefied diet; adequate thin liquid intake usually a problem; may force self to eat.

Needs tube feeding

4 Supplemental tube feedings — Oral intake alone no longer adequate; patient uses or *needs* a tube to supplement intake; patient continues to take significant (greater than 50%) nutrition orally.

3 Tube feeding with occasional oral nutrition — Primary nutrition and hydration accomplished by tube; receives less than 50% nutrition orally.

No oral feeding

2 Secretions managed with aspirator and/or medications — Cannot safely manage any oral intake; secretions managed with aspirator and/or medications; swallows reflexively.

1 Aspiration of secretions — Secretions cannot be managed noninvasively; rarely swallows.

Adapted with permission. Hillel AP and others: *Neuroepidemiology* 8:142-150, 1989.

instructed to keep a daily reporting log of the effectiveness of the medication so that the dosage can be adjusted.[20]

Nutrition. The popular press has reported on nutritional cures for ALS. To date, however, nutritional therapy has not been found effective in clinical trials. Norris and Denys[20] reported on a number of studies to determine the effectiveness of several nutrients, including vitamin E, octacosanol (long-chain alcohols reported by the ALS Society of America as helping some patients) and intravenous amino acids. They concluded that no nutritional deficiencies are related to the onset of ALS and that dietary supplements have no effect on the course of the disease. They also caution that national publicity and unwarranted anecdotal claims about improvement in function are based on a placebo effect because of the uneven progression of the disease in some patients.

Although nutritional treatment is not effective in changing the course of the disease, a nutritious diet and adequate calories must be maintained. This may be quite difficult in patients who must be fed because of quadriplegia, and particularly in patients with dysphagia. The patient should be referred for a dietary consult in cooperation with the therapist consulting on feeding and swallowing to determine the most nutritious diet possible.

Dysphagia. Patients with severe dysphagia who are no longer able to consume nutrients orally because of motor control problems and aspiration may need feedings via nasogastric tube or percutaneous gastrostomy depending on the patient's wishes for long-term care. Many patients with dysphagia also have severe problems with management of their saliva (sialorrhea) (see Chapter 26). Normal average flow is about 1 ml/minute from the parotid, submaxillary, sublingual, and minor salivary glands. With stimulation this amount can increase to 8 ml/minute. If a patient has difficulty transporting saliva back to the oropharynx for swallowing, choking and drooling are common. This is very disconcerting to a person who must constantly wipe his or her mouth or have someone do it for him or her.

In addition, secretions are also thickened because of dehydration. With pooling of the thickened saliva, the possibility of aspiration is increased. Viscosity of saliva can best be treated by hydration and in some cases with papaya tablets or papase, the enzyme in meat tenderizer.[30] Drugs such as decongestants, antidepressant drugs with anticholinergic side effects, and atropine-type drugs have been used to help control the amount of saliva. In extreme cases, various surgical procedures, such as ligation of the salivary gland ducts, severing the parasympathetic supply to the salivary glands, and excision of the salivary glands, have been used effectively with patients for whom constant drooling and aspiration are major problems.[10,24]

The progressive loss of swallowing ability accounts for considerable misery in the patient with advanced ALS, and it must be dealt with aggressively (see Chapters 6 and 26).[5] Aspiration can be the cause of sudden death in the patient

with ALS, although it is not common. With mild aspiration problems in a patient who is still able and wants to eat, dietary changes and instruction in swallowing techniques by speech, occupational, and/or physical therapists can be very helpful. If aspiration cannot be controlled, surgical interventions are sometimes necessary to make the patient's life more comfortable. Tracheostomy is often performed because it provides easy access for suctioning if aspiration occurs. Other invasive options that definitely prevent aspiration but interfere with the patient's ability to speak if still possible, are laryngectomy, tracheal diversion and epiglottic "sewdown."[11,21]

Respiratory care. Within the last 10 to 15 years, respiratory management of the patient with ALS has changed dramatically. Today, despite quadriplegia and respiratory muscle paralysis, many patients can choose long-term mechanical ventilation to prolong life. Although in the initial stages of ALS, most patients indicate that they would not want prolonged respirator dependence at home, patients may change their minds as they adapt to the disease restrictions.[17] Oliver[22] states that when counseling patients about outcome and treatment options, the "aim should be to avoid inappropriate treatment, which could cause harm to the patient, may merely prolong a poor quality of life and could lead to further distress (p. 15)." Decisions about long-term respirator use should be made by the patient and involved family, friends, or partners with input from the interdisciplinary team caring for the patient. Discussions of preferred long-term care options should be revisited as the patient's condition changes. Physicians and health care workers who may have input to the patient and family must be aware of their own feelings and beliefs about prolonging life. For example, a healthy physician or therapist who values control and an active life-style may envision a life on a ventilator as intolerable and pass that value on to the patient who may or may not have the same needs. The patient's decision or change in decision must be respected by the medical team involved in care. In medical centers using a team approach, patients and families may find support by meeting with counselors or peers with ALS who are making or have made decisions about long-term ventilator care.

If a patient decides that home ventilation is a reasonable option, it can be helpful for those involved to visit another patient who is using in-home mechanical ventilation (HMV).[24] Because the decision for home ventilation affects the life not only of the patient, but also the patient's spouse, children and extended family who may be responsible for some aspects of home care, or whose lives may be affected by the presence of in-home nurses or attendants, the decision for HMV should not be taken lightly. Extensive preparation, ongoing support, and respite options for caregivers are necessary if HMV is to be successful. Success of HMV also depends on such variables as third-party payment for home care equipment and nurse/attendant staffing, working status of the partner/spouse, age and physical fitness of spouse and children, pre-ALS family psychosocial interactions, and financial factors. HMV should be viewed as long-term, often extending for more than 1 year. In a Kaiser Foundation Hospital program from 1987 to 1992, 34 patients with ALS were discharged to HMV. On average, the patients were on the ventilator 23 hours/day and needed 24 hour, 7-day a week care (at least three trained caregivers per week). Eighty-seven percent of the patients were alive at the end of one year, 58% at 3 years, and 33% at the end of 5 years. Less than 25% of the ALS patients in the Kaiser study had elected HMV in advance of the decision to begin ventilator assistance.[24]

Approximately half the patients with ALS experience dyspnea as a secondary symptom of acute respiratory illness. When a patient presents with dyspnea, concurrent infection and disease that might respond to medication or short-term respiratory support measures must be ruled out and treatment or nontreatment, as desired by the patient, should be initiated. Scheduled, serial evaluations of respiratory status are essential so that the patient and the treatment team can make informed decisions about appropriate treatment relative to both acute illnesses and progressive respiratory difficulties.

Physiological factors indicating respiratory failure are vital capacity and maximum voluntary inspiratory and expiratory ventilation of less than or equal to 30% of predicted, hypoxemia, mild hypercapnea, and acidosis. Clinical signs are dyspnea with exertion or lying supine, weak or ineffective cough, tachycardia (also signs of pulmonary infection: fever, tachypnea, tachycardia), changes in sleep pattern, daytime sleepiness, mood changes, and morning headaches. If the dyspnea is a symptom of disease progression, the patient and family must be involved in the long-term care decisions related to instituting mechanical assistance under either emergency situations or in response to gradual deterioration. This discussion should occur before the patient develops respiratory failure (see section on psychosocial issues). Acute respiratory failure can be so frightening, however, that few patients or family members are prepared to forego intubation and artificial ventilation during the emergency. If patients have stated that they do not want mechanical ventilation, appropriate use of medications such as morphine can markedly control the person's sense of air hunger[22] during the dying process.

Progressive respiratory changes. Numerous measures can be taken to reduce respiratory discomfort before the decision for permanent ventilation must be made. Progressive respiratory failure is related to primary diaphragmatic, intercostal, and accessory respiratory muscle weakness; decreased pulmonary compliance; a weak cough; and bulbar symptoms such as a decreased gag reflex with aspiration.

Depending on the role of the physical therapist in a specific type of treatment facility—medical center, community or rural hospital or clinic—physical therapists may be involved in the treatment of respiratory changes. Postural drainage techniques with cough facilitation (suctioning if necessary) can be very helpful, especially during acute respiratory illnesses. The patient also should be taught breathing exercises, chest stretching, and incentive spirometry techniques.[16] If possible an assessment of the home environment might be helpful to identify sleeping positions and energy conservation techniques that could be incorporated into the patient's daily life. When home nursing assistance or attendants are available, they should be taught to carry out the postural drainage and breathing exercise program with the patient because few in-home care specialists are skilled at these specific techniques.

Oxygen at 2 liters or less can be used intermittently at home as can intermittent positive-pressure breathing support. Hypoventilation with a decline in oxygen saturation is common during sleeping and often results in morning confusion and irritability. In some cases, intermittent nasal ventilation,[9] the use of a Cuirass respirator (external chest unit providing intermittent negative pressure), or exsufflation or pneumobelt may be helpful.[4,24]

Therapeutic management

When determining therapeutic goals and treatment, one must consider the rate of the patient's disease progression, the extent and areas of involvement, and the stage of illness. Patients with severe respiratory and bulbar complications may not benefit as greatly from active exercise programs. With guidance and environmental adaptations, however, patients with slowly progressing weakness may be able to continue many of their activities of daily living for an extended number of years. In the final stages of the disease when the patient is bedridden, physical therapy interventions, such as stretching, will not be effective. The patient may benefit, however, from efforts to decrease muscle and joint pain related to immobility. The efficacy of therapeutic interventions is also related to the timing of interventions, the motivation and persistence of the patient in carrying out the program,[36] and support from family members.

Assessment. The extent of the therapeutic assessment of a patient with ALS depends somewhat on whether the therapist is working as a member of a neuromuscular team or as an independent or clinic-based therapist receiving a referral to evaluate and treat. The physical and occupational therapists working as team members may have a more circumscribed role related to gross motor function and activities of daily living (ADL), with other consultants focusing on bulbar, respiratory, and environmental adjustments. The therapist working in a facility without a neuromuscular disease clinic or in a community or rural environment, however, should be aware of the need to carry out a broader based assessment.

If possible, the therapist should contact the patient before the initial consult and request that the patient keep an activity log for 5 days. If an early contact is not possible, the therapist can assign that task during the initial session. The log should include 15-minute time increments in which the patient can jot down what he or she was doing during a specific time period. Space also should be included to indicate whether the patient was experiencing fatigue or pain during the activity. An example of an activity log and how it is used is shown in Fig. 13-2.

The evaluation will vary depending on the patient's situation; however, a typical initial assessment might include:

1. Review of the patient's medical and activity record.
2. Discussion of the patient's life-style, daily living tasks, fatigability, safety issues, psychosocial support issues (family and agencies), and patient goals.
3. Baseline testing of muscle strength (MMT or dynometer testing if standards are clear and can be replicated) and range of motion assessment (ROM).
4. Assessment of functional activity level. (It is preferable to use one of the standardized tests, or scc Table 13-1.)

Name: J. Costello

DATE: 5-10-92
DAY: Sun.

DAILY ACTIVITY LOG

Instructions: 1) In column I write in what you are doing during the 24 hour period. You may draw a line or an arrow to indicate when the activity occurs for more than one 15 minute time period.

2) In column II indicate whether you are lying down, sitting, standing, or moving actively (walking, etc.) during the activity.

3) In column III on a 10 point scale, indicate how fatigued you feel while performing the activity (No fatigue = 0, extreme fatigue = 10.)

4) In column IV indicate where you feel pain if any and score the intensity on a 10 point scale (No pain = 0, extreme pain = 10.)

Try to fill out your log three or four times a day so you don't forget what you have been doing. An example is shown below.

	I	II	III	IV	
	What are you doing? Type of activity	What position are you in (lying, sitting, standing, moving)	Fatigue level 0 - 10	Pain	
				Location	Intensity 0 - 10
5:30 AM	Sleep	lying	0		
45					
6:00					
15					
30	Bathroom shave etc	Standing	2	neck	3
45					
7:00					
15	Breakfast	Sitting	3	neck	3
30					
45					
8:00	Reading	sitting	3	neck shoulder	3
15					
30					
45	Walk	Standing, moving	4	neck	2
9:00					
15	Nap	lying	2	neck hips.	4
30					
45					
10:00	Reading/TV	Sitting	4	neck hips.	3
15					
30					
45					
11:00					

Fig. 13-2. Example of a log for monitoring activity level of patients with amyotrophic lateral sclerosis.

Table 13-1. Common physical findings of bulbar amyotrophic lateral sclerosis

Anatomic site	Innervation	Method of evaluation	Progression of findings	Progression of symptoms
Group I Tongue	XII	Inspect for fasciculations at rest	Fasciculations evident	Dysarthria (disturbance of lingual-alveolar consonants "t," "d," "l," etc.)
		Range of motion	Slow, incomplete lateral movements	Inability to clear buccal sulcus of food
			Loss of lateral force	Marked dysarthria (slow rate and slurring of consonants)
			Unable to reach palate with mouth open	
		Protrusion	Unable to protrude beyond lips	Oral transport difficulties Dietary changes
		Perform rapid lateral motion	Unable to protrude beyond incisors	Speech intelligiblity problems
			Atrophy evident	
			Paralysis	
Lips	VII	Suck on gloved finger	Lack of suction	Inability to whistle
		Smile or curl lips over teeth	Inability to complete a seal	Inability to use a straw
		Hold seal and blow out cheeks	Inability to purse lips	Dysarthria (loss of bilabial consonants "p" and "b")
				Drooling
Group 2 Palate	V,X,XI	Visual examination during phonation and stimulation of gag	Unsustained or slow palatal elevation	Dysarthria (hypernasal speech)
		Puff out cheeks to check for nasal air leak (hold lips closed if necessary)	Palate fails to reach Pasavant's ridge	Inability to use a straw
			Absence of palatal movement	Nasal air emission during speech
				Nasopharyngeal reflex on swallowing
Muscles of mastication Masseter/temporalis	V	Palpate during bite Visual inspection for wasting	Noticeable wasting	Chewing fatigue
				Elimination of specific, tough foods from diet
				Dietary changes (soft foods and liquids)
			Unable to palpate contraction	Mouth breathing and drying of secretions
Pterygoids		Move jaw from side to side	No observable lateral jaw movement	Unable to use dentures
Group 3 Neck and shoulder Trapezius	XI	Hold arm in coronal plane, hand externally rotated, as patient elevates arm against resistance while the trapezius is palpated	Progressive inability to raise the arm (often asymmetrical weakness)	Inability to comb hair Inability to perform facial grooming

Adapted with permission from Hillel AD and Miller RM: *Head Neck* 11(1):51-59, 1989.

Continued.

Table 13-1. Common physical findings of bulbar amyotrophic lateral sclerosis—cont'd

Anatomic site	Innervation	Method of evaluation	Progression of findings	Progression of symptoms
Group 3–cont'd				
Sternocleido-mastoid (SCM) or mounted head support		Turn the head against resistance applied to patient's opposite chin	Progressive weakness in turning the head against resistance (often asymmetrical)	Inability to lift head when supine Inability to support head while sitting. Wears neck collar, has weakness
Vocal cords	X	Mirror or fiberoptic laryngoscopy	Progressive loss of abduction of vocal cords: mild abductor weakness, near midline paralysis Paradoxical vocal cord movement	Strained-strangled voice Short of breath (SOB) (stridor usually not present due to impaired respiratory function)
Group 4				
Extraocular muscles	III,IV,VI	Assessment of extra-ocular movements	Limitation of extraocular movement	Limitation of gaze
Respiratory group				
Diaphragm	$C_{3,4,5}$	Pulmonary Function Test (PFTs) or hand-held respirometer for vital capacity	Diminishing vital capacity: 1.5-2.0 liters	SOB during exertion if patient has remained active
Intercostal	C_7-L_3			
Accessory mm of respiration	VII,XI,XII, C_{5-8}	Cough Sustain a vowel Blow against a tissue	1.0-1.5 liters 0.5-1.0 liters	Weak cough Change in speech phrasing (5-10 syllables per breath) Speech produced in syllable-by-syllable fashion (if vocal) SOB on swallowing

5. Assessment of pain (type, site and intensity; use body chart and subjective pain scale). Identify what makes pain worse, better.

6. Assessment of bulbar and respiratory function. (For an in-depth evaluation of bulbar function, the patient should be referred to an ear, nose and throat clinic or communications disorders clinic.) See Table 13-1 for bulbar and respiratory evaluation suggestions.

Treatment. Treatment goals and the recommended exercise/activity program must be based on the patient's personal goals. Treatment goals are often a difficult area for physical therapists to discuss with the patient because both know that the disease is progressive despite interventions. It is easy and most common for the patient and therapist to assume that because nothing can be done to "cure" the disease, it is kinder not to make additional demands on a patient who is already coping with daily loss. Some feel that exercise programs may create false hopes that exercise will delay progression. The literature on rehabilitation in neuro-muscular disorders, however, suggests that patients with ALS can benefit from carefully designed exercise and activity programs.

The general, broad goals for both patient and therapist are related to maintaining maximal independence in daily living for as long as possible. More specific therapeutic goals are (1) maintenance of maximal muscle strength within limits imposed by ALS and (2) prevention and minimization of secondary consequences of the disease such as contractures, thrombophlebitis, decubiti, and respiratory infections.[14,36]

When designing a treatment program, the physical therapist should know what the patient has been told about the disease process and the expected course of symptom development. If diagnostic and prognostic information is not explicit, neither therapist nor patient will be able to make appropriate goal and treatment plans. Before determining treatment goals, the therapist must consider the following:

1. The rate of the patient's disease progression
2. Distribution of weakness and spasticity, respiratory

factors leading to hypoxemia, and easy fatigability and bulbar involvement
3. Phase of the disease

Sinaki[32] has described three phases and six substages of ALS with recommended exercise levels. His work has been adapted in the accompanying box.

Two major factors to consider in stages I and II are prevention of overuse fatigue and prevention of disuse atrophy. Both patient and therapist must delicately balance the level of activity between the extremes of excessive exercise and inadequate exercise to prevent more rapid disability.

Exercise or overwork damage. The first consideration in designing a program is to "do no harm." Anecdotal evidence that muscle activity or overwork exercise can lead to a loss of muscle strength has been reported since the poliomyelitis epidemic of the 1940s and 1950s.[2] During that time physicians and therapists noted that patients with poor and fair grade muscles who exercised repeatedly or with heavy resistance following reinnervation often lost the ability to contract the muscle at all.

Reitsma[27] noted that vigorous exercise damaged muscles with less than one third of motor units functional. If more than one third of the motor units remained, exercise led to hypertrophy. Therefore the amount of strengthening attained seems to be proportional to the number of intact or undamaged motor units. Exercise at a level to elicit a training effect in normal muscle, however, may cause overwork damage in weakened, denervated muscle.

In contrast in more recent work, Sanjak and others[29] suggested that muscle damage does not necessarily result from resistance exercise testing or training, although fatigue occurs easily during both anaerobic and aerobic exercise. Exercise energy requirements during bicycle ergometry testing were greater than expected, possibly because of motor inefficiency secondary to weakness. Work capacity and Vo_2 max were decreased, but heart rate, respiratory responses, and blood pressure were within normal limits. In addition, patients in several case studies had lowered responses in force production and oxygen use related to their decreased muscle mass. Controlled case studies have shown that although the muscle may be denervating, it will respond to exercise, therefore, some form of exercise or activity that maximizes motor unit recruitment may be helpful.[8] Miller found that mild progressive resistance exercise was helpful if the patient had muscle strength in the good (4) to normal (5) range.[20]

Vignos[36] suggests that for a patient to make any gain in function, a therapist (or physician) should be prepared to accept the possible consequences of overwork weakness when establishing an exercise program. Needless to say, the therapist should carefully monitor the patient's exercise or

activity program to ensure that any decrement in strength is related to the progress of the disease rather than excessive overwork of weakened muscles. When determining the possible detrimental effects of exercise, a distinction must be made between the transient muscle fatigue that most of us feel from moderate heavy work and the prolonged, persistent decrease in muscle strength and endurance following excessive exercise of weakened muscles.[2] If a patient shows evidence of significant, persistent weakness following institution of an exercise program or persistent morning fatigue following exercise on the previous day, the therapist must carefully redesign the patient's exercise program and activity level and increase the frequency of monitoring the patient's home program.

Because the possible positive and negative effects of resistive exercises are not clear, the therapist must take an assertive yet cautious approach to exercise. Although the therapist cannot determine the number of intact motor units available to a patient or whether the patient is evoking maximal motor unit recruitment during activities, the therapist must make decisions about underwork and overwork and adjust the patient's program based on his or her response to exercise. The program must be adjusted as the disease progresses to prevent possible damage from excessive overwork and fatigue (Fig. 13-3).

Disuse atrophy. The second consideration for the therapist working with a patient with ALS is to prevent further deconditioning and **disuse atrophy** beyond the level caused specifically by the disease process. It is common for patients experiencing the decline in function of ALS to markedly decrease their activity level after diagnosis. If the patient had led a very sedentary life-style before diagnosis, the additional decrease in activity level secondary to ALS can lead quickly to marked cardiovascular deconditioning and disuse weakness. Maintenance of strength and endurance requires daily activity and repetitive muscle contractions. In normal persons, absence of muscle contraction can result in 3% to 5% decreases in muscle strength per day. If the patient's exercise level requires less than 20% of the maximal contraction strength of the muscles, a decrease in strength will occur.[19] When designing an exercise program, one must keep in mind that training for hypertrophy or prevention of atrophy in intact muscle groups depends more on the intensity of the contraction than on the duration of contraction[19] (Fig. 13-3).

Most patients need specific guidance about what type of activities and exercises they should do.[36] Although many physicians may suggest to patients that they increase their activity level, their suggestions are seldom specific. Examples of exercise advice patients have recalled are, "Try to move around as much as possible," "Walk some more," and "Be active, but don't over do it." Because it is difficult for most patients to change their typical exercise pattern even when they know it is important, referral for a physical

Exercise and rehabilitation programs for patients with ALS according to stage of disease

Phase I (independent)

STAGE I:
Patient Characteristics:
Mild weakness
Clumsiness
Ambulatory
Independent in ADLs

Treatment:
Continue normal activities or increase activities if sedentary to prevent disuse atrophy.
Begin program of ROM exercises (stretching, yoga, Thai Chi).
Add strengthening program of gentle resistance exercises to all musculature with caution not to cause overwork fatigue.
Provide psychological support as needed.

STAGE II:
Patient Characteristics:
Moderate, selective weakness
Slightly decreased independence in ADL, examples:
   difficulty climbing stairs
   difficulty raising arms or
   difficulty buttoning clothing
Ambulatory

Treatment:
Continue stretching to avoid contractures.
Continue cautious strengthening of muscles with MMT grades above F+ (3+). Monitor for overwork fatigue.
Consider orthotic support (i.e., AFOs, wrist, thumb splints).
Use adaptive equipment to facilitate ADLs.

STAGE III:
Patient Characteristics:
Severe selective weakness in ankles, wrists, and hands
Moderately decreased independence in ADLs
Get easily fatigued with long distance ambulation
Ambulatory
Slightly increased respiratory effort

Treatment:
Continue Stage II program as tolerated. Caution not to fatigue to point of decreasing patient's ADL independence.
Keep patient physically independent as long as possible through pleasurable activities, walking.
Encourage deep breathing exercises, chest stretching, postural drainage if needed.
Prescribe wheelchair standard or motorized with modifications to allow eventual reclining back with head rest, elevating legs.

Phase II (partially independent)

STAGE IV:
Patient Characteristics:
Hanging-arm syndrome with shoulder pain and sometimes edema in the hand
Wheelchair dependent
Severe lower extremity weakness (=/–spasticity)
Able to perform ADLs but fatigues easily

Treatment:
Heat, massage as indicated to control spasm.
Preventive antiedema measures.
Active assisted passive ROM exercises to the weakly supported joints—caution to support, rotate shoulder during abduction and joint accessory motions.
Encourage isometric contractions of all musculature to tolerance.
Try arm slings, overhead slings or wheelchair arm supports.
Motorized chair if patient wants to be independently mobile. Adapt controls as needed.

STAGE V:
Patient Characteristics:
Severe lower extremity weakness
Moderate to severe upper extremity weakness
Wheelchair dependent
Increasingly dependent in ADLs
Possible skin breakdown secondary to poor mobility

Treatment:
Encourage family to learn proper transfer, positioning principles, and turning techniques.
Encourage modifications at home to aid patient's mobility and independence.
Electric hospital bed with antipressure mattress.
If patient elects HMV, adapt chair to hold respirator unit.

Phase III (dependent)

STAGE VI:
Patient Characteristics:
Bedridden
Completely dependent in ADL

Treatment:
For dysphagia: soft diet long, spoons, tube feeding, percutaneous gastrostomy.
To decrease flow of accumulated saliva: medication, suction, surgery.
For dysarthria:
   palatal lifts, electronic speech amplification eye pointing electronic.
For breathing diffculty:
   clear airway, tracheostomy, respirator if elect HMV.
Medications to decrease impact of dyspnea.

Adapted with permission from Sinaki M: In Yase Y and Tsubaki T, editors: *Amyotrophic lateral sclerosis: recent advances in research and treatment*, Amsterdam, 1988, Elsevier Science.

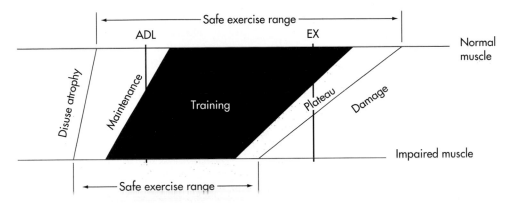

Fig. 13-3. Exercise window for normal and damaged or denervated muscles. Used with permission. Coble NO and Maloney FP: Effects of exercise on neuromuscular disease. In Maloney FP, Burks JS, and Ringel SP: *Interdisciplinary rehabilitation of multiple sclerosis and neuromuscular disorders,* New York, 1985, J.B. Lippincott Company.

therapy consult can be very helpful. In general, however, the most acceptable method of maintaining muscle strength in patients with ALS is through daily activities requiring muscular effort.[31]

The first step in working with a patient in phase I (Independent) of ALS is to determine the patient's current activity level. A program to increase activity must be designed specifically with input from the patient about willingness to participate and with knowledge of the patient's environmental situations and social support systems. In the early stages of the disease, patients should be encouraged to continue as many of prediagnosis activities as tolerated. For example, a golfer should continue to golf as long as possible. Walking the course should be encouraged if it is not too fatiguing. When walking or balance becomes difficult on uneven terrain, the golfer can use a golf cart, decrease the number of holes played, move to a par 3 course, or hit balls at a driving range. If upper extremity weakness is a major problem that interferes with swinging the club for distance shots, the player can continue playing the greens or on putting courses. Some golfers may need adaptations to club handles with sticky substances such as Velcro to prevent the club from rotating on impact.

Older, newly diagnosed patients with ALS who have led a sedentary life-style before diagnosis, should be encouraged to increase their activity level. This may include activities within or around the home such as sharing household and gardening tasks or beginning a walking program around the neighborhood. After diagnosis, some patients begin searching for in-home exercise devices such as bicycles and rowing machines. As with healthy persons who start an exercise program after the purchase of exercise equipment, it is unlikely that patients with ALS will use the equipment consistently. The "search" for a perfect exercise machine may reflect the patient's desperation to do something tangible. Without taking away the patient's motivation to

exercise, therapists can encourage patients to begin exercise programs that do not require expensive equipment, such as walking or working-out to specific exercise videos. A clever therapist can make a tape for each patient that includes stretching and strengthening exercises (using inexpensive elastic bands or small weights) with follow-up breathing, "warm-down," and relaxation exercises.

In general for most patients in the early stages of ALS, it is best to "prescribe" pleasurable, natural activities such as swimming, bowling (if shoulder strength is not yet a problem), walking, bicycling (may need three-wheeler), and yoga. Some patients prefer to exercise alone, whereas others will gain confidence and companionship by joining a group activity. It is important to listen to the patient's desires related to group activities. Among those who have been pressured to participate, the dropout rate is high. Some spouses or family members are supportive of the patient's activity needs and will join the patient in his or her regimen. If possible, the spouse and family members should be engaged in the treatment planning process.

The therapist must observe the patient completing his or her *entire* recommended activity program. It is essential to monitor the patient's response to the program because fatigue from exercise sessions can interfere with the ability to carry out other normal daily activities. If the patient becomes too exhausted at the end of a session, he or she may learn to fear exercise and may become depressed about the decreased activity status. This depression may lead to decreased activity and deconditioning.[14]

By the end of phase I (Independent) and during phase II (Partially Independent) the goal of physical therapy intervention should be to help the patient adapt to limitations imposed by weakness and spasticity, an increasingly compromised cardiorespiratory status, and possible pain from stress related to weakness or muscle imbalance. This transition stage is often frightening for patients because the decrease in function and independence becomes clear. If possible, the patient should be seen for a comprehensive physical therapy reevaluation at this time.

The first step in the reassessment is to ask the patient about his or her current activity level and to identify what the patient can and can no longer do. After a full physical assessment of the patient's motor status similar to the initial evaluation, patient, family members, and the therapist (include occupational and speech therapist if team approach is possible) should discuss treatment options and adaptive devices that might help the patient remain as independent as possible. During late phase I and during phase II, many patients show significant weakness of both upper and lower extremity musculature, but each patient has his or her own pattern and rate of progression of weakness and onset of spasticity, bulbar, and respiratory symptoms. A typical patient at this time may have marked weakness of the intrinsic muscles, shoulder muscle weakness (in some cases "hanging arm" syndrome) with shoulder pain, and generalized lower extremity weakness, in some cases more severe distally. Patients may be able to walk within the home environment, but many patients have precarious balance and fall easily because of muscle weakness. At this stage, most patients complain of fatigue with minimal work and have to rest frequently when carrying out ADLs.

CASE 1 ▾ Mr. Turner

Mr. Turner is a 45-year-old man diagnosed 2 years ago with ALS. He lives at home with his wife who works full-time and two teenaged children. Mr. Turner is a computer programmer for an engineering firm in the area. Since his diagnosis, Mr. Turner has been able to continue his full-time work schedule, although he states that he is no longer able to touch type and can type with the index fingers only. He has noticed that his shoulders and neck hurt after an hour at the computer. In the last 2 weeks he has found it very fatiguing to walk to the cafeteria for lunch, and he fears that he will be knocked down when walking in crowds. He dropped his tray last week, which was very embarrassing, so he decided to eat in his office even though he misses the socialization and opportunity to discuss work issues with his colleagues.

Mr. Turner has been able to continue most of his nonwork activities, although he is no longer able to operate his sailboat independently and is having trouble maintaining his balance when golfing. He states that his wife and children are supportive and that they have made some changes in the home environment to accommodate his increasing weakness. He also revealed, however, that his children seem frustrated with him because he is so much slower than he was before the illness.

On assessment, Mr. Turner showed marked wasting of hand intrinsics. He was unable to abduct or flex either shoulder past 90 degrees. His right shoulder showed considerable atrophy, especially of the deltoid and supraspinatus muscles. All other upper extremity movements were weakened but in the G– (4–) range. His neck posture was forward (neck extension is F+ (3+), neck flexion is G– (4–). Scapular winging was noted bilaterally. No spasticity was evident in the upper extremities.

Lower extremity musculature showed generalized weakness at about the F (3) to F+ (3+) range, left musculature weaker than right, with marked wasting of the foot intrinsics and a cavus foot position bilaterally. Spasticity was noted of the hip adductors and hamstrings on passive motion. Most obvious during gait was inadequate dorsiflexion for heel strike and no propulsion during heel-off. He showed bilateral corrected gluteus medius pattern on weight bearing. He needed to pause to lock each knee during weight bearing and at times he pushed his knee into extension with his hand. He had great difficulty ascending and descending steps in his home. There were no stairs to negotiate at work.

Until this appointment, Mr. Turner had not been willing to discuss the use of adaptive equipment or to use a wheelchair. During prior clinic visits his decisions were supported and he was told that when he was ready, therapists would work with him and his family to help with equipment decisions. (It is important that therapists present but not press adaptive equipment options to patients when they first start to show impairment in functional ability. If shown how the equipment will help them maintain independence, most patients are receptive to its use. Even when presented in a positive way, however, a wheelchair or adaptive devices may be resisted long after the adaptations would facilitate mobility and ADLs. Therapists must be very attentive to patient's feelings and fears at this time because use of a wheelchair heralds to many patients the beginning of the end.)

Mr. Turner also showed some early bulbar signs. He noted that he sometimes had to catch drool when working intensely, and that his pillow was moist in the morning. Food sometimes got stuck in his cheek area and he could not move it out with his tongue. Swallowing was still adequate for eating all foods; however, he had had a few coughing episodes when drinking coffee and wine. He showed increased use of accessory musculature when breathing but had no complaints of respiratory distress. His cough was adequate to clear secretions.

With input from the therapist, Mr. Turner and his wife identified the following general goals:

1. Increase mobility
2. Control fatigue and pain of upper extremities and neck during computer work
3. Maintain maximal muscle strength and range of motion (patient complained that he felt stiff)
4. Identify safety issues within the home and work environment and adjust household and work environment to prepare for time when Mr. Turner could not ascend and descend stairs safely

A treatment plan was discussed to achieve the following:

1. **Increase mobility.** Because of his increased walking difficulties, Mr. Turner decided to use a front-wheeled walker with a seat attachment at home. Because of his hand grip weakness, he felt most stable using attached forearm troughs. For his work site, he selected a motorized wheelchair so that he could maintain his independence at work. Although he found that he could push an ultralight manual chair, it was clear that his upper extremity strength was decreasing. To prevent overworking and further damaging weakened musculature, he was discouraged from self-propelling a manual chair because of the repetitive pushing action and the effort necessary to cope with inclines. Although most patients will need a motorized device, such as a wheelchair or scooter, to maintain independent mobility, some homes would need adaptations to allow electric wheelchair access. Some patients are initially horrified at the "appearance of disability" when using a motorized wheelchair and would prefer the electric scooter, which is more socially accepted. The scooter, however, does not provide adequate support for the patient in the later stages of the disease. Therefore its purchase should be discouraged unless the patient has adequate financial resources to make the transition later to a motorized chair.

   Factors to consider include: extent of insurance coverage or financial assistance programs for purchase of wheelchair (some policies or programs may provide only one type of wheelchair or only one wheelchair, either motorized or manual); transportability of motorized chair from home to community and work (few motorized wheelchair brands fold for stowing in car trunk and few families can afford to purchase a van that will allow patient to drive or be driven while in motor chair); reclining potential of chair back and head rest (preferably electric) to allow the patient to shift weight and rest while in the chair during later stages of the disease; removable arm rests for ease of transfer; potential for head rest attachment or extension; potential mounting area for portable respirator equipment if needed; ease with which caregiver can help patient with chair mobility, transfers. Because Mr. Turner's insurance and Medicare would not fund an additional manual chair and because the family had no way to transport the electric wheelchair, the ALS Society loaned the family a manual wheelchair for home use. Although not ideal it was functional. Mr. Turner's son made some inexpensive adjustments to adapt the chair for a head rest and his daughter and grandchildren repainted the chair to his specifications.

   Because Mr. Turner wanted to keep as active as possible and use his walker within the home, he was fitted with bilateral ankle-foot orthoses (AFOs) with a flexible ankle joint and pretibial shell to facilitate knee extension. Straps were simple overlap style because Mr. Turner had poor thumb and grasp control.

2. **Decrease fatigue and pain of upper extremities.** Mr. Turner was taught some simple self-ROM exercises of the neck and arms to carry out every half hour while working at the computer. In a simulated work environment, the therapist noted that Mr. Turner had a very forward head position when working at a computer similar to his workstation. The height of the computer was adjusted to decrease his neck strain, and the desk height was adjusted to allow his wheelchair to fit under the desk so that his arms could rest fully on the surface. He felt immediate relief with the adaptations. He was also fitted for a soft neck collar to wear when he felt he needed more neck support. (As his condition worsened, he learned to rest his head on the head rest of his chair and recline slightly for a few minutes every 15 minutes.)

3. **Maintain maximal muscle strength and ROM.** Mr. Turner was taught as many self-ranging maneuvers as possible, which he was encouraged to do in small segments frequently throughout the day. For example, his series of motions included neck rotations, side bends, and flexion and extension within strength limits, upper extremity motions, with the exception of shoulder flexion and abduction past 90 degrees, hip flexion, abduction and rotations, full knee extension, and all ankle motions. When using the walker, Mr. Turner was encouraged to extend each hip fully and to stretch his heel cords. Mrs. Turner and their adult children were taught to administer full ROM exercises, including trunk rotations with special attention to ranging of the shoulder to prevent impingement. Simple massage techniques were also taught to all family members who felt comfortable with the task.

   Maintaining maximal muscle strength is difficult because any program must be designed to prevent disuse activity *and* prevent overwork damage. No exercise program should be recommended that would cause enough fatigue to require extensive periods of postexercise rest or interfere with his participation in normal ADL. Mr. Turner had been active before the onset of ALS and he liked to exercise. Therefore he rented a portable pedaling unit to attach to a chair at home. He pedaled two to four times a day, with no additional resistance, to the point when he felt fatigue (usually 3 to 5 minutes at this stage). He carefully monitored his soreness and fatigue level after exercise and increased and decreased his pedaling depending on how he felt immediately and several days after exercise. Mr. Turner felt invigorated by this exercise, which he usually did while watching television. He was also taught a series of simple elastic band exercises, with tensile strength adjusted according to his ability to contract his muscles without fatigue. Mr. Turner was also shown a series of isometric exercises for all muscle groups to do throughout the work day. Because he had some foot and ankle edema, he was encouraged to wear lightweight pressure stockings while sitting. Mr. Turner also had access to a swimming pool, and he was encouraged to carry out walking and upper extremity exercises provided another adult was with him in the water at all times.

4. **Assess environment of home and work.** Occupational therapy input was requested to help with ADL aids such as reachers, utensil adaptors to facilitate grip, rubber pen grippers, key adaptors to permit turning, and thumb abduction splints to assist in pincer grasp. Mr. Turner's occupational therapist made several visits to his work-site and home to identify adaptations of the environment for safety and independence. His wheelchair was eventually adapted with universal joint arm troughs to decrease his effort during self-feeding and basic upper body hygiene. Ramps were recommended for home entry, and nonpermanent safety rails were placed in the

bathroom. Mr. Turner was able to assist with transfer to a shower chair and the shower head was replaced with a handheld unit.

A speech pathology consultation was also requested. Using information from the physical therapist's Manual Muscle Test (MMT), the speech pathologist carried out a thorough bulbar evaluation and provided information about swallowing techniques. The speech therapist focused on ways to decrease drooling and ways to cope with food "pocketing" (tongue mobility was impaired) using techniques such as hand pressure on the cheek to push food back to the center of his mouth. The therapist also instructed Mr. Turner and his wife how to prepare foods with textures that were easily swallowed and manipulated. Mr. Turner had lost 5 pounds during the last 6 months so he was also referred to the dietitian for information about how to maintain nutritious calorie intake.

Because Mr. Turner was cared for in a neuromotor disease clinic, he benefitted from input from multiple specialists working as a team to help him maintain his independence. Unfortunately, many patients do not have the benefit of such a coordinated treatment environment. Therefore when necessary, the therapist must be in a position to provide input on adaptive devices and safety and bulbar issues if specialist input is not available. Therapists working in smaller communities and rural areas most likely need to be chameleon-like to play many therapeutic roles when working wth the patient with ALS.

Physical and occupational therapists are usually less involved in the care of the patient in phase III (Dependent) and nursing personnel become more active. During this phase, therapists make home visits to support caregivers and respond to questions about pain control, bed mobility and positioning, ROM, and equipment adaptations. Therapists should be sure to teach all caregivers some basic body mechanics to use during lifting and patient care activities. If possible, patients should be moved from the bed to a reclining wheelchair or neurochair during specific times of the day so that they can continue to be part of the family activities. Some patients, however, feel uncomfortable with their dependency and appearance and are reasonably content to stay in their room with television and visits from family members. This often very personal decision by patients must be respected. Others elect to be in the midst of activities even when dependent on HMV. The ease of caregivers in transferring and caring for the person in the wheelchair also must be considered. The therapist should review ROM procedures with family and professional caregivers and provide splinting or positioning devices if spasticity or paralysis leads to caregiving difficulties (i.e., excessive

adductor tone and contractures interfering with hygiene and bowel care) or tissue damage and pain. If nursing care providers do not give advice on pressure relief beds or mattresses, therapists should be prepared to do so. Unfortunately, many insurance providers and Medicare may not fund special mattresses. Therapists may also need to review postural drainage techniques with caregivers.

During phase III, most patients have severe problems eating and maintaining nutrition. These problems are best handled medically, and the aggressiveness of treatment intervention depends on the patient's preference and whether he or she still wants to attempt any oral feeding (i.e., syringe feeding, oral gastric tubes, gastrostomy).

Of greatest importance at this phase is the patient's ability to communicate. Some patients with dysarthria and weakened respiratory function may benefit from palatal appliances and electronic speech amplifiers. Patients with a tracheostomy may benefit from use of the Passy-Muir speaking valve tracheostomy tube (Passy Muir Inc., Irvine, Calif.). These devices need to be recommended by communication specialists.

The simplest communication devices for the nonspeaking patient are note pads or "magic slates." Later, the patient who can no longer write may need a communication board with words, phrases, and letters to which the patient can finger point or eye point. In some cases, patients have access to augmented communication devices, such as a computerized speech synthesizer, which can be programmed with specific commands, words, and letters. These units can be set up to operate with eye pointing, infrared beams attached to the head, electrodes controlled by forehead musculature, and eye blink. Some systems can be programmed to turn on and off television, lights, and other electronic units.

Unfortunately, these devices are often very expensive and may not be available to all patients. Financial support is often not extended for "high tech" equipment by third-party payers because of the patient's limited life expectancy. The ability to communicate and to call for help, however, is of paramount importance with totally dependent patients.

Psychosocial issues

Giving the bad news of a terminal diagnosis is difficult for even the most experienced clinician. In dealing with the diagnosis of ALS, most physicians now believe that the diagnosis, prognosis, and possible patterns of progression should be shared with the patient and family or partners and caregiving friends. Only by knowing the truth can patients and families deal openly with each other and make plans for the future.[22] All information need not be given at the time of diagnosis. Rather the patient and family can be exposed to more in-depth information over a number of sessions when they have the opportunity to ask questions that occur during the assimilation process. If patients are referred to a specialty clinic from a rural area, it is absolutely imperative that patients are contacted regularly at home by phone following the initial diagnosis to allow follow-up questions and to make appropriate support referrals if needed.

Patients will progress through the diagnostic process with different responses and at different rates on a continuum from taking a very cognitive approach by asking many questions and reviewing the most current research, to the extreme of marked denial and disinterest in participating in any medical or therapeutic recommendations. Although some degree of denial can be a useful coping strategy, Oliver and Cardy[23] have found that most patients with motor neuron disease want to talk about their prognosis and future. The opportunity to express fears and concerns is essential. The overall goal of helping the patient and family members express themselves is to provide a forum for self-reflection and insight[26] about the process of living while dying. Nevertheless, the view by some health care workers that patients and families cannot deal with the disease effectively unless they express complete acceptance may be as faulty as hiding the diagnosis from the patient.

Purtillo[26] identifies four major fears of the patient who has a terminal condition: fear of isolation, fear of pain, fear of dependence, and fear of death itself. Patients with progressive diseases often see their social contacts decrease. Mr. Turner was very concerned when he was no longer able to join his colleagues in the company lunch room. After he received his motorized wheelchair he was able to continue his social contacts until his bulbar symptoms progressed to a point that he chose not to eat in public. When Mr. Turner lost the ability to speak and had to use his computerized speech system, he noticed that fewer colleagues stopped by his office to talk because of the slowness of the communication process. Although he understood the problem, Mr.

Turner mourned considerably about his loss of friendship and his loss of standing as a competent computer expert. Because of his need for social contact, Mr. Turner continued to work until he could no longer tolerate the sitting position. His fear of isolation increased when he became homebound. Although colleagues came for visits regularly at first, as Mr. Turner progressed to a near locked-in state only a few close friends came by for brief visits. Mr. Turner's greatest fear was being separated from his family and abandoned to hospital care with the usual inconsistent staffing patterns. Fortunately in his community, Mrs. Turner was able to set up visitations from several church members, clerics, and hospice volunteers.

Fear of uncontrolled pain is common among persons with terminal diseases. Patients need assurance that their pain will be controlled. Many patients can recall the postsurgical horrors of being in severe pain, but being told they had to wait another 2 hours for their next medication. Fortunately, today pain medications can be administered in many forms, dosages, and frequencies that can be tailored to the patient's specific needs. Because many patients are routinely undermedicated for pain, patients with ALS and their families need to be assertive about pain management. Keeping a pain log of intensity, type, location, and time of pain may provide the physician with information necessary to best prescribe dosages. Although sensory systems of ALS patients are essentially normal and not the cause of pain, many patients do experience significant pain from musculoskeletal sources, persistent spasms, or spasticity and pressure sores. Most of these problems can be handled with appropriate pain medications, muscle relaxants, careful positioning, frequent ROM, and tissue massage.

A major concern of patients with ALS is the dependence for ADLs associated with late phase II and phase III of the disease. Because the process is gradual, most patients have the opportunity to make adjustments. The dependency issues and resulting privacy issues are more uncomfortable for some patients than others, especially for the person who has always valued total control and independence. (See Case 1 continued on p. 392.)

Not all patients with terminal illness react the same way during the dying process. Throughout the process, patients and family members may cycle and recycle through a range of different reactions, such as the stages described by Kubler-Ross: depression, anger, hostility, bargaining, and acceptance (order is not implied).[26] How the patient coped with life's difficulties before the illness and his or her prior relationship patterns often direct how the patient will deal with the terminal illness.

Health care providers and family members often have great difficulty coping with a patient who is depressed, and they make repeated efforts to "talk the person out of" the depression. Smith[33] reminds us to distinguish between depression that can be destructive and the mourning or grieving that is a necessary and vital response to dealing with

CASE 1 ▼ **Mr. Turner—(continued)**

Mr. Turner had great difficulty adjusting to his physical dependence. Because of his very slow onset of dysphagia and his augmented communication system, he was able to continue control over his expressive, cognitive, and emotional life until the last 5 or 6 months of his life. Initially, Mr. Turner angrily resisted his wife's attempts to help him with eating and dressing tasks. This began to alienate her and the children until a family meeting was held with their medical social worker and physical and occupational therapists. All family members had the opportunity to express their frustrations. A major irritation to the children was what they perceived to be their constant waiting for their father to complete a task. Mrs. Turner was most irritated when Mr. Turner yelled at her when she attempted to help even though he frequently expressed anger about his clumsiness. Mr. Turner sadly admitted that he was having increasing difficulty with his ADLs and was sometimes too tired after dressing to participate in family activities. At the end of the meeting, the family had worked out a compromise plan. Mr. Turner would continue to do as much as possible for himself. He would specifically ask for help from Mrs. Turner when he wanted it so she did not get caught in his anger about needing help. He preferred that the children not have to take any role in his care at this point, but realized that he might need their help later. Visiting nurse support was requested twice a week to help with bathing, and the occupational therapist was requested to make another home visit to help with toileting needs. Mr. Turner felt comfortable with his wife and children carrying out ROM. A therapy home visit was arranged to review exercise/positioning program as well as respiratory exercises and postural drainage techniques.

As Mr. Turner became totally dependent, he needed 24-hour care. Professional nurses were provided through his insurance contract 14 hours a day from 6:30 AM to 8:30 PM. Family members provided care until midnight. Initially Mr. Turner was able to activate a bell at night to call for help. His wife and children followed a schedule to turn him every 3 hours throughout the night. When Mr. Turner became respi-

rator dependent and was no longer able to call for help, it became clear that the nighttime responsibilities were taking a heavy toll on his wife who worked full-time and the children who were in high school and college. Fortunately the family was able to pay for a nurse assistant to remain at Mr. Turner's bedside throughout the night, although the family members all felt that they had no privacy. Although the family was committed to having Mr. Turner remain at home until his death, all agreed that they needed respite. Thus several week-long hospitalizations were made to give the family a break in the constant care needs.

Although Mr. Turner had elected HMV, he also had signed a Durable Power of Attorney for Health Care, indicating that he did not want treatment for infections and that palliative care for comfort should direct his treatment. He had a strong lust for life, but had come to accept his impending death. He did not have a strong religious view of life, but had talked with all his caregivers and therapists about his concerns around death. He freely expressed his fear of "non-being." Because his caregivers and therapists were willing to talk about his and their own feelings, Mr. Turner came to believe that he would live on in the minds, hearts, and behavior of those he had known. This idea seemed to give him great comfort. He particularly liked to talk to others about special times they had had together and how their interactions had affected each other. To help Mr. Turner process his death, his family, friends, and medical team put together an album of pictures and statements about their time together. Mr. Turner frequently liked to have his wife read through the book with him. His family continued to carry out his ROM exercises and massage because Mr. Turner had indicated that the treatments provided him physical comfort and the spiritual closeness he needed with his family. His primary treatment during the last few days consisted of morphine to decrease his respiratory discomfort. After 5 to 6 months totally dependent for all care and respiratory function, Mr. Turner died at home in his sleep after a respiratory illness.

loss. In both states, the person may feel a level of withdrawal, sadness, apathy, loss of interest in activities, and cognitive distortions. In a depressive state, however, the patient experiences an accompanying loss of self-esteem. A person in mourning rarely experiences that loss of self-esteem essential to a diagnosis of depression. The grieving person's feelings are congruent with the degree of loss experienced. Because of the discomfort overt grieving causes onlookers, some professional caregivers try to rush the patient and family into formal counseling as soon as mourning occurs. This option should be offered, but other recommendations such as guidance from a cleric, support groups, hospice volunteers, and informal support from friends are also invaluable resources for the person uncomfortable with formal counseling situations.

With today's pressure to express oneself and talk about

one's feelings, patients are often pressed to "talk out" their problems and feelings. Although it is important for a caregiver to give a patient the opportunity to talk about dying and to feel comfortable with the topic, each patient's personal style in talking about death must be respected. For example, some persons are not comfortable sharing feelings with a professional counselor or psychologist. This is especially true for older patients or those who were raised with the view that one should maintain the appearance of control or that seeking emotional help shows weakness or defect. Pressuring a patient to see a mental health worker can lead to loss of trust. Therefore therapists and other persons involved in the care of a dying patient should feel comfortable talking with their patients about death and be prepared to suggest various options if the patient expresses the need for emotional support.

Caregiver issues

Often in the concern for the patient's needs, professionals pay little attention to the effect a person's degenerative illness has on other members of the family. ALS significantly affects the person's extended family because the patient gradually becomes increasingly dependent on family members, partners, or caregiving friends for physical care, social arrangements, cognitive stimulation, and emotional support. For some families, the spouse may have to take on additional work, return to work, or in the case of some older women, join the work force for the first time in order to deal with the financial stresses that occur when chronic illness invades the family unit. Family members must absorb the former family duties of the dependent person. For example, a husband may have to handle all the cooking and cleaning tasks; older children may have to take on the total care of younger siblings, increase household chores, or work to help support the family. All family members may have to become involved in the physical care of the increasingly dependent person with ALS.

Families have differing levels of long-term care coverage. Some families are fortunate to have excellent coverage that provides extensive home nursing support, whereas other families are unable to cope with the financial stresses and must accept public assistance during the final stages of the person's disease. For example the Springer family, consisting of the father with ALS (age 61), mother (age 59) and son (age 25), was forced to life on a combination of Supplemental Security Income, general assistance, and food stamps after the father became ill. The family had little savings and catastrophic insurance coverage that did not cover any long-term care. Mrs. Springer returned to work full-time and cared for her husband all evening. When he reached the point of needing full-time care, the wife had to quit work to care for her husband because she did not make an adequate salary to pay for nursing care and maintain the family finances. Because the son had to care for his own family of four, he was not able to help out the family financially, although both he and his wife provided several half-days of respite care for their mother so she could do shopping and spend some time out of the home. The process of "going on welfare" was very upsetting to the family. After numerous discussions about options for home care, Mr. Springer decided that continuing his life was too great a burden on his family and he requested that his life be terminated. Because that was not considered an option, his family and primary physician worked out a plan to allow a peaceful death without placing Mr. Springer on any artificial feeding, respiration, or antibiotics. He died at home 3 months after the decision was made.

In another case, a young single woman who lived alone and had no family found that she could not rely on friends for her care even though they were supportive and visited her often. When she was no longer able to care for herself safely she was admitted to a nursing home where she died 2 years later.

Children of patients with ALS also have to deal with major changes in their lifestyle. Although they may love their parent who is sick, at some level most are very frustrated with factors such as the need to provide physical care to parents (sometimes when they have not had positive relationships with that parent), the lack of privacy in their home when nursing personnel and attendants are present, changes in family mobility, interruptions in family and personal life plans, embarrassment because of the parent's appearance and dependency, lack of attention from the caregiving-working parent, and fear of financial crises (possible loss of home, no financial support for college, etc.).

The entire family is affected by the sick person's increasing dependency and impending death. The changes the family must make to anticipate and deal with the dependent person's needs have a significant emotional overlay. Anger, helplessness, frustration, sadness, or mourning for an impending loss; guilt; and remorse commonly occur and recur at different stages as the sick person and family try to adjust to the progression toward death. Weariness and exhaustion from day-to-day caregiving and frequent interactions with health and social agencies can try the soul of the most adaptable persons.[37] Fortunately, most families manage to cope with the process—the major contributing factor being the coping ability of families before the illness. To be really effective, the physical therapist working with the patient with ALS must be prepared to help families and caregivers find appropriate ways of coping with the emotional, social, and physical stress of caregiving.

POLYRADICULONEUROPATHIES

The **polyradiculoneuropathies** are often divided into the axonal neuropathies and the demyelinating neuropathies. Axonal polyneuropathies are most often related to toxic and metabolic causes such as diabetes, alcohol abuse, and less commonly chronic exposure to heavy metals and household or industrial toxins.[72]

The most common of the primary demyelinating diseases is **Guillain-Barré syndrome (GBS),** which affects the mixed peripheral nerves. The syndrome may reflect an autoimmune response, although no common antigen has been identified and no consistent predisposing factors are known. Approximately 60% of the GBS cases, however, follow a respiratory or gastrointestinal illness.[84,89] Diagnostic criteria for GBS is detailed in the box on p. 394.

Peripheral nerve biopsies are seldom indicated in GBS, but when performed show inflammatory cells, primarily lymphocytes infiltrating the interstitium and perivascular spaces with deterioration of myelin sheath.[43] Within 2 to 3 weeks of the acute demyelination process, Schwann cells proliferate to herald recovery. Because of damage to the myelin sheath, saltatory propagation of the action potential is disturbed resulting in slowed conduction, dyssynchrony of conduction, disturbed conduction of higher frequency impulses, or complete conduction block.

Common diagnostic features of Guillain-Barré Syndrome

A. Motor weakness.
   1. Progressive symptoms and signs of motor weakness that develop rapidly.
      a. Relative symmetry of motor involvement.
      b. Usual progression of weakness from distal to proximal; self-limiting to distal limbs of upper and/or lower extremities or may extend to full quadriplegia with respiratory and cranial nerve involvement.
   2. Areflexia of, at least, distal tendon responses.
B. Mild sensory symptoms or signs, particularly paresthesias and hypesthesias.
C. Autonomic dysfunction such as tachycardia and arrhythmias, vasomotor symptoms.
D. Absence of fever at onset of symptoms; history of flulike illness common.
E. Laboratory tests nonspecific but may have elevation of cerebrospinal fluid protein; cerebrospinal fluid cells at 10 or fewer mononuclear leukocytes/cubic millimeter of cerebrospinal fluid.
F. Electrodiagnostic testing, nerve conduction velocities usually abnormal.
G. Recovery usually begins 2 to 4 weeks after plateau of disease process.

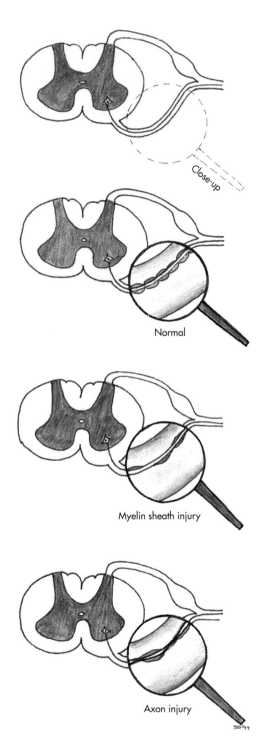

Close-up

Normal

Myelin sheath injury

Axon injury

Fig. 13-4. Drawing of peripheral nerve showing axonal degeneration and demyelination.

Although GBS is primarily considered a demyelinating disease, axonal degeneration also has been noted in many cases either as an effect of the inflammatory process against myelin or as the primary pathophysiology.[42] In axonal neuropathies, the conduction velocity is within normal limits, but the number of motor units is decreased (Fig. 13-4). For a very readable review of reactions of neurons and peripheral nerves to injury see Kandel and others[56] and refer to Chapter 12.

Clinical features

GBS in both children and adults is characterized by a rapidly evolving, relatively symmetrical ascending weakness or flaccid paralysis. Motor impairment may vary from mild weakness of distal lower extremity musculature to total paralysis of the peripheral, axial, facial, and extraocular musculature. Tendon reflexes are usually diminished or absent. Approximately 20% of patients may require assisted ventilation because of paralysis or weakness of the intercostal and diaphragm musculature. Impaired respiratory muscle strength may lead to an inability to cough or handle secretions and decreased vital capacity, tidal volume, and oxygen saturation. Secondary complications such as infections or organ system failure can lead to death in approximately 5% of patients with GBS.[70,84]

ANS symptoms are frequently noted. Low cardiac output, cardiac dysrhythmias, and marked fluctuations in blood pressure may compromise management of respiratory function and can lead to sudden death. Other typical ANS symptoms may result in peripheral pooling of blood, poor venous return, and urinary retention.

Sensory symptoms such as distal hyperesthesias, paresthesias (tingling, burning), numbness and decreased vibratory or position sense are common, but not progressive or persistent. The sensory disturbances often have a stocking and glove pattern rather than the dermatonal distribution of loss. Although the sensory problems are seldom disabling, they can be very disconcerting and upsetting to patients, especially during the acute stage. Some patients experience severe burning or hypersensitivity to touch or even air movement, which can interfere with nursing care and limit therapy interventions.[56]

Pain was identified as a significant symptom in the original articles describing GBS.[42,46] In 1949, 1963, and 1984 studies of 50, 35, and 29 patients with GBS, respectively, approximately 55% of patients reported pain preceding their illness or early during onset.[42] Seventy-two percent reported pain at some time during the full course of the disease process. When pain was prominent, patients spontaneously revealed its presence during a medical history. Therefore patients who present with the onset of low back pain not associated with known injury or stress and complaints of paresthesias and vibratory or decreased tendon reflexes should be evaluated or monitored for possible GBS.[41]

The most common description of pain was of muscle aching typically associated with vigorous or excessive exercise. Pain was usually symmetrical and reported most frequently in the large bulk muscles such as the gluteals, quadriceps, hamstrings, and less often in the lower leg and upper extremity muscles.[73] Some pain reported during late stages of the illness was described as "stiffness." Pain was consistently more disturbing at night. Location and severity of pain were not clearly related to the degree of paralysis or sensory loss. In a series of large studies of GBS, pain as a major symptom was reported less frequently. Those reports, however, were retrospective chart reviews and may not reflect the true incidence of pain associated with GBS.[42] Based on the absence of clinical sensory or electrophysiological abnormalities, Ropper and others[74] stated that GBS pain is not "neuritic" pain and that nerve or spinal ganglia inflammation is not responsible for the perceived pain. Serum creatinine kinase level was elevated in 10 of 13 patients with pain and in only one of eight patients without pain. This finding suggests that changes in muscle related to neurogenic origin may be the cause of pain.

Prognosis

In more than half the cases of GBS, weakness or paralysis has reached its nadir within the first week after diagnosis and within 3 weeks in 80% of cases. In some cases, the process of increasing weakness continues for 1 to 2 months. Onset of recovery is varied, with most patients showing gradual recovery of muscle strength 2 to 4 weeks after progression has stopped or plateaued. Although 30% of the patients may show minor neurological deficits (i.e., diminished or absent tendon reflexes) and 15% may show persistent residual deficits in function, approximately 80% become ambulatory within 6 months of onset of symptoms. The most common long-term deficits are weakness of the anterior tibial

musculature, and less often weakness of the foot and hand intrinsics, quadriceps, and gluteal musculature. Five percent of patients may die of secondary cardiac, respiratory, or other systemic organ failures.[42,84]

Until studies in the mid to late 1980s, it was difficult to determine which patients would have a complete recovery. A clear relationship between nerve conduction velocities and prognosis has not been found,[65] although poor outcome has been related to rapid progression to quadriplegia, respiratory dependence, and failure to show improvement within 3 weeks of plateau.[44,88] More recently several researchers have identified a subgroup of patients diagnosed with GBS who present with primary axonal degeneration as opposed to demyelination. Those patients tended to show a prolonged recovery period with persistent disability. For example, in the previously cited study of six children, the three children with clear axonal degeneration had persistent motor weakness 5 years after illness compared with the three children who demonstrated demyelination or mixed axonal and demyelinating processes.[42]

Medical treatment

Medical treatment depends on the rate and degree of ascending paralysis. Because most patients return to their prior functional status, excellent supportive care during the acute stage is imperative. Respiratory compromise should be expected and all patients, including those with limited paralysis and sensory dysfunction, must be closely monitored for the rapid onset of cardiopulmonary decompensation. Because of the possibility of sudden respiratory decompensation, patients with evidence of GBS must be hospitalized so that immediate cardiorespiratory support can be given if vital capacity falls below 20 ml/kg or oxygen saturation falls below 75%.[70] Patients who progress to respiratory paralysis must be treated in an intensive care environment where adequate respiratory function can be maintained, secondary infections can be prevented or limited, and metabolic functions can be carefully monitored. After extubation, aspiration can be a serious complication because of oral muscle weakness and dysphagia.

In addition to the intensive supportive care required, two more specific drug-based treatments are under investigation for their ability to decrease the duration of respirator dependence and the time to onset of improvement. Because humoral factors and an autoimmune response are thought to be involved in the process of GBS,[47,68,83] several studies have focused on the value of plasma exchange as a modulator of disease severity. Since the initial studies in 1984,[47,68] two large clinical trials (see French Cooperative Group[46] and Guillain-Barré Syndrome Study Group[48]) carried out in the United States and France have shown that patients undergoing plasmapheresis (removal of plasma from withdrawn blood with retransfusion of the formed elements back into the blood) had shorter periods on mechanical ventilation and walked earlier than subjects who did not undergo exchange. This was particularly true for

Factors to consider in evaluation of patient with Guillain-Barré syndrome

History

Pattern and sequence of symptom onset.
Recent illness, injury, prior episodes of sensory-motor problems.

Motor function

Visual inspection to identify symmetry of muscle bulk and function.
Myotatic reflexes, r/o tonic reflexes.
Manual muscle testing carefully identifying pattern of weakness (testing should be as muscle specific as possible rather than assessing muscle groups only) (use form for serial recording).
Presence of muscle fasciculations.
Cranial nerves.
Range of motion (use form for serial recording).
Equilibrium reactions sitting and standing (if testable).
Current functional status (ADL including bowel and bladder function, ambulation).

Sensory system

Identify pattern of sensory loss or changes (use body chart).
Identify specific type of sensory change (i.e., paresthesias, anesthesias, hypesthesias [use body chart]).
Identify pain type and location (use body chart). What makes it better, what makes it worse?
Identify pressure points or areas that might lead to pressure sores.

Autonomic system

Blood pressure resting and immediately following activity (prone, sitting, standing if possible).
Heart rate resting and immediately following activity, dysrhythmias.
Body temperature stability.
Bowel and bladder control.

Psychosocial systems

Identify patient and family concerns in acute circumstances and concerns about long-term issues that may affect patient and family. Your assessment need not be extensive if referral can be made for social service evaluation of patient and family financial concerns, day-to-day living problems (transportation, child care, etc.), support systems, and coping strategies.

Electrodiagnostic testing

Nerve conduction velocity (Physician will order these studies to be performed by a clinician skilled in the procedures. This may be a physical therapist, physician or technician depending on facility).

patients treated within the first week of hospitalization and those with more severe disease. Plasma exchange, however, has some serious possible complications that relate to an increased incidence of hypotension and arrhythmias, which makes it unsuitable for GBS patients with autonomic instability. The need for multiple infusion lines increases the possibility of septicemia and thrombosis. The technique is also expensive and requires highly skilled personnel and equipment.

Intravenous immunoglobulin (IVIG) also has a positive impact in the treatment of chronic inflammatory polyneuropathy. A randomized controlled trial of IVIG and plasmapheresis was conducted with 150 patients. Results indicated that IVIG was at least as effective as plasma exchange. A small 1993 study, however, has reported an incidence of relapse following IVIG. Currently an international randomized trial is underway to evaluate the two treatments.[70] Although corticosteroids were used to decrease the inflammatory process in GBS beginning in the 1960s, a clinical trial of steroid effectiveness in 1993 suggested that steroids were not useful in the treatment of GBS,[55] although they may have some place in the treatment of other chronic demyelinating polyneuropathies.[89]

Therapeutic evaluation.   A comprehensive therapeutic evaluation of the patient with GBS includes factors shown in the accompanying box.

Motor evaluation.   The extent of the evaluation depends on the patient's condition and his or her ability to participate in the assessment. In many situations, therapists carry out manual muscle testing (MMT) procedures by testing functional muscle groups. In GBS, however, it is important to test muscle strength and ROM as specifically as possible so that the patient's course of progression and improvement can be tracked, possible patterns leading to contractures can be predicted and prevented, and the appropriate level of exercise can be implemented. Because one cannot complete a full MMT every week with a debilitated patient, it is most common to select a few specific muscles (i.e., sternocleidomastoids, deltoids, triceps, flexor carpi ulnaris, lumbricals, iliopsoas, gluteus medius, anterior tibialis, flexor hallucis longus) to test weekly, with more complete testing performed once a month or for major evaluations only. Patients who report considerable pain during handling or active movement may not tolerate testing or may be unwilling or unable to cooperate with MMTs. Therefore the therapist may wish to track the patient's level of pain on a pain scale to help determine weakness related to pathology or apparent weakness secondary to pain. Changes in the patient's condition should be monitored with serial MMTs, ROM recordings, sensory testing, and functional status evaluations (see Karni and others[57] and Lewis and Bottomley[62] for suggestions on serial functional assessments). Care should be taken not to fatigue the patient in any single evaluation session.

Respiratory and dysphagia evaluation.   Although therapists are active in the treatment of a patient's movement problems, they also are involved in evaluating the patient's respiratory and swallowing dysfunction. Therapists are usually involved early in the care of patients with GBS. For patients with respiratory and/or bulbar paralysis, the physical therapist's initial contact may be in the intensive care unit. Although most hospitals have fully equipped intensive care units, a therapist working in rural or smaller community hospitals may be the first person to note a patient's changing effort-related respiratory status during evaluation and treatment sessions. Therefore the therapist must be prepared to advise nursing and medical staff about the need to test oxygen saturation levels and vital capacity. For complete information on the physical therapist's evaluation of patients in acute respiratory failure, see Chapter 15 of reference 54.

Patients with severe oral-motor problems and dysphagia should be evaluated thoroughly and treated by a therapist skilled in oral-motor dysfunction and feeding. This might be a speech therapist, occupational therapist, or physical therapist, depending on the facility. Patients with a feeding tube should receive their feedings in an relatively upright position and should remain in that position for 30 to 60 minutes after feeding to decrease the chance of aspiration. According to Longemann,[64] about 40% of patients receiving bedside swallowing assessments have undetected aspiration. Therefore the bedside evaluation should be considered only a preliminary step in the diagnostic process. In addition to careful evaluation of oral-motor control, some clinicians recommend cervical auscultation, particularly during the acute phase, to listen to swallowing sounds.

With evidence of swallowing difficulties and possible aspiration, the patient should be referred for comprehensive testing with videofluoroscopy. Swallowing also can be assessed using techniques such as fiberoptic endoscopy, ultrasound, electroglottography to determine laryngeal movement, and scintigraphy, which involves scanning a radioactive bolus during swallowing.[77]

Treatment planning. Goals for the acute care patient with GBS include the following:

1. Facilitate resolution of respiratory problems
2. Prevent decubitus ulcers
3. Minimize pain
4. Prevent contractures
5. Prevent injury to weakened or denervated muscles
6. Facilitate muscle contraction while monitoring overuse and fatigue

Positioning to prevent contractures and pressure sores. To prevent pressure sores, the physical therapist needs to be involved within the first few days of hospitalization, especially for the patient who has complete or nearly complete paralysis. A positioning program for the dependent patient is the first line of defense. The therapist should arrange for a special mattress or unit that constantly changes the pressure within the mattress or shifts the patient's position or is designed to spread pressure over wide surfaces. For patients who are slender with prominent bony surfaces,

the therapist may need to fashion foam "doughnuts" or pads or use sheepskin-type protection for pressure relief. Patients who are experiencing muscle pain may prefer to have their hips and knees flexed. In these cases, it is imperative to position the patient out of the flexed position for part of each hour.

As part of a complete positioning program, therapists should consider how to best maintain the physiological position of the hands and feet. Research has shown that mild continuous stretch maintained for at least 20 minutes is more beneficial than stronger, brief stretching exercises.[81] Therefore use of splints for prolonged positioning is superior for maintaining functional range than short bursts of intermittent manually applied passive stretching. Although some facilities still use a foot board to control passive ankle dorsiflexion, most therapists now use moldable plastic splints, which can be worn when the patient is in any position. Because ankle-foot splints often prevent visual inspection of the heel position, however, care must be taken to ensure that the heel is firmly down in the orthosis and that the strapping pattern is adequate to secure the foot. The strap system must be simple enough to be positioned properly by all staff and family members caring for the patient. The ankle-foot splint should extend slightly beyond the end of the toes to prevent toe flexion and skin breakdown from the toes rubbing on sheeting. Wrist and hand splints may be prefabricated resting style splints or molded to meet the patient's specific needs. Because increased tone is not a problem in the patient with GBS, a simple cone or rolled cloth may be adequate to maintain good wrist, thumb, and finger alignment.

Range of motion. The onset of connective tissue shortening in response to immobilization is very rapid.[38] To be effective, the ROM program must include both accessory and physiological motions to increase circulation, provide lubrication of the joints, and maintain extensibility of capsular, muscle, and tendon tissue.

ROM can usually be maintained with standard positioning and ROM programs. Nevertheless some patients, especially those who have complained of severe extremity and axial pain early during the disease process and those who have been quadriplegic and respirator dependent for prolonged periods, may develop significant joint contractures despite preventive interventions.

Soryal and others[78] reported on three patients who had marked residual contractures that limited function after strength improved. None of the patients had radiological signs of erosive arthopathy or inflammatory joint disease. Soryal and colleagues hypothesized a number of possible mechanisms for the limitations in range of motion: (1) Therapists and nurses may have been reluctant to fully range patients who complained of marked pain during passive movement; (2) the contractures may have been secondary to pain or damage caused by inappropriate excessive passive movement of hypotonic and sensory impaired joints and muscles; (3) the paralysis may have resulted in lymphatic stasis with accumulation of tissue fluid in tissue spaces and nutritional disturbances; and (4) vasomotor disturbances resulting from autonomic neuropathy may have led to adhesions and fibrosis. Although the authors found few reports describing contractures as a significant residual problem, they suggested that ROM programs must be defined precisely as to frequency and duration, particularly for patients complaining of early joint pain.

Some patients will continually position their limbs so muscle and tendons are in the shortened range in an attempt to decrease muscle pain. This may lead to contractures. The therapist should be aware of changes in "end feel" over time when ranging each joint to determine if capsular and ligamentous structures are also becoming more restricted as the muscle and tendon tissue shortens. Patients who have intact sensation of pain and temperature may respond positively to the use of heat to decrease muscle pain and to facilitate tissue elongation before stretching. Several basic studies of the relationship between load and heat, using rat tail tendon, have shown that it is possible to attain permanent length increases in collagenous tissue using a combination of heat and stretch.[61,86,87]

Based on these studies, Warren[85] suggests that stretch be combined with the highest tolerable therapeutic temperature (approximately 45° C, 113° F). He also recommends that the application of stretch should be of long duration, that moderate forces should be used, that tissue temperature should be elevated before stretching, and that elongation of tissue should be maintained for at least 8 to 10 minutes while the tissue is cooling. (**Caution:** Heat should *not* be used on a patient with a sensory deficit, particularly an inability to distinguish differences in temperature.) Because heating of deep tissue is not possible with patients, Warren's[85] suggestions may be relevant only for superficial muscle/ tendon groups. (Heating muscle and tendon tissue before sustained stretching, however, was a mainstay in prevention of contractures caused by muscle spasms secondary to poliomyelitis, and it may have a place in treatment of muscle spasm and contractions in GBS.)[79]

If pain seems to be a major factor in limiting the patient's passive or active motion, the treatment team should determine the best approach to alleviating pain. According to one study, patients with GBS did not seem to show a consistent response to any specific pain medication, although 6 of the 13 patients seemed to have a positive effect with codeine, oxycodone hydrochloride and acetaminophen (Percocet) or oxycodone and aspirin (Percodan). In several studies,[63,67,82] some patients with neuropathies have had decreased pain after using transcutaneous electrical nerve stimulation (TENS) (see Chapters 30 and 33). Although there is no study related to the effect of TENS specifically on pain associated with GBS, it might be a treatment option in patients whose pain is not controlled with passive movement or pain medications. (**Note:** Some patients who experience extreme sensitivity to light touch, such as movement of sheets, air flow, and intermittent touch contact, benefit from a "cradle," which will hold the sheets away from the body. Some find relief if the limbs are wrapped

snuggly with elastic bandages, which provide continuous low pressure while warding off light, intermittent stimuli.)

Because denervated or weakened muscles can be injured easily, it is the therapist's responsibility to ensure that joint structures are not damaged and that ROM is done with appropriate support of the limb to prevent sudden over-stretching. This is particularly true at the shoulder because many persons are not careful to rotate the shoulder externally during abduction to prevent impingement and capsular damage.[59] Caution also should be taken when ranging or stretching the ankle into dorsiflexion to ensure that the subtalar joint is in neutral or locked position so that the Achilles tendon is effectively elongated and the midfoot structures are not overstretched. In hospitals where the patient is treated by a changing therapy or nursing staff or by family members, a positioning schedule with diagrams, a splinting plan, and ROM recommendations should be presented in poster form at the patient's bedside to provide consistent treatment.

ROM of all involved joints should be performed at least twice a day, more frequently if the patient has no active movement. Patients should be encouraged to move actively when they can do so without causing pain or fatigue. They should be observed carrying out their active range to determine whether change has occurred in the quality of movement that may be related to decreasing strength. If the patient cannot complete ROM through full range independently, the therapist or nursing staff must carefully assist the patient in moving to the end range. This may not be easy if the patient experiences pain with motion. Knowing whether to "push through the pain" or stay within the limits of pain is often a great dilemma for the therapist. The therapist needs to find a balance between working for full joint range and reacting to the patient's complaints of pain.

Based on evidence that continuous passive motion (CPM) is effective in maintaining joint range in both rabbits and humans,[76] Mays[66] described a case study of a patient with GBS (quadriplegia with 7 days of mechanical ventilation) who had persistent pain and stiffness of the upper extremities and fingers approximately 3 months after the onset of GBS. Therefore CPM of the hands and fingers was added to a program of occupational therapy which included ROM, splinting and ADL. The author reported an increase in the rate of recovery of finger range and a decrease in pain following use of CPM. Numerous other studies have reported the value of CPM in maintaining or increasing ROM following hip and knee surgery. It may be a very useful adjunct to traditional therapy for patients with GBS, especially those who continue to develop contractures with intermittent ROM programs.

Massage also may play a positive role in maintaining muscle tissue mobility and tissue nutrition. A study of crush injuries of muscle in rats reported that massage may lessen the amount of fibrosis that develops in immobilized, denervated, or injured muscle.[52] The use of massage in patients with GBS has not been described; however, it makes intuitive sense that it may be a useful adjunct to ROM exercises in patients who do not have marked hypersensitivity to touch, dysesthesias, and muscle pain.

Positioning to increase tolerance to upright. Because of the autonomic lability of many patients with GBS and the effect of prolonged immobility in supine position, most patients must be placed on a graduated program to regain tolerance to the upright position. Because of possible axial muscle weakness, it is imperative to properly stabilize the patient's trunk when instituting upright sitting or standing on a tilt table. This program can be started in the intensive care environment if the patient is on a circlelectric or Nelson bed. If a "standing" bed is not available, a sitting program can be initiated as soon as it is tolerated. A tilt table progressive standing program can be instituted when the patient's respiratory and autonomic nervous systems are no longer unstable. Caution should be taken to fully stabilize the patient to limit activity in muscles below the fair range.

Programs of active exercise. Although most patients with GBS recover from the paralysis, the course and rate of recovery may vary significantly between patients. Strength usually returns in a descending pattern, the opposite of the pattern noted during onset of the disease. The most important concept to remember in designing an exercise program is that exercise will not hasten or improve nerve regeneration, nor will they affect the renervation rate during the rehabilitation process.[80] The major goal of therapeutic management therefore must be to maintain the patient's musculoskeletal system in an optimal "ready" state, to prevent overwork, and to pace the recovery process to obtain maximal function as reinnervation occurs.

The rule in developing an exercise program for patients with GBS is that muscle fatigue must be avoided and rest periods must be frequent.[51,81] Although this is a time-honored precaution, little clear physiological evidence is available to support or negate it. Studying the effect of exercise on rat muscle after nerve injury, Herbison and others[51] identified a loss of contractile proteins during initial reinnervation. After reinnervation the same amount of exercise resulted in muscle hypertrophy. Reitsma[71] noted that vigorous exercise damaged muscles if fewer than one third of motor units were functional. If more than one third of the motor units remained, exercise led to hypertrophy. Therefore the amount of strengthening attained seems proportional to the number of intact or undamaged motor units. Exercise at a level to elicit a training effect in normal muscle may cause **overwork damage** in damaged muscle. Refer to Chapter 29 for additional information. Because the therapist cannot determine the number of intact motor units available to a patient, the therapist must be cautious when initiating exercise with any patient postdenervation.

The safe exercise range differs for normal and impaired muscle, with the therapeutic window being smaller for muscles undergoing reinnervation. Refer again to Fig. 13-3, for a graphic example of the exercise "windows" for normal and damaged or denervated muscle.

Anecdotal evidence about damaging denervated muscle burgeoned during the major poliomyelitis (polio) epidemic

of the 1940s and 1950s. Physicians and therapists noted that polio patients with poor (2) and fair (3) grade muscles who exercised repeatedly or with heavy resistance after reinnervation often lost the ability to contract the muscle at all. Bensman[39] reported on eight patients who had stabilized following acute polyradiculoneuritis (among them patients with GBS). All eight patients experienced a temporary loss of function after strenuous physical exercise. Three patients apparently had significant decreases in strength. All patients were then placed on a program of passive ROM and an increase in muscle strength was noted. Recurring episodes of a temporary loss of function appeared related to strenuous exercise and fatigue. Bensman recommended that once the patient has stabilized, active exercise may begin as follows: (1) short periods of nonfatiguing exercise appropriate to the patient's strength, (2) an increase in activity or exercise level only if patient improves or if there is no deterioration after 1 week, (3) a return to bed rest if a decrease in function or strength occurs, (4) a program of exercise directed at strengthening for function rather than strength itself, and (5) a limit of fatiguing exercise for 1 year with a gradual return to sport activities and more strenuous exercise. Steinberg[80] suggested that patients be allowed to exercise to the first point of fatigue or muscle ache. Abnormal sensations (tingling, paresthesias) that persist for prolonged periods of time after exercise may also indicate that the exercise or activity level was excessive.

During the initial stages of exercise, the repetitions per exercise period should be low, and the frequency of short periods of exercise should be high.[81] As reinnervation occurs and motor units become responsive, the early process of muscle reeducation exercise used by the therapist may be similar to that used during the polio era. To encourage active contraction of the muscle the therapist should carefully demonstrate to the patient the expected movement. The therapist then passively moves the patient's limb while the patient observes. After gaining a clear picture of what movement is expected, the patient is encouraged to contract his or her muscle(s). Facilitatory techniques such as skin stroking, brushing, vibration, icing, and tapping may be used in conjunction with the muscle reeducation process. The patient is taught to reassess his or her movements and to make corrective responses. As the patient gains strength, the movements are translated into functional activities.[51]

Functionally directed exercise should be started judiciously, and the activities should be appropriate for the muscle grade of that muscle or muscle group. For example, if the patient's deltoid muscle receives a Poor (2) grade (full range of motion with gravity eliminated), the patient should be cautioned not to repeatedly attempt to elevate his or her arm against gravity (i.e., to shave or do one's hair). Exercises should be developed to allow the patient to exercise in the gravity free position (overhead slings, powder boards, pool exercises) that allow the patient to move actively through a full range until he or she can take resistance in the gravity eliminated position. Many younger patients have to be reminded to pace their activity so they do not overly fatigue and possibly injure their recovering muscles. Children, teenagers, or adults with impaired judgment often need a strict schedule of rest and activity.

Patients and staff also need to be reminded that prolonged sitting, even when supported, may tax the axial musculature and a program of gradual sitting should be instituted, with the final goal being independent, unsupported sitting with functional adaptive reactions. In busy hospitals a schedule of sitting and activity should be posted in clear view at the patient's bedside.

As reinnervation progresses and strength and exercise tolerance increases, the therapist may choose to use facilitative exercise techniques such as proprioceptive neuromuscular facilitation (PNF), which intentionally recruit maximal contraction of specific muscle groups. Although PNF techniques are excellent for eliciting maximal contraction, care must be taken not to overwork the weaker components of the movement pattern. A positive aspect of PNF techniques is that they can be tied in with functional patterns such as rolling, which is necessary for bed mobility, transitions to quadruped, kneeling, sitting and standing stability, and gait.

Although 65% to 75% or more of patients with GBS show a return to clinically normal motor function, there is anecdotal and empirical evidence that some patients continue to show deficits during strenuous exercises that require maximal endurance. Four soldiers who were considered clinically recovered from GBS (normal motor power with or without reappearance of reflexes and the absense of sensory impairment) were unable to pass the Army Physical Fitness Test (APFT), which is designed to measure a minimal acceptable age-related level of physical fitness (maximal effort to challenge respiratory and muscular endurance, strength, and flexibility). Before onset of GBS the four patients had all exceeded the APFT standards. None was able to pass the APFT as long as 4 years after the illness indicating that the sustained effort required in the fitness testing unmasked a significant, persistent deficit that interfered with their ability to continue their military careers.[40] Therefore the possibility of long-term endurance deficits should be considered when patients appear to have reached full recovery but report difficulty when returning to work or activities that require sustained maximal effort.[58]

Cardiovascular fitness also is compromised after recovery from GBS. Most patients with neuromuscular disease have lower Vo_2 max values than expected for age. This may be due to altered muscle function but is also related to deconditioning from an imposed sedentary life-style.[45] Several studies have attempted to determine the effect of endurance exercise training after GBS. One study of a 23-year-old woman with a chronic-relapsing form of GBS (usually a slow onset polyneuropathy with a remitting-relapsing course and persistent slowing of nerve conduction velocities) who had an onset at age 15, was placed on a walking and cycling program at 45% or less of her predicted maximal heart rate reserve. The low intensity exercise program was selected to prevent possible fatigue-related relapse. After the program, the subject had increased her walking time 37%, her walking distance approximately 88%, and her cycle ride time more than 100%. Although no standardized or formalized recording of functional level was recorded before and after the exercise program, the patient reported that her energy level for ADLs was a "little higher" and that stair walking was easier.[58]

In another single-subject study of a 54-year-old man three years after onset of GBS with residual weakness, the authors demonstrated similar improvements in cardiopulmonary and work capacities, as well as leg strength after a 16-week course of three times a week aerobic exercise program. The subject also reported expanded ADL capabilities. The authors suggested that their training regimen may disrupt the cycle of inactivity after recovery from GBS that leads to further deconditioning and less activity in patients with mild residual weakness.[69]

Florence and Hagberg[45] developed a cardiovascular fitness program for 12 patients with various neuromuscular diseases and demonstrated that the patients showed relatively normal physiological adaptations to training, although there were considerable variations in response depending on disease classification. No significant deleterious training effects were found, except that three patients with dystrophies did show increases in creatine kinase (CK) and myoglobin levels. In contrast to the two single-subject case studies cited earlier, patients in the Florence and Hagberg study did not report beneficial changes in ADL. As in the case studies, adaptive function was not formally assessed.

When neural recovery begins, the initiation of active exercise must be implemented with a clear understanding that excessive exercise during early reinnervation, when there are only a few functioning motor units, can lead to further damage rather than the expected exercise-induced hypertrophy of muscle.

Adaptive equipment and orthoses. Judicious use of orthotic devices and adaptive equipment should be considered an integral part of the rehabilitation process. The purpose of the orthotic and adaptive devices is twofold: (1) to protect weakened structures from overstretch and overuse and (2) to facilitate ADL within the limits of the patient's current ability. Orthotic devices and adaptive equipment should be introduced and discontinued based on the serial evaluations of strength, ROM, and functional needs. For example, a hospitalized patient who has Poor + (2+) middle deltoid strength may practice upper extremity activities such as eating while using suspension slings. A thumb position splint may be used temporarily to aid thumb control in grasping tasks.

Although most patients with GBS have a complete functional recovery, many show a more prolonged residual weakness of calf and, most commonly, anterior compartment musculature, requiring the use of an AFO. The decision whether to use prefabricated orthosis or custom appliances is not always simple. Several temporary orthotic measures can be considered. For example, if the patient shows good gastrocnemius-soleus strength with mild weakness of the dorsiflexors, a simple elastic strap attached to the shoe laces and a calf band may be sufficient to prevent overuse of the anterior compartment muscles. An old fashioned, relatively inexpensive spring wire brace, which can be attached to the patient's shoes to facilitate dorsiflexion, is a good choice for patients who complain of sensory hypersensitivity when wearing a plastic orthosis.

Most therapy units today have access to varied sizes of plastic, fixed ankle AFOs that can be used until a decision is made to have the patient fitted with custom AFOs. A newer system of prefabricated AFOs with adjustable ankle motion cams has been developed that allows the therapist to limit plantarflexion and dorsiflexion to the specific needs of the patient.* For patients with reasonable control of plantarflexion and dorsiflexion but with lateral instability because of peroneal weakness, a simple ankle stirrup device such as the Aircast Swivel-Strap stirrup splint can be used temporarily to provide lateral ankle stability.† Although very few patients with GBS need knee-ankle-foot orthoses (KAFOs) on a long-term basis, inexpensive air splints or adjustable long-leg metal splints to control knee position are sometimes helpful when working on standing weight bearing and during initial gait training. Refer to Chapter 32 for additional information on orthotics.

Most patients will need a wheelchair for several months as strength and endurance improve. A quandry for the therapist is to predict how long a wheelchair will be necessary and whether it should be rented or purchased. While moving from wheelchair mobility to independent ambulation, patients will usually progress from parallel bars, to a walker, then to crutches, or cane. Because wheelchairs, walkers, crutches, and canes, especially custom appliances, are very expensive and are not always included in insurance coverage, the therapist should carefully consider the cost to the patient during the recovery process.

Treatment of respiratory and dysphagia dysfunction. Depending on the facility, physical therapists may be involved in the respiratory care of patients with GBS. Goals of treatment are related to increasing ventilation or oxygenation, decreasing oxygen consumption, controlling secretions, and improving exercise tolerance. Readers should refer to *Cardiopulmonary Physical Therapy,*[54] 3rd edition for coverage of treatment programs and techniques for the GBS patient with acute or residual respiratory dysfunction. Chapter 15[51] provides a thorough review of postural drainage, positioning and secretion control techniques, breathing exer-

cises, including incentive spirometry methods, to minimize oxygen consumption and improve exercise tolerance. Chapter 17[50] details how to work with the patient with acute respiratory failure, and Chapter 18[53] provides extensive coverage in working with the respirator-dependent patient.

In many facilities, speech pathologists or occupational therapists are responsible for establishing a dysphagia treatment program. Therapists responsible for treatment of patients with dysphagia and swallowing problems should refer to Langmore and Longemann's classic text on the evaluation and treatment of swallowing disorders.[60] Basic treatment goals are the prevention of choking and aspiration and the stimulation of effective swallowing and eating. The act of chewing and swallowing is complex and requires coordinated reflexive and conscious action. Treatment is focused on positioning, head control, and oral-motor coordination (i.e., sucking an ice cube, stimulating the gag response, facilitating swallowing with pressure on neck and thyroid notch timed with intent to swallow). A conscious swallowing technique is introduced with thick liquids and progressed to thinner liquids after the patient's oral-motor coordination response is enough to control movement of fluids. Once the patient has good lip closure, fluids should be introduced one sip at a time from a straw cut to a short length to minimize effort. Gradually, semisoft moist foods are introduced (pasta, mashed potatoes, squash, jello). Any crumbly or stringy foods (coffee cakes, cookies, chips, celery, cheeses) should be avoided, and the patient should not attempt to talk or be interrupted during eating until choking does not occur and swallowing is comfortable and consistent.[75] Feeding training should occur during frequent, short sessions to prevent fatigue. Therapists should be prepared to use the Heimlich maneuver if choking occurs.

In summary, the rehabilitation program for a person with GBS must be graded carefully according to the stage of illness. In the acute care environment when respiratory deficits are present, the initial emphasis will be directed toward support of maximal respiratory status through postural drainage, chest stretching, and breathing exercises. Because of prolonged bed rest and immobility related to weakness, accessory and physiological ranges of motion must be maintained with around-the-clock efforts. Splinting or positioning devices are recommended to maintain functional positions during prolonged periods of immobility.

When neural recovery begins, the initiation of active exercise must be implemented with a clear understanding that excessive exercise during early reinnervation, when there are only a few functioning motor units, can lead to further damage rather than to the expected exercise-induced hypertrophy of muscle. Adaptive equipment and orthoses should be used as needed to protect weakened muscles, facilitate normal movement, and prevent fatigue during the reinnervation process. For an understanding of the clinical problem, refer to Case 2 on p. 402 followed by a complete summary of a typical therapeutic progression in the box on p. 404.

---

* The Natural Select™ Articulated Ankle Foot Orthosis. Zinco Industries, Inc, PO Box 5030, Pasadena, Calif 91117.
† Aircast, Inc, PO Box 709, Summit, NJ 07901.

CASE 2   ▼   Nancy

Nancy, a 16-year-old girl with a history of repeated hospitalizations for asthma was admitted to the hospital with tingling in the hands and feet and mild respiratory distress. Because staff thought there was a significant emotional component to her asthma attacks, her repeated complaints of paresthesias, muscle pain, and weakness were largely ignored or attributed to anxiety attacks. The day after admission, Nancy began staggering while walking and became extremely agitated and hysterical, screaming that she was dying and could not breathe. A medical assessment showed evidence of wheezing with a normal chest radiograph and decreased vital capacity. She was uncooperative during strength testing, although strength was estimated to be within normal limits except for approximately Fair +(3+) strength of the dorsiflexors and everters and Good strength of the plantarflexors. She became extremely upset when her feet were touched.

Because of her psychological history, she was referred for psychiatric assessment and was placed on an anxiolytic medication. Two hours later she suffered a full respiratory arrest and was intubated and maintained on mechanical ventilation. Over the next 3 days she developed flaccid quadriplegia and within 5 days she had complete cranial nerve involvement. She was weaned from the respirator after 29 days following several episodes of pneumonia. Postextubation, she had swallowing and speech problems that resolved by time of discharge at 3 months after onset. During the acute stage, she was catheterized because of urinary retention and was treated for a bowel obstruction. Sensation was normal for perception of temperature changes and deep pressure.

Proprioception was diminished at the ankle, knee, and fingers. Paresthesias and hypesthesias, aggravated by light touch, were present in a glovelike pattern of both hands and feet.

Nancy's physical therapy treatment began in the intensive care unit (ICU). Although her postural drainage treatment was performed by respiratory therapy in conjunction with aerosole medication by intermittent positive pressure, physical therapists began a course of chest stretching techniques in coordination with a fastidious ROM program performed twice a day by a therapist and on the evening and night shifts by a nurse. A pressure relief mattress was ordered for her bed. To prevent contracture development, an occupational therapist fabricated bilateral wrist and finger splints; a physical therapist molded ankle splints to maintain 90 degrees of dorsiflexion with neutral eversion-inversion. A positioning and range of motion schedule in poster form with pictures of positions and ROM patterns was posted at Nancy's bedside.

Because Nancy complained of severe hypersensitivity to light touch or to any passive movement of her limbs, a cradle was placed on the bed to prevent sheets from touching her and to prevent air flow changes from irritating her skin. She was fitted for above knee light pressure stockings, which seemed to decrease her sensitivity to light touch.

Progression of the GBS process seemed to plateau at approximately 15 days after onset with a very gradual return of respiratory function complicated by infections. Weaning from the respirator was difficult and the physical therapist played a major role in instructing Nancy, the staff, and her family in appropriate breathing exercises to be performed every 1 or 2 hours. Because her parents wanted to be involved with her care, they were taught ROM techniques with special attention to correct shoulder ROM techniques. The physical therapists continued to follow Nancy twice a day to ensure that accessory motions were completed with the physiological motions. Moist hot packs similar to those used during the polio era were used effectively before ROM for 1 week during which Nancy complained of severe muscle pain.

As part of her positioning program, Nancy was placed in supported semisitting position while on the respirator. As muscle control returned, a muscle reeducation program was initiated, which focused initially on head and trunk, then upper and lower extremities. Exercise periods were limited to 15 minutes twice a day. Ideally, she would have benefitted from more frequent short sessions; however, this was not possible. Therefore her parents were shown how to cautiously guide her active exercise program so that she was able to exercise more frequently at low repetitions. When each muscle group reached an MMT grade of Fair+ (3+) or greater, Nancy was allowed to use the muscles in functional activities with very proscribed limitations in activity duration. When she was able to tolerate upright sitting and had some bed mobility, Nancy was transferred to a Nelson bed in which she could begin a gradual standing weight-bearing program.

A speech therapist worked with Nancy in ICU to help her relearn safe swallowing patterns and to reintroduce her to different textured foods. A dietitian had been working with Nancy throughout her hospitalization to ensure adequate nutrition while intubated, and she worked closely with the speech therapist to progress Nancy's diet as she became able to handle liquids and solids.

After being weaned from the respirator and transferred to the general floor, Nancy was brought to the physical therapy department for treatment, which was frequently done in conjunction with occupational therapy. As strength increased, she began a program of resisted exercise. Trunk and upper and lower extremity PNF patterns were used as the primary exercise technique; however, great caution was used to avoid overworking weak muscle groups evoked during use of the PNF pattern. A full mat program with rolling and coming to sitting was also instituted. Occupational therapists focused on graduated use of Nancy's upper extremities, first using overhead slings attached to a wheelchair and later using a lap board to support her weakened shoulder musculature while practicing hand activities.

After 2 months of hospitalization, Nancy was discharged home to return for daily outpatient rehabilitation. Because Nancy appeared to be regaining strength well, she was provided with an ultralight rental wheelchair through her insurance for use until a final determination was made for long-term need. Nancy was also fitted with prefabricated adjustable AFOs, which were purchased through the physical therapy department. After 4 to 6 months a determination

Continued.

MUSCULAR DYSTROPHY

Muscular dystrophy refers to a group of hereditary myopathies characterized by progressive muscle weakness, deterioration, destruction, and regeneration of muscle fibers. During the process muscle fibers are gradually replaced with fibrous and fatty tissue. Accumulation of metabolic storage material in the muscle fibers is not found. Each of the inherited myopathies (i.e., Becker's dystrophy, myotonic dystrophy, limb-girdle dystrophy, and facioscapulohumeral) has its own unique genetic and phenotypic characteristics.

Because **Duchenne muscular dystrophy** (pseudohypertrophic) **(DMD)** is one of the most commonly known forms of the dystrophies, it will be used as a model for discussion of treatment implications for therapists. DMD is a disease of progressive muscle weakness leading to total paralysis and early death in the late teens or young adulthood. It has an incidence rate between 13 to 33/100,000 live births and a new mutation rate of approximately 1 in 10,000 (i.e., one third or more cases occur in families without a family history of DMD). In the last few years the abnormal gene for DMD has been detected on band Xp21 of the X chromosome. Because it has an X-linked, recessive pattern, the disease affects males almost exclusively. In almost 100% of patients with DMD, immunoblotting or immunostaining techniques show complete absence of dystrophin from muscle tissue. An early abnormality during the process of muscle fiber destruction is the breakdown of the muscle fiber plasma membrane. The membrane destruction results in an influx of calcium-rich extracellular fluid and complement components into the muscle fibers. In addition there is activation of intracellular proteases and complement with the ultimate removal of necrotic fibers by macrophages.[100,141]

Laboratory studies show serum CK elevated more than 100 times normal in early stages of the disease. These CK levels decrease over time with loss of muscle mass. Elevated CK is evident at birth long before symptoms are evident. Muscle biopsy data show degeneration with gradual loss of fiber, variation in fiber size, with a proliferation of connec-

tive and adipose tissue. Histochemical studies indicate loss of subdivision into fiber types, with a tendency toward type I fiber predominance. EMG studies show patterns of low amplitude, short duration, polyphasic motor unit action potentials.

Cardiac involvement is universal, although clinically significant cardiomyopathy is not common and death caused by cardiac dysfunction occurs in only about 10% of patients. Typically, the posterobasal area of the left ventricle is scarred producing ECG patterns with tall right precordial R waves and deep left precordial Q waves in 90% of patients.[142] Weakness of the respiratory muscles is usually evident by the tenth or twelfth year, although the diaphragm remains functional longer than intercostal and accessory muscle function. A progressive, sometimes severe scoliosis may contribute to respiratory compromise. Pure respiratory failure or respiratory failure secondary to infection is the usual cause of death, most commonly between the ages of 18 to 25. Other less common causes of death include gastric dilation and aspiration.[140]

The average intelligence quotient (IQ) of boys with DMD is approximately 85, with one third of the boys testing below 75. Although the relationship between lower IQ and DMD was initially thought to be related to limited life experience caused by the disease, recent studies have shown that dystrophin is also found in brain tissue. This suggests a possible relationship between the gene defect, which may cause decrease in dystrophin in brain tissue and impaired IQ. In contrast to the progressive pattern of muscle deterioration, intellectual impairment is not progressive.[140]

Clinical features

Although histological studies have indicated that DMD may be identified in the fetus as early as the first trimester, symptoms are seldom noted until the child is between 2 and 5 years of age. When recalling the child's early development, parents often state that the affected child was more placid and less physically active than expected.[91] The earliest

Medical status of patients with GBS and possible treatment outline

MEDICAL STATUS

Tracheostomy
Respirator dependent
Complete cranial nerve paralysis
Quadriplegia

Respiratory on IMV
Weaning to respirator at night by end of week 7
No active muscle contractions except eye opening, and lip movements
Dysphagia

Palpable muscle activity neck, trunk proximal musculature of upper and lower extremities

TREATMENT: (Depends on rate of recovery)

Week 1:
Postural drainage every 3 hours around the clock.
Passive ROM to all joints.
Splinting (molded plastic) of hands and feet to maintain functional position.
Positioning, splinting and ROM program schedule posted at bedside.

Weeks 2-5:
Postural drainage decreased to two times each shift (every 8 hours).
Passive ROM, physiological and accessory motions, gentle stretching of intercostal musculature, trunk rotations.
Continue splinting and positioning program.
Family education: family members taught gentle physiological ROM techniques, with attention to correct shoulder patterns and simple massage techniques.

Weeks 6-7:
Postural drainage two times each shift (every 8 hours).
Continue ROM program, splinting and positioning.
Begin to build tolerance of upright sitting with good trunk alignment.
Begin facilitation of active facial/tongue muscle activity in patterns necessary for swallowing, eating and speaking. Speech pathology, occupational therapy consult for dysphagia training.
Family members active in care with ROM, helping with ROM, splinting and positioning schedule as they choose.

Weeks 8-12:
Postural drainage one time each shift.
Chest stretching, breathing exercises.
Dysphagia program in collaboration with speech consultant.
Muscle reeducation program with EMG biofeedback progressing to gravity eliminated exercises using suspension slings attached to bed.
 Tilt table standing program to increase tolerance to upright (wearing positioning splints if necessary).
Collaborate with occupational therapy for treatment in wheel chair with suspension slings to facilitate active arm motion in gravity limited position.
Exercise, rest, positioning schedule posted.
Family, patient educated about stimulating activity level to prevent fatigue, overuse of reinnervating muscles.

obvious manifestations of DMD, however, may be the delay of early developmental milestones, particularly crawling and walking. In many cases the onset is very gradual. Parents or teachers may first identify a problem because the boy is noted to have difficulty keeping up with peers during normal play activities and to be somewhat clumsy with frequent falling when attempting to run, jump, climb structures, or negotiate uneven terrain. By age 5 years, symmetrical muscle weakness can usually be clearly identified with MMT. Deep tendon reflexes may be absent by 8 to 10 years or earlier. Sensation is normal.

The typical progression of weakness is symmetrical from proximal to distal, with marked weakness of the pelvic and shoulder girdle musculature preceding weakness of the trunk and extremity muscles. Muscles innervated by cranial nerves (except the sternocleidomastoids) are not involved, and bowel and bladder function is usually spared. Progression of weakness is slow but persistent. Marked weakness of the legs and anterior neck musculature affecting functional activities, including head control, usually precedes upper extremity muscle weakness affecting functional activities. A typical child will continue walking until about age 12 at which time use of a wheelchair becomes imperative. A rapid decrease in strength may occur after

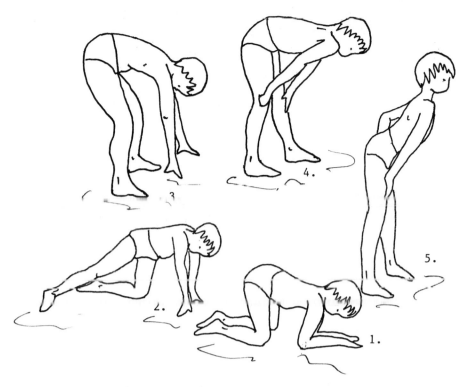

Fig. 13-5. Child demonstrating Gower's maneuvers necessary to achieve upright posture in patients with pelvic and trunk weakness.

prolonged periods of immobilization secondary to illness, injury, or surgery.[102]

Progression of lower extremity weakness. Before age 5, hypertrophy of the calf muscles is frequently noted. Pseudohypertrophy is evident as the muscle tissue is replaced by fat and fibrous tissue.[91,142] Even in the early stages of the disease, few boys with DMD walk with a normal gait pattern. Because of early pelvic girdle muscle weakness, most young boys retain a developmentally immature, wide-based gait pattern. An early distinctive feature of DMD is the Gower's maneuver in which the child gets up from the floor by using his arms to crawl up his own legs (Fig. 13-5).

Muscle imbalance occurs in typical patterns secondary to weakness and contractures. As the posterior hip muscles weaken, the child must arch his back when standing and retract his shoulder girdle to maintain the center of gravity behind the hip joint. This creates a pattern of lumbar lordosis and protrusion of the abdomen. As the quadriceps weaken, the child must maintain his knees in hyperextension to place the line of gravity anterior to the knee joint. At this point, the equinus contractures caused by a muscle imbalance between the plantar and dorsiflexors may help the child maintain knee control because the gastrocsoleus group provides a torque opposing knee flexion. If plantarflexion contractures become severe, however, the child will not be able to maintain standing balance because his base of support is too small and his ankle adaptive strategies are nonfunctional. Once the child stops weight bearing, development of severe equinovarus deformities is common. Fig. 13-6 shows a pattern of

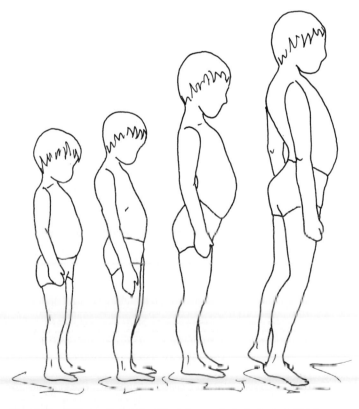

Fig. 13-6. Pattern of progression of muscle imbalance affecting trunk and lower extremities.

progression of muscle imbalance affecting the trunk and lower extremities in stance. Note the increasing lordosis and plantarflexion as the boys attempt to maintain their center of gravity posterior to the hip joint and anterior to the knee joint.

Typical gait pattern progression. The typical changes in gait pattern over time are identified in Fig. 13-7. Keep in mind that age alone is not an adequate index of predicted gait pattern. Many factors influence how long a child will be able to ambulate. Contributing factors are rate of progression of weakness; severity of contractures (hip flexion, external rotation, abduction, knee flexion, and plantar flexion-inversion contractures occur as disease progresses); effect of body weight; degree of respiratory compromise; type of treatment interventions such as bracing, surgery, and exercise; extent of family support; and the child's personal motivation to ambulate. For an extensive analysis of changes in gait pattern see Sutherland and others.[135] When the child can no longer ambulate functionally, a wheelchair must be ordered to fit the specific needs of that child within his home and community environment.

Progression of upper extremity weakness. The upper extremity pattern of weakness is similar to that of the lower extremities, with proximal musculature being affected before distal musculature. Functional changes related to weakness of upper extremity musculature, however, usually lag behind those of the lower extremities by 2 to 3 years. The early weakness of the scapular stabilization muscles interferes with controlled movement of the arms and hands during reaching. Gradually, the boy loses biceps and brachioradialis function followed by continued deterioration of triceps and more distal musculature. The marked instability of scapular musculature is clearly evident when the child tries to elevate his trunk with his arms (i.e., when attempting to use crutches) or when he is lifted from under the shoulders. A classic test of scapular stability is Meryon's sign in which the child slips from the examiner's grip as the child is being lifted from under the arms (Fig. 13-8). Typical progression of upper extremity weakness is shown by use of the reaching test (Fig. 13-9).

By the time the child reaches stage 3 of the reaching test, he needs considerable help with eating, hair care, and oral hygiene. Because of major trunk involvement and marked lower extremity weakness, the child will also be dependent for most ADLs, such as hygiene, dressing, and transferring. Typical functional stages in DMD are identified in the box on p. 408.

Medical treatment

Treatment of primary pathology. To date DMD is incurable. Some clinicians suggest that until an effective treatment can be found, the best way to decrease the number of children with DMD is through genetic counseling. Statistical tables are available to determine the risk of a mother or daughter with an affected son or brother. The risk

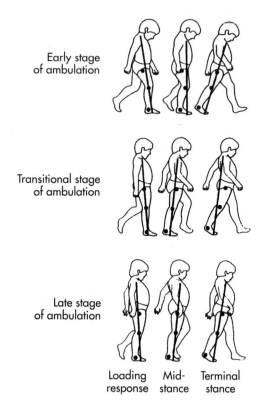

Fig. 13-7. Early through late stages of ambulation demonstrating changes in alignment at loading response, midstance, and terminal stance phases of gait. Used with permission. Hsu JD and Furumasu J: Gait and posture changes in the Duchenne muscular dystrophy child, *Clinical Orthopaedics and Related Research* 288, 1993.

factor is determined by calculating the number of normal males in the family and the CK level of the female and her mother. Serum CK is elevated in the female carriers, although its level is cyclic with a peak level occurring in the few months after the carrier's birth, then decreasing until age 4 years. Another peak in carrier CK level occurs at age 10 years and falls again at age 40 years when it begins to rise again. Genetic molecular probes of possible carriers are now available to identify deletions within the Xp21 region of the short arm of the X-chromosome at a 95% accuracy level. Of course, some families may have belief systems that do not allow consideration of pregnancy termination to prevent having a boy with possible DMD. Those views must be respected. Prenatal diagnosis of DMD for women without a family history of the disease is not yet practical.[129]

Despite much effort an effective pharmaceutical agent has not been identified to treat DMD. More recently, studies have shown that mazindol, a growth hormone inhibitor may slow weakness and contracture in DMD. In some cases, oral corticosteroids are effective to prolong ambulation,[95,100,105] although the results have been questioned because of possible problems with research bias.[112] More recently researchers have attempted to implant the normal precursor muscle cells or myoblasts directly into dystrophic mice and,

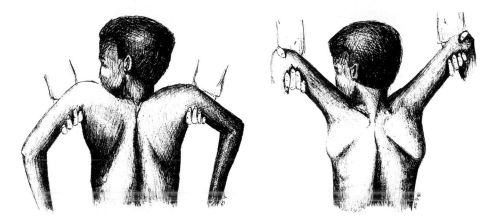

Fig. 13-8. Illustration of Meryon's sign showing lack of scapular stability in as child slips from examiner's grip when lifted from under the arms.

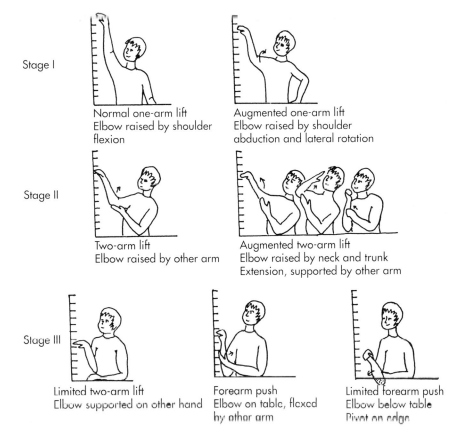

Stage I

Normal one-arm lift
Elbow raised by shoulder flexion

Augmented one-arm lift
Elbow raised by shoulder abduction and lateral rotation

Stage II

Two-arm lift
Elbow raised by other arm

Augmented two-arm lift
Elbow raised by neck and trunk Extension, supported by other arm

Stage III

Limited two-arm lift
Elbow supported on other hand

Forearm push
Elbow on table, flexed by other arm

Limited forearm push
Elbow below table
Pivot on edge

Fig. 13-9. Method of evaluating the working hand as demonstrated by the reaching test.

In several cases, into children with DMD to precipitate the proliferation of normal donor muscle cells into the host muscles of dystrophic subjects, but results have not lead to significant improvement to date.[124] Although no cure for DMD looms in the immediate future, the functional status of the patient, quality of life, and life expectancy can be influenced with thoughtful, functionally based treatment and supportive care.

Treatment of cardiopulmonary factors. Respiratory failure is the cause of death in 70% to 80% of patients with DMD. Cardiac and other causes account for the remaining deaths.[112] Because of limited activity, the cardiorespiratory fitness of children with DMD is impaired early in the disease process. Once the child becomes wheelchair dependent, his cardiorespiratory fitness deteriorates markedly. With increasing weakness of the respiratory musculature and the

Functonal transitions in muscular dystrophy

1. Ambulates with mild waddling gait and lordosis. Can run with marked effort, gait problems magnified. Can ascend, descend steps, curbs.

2. Ambulates with moderate waddling gait and lordosis. Cannot run. Difficulty with stairs and curbs. Rises from floor using Gower's maneuver. Rises from chair independently.

3. Ambulates with moderately severe waddling gait and lordosis. Rises from chair independently but cannot ascend or descend curbs or stairs, or rise from floor independently.

4. Ambulates with assistance or in some cases with bilateral KAFOs. May have had surgical releases of contractures. May need assistance with balance. Needs wheelchair for community mobility. Propels manual chair slowly. Independent in bed and self-care, although may need help with some dressing and bathing because of time constraints.

5. Transfers independently from wheelchair. Unable to walk independently, but can bear and shift weight to walk with orthoses if supported. Can propel self in manual chair but limited endurance. Motorized chair more functional. Independent in self-care with transfer assist for bath or shower.

6. Wheelchair independence in motorized chair. May need trunk support or orthosis. Needs assistance in bed and with major dressing. Can perform self-grooming but dependent for toiletting and bathing. May need alternating pressure relief mattress.

7. Wheelchair independence in motorized chair but may need to recline intermittently while in chair. Dependent in hygiene and most self-care requiring proximal upper extremity control.

8. As above and will use two hands for single hand activities—one hand supports working arm. May perform simple table-level hand activities, some self-feeding with arm support.

9. Sits in wheelchair only with trunk support and intermittent reclining or transfer to a supine position. Boys attending school may need to be on gurney for part of day. May benefit from nighttime ventilatory support or intermittent day time positive pressure breathing. (Some patients may have had an elective tracheostomy and need ventilatory support unit attached to wheelchair.) May have some hand control if arms supported. Will need help with turning at night.

10. Totally dependent. Unable to tolerate upright position, may elect home ventilatory support. Tracheostomy necessary for prolonged ventilation. Tracheostomy may be adapted for speech if oral musculature adequate. Needs 24-hour care. If around the clock home care cannot be arranged, patient must be hospitalized.

development of scoliosis, physicians must be vigilant in their treatment of respiratory infections. Physical therapy interventions, such as postural drainage and breathing exercises, are invaluable in preventing early death from respiratory failure (see *Cardiopulmonary Physical Therapy*,[115] and recommendations for respiratory physical therapy in the ALS and GBS sections of this chapter). Sleep hypoxia is common in the later stages of DMD. In some cases, intermittent positive pressure breathing (IPPB) by nasal mask has been effective in controlling oxygen desaturation at night.[112,129,130] Nighttime mechanical ventilatory support seems to provide relief for symptoms such as insomnia, progressive drowsiness, morning headaches, dyspnea, and anxiety.[94,117,125]

Several options for sustaining life in the final stages of DMD are the use of the Cuirass chest respirator and tracheostomy with mechanical ventilation. External ventilation support is initially used at night, then intermittently throughout the day until respiratory support is required at all times. As with patients with ALS, many significant treatment and ethical decisions must be made by the patient, family, and care providers when submitting to prolonged HMV.[122,131]

Cardiomyopathy frequently associated with DMD seldom becomes symptomatic because the child's decreased activity level does not stress the weakened heart muscle. In later stages of the disease, however, cor pulmonale with right heart failure may occur. Medical treatment of any cardiac symptoms generally follows the conventional interventions. Some boys with a severe scoliosis that creates cardiac compression may require correction by spinal fixation.[121]

Treatment of orthopedic factors. Scoliosis is a frequent complication of DMD, with incidence being reported from 49% to 93%. In a retrospective study of 88 patients with DMD, Lord and others[118] showed that scoliosis was age-related, being identified in 30% of boys in the 8- to 14-year age group, 92% in the 15- to 20-year age group, and 64% in boys over age 20 years. The decrease in the number of boys with scoliosis over age 20 suggested that boys without scoliosis have greater longevity, although the evidence was not conclusive. Fig. 13-10 presents an example of a boy with a moderate scoliosis affecting sitting posture.

Scoliosis tends to occur in two basic patterns: the early onset form (approximately 23%), which becomes evident before the child becomes wheelchair dependent, and the late onset form, which develops, on average, 4 years after wheelchair dependency. In the early onset form the curve usually becomes severe and progressive leading to pulmonary compromise and structural-based pain. In the late onset form the course is usually mild. The traditional view of scoliosis development has been that the child's increasing weakness leads to abnormal sitting postures, which in turn leads to severe kyphoscoliosis. Unfortunately, attempts to control sitting posture through the use of spinal orthosis and wheelchair seating inserts (i.e., inserts that place the child in

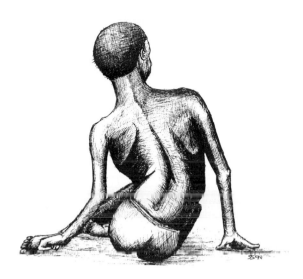

Fig. 13-10. Moderate scoliosis affecting sitting stability.

lumbar lordosis to lock facets, thereby preventing rotation and lateral collapse or, more commonly, lumbar and thoracic lateral supports) have been disappointing.[118] Although DMD is generally thought to have a symmetrical pattern of weakness, recent evidence suggests an asymmetrical paraspinous involvement, which may be the cause of the severe scoliosis seen in some boys.[134]

Miller and others[121] reported on 68 patients with DMD who underwent posterior spinal fusion with instrumentation for severe scoliosis. (Over the course of the study, several different forms of fixation were used.) Although they found that the boys who underwent spinal fixation were more comfortable in their later years and were easier to care for, deterioration of pulmonary function was not slowed after surgery. The average age of death of the boys in the study was 18.3 years. This was the same as the average age of death reported for another similar group of boys who did not have spinal surgery.

In interviews with 42 end-stage patients who underwent scoliosis surgery or their caregivers, 35 felt that the instrumentation was beneficial, 6 felt that it was not, and 1 was uncertain.[122] Of 15 patients interviewed, all felt that the surgery was helpful. Seventeen percent of the boys had pulmonary complications after surgery. Based on their experience, the authors suggest that a forced vital capacity (FVC) of at least 35% of normal is necessary before surgery can be performed. They recommend that spinal stability is best achieved with segmental fixations rather than with Harrington rods because the segmental fixation systems allow immediate postoperative mobilization of the patient, which is essential to prevent marked disuse deterioration. Attention must also be given to how the spine is positioned with fixation. If the curve cannot be completely corrected, the curves should be balanced to create a horizontal pelvis. Maintenance of some lumbar lordosis (45 degrees) and

thoracic kyphosis (25 degrees) is essential because it allows the boy to keep his head in a forward position to compensate for severely weakened anterior neck muscles. Physical therapists must play an aggressive role in treatment of children with DMD after spinal fixation. Other orthopedic interventions to improve mobility are discussed later.

Nutritional concerns.   Excessive weight gain that decreases functional ability is a frequent and difficult problem for children with DMD and their families. The typical active child needs about 2400 calories to maintain weight and grow. The child with DMD who is more sedentary or wheelchair dependent may need 1200 or fewer calories to maintain weight. A healthy low-fat diet should be encouraged with adequate bulk foods and fluids to facilitate bowel function and motility. Problems with obesity are often related to the family's typical pattern of eating and nurturing. It is not uncommon for the child and family members to "feed" their anxiety or depression about the disease.[129] In many cases family members and friends feel that the child's only pleasure may be eating. Although this may seem true, caring for a totally dependent obese teenager or young adult can become problematic for both the child and the caregivers. Before obesity becomes an issue, the child and his family should be referred for comprehensive nutritional advice from a specialist experienced in dealing with childhood obesity. Suggestions for adapting eating behavior and food choices will not be followed if they are too restrictive or unreasonable for the child's social situation.[103,108]

As the disease progresses, some children develop problems swallowing. To decrease the possibility of aspiration, careful attention must be paid to food textures and chewing and swallowing functions (see section on ALS for information on dealing with bulbar symptoms). Depending on the patient's and family's decisions about prolongation of life, some patients choose to supplement or receive their nutrition via nasogastric or orogastric tube or elect to have a permanent percutaneous gastrostomy placed.

Therapeutic intervention

Therapeutic assessment.   Ideally, a team of specialists should be involved in the long-term care of a child with DMD and his family. The therapist's primary role is twofold: to perform serial evaluations of the child's movement capabilities and to adjust the child's intervention program accordingly to maximize function as the disease progresses. A typical physical therapy evaluation should include assessment of muscle strength, ROM, and functional status. In some facilities the physical therapist also collects data on the child's pulmonary status (see *Cardiopulmonary Physical Therapy*, Chapter 15 for assessment information[115]).

Manual muscle testing.   MMT is a reasonably reliable technique for measuring muscle strength of children with DMD if consecutive evaluations are made by the same rater. Reliability of scores in the gravity eliminated position was highest.[106] In DMD, there is a linear pattern of decreased muscle strength without marked changes in the rate of deterioration in strength over time. The rate of muscle weakness is not influenced by bracing programs or wheelchair use,[90] although functional status may change. Manual muscle testing after prolonged periods of immobility, however, may reflect increased weakness from disuse atrophy rather than the disease progress. Therefore marked, precipitous decreases in MMT scores may reflect a transitory situation that will respond to increased activity and exercise.

Range of motion.   As with MMTs, serial ROM evaluations should be completed by the same therapist because intrarater reliability is higher than interrater reliability.[123] Careful tracking of ROM is imperative because the development of contractures of the hip, knee, and ankle caused by muscle imbalance is a more common reason for early loss of ambulation than actual muscle weakness.[127]

Functional status.   The child's functional status continues to be relatively stable for some time even when MMT indicates that the child is losing strength. Because the weakness is gradual, many children develop remarkably adaptive adjustments in movement patterns to cope with the loss of strength. Brooke and others[96] describe a functional scale for determining the child's status and for predicting appropriate care (also see Vignos and others[137]).

Respiratory function.   The physical therapist's role in evaluating respiratory status in children with DMD will vary depending on the facility and area of the nation in which the therapist works. For information on a full evaluation see *Cardiopulmonary Physical Therapy,* Chapter 15[113] and refer to the section on ALS in this chapter. At minimum, the therapist should evaluate bulbar function, cough effectiveness, and vital capacity (a simple spirometer available in most clinics is adequate). For more sophisticated testing, the child should be seen by a pulmonary function specialist. In addition, the therapist may find it helpful to test the child's energy cost during ambulation using the Energy Expenditure Index described by Rose and others[126] which divides walking heart rate minus resting heart rate by walking speed (EEI = WHR − RHR/D/T). This technique was adapted for use in the clinic by using a simple exercise watch pulsimeter (Hallum, unpublished data). By determining the child's work efficiency using this simple method, it may be possible for clinicians to help the child, family, and treatment team to determine when it may be best to make the transition to a wheelchair.

Goals.   The basic goals for a therapeutic program are very straight forward: (1) maintain full ROM, (2) prevent contractures that can lead to further disability and pain, (3) maintain maximal strength/prevent disuse atrophy, (4) facilitate maximal functional abilities using appropriate adaptive equipment, (5) maintain maximal respiratory muscle strength and movement of secretions, and (6) foster realistic child and family expectations within the context of the environment. These broad based goals, however, may not be adequate for today's third-party payers, and the therapist will need to write more specific, time-oriented goals.

Therapy treatment.   In today's health care environment, therapists act primarily in the role of consultant rather than direct service provider. Much of the child's exercise program must be carried out at home by caregivers. Because both parents often work today, or because the child lives in a single parent home with a working parent, compliance with home programs is problematic. If possible, as many exercise activities as possible should be encouraged within the child's school day so that parents can focus on nurturing, general caregiving, and simple positioning and bedtime exercises. Under the supervision of a consulting therapist, the child's therapy often can be provided in some form at the child's school if on-site therapists, personal attendants, or adapted physical education teachers are available.

Respiratory care.   Although physical therapists most often focus on mobility issues, they also should be prepared to provide the child and family with methods to improve breathing efficiency. In the early stages of the disease, the child and family can be taught simple breathing exercises stressing diaphragmatic breathing, full chest expansion, air shifts, and rib cage stretching. Most children enjoy playing with hand-held incentive spirometer units and playing blowing games (e.g., bubbles, pinwheels). Once the child begins to have difficulty clearing secretions, the family should be taught postural drainage and coughing techniques such as "huffing" and manual coughing assists (see *Cardiopulmonary Physical Therapy,* Chapter 25 for information on techniques that can be adapted for DMD).[139] These techniques should be reviewed and used aggressively whenever the child is bed-bound for more than a day or two and before and after all surgical procedures.

Respiratory muscle exercises increase strength and endurance in subjects with and without pulmonary disease.[92] Preliminary evidence suggests that respiratory endurance can be improved in children with DMD.[101] More recently in a study of 18 boys with DMD to determine the efficacy of respiratory endurance and strength training programs, the authors found improvement in ventilatory muscle endurance, but not in respiratory muscle strength.[120] Although respiratory exercise cannot reverse the process of respiratory failure, attention to pulmonary hygiene and breathing exercise can help the child cope more effectively with respiratory infections and the discomfort accompanying respiratory compromise.

Prevention of contractures.   The two-joint muscles are most prone to developing significant contractures. Early in the course of the disease process, a home program must be instituted to include ROM, stretching, and positioning. Both parents and the child must be educated about the expected changes in muscle balance and how they can play an active role in preventing or limiting the impact of contractures secondary to muscle imbalance.

Initially, the child should be encouraged to move his own limbs actively through full range. At the first sign of loss of end-range of motion, the physical therapist should adjust the child's program to include specific stretches. As active ROM becomes more difficult, parents will need to assist the child to move his limbs to the end ranges of all motions to stretch the muscles and periarticular structures. The stretching program should use static stretching techniques with prolonged, mild tension to affect both the viscoelastic and plastic properties of the muscle.[143] Although studies to show the best length of time to stretch muscles with contractures have not been performed, a stretch of 15 seconds increased ROM in persons with normal muscle tissue.[119] If the child can actively contract the contractured muscle, hold-relax or contract-relax, PNF techniques may be useful to increase ROM. Joint mobilization techniques should be included in the treatment program before capsular contractures occur. Intuitively, one would expect that to decrease contractures, the length of stretching time should be prolonged, and the increased range should be maintained with positioning or bracing. The best approach to contractures, however, is to prevent them. (Also see Grossman and others[109] for a review of effect of immobilization on muscle and appropriate therapy interventions.)

Because the development of contractures follow a predictable pattern, a positioning program should be started before contractures are evident. For example, the child can be encouraged to watch television while lying prone with legs aligned out of the common "frog leg" pattern. Once a child has significant hip flexor or iliotibial band contractures, stretching techniques must be very specific because simple prone positioning can force the lumbar spine into excessive lordosis. Although difficult to accomplish in some mainstreamed school environments, positioning the child in a standing frame during several class periods helps provide prolonged stretch to hip, knee, and ankle musculature. Some children will tolerate night splinting to control plantar flexion contractures; however, few children will tolerate wearing long-leg splints at night to prevent knee flexion contractures or to align the hips (additional bar between legs to control rotations). Research supports the view that the combination of stretching, positioning, and splinting should begin before contractures exist. If night ankle splints are worn consistently in combination with stretching, the rate of progression of contractures can be minimized.[97] In a prospective study of prevention of deformity in DMD, Scott and others[127] found that boys who had consistent treatment with AFOs (splints) and daily stretching were able to continue walking longer than boys who did not have a stretching and splinting program.

Maintenance of maximal functional level. Ideally, the child with DMD should be as active as possible to prevent disuse weakness not directly related to the disease process. Studies on the value of active exercise on dystrophic muscles have shown varied results. In animal studies, dystrophic

mice trained on a treadmill showed increased damage to muscle tissue,[136] whereas forced swimming in dystrophic mice had no adverse effect.[140] In a more recent study of endurance training of dystrophic hamsters, Elder[104] concluded that increased contractile activity associated with treadmill exercise had no detrimental effect on developing muscle and may have had a beneficial effect in young animals by improving fiber hypertrophy, increasing maximal tetanic force, and decreasing fiber degeneration.

Studies of humans with muscular dystrophy have also shown mixed results. In a case review of three generations of patients with facioscapulohumeral muscular dystrophy (seven cases and one suspected case), Johnson and Braddom[116] noted asymmetrical weakness of the upper extremities, which they related to patterns of overuse (dominant side or side used most often in work activities). Based on their information and additional evidence that muscle-derived enzymes (CK and myoglobin concentrations in blood) were markedly elevated in patients with DMD after prolonged exercise,[107] Johnson and Branddom[116] suggested that endurance exercise may be contraindicated.

In another study boys exercised one quadriceps isokinetically for 6 months. The contralateral leg was used as a control. At the end of the study, no evidence of overwork weakness was noted. There was a nonsignificant increase in muscle strength of the exercised quadriceps over the nonexercised contralateral muscle, which was maintained for 3 months after cessation of exercise. The authors concluded that submaximal exercise did not negatively effect muscle tissue, but it may be of limited value in increasing strength.[99]

Other research has shown that judicious exercise may have a positive effect on function. For example, Vignos and Watkins[138] in 1966 compared two groups of boys with DMD. One group participated in a 12-month home-strengthening program using graduated weights for maximal resistance. The control group continued their normal activities but did not participate in the exercise program. The muscle strength of both groups had showed a decline during the year before the study. At the end of the study, the control group showed continued decline. The exercise group, however, showed a small increase in strength as measured by MMT. Because the initial strength of the muscles before the program was positively related to improvement, the authors suggested that the exercise program should be started during the initial stages of the disease rather than waiting until the child has quit ambulating.

In addition to active and resistive exercise programs, Scott and others[128] completed a small study of the effect of intermittent chronic low frequency electrical stimulation (ES) on dystrophic anterior tibialis muscles. They demonstrated a significant increase in mean voluntary contraction force and suggested that ES can have a beneficial effect if used with children whose muscles are not already markedly weakened.

Overall, the data from animal and human studies suggest that submaximal exercise is not harmful and may be helpful in maintaining maximal movement function if the patient does not exercise into marked fatigue. Hasson[111] in his review of exercise studies of patients with muscular dystrophy, concluded that exercise consisting of brief periods of low or high-intensity activity can improve strength for patients with minimal to moderate weakness, but that exercise programs have no effect on strength of muscles already severely weakened. Oxygen consumption also improved with endurance training, although it is not clear whether repetitive endurance training at moderate or high intensity (70% of Vo_2max) may cause muscle damage. Increased recruitment of motor units from training effects also may improve muscle coordination and reduce disuse atrophy. See Fig. 13-11 for a graphic example of responses of normal and impaired muscle to exercise.

Ideally, the child's exercise needs can be incorporated into pleasurable activities adapted for children with movement and weakness-related balance problems. Because endurance is a problem, aerobic-type programs are not appropriate in most cases, with the exception of respiratory endurance programs previously noted.[101] Many ambulatory children, however, enjoy ball activities, walking-based, simple obstacle courses, parachute games, table tennis, cycling (preferably tandem), and especially swimming. Swimming is an excellent exercise for children with DMD because they often are quite buoyant due to their increased fat/muscle ratio. Many children can continue to float or swim independently on their backs well into the time they are able to move only distal muscle. All activity programs should have structured rest periods. A safe indicator of extent and intensity of exercise is that the patient should recover from exercise fatigue after a night's rest. An active exercise program did not benefit patients who were in later, dependent stages of DMD.[111]

Maintenance of ambulation. As the DMD progresses, the child's posture and gait pattern become extreme and he must work harder to maintain balance while walking. Most children gradually discontinue walking about a year after they lose their ability to deal with stairs or when daily ambulation time decreases to less than one-half hour per

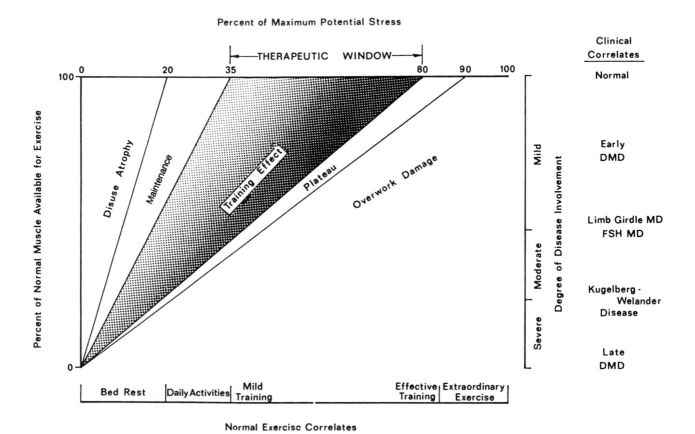

Fig. 13-11. Idealized response of normal and impaired muscle to exercise. The therapeutic window of safe exercise narrows progressively. Activities (lower X axis) causing normal exercise effects in normal muscle (upper X axis) correlate to different effects in impaired muscle. Used with permission. Coble NO and Maloney FP: Effects of exercise on neuromuscular disease. In Maloney FP, Burks JS, and Ringel SP: *Interdisciplinary rehabilitation of multiple sclerosis and neuromuscular disorders,* New York, 1985, J.B. Lippincott Company.

day.[138] Toward the end of the child's independent walking stage, he has a marked anterior pelvic tilt with lordosis and a protuberant abdomen. His shoulders are retracted and he may hold his hands behind his hips or elevated in a mid-guard position to stabilize his hips. He has a severe waddling gait with a shortened stride and he must carefully lock his knees at each step. He falls frequently. Fig. 13-12 shows the typical walking pattern of a boy who is being considered for release of contractures and bracing.

If the child and his family have followed an aggressive ROM, positioning, and activity program, the child's walking time may be extended by months. In most cases, however, the contractures from muscle imbalance continue relentlessly and the child begins to need support when walking. When contractures at the hip, knee, and ankle show evidence of interfering with the child's ability to stabilize each joint during stance, most children are referred for surgery to restore functional joint motion.

Bach and McKeon[93] studied 13 boys with DMD who had surgery to release lower extremity contractures. Seven boys were ambulating independently before surgery (early surgery group) and six boys were preparing to use or had begun using a wheelchair before surgery (late surgery group). Depending on the child's contracture patterns, the boys underwent surgical procedures that typically included subcutaneous releases of the Achilles tendons and hamstring

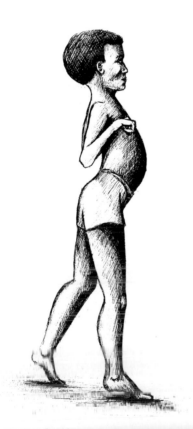

Fig. 13-12. Illustration showing typical walking pattern of a boy who is being considered for release of contractures and bracing.

muscles and fasciotomies of the iliotibial bands. Four patients had rerouting of the posterior tibialis to the dorsal surface of the second or third cuneiform to balance the foot and prevent the often severe varus position of the foot. Boys in the late surgical group required more extensive inpatient rehabilitation, whereas boys in the early surgical group were treated as outpatients after a short in-hospitalization.

Physical therapy was started on the second postoperative day. The program consisted of general conditioning exercises of the trunk and extremities (i.e., rolling, trunk stabilization, neck and head control), stretching exercises, and intensive weight bearing in standing while wearing bilateral long-leg casts or below knee casts depending on the surgery. One child participated in a pool therapy program.

Based on their results, Bach and McKeon[93] suggest that early surgery for contractures followed by intensive physical therapy can prolong brace-free ambulation. The number of falls experienced by the boys decreased markedly after the surgery and rehabilitation period. Boys in the early intervention groups benefited from the surgical interventions more than the boys in the later intervention groups. All patients and their families in the early surgery group thought that the procedures were helpful. Boys in the late surgery group, however, stated either that they would not have had the surgery if they had a chance to decide again or that they had no opinion (also see Bach and McKeon[93] for succinct review of orthopedic treatment to prolong ambulation).

In current standard treatment protocols for children with DMD, bilateral KAFOs are used in conjunction with surgical release of contractures. Surgery is followed by an aggressive therapy program. The main criterion for the surgery-bracing program is the child's impending loss of ability to walk independently. When this occurs, the child has usually lost about 60% of his muscle mass,[132] and he has a pattern of contractures that magnifies the effect of the weakness. Ideally, the KAFOs should be measured and fitted in final form before the surgery so the child can begin upright weight bearing in the KAFOs the day after surgery. The KAFOs are commonly fabricated of molded plastic thigh units (ishial weight-bearing quadrilateral socket) with metal joints at the knee (drop locks) and ankle (or a flexible plastic ankle component)[114] (see Fig. 13-13). If the orthoses are not immediately available, the child can begin the standing program in long-leg casts.

In the hospital, standing in bilateral KAFOs can be initiated on a tilt table. Most children are quite fearful after surgery and complain of significant pain when their legs are moved or if they are placed upright. For therapy to be successful during this early standing stage and during passive ROM exercises, the child must have adequate pain medication. If the child is not properly medicated in the first few days after surgery, the therapist may have to deal with very difficult, resistant behaviors of the child, which persist long after the pain should have subsided. Pain protocols must be discussed before the child's surgical procedures. The

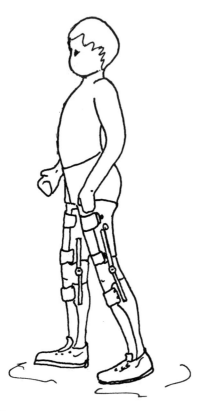

Fig. 13-13. Example of boy walking in KAFOs showing ishial weight bearing quadrilateral socket, knee drop locks, and plastic ankle component.

child should be medicated at least one-half hour before the therapist's visit.

Gait training is usually begun within 48 hours after surgery. Initial work focuses on helping the child regain his sense of standing balance because his old patterns of equinus, lordosis, and shoulder retraction may no longer be adaptive. The child should be allowed to find his own best center of balance, and he should be allowed to use compensatory gait deviations necessary to allow the best mobility and stability. Depending on the child's upper extremity strength and control, he may progress from parallel bars for balance assist, to pushing a wheelchair or weighted walker, to balance assist from a therapist using a safety strap to prevent falls. Some children who seem to need a walker for balance transition do best if they use a walker with forearm rests and vertical hand grips, which seems to help them stabilize their arms more effectively than a standard walker. Fortunately, most children do learn to walk independently without support again after surgery, although they are unable to negotiate steps or inclines or rise from the floor independently.[110]

Hyde and others[114] reported that 24 of 30 boys treated with KAFOs were able to achieve functional ambulation again. In another study, 15 of 17 boys with DMD who had ceased walking were able to ambulate again after release of

contractures followed by use of KAFOs and physical therapy. Even though the children's walking speed was decreased after bracing and the children were not able to rise from the floor or negotiate stairs, the children's ability to move about independently at home or around the classroom was considered invaluable for their independence.[132] Unfortunately, none of the studies on bracing included formalized evaluations of the children's level of satisfaction with the surgical treatment, bracing, and rehabilitation process. In addition to gait training, the physical therapist should work with the child to help him learn to fall as safely as possible. Even though practice falls do not duplicate the sudden crash from unexpected falls, most children develop a stronger sense of confidence if they have worked on falling techniques.

Use of swivel walkers has been recommended by some therapists and physicians because the child does not need upper extremity control for support. Although the concept of hands-free walking seems logical, boys with DMD had more difficulty using the walkers when compared to children with paraplegia because of the more delicate postural adjustments needed by children with dystrophy and their greater sensitivity to the motion restriction of the swivel walker. Some therapists have reported success using the ORLAU VCG (variable center of gravity) walker[133]; however, support for its use is not widespread.

Because most children with DMD today are discharged home within a few days after surgery, physical therapists must provide options for continuing the standing within the home. Standing frames are often available through the child's school district or therapy unit. If they are not, the therapist can help the family build a simple standing frame for home. This frame often can be made from a piece of plywood, or a gluteal strap system can be attached to a table at home. If possible the child should be positioned just forward of the line of gravity to encourage back extension with facet stability and to allow the child better head control (remember the weak anterior neck muscles).

Transition to wheelchair. Although surgical and orthotic interventions may prolong ambulation within the home and classroom past the predicted time for cessation of independent walking (8 to 12 years), most children begin to use a wheelchair for community mobility and long distances before this time. When children begin to spend more time in their chair, the rate of development of contractures, disuse weakness, and obesity increases.[114,132] Because of this more rapid deterioration in the child's functional skills, professionals and parents often discourage the child from using a chair for mobility. Children, however, tend to welcome use of the chair because they have more energy for their social interactions and learning tasks.[114]

Selection of the appropriate wheelchair is often difficult for the patient and family because of the multiple decisions that must be made. Few children with DMD can propel a manual wheelchair for more than a few years because of their increasing upper extremity weakness. In addition, their propulsion speed in their manual chair is seldom adequate to keep up with their peers. Eventually, the child will need a motorized chair. Although this provides tremendous freedom for the child, a motorized chair presents problems to many families because transporting the chair requires a van and lift unit, which are seldom funded by insurance or donations. Ideally, the child should have both a manual and motorized chair; however, in today's health policy climate, parents often have to engage in protracted efforts to attain adaptive equipment for their child.

An important consideration when purchasing a wheelchair is the trunk support system. Traditionally, boys with DMD are thought to develop a gravity collapse of the spine related to their functional sitting posture. To control the collapsing spine, spinal orthosis and seat inserts to lock the spine in extension (to prevent lateral bending and rotation) are frequently recommended. Unfortunately, the effectiveness of positioning devices to control the development of scoliosis has been disappointing.[118] Although Drennan[102] suggests that spinal fixation is necessary to control scoliosis, all children are not candidates for surgery. The therapist, therefore should work with the child, family, and the orthopedist to determine the best system to maintain optimal spinal alignment and trunk stability as the child weakens. In addition, as the child becomes more physically dependent, the chair may need to be fitted with pressure relief seat cushions, elevating leg rests, and a reclining back with a head rest.[110]

Because of the problems associated with increased wheelchair use, the therapist must work closely with the family and any school-based personnel to design a realistic plan to prevent rapid deterioration once the child begins to spend more time in the chair than walking. If possible, the child's standing program in KAFOs should be continued at school and at home as long as possible, with a goal of 3 to 5 hours of standing per day. With mainstreaming, however, continuing a standing program at school is sometimes difficult because attendants and equipment are not available, the child may need to move from room to room for different classes, and the child may not like being singled out for special treatment. It is helpful to caregivers if the child continues to wear his KAFOs when using the chair until he is totally dependent for transfers and can no longer be pivoted from chair to another surface.

If the child uses a motorized wheelchair, directional control systems must be adapted to each child's needs. Most young people with advanced DMD do well for years with a hand control system; however, some young people need control systems that can be operated by head, tongue, or breath movements. A patient using a respiratory support system will need his wheelchair adapted to accommodate the ventilation unit.

When the child can no longer tolerate the sitting position, some children have continued to attend school on a gurney.

Another option to consider for use at home or at school is the neuro chair used in many hospitals, which can be adjusted from a horizontal position to various sitting angles. Caregivers often find this highly adjustable chair invaluable, because the bedridden patient can be transferred directly from bed to the horizontal chair surface with a slide pull rather than a lift. Once the patient is on the unit in its horizontal position, it can be adjusted to any upright position that is tolerated by the patient. (This chair is also useful for patients with ALS and GBS.)

Psychosocial issues

Psychosocial issues related to DMD are family issues. At the time of the child's diagnosis, the parents are often emotionally devastated and cycle back and forth through many phases of denial, anger, sadness, and active coping. This process tends to recur when the child does not meet expected normal physical and social milestones or when he reaches predicted stages of deterioration, such as the transition to a wheelchair. Early in the child's life, the family should be guided to encourage the child's independence and to discourage overprotection. Therapists can play an important role in helping the child and family identify realistic goals for independence.

Psychosocial support should be made available to the child and family during predictable times of crisis. Major times of crisis occur around the age of 5 years when the child begins to realize his differences, between the ages of 8 to 12 years when the child loses the ability to walk independently, during the adolescent years when social interactions become restricted, and around the time of high school graduation when the child and family must face vocational limitations and almost certain death within the next decade. Transition times are often accompanied by depression, withdrawal, and anxiety in the child and family members. Parents had a marked preoccupation with their sons and a diminished expression of enjoyment.[141]

In a pilot study, 43 boys with DMD between the ages of 4 ½ and 15 years completed human figure drawings (HFDs). HFDs have been used for 75 years as a projective tool to identify emotional factors that may not be verbalized clearly by the child. Using the process, the authors found that the children's drawing were characterized by emotional indicators suggesting physical inadequacy, body inadequacy, immaturity, and insecurity. Adolescents with DMD felt significantly isolated from the mainstream of life.[141] Predictably, the integrity, strength, and intragenerational and intergenerational function and coping styles of the child's family contribute a great deal to the way the family responds to the child's progressive deterioration. Extended periods of anxiety and depression should be treated vigorously with cognitive interventions, support groups, respite care, and when appropriate short term anxiolytics and antidepressants. Parents and the child should be given the opportunity to discuss the impending death in an accepting environment

CASE 3 ▼ Jeremy

Jeremy was 3 years old when he was diagnosed with DMD. He lived at home with his mother and a 5-year-old sister. There was no known family history of DMD, although family lore suggests that a cousin died very young from pneumonia and a "wasting disease." Jeremy was referred for a medical evaluation when a playground supervisor at his preschool noted that he was very clumsy when running and that he had difficulty on the playground climbing equipment and the slide. He also had difficulty rising from the ground and needed to hold a railing when stepping up a stair.

During a medical history, Jeremy's mother said that she had noticed that he was "slow to develop" but was not worried because she thought he was just "a late bloomer." A muscle biopsy was positive for a diagnosis of DMD. A physical therapy evaluation 3 months after diagnosis showed ROM to be within normal limits for all joints. Muscle weakness was evident on MMT with G− (4−) hip abduction and extension and quadriceps strength bilaterally. Hip flexion, knee flexion, dorsiflexion, and toe extension were in the G (4) range. Plantar flexion was G+ (4+) with evident hypertrophy. Shoulder abduction and flexion was in the G (4) range, although he had difficulty sustaining abduction for more than 5 seconds.

Jeremy had a moderate head lag when moving from supine to sitting due to G− (4−) anterior neck muscles. The therapist made an on-site school visit to help the teachers identify obstacles to Jeremy's full integration with his classmates. The school custodian built some ramps to help Jeremy use the playground equipment.

Jeremy ambulated independently until age 8 years. His gait pattern was typical of late stage ambulation (marked equinus, knee hyperextension during stance, bilateral Trendelenburg on stance, marked lordosis with a protuberant abdomen with arms held posterior to hips). He had 40-degree hip flexion contractures with iliotibial band tightness, no knee contractures, and 25-degree plantarflexion contractures. MMTs showed the expected decrease in strength, with pelvic and shoulder girdle muscles being weaker than more distal musculature, except anterior tibialis and the peroneals were F+ (3+). He was unable to rise independently from the floor and needed assistance with stairs. Because his gait pattern was very slow and he needed to rest frequently when walking more than 20 feet at school, Jeremy had been using a manual wheelchair for long distance mobility since the age of 7 years.

On the recommendation of orthopedist consultants, Jeremy underwent bilateral percutaneous hip flexor lengthenings, iliotibial band fasciotomies, and heel cord releases. Bilateral KAFOs had been fitted before surgery, and Jeremy was placed in the braces after surgery. No casting was done. Despite his complaints, he was gradually brought to the full weight-bearing standing position by late afternoon on the day after surgery. Adjustments were made in his pain medication schedule to allow him to tolerate the process more comfortably. By the third hospital day, Jeremy participated in two therapy sessions per day and was standing in the parallel bars where he was taught lateral and anteroposterior weight shifting in preparation for ambulation. Active assisted and passive ROM exercises were performed without the KAFOs twice a day. On the fourth hospital day, Jeremy began to take short steps using the parallel bars for balance. His mother was also taught his exercises so that Jeremy could have more than two therapy sessions a day. On the fourth day, he practiced walking for 10 minutes six times a day with full physical therapy treatment twice a day.

Because Jeremy was from a rural area and daily physical therapy would not be available on discharge, he was kept in the hospital for three additional days for intensive rehabilitation. An occupational therapist worked with Jeremy to provide adaptive equipment for reaching, self-care, and eating (he was unable to raise his arms above 45 degrees and needed his left arm to assist the right when reaching). He was discharged home on the eighth day. An Elks Traveling Therapist arranged to visit the family once a week for the next month to continue ambulation training and to guide the mother in a home positioning and ROM program. The therapist also helped the mother adapt the home environment and his school to adjust expectations of Jeremy so he was less prone to falling and excessive fatigue.

The family was lost to follow-up, but by report, Jeremy continued to ambulate in his KAFOs for approximately 9 months after surgery when he chose to use his wheelchair full-time. A motorized wheelchair was recommended; however, his mother felt that it was easier to handle Jeremy in his manual chair. The Muscular Dystrophy Association loaned Jeremy a motorized wheelchair for school use. He had developed a moderate scoliosis, but did not complain of pain. He refused to wear a molded spinal corset, but the padded thoracic pads fitted to his chair increased his comfort. By age 15, Jeremy was dependent for all care except feeding. He was able to sit with support in a large living room chair and he enjoyed watching television and playing card games with a few friends who visited his home. He was disinterested in continuing school and missed more days than he attended. He was not cooperative with his home-based teacher.

During his fifteenth year, Jeremy had repeated episodes of chest congestion and difficulty handling stringy foods. The visiting therapist taught his mother some postural drainage and breathing exercises for Jeremy; however, the mother did not follow through with the recommendations. Because his mother had to work full-time, a public agency provided in-home care during the days when Jeremy was not at school or after he returned from school. The mother refused in-home nursing care, preferring to continue with the attendant who was not comfortable carrying out Jeremy's exercises or pulmonary care. The family refused counseling or support from parents of other children with disabilities. Jeremy died at home after a brief bout with pneumonia.

with persons who are experienced dealing with degenerative diseases. Because the child and family have long anticipated the child's death and have made transitions through many levels of grieving, the process of separation and mourning may have occurred before the child's death. Each child and family member, therefore, should be helped to deal with the process according to his or her own pace and in response to individual needs.

The child's death is sometimes considered a welcomed relief.[98] This feeling of relief, however, is often accompanied by survivor guilt and a tremendous sense of loss of life focus for the family members whose lives have been so intertwined with that of the child's. Ideally, arrangements should be made for the family to meet with the professionals with whom they feel most comfortable several weeks after the child's death and again several months later so that the family (and caregivers) can deal with their thoughts and feelings. (See Case 3 on p. 416.)

SUMMARY

Three very different diseases have been described to depict the varied effects of neuromuscular pathology on a person's day-to-day function. Amyotrophic lateral sclerosis is an adult-onset degenerative disease of the upper and lower motor neurons; Guillain-Barré syndrome is an inflammatory process affecting the peripheral nervous system of children and adults; Duchenne muscular dystrophy is an inherited degenerative disease presenting in childhood that affects muscle tissue.

In all three conditions, the therapist is challenged to design a therapy program that will provide the patient with the impetus to become or remain as active as possible without causing possible muscle damage from excessive exercise demands or overwork. Two even more difficult tasks are (1) to help the patient and family identify realistic goals and (2) to help the patient find a balance between struggling to maintain his or her functional level and adapting to the inevitable changes in level of independence.

Therapists must also be aware of their own feelings and reactions to patients with severe neuromuscular diseases. Working with patients wth GBS is usually a positive experience because the majority of patients attain full recovery despite their often severe disability during the acute illness and long recovery period. Working with patients with degenerative terminal diseases, however, draws deeply on the therapist's emotional and spiritual strength.

A typical response of health care professionals is to view these patients' conditions as hopeless and to assume that the patients must also perceive their existence as hopeless, depressing, and without value. Research does suggest that there is an increased incidence of depression and demoralization in patients with degenerative, terminal diseases when compared with nonaffected populations. Other research, however, has indicated that many patients perceive their own life satisfaction much more positively than professionals

would believe.[93] Therefore therapists must tap into the patients' positive energy to design treatment programs that respect patients' goals and life plans within the context of their environments.

ACKNOWLEDGMENTS

Thanks to Gretchen Nelson and David Newman, student assistants, for their support services and to the many colleagues who commented on the text during its development.

REFERENCES
Amyotrophic Lateral Sclerosis

1. Appel SH and Smith GR: Can neurotrophic factors prevent or reverse motor neuron injury in amyotrophic lateral sclerosis? *Exp Neuro* 124:100, 1993.
2. Bonnett RI and Knowlton GC: Overwork weakness in partially denervated skeletal muscle, *Clin Orthop* 12:22, 1958.
3. Brooks BR and others: Design of clinical therapeutic trials in amyotrophic lateral sclerosis. In Rowland L, editor: *Advances in neurology,* vol 56, New York, 1991, Raven Press.
4. Caroscio JT: Amyotrophic lateral sclerosis: the disease. In Caroscio JT, editor *Amyotrophic lateral sclerosis,* New York, 1986, Thieme Medical Publishers.
5. Carpenter RJ, McDonald TJ, and Howard FM: The otolaryngologic presentation of amyotrophic lateral sclerosis, *ORL* 86:479, 1978.
6. Chou SM: Pathology of intraneuronal inclusions in ALS. In Tsubaki T and Toyokura Y, editors: *Amyotrophic lateral sclerosis,* Baltimore, 1979, University Park Press.
7. Daube JR and others: Classification of ALS by autonomic abnormalities. In Tsubaki T and Yase Y, editors: *Amyotrophic lateral sclerosis,* Amsterdam, 1987, Elsevier Science Publishers.
8. Hasson SM: Progressive and degenerative neuromuscular diseases and severe muscular dystrophy. In Hasson SM: *Clinical exercise physiology,* St Louis, 1994, Mosby.
9. Heckmatt JZ, Loh L, and Dubowitz V: Night-time nasal ventilation in neuromuscular disease, *Lancet* 335:579, 1990.
10. Hillel AD and Miller RM: Bulbar amyotrophic lateral sclerosis: patterns of progression and clinical management, *Head Neck* 11(1): 51-59, 1989.
11. Hillel AD and Miller RM: Management of bulbar symptoms in amyotrophic lateral sclerosis. In Cosi V and others: *Amyotrophic lateral sclerosis. Therapeutic, psychological and research aspects.,* New York, 1987, Plenum Press.
12. Hillel AD and others: Amyotrophic lateral sclerosis severity scale, *Neuroepidemiology* 8:142, 1989.
13. Hirano A: In pursuit of the early pathological alterations in ALS. In Tsubaki T and Yase Y, editors, *Amyotrophic lateral sclerosis,* Amsterdam, 1988, Elsevier Science Publishers.
14. Hoberman M: Physical medicine and rehabilitation: its value and limitations in progressive muscular dystrophy, *Proceedings of the Third Medical Conference of the Muscular Dystrophy Association of America* 1954, pp. 109-115.
15. Houpt JL, Gould BS, and Norris FH: Psychological characteristics of patients with amyotrophic lateral sclerosis, *Psychosom Med* 39:299, 1977.
16. Humberstone N: Respiratory assessment and treatment. In Irwin S and Tecklin JS, editors, *Cardiopulmonary physical therapy,* Philadelphia, 1990, Mosby.
17. Moss AH and others: Home ventilation for amyotrophic lateral sclerosis patients: outcomes, costs and patient, family and physician attitudes, *Neurology* 43:438, 1993.
18. Mulder DW and Kurland LT: Amyotrophic lateral sclerosis (motor neuron disease): four clinical questions. In Tsubaki T and Yase Y, editors: *Amyotrophic lateral sclerosis,* Amsterdam, 1987, Elsevier Science Publishers.

19. Muller EA: Influence of training and of inactivity on muscle strength, *Arch Phys Med Rehabil* 51:449, 1970.

20. Norris FH and Denys EH: Nutritional supplements in amyotrophic lateral sclerosis. In Cosi V and others: *Amyotrophic lateral sclerosis. Therapeutic, psychological and research aspects,* New York, 1987, Plenum Press.

21. Norris FH, Smith RA, and Denys EH: The treatment of amyotrophic lateral sclerosis. In Cosi V and others: *Amyotrophic lateral sclerosis. Therapeutic, psychological and research aspects,* New York, 1987, Plenum Press.

22. Oliver D: Ethical issues in palliative care—an overview, *Palliat Med* 7 (suppl 2):15, 1993.

23. Oliver D and Cardy P: *Motor neurone disease: death and dying,* North Hampton, 1991, Motor Neurone Disease Association.

24. Oppenheimer EA: Decision-making in the respiratory care of amyotrophic lateral sclerosis: should home mechanical ventilation be used? *Palliat Med* 7 (suppl 2):49, 1993.

25. Pradas J and others: The natural history of amyotrophic lateral sclerosis and the use of natural history controls in therapeutic trials, *Neurology* 43:751, 1993.

26. Purtillo R: *Health and professional and patient interaction,* ed 4, Philadelphia, 1990, WB Saunders.

27. Reitsma W: Skeletal muscle hypertrophy after heavy exercise in rats with surgically reduced muscle function, *Am J Phys Med* 48:237, 1969.

28. Ringel SP and others: The natural history of amyotrophic lateral sclerosis, *Neurology* 43:1316, 1993.

29. Sanjak M, Reddan W, and Brooks BR: Role of muscular exercise in amyotrophic lateral sclerosis, *Neurol Clin* 5:251, 1989.

30. Scott A and Heughan A: A review of dysphagia in four cases of motor neurone disease, *Palliat Med* (suppl 2):41, 1993.

31. Siegel IM: The management of muscular dystrophy: a clinical review, *Muscle Nerve* 1:453, 1978.

32. Sinaki M: Exercise and rehabilitation measures in amyotrophic lateral sclerosis. In Yase Y and Tsubaki T, editors: *Amyotrophic lateral sclerosis: recent advances in research and treatment,* Amsterdam, 1988, Elsevier Science.

33. Smith EWL: A gestalt therapist's perspective on grief. In Stern EM, editor: *Psychotherapy and the grieving patient,* New York, 1985, Harrington Park Press.

34. Sobue G and others: Degenerating compartment and functioning compartment of motor neurons in ALS: possible process of motor neuron loss, *Neurology* 33, 654, 1983.

35. Tashiro K and others: Sensory findings in amyotrophic lateral sclerosis. In Tsubaki T and Yase Y, editors: *Amyotrophic lateral sclerosis,* Amsterdam, 1988, Elsevier Science Publishers.

36. Vignos PJ: Physical models of rehabilitation in neuromuscular disease, *Muscle Nerve* 6:323, 1983.

37. Vine P: *Families in pain,* New York, 1982, Pantheon Books.

Guillain-Barré Syndrome

38. Akeson WH and others: The connective tissue response to immobility: an accelerated aging response? *Exp Gerontol* 3:289, 1968.

39. Bensman A: Strenuous exercise may impair muscle function in Guillain-Barré patients, *JAMA* 214:468, 1970.

40. Burrows DS and Cuetter AC: Residual subclinical impairment in patients who totally recovered from Guillain-Barré syndrome: impact on military performance, *Mil Med* 155:438, 1990.

41. Clague JE and MacMillan RR: Backache and the Guillain-Barré syndrome: a diagnostic problem, *Br Med J* 293:325, 1986.

42. Currie DM and others: Guillain-Barré syndrome in children: evidence of axonal degeneration and long-term follow-up, *Arch Phys Med Rehabil* 71:244, 1990.

43. Drennan JC: Neuromuscular disorders. In Morrissy RT: *Pediatric orthopaedics,* ed 3, Philadelphia, 1990, JB Lippincott.

44. Eberle E and others: Early predictors of incomplete recovery in children with Guillain-Barré polyneuritis, *J Pediatr* 86:356, 1975.

45. Florence JM and Hagberg JM: Effect of training on the exercise responses of neuromuscular disease patients, *Med Sci Sports Exer* 16(5):480, 1984.

46. French Cooperative Group on Plasma Exchange in Guillain-Barré Syndrome: Efficiency of plasma exchange in Guillain-Barré syndrome: role of replacement fluids, *Ann Neurol* 22:753, 1987.

47. Greenwood RJ and others: Controlled trial of plasma exchange in acute inflammatory polyradiculoneuropathy, *Lancet* 1:877, 1984.

48. Guillain-Barré Syndrome Study Group: Plasmapheresis and acute Guillain-Barré syndrome, *Neurology* 35:1096, 1985.

49. Guillain G, Barré JA, and Strohl A: Sur un syndrome de radiculo-nevrite avec hyperalbuminose du liquide cephalo-rachidien sans reaction cellulaire: remarques sur les caracteres cliniques et graphiques des reflexes tendineux, *Bull Mem Soc Med Hop Paris* 40:1462, 1916.

50. Hammon WE: Physical therapy for the acutely ill patient in the respiratory intensive care unit. In Irwin S and Tecklin JS, editors: *Cardiopulmonary physical therapy,* St Louis, 1990, Mosby.

51. Herbison and others: Exercise therapies in peripheral neuropathies, *Arch Phys Med Rehabil* 64:201, 1983.

52. Hertling D and Jones D: Relaxation. In Kessler RM and Hertling D: *Management of common musculoskeletal disorders: physical therapy principles and methods,* Philadelphia, 1983, Harper & Row.

53. Holtacker TR: Physical rehabilitation of the ventilator-dependent patient. In Irwin S and Tecklin JS, editors: *Cardiopulmonary physical therapy,* St Louis, 1990, Mosby.

54. Humberstone N: Respiratory assessment and treatment. In Irwin S and Tecklin JS, editors: *Cardiopulmonary physical therapy,* St Louis, 1990, Mosby.

55. Irani DN and others: Relapse in Guillain-Barré syndrome after treatment with human immunoglobin, *Neurology* 43:872, 1993.

56. Kandel ER and others, editors: *Principles of neural science,* ed 3, Connecticut, 1991, Appleton & Lange.

57. Karni Y and others: Clinical assessment and physiotherapy in Guillain-Barré syndrome, *Physiotherapy* 70:288, 1984.

58. Karper WB: Effects of low-intensity aerobic exercise on one subject with chronic-relapsing Guillain-Barré syndrome, *Rehabil Nurs* 16:96, 1991.

59. Kessler RM: The shoulder. In Kessler RM and Hertling D: *Management of common musculoskeletal disorders: physical therapy principles and methods,* Philadelphia, 1983, Harper & Row.

60. Langmore SE and Longemann JA: After the clinical bedside swallowing examination: what next, *Am J Speech-Language Pathol* 1:13, 1991.

61. Lehmann JF and others: Effect of therapeutic temperature on tendon extensibility, *Arch Phys Med Rehabil* 51:481, 1970.

62. Lewis CB and Bottomley JM, editors: *Geriatric physical therapy. A clinical approach,* Norwalk, 1994, Appleton & Lange.

63. Long DM and others: Transcutaneous electrical stimulation for relief of chronic pain, *Adv Pain Res Ther* 3:593, 1979.

64. Longemann J: *Evaluation and treatment of swallowing disorders,* San Diego, 1983, College-Hill Press.

65. McLeod JG: Electrophysiological studies in the Guillain-Barré syndrome, *Ann Neurol* 9 (Suppl):20, 1981.

66. Mays ML: Incorporating continuous passive motion in the rehabilitation of a patient with Guillain-Barré syndrome, *Am J Occup Ther* 44:750, 1990.

67. Melzack R: Prolonged relief of pain by brief, intense, transcutaneous somatic stimulation, *Pain* 1:357, 1975.

68. Osterman PO and others: Beneficial effects of plasma exchange in acute inflammatory polyradiculoneuropathy, *Lancet* 2:1296, 1984.

69. Pitetti KH and others: Endurance exercise training in Guillain-Barré syndrome, *Arch Phys Med Rehabil* 74:761, 1993.

70. Rees J: Guillain-Barré syndrome: the latest on treatment, *Br J Hosp Med* 50:226, 1993.
71. Reitsma W: Skeletal muscle hypertrophy after heavy exercise in rats with surgically reduced muscle function, *Am J Phys Med* 48:237, 1969.
72. Ringel SP and Cooper WH: Classification of neuromuscular disorders. In Maloney FP and others, editors: *Interdisciplinary rehabilitation of multiple sclerosis and neuromuscular disorders,* Philadelphia, 1985, JB Lippincott.
73. Ropper AH and others: Pain in Guillain-Barré syndrome, *Arch Neurol* 41:511, 1984.
74. Ropper AH and others: Severe acute Guillain-Barré syndrome, *Neurology* 36:429, 1986.
75. Ruttenberg N: Assessment and treatment of speech and swallowing problems in patients with multiple sclerosis. In Maloney FP, and others: *Interdisciplinary rehabilitation of multiple sclerosis and neuromuscular disorders,* Philadelphia, 1985, JB Lippincott.
76. Salter R: Clinical application of basic research on continuous passive motion for disorders and injuries of synovial joints: a preliminary study, *J Orthop Res* 1:325, 1984.
77. Sonies BC: Instrumental procedures for dysphagia diagnosis, *Semin Speech Lang* 12:185, 1991.
78. Soryal I and others: Impaired joint mobility in Guillain-Barré syndrome: a primary or a secondary phenomenon? *J Neurol Neurosurg Psychiatry* 55:1014, 1992.
79. Spencer WA: *The treatment of acute poliomyelitis,* Springfield, Ill., 1954, Charles C. Thomas.
80. Steinberg JS: *Guillain-Barre syndrome (acute idiopathic polyneuritis): an overview for the lay person,* Wynnwood, PA, 1987, The Guillain-Barré Syndrome Support Group International.
81. Stillwell GK: Rehabilitative procedures. In Dyck PJ and others, editors: *Peripheral neuropathy,* ed 2, Philadelphia, 1984, WB Saunders.
82. Thorsteinsson G and others: Transcutaneous electrical stimulation: a double blind trial of its efficacy for pain, *Arch Phys Med Rehabil* 58:8, 1977.
83. Toyka KV and Heininger K: Humoral factors in peripheral nerve disease, *Muscle Nerve* 10:222, 1987.
84. Van der Meche FGA and others: A randomized trial comparing intravenous immune globulin and plasma exchange in Guillain-Barré syndrome, *N Engl J Med* 326:1123, 1992.
85. Warren CG: The use of heat and cold in the treatment of common musculoskeletal disorders. In Kessler RM and Hertling D: *Management of common musculoskeletal disorders: physical therapy principles and methods,* Philadelphia, 1983, Harper & Row.
86. Warren CG and others: Elongation of rat tail tendon: effect of load and temperature, *Arch Phys Med Rehabil* 52:465, 1971.
87. Warren CG and others: Heat and stretch procedures: an evaluation using rat tail tendon, *Arch Phys Med Rehabil* 57:122, 1976.
88. Winter JB and others: Prognosis in Guillain-Barre syndrome, *Lancet* 1:1202, 1985.
89. Wyngaarden JB and Smith LH: *Cecil textbook of Medicine,* ed 18, Philadelphia, 1986, WB Saunders.

Muscular Dystrophy

90. Allsop KG and Ziter FA: Loss of strength and functional decline in Duchenne dystrophy, *Arch Neurol* 38:406, 1981.
91. Appel SH: The muscular dystrophies, *Neurol Clin* 1(1):7, 1979.
92. Asher MI and others: The effects of inspiratory muscle training in patients with cystic fibrosis, *Am Rev Respir Dis* 126:833, 1982.
93. Birch JR and McKean J: Orthopedic surgery and rehabilitation for the prolongation of brace free ambulation of patients with Duchenne muscular dystrophy, *Am J Phys Med Rehabil* 70(6):323, 1991.
94. Bach JR and others: Management of end stage respiratory failure due

to late stage Duchenne muscular dystrophy, *Arch Phys Med Rehabil* 10:177, 1987.
95. Brooke MH and others: Clinical investigation of Duchenne muscular dystrophy. Interesting results in a trial of prednisolone, *Arch Neurol* 44:812, 1987.
96. Brooke MH and others: Clinical investigations in Duchenne muscular dystrophy. Part 2. Determination of the "power" of therapeutic trials based on the natural history, *Muscle Nerve* 6:91, 1983.
97. Brooke MH and others: Duchenne muscular dystrophy: patterns of clinical progression and effects of supportive therapy, *Neurology* 39:475, 1989.
98. Childress J: The dying child. In Kruger DW: *Rehabilitation psychology,* Rockville, MD, 1984, Aspen Publishers.
99. de Lateur BJ and Giaconi RM: Effect on maximal strength of submaximal exercise in Duchenne muscular dystrophy, *Am J Phys Med* 58(1):26, 1979.
100. De Silva S and others: Prednisolone treatment in Duchenne muscular dystrophy, *Arch Neurol* 44:818, 1987.
101. Di Marco AF and others: Respiratory muscle training in muscular dystrophy, *Clin Res* 30:427, 1982.
102. Drennan JC: Neuromuscular disorders. In Morrissy R, editor: *Pediatric orthopaedics,* ed 3, Philadelphia, 1990, JB Lippincott
103. Edwards RHT: Weight reduction in boys with muscular dystrophy, *Dev Med Child Neurol* 26:384, 1984.
104. Elder GCB: Beneficial effects of training on developing dystrophic muscle, *Muscle Nerve* 15:672, 1992.
105. Fenichel G and others: Long-term benefit from prednisone therapy in Duchenne muscular dystrophy, *Neurology* 41:1874, 1991.
106. Florence J and others: Intrarater reliability of manual muscle test grades in Duchenne muscular dystrophy, *Phys Ther* 72:115, 1992.
107. Fowler WM and others: The effect of exercise on serum enzymes, *Arch Phys Med* 49:554, 1968.
108. Griffith R and Edwards RHT: A new chart for weight control in Duchenne muscular dystrophy, *Arch Phys Med Rehabil* 63:1256, 1988.
109. Grossman MR, Sahrmann SA, and Rose SJ: Review of length associated changes in muscle: experimental evidence and clinical implications, *Phys Ther* 62:1799, 1982.
110. Harris SE and Cherry DB: Childhood progressive muscular dystrophy and the role of physical therapy, *Phys Ther* 54(1):4, 1974.
111. Hasson SM: Progressive and degenerative neuromuscular disease and severe muscular dystrophy. In Hasson SM: *Clinical exercise physiology,* St Louis, 1994, Mosby.
112. Heckmatt J and others: Management of children: pharmacological and physical, *Br Med Bull* 45(3):788, 1989.
113. Humberstone N: Respiratory assessment and treatment. In Irwin S and Tecklin JS, editors: *Cardiopulmonary physical therapy,* St Louis, 1990, Mosby.
114. Hyde SA and others: Prolongation of ambulation in Duchenne muscular dystrophy by appropriate orthoses, *Physiotherapy* 68(4):105, 1982.
115. Irwin S and Tecklin JS, editors: *Cardiopulmonary physical therapy,* St Louis, 1990, Mosby.
116. Johnson EW and Braddom R: Over-work weakness in facioscapulohumeral muscular dystrophy, *Arch Phys Med Rehabil* 52:333, 1971.
117. Leger P and others: Home positive pressure ventilation via nasal mask for patients with neuromuscular weakness or restrictive lung or chest-wall disease, *Respir Care* 34:73, 1989.
118. Lord J and others: Scoliosis associated with Duchenne muscular dystrophy, *Arch Phys Med Rehabil* 71:13, 1990.
119. Maddling SW and others: Effect of duration of passive stretch on hip abduction range of motion, *J Orthop Sports Phys Ther* 8(8):409-416, 1987.
120. Martin AJ and others: Respiratory muscle training in Duchenne muscular dystrophy, *Dev Med Child Neurol* 28:314, 1986

121. Miller Γ, Moseley CF, and Koreska J: Spinal fusion in Duchenne muscular dystrophy, *Dev Med Child Neurol* 34:775, 1992.
122. Miller JR, Colbert AP, and Schock NC: Ventilator use in progressive neuromuscular disease: impact on patients and their families, *Dev Med Child Neurol* 30:200, 1988.
123. Pandya S and others: Reliability of goniometric measurements in patients with Duchenne muscular dystrophy, *Phys Ther* 65:1339, 1985.
124. Partridge TA: Myoblast transfer: possible therapy for inherited myopathies, *Muscle Nerve* 14:197, 1991.
125. Rideau Y and others: Prolongation of life in Duchenne's muscular dystrophy, *Acta Neurologica* 38:118, 1983.
126. Rose J and others: The energy expenditure index: a method to quantify and compare walking energy expenditure for children and adolescents, *J Pediatr Orthop* 11:571, 1991.
127. Scott OM and others: Prevention of deformity in Duchenne muscular dystrophy, *Physiotherapy* 67(6):177, 1981.
128. Scott OM and others: Responses of muscles of patients with Duchenne muscular dystrophy to chronic electrical stimulation, *J Neurol Neurosurg Psychiatry* 49:1427, 1986.
129. Siegel IM: Update on Duchenne muscular dystrophy, *Comp Ther* 15(3):45, 1989.
130. Smith PEM, Calverly PMA, and Edwards RHT: Hypoxia during sleep in Duchenne muscular dystrophy, *Am Rev Respir Dis* 137:884, 1988.
131. Smith PEM and others: Practical problems in the respiratory care of patients with muscular dystrophy, *N Engl J Med* 316:1197, 1987.
132. Spencer GE and others: Bracing for ambulation in childhood progressive muscular dystrophy, *J Bone Joint Surg* 44-A(2):234, 1962.
133. Stallard J and others: The ORLAU VCG (variable centre of gravity) swivel walker for muscular dystrophy patients, *Prosthet Orthop Int* 16:46, 1992.
134. Stern LM and Clark BE. Investigation of scoliosis in Duchenne dystrophy using computerized tomography, *Muscle Nerve* 11:775, 1988.
135. Sutherland DH, Olshen R, Cooper L: The pathomechanics of gait in Duchenne muscular dystrophy, *Dev Med Child Neurol* 23:3, 1981.
136. Taylor DC and others: Viscoelastic properties of muscle-tendon units: the biomechanical effects of stretching, *Am J Sports Med* 18:300, 1990.
137. Vignos PJ, Spencer GE, and Archibald KC: Management of progressive muscular dystrophy of childhood, *JAMA* 184:89, 1963.
138. Vignos PJ and Watkins MP: The effect of exercise in muscular dystrophy, *JAMA* 197(11):121, 1966.
139. Wetzel JL and others: Respiratory rehabilitation of the patient with a spinal cord injury. In Irwin S and Tecklin JS, editors: *Cardiopulmonary physical therapy,* St Louis, 1990, Mosby.
140. Wilson J and others, editors: *Harrison's principles of internal medicine,* ed 12, New York, 1991, McGraw-Hill.
141. Witte RA: The psychosocial impact of a progressive physical handicap and terminal illness (Duchenne muscular dystrophy) on adolescents and their families, *Br J Med Psychol* 58:179, 1985.
142. Wyngaarden JB and others, editors: *Cecil textbook of medicine,* ed 19, Philadelphia, 1992, WB Saunders.
143. Zachazewski JE: Improving flexibility. In Scully RM and Barnes MR, editors: *Physical therapy,* Philadelphia, 1989, JB Lippincott.

CHAPTER 14

Head Injury

Patricia A. Winkler

LEARNING OBJECTIVES

After reading this chapter the student/therapist will:

1. Have an understanding of current concepts in motor control and motor learning theories.
2. Understand the meaning of impairment, disability, and handicap and their interrelationships.
3. Be knowledgeable in methods of evaluating, assessing, and treating head-injured clients based on impairment and disability analysis.
4. Be able to differentiate between development of basic movement patterns and motor skills.
5. Understand the role of synergy formation, synergy selection and modification, anticipatory and feedback information as used in motor skills.
6. Be familiar with the learning concepts of knowledge of results, whole task practice, and breaking tasks into natural subtasks.

KEY TERMS

traumatic head injury	learning theory
motor skill	systems theory
plasticity	synergy
motor learning	anticipatory responses
motor control	knowledge of results

Traumatic head injury is an insult to the brain . . . caused by an external physical force, that may produce a diminished or altered state of consciousness, which results in impairment of cognitive abilities or physical functioning. It can also result in the disturbance of behavioral or emotional functioning. These may be either temporary or permanent and cause partial or total functional disability or psychological maladjustment.[73]

AN OVERVIEW OF HEAD INJURY
Epidemiology of traumatic head injury

Every 5 minutes in the United States one person will die and another will become permanently disabled as a result of a traumatic head injury. Two million head injuries occur every year, with 500,000 severe enough to require hospitalization. Head injury has become the leading killer and disabler of children and young adults. Other industrialized countries have similar appalling statistics. Motor vehicle crashes cause 50% of all traumatic brain injuries, falls account for 21%, violence accounts for 12%, and sports and recreation are responsible for 10%. Child abuse accounts for 64% of infant brain injuries, and 50,000 children sustain bicycle-related brain injuries; 400 of these children die.[20]

Population of head-injured clients

The incidence of head injuries is higher for males than for females by more than 2 to 1. The majority of those injured are between 15 and 24 years.[55]

Cost

The estimated lifetime cost for each severely brain-injured individual exceeds $4 million, with a total cost of nearly $25 billion a year.

Mechanisms of injury

Acceleration, deceleration, and rotational forces act on the head at the time of impact, resulting in a temporary deformation of the skull. Brain damage is caused by tissue compression, tension, shearing, or a combination of these mechanisms.[35] Injuries to the brain can be both coup (injuries at the site of impact) and contrecoup (injuries distant from the part of the brain sustaining the blow).

Types of head injuries

To determine the medical treatment regime, the physician must distinguish between primary (impact) and secondary brain damage. Primary damage includes skull fractures, contusions of the gray matter, and diffuse white-matter lesions. Secondary damage includes brain swelling, intracranial hematoma, cerebral hypoxia, and ischemia. The objective, of course, is to prevent or minimize secondary brain damage. The secondary damage can develop as rapidly as within an hour of injury.[55] Thus by the time the therapist initiates treatment, a combination of primary and secondary sequelae has developed.

Gilroy and Meyer[35] describe different types of traumatic head injuries. Their list, discussed below, includes skull fractures, closed head injuries, penetrating wounds of the skull and brain, and traumatic injury to extracranial blood vessels.

Skull fractures. Linear or comminuted fractures generally result from low-velocity objects, and depressed fractures generally result from higher-velocity objects. Impact damage can be direct or remote. Linear fractures can produce contusions, lacerations, traumatic aneurysms, and cranial nerve damage. Depressed fractures decrease the volume of the cranial cavity and can produce uncal or lower-brainstem herniation, in addition to cranial nerve damage, contusions, and lacerations. Compound, depressed skull fractures are considered open head injuries. Skull fractures also can occur without subsequent brain damage.[35]

Closed head injuries. Persons sustaining closed head injuries without a fracture can experience minor injury, or they can experience severe and irreversible brain damage. Damage suffered from closed head injuries includes brainstem damage, contusions, diffuse white-matter lesions, injury to blood vessels, damage to cranial nerves, and traumatic cerebrospinal fluid rhinorrhea.

Brainstem damage can be primary or secondary. Primary damage can be the result of an acceleration or deceleration pressure wave causing a downward displacement of the brainstem through the foramen magnum.[35] However, it is doubtful that primary brainstem damage occurs except in conjunction with more extensive cortical and subcortical destruction.[55] Secondary damage can result from the development of brain swelling or intracranial hemorrhage, which increases the bilateral or unilateral volume of the supratentorial contents. Because the supratentorial contents are contained within a rigid structure, increased pressure can result in cingulate herniation, uncal herniation, and central (or transtentorial) herniation, with progressive brainstem dysfunction.[35]

Contusions of the gray matter can occur beneath the site of impact or remote from it. Occipital blows are more likely to produce contusions than are frontal or lateral blows. Contusions of the undersurface of the temporal and frontal lobes and on the anterior poles of the temporal lobes are common because of the irregular surface of the cranial vault in these areas. Cerebral contusions are not necessarily associated with a loss of consciousness, but they can initiate the processes of secondary brain damage.[55]

Diffuse damage to the white matter involves severance of axons because of shearing forces at the time of impact.[98] Lesions frequently occur in the splenium of the corpus callosum and diffusely in the white matter elsewhere in the brain.[35,55] Diffuse white-matter damage can result in a sudden loss of consciousness with bilateral extensor rigidity of the extremities and usually with some autonomic dysfunction. Clinically, these signs are frequently attributed to "primary brainstem damage." At autopsy, however, the lesions are not confined to the brainstem.[55]

Traumatic injury to blood vessels also can occur with closed head injury. Examples of damage to blood vessels include weakening of and damage to arterial walls by contact with bony prominences (such as damage to the internal carotid artery at the point where it enters the skull through the carotid canal), torn cortical veins (resulting in hematoma), and ruptured capillaries (which produce hemorrhages).[35]

Direct trauma, brainstem damage, avulsion, contusion, or increased intracranial pressure can damage cranial nerves. All of the cranial nerves are susceptible to injury, but damage to the optic, vestibulocochlear, oculomotor, abducens, and facial nerves is more common. Lesions of the olfactory nerve may or may not be detected. Statistics on cranial nerve involvement, however, vary with the source.

Closed head injury is one cause of cerebrospinal fluid rhinorrhea. Shearing forces or a sudden increase of intracranial pressure can cause this complication. However, cerebrospinal fluid rhinorrhea occurs more frequently with fractures of the posterior wall of the frontal sinus, with tearing of the dura and arachnoid. A persistent or intermittent clear fluid discharge from the nose should be reported. This drainage is increased by neck flexion, coughing, or straining.[35]

Penetrating wounds of the skull and brain. A variety of both high- and low-velocity objects can penetrate the skull. High-velocity penetration, or missile injury, is likely the result of a gunshot wound. Metallic objects, sticks, and sharp toys are capable of puncture wounds. Bone fragments may penetrate the dura in nonmissile injuries. In an interesting case, damage was caused by a fall on a kite stick that penetrated the brain through the orbit. Location, pathway, depth of penetration, and the subsequent secondary complications determine the ensuing brain damage.[35] In addition, there is the risk of intracranial infection with open injuries.

Traumatic injury to extracranial blood vessels. Gunshot wounds, blows to the neck, injuries to the face, or cervical hyperextension can damage the internal carotid artery.[35] The vertebral artery can be injured during cervical manipulation,[69] cervical traction, or sudden hyperextension or rotation of the neck.[44] Insufficiency or infarction can occur in such cases. The consequences of any of these types of injuries vary, but they might include neuronal loss, axonal degeneration, diffuse brain atrophy, hydrocephalus, scar tissue formation, and abnormal neuronal activity.[35]

Additional types of head injuries and other traumatic and disease entities involving the brain can exhibit clinical manifestations approximating those found in severe head trauma. In some open injuries, portions of the skull and brain are actually abolished. Drug overdoses, tumors, certain cerebral hemorrhages, and a variety of hypoxic conditions, such as near-drownings, may clinically fall into the category of brain injuries.

Immediate clinical aspects

The immediate clinical aspects of traumatic head injury can include alterations in autonomic function, consciousness, motor function, pupillary responses, ocular movements, and other brainstem reflexes. Each of these aspects is discussed briefly here.

Alterations in autonomic function can occur, and one vital sign may change without affecting the others. The pulse and respiratory rates can be slow, normal, rapid, irregular, or otherwise abnormal. Temperature can be elevated. Blood pressure can be low, normal, or elevated. Other disturbances

in autonomic function also can be present, including excessive sweating, salivation, lacrimation, and sebum secretion.[17]

Consciousness may or may not be altered. Plum and Posner[79] provide an in-depth account of this fascinating area. Conscious behavior is determined by content and arousal. Content is the sum of cognitive and affective functions. Arousal is associated with wakefulness and depends on an intact reticular formation and upper brainstem that function in collaboration with other parts of the brain. Content (or cognition) and arousal may be individually impaired, or a combination of impairments of both of these physiological components may be present. For example, arousal does not guarantee cognition, a circumstance that is clinically observable.

Alterations in consciousness result from conditions in which there is diffusely extensive and bilateral cerebral hemispheric depression of function, direct depression or destruction of the brainstem-activating mechanisms responsible for consciousness, or a combination of the two effects. Stupor and coma indicate advanced brain failure, and the more prolonged the failure, the more guarded the prognosis.[79]

In mild concussion the loss of consciousness lasts a relatively short time, and there is little or no retrograde amnesia. The client may be irritable or distractable and have difficulty with reading and memory. There may be complaints of headache, fatigue, dizziness, and changes in personality and emotional disposition. This group of symptoms constitute what is called *posttraumatic neurosis* or *syndrome*. Whether these symptoms are organic or psychogenic is unclear.[35]

In moderate or severe head injury, unconsciousness can be prolonged. A variety of terms are used to label gradations of consciousness; many of them are conflicting. There is agreement that clear-cut criteria for levels of consciousness are difficult to establish. As a result, it is probably more accurate and helpful to disregard the various labels and to describe the client's levels of arousal and cognition. Therefore in the interest of clarity, levels of consciousness are discussed separately from levels of cognitive functioning.

Plum and Posner's definitions[79] of various stages of acutely altered consciousness are briefly presented, intermingled with some insights from the descriptions offered by Gilroy and Meyer.[35] One difference between these two continua is that Plum and Posner[79] do not equate the presence or absence of motor responses with the depth of coma. These authors point out that the neural structures regulating consciousness differ from and are more anatomically distant from those regulating motor function.

Coma is defined as a complete paralysis of cerebral function, a state of unresponsiveness. The eyes are closed, and there is no response to painful stimuli. Within 2 to 4 weeks, nearly all clients in coma begin to awaken. *Stupor* is a condition of general unresponsiveness. However, the client, who is usually mute, can be temporarily aroused by vigorous and repeated stimuli. *Obtundity* describes a client who sleeps a great deal and who, when aroused, exhibits reduced alertness, disinterest in the environment, and slow responses to stimulation. *Delirium* is often observed in recovery from unconsciousness after severe head injury. This state is characterized by disorientation, fear, and misinterpretation of sensory stimuli. The client is frequently loud, agitated, and offensive. *Clouding of consciousness* is a state of quiet confusion, distractibility, faulty memory, and slowed responses to stimuli. Recovery to *consciousness,* if it occurs, includes a gradual recovery of orientation and recent memory.[79] The duration of each of these stages is variable and can be prolonged. Improvement can be arrested at any point.

Motor abnormalities after severe head trauma are common. Reflex motor responses in unconscious clients are tested by applying a noxious stimulus, such as pressure on a nail bed using a pencil or supraorbital pressure, and observing the response. Internal stimuli can also elicit tonic spasms. Motor responses generally fall into three categories: appropriate, inappropriate, or absent.[79]

The usual abnormalities include monoplegia or hemiplegia and abnormal reflexes. Great variance exists. Initial flaccidity can gradually become spasticity or rigidity. The terms *decorticate* or *decerebrate rigidity* are often used to denote abnormal posturing. As with other labels, however, these are not always well defined, and a description of the abnormalities is preferred. Examples of typical motor disturbances include abnormal flexor responses in the upper extremities and extensor responses in the lower extremities (decorticate), abnormal extensor responses in upper and lower extremities (decerebrate), abnormal extensor responses in the upper extremities with flaccid or weak flexor responses in the lower extremities, absence of motor responses (flaccid), or a mixture of these. Responses can be bilateral or unilateral. Furthermore, the same client can initially display flexor responses in the arms that can later change to extensor responses. These shifts possibly reflect the physiological effects of changes in the amount of tissue compression or irritation.[79]

Pupillary responses and ocular movements can become pathological signs in coma because the brainstem areas controlling consciousness are adjacent to those controlling the pupils and ocular motility. Abnormalities in pupil size, shape, and light reflexes can be manifested unilaterally or bilaterally. Eye movements in coma can be abnormal, as can the oculocephalic and oculovestibular reflexes. Oculomotor and pupillary signs are valuable in assisting with the diagnosis, localizing brainstem damage, and determining the depth of coma.[79] Interpretation can be difficult, partially because of the variety of influences on these signs.[55]

Other brainstem responses might include grimacing to pain, which is frequently associated with a flexor or localizing motor response. The pharyngeal reflex may also be absent; the implications of this are obvious. Absence of brainstem reflexes usually indicates a poorer prognosis, but this is not necessarily a predictor of ultimate outcome.[17]

Diagnostic monitoring procedures and medical management

In addition to the traditional neurological examination that the physician performs, a variety of diagnostic and monitoring procedures may be ordered for the recently injured client. The selection of the tests depends on the availability of the special equipment required for testing and on the perceived need for the tests. Although therapists are not educated in the interpretation of these procedures, a general understanding of their purposes is useful. In addition to the primary aim of guiding the physician, the results of some of these procedures may secondarily aid the therapist in the selection of intervention strategies. Conversely, other monitoring procedures may restrict the choice of therapeutic approaches.

A list of the more common procedures might include the Glasgow Coma Scale (GCS) and additional neurological assessments, radiographic examination, computed axial tomography (CT) scanning, magnetic resonance imaging (MRI), cerebral angiography, positive emission tomography (PET), radioisotope imaging, ventriculography, echoencephalography, monitoring of intracranial pressure and cardiorespiratory and cardiovascular function, measurement of cerebral blood flow and metabolism, electroencephalography (EEG), cerebral spinal fluid and other biochemical studies, and evoked potential studies of the visual, auditory, and somatosensory systems. A third of the clients hospitalized with head injuries have extracranial injuries, which are explored with a physical examination and appropriate special tests.[55]

It is neither our intent nor within the scope of this chapter to report on the potential diagnostic, monitoring, and prognostic capabilities of specific procedures. References on these techniques are abundant; for example, a brief overview is available in Jennett and Teasdale's *Management of Head Injuries.*[55] Three of these monitoring procedures, however, deserve mention here: the GCS, CT scanning, and evoked potential studies.

The GCS (see box on p. 425), introduced in 1974, is designed to assess and monitor the level of consciousness. Three aspects of coma are observed independently: eye opening, best motor response, and verbal performance. Each of these components has a numerical scale. An overall coma score is obtained by adding the numerical value assigned to each of the three components. Coma scores range from 3 (least responsive) to 15.[55] According to Jennett and Teasdale's definition of coma ("not obeying commands, not uttering words, and not opening the eyes"),[55] a Glasgow total score of 8 or less defines coma in 90% of cases. Pupillary reactivity, spontaneous eye movements, and oculovestibular responses are additional neurological assessments used

Glasgow Coma Scale

Eye opening	E
Spontaneous	4
To speech	3
To pain	2
Nil	1

Best motor response	M
Obeys	6
Localizes	5
Withdraws	4
Abnormal flexion	3
Extensor response	2
Nil	1

Verbal Response	V
Orientated	5
Confused conversation	4
Inappropriate words	3
Incomprehensible sounds	2
Nil	1

Coma Score (E + M + V) = 3 to 15

From Jennett B and Teasdale G: *Management of head injuries,* Philadelphia, 1981, FA Davis.

in conjunction with the GCS. Spontaneous eye movement classifications can include visual fixation, conjugate, roving dysconjugate, nystagmus, and no movement. The oculovestibular reflex is tested using ice water irrigation, and the responses can include conjugate eye movements, dysconjugate eye movements, nystagmus, or no response. One importance of the GCS is that both the coma score and the grades of response on each component of the scale have been demonstrated in some studies to correlate with outcome[45,55] (discussed later in this chapter). However, Van Den Berge and others[104] found difficulties with interrater reliability in assessing oculocephalic responses. Also, the relative value of each component of the scale differs according to the time interval elapsed.[67] Another concern is the practice of adding the scores on this scale, which is an ordinal level scale.

CT scanning and MRI are radiological techniques that permit visualization of intracranial structures. They make "it possible to observe the presence, evolution, and resolution of lesions that could previously only be presumed on the basis of clinical features or deduced indirectly . . ." (p. 114).[55] Sequential CT scanning is frequently used with head injured clients to follow their course of recovery. CT scanning reveals the current status of the lesion. With the possible exception of the diagnosis and, hence, prognosis of diffuse white-matter impact damage,[118] the Glasgow study[94] and the other studies[64,118] reviewed by Jennett and Teasdale indicate that prediction of outcome should not be based on CT scanning or MRI alone.

Changes in electrocerebral potentials that occur in response to specific stimuli also are studied. Visual, auditory, and somatosensory evoked potential examinations are used with brain-injured clients. Evoked responses may yield more information than the clinical neurological examination alone and may also assist in localizing the structural damage. Evoked potential studies may aid in prognosis[42,79]; however, the usefulness and significance of evoked potential studies with these clients is still being investigated. (Refer to Chapter 29 for additional information.)

On admission to the hospital, a neurosurgeon usually assumes initial and primary responsibility for the client. The first priority in medical care is resuscitation, after which baseline assessments are made and a history obtained. Immediate surgery may or may not be indicated. Early concerns may include the management of respiratory dysfunction, cardiovascular monitoring, treatment of raised intracranial pressure by means of pharmacological, mechanical, or surgical procedures,[17] and general medical care. Examples of general medical care are familiar: maintenance of fluid and electrolyte balance, nutrition, eye and skin care, prevention of contractures, postural drainage, and possibly restraints.[55] This type of care gradually lessens as the client responds, or it may continue if unconsciousness persists.

Pharmaceutical agents are prescribed as an adjunct to care for a variety of reasons. Antibiotics may be used with respiratory complications or with compound fractures. Anticonvulsants may be prescribed for treatment or prophylaxis of seizures. Raised intracranial pressure might be treated with diuretics or barbiturates.[17,33] Traumatically acquired neuroendocrine dysfunctions, such as hyperphagia and thermal regulation, may be treated with pharmacological agents.[37]

Medications also may be prescribed to decrease spasticity. Diazepam (Valium) initially was the drug most commonly administered. However, diazepam also promotes drowsiness and decreased responsiveness and can increase muscle weakness and ataxia.[117] These side effects actually hinder rather than assist in rehabilitation. Glenn and Wrobewski[38] conclude that, "rarely, if ever, are the benefits of diazepam's antispasticity effect great enough to justify its use in the brain-injured population" (p. 71). Baclofen is now used more frequently with brain-injured clients; however, baclofen also can produce lethargy, confusion,[117] and reduction in attention span[38] in some clients. Dantrolene sodium is another medication used to decrease spasticity. This drug works directly at the muscle level and therefore is less likely to cause cognitive disturbances, but more likely to cause generalized weakness.[116]

Sedative drugs ordered in an attempt to control delirium may add to the client's confusion[33] and may also contribute to a decreased responsiveness. Later in the rehabilitative process, various antidepressants may be used to treat aggressive and disruptive behaviors. These, too, may have deleterious side effects.

Thus although therapists are not directly concerned with drug therapy, awareness of the effects of drugs on a specific client is a necessity. If a drug is perceived as interferring with the goals of therapy, this can be discussed with the physician or nurse. Perhaps the dosage can be adjusted or an alternative drug prescribed, or perhaps the drug (or the therapy) can be administered at a different time of day.

Sequelae and complications

Roughly four categories of sequelae from the head injury itself can be identified: physical, cognitive, behavioral, and medical. These are not meant to diminish the significance of the social and economic sequelae, which are considered elsewhere. The types and frequencies of deficits in each category are largely a matter of speculation. Reports of sequelae are influenced by the time that has elapsed since the injury, the skill of the examiner, and the assessment equipment available.

Motor disturbances resulting from head injury generally have a good prognosis.[17] Of the physical deficits encountered, dysfunctions in the cerebral hemispheres and of the cranial nerves are the most common disorders, and these may partially resolve. In a Glasgow study some degree of hemiparesis was present 6 months after injury in 49% of the 150 clients who regained consciousness after severe head injury.[55] The specific manifestations of the hemiparesis can include a wide range of deficits, such as loss of selective motor control, balance, primitive reflexes and sensation, as well as the presence of abnormal tone. Combinations of asymmetrical cerebellar and pyramidal signs and of bilateral pyramidal and extrapyramidal signs have been reported.[81] In at least two studies[55,81] a quarter of the cases had no neurophysical sequelae.

As already mentioned, damage to one or more cranial nerves is not uncommon. Recuperation tends to occur with the exception of the complete recovery of hearing, vestibular function, and smell. These losses can be more permanent.[17,55]

Aphasia, dysarthria, dysphagia, and visuospatial and perceptual motor difficulties can occur because of focal lesions. Posttraumatic epilepsy is also a possible sequela. More severe head injuries tend to manifest more persistent physical problems.[55]

Either temporary or permanent disorders of intellectual function and memory are frequent. Mental (cognitive and behavioral) sequelae can result from generalized or focal brain injuries. Decreased attention span, perseveration, reduced problem-solving ability, lack of initiation, and loss of reasoning and abstract thinking are signs commonly observed by therapists. Formal testing of intellectual function can be hampered by inadequate perceptual, visual, and motor performance.

Memory impairments are an aftermath of generalized lesions. Two types of amnesia are frequently associated with head injury. *Retrograde amnesia* is defined by Cartlidge and Shaw[17] as a "partial or total loss of the ability to recall events that have occurred during the period immediately preceding brain injury." The existence of a correlation between the severity of the injury and the length of retrograde amnesia is controversial. The duration of the retrograde amnesia may progressively decrease. *Posttraumatic amnesia* is defined "as the time lapse between the accident and the point at which the functions concerned with memory are judged to have been restored" (p. 55).[17] The duration of posttraumatic amnesia is considered a clinical indicator of the severity of the injury.[17] An additional deficit can be the inability to form new memory, referred to as *anterograde memory*. This could result in decreased attention or inaccurate perception. The capacity for anterograde memory is frequently the last function to return following recovery from loss of consciousness.[85] The client's inability to develop ongoing short-term memory can be quite frustrating for the rehabilitation team.

For the family, behavioral sequelae are perhaps the most devastating feature of head injury. Personality changes nearly defy measurement and may be apparent only to those closest to the client. Behavioral changes can be present even without cognitive and physical deficits. Frontal lobe lesions are a common cause of alterations in behavior. Irritability and aggressiveness are possible manifestations, as are losses of inhibition and judgment. A client may become anxious, euphoric, apathetic, or emotionally labile. Personal hygiene may be neglected. With some clients there is a general reluctance to change. This reluctance seems to parallel that found among the geriatric population. Although actual psychoses can be sequelae, they appear to be neither common nor definitively related to the head injury. The depression encountered seems to be reactive rather than endogenous.[17,55]

The social consequences of inappropriate behavior can be disastrous and a stumbling block to achieving therapy goals. A correlation between preinjury personality and postinjury changes has not been established.[55] It does seem reasonable, however, that factors within an individual's psychological makeup may affect reaction to the injury. Head trauma frequently happens to adolescents—an age group fraught with its own problems that may be aggravated by the injury.

Medical disorders in other bodily systems can be caused by damage to the brain. These disorders include metabolic, neuroendocrine, cardiovascular, gastrointestinal, respiratory, and hematological disorders. Headaches are also a postinjury complaint.[17]

Finally, no discussion of the sequelae of head injury would be complete without mention of those unfortunate enough to remain in a "persistent vegetative state" (PVS). This state is characterized by a wakeful, reduced responsiveness with no evident cerebral cortical function. The vegetative state can result from diffuse cerebral hypoxia or from severe, diffuse white-matter impact damage. The brainstem is usually relatively intact. Clients may track with their eyes and show minimal spontaneous motor activity, but they do not speak, nor do they respond to verbal stimulation.[53] Life expectancy can be weeks, months, or years.[55,84] Brain-injured clients who remain vegetative for 3 months rarely achieve an independent outcome. However, the term "persistent" should not be added to "vegetative state" until the injury has stabilized or lasted for approximately 1 year.[9]

In the early weeks after injury, certain behaviors exhibited may lead to what later turns out to be false optimism. For example, one young woman who has seemingly remained in a vegetative state for over 3 years has been known to pedal a bicycle when placed and held on it, to turn pages of a magazine, to flip the photographs in a picture-display caddy, and to pet a horse. Yet she has no head control, no balance, no definitive response to verbal stimulation, and no communication of any kind. The motor behaviors could be automatic, triggered by the stimulus. Perhaps she was too easily classified as "vegetative." In this case, however, the distinction between severely disabled and vegetative is subtle, because no intellectual contact has been established with this client.

A list of the complications that could accompany head injury would be limitless. In addition to any concomitant injuries, some of the diagnostic, monitoring, and therapeutic procedures themselves carry hazards. So does prolonged bed rest. Catheters, nasogastric tubes, and tracheostomies can cause iatrogenic injuries. Infections, contractures, skin breakdown, thrombophlebitis, pulmonary problems, heterotopic ossification, and surgical complications are but a few risks.

Prognostic indication

Numerous problems are encountered in trying to predict outcome. Included among these problems are the accuracy and reliability of appraisal of factors by a number of different observers, the uniform implementation and interpretation of predictive factors, the percentage of error in prediction, the possible effects of intervention strategies and bias in treatment based on predictions, and, finally, the definition of what constitutes a "successful" outcome. Understanding these problems is imperative because the therapist can provide persuasive suggestions as to the type and intensity of rehabilitative care after injury. Consequently, the following discussion of prediction precedes a presentation of some possible prognostic indicators.

If indeed there are factors or tests that have predictive value, then they need to be administered, compared, and interpreted uniformly. The differences in operational definitions, types and sizes of populations, and length of time after injury when outcome assessment was made contribute to the lack of consistency in studies of predictive factors. For example, several authors have found that clients under age 20 usually recover,[7,55,96] however, even this has not been uniformly confirmed.[33] One study of the Glasgow Coma Scale[52] indicates that this scale is a simple and consistent outcome predictor. Other studies,[67,104] however, have not

confirmed the scale's reliability and suggest that the criteria may not be standardly applied.

Another concern is the percentage of error in prediction. If prediction is 80% or even 90% accurate, there are still 10% to 20% of the clients with head trauma whose outcome may be predicted incorrectly. Even if the statistics are significant, one may feel very differently if the client whose future is misinterpreted is a family member.

A potentially greater problem in prognosis is defining what constitutes a successful and worthwhile outcome. Therapists accustomed to working with children who may from birth be profoundly mentally retarded and multiply handicapped have perhaps learned to measure improvement in minute increments over a period of time. Perhaps through dealing with C2-3 quadriplegic clients, therapists have come to believe that life is more than independence in activities of daily living (ADL) and gainful employment. The definitions of "successful rehabilitation" and "severely disabled" are relative. Each element of disability, whether cognitive, behavioral, social, or physical, follows its own, but interrelated, course of recovery. Outcome for each area may be different and of differing significance to the client, family, and rehabilitation team members. Clarification of expectations is needed so that physicians, families, clients, and health professionals can better communicate.

Predicting outcome is an important goal for which research is beginning to supply possible answers. In general, however, these predictors are more reliable with *groups* of head-injured clients than with *individual* clients. For the individual client, predictors are best used as guidelines (see the textual discussion and the accompanying box on p. 428 on factors influencing management and recovery after a traumatic head injury).

Prognostic indicators may be divided into two major categories: preinjury characteristics and postinjury characteristics. Postinjury characteristics can be arbitrarily subdivided into static and dynamic characteristics. Many of the factors that may influence management and outcome are self-explanatory. Those that are more indicative of outcome include pretraumatic intelligence and personality, age, cause and type of injury, immediacy of injury, length of retrograde amnesia, duration of posttraumatic amnesia, depth and duration of coma, posttraumatic cognitive and behavioral changes, family adjustment and support, and pattern and quality of sensory/motor recovery. These factors are briefly discussed here.

Only under rare circumstances (usually in the military) are objective measures of the client's preexisting intellectual and behavioral characteristics available. Pre- and post-injury impressions of the client's personality are useful but certainly cannot be considered objective. Thus there is a paucity of studies linking outcome to the preexisting personality. However, preinjury mental characteristics are generally believed to contribute to outcome. That is, those persons with a history of low intellectual ability, difficulty

---

Factors that can influence management and recovery after a traumatic head injury

Preinjury characteristics

A. Cognitive factors
   1. Intelligence*
   2. Memory
   3. Level of education
B. Behavioral factors
   1. Personality*
   2. Psychological status
C. Social factors
   1. Vocational skills
   2. Avocational skills
   3. Interpersonal skills
   4. Family/friends support systems
D. Physical factors
   1. Age*
   2. General health and physical fitness
   3. Existing physical deficits
   4. Morphology
   5. Level of **motor skill** development and capacity for motor learning

Postinjury characteristics

A. Static factors
   1. Trauma factors (neurological)
      a. Location(s) and extent of injury
      b. Cause and type of injury*
      c. Immediacy of injury*
   2. Cognitive factors
      a. Ultimate duration of retrograde amnesia (RA)*
      b. Ultimate duration of posttraumatic amnesia (PTA)*
   3. Physical factors: extracranial injuries

B. Dynamic factors
   1. Trauma factors (neurological)
      a. Depth and duration of coma*
      b. Secondary brain damage
      c. Brainstem reflexes
      d. Special investigations (radiological and laboratory tests)
   2. Cognitive factors
      a. Rate of recovery of intellectual and memory functions*
      b. Quality of recovery of intellectual and memory functions*
      c. Communication disorders
   3. Behavioral factors
      a. Primary personality changes*
      b. Secondary personality changes*
      c. Psychological status
   4. Social factors
      a. Opportunity to reenter occupation/school
      b. Avocational reintegration abilities
      c. Reaction to family/friends
      d. Family adjustment and support capabilities*
   5. Physical factors
      a. Pattern and quality of sensory/motor recovery*
      b. Rate of recovery of sensory/motor function*
      c. Range of motion and muscle flexibility
      d. Cranial nerve deficits
      e. Concomitant disabilities
   6. Environmental factors
      a. Staff/facilities/equipment available
      b. Attitude of health care providers
      c. Expertise of health care providers
      d. Room/housing and treatment settings

*Discussed in the text.

---

with interpersonal relationships, and emotional disturbances have fewer resources with which to cope with injury than those who are more self-confident, ambitious, vital, well-educated, intelligent, and emotionally stable.

Numerous researchers[7,38,62] have reported age as an important factor influencing both mortality rate and functional recovery; it is a single factor with predictive power. Generally, younger clients (under 20 years of age) make a better recovery even after deeper or more prolonged unconsciousness.[55] However, long-term follow-up to prove or disprove this hypothesis does not exist. Perhaps the immediate improvement is greater, but is the *capacity* for learning affected? Recent evidence suggests that although children may experience fewer cognitive and physical deficits, they may have more behavioral problems.

The cause and type of head injury are also indicative of prognosis. For example, clients with subdural hematomas have a poor outcome, whereas clients with epidural hematomas have demonstrated good to moderate recoveries.[31]

Hypoxic or ischemic damage, such as occurs with near-drownings, late resuscitative efforts, and as a complication of the primary injury, suggests a poor outcome.[9]

Most recovery occurs within the first 6 months after injury—a finding of data bank study of more than 500 brain-injured survivors.[55] This does not imply, however, that recovery does not continue after 6 months, only that the rate of improvement progressively slows. Therefore the time at which the client is assessed will influence the prognosis. It should also be noted that death as a direct result of the brain injury usually occurs within the first 2 to 3 days after injury.[16] An additional time-related factor in outcome may be the interval between the injury and the start of a rehabilitation program. Gogstad and Kjellman[39] in Sweden report that "continuous and rapid rehabilitation gives better responses than late introduced efforts, evidently through preventing social and psychological complications" (p. 283). Prevention of physical complications could be added to their list.

The duration of retrograde amnesia, defined earlier in this

chapter, is considered an indicator of the severity of the injury in head trauma.[17,35] Posttraumatic amnesia marks the duration of altered consciousness[55] and also has been demonstrated to correlate with the severity of injury.[28,34] However, because these are retrospective indicators and because they are difficult to assess in clients with severe neurological deficits, their value in influencing management decisions is questionable.

The most important factor in determining prognosis is the degree of brain damage sustained. This is indicated by the depth and duration of coma, and it has been related to outcome.[16,33,97] The definition of what constitutes coma varies considerably, and as noted in a previous example, observer accuracy and reliability are not always optimal. Although coma duration cannot be determined initially, it can be a useful guide for prognosis relatively early during the course of recovery. Stover and Zeiger[97] report that coma lasting more than 1 week is usually associated with either some permanent mental or physical disability or both.

The Glasgow Coma Scale, designed to reliably assess and monitor the degree of impairment of consciousness,[54] allows more objective observation of coma depth and duration.[55] When a client is assessed during the first week after trauma, the overall coma score and the best response grades on each component of the scale correlate with outcome at 6 months.[56] This scale may be a useful predictor because of its reported reliability and its availability; however, it is not without limitations. One problem is that data collection does not begin until 6 hours after trauma.

Outcome, as classified by Jennett and Bond[52] (see box on the Glasgow Outcome Scale), is used in statistically correlating early clinical features with outcome. An extended scale with more discriminating categories is needed for analyzing the rate and degree of recovery,[55] for assessing the efficacy of treatment strategies, and for justifying continued formal treatment. Also, for the purpose of further assessing outcome, it is useful to determine the component disabilities (cognitive, physical, behavioral, and social) that are present and the relationship of each to the overall outcome.[11] For example, a client may be dependent because of cognitive or behavioral (rather than physical) dysfunction. Rappaport's Disability Rating Scale[80] may be a more sensitive scale for clients in long-term rehabilitation programs, however, further study is indicated.[27]

Other aspects of coma, in addition to the response score and coma duration, are important in reflecting brain dysfunction.[45] Favorable clinical signs include pupillary reactivity, evidence of intact brainstem function, and reflexive and spontaneous eye movements. On the other hand, nonreactive pupils, absent eye movements, and abnormalities in brainstem function indicate greater brain dysfunction. These signs may signify a prognosis that is poorer than it is for those clients who do not exhibit these negative signs. However, negative signs per se do not necessarily indicate that the clients will be unable to successfully reintegrate into

> ## Glasgow Outcome Scale
>
> **Vegetative state**
>
> A persistent state characterized by reduced responsiveness associated with wakefulness. The client may exhibit eye opening, sucking, yawning, and localized motor responses.
>
> **Severe disability**
>
> An outcome characterized by consciousness, but the client has 24-hour dependency because of cognitive, behavioral, or physical disabilities, including dysarthria and dysphasia.
>
> **Moderate disability**
>
> An outcome characterized by independence in ADL and in home and community activities but with disability. Clients in this category may have memory or personality changes, hemiparesis, dysphagia, ataxia, acquired epilepsy, or major cranial nerve deficits.
>
> **Good recovery**
>
> Client able to reintegrate into normal social life and could return to work. There may be mild persisting sequelae.

Modified from Jennett B and Bond M: *Lancet* 1:480, 1975.

society, particularly if they are young and if these signs are interpreted early. Outcome predictions based on very early assessments can be excessively pessimistic.[56] Nonetheless, the pattern of posttraumatic consciousness remains an important variable for predicting the outcome after head injury and for judging progress.

The rate and quality of return of intellectual and memory function may also affect ultimate outcome and the occupational outlook. Generally, the faster and more complete the improvement in mental factors, the better the prognosis. In the Gilchrist and Wilkinson[33] study of 84 clients, the degree of mental involvement affected the capacity to return to work. Of their clients, 62% with no changes or mild mental changes returned to work, whereas only 23% of their clients with moderate or severe impairments returned to work. Cognitive disability can greatly interfere with recovery because independent function cannot occur when cognition remains greatly decreased. This is particularly true when there is an impaired rate and ability to learn. Observation of the speed with which a client moves through stages of consciousness may assist in ascertaining the rate of cognitive return. Communication of any kind is a positive sign, as are signs that the client is understanding communication, such as appropriate facial expression.

Lesions causing behavioral changes—such as loss of insight, disinhibition, aggression, depression, impaired judgment, apathy, or hyperactivity—can interfere with rehabilitation and social reentry. In one study the group of clients who were unaware of their own condition tended to be those who experienced the behavioral disturbances. This lack of insight persisted even at their 2-year follow-up. Interestingly, a substantial number of these clients also had posttraumatic epilepsy.[43] The fewer the personality changes, the easier for all involved. Early observations of the client progressing through various phases of consciousness may give clues as to the extent and persistence of personality changes.

There is little doubt that when the client is beyond the vegetative state, the level of family support and adjustment to the loved one affects outcome to some extent. The family can assist or hinder the client in the adjustment process. Work by Bond[12] in Glasgow suggests that positive reactions by families of clients with head injuries include insight, acceptance of rehabilitation goals, willingness to share responsibilities necessary to attain goals, resourcefulness, and tolerance of increased stress. Lack of insight, denial, nonacceptance of rehabilitation, dependence on professionals, hostility, overly ambitious expectations, overprotectiveness, depression, and a low level of intelligence are among the negative family factors. In most families there tends to be a mixture of both positive and negative factors in the members' reactions.[12] Fostering family interest, involvement, and concern is a critical part of the treatment.

Not only is each of the variables a consideration when the therapist determines goals of treatment, but the interplay among the variables is also important. Although it is tempting to search for the *one* reliable and accurate outcome predictor, prognosis most probably depends on multiple predictor variables. For example, a combination of the GCS score, oculocephalic response, and age predicted outcome with 80% accuracy.[18] Different predictive factors also may be more or less significant to each individual client. Perhaps Evans[28] still has the most accurate categories for depicting the outcome of the acute head injury: "death, rapid complete recovery, or anything else." Rehabilitation programs must select from the group of clients classified as "anything else." Recognition of prognostic indicators and the outcome predictors assists in directing clients to facilities that best meet their needs and serves as the background to develop realistic treatment goals.

CONCEPTUAL FRAMEWORK FOR PHYSICAL THERAPY TREATMENT

The therapist is concerned with multiple problems following head injury. A partial list of the most common are in the box.

Information regarding the nature or cause of these problems is scant. Sahrmann and Norton[88] showed that the slowed movement seen in patients with spastic biceps is due to inadequate force production. Spatial disorganization in normal synergies was reported by Bourbonnais and others.[13] In their study, the spastic biceps of stroke patients showed a shift of 90 degrees or more in the angle of peak electromyographic (EMG) output when compared to normal. Similarly,

---

Problems following head injury

Weakness and inability to develop normal force
Changes in muscle elastic properties
Abnormal sequencing and timing of motor functions
Tone changes
Velocity of movement problems
Lack of control of the infinte degrees of freedom for producing coorindated movement
Inability to physically adapt to new challenges
Loss of anticipatory ability
Changes in sensory systems
Poor cognition
Loss of integration skills

Nashner and others[72] reported disturbances in temporal organization of muscle firing in response to perturbations during standing in cerebral palsy clients. Horak[47] showed normal balance synergies but problems with scaling of amplitudes in clients with cerebellar dysfunctions. Watkins and others[107] reported that clients with cerebral vascular accident (CVA) take longer to produce tension in involved muscles and have a longer interval between reciprocal contractions.

Function-induced plasticity

Therapists believe that the human brain shows **plasticity** after injury, a concept also widely accepted in the medical community. More controversial, however, is the concept that neurological recovery is driven from the periphery; that is, that activities in which a client participates change brain structure and organization. The concept that structural neural changes are influenced by the external environment is basic to physical therapy treatment.

Evidence that mammalian brain anatomy and function are modifiable by environmental factors was first irrefutably demonstrated by Wiesel and Hubel[109] who described the importance of environmental experience on functional development of brain cells in the visual cortex of kittens. Normal development of neurons in the visual system of a cat depends on its visual experiences as a kitten. In their experiments, Hubel and Wiesel sutured one eye of kittens shut. The kittens failed to develop binocular vision in visual cortex cells, which normally are driven by either eye. These experiments showed that visual experiences determine the synaptic organization of neurons in the visual cortex.

Devor[23] demonstrated plasticity in the sensory system. After nerve transection of dorsal horn cells, he found that sensory receptive fields reorganized so that new dorsal horn cells now represented skin areas previously represented by the injured dorsal horn cell.

Active participation is also important in **motor learning**. Held's[46] experiments showed that kittens who pull carts carrying other kittens learned a maze task better than the kittens who were pulled (visual versus sensory-motor experience).

The difference that physical intervention makes in recovery after head injury has been shown in several studies. Black and others[10] showed an 82% recovery in monkeys who had early physical training and a 67% recovery in those whose training did not start for 4 months after their lesions developed. In the kitten deprivation studies of Mitchell and others[70] recovery occurred in the sutured eye only if the animal was forced to use that eye. Wolf and others[113] and Taub and others[101] showed that function in hemiplegic upper extremities is improved by forced use of the involved arm. Their experiments restricted use of the uninvolved side. Tower[103] demonstrated that when brain lesions caused limb dysfunction, monkeys did not use the involved limb, but if the remaining useful limb was restrained, the monkeys then began using the first "useless" limb for climbing and other activities.

Recovery after head injury

Plasticity in the normal central nervous system (CNS) is well established. The mechanisms thought responsible for CNS recovery[58] after injury are of two types: those that change the neuronal level and those that substitute for lost function. Changes at the neuronal level include the following:

- Development of supersensitivity of postsynaptic membranes
- Recruitment of previously silent synapses
- Sprouting of side branches in cut axons and new side branch growth of uninjured axons to synapse at sites vacated by injured axons

Substitutions may occur through the following:

- Vicarious function in which another part of the nervous system can take over function performed by the damaged area
- Hyperinnervation where "extra" cells in the brain assume function for lost cells (There are many more neurons present than the mature brain needs.)

Reorganization and regeneration recovery mechanisms are the likely areas for intervention by the therapist. These represent mechanisms that are influenced by the environment and can be altered by learning. Treatment by manipulation of the environment can lead to improved recovery. Bach-y-Rita[2,3] states that long-term rehabilitation is key to improved motor control and that recovery can continue to occur as long as the brain is challenged.

Motor learning theories

Current research establishes a CNS that becomes more efficient at the muscle and brain level as motor learning proceeds. Factors affecting effectiveness and speed of motor learning are discussed in the conceptual framework section

of this chapter. Evaluation and treatment techniques sections are based on that framework.

To produce motor patterns more efficiently, the CNS must have an intricate understanding of the smallest details of how the musculoskeletal system works as well as the constraints placed on movement. Constraints are determined by the task to be accomplished, time, and the laws of physics. Motor **learning theories** try to explain how the CNS accomplishes the miracle of coordinated, meaningful movement.

Systems theory. Motor learning theory has evolved in the last few years from a concept of a hierarchically organized brain, in which higher centers have dominance over lower centers, to the **systems theory**, in which multiple centers interact. Systems theory views movement as a result of peripheral and CNS influence contributing different aspects to motor control. Different motor responses can occur in response to identical situations. For example, systems theory is compatible with the research showing that the upper extremity motor pattern used to pick up a pen varies depending on what is to be done with the pen: Will it be used to write, or will it be handed to another person? The systems model states that movement is based on the task or goal to be accomplished, not, as in hierarchical models, on a response to a particular sensory stimulus.

The systems model of motor control may have been first proposed in the 1930s by Bernstein[8] who stated that movement is a result of many different systems interacting and that each area of CNS influence could be enhanced or diminished depending on the task to be accomplished.

In the systems model many of the behaviors and "patterns" after head injury are seen as attempts by the CNS to compensate for loss. For example, spasticity may be the result of an attempt to increase force. When the amplitude of a contraction cannot be increased due to injury, the CNS may increase the length of time the muscle fires or may recruit muscles not normally used in a particular pattern of movement.

Although debate is ongoing as to whether many of the abnormal functions seen after head injury result from loss of functions or from an attempt to compensate for the lost functions, the goal of intervention is the same: *to help a client work in the environment to produce movements that are efficient, successful, and to some extent socially acceptable.*

Synergistic organization. Synergies, or motor patterns, are seen as the basis of movement in the systems theory. Synergies are defined as a fixed set of muscles contracting with a preset sequence and time of contraction. The need for the brain to use synergistic organization comes from the infinite number of movement combinations that are available. The possible movements at a joint are defined as the degrees of freedom. For example, the hip has three degrees of freedom or three spatial dimensions into which it can move the thigh: flexion, abduction, and rotation. When combined with remaining lower limb joints, many different ways of placing the foot on the floor during walking are possible. There can be more hip flexion and less knee and foot flexion. There can be circumduction at the hip with little knee or foot flexion. Even with the many possibilities, the foot still lands at exactly the same point in space.

These multiple movement options give the system flexibility, but the brain now has an inordinate amount of movement possibilities available and would have to calculate all possible solutions for each desired movement. The rapid response time needed to be effective is short for many movements, such as balance reactions, emphasizing the need for the brain to organize movement into quick response groups. By use of synergies, flexibility is maintained but speed and efficiency are added. Force (amplitude) of contraction, velocity, and timing can be changed to meet task demands.

Synergies are shaped through experience. They are developed before (innate) and after birth (learned). Some of the developed synergies may be combinations of innate synergies. Anatomically, the central generator of patterns appears to be the kinetic system (basal ganglia and spinal cord). The cerebellum is proposed as the system that smooths out the synergies through modification of amplitude of contraction, timing, and coordination within the synergy.

Early experiments on motor control demonstrated how synergies develop. Payton and Kelley[78] showed that with practice of a novel motor task, movements became more organized. On EMG studies, less electrical activity occurred and there was less time to peak activation of the muscle in a motor task after it had been learned. Recently, PET scans, which show brain cell activity levels, have demonstrated the same phenomenon in the brain. As a group of subjects practiced a motor skill, initially large areas of brain cells fired (light areas on the scan) but, as skill developed, fewer and fewer bright areas were illuminated. Synergies appear to develop as a means of motor output for nearly all learned motor activities.

The best understood synergies are the balance and reaching patterns. Both appear to be basic innate synergies. Quiet standing in humans is maintained by proprioceptive, visual, and vestibular inputs. It requires the coordination of many muscles, especially those of the hips, knees, and ankles to maintain the body's center of gravity over its base of support. This complex coordination of muscle control is accomplished by sequences of stereotyped patterns mediated via the brainstem, cerebellum, and spinal cord. Mechanoreceptor input in response to movement or body sway stimulates the response in which posture is stabilized by small changes in the angle between the foot and the leg. For example, when length, force of contraction, or movement velocity of the calf muscles exceeds the threshold of mechanoreceptors in the muscles, skin, or joints, mechanoreceptor signals initiate rapid postural readjustments by triggering a synergistic response.

For small center of gravity movements, these synergies are sequenced in a distal to proximal manner. The direction of sway determines the particular synergy elicited to correct for the shift in the center of gravity. In forward losses of balance the posterior extensor muscles of the legs and trunk respond in about 100 msec. In backward losses, the anterior muscles respond including anterior tibialis, hip flexors, and abdominals. Contraction (temporal sequencing) is in a distal to proximal manner starting with the gastroc/anterior tibialis, quadriceps/hamstring and back extensors/abdominals.

The timing between muscle contractions and the proximal to distal sequence are preset. The amplitude of contraction varies with the environmental demands. In greater losses of balance, a different synergy is used in which the client might bend at the hip and knees. If the balance loss is great enough, a person takes a step to maintain upright balance.[71] For additional information refer to Chapter 28 on balance.

Weight shifts from one leg to the other and stability after the weight shift are other aspects of dynamic balance performed through synergies. The movement pattern of the swing leg in gait is limited in number of degrees of freedom at each joint and sequence of movement by synergies. There is also a specific coordination and timing of swing leg movement in relation to the stance leg movement (interlimb timing and coordination).

In walking, the sequence of contraction of the leg muscle from ankle to hip, the time of onset of the contraction of each muscle, and a ratio of force for each muscle are all preset in the motor control program of the brain or spinal cord. If an increase in speed is needed, force can be increased within the synergy, but the basic synergies, or motor programs, are what give identity to a gait pattern. Whether you are walking fast or slow, there is an individually recognizable pattern.

In the reaching and grasping pattern, three components have been identified: the reaching portion, the grasping or prehension portion, and the maintenance of balance. The reaching and maintenance of balance are synergies.[32,41] The reaching pattern is determined by the target. Again, there is a distal to proximal sequence of firing. Movement is in a straight line and the velocity curve is always bell-shaped.[68]

The characteristics of hand control differ from control of many other parts of the body. It is not a synergistic movement. Unlike other motor acts, the motor/sensory cortex helps with force production and selection of muscles[30] during hand movement. This may be why more severe deficits are seen in the hand after cortical injury.

In summary, the CNS has solved movement tasks by decreasing the amount of decision making for each movement. It packages movements into synergies that have fixed relationships to other body movements and that can be modified to meet environmental demands.

Anticipatory and feedback mechanisms for synergy modification.   Movement, to be purposeful, must match the environment. For example adjustments are made for walking on grass, a surface that may be both soft and irregular. The normal gait synergy changed, but how did this happen before the movement? In the case of grass, the visual system provided information about the environment before movement so the CNS could anticipate what changes were needed in the synergy. The walking pattern can adapt to environmental constraints such as obstacles, uneven surfaces, or speed demands by modifying the basic synergies' velocity, intensity, and duration of contractions. Balance responses can also be anticipatory, as when they precede movement, for example, the body moves backward before reaching forward.[49]

Feedback through sensory information helps fine tune the subsequent steps in the walking example. When movement of the head occurs, the visual array moves in the peripheral visual field, the joints and muscles move and the semicircular canals fire. These sensory impulses result in motor system adaptations to the environment. At the same time, the different sensory inputs are checked against each other for clarification of any ambiguous information. If the visual array is moving but the vestibular and mechanoreceptive systems perceive no movement, the brain interprets this combination of information as an object moving past the person, not body movement; therefore no balance adjustments are made.

In the reaching/prehension pattern, target location is coded by the visual system. Both the spatial and temporal conditions are present before the movement begins. Once the hand is at the target, the hand has already been shaped for prehension. Initially, grip is determined by the visual system (anticipatory) and past memory (learning) of the characteristic of the object to be picked up. Tactile input from the finger tips (feedback) is then used to make adjustments in grip force if the initial grip was not effective. Once movement occurs, there is a final comparison of the original planned pattern with the executed pattern to see if they matched.

In summary, to meet the motor task (external) requirements, synergies are used and modified through a feedforward and feedback system of control. Feedforward, or **anticipatory responses** (often from vision and past memory of successful movements), are used for the initial movement. Feedback is used to check the effectiveness of the response and modify it, if needed. A final check is made to determine whether the motor pattern matched the original "planned" pattern after movement occurred.

Dynamic pattern theory. The dynamic pattern theory[59,92] addresses problems of when motor behavior changes and also uses concepts of basic patterns of movement. The theory states that certain patterns are very stable or unstable and that transition between patterns or to a new pattern depends on pattern stability. (See Giuliani[36] for a summary of this theory.) The challenge for the physical therapist is to identify what makes these "stuck" behaviors become more unstable and perhaps amenable to change. Patterns that are very "set" are much more difficult to change than those who are more variable. In fact phase

transitions between old and new patterns are noted by periods of increased variability. The client appears to vacillate between the old and the new behaviors during transition phases and before new behavior establishment points. Repetition is important to develop more consistent motor patterns and new establishment points.

Motor skill acquisition and feedback. *The goal of the physical therapist's treatment is to produce a task-oriented behavioral change that becomes permanent without continued therapist help or intervention.* Often the client performs well during therapy but does not seem to carry the improved performance outside the clinic. This difference between performance and learning is discussed by Schmidt.[91] Motor learning, as he defines it,[90] is "an area of study focusing on the acquisition of skilled movements as a result of practice." Differentiation must occur between performance, which can be temporary, and learning, which is longer term. Many therapy techniques that improve a client's performance inhibit learning because they are based on the external controls and support provided by the physical therapist's manipulations. The type of feedback and the method in which it is provided are critical to learning new motor skills. For example when the hip stabilization component of walking is externally provided by the therapist during gait training, the client has no need to develop his or her own hip stabilization patterns.

Knowledge of results, i.e., information on how successful the movement was in meeting the task goals, is also considered basic to learning. Knowledge of results is extrinsic information over and above that proved by the task itself.[91] During the practice portion in most tasks, increasing any type of feedback appears to improve task performance.[75] But long-term learning may occur better with knowledge of results (KR) provided less often. The relative frequency with which KR is provided in relation to the number of trials is important in learning. Bandwidth knowledge of results, in which information is given about trials falling outside a certain range, appears the most effective for learning. Delaying KR also improves learning.

Changing motor function with adaptive and part-task training. The commonly used techniques of teaching a task by practicing at a slower speed or practicing a part of a motor task is not effective. For example, to make walking easier, a physical therapist may have the client practice the stepping component of gait while providing balance support for the client. Weight shifting is often practiced as a component of gait before walking is initiated. In a study by Man and others,[66] a complex task was broken down into adaptive training methods (e.g., slower motions) and part task training (on components of the task). Those practicing the whole task did as well or better than either experimental group. This may explain why Winstein and others[117] found no carry-over of successful weight shifting training in standing to weight shift in walking in a group of hemiplegic clients. A finding that practicing small components of a task does not make one better at the whole task is not too surprising. Many of us can jump, have good shoulder power, and can throw overhead but cannot, without practice, put this together to play basketball. A minimum basic amount of strength, range of motion (ROM), and interlimb sequencing is necessary to play basketball, but is not adequate to play without the actual practice of the sport.

But practicing other than the whole task may be possible. Using the same task as Man and others,[66] Newell[74] showed that part-task training was effective when it was conducted in natural subtasks of the whole. These subtasks are part of the whole task but are distinguished by changes in speed or direction. This area of skill acquisition has not been studied adequately.

To review, the conceptual framework for the evaluation and treatment of head injury clients is based on systems theory, which states that movement is goal-oriented and a result of combined systems working together to produce synergistic movement. Synergistic movement is anticipatory in nature with sensory feedback and previous experience contributing to task accomplishment. Changes in motor behavior are determined by how "set" patterns (dynamic pattern theory) are influenced by the type of practice, knowledge of the effectiveness of the results, and how the motor skills are broken down for practice.

EVALUATION, MEASUREMENT, AND ASSESSMENT
General considerations

Most of this section describes motor function; however, motor function is only a small part of the problem of the head-injured client. Social and family problems will likely be the most devastating in the long term. Motivation, attention skills, emotional instability, memory and learning, and social deficits are all cognitive processes that prevent or retard clients' progress in the physical therapy program. Working with professionals who specialize in these areas will improve the client's chances to escape deficits that are permanently handicapping. These programs can make a difference. Brotherton and others[14] documented long-term social behavior improvement in four severely head-injured clients who had undergone traditional social skills training programs.

Working on client goals helps to establish motivation. Client goals that seem unrealistic should not be dismissed as inappropriate. The high school athlete who wants to play football next week and presently has no postural control can be approached about discussing how he will learn to sit, stand, walk, and run. Most clients who go through rehabilitation programs begin to assess their own potential more appropriately once they have worked through part of their program. Many people think that the brain heals like any other part of their body and expect full recovery. Sometimes giving clients time out of therapy to experience everyday life at home and work helps them determine their own goals and

---

Rancho Los Amigos Hospital scale of cognitive function

I. No response
II. Generalized response
III. Localized response
IV. Confused–agitated
V. Confused–inappropriate
VI. Confused–appropriate
VII. Automatic–appropriate
VIII. Purposeful–appropriate

---

needs and to set priorities. The client who couldn't see doing "silly exercises" comes back asking to learn ADLs. In many cases it is the families who need help understanding their family member's social and behavioral changes.

Cognitive measurement tool. Numerous observations of clients with head injuries at Rancho Los Amigos Hospital resulted in a descriptive categorization of various stages of "cognitive function" as shown in the box above.

Although termed a cognitive scale, this scale actually includes both cognitive and behavioral components of general cerebral function. Even before this categorization was developed, physical therapists experienced with clients with head trauma had observed that mental recovery was characterized by a progression through a series of stages. The publication of these observations by the Professional Staff Association at Rancho offers more uniform assessment, documentation, and prediction of these stages.

Scales such as this one provides a common ground for communication. Perhaps as knowledge of the development and the redevelopment of cognitive and behavioral functions increases, so will sophistication of the scales. This would permit a more independent evaluation of these two related yet separate cortical functions. Fig. 14-1 depicts the close association of cognitive, behavioral, and physical functioning soon after injury. The three domains gradually become more distinguishable in later stages of recovery and can be assessed more independently; however, their interrelationships remain exceedingly complex.

Motor-sensory evaluation and measurement format. The purpose of the evaluation and assessment is to determine what prevents the client from performing in a functional, acceptable manner as identified by the client, the therapist, and the society. (For the components of evaluation, see the box on p. 435.)

Physical therapy evaluation identifies the problems that can be managed by the physical therapist and to "tease" out those factors that influence or restrict the choice of therapeutic approaches. Measurement establishes a baseline on which to judge future improvement or lack thereof. This baseline should be quantified to permit measurement of the effectiveness of the intervention strategies. Assessment provides a qualitative aspect of determining reasons why a

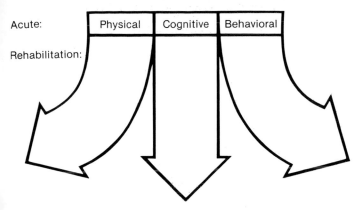

Acute: Physical | Cognitive | Behavioral

Rehabilitation:

Fig. 14-1. Schema representing the close association of cognitive, behavioral, and physical functioning soon after injury. The three domains gradually become more distinguishable in the later stages of recovery.

problem is present. Assessment would examine the various possible causes of the problem and determine which are most critical. The assessment thus determines treatment goals.

An example of evaluation, measurement, and assessment would be as follows. A client falls several times a week. Evaluation shows inadequate balance. Measurements might include strength, ROM, tone, balance synergies, etc. Assessment shows that the 20-degree hip flexion contracture and P+ ankle strength together prevent the client from using normal ankle balance strategies, which results in balance losses and falling. Long-term treatment goals might be to decrease falling by achieving the short-term goals of neutral hip extension and ankle strength at the G level.

The World Health Organization's International Classification (ICIDH)[114] of impairment, disability, and handicap can be useful for evaluation. This model links physical changes at the individual level (those changes within the body) to functional deficit (how the physical change results in abnormal function of the body within the environment) and to society (e.g., how the functional changes make a person unable to hold a job or drive). In the ICIDH model, impairment is the result of the disease at the organ level. Disability results from the impairment at the functional or skill level. Handicap is the consequence at the societal level.

In using this type of evaluation more emphasis is placed on functional skills than physical normalcy. There is much debate by the insurance industry, case managers, and therapists about a client's right to have a physical therapist reestablish normal movement rather than functional skill. Until societies truly accept people whose physical movements vary from "normal," however, there will be deficits in the handicap area, even for those who have no functional deficits. Societies have been unable so far to accept people with physical disabilities such as paralysis, ataxia, and dysarthria as fully capable.

The method of evaluation should lead to understanding

Components of evaluation

I. Medical record data
II. Nursing observations
III. Client/family data
    A. Subjective data: personal factors and goals
    B. Objective data
        1. General observations
        2. Screening of systems
            a. Respiratory
            b. Circulatory
            c. Integumentary
            d. Musculoskeletal
            e. Bowel and bladder
        3. Cerebral function
            a. General cerebral function (e.g., cognition)
            b. Specific cerebral function (e.g., language)
        4. Autonomic nervous system function
        5. Sensory function
            a. Primary sensations
            b. Cortical or integrative sensations
        6. Motor performance—impairments
            a. Complex motor activities
                1) Basic synergies
                2) Modifies synergies
                3) Anticipatory reactions
                4) Uses feedback correctly
                5) Shows variability in motor performance
            b. Components, or basic element, of motor performance
                1) Tone
                2) Muscle strength
                3) Muscle length/flexibility
                4) Response speed
                5) Movement speed
                6) Muscular endurance
                7) Vision
                8) Vestibular
        7. Disabilities
        8. General cardiovascular endurance/fitness
        9. Social/economic/family factors-handicaps
IV. Physician and other team member assessments

the underlying causes of the disabilities and should be the basis of the treatment program. Starting at the disability level is most useful. Disability is a functional or performance limitation. Performance deficits are what bring the client into the clinic in the first place. Impairment is the underlying deficit that causes a disability.[63] It is determined through the traditional physical therapy measurements of strength, speed, ROM, timing, sequencing, velocity, endurance, etc. Impairments of components of movements can be assessed in light of their contribution to the disability.[58] For example, a particular disability may be the result of multiple impairments, but certain critical components appear to have more influence on a function. In gait disabilities in children with cerebral palsy, Olney and others[77] demonstrated that poor force output by ankle plantar flexors during the push-off phase of gait was the most important factor in their poor gait performance. Therefore weakness in the gastrocnemius area might be considered a critical impairment in these clients. In deficient standing balance, break down in the sequencing of lower extremity muscle contractions may be the crucial impairment. In grasping activities, arm movement, prehension, and maintenance of balance comprise the task. Deficiencies of timing, strength, or sequencing can contribute to poor hand function. Sensory deficits at the hand level, however, may be the critical impairment related to poor manipulation skills. Additionally, deficits in the circulatory, respiratory, integumentary, as well as the musculoskeletal systems can account for poor function in the head-injured client (Fig. 14-2).

The therapist's assessment determines relative contributions of the impairments to disability, which then focuses the treatment program. Not all impairments can be eliminated. It is the therapist's task to find alternatives for the client to perform functional activities when the impairment cannot be restored.

When resolving problems at the impairment level is not possible, the ICIDH evaluation system helps the physical therapist identify substitutions that would achieve the same functional goals (e.g., use of a wheelchair for the client who will not be able to walk, or use of a feeding cuff for a client who will not develop adequate motor function in the hand for feeding).

Evaluation of motor performance in the head-injured client

Disabilities. Disability can be assessed with formal measurement tools. Wade[106] provides an in-depth presentation of evaluations for this level. The Barthel Index (Appendix Chapter 25) is an example of a very simple tool for gross assessment of overall disability.[65] It simply asks whether functional skills can be performed within a reasonable time limit. These types of indexes should be chosen to address what abilities the client can accomplish and are not treatment tools. Their sole purpose is to identify disabilities.

Impairment. In head-injured clients, the focus of treatment is often at the impairment level. Impairment can be assessed at the component and complex task levels.

The physical therapist has a multilevel assessment task, which includes (1) identification of the components that

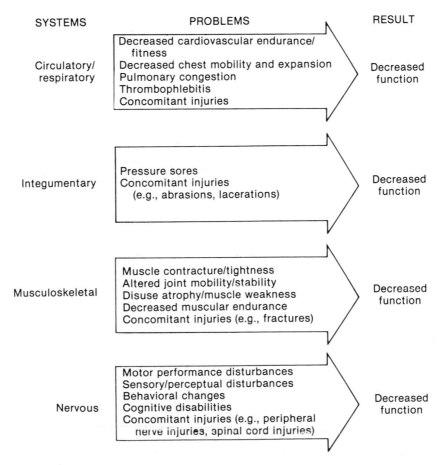

Fig. 14-2. Therapists develop intervention strategies to deal with functional deficits that may result from a variety of problems occurring primarily in one or more of the body systems depicted.

compose a complex task or disability, (2) assessment of the degree to which a component's deficit contributes to the disability, and (3) assessment of the ability to recover the necessary improvement in a component.

Impairment at the basic component level of performance.   Breaking motion down to its most basic components may be helpful, but two caveats are necessary. First, improvement in abnormal components may not lead to improvement in disabilities. Second, treating the individual impairments will not necessarily result in learning a skill. Skills result from an organization of many motor functions together. Conversely, not having a critical component, such as arm strength, may be the one factor preventing a person from learning to perform a skill (e.g., enough force can't be generated to throw a ball 5 feet in the air to hit a basket).

Existing physical therapy evaluation and measurement tools often address the impairment level. These include muscle strength tests, flexibility (ROM) tests, speed of motion, reaction time, sensation, vision, vestibular, tone, and proprioceptive evaluations.

Strength or force production.   Weakness may occur in any muscle affected by paralysis. Individuals with brain damage show atrophy in motor units, as well as motor units that fatigue easily.[25,26] Disuse, cast immobilization, joint dysfunction, improper nutrition, drugs, and aging can cause differential weakness with altered morphological, biochemical, and physiological characteristics within the muscle.[82] EMG studies by numerous investigators[83,99] suggest that reduced activity alters motor unit properties, discharge frequency, and recruitment patterns. Loss of motor units also has been reported.[44]

Changes in muscle length affect strength. In clients with CVA, shortened muscles tend to be strong in short ranges, and lengthened muscles are strongest in lengthened ranges but weak in shorter positions when compared to the strength-length curves of normal muscles.[87]

Strength or force at the component level may be assessed functionally (e.g., the client has enough strength to lift the arm overhead, out to the side, and up to the mouth). In other cases, such as an inability to perform balance reactions, individual strength of muscles may be important. Using either traditional manual muscle testing, force transducers, or strength testing with isokinetic testing throughout the range provides good strength information. The level of testing chosen should be consistent with the deficit and the therapist's perception of its importance in contributing to disability.

Flexibility.   Flexibility at the muscle and joint level is important. Tardieu and others[100] showed that muscles lose sarcomeres rapidly when consistently held in a shortened position. This loss results in a stiffening of the muscle due to mechanical changes. Increased tone at a joint may also produce functional range limitations. Assessments should determine the contribution of both tone and tissue factors in

limiting flexibility. Active and passive motion should be compared because stiffness (not contracture) often prevents good function. For example active dorsiflexion is often limited in clients who have full passive ROM because stiffness begins at neutral level or below. The functional result of this is foot drop or toe catch in the swing phase of gait because the tibialis anterior cannot generate adequate strength to overcome the stiffness. This restriction also may limit the body moving forward over the foot during the stance phase of gait resulting in hip retraction or an apparent balance loss. Knee hyperextension also can result from lack of forward motion of the tibia.

Tone.   The underlying neurophysiological mechanism of increased tone after head injury is not known. The components that are known are very complex (See Craik[22] for a review of these concepts from a physical therapy application). Research does not support the previously held theory that gamma motor activity is responsible for resting tone or that the stretch reflex is purely monosynaptic through the Ia afferents from a single muscle.

Variability of findings in the literature on what spasticity is and when it occurs continues to be confusing. Present discussion involves whether spasticity is more than one phenomenon neurophysiologically, and whether it is an abnormal input, or a processing problems at the spinal cord level or supraspinal level. Perhaps increased tone occurs because muscles not normally used in a synergy try to substitute for muscles that are unable to produce adequate force.[88] Limited ability (1) to produce higher speeds of motion, (2) to adequately activate antagonists during motion, and (3) to coactivate agonist and antagonists and larger intervals between reciprocal contractions have all been reported in spastic clients.[4,24,60] The question of abnormal tone production may not be solved until it is determined whether tone and force are independent of each other. Whatever the cause of increased tone, the physical therapist can evaluate tone at two levels: Is it interfering with function and, if so, can it be changed?

Evaluation begins with identifying whether there is increased or decreased muscle tension at rest. If it is increased, is the tension at the muscle level (stiffness or sarcomere involvement) or the neurological level? Muscle stiffness secondary to tissue changes are common in the head-injured client. If there is increased tone during movement, EMG may be beneficial to determine the nature of the tone. Is it a problem of cocontraction of agonist and antagonist at a joint? A problem of prolonged contraction? Or is it poor sequencing, either temporally or spatially, of other muscles involved in the movement?

Spatial sequencing of movement involves the contraction of a preset group of muscles. Temporal sequencing involves muscles contracting in a fixed sequence. EMGs and videoanalysis provide additional depth of information regarding the sequence and timing of movement patterns (Fig 14-3). For example is the normal temporal sequencing in the

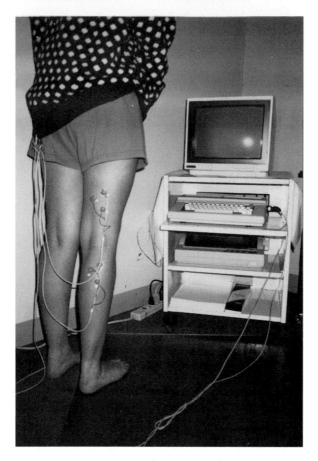

Fig. 14-3. Measurement of the sequence of contraction of gastrocnemius and hamstring in forward perturbation using dual channel EMG with surface electrodes.

distal to proximal manner present in the upper extremity during a reaching task? In a balance reaction, are the ankle, hip, and back extensors (spatial sequencing) all contracting in response to a forward perturbation? (See Treatment for a discussion of modifying tone-related components.)

Speed of motion. Research shows that seemingly very different movements may actually be spatially the same (same muscles involved) but appear different because of pauses within the movements, velocity, or speed.[40]

Measurements include how quickly a joint can be moved. Recording the number of repetitions of a movement in a specific time frame provides an easy clinical measurement. Instruments can measure partial and whole extremity motion speed. Speed of movement at each joint in a synergistic movement (videotaped) can help to analyze function. Is poor performance due to speed of movement problems in just one part of the synergy, or in all parts?

Reaction time. How fast can the client begin motion? This parameter can be measured by EMG or with other computerized equipment.

Reaction time assessment gives insight into the time of processing as it entails the time from a stimulus to a response. Quick reaction time may be critical for more automatic patterns, such as balance responses, to be effective.

Endurance. Muscle endurance refers more to the ability at the muscle level to produce the same level of contraction over time. It may be measured by repeating muscle testing before and after using the muscle for a set time or by EMG using medium frequency analysis.

Cardiovascular endurance determines how effectively the body can use oxygen and how soon fatigue sets in. This type of endurance can be measured with several bicycle tests,[115] and with treadmills using a Bruce[15] protocol. A simple test is heart rate before and after activity; the less change and more rapid the return to resting rate, the better the fitness level.

Fatigue, which is separate from endurance, may result from increased energy requirements resulting from less efficient motor patterns or more CNS activity.

Sensory function. Various sensations can be impaired. Problems in the sensory system are often reflected in the motor system, creating distorted movement through faulty information in the feedforward or feedback processes.

Two broad categories of sensations can be defined based on type of information: primary sensations and cortical (or integrative) sensations. This arbitrary division is useful functionally but is not anatomically based. Primary sensations include exteroception and proprioception. The exteroceptors of smell, sight, and hearing are sometimes referred to as teloreceptors. Vision, hearing, olfaction, gustation, pain, touch, temperature, position sense, and kinesthesia are commonly checked primary sensations. Sensations cannot be tested definitively clinically without client participation. Further evaluations of sensation are provided in specific systems.

PROPRIOCEPTION, LIGHT TOUCH, TWO-POINT DISCRIMINATION AND STEREOGNOSIS. Traditional evaluations of proprioception include the ability to distinguish motion and motion direction at each joint. Some clients who cannot distinguish direction or movement still function well. They may have proprioceptive function at the unconscious level (e.g., cerebellar) while not perceiving the input at the parietal (cortical) level. Light touch is tested with a brush for localization and quality of sensation. Two-point discrimination can be tested using instruments specifically designed to measure how far apart two separate spots of contact need to be to identify them as distinct. Stereognosis, the ability to identify objects placed in the hand without visual assistance, may be critical to normal hand use.

VISION AND VISUAL PERCEPTION. Vision is critical in recovery of many motor functions because it is responsible for much of the feedforward or anticipatory control of movement. For example, balance can be maintained through the visual system by modifying the synergy before perturbation occurs. Feedback through the peripheral field visual array movement can also trigger balance synergies.

General visual functions can be screened by the physical therapist as follows:

1. Tracking is assessed through the whole visual field, observing for any nystagmus or multiple saccades.
2. Focus can be checked by observing for constriction and dilation of the pupil, which should occur as an object is moved to and from the nose.
3. Binocular vision is controlled through retinal slip. This reflex signals whether the eyes and fovea are focused on a single point or target; do the images in both eyes match? A "jump test" can screen binocular vision. The client stares at an object at about 18 inches from the nose. The therapist covers one eye. If there is movement to adjust the remaining uncovered eye back to the object, both retinas may not be focusing on one point (this usually results in diplopia or blurred vision). Observing whether light reflections fall on exactly the same place on both pupils is also useful in evaluating binocular eye focus.
4. Peripheral visual movement receptors are stimulated with an optokinetic drum. This may provide insight into the peripheral visual field's perception of movement. Much of visual balance control is through the peripheral field.
5. Visual fields can be grossly tested by having the client look forward at a point (observer sits in front of the client to be sure client remains focused on a point) (Fig. 14-4). The client indicates when he or she first sees an object coming into the peripheral field from behind or a "spotter" notes when the client looks toward the object.
6. Visual interactions with the vestibular system are assessed through the vestibularocular reflex (VOR). This reflex maintains a fixed gaze on a target as the head moves.
7. Perceptual tests that evaluate how visual information is used include visual memory tests and figure-ground tests, etc.

Optometrists and ophthalmologists are appropriate referrals for clients needing in-depth visual workups, especially when visual perception is involved. Refer to Chapter 27 for additional information on vision and visual testing.

VESTIBULAR SYSTEM. The vestibular system monitors position of the head in space and helps distinguish when the body is moving versus when the visual surround is moving. Vertigo, eye/head incoordination, and postural and balance complications occur as a result of problems in the vestibular cerebellar systems.

Vertigo or dizziness involves the client's perception of abnormal motion, which may include self or object motion. Dizziness, nausea, and disorientation are thought to be stimulated by a sensory conflict between vestibular, mechanoreceptive, and visual information. When the vestibular system reports information (e.g., you are moving), the

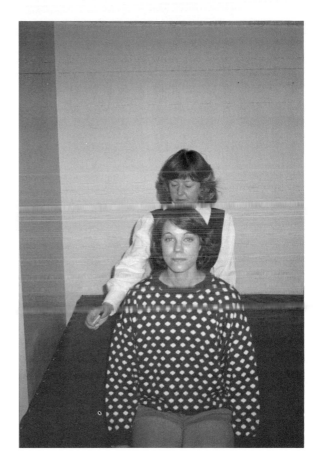

Fig. 14-4. Testing of peripheral visual fields from behind the client.

information is checked against the visual field flow and muscle and joint information to confirm movement. If the remaining two systems report different or no movement, then a sensory conflict results.

Eye/head problems can involve eye movement problems of saccades, which are used to bring objects onto focus on the fovea, poor smooth pursuit movement in tracking of moving objects, inability to hold an image steady on the retina during head movement (resulting in blurred or double vision), and finally an inability to coordinate head and eye motion while looking at still or moving objects.

Postural control deficits include inappropriate selection of balance using ankle, hip, or suspension strategies for the environmental demands, poor scaling of strategies, and poor adaptation to environmental conditions.[47]

Vestibular tests can be performed at the screening level to note dizziness with body, head or eye motions. Symptoms occurring only with specific head positions can be an indicator of problems in the semicircular canals. In-depth evaluation tools may be used when clients are symptomatic. A vestibular assessment, such as the one presented by Horak,[48] provides comprehensive information on vestibular functioning for the physical therapist. This type of testing assesses oculomotor function, balance and coordination, and sensory conflicts. (Refer to Chapter 28 for additional information on balance.)

Tests by other professionals for peripheral versus central vestibular dysfunction can include electronystagmography (ENG) using calorics to stimulate one ear with ice water for detecting asymmetries, positional tests to confirm nystagmus in differing head positions, and the rotational chair to stimulate the vestibularocular reflex for eye movement compensation during head and body rotation. Audiograms and auditory brainstem responses establish hearing abnormalities. Tympanometric fistula tests use pressurized air in the external ear canal to identify fistulas.

When dizziness or disorientation occurs evaluation helps determine the treatment process. A practical division includes testing in lying, sitting, and standing. Positive test in these positions include symptoms occurring when the head is fixed with eyes moving, eyes fixed with head moving, head on body motions, body on body motions, or body moving in space.

Certain questions posed by the therapist help direct problem-solving strategies. Do symptoms occur mainly when the client moves, or do they occur mainly when objects move in the client's visual periphery? These tests answer questions about the most dominant of the systems. Testing of vestibular function with the eyes closed and on moving or soft surfaces helps evaluate the influence of the vestibular rather than the visual and proprioceptive systems. If the client falls when the eyes are closed or is unstable on soft or moving surfaces, the client may be dominated by visual or proprioceptive systems, and the vestibular system may be contributing little input to functioning.

Impairment at complex task level. Once the basic components of performance have been evaluated, the task is to determine which aspects of poor performance are associated with lack of a component and which aspects are related to the use of these components in combined manners or synergies. Complex task evaluation asks different questions than component evaluation and requires extensive knowledge of abnormal and normal movement.

Complex task evaluation and assessment may be considered from the point of view of the dynamical systems theory as follows:

1. *Are those innate programs thought to be present at birth working? At what level?*

This level of evaluation asks whether basic motor patterns are available, accessible, and used appropriately. Are basic reflexes intact? Do movement patterns show basic synergies such as in standing and reaching? Are swallowing, eye tracking, smiling, withdrawal reflexes, and the ability to voluntarily move the trunk, head, and limbs present? Does the client appear to have the ability to coordinate motions (decrease the degrees of freedom)? Injury at this level might most affect basic synergy production and sequencing. The kinetic system involving the basal ganglia is presently most associated with these functions.

2. *Are the basic synergies being selected or modified to meet specific task requirements?* These functions are presently associated with the synergic or cerebellar functions, which provide tone, timing, coordination, and amplitude of motions. The synergistic system smooths out the motor program and provides adaptability. Is the client able to use the basic synergies in a useful manner? Is the client able to modify and then accomplish activities such as walking and ball catching? Is there good interlimb coordination? Does the client respond correctly to environmental changes or stimuli? When synergies are used, are they appropriate for the stimulus? For example, many clients inappropriately use the hip strategy in response to all losses of balance.

3. *Does the client show anticipatory reactions?* These reactions are dependent on learning. Anticipatory reactions require combining past information with present information to make motor responses appropriate to internal and external needs. For example does the gastrocnemius contract before forward-reaching activities? Does the client step over objects, shape the hand for picking up objects? Almost all motor functions have an anticipatory component. Counterforces to our movements that must be anticipated are almost always present. The sensory systems modify performance at this level of functioning. Component evaluation of visual, vestibular, and mechanoreceptive systems may lead to understanding deficits at this level.

4. *Does the client use feedback correctly?* Feedback is used to modify and fine tune responses. Is activity corrected to meet changing environmental conditions? When not successful at task performance, does the client use this information to modify subsequent responses? Is the modification appropriate, or does it result in poorer performance?

5. *Does the client show variability of performance?* The plastic nervous system can adapt and change its motor output to meet different requirements.

VanSant[105] showed that children and adults vary the way they stand from supine, even under the same environmental conditions. She states that, indeed, the most striking observation in normal individuals is this variability of performance. The lack of variability has been suggested by many[89] as a sign of system damage. When assessing the head-injured client, look for variability of performance in basic motor acts. Can the client accomplish the same task in several ways? Can the client adapt to different task demands?

As the complex task is being performed, keep in mind that the extent of deficit is important. To what extent is the observed motor behavior involved? Is the behavior totally absent? Is it deficient, or are there signs of substitution of function or adaptation? Spasticity, cocontraction, and reversed sequences might be CNS efforts to substitute for lost functions.

Let's use walking as an example of the evaluation process

thus far. The activity of walking requires three complex elements: postural control, balance, and extensor strength.[102] Are the basic components to achieve each complex task adequate in the client? The client needs enough strength to hold the weight of the body against gravity, plus adequate ROM to achieve an upright position. Speed of motion and reaction times for initiation of motion are important.

In complex task analysis, postural control requires the client to be able to support the body in an upright position from the head down. Is there coordination between body segments? Balance uses basic synergies to control sway. Is the client using balance synergies with a temporal sequence of distal to proximal contraction in the lower extremities during small perturbations? Or is the client cocontracting, indicating a temporal or spatial sequencing problem in the synergy? Does the client use only the appropriate muscles in balance responses (spatial sequence)? Does he or she appropriately use a hip or knee flexion response to larger perturbations (adaptability of response)? Is there efficient movement in the swing leg? Does it move in a straight line and is foot placement on the floor appropriate (coordinated movement)? If not, does closing the eyes change the character of the movement? If it does, the client may be dominated by the visual system and may be having difficulty using mechanoreceptor synergies for movement and may be more visually dominated. Is interlimb timing good? Does the client step over a small object? If not, was it because the client misjudged the height of the object (visual anticipatory responses) or misjudged the distance to move the leg (modification of the locomotion synergy at the amplitude level)? Or is movement too disorganized to clear the object (problem with control of the degree of freedom, timing, or perhaps a lack of basic locomotor synergy)?

TREATMENT

Because the therapist can identify a deficit during the evaluation does not mean the deficit can be fixed. Based on assessment, two levels of treatment are likely to be ongoing. At the impairment level, basic components of performance that are faulty and are contributing to lack of motor performance can be addressed. Loss of complex movements and synergies also will be part of the rehabilitation targets. At the disability level, substitutions such as bracing, wheelchairs, functional electrical stimulation, ambulation devices and environmental changes such as ramps, chairs, bath benches, and reachers provide immediate change and improve the disability rating.

Using the ICIDH model of impairment, disability, and handicap, the therapist determines whether improvement is possible at the level of impairment and addresses the specific impairments. For example in the weak, contracted client who is unable to roll over, strengthening and stretching may be done. In the client with a permanent contracture or paralysis, a cloth loop may be provided to allow turning over by pulling with the arm.

Disability: not able to walk	
Impairment: P+ lower extremity extensor strength	
Can improve	Use weights, resistive exercises, anti-gravity work, etc.
Cannot improve (significantly)	Address at disability level; use wheelchair, cane, walker, bracing, etc.
Impairment: Disrupted sequence of muscle contraction	
Can improve	Use exercises to sequence muscles distally to proximally; use EMG feedback, etc.
Cannot improve	Use bracing, electrical stimulation for bracing, wheelchair

An example of the ICIDH treatment model for walking is presented in the box above.

Whether head-injured clients can relearn motor skills in the normal manner is controversial, evidence to direct us to better approaches is lacking. One difference between normal persons learning motor skills and head-injured clients relearning motor skills may be that basic components of movement such as strength and ROM may contribute significantly to loss of the motor function in head-injured clients and impede their ability to relearn functional skills.

The ability to "fix" an impairment does not depend solely on the therapist's skills, but includes inherent properties within the client such as the amount of physical damage, cognition, and motivation. Just as critical are external constraints, for example, the availability of treatment devices such as EMG for biofeedback, stimulation devices, pools, and other equipment, travel to and from treatment, availability of qualified providers of care, as well as financial constraints on treatment.

Component level treatment of impairment

At the component level are numerous and well-known approaches to treatment. A quick review of some of the current basis of component treatment and more nontraditional approaches may be useful.

Strength. Muscle tension is increased by increasing both the number of motor units firing (spatial summation) and the rate at which they are fired (temporal summation). Improvements in strength are usually speed specific, so use of resistance at different speeds is critical. Body position in space may also be related to differences in force production. Present thought is that the brain uses different spatial maps for movement; therefore, use of the extremities and trunk in multiple positions is important to address all different types of patterns of muscle activation. Production and practice of eccentric contractions are important in controlling speeds of movement and achieving accuracy of movement, especially in gait and upper extremity reaching tasks. Morphological constraints such as weight, height, limb length, sex, and age also should be considered.

Flexibility. Flexibility can be addressed with traditional orthopedic techniques, including joint mobilization, stretching, and dynamic splinting. Additionally, electrical stimulation[6] is extremely effective in improving flexibility, especially in dorsiflexion. For example, a small spot electrode placed over the peroneal nerve at the fibular head and a 2-inch square electrode medial to the lateral hamstring about 2 to 3 inches above the knee works well. Using this technique 10 to 20 minutes a day is usually adequate (Fig. 14-5). Wrist flexor tightness has been treated in the same manner with good results.

Speed of movement. Speed of movement may be trained with isokinetic equipment, manually during resistive exercises, or with computerized equipment such as force platforms. Varying speed is important with activities. Knowledge of results is imperative for progress.

Reaction time. Reaction time training also can be done on force platforms. In a pilot study by South Valley Rehabilitation in Englewood, Colorado, exercise performed while standing on foam pads (10 inches thick of medium density (Fig. 14-6) improved reaction time in a group of eight clients with neurological deficits. Work on compliant surfaces may require earlier corrections to avoid falling.

Endurance. Use of repetitions, increasing duration, intensity, and type of movement training can improve endurance. Upper extremity use can enhance cardiovascular conditioning in clients who are unable to walk or ride bicycles.

Tone. Problems in spatial and temporal sequencing seem better addressed with multiple channel surface EMG (Fig. 14-7). The client can see both the level of muscle recruitment and the sequence in which the muscles function if dual channels are used (see Fig. 14-3). Cocontraction can be decreased during gait or reaching using EMG biofeedback. Activation of muscles omitted in the gait or reaching patterns can be worked on. In clients unable to use EMG biofeedback information to make changes, functional electrical stimulation may achieve some of the goals (see Fig. 14-5). For example, gait training using an electrical stimu-

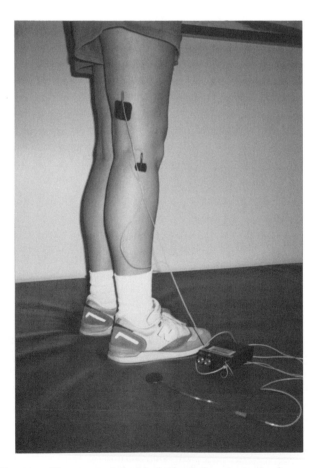

Fig. 14-5. Placement of electrical stimulation electrodes for peroneal nerve to attain dorsiflexion for stretching a tight gastrocnemius or for electrical bracing when used with a heel switch.

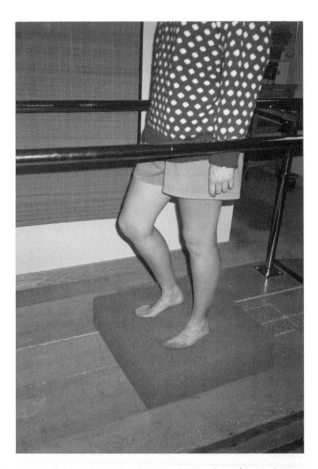

Fig. 14-6. Foam block to improve speed of motion and reaction time.

lator on the dorsiflexors and/or plantar flexors can achieve more normal activation patterns of the foot while providing some internal feedback information about sequencing. A heel switch and unit with separate channel controls and ramp adjustment is necessary. Using electrical stimulation on the gastrocnemius and hamstrings, with a slight delay of hamstring activation, has been effective. The second channel current can be ramped slightly to delay its onset for hamstring contraction. The goal is to slowly remove the "artificial" assistance over time.

Vestibular.   Basic research has indicated good response to treatment, especially for peripheral vestibular dysfunction.[63] Clients with sensory mismatches such as clients with vestibular dysfunction, may require work during which they have enhanced input from the two normally functioning systems to adapt or retrain the faulty vestibular system. For example, the client who is dizzy when moving the head may need increased mechanoreceptive input to provide information of the specific body motion that is occurring. The client can perform head motion in supine or sitting with feet and arms well supported (proprioceptive and tactile input) and eyes open. Progress in treatment

occurs by decreasing the additional input as symptoms decrease so that the client is finally in standing position and increasing the amount of movement. Visual cues can be altered by adding movement in the peripheral visual area (movement in the visual surround). This causes the visual system to perceive body motion when there is none and forces the use of the mechanoreceptive and vestibular systems to determine the real motion. Work on visual and vestibular enhancement is often done on balance boards (Fig. 14-8). Wearing bicycle glasses or taping the medial aspects of glasses can reduce peripheral visual input, enhancing vestibular and mechanoreceptive input in clients with dizziness caused by visual movement or visual-vestibular conflicts. In clients whose vestibular systems no longer function, enhancing visual and proprioceptive information is critical.

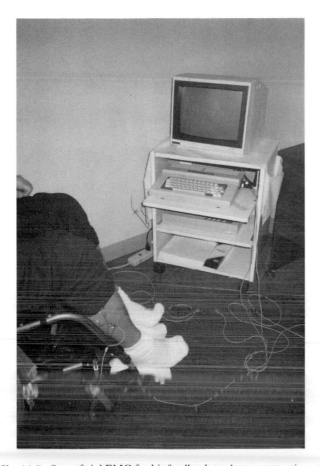

Fig. 14-7. Superficial EMG for biofeedback to shape contraction at onset and offset.

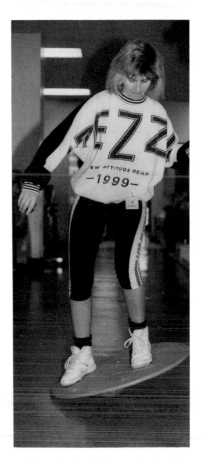

Fig. 14-8. Providing the appropriate sensory input is critical to stimulating the correct movement synergy or balance response. Although treatment of mechanoreceptive balance problems requires using flat, firm surfaces, visual and vestibular balance problems are best treated on irregular, compliant, or moving surfaces, such as the multidimensional balance disk shown. The client should not be permitted to hold onto the therapist or to assistive devices because use of the arms changes the balance responses.

Complex level treatment of impairment

Synergies. In clients who have available component function, establishing basic synergies should be based on whole task and natural subtask work. As stated earlier, subtasks of skills improve performance as Newell[74] reported. Identifying natural subtasks is difficult. Winstein[110] suggests that "natural breaks in the resultant velocity profile of a multisegment movement may signify the end of one subunit and may identify natural subtasks of a movement."

The variability shown in the task performance by normal subjects also may help elucidate subtasks. Assessment of a task, as done by VanSant[105] in her supine to stand studies, may provide a model to identify subtasks. In VanSant's study, the upper extremity patterns varied in six ways: push and reach to bilateral push, asymmetrical push, symmetrical push, symmetrical reach, asymmetrical push with thigh push, push and reach to bilateral push with thigh push. The head and trunk movement patterns varied in five ways: full rotation abdomen down, full rotation abdomen up, partial rotation, etc., and the lower extremity patterns varied in five ways: kneel, jump to squat, half kneel, asymmetrical squat, symmetrical squat. An exercise program to teach a client to get up from supine might work on upper extremity patterns as a subtask, trunk patterns as a subtask, lower extremity patterns as a subtask, and then on the whole task. Natural subtask work probably will be more effective if performed in the environment in which the pattern is normally used.

Ambulation training requires working in the upright position. This task might be broken down into more natural subtasks of gait, for example, working on half a gait cycle by moving the stance hip from the full backward to full forward position during opposite leg swing and ending with weight shift to the swing leg.

Goal-oriented tasks are mandatory in working with upper extremity losses (Fig. 14-9). Many clients with minimal function can pick up and carry boxes. Often grip, but not release, often is present. Again, EMG biofeedback is useful in helping develop release.[21] Functional release in clients with grip can be achieved by using an electrical stimulator on the finger extensors and using a hand switch. Some clients respond to a continuous low level stimulation of the finger extensors and can learn to release by relaxing their grip. The upper extremity also appears to select specific synergies for hand use in different positions. Clients often can open their hands in forward-reaching position but not with the elbow bent. Many clients with minimal functioning can be fitted with a utility cuff to hold writing instruments and write on boards or on tables while standing. This technique assists the shoulder in producing appropriate movement sequences for hand use but does not facilitate hand function. The treatment, however, does provide whole task practice even though some basic components are compensated through substitution. The therapist also might consider using a restraining device on the uninvolved side (with the client's permission) to force use of the involved extremity.

The importance of whole task practice at each treatment session is critical for two reasons. First, it is the only legitimate feedback of performance. For example, when teaching a throwing motion for basketball, if practice of the arm motion and ball throwing is without a target, feedback may indicate that ball release is adequate. The skill of shooting the ball into the basket is placing the ball at a specific point in space. The feedback that the ball hit the target is what determines the accuracy of the motion. Throwing the ball into the air is not the same task and uses different motor and sensory information than does basket shooting. Second, the forced use studies of Wolf and others[113] and Taub and others[101] demonstrate that motor skills improve better with functional use (whole task practice). When they restrained the unaffected arm in clients with CVA and monitored improvement in the involved arm, they found significant improvement in function in clients who had previous traditional arm rehabilitation.

Whole task practice in the head-injured client leads to the question of safety. How do I allow a client who cannot walk without falling to practice walking in light of research indicating that holding onto or using assistive devices changes the very skill I am trying to teach? If the deficit is

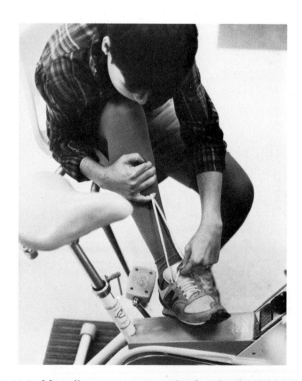

Fig. 14-9. Most clients seem to respond to functional activities such as dressing. Sitting, leaning forward (as to put on shoes) simulates the inverted position and actively involves the client in the treatment. This is also an example of integrating components of movement into a meaningful activity and using the same activity to further develop motor components.

in balance, then walking without assistance may be critical to progress. The best we may be able to do is to change the environment. Allowing a client to walk between parallel bars increases the likelihood he or she will either catch himself or herself or that the therapist can catch the client during falls. Walking on mats may allow for both environmental stimulus for soft, uneven surface work and for safer falling. Falling may be critical in relearning ambulation. Little research is available in this area, but in a study by Cintas,[19] children who pushed themselves more fell more (more problem solving experiences?) but gained more gait skills.

Modification of synergies. Reversing tasks in some clients allows them to develop increased control but requires modifying a task or synergy. For example, slowly lowering a spoon from the mouth may improve lifting the spoon to the mouth. Changing control by having clients stop and start at different points in an activity or changing directions also develops improved responses as well as flexibility. The client is asked to stop without taking another step, to turn right, or to step backward during ambulation. These techniques provide external influences on motor activities, helping to establish flexibility into responses. Adding objects to the environment and exposing the client to changing environments also develop adaptations to synergies.

Anticipatory responses. More complex activities such as postural stability require work at the anticipatory response

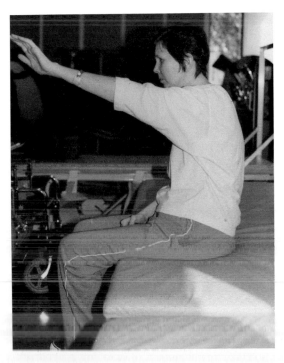

Fig. 14-10. Anticipatory trunk movements are essential to provide postural stability immediately before some extremity movements. For example, spinal extension and an anterior pelvic tilt usually accompany elevating an arm overhead. However, head-injured clients frequently lack adequate preparatory movements and typically maintain trunk flexion while attempting this activity.

level as well as the stability level. Moving the extremities (Fig. 14-10), adding weights to extremities during forward movement, and changing motion speeds are effective techniques. Pulling and pushing activities require an anticipatory set.

More dynamic movement may be practiced with ball activities. Using punching, catching, throwing and kicking activities with weight balls as well as regular balls will change the force and speed requirements at the same time requiring the client to adapt responses to the changing environmental demands. Treadmills help clients to adapt their motion to the environmental changes and make anticipatory responses.

Variability. VanSant[105] also stated that variability of performance in her study had "some to do with body size, strength and ROM." Since force production (strength) and ROM might be critical components in variability, work in water or with weight to change force production and ROM may also enhance different responses. It is important to build environmental constraints so that clients can perform functional movements in alternative ways.

Learning, practice and feedback. According to Winstein,[111] "KR (knowledge of results) research presently suggests a need to reexamine treatment approaches that advocate performance accuracy, strong guidance (either manual, tactile, or verbal), frequent and continuous feedback, and avoidance of errors or 'abnormal' movements." The KR research findings are consistent with the dynamic systems model that requires the client to be actively involved in problem solving through trial and error and adapting to new environmental situations. The higher level client needs help to solve his or her own motor problems and thus less physical support but expanded environmental experiences.

Conversely, the client with minimal motor function or the client who is in an early recovery state may require a great deal of external help with basic components of movement before learning how to access or develop basic synergies and skill. Assisting movement is appropriate for the level of this client's functioning.

Because feedback is so critical to learning and improving motor performance, especially at the higher levels of functioning, the method of treating clients by assisting motion comes into question. What happens when the therapist holds on to a client and guides him or her through more normal movement? The client is able to experience what normal motion feels like. However, normal movement is unique in that it will change depending on the context in which it is performed and the task constraints. The client being assisted in ambulation will not be making balance responses when falling if the therapist is providing balance support. The same problems may be inherent in using assistive devices such as canes and walkers. For example Horak[48] showed that using a cane for balance disrupts the normal distal to proximal sequence in the lower extremities.

and much of the balance responses are transferred to the arm, shoulders, and trunk. One might suspect the same to be true of many externally guided motions. The therapist must provide the client with opportunities to practice all parts of the complex motor tasks, or the task requirements are not the same. Practice needs to be task specific, but flexibility of response can be built in by changing environmental and task constraints.

Summary of treatment concepts

In general lower level functioning clients (those with losses of basic synergies, component impairments, or cognitive changes) need more hands-on help from the therapist trying to develop a basic motor program. Treatment may need to focus at the component level, establishing strength, flexibility, timing, and sequencing of movements. In higher level clients who are able to accomplish complex level work, if the client cannot manage multiple tasks, such as balance and anticipatory reactions, the therapist may choose to work in subtasks. For example, body positioning and stabilization may be critical for developing adequate head stabilization and mobility in sitting. Additional requirements of balance can be added later. When head control is emerging, it may be appropriate to work on anticipatory reactions by requiring the client to move the head and not fall over. Visual control of head motion can be used. Whenever possible it is important to add whole task practice of sitting unsupported.

Much higher level clients benefit from high level functional activities. Square dancing, line dancing, karate, Tai Chi, handball, and other sports often promote additional progress in balance, sequencing, and speed of movement. The clever therapist will tease out those components of these activities that best address the deficits in the client and structure fun activities that provide specific training for the deficits in balance, gait, upper extremity use, etc.

Don't throw out the baby with the bath water. While present research does not support the hierarchical theories on which previous treatments were based, specific treatment techniques themselves often produced good results. Using the treatment techniques in light of systems theory application may result in better outcomes. We can lose the rigid sequencing of treatment and keep the techniques that work. For example, practicing sitting to stand could be expanded to include the weight shift forward in preparation for standing. This activity appears to be one of the natural subtasks of coming to standing from lying down on a bed.

SUMMARY

The following 12 concepts summarize the theory, research, and treatment concepts presented in this chapter.

1. Physical therapy treatment is based on the nervous system's ability to learn through environmental influences.

2. As a starting point the disability should be evaluated.
3. The impairments that are the major contributors to the disability must be identified.
4. Once components of movement are in place, the use of synergies should be stressed through repetition of functional activities.
5. Treatment should be performed with the goal of the movement incorporated into the treatment.
6. Practice is necessary in multiple environments.
7. The client should be allowed to problem solve.
8. Assistance by the therapist should be kept to a minimum; variability in performance is normal.
9. EMG biofeedback, functional electrical stimulation, and isokinetic methods, as well as kinamatics, should be used to modify responses that appear more resistant.
10. Situations that cause changes in responses should be identified.
11. Feedback should be provided more randomly and summarized when the client falls outside a specified margin.
12. Substitution devices, assistive devices, and environmental changes should be provided for those clients who will not recover from disability impairments.

Remember, the therapist's uniqueness lies in the ability to do assessment and effective treatment, not measurement.

Quality of life

A life has been saved. The job of the rehabilitation team is to help improve the quality of that life. But what is quality of life? Family members knew the client before injury. The "rehabilitated" client may be dramatically different from their expectation. The rehabilitation team members, who can contrast the client's progress only since injury, may be quite pleased. Is quality measured by past performance, past potential, present performance, or future potential? Clients themselves may or may not have insight into past, present, or future performance and potential. What are the standards by which quality of life is measured? Is it income, reduction of dependency, contribution to society, or social interaction? Each of these indicators has been used as a standard. Ultimately, the determination of successful rehabilitation relies on the answer to these questions. Jennett and Teasdale[55] suggest six aspects of living: ADL, mobility and life organization, social relationships, work or leisure activities, present satisfaction, and future prospects. Most of these factors, while helpful, cannot be quantitatively measured, and they do not entirely answer the question of quality of life. However one estimates the quality of life, those who have chosen to help rehabilitate clients with head injury continue to pursue an ideal of quality for each life that has been saved and may, by doing so, enhance the quality of their own.

CASE 1 ▼ Mrs. E. K.

Mrs. E.K. is a 60-year-old woman who sustained a head injury in a fall. Injury in the cerebellum and midbrain resulted in left-sided body involvement. Mrs. E.K. walks with circumduction during swing phase on the left side with minimal knee bend and slowed dorsiflexion. The left arm is held tightly against her chest with the elbow in flexion and the hand in full supination. Client goals included being able to sew again and to square dance with her club.

Evaluation:
I. Disabilities
  1. Unsafe walking with frequent falls
    A. Impairments—component
      1. Strength F+ left hip extensor, hamstring and gastrocnemius; otherwise WNL in lower extremities.
      2. Flexibility—left rectus femoris tight at 100 degrees in prone.
      3. Tone—Ashworth level 3 left quad.
      4. Reaction time to weight shift delayed in left leg.
      5. Speed of motion slowed in left knee extension and flexion and left foot dorsiflexion.
    B. Impairments—complex
      1. Innate synergies are poor in trunk. There is no trunk rotation during walking and a proximal to distal balance responses during small perturbations (EMG). Visual-vestibular control of balance was poor, cannot stand on 12-inch thick foam pad without balance loss, cannot maintain narrow base stance with eyes closed.
      2. Anticipatory responses are poor on soft and irregular terrain.
      3. Feedback from lower extremity propioceptors is generally ignored in balance and gait.
Assessment: Poor walking and balance secondary to decreased use of proprioceptive information, weakness in the hip extensors, and increased tone in the quadriceps.
  2. Poor reaching and manipulation skills in the left upper extremity
    A. Impairments—component
      1. Tone—cocontraction of anterior and posterior deltoid; biceps and triceps in forward reaching; tremor of high frequency in the scapular stabilizers, especially the external rotators at rest and with movement; there is slower frequency tremors of larger amplitude in the wrist flexors and extensors during voluntary motion.
    B. Impairments—complex
      1. Modification of synergies is poor for upper extremity reaching. Amplitudes of movement are far too large for tasks. During walking, if the left arm is placed at the left side it flails wildly, knocking Mrs. E.K. off balance.

Assessment: Upper extremity is not being used functionally due to tremor and large amplitude of motion coming mainly from the scapular and shoulder muscles during activities. The arm is held in cocontraction during walking and other activities to decrease the instability in balance caused by large movements.
II. Handicap—decreased social interaction with friends

Mrs. E.K. lived 70 miles from the treatment clinic. Most of her treatment consisted of a home program. She was seen in the clinic once every 3 weeks for 3 months, then once a month for a year.

The initial home program focused on the basic impairments of reducing quadriceps tightness and increasing hip extensor and gastrocnemius strength in the lower extremity. To reestablish some control of amplitude of motion in the left arm, gross movement activities using the hand with the elbow stabilized and a wrist splint were initiated for the left upper extremity and included drawing large circles with a pen in a fisted hand and pulling yarn through some large holes. She also used her left elbow to stabilize paper while writing. Strength and flexibility improved to within normal limits.

The remaining program focused on hand-guided movement activities such as sewing with yarn on a large (3/8-inch squares) mat, writing, combing hair, molding clay, playing the organ, etc. These activities were first performed with the elbow stabilized and a wrist splint, then the elbow not stabilized, and finally without the wrist splint.

Lower extremity work included trying to improve the use of proprioceptive function. Standing exercises with the eyes intermittently closed and open and glasses that had vasoline on them were used to decrease visual inputs. Quickness of motion was promoted through rapid walking while the client's husband told her to stop abruptly and the client tried not to take a second step after the command. Speed of dorsiflexion was facilitated through use of a rocker board (without holding on), jumping on foam, and walking with a longer step on the right.

As the amplitude of arm motion decreased with use, Mrs. E.K. was able to walk with her hands clasped behind her back and worked on trunk rotation coordinated with gait. When this was accomplished, she was able to allow her arm to hang freely at her side and had a natural trunk rotation in walking. A videotape with beginning line dancing was used at home for higher level balance exercises and for enjoyment.

At discharge, Mrs. E.K. had good synergies and improved pattern of motion in the left lower extremity. An articulated ankle-foot orthosis was used for long walks or when she was very fatigued. She was able to sew and use the left arm for most activities, although a much smaller tremor persisted with volitional movement.

CASE 2 ▼ Severely Involved Client

P.H., a 21-year-old woman was in an auto accident and sustained a severe head injury and fractures of the left scapula, left radius, right ankle (fused), and jaw. She developed heterotrophic ossification in the right elbow. P.H. was in a coma for 1 month and a stupor for 2 more months.

Expressive language was minimal with severe aphasia. The few words said were dysarthric. P.H. appeared to understand well, following directions and nodding appropriately to questions.

Behavior was immature. For example, she continuously hugged and kissed her boyfriend when he was in the room. P.H. was easily frustrated by difficult tasks. At these times she became extremely agitated and scratched herself to the point of bleeding.

Mobility was by wheelchair. P.H. was independent in transfers. She could roll and come to sit independently, but needed moderate assist to kneel and come to stand and maximal assist to walk.

Evaluation:
I. Disabilities
  1. Unable to do self-care; personal grooming hygiene; or dress
    A. Impairments—components
      1. Strength—right arm fairly normal strength; left arm—not able to actively abduct shoulder but able to actively hold if placed at 90 degrees; external rotation and flexion—fair; active elbow flexion and extension through available range; wrist extension through half range and flexion through full range; gross and fine finger control present. Head was held in extreme forward position and flexed; normal head position could be maintained only 2 to 3 seconds. Trunk was in flexed position and normal extension also held no longer than 2 to 3 seconds.
      2. Flexibility—left shoulder limited to 120-degrees flexion and abduction; 45-degrees external rotation; left forearm supination +10 degrees; right elbow 90-degrees flexion; −20-degrees extension.
      3. Tone—cervical hypotonia; left biceps, triceps, wrist flexor and finger flexors are 3 (Ashworth scale). The tone in the left arm was of a cocontraction nature at the elbow; there was poor spatial sequencing throughout the limb.
      4. Speed of movement was extremely delayed throughout the left upper extremity; normal in the right.
      5. Reaction time was decreased in all left arm movements, normal right (using a touch plate).
      6. Endurance—cervical and trunk extensors and the left scapular muscles had poor muscular endurance with decreasing active range after three to five contractions. Cardiovascular fitness was poor, P.H.'s heart rate was 135 beats/minute after mild exercise of 5 minutes.

      7. Sensory—light touch intact in both upper extremities, proprioception within normal limits both arms except for the left hand where movement was perceived correctly but direction was not consistent. Identified 4 of 10 objects placed in the hand. The visual system showed lateral deviation to the left in the left eye and a dilated left pupil. Visual tracking was poor; P.H. stopped tracking at mid-line going toward the left. She did not use saccadic motion when trying to read and had intermittent diplopia.
        Vestibular function appeared intact except for possible abnormality in perception of vertical (this did not appear as a visual problem as eyes closed did not change off vertical position).
    B. Impairments—complex
      1. Innate synergies appear intact except for in the cervical area where the head is not held upright to maintain the eyes level.
      2. Modification of synergies is poor in the left arm where movement patterns were gross and poorly refined, and interlimb coordination was poor.
      3. Anticipatory responses were present in the trunk in sitting and reaching forward; they were not present during grasp of objects; hand size and grip were not matched to objects being picked up.
      4. Variability of performance—P.H. was able to reach and grasp as well as bend in many different ways with the right arm but had mainly an adducted, internal rotation pattern with elbow flexed on the left.

Assessment: Poor motor manipulation and prehension synergies in the left upper extremity resulted in nonuse of the left hand. Precision in grip was impaired by poor feedback from the fingers. Contributing to the lack of use of the hand was poor strength in the scapular stabilizers secondary to the scapular fracture and injury. Lack of adequate elbow ROM secondary to heterotrophic ossification (H.O.) in the right elbow prevented grooming, personal hygiene such as teeth brushing, and applying makeup with the right arm, which had fairly normal function. Prolonged bed rest had resulted in poor trunk postural muscle endurance and a forward lean when standing. Visual and synergy dysfunctions result in flexed forward head position. Perception of vertical was abnormal perhaps due to vestibular-cerebellar dysfunction.

  2. Unable to walk
    A. Impairments—components
      1. Strength—fair to good strength left leg except poor in the gastrocnemius; good strength right leg except fair in the right gastrocnemius and trunk extensors were fair.
      2. Flexibility—trunk flexion is limited to about half normal lumbar flexion by tight back

CASE 2   Severely Involved Client—cont'd

extensors, gastrocnemius are tight at neutral on the left. Fusion right ankle at +5 degrees of dorsiflexion.

3. Tone—Ashworth 3 in the left quad and gastrocnemius.
4. Reaction time in gastrocnemius and dorsiflexors were significantly delayed (force platform).
5. Speed of left dorsiflexion was poor in swing phase dorsiflexion.
6. Endurance poor in trunk and lower extremity muscles; there was a reduction in amount of resistance tolerated after approximately 10 repetitions using isolated muscle testing.
7. Sensory systems—lower extremity light touch and proprioception intact in the right lower extremity; decreased proprioception (needs larger movement for accuracy) in the left lower extremity. Vision, vestibular systems were addressed under the disability #1.

B. Impairments—complex
1. Innate synergies—appear intact in the right lower extremity, but ankle strategy is absent in the left.
2. Modification of synergies—right lower extremity shows a poor ability to modify walking patterns resulting in large amplitude movements at the hip and knee during walking. The left lower extremity shows modification of the hip strategy for different surfaces. Interlimb coordination in the lower extremities is poor.
3. Anticipatory responses were generally absent in the left lower extremity and trunk during standing when right leg lifting. Anticipatory reactions did occur in the right leg when lifting the left leg forward.
4. Use of feedback was present when tactile or auditory. Poor use of visual feedback in modification of walking or standing in both lower extremities.
5. There appeared to be poor ability to vary the movement pattern in the right lower extremity during balance and walking (in the parallel bars). Variability of response was present depending on verbal cues but not spontaneously present in response to environmental cues. Pattern was fairly fixed and of a steppage-type gait.

Assessment: P.H. appears unable to walk without moderate to maximum assistance due to lack of higher level balance synergies and lack of anticipatory responses to movements of her center of gravity. Poor gastrocnemius strength also probably contributed to lack of ankle strategy. Poor quality of movement in the right leg was secondary to inability to modify underlying synergies.

3. Postural disability—unable to hold head up, stands with weight on right leg leaning about 15 degrees to the right

A. Impairments—components
1. Strength is fair in the extensors of the mid and lower trunk muscles, poor in cervical extensors.
2. Flexibility—forward flexion is limited to 50% of normal by tightness in the lumbar extensors.
3. The left lumbar extensors have above normal tone and often elicited an extensor spasm during forward bending.
4. Sensory—right tilt off vertical 15 degrees.

B. Impairments—complex
1. Balance synergies show proximal to distal firing beginning in the trunk flexors and extensors during small perturbations in normal standing. Occluding vision during normal standing does not change balance and only slightly degrades balance when on foam.
2. Modification of upright balance is poor with the visual and/or proprioceptive feedback.

Assessment: P.H. has problems perceiving the vertical position in sitting and standing secondary to visual and proprioceptive losses. She has poor muscular endurance secondary to prolonged bed rest, slowed movement, and decreased activity level over months. Walking is with hip strategy of knees and hips bent due to poor production of torque on floor by the gastrocnemius muscles and delayed responses to movement. Anticipatory responses for ambulation are minimal and secondary to lack of accurate visual input.

II. Handicap: Immature behavior resulting in loss of friends and inability to hold a job.

Long-term goals were independent ambulation without an assistive device for household and with a cane for community. Independence in all self-care and ADLs.

Treatment: Initial goals included improving those impairments in the basic component level that did not allow higher levels of functioning. These were neck and trunk strength and endurance, left scapular and shoulder muscle strength and flexibility, improving gastrocnemius strength and flexibility; visual skills particularly in gaze stabilization and tracking; awareness of vertical. P.H.'s attention span was slightly shorter than normal.

Functional electrical stimulation (FES) to the posterior cervical muscles, intermittent use of a supportive collar to take the extensor muscles off stretch, and eye fixation exercises to focus on a single point were used to encourage visual control of head position.

Complex neck activities to encourage basic synergy use and modification included seated activities in which P.H. wore a "hat" with a flat top from which she tried to prevent an object from falling off (first flat stable objects and later more rounded objects). This exercise was performed first on a firm, flat seated surface and progressed to sitting on an exercise ball. The ball promoted automatic neck muscle synergies in which the body moves and the head is kept upright and still.

Traditional basic left upper extremity strengthening

Continued.

CASE 2 ▼ Severely Involved Client—cont'd

exercises included use of Theraband. Functional activities that required scapular use such as emptying the dishwasher with the left hand were assigned homework.

Electrical stimulation twice a day for 15 minutes to the right triceps gained 20 degrees of extension and 100 degrees of flexion. Active extension exercises were also given. In the clinic, P.H. worked on picking up and manipulating objects of different sizes and shapes, throwing balls at targets, two-handed carrying, etc.

P.H. enjoyed cooking, so tasks were given that used right elbow extension, such as rolling cookie dough. Exercises such as washing the dishes with hands in soapy water for proprioceptive feedback and enhancement of feedback through the finger tips for grip were used. Setting the table with the left hand helped establish better functional use (plastic dishes).

Complex functions in manipulation with the left arm were facilitated by doing two-hand activities. P.H. used large mats to hook a small rug, and she had a list, as mentioned earlier, of chores to do that required lifting and manipulating with both hands. When able, she began trying two-hand typing. One of the most motivating activities was applying makeup and contact lenses.

Visual treatment used exercises that required visual fixation at different points in space and at different distances using letters and objects, with the goal of seeing only one image. These exercises advanced to include moving objects and head moving with a fixed object, and progressed to both the object and head moving while maintaining a single image. Finally, full body movement with eyes fixed on moving object was accomplished.

Improved use of vestibulocerebellar function was promoted through use of foam, standing on narrow beam, and walking on ramps and grass, activities that require the use of the visual and vestibular systems.

Spasticity was addressed with exercises to promote less cocontraction and distal to proximal sequencing in both the left leg and left arm. EMG biofeedback with a two-channel setup on the triceps/biceps and wrist flexors/wrist extensors was used to teach decreased cocontraction during activities such as reaching and lifting. This was carried over to the home program.

P.H. used a Nordic Track for general cardiovascular fitness work. The gliding motion with toe loops allowed her to keep her feet near the ground when moving forward and the arm work encouraged free movement of the trunk in rotation.

In the lower extremity program gastrocnemius strengthening concentrated on standing exercises such as heel lifts and toe walking along. Speed of motion exercises were performed with left foot back and pulling forward quickly.

Exercises were not popular. The goal P.H. had when first starting therapy was "to dance with my boyfriend." To encourage functional use of postural and balance synergies, dancing was used. She started first with slow dancing with her boyfriend. Gradually, she was able to dance to faster music without being held, by using trunk and arm motion and a side-stepping motion. Finally, forward-backward movements and turning and bending were added. Additionally, P.H. agreed to model in the head-injury fashion show, which provided motivation to walk independently.

Balance exercises such as swaying around the ankles, getting from kneeling to standing, and working on a force platform for attaining and feeling vertical were successful. A videocamera was used from behind to get P.H. to lift her foot so that "she could see her sole on the left foot" and resulted in increased left knee flexion in her gait pattern. Walking was started with a full step program on each foot. Goals were to keep the light at her waist from moving more than 2 inches side to side. This was also facilitated by moving the parallel bars extremely close together and asking P.H. not to touch the bars with either hip as she practiced stepping.

Trunk and anticipatory responses early on used a Gymnastik ball as well as weighted and reaching exercise, ball kicking to a goal, ball catching, and ball throwing to a target. P.H. practiced walking over and around various objects.

A behavioral modification program was established so that P.H. was given control to stop activities that were too stressful for her; and she participated in a volunteer program on a farm feeding and watering animals two to three times a week on a fixed schedule to establish personal responsibility and provide a positive learning environment.

P.H. reached the goals of independent household ambulation and community ambulation with a cane. She had normal posture and good assistive and gross independent use of the left hand and arm. Tone in the left arm and left quadriceps were at a level 2 at discharge.

ACKNOWLEDGMENT

Thank you to Susan Smith, the previous author of this chapter, for much of the basic information on the fundamentals of head injuries.

REFERENCES

1. Astrand P: Astrand test, *Acta Physiol Scand* 49 (suppl 169).1960.
2. Bach-y-Rita P: Brain plasticity as a basis for therapeutic procedures. In Bach-y-Rita P, editor: *Recovery of function: theoretical considerations for brain injury rehabilitation,* Baltimore, 1980, University Park Press.
3. Bach-y-Rita P: Brain injury, *Wall Street Journal,* Oct. 12, 1993.
4. Badke MB and Duncan PW: Patterns of rapid motor response during postural adjustment when sitting in healthy subjects and hemiplegic patients, *Phys Ther* 63:13, 1983.
5. Baker LL and Parker K: Neuromuscular electrical stimulation for the head injured patient. *Phys Ther* 63:[12]1967-1974, 1983.
6. Benton L and others: *Functional electrical stimulation: a practical clinical guide,* Downey, Calif., 1981, Rancho Los Amigos Rehab. Engineering Center.
7. Berger MS and others: Outcome from severe head injury in children and adolescents, *J Neurosurg* 62:194, 1985.

8. Bernstein N: *Coordination and regulation of movements,* New York, 1967, Pergamon Press.

9. Berrol S: Evaluation and the persistent vegetative state, *Head Trauma Rehabil* 1:7, 1986.

10. Black P and others: Recovery of motor function after lesions in motor cortex of monkey. In Black P: *Outcome of severe damage to the central nervous system,* New York, 1975, Elsevier, pp. 65-83.

11. Bond MR: Assessment of psychosocial outcome of severe head injury, *Acta Neurochir* 34:57, 1976.

12. Bond MR: Outcome as a reflection of the interaction of the brain-injured and their families. Presented at the Sixth Annual Postgraduate Course on the Rehabilitation of the Brain-injured Adult. Williamsburg, Va., June 10, 1982.

13. Bourbonnais D and others: Abnormal spatial patterns of elbow activation in hemiparetic human subjects, *Brain* 112:85, 1989.

14. Brotherton J and others: Social skills training in the rehabilitation of patients with traumatic closed head injury, *Arch Phys Med Rehabil* 69:827, 1988.

15. Bruce RA: Exercise testing of patients with coronary artery disease, *Ann Clin Res* 3:323, 1971.

16. Carlssen CA and others: Factors affecting the clinical course of patients with severe head injuries. I. Influence of biological factors: II. Significance of posttraumatic coma, *J Neurosurg* 29:242, 1968.

17. Cartlidge NEF and Shaw DA: *Head injury,* London, 1981, WB Saunders.

18. Choi S and others: Chart or outcome predication in severe head injury, *J Neurosurg* 59:294, 1983.

19. Cintas H: The relationship of motor skill level and risk-taking during exploration in toddlers, *Pediatr Phys Ther* 165, 1992.

20. Colorado Head Injury Foundation, Inc. 1993. Brochure.

21. Cozean C and others: Biofeedback and functional electric stimulation in stroke rehabilitation, *Arch Phys Med Rehabil* 69:401, 1988.

22. Craik R: Abnormalities of motor behavior. In Lister M, editor: *Contemporary management of motor control problems,* Alexandria, Va., 1991, American Physical Therapy Association.

23. Devor M and others: Dorsal horn neurons that respond to stimulation of distant dorsal roots, *J Physiol* (London) 270:519, 1977.

24. Dietz V and Berger W: Interlimb coordination of posture in patients with spastic paresis: imperial functions of spinal reflexes, *Brain* 107:965, 1984.

25. Dietz V and others: Motor unit involvement in spastic paresis: relationship between leg muscle activation and histochemistry, *J Neurol Sci* 75:89, 1986.

26. Edstrom L and others: Correlation between recruitment order of motor units and muscle atrophy pattern in upper motorneurone lesion: significance of spasticity, *Experimentia* 29:560, 1973.

27. Eliason MR and Topp BW: Predictive validity of Rappaport's disability rating scale in subjects with acute brain dysfunction, *Phys Ther* 64:1357, 1984.

28. Evans CD: Assessment of disability after head injury, *Rheumatol Rehabil* 15:168, 1976.

29. Evans CD and others: Rehabilitation of the brain-damaged survivor, *Injury* 8:80, 1976.

30. Evarts EV: Role of motor cortex in voluntary movements in primates. In Brookhart JM and others, editors: *Handbook of physiology, the nervous system—motor control,* Bethesda, 1981, American Physiological Society.

31. Gennarelli TA and others: Influence of the type of intracranial lesion on the outcome from severe head injury, *J Neurosurg* 56:26, 1982.

32. Georgopolous AP: On reaching, *Annu Rev Neurosci* 9:147, 1986.

33. Gilchrist E and Wilkinson M: Some factors determining prognosis in young people with severe head injuries, *Arch Neurol* 36:355, 1979.

34. Gillingham FJ: The importance of rehabilitation, *Injury* 1:142, 1969.

35. Gilroy J and Meyer JS: *Medical neurology,* ed 3, New York, Macmillan.

36. Giuliani C: Theories of motor control. In Lister M, editor: *New concepts for physical therapy in contemporary management of motor control problems,* Va, 1991, American Physical Therapy Association.

37. Glenn MB: Update on pharmacology: pharmacology: antispasticity medications in the patient with traumatic brain injury. Part I, *J Head Trauma Rehabil* 3:87, 1988.

38. Glenn MB and Wrobewski B: Update on pharmacology: antispasticity medications in the patient with traumatic brain injury, *J Head Trauma Rehabil* 1:71, 1986.

39. Gogstad AC and Kjellman AM: Rehabilitation prognosis related to clinical and social factors in brain injured of different etiology, *Soc Sci Med* 10:283, 1976.

40. Golani I and Fentress JC: Early ontogency of face grooming in mice, *Dev Psychobiol* 18:529, 1985.

41. Gordon J: Anticipatory guidance from a motor control perspective. Presented at *Annual Sensorimotor Integration Symposium,* San Diego, July 10-12, 1992.

42. Greenberg R and others: Prognostic implications of early multimodality evoked potentials in severe head injury patients: a prospective study, *J Neurosurg* 55:227, 1981.

43. Groswasser Z and others: Closed cervical cranial trauma associated with involvement of the carotid and vertebral arteries, *Laryngoscope* 81:1381, 1971.

44. Gurdjian ES and others: Closed cervical cranial trauma associated with involvement of the carotid and vertebral arteries, *Laryngoscope* 81:1381, 1971.

45. Heiden JS and others: Severe head injury: clinical assessment and outcome, *Phys Ther* 63:1946, 1983.

46. Held R: Plasticity in sensory-motor systems, *Sci Am* 213:84, 1967.

47. Horak FB: Comparison of cerebellar and vestibular loss on scaling of postural responses. In Brandt T and others, editors: *Disorders of posture and gait,* New York, 1990, Georg Thieme Verlag.

48. Horak FB: Determinants of movement in central nervous system damage: implications for assessment and treatment of children and adults. Presented at Symposia, Denver, July 27-29, 1984.

49. Horak FB and others: The effects of movement velocity, mass displaced, and task certainty on associated postural adjustments made by normal and hemiplegic individuals, *J Neurol Neurosurg Psychiatry* 47:1020, 1984.

50. Horak FB and Shumway-Cook A: Vestibular rehabilitation, Unpublished paper, course notes, Dallas, November, 1992.

51. Hubel DH and Wiesel TN: The period of susceptibility to the physiological effects of unilateral eye closure in kittens, *J Physiol* 206:419, 1970.

52. Jennett B and Bond M: Assessment of outcome after severe brain damage: a practical scale, *Lancet* 1:480, 1975.

53. Jennett B and Plum F: Persistent vegetative state after brain damage: a syndrome in search of a name, *Lancet* 1:734, 1972.

54. Jennett B and Teasdale G: Aspects of coma after severe head injury, *Lancet* 1:878, 1977.

55. Jennett B and Teasdale G: *Management of head injuries,* Philadelphia, 1981, FA Davis.

56. Jennett B and others: Prognosis of patients with severe head injury, *Neurosurgery* 4:283, 1979.

57. Johansson RS and Westling G: Signals in tactile afferents from the fingers eliciting adaptive motor responses during precision grip, *Exp Brain Res* 66:141, 1987.

58. Johnson D and Almi CR: Age, brain damage and performance. In Finger S, editor: *Recovery from brain damage,* New York, 1978, Plenum Press.

59. Kelso JAS and Schoner G: Self-organization of coordinative movement patterns, *Hum Move Sci* 7:27, 1988.

60. Knutsson E and Martensson A: Dynamic motor capacity in spastic paresis and its relationship to prime motor dysfunction, spastic reflexes and antagonistic coactivation, *Scand J Rehabil Med* 12:93, 1980.

61. Kondraske GV: Measurement science concepts and computerized methodology in the assessment of human performance. In Munsat TL, editor: *Quantification of neurologic deficit,* Stoneham, Mass, 1989, Butterworth.

62. Kondraske GV and others: Human performance measurement: some perspectives, *IEEE Eng Med Biol Soc Mag* 7:11, 1988.

63. Konrad H and others: Rehabilitation therapy for patients with disequilibrium and balance disorders, *Otolaryngol Head Neck Surg* 107:107, 1992.

64. Lanksch W and others: Correlations between clinical symptoms and computer tomography findings in closed head injuries. In Frowein RA and others, editors: *Advances in neurosurgery* 5, Berlin, 1978, Springer-Verlag.

65. Mahoney FI and Barthel DW: Functional evaluation: the Barthel Index, *Md State Med J* 14:61, 1965.

66. Man AM and others: Adaptive and part-whole training in the acquisition of a complex perceptual-motor skill, *Acta Psychol* (Amsterdam) 71:179, 1989.

67. Marrubini MB: Classification of coma, *Intens Care Med* 10:217, 1984.

68. Martenicuk RG and others: Constraints on human arm movement trajectories, *Can J Psychol* 41:365, 1987.

69. Mehalis T and Farhat SM: Vertebral artery injury from chiropractic manipulation of the neck, *Surg Neurol* 2:125, 1974.

70. Mitchell DE and others: Recovery from the effects of monocular deprivation, *J Comp Neurol* 176:53, 1977.

71. Nashner LM: Organization and programming of motor activity during posture control, *Prog Brain Res* 50:177, 1979.

72. Nashner LM and others: Stance posture control in select groups of children with cerebral palsy: deficits in sensory organization and muscular coordination, *Exp Brain Res* 49:393, 1983.

73. National Head Injury Foundation, Annual Report, 1985-1986.

74. Newell KM: Knowledge of results and motor learning, *J Motor Behav* 4:235, 1974.

75. Newell KM and others: Whole-part training strategies for learning the response dynamics of microprocessor driven simulator, *Acta Psychol* (Amsterdam) 71:197, 1989.

76. Oldendorf WH: The quest for an image of brain: a brief historical and technical review of brain imaging techniques, *Neurology* 28:517, 1978.

77. Olney S and others: Mechanical energy patterns in gait of cerebral palsied children with hemiplegia, *Phys Ther* 67:1348, 1987.

78. Payton O and Kelley D: Electromyographic evidence of the acquisition of a motor skill: a pilot study, *Phys Ther* 52:3:261, 1987.

79. Plum F and Posner JB: *The diagnosis of stupor and coma,* ed 3, Philadelphia, 1980, FA Davis.

80. Rappaport M and others: Disability rating scale for severe head trauma: coma to community, *Arch Phys Med Rehabil* 63:118, 1982.

81. Roberts AH: Long-term prognosis of severe accidental head injury, *Proc R Soc Med* 69:137, 1976.

82. Rose SJ and Rothstein JM: Muscle mutability. I. General concepts and adaptations to altered patterns of use, *Phys Ther* 62:1773, 1982.

83. Rosenfalck A and Andreassen S: Impaired regulation and firing pattern of single motor units in patients with spasticity, *J Neurol Neurosurg Psychiatry* 43:907, 1980.

84. Rosin AJ: Very prolonged unresponsive state following brain injury. *Scand J Rehabil Med* 10:33, 1978.

85. Russell WR: Cerebral involvement in head injury: a study based on the examination of two hundred cases, *Brain* 55:549, 1932.

86. Sahrmann SA: Diagnosis by the physical therapist—a prerequisite for treatment: a special communication, *Phys Ther* 68:1703, 1988.

87. Sahrmann SA: Posture and muscle imbalance: faulty lumbar-pelvic alignment and associated musculoskeletal pain syndromes. In *Postgraduate advances in physical therapy: a comprehensive independent learning office study course,* Alexandria, VA, 1987, American Physical Therapy Association.

88. Sahrmann SA and Norton BJ: The relationship of voluntary movement to spasticity in the upper motor neuron syndrome, *Ann Neurol* 2:460, 1977.

89. Schmidt RA: A Schema theory of discrete motor learning, *Psychol Rev* 82:225, 1975.

90. Schmidt RA: *Motor control and learning: a behavioral emphasis,* Champaign, Ill, 1988, Human Kinetics Publishers.

91. Schmidt RA: Motor learning principles for physical therapy. In Lister M, editor: *Contemporary management of motor control problems,* Proceeding of the II Step Conference, Norman, OK, 1991, American Physical Therapy Association.

92. Schoner G and Kelso JAS: Dynamic pattern generation in behavioral and neural systems, *Science* 239:1513, 1988.

93. Shapiro DC and others: Evidence for generalized motor programs using gait patterns analysis, *J Motor Behav* 13:33, 1981.

94. Snoek J and others: Computerized tomography after recent severe head injury in patients without acute intracranial hematoma, *J Neurol Neurosurg Psychiatry* 42:215, 1979.

95. Spans F and Wilts G: Denervation due to lesions of the central nervous system, *J Neurol Sci* 57:291, 1982.

96. Stewart WA and others: A prognostic model for head injury, *Acta Neurochir* 45:199, 1979.

97. Stover SL and Zeiger HE: Head injury in children and teenagers: functional recovery correlated with the duration of coma, *Arch Phys Med Rehabil* 57:201, 1976.

98. Strich SJ: Lesions in the cerebral hemispheres after blunt head injury, *J Clin Pathol* 23 (suppl 4):154, 1970.

99. Tang A and Rymer WZ: Abnormal force-EMG relations in paretic limbs of hemiparetic human subjects, *J Neurol Neurosurg Psychiatry* 44:690, 1981.

100. Tardieu C and others: For how long must the soleus muscle be stretched daily to prevent contracture? *Dev Med Child Neurol* 30:3, 1988.

101. Taub E and others: Technique to improve chronic motor deficit after stroke, *Arch Phys Med Rehabil* 74:247, 1993.

102. Thelen E: Evolving and dissolving synergies in the development of leg coordination. In Wallace SA, editor: *Perspectives on the coordination of movement,* New York, 1991, Elsevier.

103. Tower SS: Pyramidal lesions in the monkey, *Brain* 63:36, 1940.

104. Van Den Berge JH and others: Interobserver agreement in assessment of ocular signs in coma, *J Neurol Neurosurg Psychiatry* 42:1163, 1979.

105. VanSant A: Rising from a supine position to erect stance: description of adult movement and a developmental hypothesis, *Phys Ther* 68:185, 1988.

106. Wade D: *Measurement in neurological rehabilitation,* New York, 1992, Oxford University Press.

107. Watkins MP and others: Isokinetic testing in patients with hemiparesis: a pilot study, *Phys Ther* 64:184, 1984.

108. Wiesel TN and Hubel DH: Comparison of the effects of unilateral and bilateral eye closure on cortical unit responses in kittens, *J Neurophysiol* 28:1029, 1965.

109. Wiesel TN and Hubel DH: Single-cell responses in striate cortex of kittens deprived of vision in one eye, *J Neurophysiol* 26:1003, 1963.

110. Winstein C: Designing practice for motor learning. In Lister M, editor: *Clinical implications in contemporary management of motor control problems,* Proceedings of the II STEP Conference, Alexandria, Va, 1991, American Physical Therapy Association.

111. Winstein C: Knowledge of results and motor learning, implications for physical therapy. In *Movement science, a monograph of the American Physical Therapy Association,* Alexandria, Va, 1991, The Association.

112. Winstein CJ and others: Standing balance training: effect on balance and locomotion in hemiparetic adults, *Arch Phys Med Rehabil* 70:755, 1989.

113. Wolf SL and others: Forced use of hemiplegic upper extremities to

reverse the effect of learned nonuse among stroke and head-injured patients, *Exp Neurol* 104.125, 1989.

114. World Health Organization: International classification of impairments, disabilities and handicaps, Geneva Switzerland, 1980, World Health Organization.

115. World Health Organization: The 3-step ergometer test, Geneva, Switzerland. In The junture fitness measurement guide untamontatee, 2SG-20502 Turkce 52, Ginland.

116. Young RR and Delwaide PJ: Drug therapy: spasticity part I, *N Engl J Med* 304:96, 1981.

117. Young RR and Delwaide PJ: Drug therapy: spasticity, part 2, *N Engl J Med* 304:96, 1981.

118. Zimmerman RA and others: Computed tomography of shearing injuries of the cerebral white matter, *Radiology* 127:393, 1978.

CHAPTER 15

Congenital Spinal Cord Injury

Jane W. Schneider, Kristin Krosschell, and Kathryn L. Gabriel

KEY TERMS

spina bifida occulta	hydrocephalus
spina bifida cystica	Chiari malformation
myelomeningocele (MM)	tethered spinal cord
myelodysplasia	standing A-frame
diastematomyelia	reciprocating gait orthosis
lipomeningocele	(RGO)
sacral agenesis	crouch-control AFO

LEARNING OBJECTIVES

After reading this chapter the student/therapist will:
1. Describe the various types of spina bifida.
2. Discuss the incidence and etiology of spina bifida.
3. Describe the clinical manifestations of myelomeningocele including neurological, orthopedic, and urologic sequelae.
4. Describe medical management in the newborn period and beyond.
5. Discuss physical therapy evaluations including manual muscle testing, range of motion, sensory testing, reflex testing, developmental/functional assessments, perceptual/cognitive evaluations.
6. List the major physical therapy goals and appropriate physical therapy management for each of the following stages: 1: before surgical closure of sac, 2: after surgery during hospitalization, 3: preambulatory, 4: toddler through preschool age, 5: primary school through adolescence.
7. Discuss psychological adjustment to congenital spinal cord injury.

A spinal cord injury is a complex disability. When a spinal cord lesion exists from birth, an additional complexity is added. This congenital condition predisposes that many areas of the central nervous system (CNS) may not develop or function adequately. In addition all areas of development (physical, cognitive, and psychosocial) that depend so heavily on central functioning will likely be impaired. The clinician therefore must be aware of the significant impact this neurological defect has not only on motor function, but also on a variety of related human capacities.

A developmental framework has been used to aid in understanding the sequential problems of the child with spina bifida. The developmental model, however, must always stay in line with the functional model for adult trauma, because the problems of the congenitally involved child grow quickly into the disabilities of the injured adult. With concentration on the present but with an eye to the future, appropriate management goals can be achieved.

AN OVERVIEW OF CONGENITAL SPINAL CORD INJURY

A congenital spinal cord lesion occurs in utero and is present at the time of birth. To understand how this malformation develops, one needs an appreciation of normal nervous system maturation.

The nervous system develops from a portion of embryonic ectoderm called the neural plate. During gestation, the neural plate develops folds that begin to close, forming the neural tube (Fig. 15-1). The neural tube differentiates into the CNS, which is composed of brain and spinal cord tissue.[92]

In the normal embryo, neural tube closure begins in the cervical region and proceeds cranially and caudally. Closure is generally complete by the twenty-sixth day.[92]

Types of spina bifida

In spina bifida there is a defect in the neural tube closure and the overlying posterior vertebral arches. The extent of the defect may result in one of two types of spina bifida—occulta or cystica.

Spina bifida occulta is characterized by a failure of one or more of the vertebral arches to meet and fuse in the third month of development. The spinal cord and meninges are unharmed and remain within the vertebral canal (Fig. 15-2, A). The bony defect is covered with skin that may be marked by a dimple, pigmentation, or patch of hair.[111] The common site for this defect is the lumbosacral area, and it is usually associated with no disturbance of neurological or musculoskeletal functioning.[83]

Spina bifida cystica results when the neural tube and overlying vertebral arches fail to close appropriately. There is a cystic protrusion of the meninges or of the spinal cord and meninges through the defective vertebral arches.

The milder form of spina bifida cystica, called meningocele, involves protrusion of the meninges and cerebrospinal fluid (CSF) only into the cystic sac (Fig. 15-2, D). The spinal cord remains within the vertebral canal, but it may exhibit abnormalities.[79] Clinical signs vary (according to spinal cord anomalies) or may not be apparent. This is a relatively uncommon form of spina bifida cystica.

A more severe form of spina bifida cystica, called myelocele or myelocystocele, is present when the central canal of the spinal cord is dilated producing a large skin-covered cyst. The neural tube appears to close normally but is distended from the cystic swelling. The CSF may ceaselessly expand the neural canal. Prompt medical attention is mandatory. This form of spina bifida is also rare.[45]

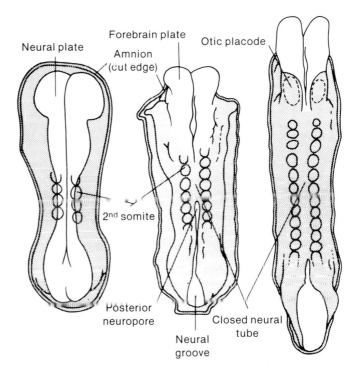

Fig. 15-1. Neural tube forming. (From Stark, GD: *Spina bifida problems and management,* London, 1977, Blackwell Scientific Publications Inc.)

The more common and severe form of the defect is known as **myelomeningocele (MM)** in which both spinal cord and meninges are contained in the cystic sac (Fig. 15-2, C). Within the sac, the spinal cord and associated neural tissue show extensive abnormalities. In incomplete closure of the neural tube (dysraphism), abnormal growth of the cord and a tortuous pathway of neural elements make normal transmission of nervous impulses abnormal. The result is a variable sensory and motor impairment at the level of the lesion and below.[111] In an open myelomeningocele, nerve roots and spinal cord may be exposed with dura and skin evident at the margin of the lesion.

Although spina bifida cystica can occur at any level of the spinal cord, meningoceles are most common in the thoracic and lumbosacral regions. Two thirds of open lesions involve the thoracolumbar junction.[111]

Because myelomeningocele occurs in 94% of the cases of spina bifida cystica and because these cases most often require rehabilitation, the terms *spina bifida*, **myelodysplasia,** and *myelomeningocele* are frequently used interchangeably.[79]

Other forms of spinal dysraphism include diastematomyelia, lipomeningocele and sacral agenesis. **Diastematomyelia** is present in 30% to 40% of patients with myelomeningocele and is secondary to partial or complete clefting of the spinal cord.[10] **Lipomeningocele,** another form of spina bifida cystica, is usually due to a vertebral defect associated with a superficial fatty mass (lipoma or fatty tumor) that

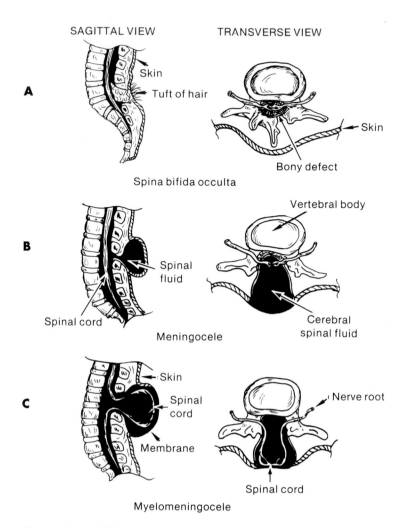

Fig. 15-2. Types of spina bifida. **A,** Spina bifida occulta. **B,** Meningocele. **C,** Myelomeningocele. (From McLone DG: *An introduction to spina bifida,* Chicago, 1980, Children's Memorial Hospital, Northwestern University.)

merges with the lower level of spinal cord. There is no associated hydrocephalus, and neurological deficit is generally minimal; however, problems with urinary control and motor control of the lower extremities may be noted.[98] Neurological tissue invasion may be secondary to a tethered spinal cord; therefore early lipoma resection is indicated not only for cosmesis but also to minimize neurological sequelae. Lumbosacral or **sacral agenesis** may occur and is due to an absence of the caudal part of the spine and sacrum. Children with this form of dysraphism may present with narrow flattened buttocks, weak gluteal muscles, and a shortened intergluteal cleft. The normal lumbar lordosis is absent, although the lower lumbar spine may be prominent. Calf muscles may be atrophic or absent. The pelvic ring is completed with either direct apposition of the iliac bones or with interposition of the lumbar spine replacing the absent sacrum. These children may have scoliosis, motor and sensory loss, and visceral abnormalities including anal

atresia, fused kidneys, and congenital heart malformations. Management is started early and is symptomatic for each system.[28]

Failure of fusion of the cranial end of the neural tube results in a condition known as anencephaly. In this condition, some brain tissue may be evident, but forebrain development is usually absent.[83] Because sustained life is not possible with this neural tube defect, anencephaly will not be discussed further.

Incidence and etiology

Statistics about the incidence of spina bifida vary considerably in different parts of the world. In the United States the incidence is approximately 2 per 1000 births.[60] This is about midrange in world statistics, considering a spina bifida birth rate of 0.3 per 1000 in Japan and 4.5 per 1000 in certain parts of the British Commonwealth.

There is some evidence of seasonal variation, suggesting

a positive relationship between the occurrence of spina bifida and conceptions in March to May.[14,104,111]

Spina bifida is thought to be more common in females than in males, although some studies suggest no real sex difference.[2,56,79,111] The incidence of spina bifida is higher in those of Celtic origin and lower in blacks and Asians.[14,76] A study of the association of race and gender with different neurological levels of myelomeningocele reported the proportions of whites and females to be significantly higher in thoracic level patients.[45] A significant relationship also has been noted between social class and spina bifida: the lower the social class, the higher the incidence.[86,87]

Genetic factors seem to influence the occurrence of spina bifida. The chances of having a second affected child are between 1% and 2%, whereas in the general population the percentage drops to one fifth of 1%.[63,66]

While these factors are related to the incidence of spina bifida, the cause of this defect remains in question. Environmental conditions, such as hyperthermia in the first weeks of pregnancy, or dietary factors, such as canned meats, potatoes, or tea, have been implicated but not substantiated.[14,54,55] In addition, nutritional deficiencies, such as folic acid and vitamin A, have been implicated as a cause of primary neural tube defect.[67,108] Genetic considerations, such as an Rh blood type, a specific gene type (HLA-B27), and an X-linked gene, have been implicated, but not conclusively.[7,17,94] It appears that environmental factors combined with genetic predisposition may trigger the development of spina bifida, although definitive evidence is not available to support this claim.[76,111]

The incidence of spina bifida can be expected to decline with the advent of amniocentesis, a procedure used to detect a variety of congenital abnormalities. The presence of significant levels of alpha-fetoprotein (AFP) in the amniotic fluid has led to the detection of large numbers of affected fetuses.[43] Currently, maternal serum AFP levels have been effective in detecting approximately 80% of neural tube defects.[34] Prenatal screening can be most effective when a combination of serum levels, amniocentesis/amniography, and ultrasonography is used.[20,46] While this screening is not yet performed routinely, it is suggested for those at risk for the defect. Knowledge of the defect allows for preparation for cesarean birth and immediate postnatal care. This includes mobilization of the interdisciplinary team who will continue to care for the child. For parents who decide to carry an involved fetus to term, their adjustment to their child's disability can begin before birth, which includes mobilizing their own support system. Education from an integrated team regarding what will follow after delivery and neurosurgical closure is imperative to aid families in decision making and to allow families to assess and understand the child's disability and future care options.

Other advances in the field of prenatal medicine include the in utero treatment of hydrocephalus. It can be expected that treatment such as this, in conjunction with prenatal diagnosis, will have a positive impact on the incidence and severity of complications of congenital abnormalities, such as spina bifida.

Clinical manifestations

The most obvious clinical manifestation of myelomeningocele is the loss of sensory and motor functions in the lower limbs. The extent of loss, while primarily dependent on the degree of the spinal cord abnormality, is secondarily dependent on a number of factors. These include the amount of traction or stretch resulting from the abnormally tethered spinal cord, the trauma to exposed neural tissue during delivery, and postnatal damage resulting from drying or infection of the neural plate.[111]

The above factors indicate that determining neurological involvement is not as straightforward as it would seem. At birth, two main types of motor dysfunction in the lower extremities have been identified. The first type involves a complete loss of function below the level of lesion, resulting in a flaccid paralysis, loss of sensation, and absent reflexes.[14,111] The extent of involvement can be determined by comparing the level of lesion with a chart delineating the segmental innervation of the lower limb muscles (Fig. 15-3). Orthopedic deformities may result from the unopposed action of muscles above the level of lesion. This unopposed pull leads commonly to hip flexion, knee extension, and ankle dorsiflexion contractures.

When the spinal cord remains intact below the level of lesion, the effect is an area of flaccid paralysis immediately below the lesion and possible hyperactive spinal reflexes distal to that area.[14,111] This condition is very similar to the neurological state of the severed cord seen in traumatic injury. This second type of neurological involvement again results in orthopedic deformities, depending on the level of the lesion, the spasticity present, and the muscle groups involved.

The orthopedic problems seen in myelomeningocele may be the result of (1) the imbalance between muscle groups; (2) the effect of stress, posture, and gravity; and (3) associated congenital malformations. Decreased sensation and neurological complications also may lead to orthopedic abnormalities.[118]

Besides the obvious malformation of vertebrae at the site of the lesion, hemivertebrae and deformities of other vertebral bodies and their corresponding ribs also may be present.[14,102,118] A lumbar kyphosis may be present as a result of the original deformity. In addition, as a result of the bifid vertebral bodies, the misaligned pull of the extensor muscles surrounding the deformity, as well as the unopposed flexor muscles, contribute further to the lumbar kyphosis. As the child grows, the weight of the trunk in the upright position also may be a contributing factor.[14,102] Scoliosis may be present at birth because of vertebral abnormalities or may become evident as the child grows older. There is a low incidence of scoliosis in low lumbar or sacral level

CHILDREN'S MEMORIAL HOSPITAL
MUSCLE EXAMINATION
PHYSICAL/OCCUPATIONAL THERAPY

Patient Name:_____ Medical Record #:_____

Attending Physician(s):_____ Patient Date of Birth:_____

Left				Comments / Muscle			(C_1), 2, 3	$T_{1, 2, 3, 4}$	$T_{5, 6}$	$T_{7, 8}$	$T_{9, 10, 11}$	T_{12}	L_1	L_2	L_3	L_4	L_5	S_1	S_2	S_3	Right			
Comments	+ (*)	+ (*)		* Enter initials of examiner / + Enter date of examination																	+ (*)	+ (*)	Comments
			Neck	Flexors	Sternocleidomastoid		•																	
				Extensor Group	$C_{1, 2, 3, 4, 5, 6, 7, 8}$, T_1																		
			Truck	Extensors	Thoracic Group		•	•	•	•														
					Lumbar Group		•	•	•	•														
				Flexors	Rectus Abdominis			•	•	•														
					Lt. Int. Obl. Rt. Int. Obl.				•	•	(•)													
				Rotators	Rt. Ext. Obl. Lt. Ext. Obl.				•	•	•	1	(2)											
				Pelvic Elev.	Quadratus Abdom.						•	1	2	3										
			Hip	Flexors	Iliopsoas							1	2	3	4									
					Sartorius								2	3	(4)									
				ADDuctor Group									2	3	4									
			Knee	Extensors	Quadriceps								2	3	4									
			Hip	ABDuctors	Gluteus Medius											5	1							
					Tensor Fasciae Latae										4	5	1							
				IR Group											4	5	1							
			Foot	Inv. Dorsfl.	Tibialis Anterior										4	5	1							
				Evertors	Peroneus Brevis										4	5	1							
					Peroneus Longus										4	5	1							
			Hallux	M.P. Ext.	Ext. Hall. Br.										4	5	1							
				I.P. Ext.	Ext. Hall. L.										4	5	1							
				M.P. Flexor	Flex. Hall. Br.										4	5	1							
			Toes	I.P. Flexors	Flex. Digit. Br. 1										4	5	1							
					2										4	5	1							
					3										4	5	1							
					4										4	5	1							
				M.P. Extensors	Ext. Digit. Br. 1										4	5	1							
					2										4	5	1							
					3										4	5	1							
					4										4	5	1							
				I.P. Extensors	Ext. Digit. L. 1										4	5	1							
					2										4	5	1							
					3										4	5	1							
					4										4	5	1							
			Hip	E.R. Group											4	5	1	2	(3)					
			Foot	Invertor	Tibialis Posterior										(4)	5	1							
			Hip	Extensor	Gluteus Maximus											5	1	2						
			Ankle	Plantar Flexors	Soleus											5	1	2						
					Gastrocnemius												1	2						
			Hallux	I.P. Flexors	Flex. Hall. L.											5	1	2						
			Knee	L. Flexor	Biceps Femoris											5	1	2	3					
			Knee	M. Flexors	Inner Hamstrings										(4)	(5)	1	2						
			Toes	I.P. Flexors	Flex. Digit. L. 1											5	1	(2)						
					2											5	1	(2)						
					3											5	1	(2)						
					4											5	1	(2)						
			Toes	M.P. Flexors	Lumbricales 1										4	5	1							
					2										(4)	(5)	1	2						
					3										(4)	(5)	1	2						
					4										(4)	(5)	1	2						

X	Present	Unable to be graded
N	Normal	Complete range of motion against gravity with full resistance
G	Good	Complete range of motion against gravity with moderate resistance
F+	Fair Plus	Complete range of motion against gravity with slight resistance
F	Fair	Complete range of motion against gravity
F−	Fair Minus	Incomplete range of motion against gravity
P	Poor	Complete range of motion with gravity eliminated
P−	Poor Minus	Incomplete range of motion with gravity eliminated
T	Trace	Contraction is felt but there is no visible joint movement
0	Zero	No contraction felt in the muscle
R	Reflexive	Contraction is a stereotypic movement in response to one specific stimulus
S	Spasticity	Increased tone noted during active or passive movement

Form No. 77053

Fig. 15-3. Muscle examination form. (Courtesy Josefina Briceno, PT, Children's Memorial Hospital, Chicago.)

Patient Name: _____ Medical Record #: _____

Left Comments	+	+	* Enter initials of examiner / + Enter date of examination (Region)	Action	Muscle	#	C1	C2	C3	C4	C5	C6	C7	C8	T1	+	+	Right Comments
			Scapula	Elevator	Upper Trapezius			2	3	4								
				Depressor	Lower Trapezius			2	3	4								
				ADDuctors	Middle Trapezius			2	3	4								
					Rhomboids					4	5							
			Shoulder	ABDuctors	Middle Deltoid					4	5	6						
					Supraspinatus					4	5	6						
				Ext. Rotator	Infraspinatus					(4)	5	6						
					Teres Minor					(4)	5	6						
				Flexor	Anterior Deltoid						5	6						
					Posterior Deltoid						5	6						
			Elbow	Flexors	Biceps Brachii						5	6						
					Brachioradialis						5	6						
			Shoulder	Extensor	Teres Major						5	6	7					
				Horiz. Add.	Pectoralis Major						5	6	7					
				Internal Rotator	Subscapularis						5	6	7					
			Forearm	Supinator	Supinator						5	6	7					
			Scapula	ABDuctor	Serratus Anterior						5	6	(7)	8				
			Wrist	Extensor	Ext. Carpi Rad. L. & Br.						5	6	(7)	8				
			Forearm	Pronation	Pronator Group							6	7					
			Shoulder	Extensor	Latissimus Dorsi							6	7	8				
			Wrist	Flexors	Flex. Carp. Rad.							6	7	8				
				Extensor	Ext. Carp. Uln.							6	7	8				
			Finger	M.P. Extensor	Ext. Digit. Com.	1						6	7	8				
						2						6	7	8				
						3						6	7	8				
						4						6	7	8				
			Thumb	M.P. Extensor	Ext. Poll. Br.							6	7	8				
				I.P. Extensor	Ext. Poll. L.							6	7	8				
				ABDuctor	ABD. Poll. L.							6	7	8				
			Elbow	Extensor	Triceps							6	7	8				
			Wrist	Flexors	Palmaris Longus							(6)	7	8				
			Fingers	M.P. Flexors	Lumbricales	1						(6)	7	8	1			
						2												
			Thumb	M.P. Flexor	Flex. Poll Br.							6	7	8	1			
				I.P. Flexor	Flex. Poll. L.							(6)	7	8	1			
				ABDuctor	ABD. Poll. Br.							6	7	8	1			
				Opponens	Opponens Poll.							6	7	8	1			
			Wrist	Flexor	Flex. Carpi Uln.								7	8	1			
			Fingers	M.P. Flexors	Lumbricales	3							(7)	8	1			
						4							(7)	8	1			
				I.P. Flexors (1st)	Flex. Digit. Sub.	1							7	8	1			
						2							7	8	1			
						3							7	8	1			
						4							7	8	1			
				I.P. Flexors (2nd)	Flex. Digit. Prof.	1							7	8	1			
						2							7	8	1			
						3							7	8	1			
						4							7	8	1			
				ABDuctors	Palmer Interossei	1								8	1			
						2								8	1			
						3								8	1			
						4								8	1			
				ADDuctors	Dorsal Interossei	1								8	1			
						2								8	1			
						3								8	1			
						4								8	1			
			Thumb	ABDuctors	ABDuctor Pollicis									8	1			

Fig. 15-3, cont'd. For legend see opposite page.

deformities.[85,102] Scoliosis may also be neurogenic, secondary to weakness or asymmetrical spasticity of paraspinal muscles, tethered cord syndrome or hydromyelia.[1] A lordosis or lordoscoliosis is often seen in the adolescent and is usually associated with hip flexion deformities and a large spinal defect.[14,79,102]

Many of these trunk and postural deformities exist at birth, but are exacerbated by the effects of gravity as the child grows. They can compromise vital functions (cardiac and respiratory) and therefore should be closely monitored by the therapist and the family.

As has been alluded to previously, the type and extent of deformity in the lower extremities depend on the muscles that are active or inactive. In a total flaccid paralysis, in utero deformities may be present at birth, resulting from passive positioning within the womb. Equinovarus (clubfoot) or "rocker-bottom" deformity are two of the most common foot abnormalities. Knee flexion and extension contractures also may be present at birth. Other common deformities are hip flexion, adduction, and internal rotation, usually leading to subluxed or dislocated hip.[14] Although many of these problems may be present at birth, it is of utmost importance to prevent positional deformity (such as the frog-leg position), which may result from improper positioning of flaccid extremities.[38]

Because the paralyzed limbs of the child with spina bifida have increased amounts of unmineralized osteoid tissue, they are prone to fractures, particularly after periods of immobilization.[30,96] Early mobilization and weightbearing can aid in decreasing osteoporosis.[102] Fortunately, these fractures heal quickly with appropriate medical management.

Hydrocephalus develops in 80% to 90% of children with myelomeningocele.[66,76] Hydrocephalus results from a blockage of the normal flow of CSF between the ventricles and spinal canal. The most obvious effect of the buildup of CSF is abnormal increase in head size, which may be present at birth because of the great compliance of the cranial sutures in the fetus, or may develop postnatally. Other signs of hydrocephalus include bulging fontanels and irritability. Internally, there is usually a concomitant dilation of the lateral ventricles and thinning of the cerebral white matter. Without reduction of the buildup of CSF, increased brain damage and death may result.

Patients with myelomeningocele have a 99% chance of having an associated Chiari II malformation.[19] This malformation is a congenital anomaly of the hindbrain in which there is herniation of the medulla and at times the pons, fourth ventricle, and inferior aspect of the cerebellum into the upper cervical canal (usually between C1 and C4 but the herniated contents may extend down to T1). Not all **Chiari II malformations** are symptomatic.

Secondary to a symptomatic Chiari malformation, problems with respiratory and bulbar function may be evident in the child with spina bifida.[14,76,111] Paralysis of the vocal cords occurs in a small percentage of patients and is associated with respiratory stridor. Apneic episodes also may be evident, although their direct cause remains in question. Children with spina bifida also may exhibit difficulty in swallowing and have an abnormal gag reflex.[111] Problems with aspiration, weakness and cry, and upper extremity weakness also may be present in children with a symptomatic Chiari II malformation.[81,117] Thus depending on the orthopedic deformities present and the neurological involvement, there is a potential from both sources for severe respiratory involvement in the affected child. These symptoms may be due to significant compression of the hindbrain structures or to dysplasia of posterior fossa contents, which can also occur in patients with Chiari II malformation.[19,89] This complex hindbrain malformation is a common cause of death in children with myelomeningocele despite surgical intervention and aggressive medical management.[71] Other common neurological problems for children with spina bifida include hydromyelia, and tethered cord.

Between 20% and 80% of patients with myelomeningocele may present with hydromyelia.[19,116] Hydromyelia signifies dilation of the center canal of the spinal cord as hydrocephalus signifies dilation of the ventricles of the brain. The area of hydromyelia may be focal, multiple, or diffuse extending throughout the spinal cord. The hydromyelia may be a consequence of untreated or inadequately treated hydrocephalus with resultant transmission of CSF through the obex into the central canal, with distension secondary to increased hydrostatic pressure from above.[19,116] The increased collection of fluid may cause pressure necrosis of the spinal cord leading to muscle weakness and scoliosis.[21] Common symptoms of hydromyelia include rapidly progressive scoliosis, upper extremity weakness, spasticity, and ascending motor loss in the lower extremities.[19,49,116] Aggressive treatment of hydromyelia at the onset of clinical signs of increasing scoliosis is mandatory and may lead to improvement in or stabilization of the curve in 80% of cases. Surgical interventions may include revision of a CSF shunt, posterior cervical decompression, or a central canal to pleural cavity shunt with a flushing device.[19,89]

Tethered spinal cord is defined as a pathological fixation of the spinal cord in an abnormal caudal location, which produces mechanical stretch, distortion, and ischemia with daily activities, growth, and development.[97] The presence of tethered cord syndrome should be suspected in any patient with abnormal neurulation (including patients with myelomeningocele, lipomeningocele, dermal sinus, diastematomyelia, myelocystocele, tight filum terminal, and lumbosacral agenesis). Presenting symptoms may include decreased strength (often asymmetrical), development of lower extremity spasticity, back pain at the site of sac closure, early development of or increasing degree of scoliosis (especially in the low lumbar or sacral level child) or change in urological function.[39,69,97] This clinical spectrum may be primarily associated with these dysraphic lesions or may be secondary to spinal surgical procedures.[97] The cord may be tethered by scar tissue or by an inclusion epidermoid or lipoma at the repair site.[19] Surgery to untether the spinal cord is done to prevent further loss of muscle function, to decrease the spasticity, to help control the scoliosis, or relieve back pain.[69]

The effectiveness of surgical untethering of the spinal cord has been demonstrated by an increase in muscle function, relief of back pain, and stabilization or reversal of scoliosis. Spasticity, however, is not always alleviated in all patients.[72] Selective posterior rhizotomy has been advocated for patients whose persistent or progressive spastic status after tethered cord repair continues to interfere with their mobility and functional independence.[113,114]

Because of the usual involvement of the sacral plexus, the child with spina bifida must commonly deal with some form of bowel and bladder dysfunction. Besides various forms of incontinence, incomplete emptying of the bladder remains a constant concern because infection of the urinary tract and possible kidney damage may result.[3] Regulation of bowel evacuation must be established so that neither constipation nor diarrhea occur.

The last major clinical manifestation resulting from the neurological involvement of myelomeningocele is that of impaired intellectual function. Although children with spina bifida without hydrocephalus may show normal intellectual potential, children with hydrocephalus, particularly those who have shunt infections, are likely to have below-average intelligence.[14,15,74,95,111]

These children often demonstrate learning disabilities and poor academic achievement. Even those with a normal IQ show moderate to severe visual-motor perceptual deficits.[76] This inability to coordinate eye and hand movements not only affects learning but also may interfere with activities of daily living, such as buttoning a shirt or opening a lunch box.[41] Difficulties with spatial relations, body image, and development of hand dominance may also be evident.[41,111] (Chapter 11 should be of great assistance when dealing with these problems in the child with spina bifida.)

The impairment of intellectual and perceptual abilities has been linked to damage to the white matter caused by ventricular enlargement.[14,111] This damage to association tracts, particularly in the frontal, occipital, and parietal areas, could account for the often severe perceptual-cognitive deficits noted in the child with spina bifida. Lesser involvement of the temporal areas may account for the preservation of speech, while the semantics of speech, dependent on association areas, is impaired. It is easy to be fooled by the "cocktail party speech" of children with spina bifida, because they generally use well-constructed sentences and precocious vocabulary.[14,119] A closer look, however, reveals a repetitive, inappropriate, and often meaningless use of language certainly not associated with higher intellectual functioning.

Latex allergy has been noted with increasing frequency among children with myelomeningocele, with frequent reports of intraoperative anaphylaxis.[8,42,105,107] A 1991 Food and Drug Administration Medical Bulletin estimated that 18% to 40% of patients with spina bifida demonstrate latex sensitivity.[38] Within latex is 2% to 3% of residual-free protein material that is thought to be the antigenic agent.[105] Frequent exposure to this material results in the development of the IgE antibody. Children with spina bifida are more likely to develop the IgE sensitivity due to repeated parental or mucosal exposure to the latex antigen.[106] Because of the risk of an anaphylactic reaction, exposure to any latex-containing products such as rubber gloves, balls, or Thera-Band should be avoided.

Considering all the clinical manifestations resulting from this congenital neurological defect, there is no doubt that social and emotional difficulties will arise for these children and their families. These will be considered as appropriate when discussing the stages of recovery and rehabilitation from birth through adolescence.

The preceding discussion concerning the clinical problems of the child with spina bifida was intended to inform, not overwhelm, the clinician. With a firm understanding of the difficulties to be faced, evaluation and intervention can be more efficient and effective.

Medical management

Before surgical closure of myelomeningocele. At birth, the myelomeningocele sac presents a dynamic rather than static disability. The residual neurological damage will be contingent on the early medical management that the newborn receives.

Since the early 1960s the presence of a myelomeningocele has been treated as a life-threatening situation, and sac closure now takes place within the first 24 to 48 hours of life.[93,111] The aim of this surgery is to replace the nervous tissue into the vertebral canal, cover the spinal defect, and achieve a water-tight sac closure.[70] This early management has decreased the possibility of infection and further injury to the exposed neural cord.[68,70,75,76]

After surgery, during hospitalization. Progressive hydrocephalus may be evident at birth in a small percentage of children born with myelomeningocele. A greater majority, however, develop hydrocephalus 5 to 10 days after the back lesion is closed.[75,112] With the advent of computed axial tomography (CT), early diagnosis of hydrocephalus can be made in the newborn without the need for clinical examination.

Although clinical signs are not always definitive, hydrocephalus may be suspected if (1) the fontanels become full, bulging, or tense; (2) the head circumference increases rapidly; (3) there is a palpable separation of the coronal and sagittal sutures; (4) the infant's eyes appear to look downward only, with the cornea prominent over the iris (sun-setting sign); and (5) the infant becomes irritable or lethargic and has a high-pitched cry, persistent vomiting, difficult feeding, or seizures.[51,66]

If the results of the CT scan confirm hydrocephalus, a ventricular shunt is indicated. This procedure involves diverting the excess CSF from the ventricles to some site for absorption. In general, two types of procedures—the ventriculoatrial (VA) and ventriculoperitoneal (VP) shunt—are currently used, the latter being the most common[104] (Fig. 15-4). The shunt apparatus is constructed from Silastic tubing and consists of three parts: a proximal catheter, a distal catheter, and a one-way valve.[36] As CSF is pumped from the ventricles toward its final destination, back flow is prevented by the valve system. In this manner intercranial pressure is controlled, CSF is regulated, and hydrocephalus is prevented from causing damage to brain structures.

Unfortunately for children with spina bifida, their problems do not end after the back is closed and a shunt is in place. Shunt complications occur frequently and require an average of two revisions before age 10.[76] The most common causes of complications are shunt obstruction and infection.[14,111] Obstructions can be cleared by revising the blocked end of the shunt. Infections may be handled by external ventricular drainage and courses of antibiotic therapy followed by insertion of a new shunting system.[111] The problem of separation of shunt components has been largely overcome by the use of a one-piece shunting system. The single-piece shunt decreases the complications of shunting procedures.

Prophylactic antibiotic therapy 6 to 12 hours before surgery and 1 to 2 days postoperatively is effective in controlling infection for both sac repair and shunt insertion.[23,76] This brief course of antibiotics has not led to resistant organisms. The main cause of death in children with myelomeningoceles remains increased intercranial pressure and infections of the CNS.[76] With the use of antibiotics, shunting, and early sac closure, the survival rate has increased from 20% to 85%.[74]

Initial newborn workup should include a urological assessment. It is the aim of the urology team to preserve renal function and to promote efficient bladder management.[66] Initially a renal and bladder ultrasound is done to assess those structures.[57] Radiographic tests such as the voiding

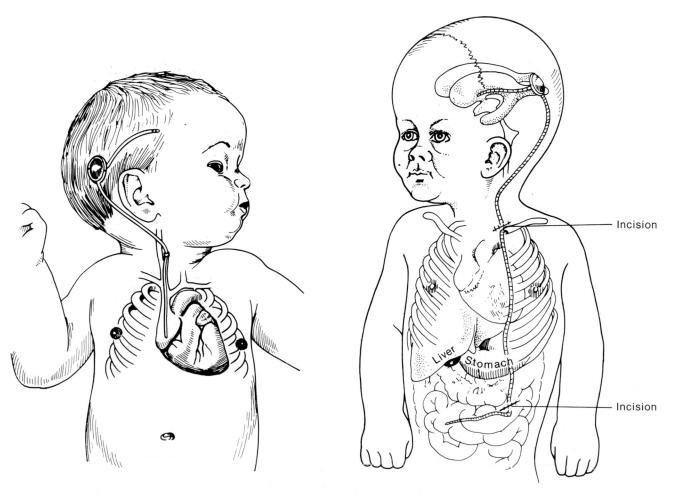

Fig. 15-4. A, Ventriculoatrial shunt *(VA).* **B,** Ventriculoperitoneal shunt *(VP).* (From Stark GD: *Spina bifida problems and management,* London, 1977, Blackwell Scientific Publications.)

cystourethrograms or a cystometregram can be performed to determine any blockage in the lower urinary tract. Functioning of the bladder outlet and sphincters, as well as ureteric reflux, also can be evaluated.[14,66,111]

These tests, plus clinical observations of voiding patterns, help the urologist classify the infant's bladder function. If the bladder has neither sensory nor motor supply, there will be a constant flow of urine. In this case infection is rare, because the bladder does not store urine and the sphincters are always open.[21]

If there is no sensation but some involuntary muscle control of the sphincter, the bladder will fill, but emptying will not occur properly. Overflow or stress incontinence results in dribbling urine until the pressure is relieved. Because of constant residual urine, infection is a potential problem and kidney damage may be the sequela.[21]

When some voluntary muscle control but no sensation is present, the bladder will fill and empty automatically. The child can eventually be taught to empty the bladder at regular intervals to avoid unnecessary accidents.

Regardless of the type of bladder functioning, urine specimens are taken to check for infection, and blood samples are taken to determine the kidney's ability to filter the body's fluids. Based on clinical findings, the urologist will suggest the appropriate intervention.

A program of clean intermittent catheterization (CIC) done every 3-4 hours prevents infection and maintains the urological system.[3,29] Parents are taught this method and can then begin[29] to take on this aspect of their child's care.

At the age of 4 or 5 years, children with spina bifida can be taught CIC. By doing so, they have become independent in bladder care at a young age. Achieving this form of independence adds to the normal psychological development of these children.

Some children may require urinary diversion through the abdominal wall (ilealconduit) or other less common methods such as intravesical transurethral bladder stimulation to handle their urinary problems.[3] Although CIC is not possible for all children with spina bifida, it remains the method of choice for bladder management.

Orthopedic management of the newborn with a myelomeningocele will generally concentrate on the feet and hips. Soft tissue releases of the feet may take place during surgery for sac closure. Casting the feet also has been effective in reducing clubfoot deformities (Fig. 15-5). Early aggressive taping for club foot also is effective in the management of clubfoot deformities.[52] Short leg posterior splints (AFOs) may be used to maintain range and prevent foot deformities.

The orthopedist also will evaluate the stability of the hips. In children with lower-level lesions, attempts to prevent dislocation are made by using a hip abductor brace (Fig. 15-6, *A*) or a total body splint (TBS) (Fig. 15-6, *B*) for a few months after birth (Fig. 15-6, *A* and 15-6, *B*). With higher-level lesions, dislocated hips are no longer treated because they do not appear to have an effect on later rehabilitation efforts.[3,32,51,61]

PHYSICAL THERAPY EVALUATIONS

In attempting to evaluate the child with spina bifida, there are any number of evaluations from which to choose, each designed to test specific, yet perhaps unrelated, components of function. The following section discusses those test procedures or specific standardized tests that would best define the complexity of the problem.

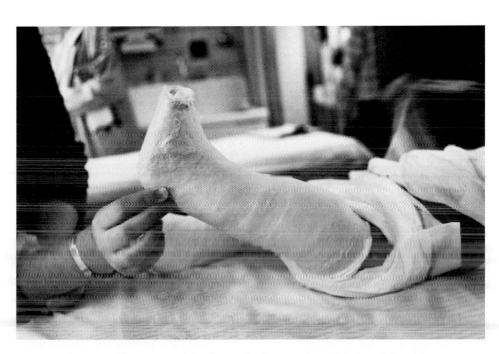

Fig. 15-5. Plaster cast of the foot and ankle to reduce club foot deformities.

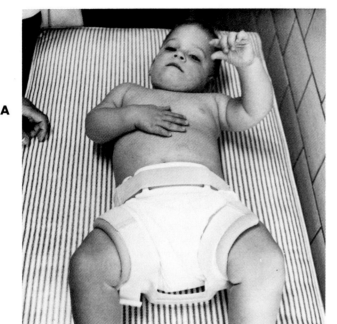
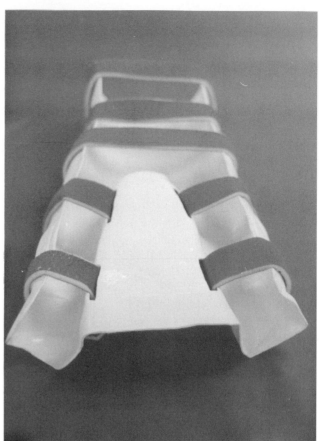

Fig. 15-6. A, Hip abductor brace. **B,** Total Body Splint.

Manual muscle testing (MMT)

The first and most obvious request for evaluation may be to determine the extent of motor paralysis. In the newborn, testing may be done in the first 24 to 48 hours before the back is surgically closed. In this case, care must be taken not to injure the exposed neural tissue during testing. Prone and sidelying to either side offers the most convenient and safe position for evaluation during this time. Subsequent testing is done soon after the back is closed and as indicated throughout childhood.

The traditional form of MMT is not appropriate or possible for the infant or young child. The following is a discussion of how muscle testing can and must be adapted for this age group.

In evaluating the newborn, the importance of state is paramount. A sleeping or drowsy baby will hardly respond appropriately during the evaluation. It is essential that the infant be in the alert or crying state to elicit the appropriate responses. There is an advantage to testing hungry or crying babies, because they are likely to demonstrate more spontaneous movements in these behavioral states.

The cumulative effect of a variety of sensory stimuli may

be more effective than using one mode in isolation. For example, the infant may be picked up and rocked vertically to allow maximum stimulation to the vestibular system and to help bring the child to an alert state. In addition, the therapist may talk to the child to help him or her fixate visually on the therapist's face. Tactile stimuli above the level of the lesion further add to the child's level of arousal, thus contributing to more conclusive test results. In this way, the CNS receives an accumulation of information from a variety of sensory systems, rather than relying on transmission from one system that may be weak or inefficient.

As the child is aroused, spontaneous movements can be observed and muscle groups palpated. Additional methods to stimulate movement may be necessary. For example, "tickling" the baby generally produces a variety of spontaneous movements in the upper and lower extremities. Passive positioning of children in adverse positions may stimulate them to move. For example, if the legs are held in marked hip and knee flexion, the baby may attempt to use extensor musculature to move out of that position. If the legs are held in adduction, the child may abduct to get free. Holding a limb in an antigravity position may elicit an automatic "holding" response from a muscle group when spontaneous movements cannot be obtained in any other way.[121]

Although none of these methods are fail-safe, they may be helpful in adapting a muscle test to a newborn or young infant. Repeated evaluation may be necessary to get an accurate picture of muscle function.

In grading muscle strength, it is important to differentiate between spontaneous, voluntary movement, and reflexive movement. After severing of a spinal cord, distal segments of the cord may respond to stimuli in a reflexive manner. This results from the preservation of the spinal reflex arc and is known as *distal sparing*. If distal sparing of the spinal cord is present, the muscles may respond to stimulation or muscular stretch with reflexive, stereotypical movement patterns. The quality of this reflexive movement will be different from that of spontaneous movement and must be distinguished when testing for level of voluntary muscle functioning.

Muscle strength is generally graded for groups of muscles and can be graded by using either a numerical or alphabetical designation (Fig. 15-7) or simply by noting presence or absence of muscular contraction. Initially, this latter method may be sufficient, but as the child matures a more definitive muscle grade should be determined.

By using an MMT form that lists the spinal segmental level for each muscle group, one can determine the level of lesion from the test results (Fig. 15-3, Fig. 15-7). If reflex activity is also noted on the form, the presence of distal sparing of the spinal cord can be determined. Muscle testing of the newborn gives the clinician not only an appreciation of muscle function and possible potential for later ambulation but also an awareness of possible deforming forces. For example, if hip extensors or abductors are not functioning, then the action of hip flexors and adductors must be countered to prevent future deformities.

Muscle testing of the toddler or young child may require some of the techniques described previously. In addition, developmental positions can be used to assess muscle strength in an uncooperative youngster. For example strength of hip extensors and abductors can be assessed as a child attempts to creep up steps or onto a low mat table. By adding resistance to movements, fairly accurate muscle grades can be determined. Ingenuity and creativity are certainly prerequisites for muscle testing in the young child.

By the age of 4 or 5 years, muscle grades can generally be determined through traditional testing techniques, although the reliability of the test results will increase with the age of the child.

Muscle testing is indicated before and after any surgical procedure and at periodic intervals of 6 months to 1 year to detect any change in muscle function. The level of innervation should not decrease throughout the life of the child with spina bifida. In the growing child or adolescent, an increasing weakness resulting from shunt malfunction,

tethering of the spinal cord, or hydromyelia frequently can be substantiated by a muscle test of the lower extremities.

Range of motion evaluation

A complete range of motion (ROM) evaluation of the lower extremities is indicated for the newborn with spina bifida. The therapist must be aware of normal physiological flexion that is greatest at the hip and knees. In the normal newborn these apparent "contractures" of up to 35 degrees are eliminated as the child gains more control of extensor musculature and kicks more frequently into extension.

In the child with spina bifida, contractures may be evident at birth because of unopposed musculature. Hip adduction should not be tested beyond the neutral position to avoid dislocation of hips that are often unstable. Range should be done slowly and without excessive force to avoid fractures so often experienced in paralytic lower extremities. ROM should be checked with the same frequency as muscle testing.

Active ROM of the upper extremities can be assessed by observation and handling the infant. A formal ROM evaluation for the upper extremities is not usually indicated. A baseline ROM and tone assessment of the upper extremities should be completed.

Sensory testing

Sensory testing of the infant and young child is simplified to determine the level of sensation as accurately as possible, with a minimum amount of testing. Full sensory tests are not possible until the child has acquired sufficient cognitive and language abilities to respond appropriately to testing.

In the newborn, sensory testing can best be done if the child is in a quiet state.* Beginning at the lowest level of sacral innervation, the skin is stroked with a pin or other sharp object until a reaction to pain is noted. Because of dermatome innervation the pin is usually drawn from the anal area, across the buttocks, down the posterior thigh and leg, then to the anterior surface of the leg and thigh, and finally across the abdominal muscles. Reactions to be noted are a facial grimace or cry, which indicates that the painful sensation has reached a cortical level. Care must be taken to see that each sensory dermatome has been evaluated. Results can be recorded by shading in the dermatomes where sensation is present (Fig. 15-8).

The therapist may be called on to evaluate the newborn before surgical closure of the spinal meningocele. Although sensory and motor levels can be determined as previously described, it is important to consider the infant's general condition when interpreting test findings. Any modification

---

* If the infant is initially quiet, evaluation should begin with a sensory test. This test usually brings the child to an alert or crying state, which is optimal for muscle testing.

THE CHILDREN'S MEMORIAL HOSPITAL
PHYSICAL / OCCUPATIONAL THERAPY

MUSCLE EXAM - MM

PATIENT NAME _____   M.R. # _____

ATTENDING M.D. _____   PT. D.O.B. _____

DIAGNOSIS _____

_____

DATE: _____

P.T. NAME: _____

	*	LEFT	RIGHT	*	COMMENTS: (Include ROM limitations, spasticity, reflexive movements, etc.)
ILIOPSOAS (L_1 - 2)					
SARTORIUS (L_1, 3)					
HIP ADDUCTORS (L_2 - 4)					
TENSOR FASCIA LATA					
GLUTEUS MEDIUS (L_4 - S_1)					
GLUTEUS MAXIMUS (L_5 - S_1)					
QUADRICEPS (L_2 - 4)					
MEDIAL HAMSTRINGS (L_4 - S_2)					
LATERAL HAMSTRINGS (L_4 - S_1)					
ANTERIOR TIBIALIS (L_4 - L_5)					
POSTERIOR TIBIALIS (L_4 - L_5)					
PERONEUS LONGUS (L_5 - S_1)					
PERONEUS BREVIS (L_5 - S_1)					
GASTROC - SOLEUS (S_1 - S_2)					
EXT. HALLUCIS LONGUS (L_5 - S_1)					
FLEX. HALLUCIS LONGUS (S_1 - S_2)					
EXT. DIGITORUM LONGUS (L_4 - S_1)					
EXT. DIG. B. (L_4 - S_1)					
FLEX. DIGITORUM LONGUS (L_4 - S_1)					
FLEX. DIG. B. (L_4 - S_1)					
LUMBRICALES					

*INDICATE INCREASE (↑) OR DECREASE (↓) IN STRENGTH IN COMPARISON TO PREVIOUS TEST DATED _____

PLEASE NOTE ANY SIGNIFICANT INFORMATION ON OTHER MUSCLE GROUPS UNLISTED ABOVE (i.e., EHB; Flex. HB; Internal or External Rotators)

X	PRESENT	UNABLE TO BE GRADED
N	NORMAL	COMPLETE RANGE OF MOTION AGAINST GRAVITY WITH FULL RESISTANCE
G	GOOD	COMPLETE RANGE OF MOTION AGAINST GRAVITY WITH MODERATE RESISTANCE
G-	GOOD MINUS	COMPLETE RANGE OF MOTION AGAINST GRAVITY WITH SOME RESISTANCE
F+	FAIR PLUS	COMPLETE RANGE OF MOTION AGAINST GRAVITY WITH SLIGHT RESISTANCE
F	FAIR	COMPLETE RANGE OF MOTION AGAINST GRAVITY
F-	FAIR MINUS	INCOMPLETE (GREATER THAN 1/2 WAY) RANGE OF MOTION AGAINST GRAVITY
P+	POOR PLUS	LESS THAN 1/2 WAY AGAINST GRAVITY OR FULL ROM GRAVITY ELIMINATED PLUS SL RESISTANCE
P	POOR	COMPLETE RANGE OF MOTION WITH GRAVITY ELIMINATED
P-	POOR MINUS	INCOMPLETE RANGE OF MOTION WITH GRAVITY ELIMINATED
T	TRACE	CONTRACTION IS FELT BUT THERE IS NO VISIBLE JOINT MOVEMENT
O	ZERO	NO CONTRACTION FELT IN THE MUSCLE

FORM 354042790

Fig. 15-7. Muscle examination form using alphabetical designation. (Courtesy Josefina Briceno, PT, Children's Memorial Hospital, Chicago.)

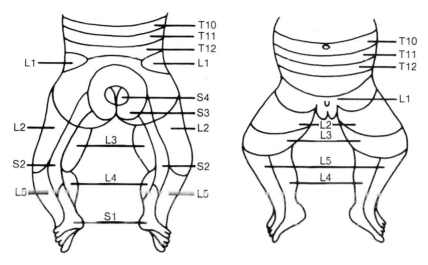

Fig. 15-8. Lower limb dermatomes. (From Brocklehurst G: Spina bifida for the clinician, *Clin Dev Med* 57:53, Philadelphia, 1976, JB Lippincott.)

taken by the mother during labor and delivery may influence the neonate's performance and thus should be noted. In addition, the physiological disorganization, normally seen in all infants during the first few days after birth, also may affect testing.[13] At best, this presurgical evaluation establishes a tentative baseline, and significant changes in the infant's neurological status in the first few weeks of life should not be surprising to the clinician.

In the young child from 2 to 7 years of age, light touch sensation and position sense can be tested in addition to pain sensation. Again, the ingenuity of the therapist will be called forth to elicit an appropriate response and reliable test results. Using games, such as "Tell me when the puppet touches you," or behavior modification techniques, like "Put your hand out for candy when I touch you," may be more effective for the young child than traditional testing methods.

From 7 years through adolescence, additional sensory tests of temperature and two-point discrimination may be added. Usually, traditional methods are sufficient to ensure reliable testing, but a more behavioral approach may be indicated, depending on the individual's cognitive functioning.

Following testing, a survey of the sensory dermatome chart should indicate whether sensation is normal, absent, or impaired.

Reflex testing

The purpose of reflex testing is twofold: to check for the presence of *normal* reflex activity and to check for the integration of primitive reflexes and the establishment of more mature reactions.[36] In the newborn, for example, one would expect strong rooting and sucking reflexes. In the child with spina bifida, because of possible involvement of the CNS as described previously, these reflexes may be

depressed or absent. Because these reflexes play an integral part in obtaining nutrients for the infant, their value is obvious.

On the other hand, primitive reflexes, which persist past their expected span, also may indicate abnormality. For example, if the asymmetrical tonic neck reflex persists past 4 months, it will limit the infant's ability to bring the hands to midline for visual and tactile exploration.

As the primitive reflexes (initially needed for survival and to experience movement) become integrated, they are replaced by more mature and functional reactions. The righting and equilibrium reactions help the child attain the erect position and counteract changes in the center of gravity. Because these reactions depend on an intact CNS, as well as a certain level of postural control, they may be delayed, incomplete, or absent in the child with spina bifida. For example, a child with a low thoracic spinal cord lesion may show an incomplete equilibrium reaction in sitting. This may be caused by the lack of a stable postural base or by lack of initiation of the reaction centrally. Both the neurological and muscular components of these reactions must be considered.[37]

Reflex testing for the child with spina bifida may not be as intensive as that for a child with cerebral palsy. It may, however, provide a check on the progress of normal development and as such reflect the integrity of the CNS.

Developmental/functional evaluations

Besides being aware of a child's sensory and motor levels, it is also important to assess the functional level. Two important questions need to be asked—"Does the child show normal components of posture and movement patterns?" and "What is the child's level of mobility?"

Several developmental and/or functional evaluations can

be adapted for the child with spina bifida. The following are some suggestions for evaluation approaches or specifically designed tests to assist in assessment of this area.

Initially, a developmental sequence may be used to assess how a child is functioning. In each position used, both posture and movement will be evaluated. The goals in using this type of assessment are to determine what a child can and cannot do, the quality of the action, and what is limiting the child. The progression would begin in the supine position, rolling to prone, prone-on-elbows, prone-on-hands, up-to-sitting, hands-knees, kneeling, half-kneeling, standing, and walking. Both the ability to obtain and the ability to maintain the positions should be assessed.

It is not merely the accomplishment of the task that must be evaluated but, simultaneously, the *way* in which it is accomplished. For example, in rolling, is head righting sufficient to keep the head off the supporting surface? From the hands-knees position, can reciprocal crawling be initiated without the lower extremities being held in wide abduction? Can the child pull to stand easily by using trunk rotation? Assessing the quality of the child's abilities will assist the clinician in determining where therapeutic measures should begin and what the goals of such intervention will be.[24]

The Milani-Comparetti motor development screening test may prove useful in assessing the functional level of the child with spina bifida. This screening examination is designed to evaluate motor development from birth to 2 years of age (Fig. 15-9).[80] It requires no special equipment and can be administered in 4 to 8 minutes. The test evaluates both spontaneous behavior and evoked responses. Spontaneous behavior includes postural control of the head and body in various positions, as well as a sequence of active movement patterns. Primitive reflexes, righting, and equilibrium reactions comprise the evoked responses. The Milani-Comparetti test should assist the clinician in evaluating each child's underlying postural mechanisms and his or her ability to attain the erect position. Refer to the test manual for special examination procedures and scoring.[80]

The Peabody Developmental Motor Scales (PDMS)[37a] is a recently standardized assessment that may prove helpful in evaluating a child with congenital spinal cord injury. The PDMS consists of gross and fine motor scales from birth through 83 months. The two scales allow a comparison of the child's motor performance with a normative sample of children at various age levels. Although the disabled child would not be expected to pass many of the gross motor items at the later age levels, the scale still serves as a reminder of expected gross motor performance at each age. The fine motor scale offers a chance to assess fine motor performance of children with congenital spinal cord injury. This area has been frequently overlooked with children with myelomeningocele. Fine motor development, however, may be affected because of congenital abnormalities in brain development associated with myelomeningocele, or related to

tethering of the spinal cord that can result in fine motor paresis. In addition, the PDMS offers guidelines for administering the test to handicapped children.[37a]

Finally, the Pediatric Evaluation of Disability Inventory (PEDI)[48] is a comprehensive assessment of function in children aged 6 months to 7 years. The PEDI measures both capability and performance of functional activities in three areas: (1) self-care, (2) mobility, and (3) social function. Capability is a measure of the functional skills for which the child has demonstrated mastery. Functional performance is measured by the level of caregiver assistance needed to accomplish a task. A modifications scale provides a measure of environmental modifications and equipment needed in daily functioning. The PEDI has been standardized on a normative sample of children, but some data from clinical samples are also available. The PEDI can be administered in about 45 minutes by clinicians or educators familiar with the child, or by structured interview of the parent. The PEDI should provide a descriptive measure of the functional level of the child with MM, as well as a method for tracking change over time.

Perceptual/cognitive evaluations

In evaluating these children, it is important to include some assessment of perceptual/cognitive status. The appropriate assessment depends largely on the age of the child.

For the newborn from 3 to 30 days old, the Brazelton Neonatal Behavioral Assessment scale may be adapted to assess the infant's organization in terms of physiological response to stress, state control, motoric control, and social interaction. Ideally, the infant should be medically stable and free from CNS-depressant drugs before evaluation. Generally, this evaluation will occur after the back lesion is closed, and a shunt is positioned to relieve the hydrocephalic condition.

While test results may not have prognostic value because of the plasticity of the nervous system at this young age, they supply the clinician with information concerning the current status of the child. This information can be conveyed to the infant's caregivers—both medical personnel and parents—so that strengths can be appreciated and weaknesses anticipated and handled appropriately. Helping parents to identify that their infant has his or her own unique characteristics and assisting them in dealing with these characteristics does a great deal to strengthen already precarious parent-infant bonding.

Repeated administration of the Brazelton Neonatal Behavioral Assessment scale in the first month of life may help monitor the infant's progress in organization and reflect the curve of recovery. Although the manual for this behavioral assessment is quite complete, proper administration scoring and interpretation require direct training with someone already proficient in using the scale.[13] Excellent training films for the Brazelton Neonatal Behavioral Assessment scale are available for purchase or through your local

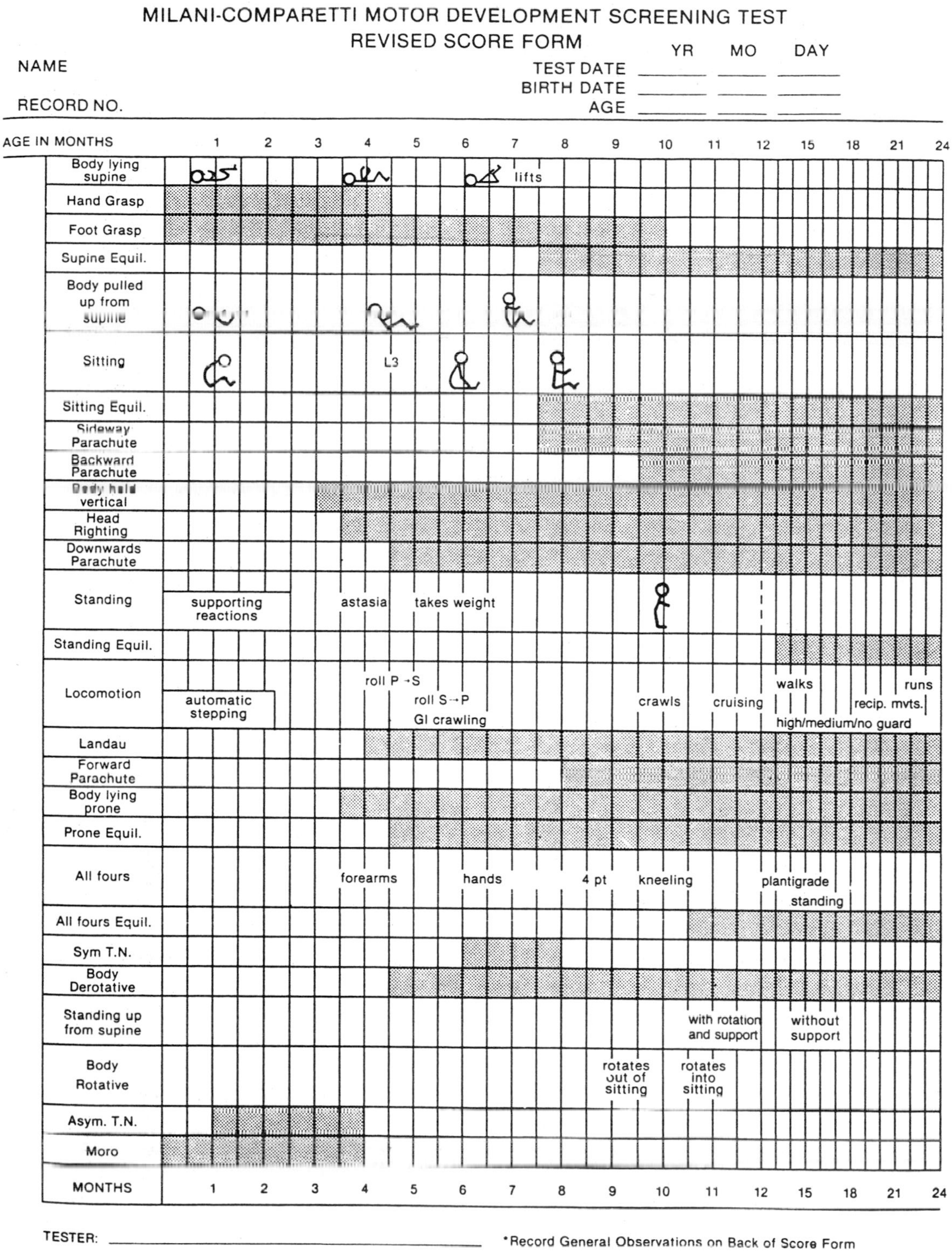

MILANI-COMPARETTI MOTOR DEVELOPMENT SCREENING TEST
REVISED SCORE FORM

	YR	MO	DAY
TEST DATE	___	___	___
BIRTH DATE	___	___	___
AGE	___	___	___

NAME

RECORD NO.

AGE IN MONTHS: 1 2 3 4 5 6 7 8 9 10 11 12 15 18 21 24

Body lying supine	lifts
Hand Grasp	
Foot Grasp	
Supine Equil.	
Body pulled up from supine	
Sitting	L3
Sitting Equil.	
Sideway Parachute	
Backward Parachute	
Body held vertical	
Head Righting	
Downwards Parachute	
Standing	supporting reactions / astasia / takes weight
Standing Equil.	
Locomotion	automatic stepping / roll P→S / roll S→P / GI crawling / crawls / cruising / walks / runs / recip. mvts. / high/medium/no guard
Landau	
Forward Parachute	
Body lying prone	
Prone Equil.	
All fours	forearms / hands / 4 pt / kneeling / plantigrade standing
All fours Equil.	
Sym T.N.	
Body Derotative	
Standing up from supine	with rotation and support / without support
Body Rotative	rotates out of sitting / rotates into sitting
Asym. T.N.	
Moro	

MONTHS: 1 2 3 4 5 6 7 8 9 10 11 12 15 18 21 24

TESTER: _____   *Record General Observations on Back of Score Form

Fig. 15-4 Milani-Comparetti Motor Development Screening Test Revised Score Form.

university's learning resource center (see the appendix at the end of the chapter).

Two full developmental evaluations, appropriate for the infant and toddler with spina bifida, are the Bayley Scales of Infant Development, 2nd edition (BSID-II)[10] and the Revised Gesell Developmental Assessment.[59] Each evaluation contains information on gross motor, fine motor, language, personal-social, and cognitive development.

The Bayley Scales, consisting of a mental and motor scale and a behavioral rating scale, can be used to test children from one month to 42 months. The BSID–II is well standardized and reliable and takes about 45 minutes to administer. It is not an easy test to learn and would initially require supervision of an experienced tester. This new edition of the Bayley provides new normative data, extended age range, expanded content coverage, and improved psychometric qualities.

The revised Gesell can be used to evaluate an infant from 4 weeks to 36 months and requires 20 to 40 minutes to administer. It has recently been restandardized and in its present form is a fairly reliable and valid instrument. The manual accompanying this assessment is complete, although somewhat complicated. The novice examiner is advised to seek assistance in learning to use this tool.

Either the Bayley or the revised Gesell will provide the clinician with a broader view of the child's total development. The gross motor information from these developmental assessments will not be specific enough for a therapist evaluating a child with spina bifida. The additional information on fine motor, language, personal-social, and cognitive development, however, is sufficient and will be most important in planning an effective intervention program.

Various tests are available as screening tools to test visual motor integration and perception.[10]

The Developmental Test of Visual-Motor Integration (V.M.I.) is an early screening tool to aid in diagnosis of learning problems in children. It assesses integration of visual perception and motor control. The test takes 10 to 15 minutes to complete and requires the child to be able to copy designs. It is norm referenced and is available for use with children from 2 years 6 months to 19 years 0 months. Extensive standardization throughout the United States has occurred.[11]

The Motor- Free Visual Perception Test (MVPT) and the Test of Visual Perceptual Skills (TVPS) can be used to determine the child's visual perceptual processing skills based on a nonmotor assessment of these skills. Both tests evaluate visual discrimination, visual memory, spatial relations, figure/ground, and visual closure. The TVPS also evaluates form constancy and sequential memory. The MVPT can be used with children from 4 to 8 years of age, and the TVPS can be used with children from 4 to 12 years of age. Both tests are easy and quick to administer (less than 15 minutes) and, based on the examiner's experience and training, interpretations can be made with prescription for remediation. The MVPT was standardized on a large sample of children in 22 states, and the TVPS was standardized on a sample of children in San Francisco.[25,40]

The Bruininks-Oseretsky Test of Motor Proficiency can be used to evaluate the higher level child with spina bifida. Fine Motor subtests of response speed, visual motor control, and upper limb speed and dexterity, can be used to assist in evaluating areas of fine motor control and coordination difficulties. This test has been standardized on a large sample of children from 4½ through 14½ years of age.[16]

The Sensory Integration and Praxis Tests (SIPT),[6] formerly the Southern California Sensory Integration Tests (SCSIT), may be used to assess the older child's sensorimotor function. Although these tests were designed to detect the presence of learning disabilities, they can be used with the child with spina bifida to document learning difficulties and the extent of impairment of the sensory systems. They often can be used to reassure the classroom teacher and parents that learning problems do indeed exist and have a suspected neurological base. These tests were standardized on 4- to 10-year-olds and will have limited value if used on children much older or those with severe perceptual or fine motor involvement. The SIPT battery can be given only by certified examiners, usually occupational or physical therapists.[4]

With a firm database provided by a thorough physical/occupational therapy evaluation and referrals to other professionals as appropriate, a reasonable treatment plan can be established and updated as necessary.

TREATMENT PLANNING AND REHABILITATION RELATED TO SIGNIFICANT STAGES OF RECOVERY
Newborn to toddler (preambulatory phase)

Stage 1: before closure of myelomeningocele—newborn. Physical therapy management of the infant in stage 1 is limited by his or her medical condition (Table 15-1). Attempts can be made, however, to prevent deformity and to maintain ROM while giving stimulation to provide as normal an environment as possible.

In addition to evaluation, the therapist may begin some early intervention measures that can be continued and expanded postsurgically. ROM and positioning in prone or sidelying may be initiated to prevent or decrease contractures in the lower extremities. If club feet are present, soft tissue stretching may be indicated. Stretching begins distally on the soft tissue of the forefoot and proceeds proximally toward the calcaneus. This is done to take advantage of the pliability of soft tissue structures and to minimize fixed deformity later. In addition, taping may be used to maintain optimal ROM and alignment between periods of stretching.[52] When treating the newborn before surgery, great care must be taken to avoid contaminating an open sac, which is usually covered with a sterile dressing and kept moist with a saline solution.[76]

Stage 2: after surgery, during hospitalization—newborn to infant. Therapeutic intervention during stage 2 will be more aggressive than before surgery but will often be limited by the infant's neurological and orthopedic status. A major goal during this stage is to prevent contracture and to maintain ROM.

Traditional ROM can be taught to nursing staff and family. It also can be carried out while the child is being held at the adult's shoulder or prone over the adult's lap. These positions allow closeness between the caregiver and infant,

Table 15-1. Summary of treatment planning and rehabilitation related to significant stages of recovery

Stage of recovery	Major physical therapy goals	Physical therapy management
Stage 1: before surgical closure of sac	Prevent contractures and deformity	ROM, positioning
	Encourage normal sensorimotor development	Graded auditory and visual stimuli
Stage 2: after surgery during hospitalization	Prevent contracture and deformity	ROM taught to hospital personnel and family Positioning in prone and side-lying
	Encourage normal sensorimotor development	Providing toys of various colors, textures, and shapes Graded auditory and visual stimuli—music boxes, squeaky toys, brightly colored objects Therapeutic handling to encourage good head and trunk control
Stage 3: condition stabilized, preambulatory	Encourage normal development sequence	Work in sitting on head righting and equilibrium reactions Eye-hand coordination activities Early weight bearing on lower extremities Encourage prone progression Weight shifting in standing frame Comprehensive home program
Stage 4: toddler through preschool	Begin ambulation	Choose appropriate orthotic device Gait training Development and strengthening of righting and equilibrium reactions
	Continue development in cognitive and psychosocial areas	Consider placement in 0-3 stimulation group Public preschool program Continue home program
	Collaborate goals with other team members	Open communication with other team members
Stage 5: primary school through adolescence	Reevaluate ambulation potential	Replace orthotic device as necessary Wheelchair prescriptions as necessary
	Maintain present level of functioning	Teach locomotion activities Maintain strength in trunk and extremities
	Prevent skin breakdown as child becomes more sedentary	Teach skin care
	Promote independence in self-care skills	Work with team members to teach dressing, feeding, hygiene, and bowel and bladder care
	Remediate any perceptual-motor problems	Provide program/activities for sensorimotor integration
	Provide appropriate adaptive devices	Check for fit and proper use of adaptive devices
	Promote self-esteem and social-sexual adjustment	Collaborate with other team members in counseling efforts

thus encouraging maximum relaxation and interaction between them.

Because of their medical conditions, hospitalized infants often experience early separation from their parents. Teaching the family to handle the child as described above may enhance parent-infant bonding. Adequate bonding is essential for normal psychosocial development to occur.

When the child is not being handled, resting positions can be used to maintain ROM and enhance development. The prone position is the most advantageous, because it prevents hip flexion contractures and encourages development of extensor musculature as the child lifts his or her head. Side-lying, which allows the hands to come to midline and

generally encourages symmetrical posture, can be used for alternating positioning. As much as possible, the supine position should be avoided because the child is most dominated by primitive reflexes and the effects of gravity in this position. For example, for the child with spina bifida with CNS involvement in addition to the spinal cord lesion, the effects of the tonic labyrinthine reflex combined with paralytic lower extremities make movement from the supine position extremely difficult.

A normal sensory experience should be presented to the child in spite of the hospital setting. Toys of various colors, textures, and shapes should be available. Musical mobiles held low enough for the child to reach provide a variety of sensory experiences. Stimuli such as squeaky toys or the human face and voice can be used to encourage visual and auditory tracking. Controlled stimulation relevant to the infant's neurological state, rather than overstimulation, should be the rule. Depending on the age of the child, appropriate learning situations must be presented to provide the child with as normal an environment as possible for perceptual and cognitive growth.

A major physical therapy goal will be to guide the child through the developmental sequence, ultimately preparing him or her to assume the upright posture. In this immediate postsurgical stage, primary emphasis will be on attaining good head and trunk control and eliciting appropriate righting reactions. For example, the child can be seated on the therapist's lap, facing the therapist, and alternately lowered slowly backwards and side-to-side. This will help to stimulate head righting and strengthen neck and abdominal muscles. Weight shifting in the prone-on-elbows position is another good activity for enhancing development of head and trunk control.

Developmental handling may be limited by frequent shunt revisions that require the infant to be kept flat for days. Increased muscle tone caused by CNS involvement must also be normalized before appropriate developmental steps can be achieved. For example, when increased tone is evidenced by shoulder girdle retraction, inhibitory techniques must be applied before normal head control can be established. The arms must be moved forward, out of the abnormal retracted position, while rotation of the shoulder girdle on the pelvis is initiated. (For additional information on normalization of tone, refer to Chapters 6, 8, and 9.)

This second stage ends as the child is discharged from the hospital. The child will be followed closely by the rehabilitation team, which may include a neurosurgeon, an orthopedist, a urologist, a nurse clinician, a physical therapy/occupational therapy (PT/OT) team, and a social worker. Before discharge, a definitive home program as well as referral to a local PT/OT/0-3 program should be given to the family, as the child will most likely require ongoing therapy.

Stage 3: condition stabilized—infant to toddler. In this stage of rehabilitation, the major emphasis is on preparing the child mentally and physically for walking. Goals of preventing contractures and maintaining ROM will remain throughout the child's life. Unless this is done, ambulation not only becomes more difficult but often impossible. If possible, prone positioning during play and sleeping assists greatly in stretching tight musculature. Resting splints for the lower extremities or a total body splint (TBS) can be used as necessary to position and maintain ROM and alignment.

Assuming that the child has previously gained good head and trunk control, the next step would be development of sitting equilibrium reactions. As sitting balance improves, fine motor and eye-hand coordination activities should be introduced. Upper extremity functioning is often overlooked in the child with spina bifida, whose problems appear to be concentrated in the lower extremities. Because most spina bifida children show decreased fine motor coordination,[76] this problem should be addressed as developmentally appropriate. The normal infant begins to reach and grasp by 6 months of age;[24] therefore the child with spina bifida must be given ample opportunities to practice and to perfect these skills at an early age. Referral to and consultation with occupational therapy at this age is highly recommended.

Early weight bearing is also of utmost importance, both physiologically and psychologically.[103] The upright position has beneficial effects on circulation and renal and bladder functioning, as well as on the promotion of bone growth[47] and density.[101] Psychologically, weight bearing in an upright posture allows a normal view of the world and contributes to more normal perceptual, cognitive, and emotional growth. One way to achieve this weight bearing is in the kneeling position. This is developmentally appropriate, because children 8 to 10 months old frequently use kneeling as a transition from all fours to standing.

Because young infants are frequently held in the standing position and bounced on their parents' laps, it is appropriate to introduce this form of weight bearing on the lower extremities from birth onward. Failure to do so will deprive the spina bifida child of the normal experience of standing at a very early age. When standing these children, however, care must be taken to see that the lower extremities are in good alignment and that undue pressure is not exerted on them (Fig. 15-10). In this way the risk of fractures is

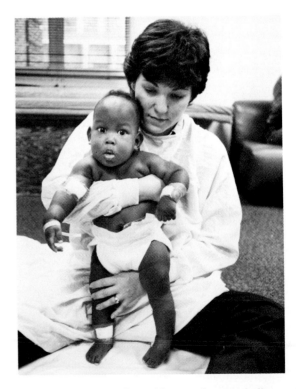

Fig. 15-10. Assisted standing with normal postural alignment.

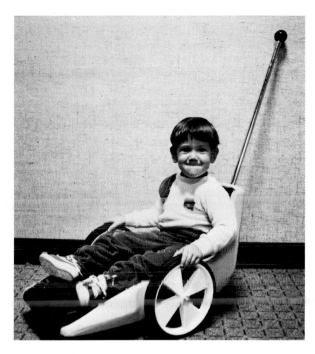

Fig. 15-11. Caster cart used for independent mobility.

minimized, and a normal weight-bearing experience is provided.

Following a normal developmental sequence, the child with spina bifida will usually begin some form of prone progression as trunk and upper-extremity stability improve. This is a significant phase of development, because it allows for the development of a sensorimotor base, as the child expands environmental horizons.[60] During this phase of high mobility, anesthetic skin must be checked for injury frequently and often protected by heavier clothing. This may help to prevent any major skin breakdown, which could significantly delay the rehabilitation process.

For some children with high-level lesions where prone mobility is not safe or practical for long distances, a caster cart (Fig. 15-11) may be used.[60] This provides the child with a means of exploring the environment safely but independently.

When the child attempts to pull to a standing position or would be expected to do so normally (at 10 to 12 months of age), the use of a standing device is indicated. Generally, a **standing A-frame** is the first orthosis chosen.[60] This is a relatively inexpensive tubular frame to which adjustable parts are attached (Fig. 15-12). Because it is not custom made, it can be fitted fairly quickly, although adjustments may be necessary to accommodate spinal deformities. This standing device offers support of the trunk, hips, and knees and leaves the hands free for other activities. Time spent in

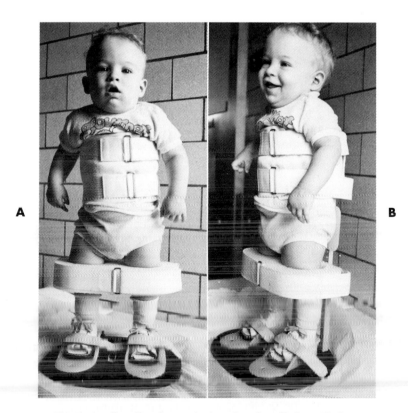

Fig. 15-12. Standing frame. **A,** Anterior view. **B,** Lateral view.

the standing frame should be increased gradually. This will allow the child to adjust to the upright position in terms of muscle strength, endurance, blood pressure, and pressure on skin surfaces.

After children have built up a tolerance for standing, they may be taught to move in the device by shifting their weight from side to side. Initial shifting of weight onto one side of the body is necessary to allow the other side to move forward. This preliminary weight shift is also a prerequisite for developing equilibrium reactions in the standing position and thus will prepare the child for later ambulation. As the child shifts weight, the trunk musculature on the weight-bearing side should elongate and shorten on the non-weight-bearing side as muscle strength allows. This normal reaction to weight shifting also includes righting of the head and should be monitored closely by the therapist for completeness.

During this preambulatory stage therapy goals may be accomplished through a comprehensive home program, with frequent checks to note progress or problems and to change the program accordingly. For the more involved child, increased frequency of direct intervention may be indicated to achieve optimal developmental progress.

The program often must be reevaluated and goals changed, if conditions such as shunt malfunctions or fractures occur. The warning signs for shunt dysfunctions are generally those previously described for suspected hydrocephalus. In addition, swelling along the shunt site may indicate a malfunction. Swelling and local heat or redness of a limb are the usual signs of a fracture. The limb may also look out of alignment. Fever may accompany a fracture. As mentioned previously, these fractures generally heal quickly with proper medical intervention and interrupt rehabilitation efforts minimally.

Toddler through adolescent (ambulatory phase)

Stage 4: toddler through preschool. This period in development marks the end of infancy and the beginning of childhood. For the normal child who has developed a strong sensorimotor foundation, physical development will be marked by increased coordination and refinement of movement patterns. In addition, a great variety of motor skills will be achieved as the normal child learns to throw, catch, run, hop, and jump. This is also a period of great cognitive growth, as children's use of mental imagery and physical knowledge of their environments expand. Concepts of size, number, color, form, and space are all developing. Emotionally, most children are becoming more independent and begin to break away from the sheltered environment of the home. They are now more interested in interacting with others and become social beings to a greater extent.

All of these changes in physical, cognitive, and emotional development will be evident in the child with spina bifida, although the degree depends on the extent of the disability. It is of utmost importance to be aware of the characteristics of normal development, so that they can be nurtured and enhanced in the disabled child.[90]

Goals for this as for any other stage must address not only physical but cognitive and emotional development. The most obvious goal at this stage is to progress the child who is already standing to an ambulatory status. Even the child with a low thoracic lesion can usually manage some form of ambulation.

Thus far, the child has learned to shift weight in the standing frame. By rotating the trunk toward the weighted side, the non-weight-bearing side can be shifted forward (Fig. 15-13). By reversing the weight shift, the opposite side can be moved forward and a type of "pivoting-forward" progression can be accomplished. To maintain balance while shifting, the child may initially use a two-wheeled walker. The therapist may help initiate weight shift and trunk rotation by alternately pulling the arms forward.[44]

Once the child has gained this form of mobility, the type of permanent bracing chosen will depend on the level of the lesion. For thoracic and high-level lumbar lesions, a parapodium is often chosen. The parapodium was developed by the Ontario Crippled Children's Center in 1970 and is similar to the standing frame, except that hinges at the hips and knees allow for sitting and standing.[44] It too can be adjusted for growth and can accommodate orthopedic deformities. As with the standing frame, proper alignment of the parapodium is critical. The therapist, in conjunction with the orthotist, should check for correct standing alignment. The prevention of additional orthopedic deformities, development of good muscular control, and normal body image depend on a good-fitting orthosis.

After a pivoting gait is learned with the parapodium, a

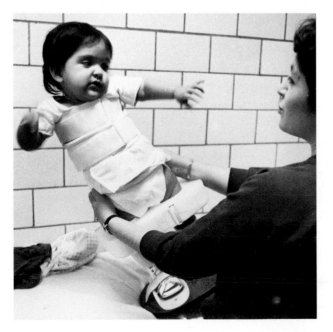

Fig. 15-13. Weight shift and forward rotation in standing frame.

swing-to or swing-through gait can be attempted. By 4 to 5 years of age, a swing-through gait, with the child using Lofstrand crutches, can usually be accomplished.[44]

Variations of the parapodium are appearing that allow for easier locking and unlocking of hip and knee joints.[15] A swivel or pivot walker also may be attached to the foot plate to allow for crutchless walking.

Another type of orthosis for the child with a thoracic or high lumbar lesion is the Orlau swivel walker. It consists of modular design similar to the standing frame, with a chest strap and knee blocks attached to swiveling foot plates.[18] Rather than the whole base moving forward, as when weight is shifted in the parapodium, in the swivel walker each foot plate is spring loaded and is able to swivel forward independently. This allows for independent balance on one foot and therefore crutchless ambulation. The Orlau swivel walker is manufactured in Shrewsbury in the United Kingdom, and kits to be assembled may be obtained from there (see Appendix B).[110]

Both the parapodium and swivel walker have had some problems with instability, ease of application, and cosmesis. New designs attempt to correct these problems. Nevertheless, existing limitations in the parapodium and swivel walker, particularly energy cost of walking, slow rate of locomotion, and cosmesis, have limited their use, primarily to the younger child.[100] These devices, however, remain an effective means of preventing musculoskeletal deformities caused by wheelchair positioning. They also enhance social-emotional development gained from the upright position.[18] Another option for the higher-level child with good sitting balance is the **reciprocating gait orthosis (RGO).**[31] This brace consists of bilateral long-leg braces with a pelvic band and thoracic extension if necessary. The hip joints are connected by a cable system that can work in two ways: If the child has active hip flexors, he or she can activate the cable system by shifting weight and flexing the non-weight-bearing extremity. This brings the weight-bearing extremity into relative extension in preparation for the next step. Without hip flexors, the child extends his or her trunk over one extremity, thus positioning it in relative extension. By virtue of the cable system, the non-weight-bearing extremity moves into flexion, thus initiating a step.[65] Several types of the RGO are in use including the dual cable LSU or the single cable Jim Campbell type.[84]

Most recently the Isocentric Reciprocal Gait Orthosis (I-RGO) has been used for children with high level spina bifida. It has a more cosmetic and efficient design as compared to the LSU or dual cable type RGO. This new "cable less" brace has two to three times less friction and therefore is more energy efficient. The brace stabilizes the hip, knee, and ankle joints and balances the person enabling him or her to stand "hands free" without the use of crutches or a walker. The I-RGO was designed by Wallace Motloch, CO, and is manufactured in Redwood City, California, at the Center for Orthotics Design, Inc. (Fig. 15-14).[84]

A more common means of maintaining the upright position has been through the use of long- or short-leg metal braces. In the 1970s conventional metal bracing was largely replaced by polypropylene braces. These plastic orthoses are considerably lighter than metal bracing and therefore reduce the energy cost of walking for the child with spina bifida.[62] They allow close contact and can be slipped into the shoe rather than being worn externally, thus affording the patient a better fitting, more cosmetic orthosis. These polypropylene braces are generally most effective with lower lumbar lesions where only short-leg bracing is required (Fig. 15-15). Although these braces cannot be worn by everyone, they have greatly improved the rehabilitation potential of those able to use them.

The type of orthosis chosen (long-leg, with or without pelvic band, or short-leg) depends on the level of the myelomeningocele and the muscle power within that level. Because lesions are frequently incomplete, muscle strength must be assessed accurately before bracing is prescribed. Independent sitting balance with hands free also is a prerequisite for use of long- or short-leg braces. Even children with L3-L4 lesions, who demonstrate incomplete knee extension, may be able to use a short-leg brace with an

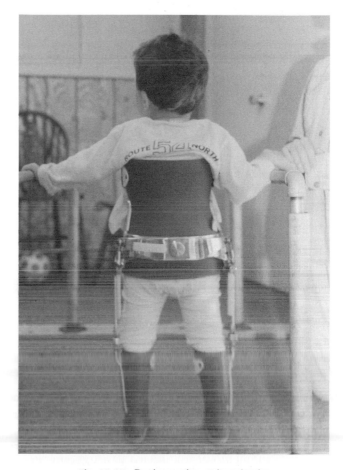

Fig. 15-14. Reciprocating gait orthosis.

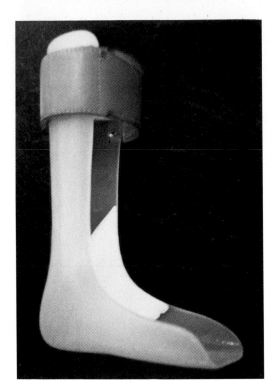

Fig. 15-15. Polypropylene ankle-foot orthosis.

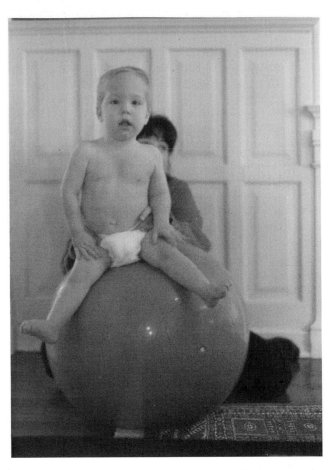

Fig. 15-16. Balance and strengthening exercises done on a movable surface.

anterior shell rather than requiring long-leg bracing.[26] This **crouch-control AFO** (CCAFO) will prevent a "crouch" gait pattern by improving knee extension during gait[12] (Fig. 15-14, *A*) The physical therapist must work in conjunction with the orthopedist and orthotist to have each child fitted with the minimum amount of bracing, which allows for joint stability and a good gait pattern (see Chapter 32).

Children ambulating with ankle-foot orthoses often show excessive rotation at the knee because of the lack of functioning lateral hamstrings. Rather than going to a higher level of bracing, a twister cable can be added, which often decreases the rotary component during gait.[26] Twister cables can be heavy duty torsion or more flexible elastic webbing depending on function. Typically, the young child who is just beginning to pull to stand and remains reliant on floor mobility as the primary means of mobility should have elastic twisters prescribed to allow for ease of creeping and transitions. The older and more active child will require heavy duty torsion cables.

For children with a low lumbar or sacral lesion, often a polypropylene shoe insert to control foot position is the only bracing needed. These inserts fit snuggly inside the shoe and help to control calcaneal and forefoot instabilities.[60]

Gait training, begun as the child first starts to stand, can now continue in a more formalized manner. Using the appropriate orthosis and assistive devices (walker, crutches, or cane), each child must be helped to achieve the most efficient and effective gait pattern possible. As a part of gait

training, the child should be taken out of the bracing and "challenged" so that righting and equilibrium reactions can be developed to their maximum. For example, having a child maintain balance while sitting on a ball or other movable surface (tilt board, trampoline) requires the participation of all available musculature (Fig. 15-16). These unconventional "gait-training" techniques can be used to improve muscle strength in general and to improve the gait pattern when bracing is reapplied.

Various forms of therapeutic exercise can be used with the spina bifida child to strengthen existing musculature. The work of Sullivan and others[115] can assist the therapist in this regard. These authors approach exercise from a developmental proprioceptive neuromuscular facilitation (PNF) point of view. A more traditional approach to therapeutic exercise can be found in Basmajian's work.[9] It includes a chapter on exercises in water, which may add an interesting adjunct to the therapeutic program for the child with spina bifida. Pearson and Williams[92] give the therapist a variety of therapeutic approaches that could be applied to the child with spina bifida. Finally, Williamson[119] provides a comprehensive overview of children with spina bifida. Especially pertinent is the chapter on sensorimotor assessment and intervention.

Regardless of the strengthening program chosen, the pediatric therapist has the special task of using creativity to involve the child in therapeutic "play activities." For example, when doing resisted rolling, a child could pretend to be trying to get away from attacking alligators. The ideas for creative activities are limitless, but essential, for combining therapy with age-appropriate cognitive abilities.

Gait training and muscle strengthening are not the only consideration of the therapist. How cognitive and psychosocial development can be enhanced during this stage of the child's development is also important. One appropriate solution is to place the child in a 0- to 3-year stimulation group. While these groups may vary in the services they provide, most usually include age-appropriate play activities and some type of parental counseling. In addition, many offer therapeutic intervention from physical, occupational, and speech therapists. This intervention may occur in groups or individually.

Besides the socialization that 0- to 3-year groups provide for the disabled child, they also teach the child age-appropriate activities of daily living (ADL), such as dressing and undressing. At this age ADL skills are more appropriately taught in a group setting than individually. For many children the 0-to-3 program, along with individualized therapy, is sufficient to enhance development in the physical, cognitive, and psychosocial realms.[120]

Presently, when children reach age 3, public school education becomes available to them. The preschool program continues to offer the same fundamental benefits as the 0-to-3 program. It is the role of the hospital-based therapist to communicate the specific needs of each child entering the public school system. In this way continuity in the child's rehabilitation program is preserved.

The rehabilitation team, usually headed by a pediatrician or clinical nurse specialist, continues to follow the child closely during this stage. The neurosurgeon will check shunt functioning and perform revisions as necessary. The orthopedist will supervise bracing efforts to prevent and correct deformities in the spine and lower extremities. Well-child care and general medical treatment is the responsibility of the pediatrician on the team. The urologist continues to monitor renal functioning while keeping the child dry and free of infection. At this stage, bowel and bladder training will usually be taught to the child and family by the clinical nurse specialist. This clinician generally initiates this training, following age-appropriate developmental guidelines.

Bladder training usually consists of transferring the job of intermittent catheterization from the parents to the child. Children as young as 3 years, but certainly by the age of 5, can learn CIC in a short period of time.[9] Children may first practice on dolls with male and female genitalia. Next, using mirrors to understand their own genitalia anatomy, they are able to accomplish the technique on themselves. CIC in conjunction with pharmacotherapy is useful in achieving continence in spina bifida children.[9] Another method of bladder training recently being used in the United States is intravesical transurethral bladder stimulation. This technique has allowed children with neurogenic bladder to rehabilitate their bladder function so that they can detect bladder fullness and generate effective destrusor contractions leading to improved continence.[57,58]

Bowel training can be achieved through proper diet, regular evacuation times, and appropriate use of stool softeners and suppositories.[57,66] Constipation (and resulting bypass diarrhea) can be prevented by proper habit training and use of fiber supplements. Stool softeners (not laxatives and enemas) and suppositories should be used to keep the stools soft and to help stimulate evacuation. Finally, toilet training, which amounts to scheduled toileting in time with the stool stimulants, usually achieves bowel continence. Consistency at each step along the way is the key to successful bowel training. A therapist may be called on to assist the parents and child in obtaining independence in this ADL activity.

Other members of the team, such as a psychologist, pedodontist, social worker, and dietitian, continue to function in their appropriate roles, interacting with the child and family as necessary. Physical and occupational therapists, as members of the team, must be sure that their treatment plans collaborate with the efforts of other team members.

Stage 5: primary school through adolescence. This stage of development is marked by less rapid growth than earlier childhood but ends with a period of rapid physiological growth.[90] Children in the 6- to 10 age group are interested in a wider variety of physical activities as they challenge their bodies to perform. The adolescent, however, is going through a period of great sexual differentiation as primary and secondary sexual characteristics develop more fully.

Cognitively, children are able to solve problems in a more sophisticated manner, although they revert to illogical thinking with complex problems. As they reach adolescence, they become capable of hypothetical reasoning, and their thought processes approach that of adults.[90]

Emotionally, the 6- to 10-year-old is in a period of relative calm. Children are very interested in school work and are eager to produce. During this period, they are building the skills of the future, preparing them for adult work.

Adolescence is a stormy emotional period. Adolescents remain in turmoil as they seek their identities through social, social, and vocational activities. As their value systems develop, they feel less ambivalence between remaining as children or striving for independence.

A therapy program must be designed to meet the individual's needs in each area. Age alone does not determine the appropriate therapeutic goals. Goals that are not suited for the child's cognitive and emotional needs, in addition to physical needs, will be doomed to failure before they are attempted. For example, an 18-month-old may have the physical capabilities to ambulate independently with crutches and braces. The child may not, however, have the cognitive skills necessary to learn a 4-point gait or be ready emotionally to separate from his or her mother for intensive therapy sessions. A more realistic goal may be to let the child walk, holding onto furniture (cruising) while a wheeled walker for more independent ambulation is slowly introduced. Another alternative to using a conventional walker is to encourage the child to play with push-toys such as grocery carts and baby buggies.

As the energy cost of walking becomes too high, it often becomes appropriate for the adolescent to use a wheelchair for locomotion. To a teenager whose emotional needs include a strong peer identity, being confined to a wheelchair may be devastating. Appropriate alternatives may be to delay the decision to use a wheelchair full-time or to limit ambulation to short distances or to those places most important to the child. Again, goals must be tailored to the child's needs and encompass his or her whole being.

In accordance with the child's growth spurts, frequent adjustment or reordering of bracing will be necessary. Continual reevaluation of orthotic needs may reveal that the level of bracing may decrease as the child grows and becomes stronger; the opposite development is also a possibility.

Usually during this stage, if it has not occurred previously, the evaluation of future ambulation potential will occur. This evaluation is frequently requested by the child whose larger size and limited abilities make ambulation more difficult each day. It must be remembered that strength does not increase in the same proportion as body weight.[93] Ambulation, although possible for the young child, may be impossible for that same person as a young adult.

While no guidelines will include every patient, generally children with thoracic-level lesions are rarely ambulators by the late teens.[32,60,76] Those with upper lumbar lesions may be household ambulators with long-leg bracing but will require wheelchairs for quick mobility as adults. With low lumbar lesions, most adults can become community ambulators. Patients with sacral-level lesions are usually able to ambulate freely within the community. Many require minimal bracing and ambulate without assistive devices.[32,60,76] It must be remembered that ambulatory status is not determined by level of the lesion alone. The muscle power available, degree of orthopedic deformity, age, height, weight of the patient, and of course motivation are also determining factors.[26,35,60,61,103]

Because a large number of older spina bifida children will become wheelchair dependent, potential problems connected with a sedentary existence must be explored. Skin care, always a concern for the child with spina bifida, becomes a priority for the constant sitter. Mirrors may be used for self-inspection of the skin twice daily.[51] Well-constructed foam, gel, or air cell seat cushions are essential for distributing pressure evenly. Children should be taught frequent weight shifting within the chair to relieve pressure areas. Clothing should not be constricting but heavy enough to protect sensitive skin from wheelchair parts. Children must also be taught to avoid extremes of temperature and environmental hazards such as radiators, sharp objects, and abrasive surfaces.[51] The therapist must reinforce the importance of skin care to prevent setbacks in the rehabilitation process that may result when skin breakdown develops.

Children with higher-level lesions may need spinal support to prevent deformities. Polyethylene body jackets can be used to provide this support and, hopefully, prevent the progression of any paralytic deformities.[60] Whatever type of device or wheelchair padding is used, the therapist must check to see that weight is distributed equally through both buttocks and that the spine is supported as necessary.

Part of the therapeutic intervention will be to provide strengthening exercises or activities to be done out of the supporting orthosis. This is necessary to maintain existing trunk strength and to preserve the child's present level of functioning.

Generally, in late childhood or early adolescence, orthopedic deformities that have been gradually developing require surgical intervention. Progressive scoliosis or kyphosis may require internal fixation when conservative methods fail.[78] Often sectioning of contracted muscles at the hip and knee is required.[32] The iliopsoas, adductors, and hamstrings are frequently the offending muscles. These surgeries, followed by strengthening exercises and gait training, often add to the ambulatory life of the child with spina bifida. For example in a child who displays an extreme lordotic posture, hip flexors may be contracted and require surgery to lengthen them. A postoperative therapeutic program might include periods of prone lying to prevent future contractures and strengthening of hip extensors and abdominals that were previously overstretched by the lordotic position.

Of primary importance during this stage is preparing the child for independence in ADL, which may be broken down into self-care, locomotion-related, and social interaction activities.[109]

In conjunction with the nurse and occupational therapist, self-care skills of dressing, eating and food preparation, general hygiene, and bowel and bladder care can be addressed. Because the adolescent is so concerned with achieving independence, he or she is more likely to comply with a regimen of strengthening exercises, if shown how they relate to functional independence. A creative therapist may, for example, incorporate trunk stability and upper-extremity strengthening work in activities such as gourmet cooking or getting ready for a dance.

Locomotion activities should include all gait-related skills, such as falling down, getting up, or ambulation on various terrains. Transfers of all types are also included in locomotion activities. Again, a creative therapeutic program helps to make achievement of skills more palatable. For example, school-aged children may enjoy a competitive relay race situation, where each child falls, gets up, walks across the room, and sits down in a chair safely. This type of activity combines gait-training activities with group socialization and may meet a variety of goals (motor and psychosocial) at the same time.

Achievement of independence in ADL for the child and adult with spina bifida does not depend solely on the level of paralysis.[109] Also important are psychosocial and environmental factors. Mean ages for the achievement of various ADL activities have been developed and may assist the therapist in establishing realistic therapeutic goals in this area.[109]

Often during this stage of recovery, the therapist may be asked to assist in assessing cognitive functioning. The perceptual/cognitive evaluations referred to earlier may be administered and the results interpreted for parents and school personnel.

As previously discussed, children with spina bifida have a general perceptual deficit,[29] which can be manifested in a variety of ways. First, the child may have difficulty recognizing objects and the relationships that they have to each other. They may therefore perceive their world in a distorted manner, thus making their reactions unstable and unpredictable. These perceptual difficulties will most likely affect academic learning and may associate failure with the learning process. Difficulties in attaining independence in ADL activities are also linked to perceptual problems. Finally, emotional disturbances may be attributed in part to the perceptual difficulties of the child with spina bifida.[41]

Remedial programs, such as the Frostig Program for the Development of Visual Perception, have been effective in improving the visual perception of spina bifida children.[41] Programs of this type are most effective when remediation begins early, preferably at or before the time the child enters school.

Children requiring programs for sensorimotor integration should be referred to a therapist certified in this area. If one is not available, many appropriate activities for sensorimotor integration may be adapted from Ayres[5] or Montgomery and Richter.[82]

Regardless of the school setting chosen for the child, the therapist should be able to serve the classroom teacher as a consultant. Advice on adaptive seating and therapeutic goals appropriate for the classroom will help ensure that the rehabilitation process will continue in the classroom, as well as promoting optimal conditions for learning.

When a child is going from a special to a regular school setting, the support of the therapeutic team is essential and invaluable. Teachers in the public school setting have had little exposure to handicapped children.[53] The teacher's expectations, as created by the therapist regarding the spina bifida child's special needs and abilities, often spell the difference between success and failure of this attempt at integration both academically and psychosocially. Even though the child may no longer require direct therapeutic intervention, periodic checks, including site classroom visits, are recommended to prevent minor problems from erupting into major ones. For example, bowel and bladder accidents can be avoided by scheduling regular times for toileting. The teacher may be able to make minor adjustments in the teaching schedule to accommodate for this scheduling. Also, full-control braces (from hip to ankles) may seem overwhelming to the layperson. If the teacher is shown how the braces lock and unlock to allow the child to sit or stand to walk, he or she may feel more at ease if ever called on to assist the child.

Physical therapy goals in this stage will be colored by the psychological perspective of the child. As the child nears adolescence, these psychosocial aspects become of paramount importance. While the physical therapist should not take on the role of the psychologist, collaborative efforts in the area of counseling will be necessary. Questions will arise many times during the physical/occupational therapy sessions, requiring factual answers that the therapist can and should provide.

Adolescents with spina bifida show great concern about self-esteem and social-sexual adjustment.[50] These concerns appear directly related to efficient bowel and bladder management.[64] Strategies to cope with bowel and bladder difficulties, as previously outlined, combined with appropriate emotional support from family and medical personnel will help to alleviate this concern.

Questions about sexuality may be brought up by either the parents or the child. Parents of children with spina bifida realize the need to teach their children about sexuality, feel inadequate about doing so, and are often reluctant to bring up questions to health professionals.[91] The therapist must be open, informed, and able to provide resources to both parents and children.

Generally, the sexual capacity of the female with spina bifida is near normal; that is, she has potential for a normal orgasmic response, is fertile, and can bear children.[22,55,76] The pregnancy, however, may be considered high risk, depending on existing orthopedic abnormalities. Affected males are frequently sterile and have small testicles and penises. Their potential for erection and ejaculation will depend on the level of the lesion.

In many cases psychological problems may be a primary cause of sexual failure.[76] It must be remembered that sexuality is not merely a process involving the genitals but depends on a positive body image and a feeling of self-esteem that is nurtured from birth.[27,61]

PSYCHOSOCIAL ADJUSTMENT TO CONGENITAL CORD LESIONS

The previous sections on goal setting and rehabilitation of the child with spina bifida have covered birth through adolescence. After adolescence, rehabilitation can be handled in much the same manner as an adult spinal cord injury. It will be important, however, to keep in mind the global effects of spina bifida on the growing child as he or she approaches adulthood.

Because of the congenital nature of spina bifida, psychological adjustment will be somewhat different than adjustment to a traumatic spinal cord injury. The psychological adjustment to this congenital disability must be considered from the perspective of the parents, the family, and of course the child.

A longitudinal study concerning the psychological aspects of spina bifida shows that the parents go through a series of steps in the adjustment process. From birth to about 6 months of age, the parents experience shock and bewilderment. Information given during this time may be rejected or misinterpreted. Health professionals therefore must be ready to repeat the same information to parents on several occasions during the first few years of the rehabilitation process.

The period of 6 to 18 months of the child's life may be the most stressful on parents. Frequent hospitalizations during this time place increased pressure on the whole family. Parents, now able to fully comprehend the implications of their child's disability, begin to worry about the future and the impact of the disability on the rest of the family structure.

The period from age 2 years through the preschool years is relatively peaceful. The parents are more concerned with toilet training, social acceptability, and general information on child rearing. They seem less aware of their child's mental limitations as he or she continues to develop into a relatively happy, well-adjusted child.

By the age of 6 years children are becoming more aware of their disabilities, and parents are concerned about problems that may arise as their children enter primary school. The child's psychological adjustment will depend, not on the severity of the disability, but primarily on the attitude of the parents and family and on the environmental conditions to which he or she is exposed.[64,88,99]

Some evidence indicates that children with spina bifida may grow up in extreme social isolation.[93] Being placed in special schools, they have little interaction with normal children their own age. Because of their disabilities, they are often denied small tasks or chores that promote a sense of responsibility in the growing child.[50,93] To promote emotional growth and psychological well-being, caregivers must be persuaded to "let go." Children with spina bifida must develop responsibility and independence by being given the chance to interact and even compete with their peers. As they approach adulthood, concerns of independent living situations and vocational placement must be addressed. With a foundation of strong support systems fostering emotional maturity, the future can be bright for the child with congenital spinal cord injury.

REFERENCES

1. Alexander MA and Steg NL: Myelomeningocele: comprehensive treatment, *Arch Phys Med Rehabil* 70:637-641, 1989.
2. Altshuler A and others: Even children can learn to do clean self-catheterization, *Am J Nurs* 77:97-101, 1977.
3. American Academy of Pediatrics, Action Committee on Myelodysplasia, Section on Urology: Current approaches to evaluation and management of children with myelomeningocele, *Pediatrics* 63(4):663-667, 1979.
4. Ayres AJ: *Southern California Sensory Integration Tests Manual,* Los Angeles, 1972, Western Psychological Services.
5. Ayres AJ: *Sensory integration and the child,* Los Angeles, 1979, Western Psychological Services.
6. Ayres AJ and Mailloux Z: *The Sensory Integration and Praxis Tests manual,* Los Angeles, 1988, Western Psychological Services.
7. Baker DA and Sherry CJ: Spina bifida and maternal Rh blood type, *Arch Dis Child* 54(7):567, 1979 (letter).
8. Banta JV, Benanni C, and Prebluda J: Latex anaphylaxis during spinal surgery in children with myelomeningocele, *Dev Med Child Neurol* 35:540-548, 1993.
9. Basmajian JV: *Therapeutic exercise,* ed 3, Baltimore, 1978, Williams & Wilkins.
10. Bayley N: *Manual for the Bayley Scales of Infant Development,* ed 2, San Antonio Tx, 1993, The Psychological Corp.
11. Beery KE: *The developmental test of visual-motor integration,* Cleveland, 1989, Modern Curriculum Press.
12. Berard C and others: Anticalcaneus carbon fibre orthosis for children with myelomeningocele, *Rev Chir Orthop* 76:222-225, 1990.
13. Brazelton TB: Neonatal Behavioral Assessment Scale, ed 2. In *Clinics in developmental medicine,* vol 88, Philadelphia, 1984, JB Lippincott.
14. Brocklehurst G: Spina bifida for the clinician. In *Clinics in developmental medicine,* vol 57, Philadelphia, 1976, JB Lippincott.
15. Brown JT and McLone DG: The effect of complications on intellectual function in 167 children with myelomeningocele, *Z Kinderchir* 34(2):117-120, 1981.
16. Bruininks RH: *Bruininks-Oseretsky test of motor proficiency examiner's manual,* 1987, Circle Pines, MN, American Guidance Service.
17. Burn J and Gibben D: May spina bifida result from an X-linked defect in a selective abortion method, *J Med Genet* 16(3):210-214, 1979.
18. Butler PB and others: Use of the Orlau Swivel Walker for the severely handicapped patient, *Physiotherapy* 88(11):324-326, 1982.
19. Byrd SE and Radkowski, MA: The radiological evaluation of the child with a myelomeningocele, *J Natl Med Assoc* 83(7):608-614, 1991.
20. Carstens C and Niethard FU: The current status of prenatal diagnosis of myelomeningocele-results of a questionnaire (German), *Geburtshilfe Frauenheilkd* 53(3):182-185, 1993.
21. Cash J: *Neurology for physiotherapists,* ed 2, Philadelphia, 1977, JB Lippincott.
22. Cass AS and others: Sexual function in adults with myelomenigocele, *J Urol* 136:425-426, 1986.
23. Charney EB, Melchionni JB, and Antonucci DL: Ventriculitis in newborns with myelomeningocele, *Am J Dis Child* 145(3):287-290, 1991.
24. Colangelo C, Bergen AS, and Gottlieb L: *A normal baby: the sensory-motor processes of the first year,* ed 2, Valhalla, NY, 1986, Valhalla Rehabilitation Publications.
25. Colarusso RP and Hammill DD: *Motor-free visual perception test manual,* revised Novato, Calif, 1995, Academic Therapy Publications.
26. De Souza LJ and Carroll N: Ambulation of the braced myelomeningocele patient, *J Bone Joint Surg* 58A(8):1112-1118, 1976.
27. Dorner S: Sexual interest and activity in adolescents with spina bifida, *J Child Psychiatry* 18:229-237, 1977.
28. Dounes E: Sacrococcygeal agenesis: a report of four new cases, *Acta Orthop Scand* 49:475-480, 1978.
29. Drago JR and others: The role of intermittent catheterization in the

management of children with myelomeningocele, *J Urol* 118:92-94, 1977.

30. Drummond DS and others: Post-operative neuropathic fractures in patients with myelomeningocele, *Dev Med Child Neurol* 23:147-150, 1981.

31. Durr-Fillaver Medical, Inc—Orthopedic Division: *LSU Reciprocating Gait Orthosis: a pictoral description and application model*, Chattanooga, Tenn, 1983.

32. Feiwell E: Surgery of the hip in myelomeningocele as related to adult goals, *Clin Orthop* 148:87-93, 1980.

33. Feiwell E and others: The effects of hip reduction on function in patients with myelomeningocele, *J Bone Joint Surg* 60A(2):169-173, 1978.

34. Ferguson-Smith MA and others: Avoidance of anencephalic and spina bifida births by maternal serum-alphafetoprotein screening, *Lancet* 1(8078):1330-1333, 1978.

35. Findley TW and others: Ambulation in the adolescent with myelomeningocele. I. Early childhood predictors, *Arch Phys Med Rehabil* 68:518-522, 1987.

36. Fiorentino MR: *Normal and abnormal development: the influence of primitive reflexes on motor development*, Springfield, Ill, 1972, Charles C Thomas.

37. Fiorentino MR: *Normal and abnormal development: the influence of primitive reflexes on motor development*, ed 2, Springfield, Ill, 1980, Charles C Thomas.

37a. Folio MR and Fewell RR: *Peabody Developmental Motor Scales and Activity Cards*, Allen, Tex, 1983, DLM Teaching Resources.

38. Gelb LN, editor: *Food and Drug Administration medical bulletin*, July 1991.

39. Gabrieli AP and others: *Tethered cord syndrome in myelomeningocele: surgical treatment and results*, International Spina Bifida Symposium, Chicago, Ill, May 1990.

40. Gardner MF: Test of visual-perceptual skills (non-motor) manual, San Francisco, 1988, Health Publishing.

41. Gluckman S and Barling J: Effects of a remedial program on visual-motor perception in spina bifida children, *J Genet Psychol* 136:195-202, June 1980.

42. Gold M and others: Intraoperative anaphylaxis: an association with latex sensitivity. *J Allergy Clin Immunol* 87:662-666, 1991.

43. Goldberg MF and Oakley GP Jr: Interpreting elevated amniotic fluid alpha-fetoprotein levels in clinical practice: use of the predictive value positive concept, *Am J Obstet Gynecol* 133(2):126-132, 1979.

44. Gram MC: *Using the parapodium: a manual of training techniques*, Rochester, NY, Eterna Press.

45. Greene WB and others: Effect of race and gender on neurological level in myelomeningocele, *Dev Med Child Neurol* 33(2):110-117, 1991.

46. Griscom NT and others: Amniography in second trimester diagnosis of myelomeningocele, *AJR* 133(6):1151-1156, 1979.

47. Guttman L: *Spinal cord injuries: comprehensive management and research*, ed 2, Oxford, 1976, Blackwell Publisher.

48. Haley SM and others: *Pediatric evaluation of disability inventory (PEDI): development, standardization and administration manual*, Boston, 1992, New England Medical Center Hospitals and PEDI Research Group.

49. Hall P and others: Scoliosis and hydrocephalus in myelomeningocele patients: the effect of ventricular shunting, *J Neurosurg* 50:174-178, 1979.

50. Hayden PW and others: Adolescents with myelodysplasia: impact of physical disability on emotional maturation, *Pediatrics* 64(1):53-59, 1979.

51. Hendry J and Geddes N: Living with a congenital anomaly, *Can Nurse* 74(6):29-33, 1978.

52. Hensinger RN and Jones ET: *Neonatal orthopedics*, New York, 1981, Grune & Stratton.

53. Hunt GM: Spina bifida: implications for 100 children at school, *Dev Med Child Neurol* 23:160-172, 1981.

54. Hyperthermia and meningomyelocele and anencephaly, *Lancet* 1(8067):769-770, 1978 (letter).

55. Hyperthermia and the neural tube, *Lancet* 2(8089):560-561, 1978 (editorial).

56. James WH: The sex ratio in spina bifida, *J Med Genet* 16(5):384-388, 1979.

57. Kaplan WE: Management of the urinary tract in myelomeningocele, *Prob Urol* 2(1):121-131, 1988.

58. Katona F and Berenyi M: Intravesical transurethral electrotherapy in meningomyelocele patients, *Acta Paediatr Hung* 16(3-4):363-374, 1975.

59. Knobloch H and others: *Manual of developmental diagnosis*, Hagerstown, Md, 1980, Harper & Row.

60. Kupka J and others: Comprehensive management in the child with spina bifida, *Orthop Clin North Am* 9(1):97-113, 1978.

61. Lee EH and Carroll NC: Hip stability and ambulatory status in myelomeningocele, *J Pediatr Orthop* 5:522-527, 1985.

62. Lindseth RE and Glancy J: Polypropylene lower extremity braces for paraplegia due to myelomeningocele *J Bone Joint Surg* 56A:556-563, 1974.

63. Lippman-Hand A and others: Indications for prenatal diagnosis in relatives of patients with neural tube defects, *Obstet Gynecol* 51(1):72-76, 1978.

64. McAndrew I: Adolescents and young people with spina bifida, *Dev Med Child Neurol* 21(5):619-629, 1979.

65. McCall RE and Schmidt WT: Clinical experience with reciprocal gait orthosis in myelodysplasia, *J Pediatr Orthop* 6:157-161, 1986.

66. McLone DG: *An introduction to spina bifida*, Chicago, 1980, Children's Memorial Hospital Myelomeningocele Service.

67. McLone DG: Results of treatment of children born with a myelomeningocele, *Clin Neurosurg* 30:407-412, 1983.

68. McLone DG: Treatment of myelomeningocele: arguments against selection, *Clin Neurosurg* 33:359-370, 1986.

69. McLone DG: Spina bifida today: problems adults face, *Semin Neurol* 9(3):169-175, 1989.

70. McLone DG and Dias, MS: Complications of myelomeningocele closure, *Pediatr Neurosurg* 17(5):267-273, 1991-1992.

71. McLone DG and Knepper PA: The cause of Chiari II malformation: a unified theory, *Pediatr Neurosci* 15:1-12, 1989.

72. McLone DG and Naidich TP: Tethered cord. In McLauren RL and others: *Pediatric neurosurgery*, ed 2, 1989.

73. McLone DG and others: *An introduction to hydrocephalus*, Chicago, 1982, Children's Memorial Hospital.

74. McLone DG and others: Neurolation: biochemical and morphological studies on primary and secondary neural tube defects, *Concepts Pediatr Neurosurg* 4:15-29, 1983.

75. McLone DG and others: Central nervous system infections as a limiting factor in the intelligence of children with myelomeningocele, *Pediatrics* 70(3):338-342, 1982.

76. McLaughlin JF and Shurtleff DB: Management of the newborn with myelodysplasia, *Clin Pediatr* 18(8):463-476, 1979.

77. McLaurin RL: *Myelomeningocele*, New York, 1977, Grune & Stratton.

78. Menelaus MB: Orthopaedic management of children with myelomeningocele: a plea for realistic goals, *Dev Med Child Neurol* 6(suppl 37):3-11, 1976.

79. Menelaus MB: *The orthopaedic management of spina bifida cystica*, ed 2, New York, 1980, Churchill Livingstone.

80. The Milani-Comparetti Motor Development Screening Test. *Test Manual*, ed 3 revised Meyer Children's Rehabilitation Institute, Omaha, Neb, 1992, University of Nebraska Medical Center.

81. Milerad J, Lagercrantz H, and Johnson P: Obstructive sleep apnea in Arnold Chiari malformation treated with acetazolamide, *Acta Pediatr* 81(8):609-612, 1992.

82. Montgomery MA and Richter E: Sensorimotor integration for

developmentally delayed children: a handbook, Los Angeles, 1977, Western Psychological Services.

83. Moore KL: *Before we are born: basic embryological and birth defects, revised reprint,* Philadelphia, 1974, WB Saunders.

84. Motloch W: Isocentric Reciprocal Gait Orthosis (I-RGO), Handout from the Center for Orthotics Design, Inc, Redwood City, California.

85. Muller EB and Nordwall A: Prevalence of scoliosis in children with myelomeningocele in western Sweden, *Spine* 17(9):1097-1102, 1992.

86. Nesbit DE and Ziter FA: Epidemiology of myelomeningocele in Utah, *Dev Med Child Neurol* 21(6):54-57, 1979.

87. Nevin NC and others: Influence of social class on the risk of recurrence of anencephalus and spina bifida, *Dev Med Child Neurol* 23:155-159, 1981.

88. Nielsen HH: A longitudinal study of the psychological aspects of myelomeningocele, *Scand J Psychol* 21:45-54, 1980.

89. Oakes WJ: Developmental anomalies and neurosurgical diseases in children, Chiari malformations, hydromyelia, syringomyelia, 2102-2124.

90. Papalia DE and Olds SW: *Human development,* New York, 1981, McGraw-Hill.

91. Passo S: Parents' perceptions, attitudes and needs regarding sex education for the child with myelomeningocele, *Res Nurs Health* 1(2):53-59, 1978.

92. Pearson PN and Williams CE: *Physical therapy services in developmental disabilities,* Springfield, Ill, 1976, Charles C Thomas.

93. Perspectives in spina bifida, *Br Med J* 2(6142):909-910, 1978 (editorial).

94. Pietrzyk JJ and Turowski G: Immunogenetic bases and congenital malformations: association of HLA-B27 with spina bifida, *Pediatr Res* 13(8):879-883, 1979.

95. Raimondi AJ and Soare P: Intellectual development in shunted hydrocephalic children, *Am J Dis Child* 127:664-671, 1974.

96. Ralis ZA and others: Changes in shape, ossification and quality of bones in children with spina bifida, *Dev Med Child Neurol* 18(6; suppl 37):29-41, 1976.

97. Riegel DH: Diagnoses and surgical treatment of tethered cord. Allegheny General Hospital, Pittsburgh Pa. Presented at the International Spina Bifida Symposium, Chicago, May, 1990.

98. Riegel DH: Lipomeningocele, surgical indications and results. Allegheny General Hospital, Pittsburg, Pa., Presented at International Spina Bifida Symposium, Chicago, May 1990.

99. Rogers BM: Comprehensive care for the child with a chronic disability, *Am J Nurs* 79(6):1106-1108, 1979.

100. Rose GK and Henshaw JT: *Swivel walkers for paraplegics—considerations and problems in their design and application,* Bull Prosthet Res 10(20):62-74, 1973.

101. Rosenstein BD and others: Bone density in myelomeningocele: the effects of ambulatory status and other factors, *Dev Med Child Neurol* 29:486-494, 1987.

102. Schaffer MF and Dias LS: *Myelomeningocele: orthopedic treatment,* Baltimore, Md, 1983, Williams & Wilkins.

103. Schopler SA and Menelaus MB: Significance of the strength of the quadriceps muscles in children with myelomeningocele, *J Pediatr Orthop* 7(5):507-512, 1987.

104. Singer HA and others: Spina bifida and anencephaly in the cape, *S Afr Med J* 53(16):626-627, 1978.

105. Slater JE: Rubber anaphylaxis, *N Engl J Med* 320:1126-1130, 1989.

106. Slater JE and others: Rubber specific IgE in children with spina bifida, *J Urol* 146:578-579, 1991.

107. Slater JE and others: Type 1 hypersensitivity to rubber, *Ann Allergy* 65:411-414, 1990.

108. Smithells RW and others: Apparent prevention of neural tube defects by periconceptional vitamin supplementation, *Arch Dis Child* 56:911-918, 1981.

109. Sousa JC and others: Developmental guidelines for children with myelodysplasia, *Phys Ther* 63(1):21-29, 1983.

110. Stallard J and others: Engineering design considerations of the Orlau Swivel Walker, *Eng Med* 15(1):3-8, 1986.

111. Stark GD: *Spina bifida: problems and management,* Boston, 1977, Blackwell Scientific Publications.

112. Stein SC and Schut L: Hydrocephalus in myelomeningocele, *Childs Brain* 5(4):413-419, 1979.

113. Storrs B: Selective posterior rhizotomy for treatment of progressive spasticity in patients with myelomeningocele, *Pediatr Neurosci* 13:135-137, 1987.

114. Storrs BB and McLone DG: Selective posterior rhizotomy in treatment of spasticity associated with myelomeningocele. In Marlin AE, editor: *Concepts Pediatr Neurosci* 9:173-177, 1989.

115. Sullivan PE and others: *An integrated approach to therapeutic exercise,* Reston, Va, 1982, Reston Publishing Co.

116. Tappit-Emas E: Spina bifida. In Tecklin JS, editor: *Pediatric physical therapy,* New York, 1989, JB Lippincott.

117. Vandertop P and others: Surgical decompression for symptomatic Chiari II malformation in neonates with myelomeningocele, *J Neurosurg* 77(4):541-544, 1992.

118. Wescott MA and others: Congenital and acquired orthopedic abnormalities in patients with myelomeningocele, *Radiographics* 12(6):1155-1173, 1992.

119. Williamson GG: *Children with spina bifida: early intervention and preschool programming,* Baltimore, Md, 1987, Paul H Brooks.

120. Wolf L: Development of self-care assessment tool for children with meningomyelocele, *Dev Disabilities* 10(2):2-6, 1987.

121. Zausmer E: Evaluation of strength and motor development in infants, *Phys Ther Rev* 33(12):621-628, 1953.

APPENDIX A   *AUDIOVISUAL RESOURCES*

Brazelton Neonatal Behavioral Assessment (16 mm films)
Part 1 Introduction
Part 2 Self-scoring exam
Part 3 Variations in Normal Behavior
  Educational Development Center
  55 Chapel Street
  Newton, MA 02160

APPENDIX B   *ORLAU SWIVEL ROCKER DISTRIBUTORS*

UK

  J Stallard
  Technical Director
  ORLAU
  Orthopaedic Hospital
  Oswestry
  Shropshire, SY107AG
  UK

US

  Mopac Ltd
  206 Chestnut Street
  Eau Claire, WI 54703
  715-832-1685

CHAPTER 16

Traumatic Spinal Cord Injury

Myrtice B. Atrice, Maureen Gonter, Doris A. Griffin, Sarah A. Morrison, and Shari L. McDowell

OUTLINE

Spinal cord lesions
  Tetraplegia
  Paraplegia
  Complete and incomplete lesions
  Clinical syndromes
Associated injuries
Mechanism of injury
Demographics
Acute medical management of SCI
  Pharmacological management
  Surgical stabilization
Complications
  Respiratory complications
  Skin compromise
  Orthostatic hypotension and edema
  Deep vein thrombosis and pulmonary embolism
  Apneic bradycardia
  Autonomic dysreflexia
  Thermoregulation
  Spasticity
  Flaccidity
  Pain
  Degenerative joint changes
  Urinary tract infection
  Contractures
  Heterotopic ossification

Osteoporosis
Spinal deformity
Gastrointestinal complications
Metabolic and endocrine changes
Rehabilitation
  Phases of rehabilitation
  Evaluation
  Goal setting
  Principles of treatment planning
  Acute rehabilitation
  Rehabilitation: achieving functional outcomes
  Rehabilitation: measuring functional outcomes
  Equipment
  Education
  Psychosocial issues in SCI rehabilitation
  Sexual issues
  Discharge planning
Outpatient services
Additional clinical considerations
  Lower extremity orthotic disposition
  Functional electrical stimulation for standing and
    ambulation
  Seating principles
Conclusion
Case 1 C5-C6 fracture

KEY TERMS

spinal cord injury (SCI)
tetraplegia
paraplegia
complete lesion
incomplete lesion
acute
autonomic dysfunction
decubitus ulcer
orthostatic hypotension
deep vein thrombosis (DVT)

pulmonary embolism (PE)
autonomic dysreflexia
spasticity
flaccidity
scoliosis
kyphosis
rehabilitation
outpatient
inpatient
orthotics

LEARNING OBJECTIVES

After reading this chapter, the student/therapist will:

1. Describe the etiology and demographics of spinal cord injury (SCI).
2. Discuss the pharmacological and acute medical management, and surgical stabilization of the SCI patient.
3. Describe the secondary complications of SCI, the appropriate interventions, and the impact of complications on the rehabilitation process.
4. Identify the basic components of the evaluation process.

5. Identify problems based on the evaluation, set appropriate goals, and plan an individualized treatment program to reach the goals.
6. Discuss patient progression and the process of discharge planning throughout the rehabilitation phases.
7. Identify equipment needs for a given SCI lesion.

Spinal cord injury (SCI) is a catastrophic condition that, depending on its severity, may cause dramatic changes in the victim's life. The effects of SCI not only have an impact on the lives of the patient and family, but society as a whole. SCI usually happens to active, independent people who at one moment are in control of their lives and in the next moment are paralyzed with loss of sensation and loss of bodily functions and dependence on others for their most basic needs. Patients need a well-coordinated, specialized rehabilitation program consisting of a team of physicians and health professionals to provide the tools necessary to develop a satisfying and productive postinjury lifestyle.[22,121]

This chapter provides a general overview of the management of the patient with SCI within the acute, rehabilitation, and postrehabilitation phases. The information is intended to aid health professionals in the treatment of individuals with SCI by providing guidelines to maximize effective intervention. These guidelines must be modified with each patient's input in order for the rehabilitation program to be truly successful in meeting individual needs.

SPINAL CORD LESIONS

SCI occurs when the spinal cord is damaged as a result of trauma, disease processes, or congenital defects. The clinical manifestations of the injury vary depending on the extent and location of the damage to the spinal cord.

Tetraplegia

Tetraplegia (quadriplegia) refers to impairment or loss of motor and/or sensory function due to damage of the cervical segments of the spinal cord.[103] Function in the upper extremities, lower extremities, and trunk is affected.[103]

Paraplegia

Paraplegia refers to impairment or loss of motor and/or sensory function due to damage of the thoracic, lumbar, or sacral segments of the spinal cord. Depending on the level of the damage, function may be impaired in the trunk and/or lower extremities. This term does not refer to lumbosacral plexus lesions.[103]

Complete and incomplete lesions

In a **complete lesion,** there is total absence of sensory and motor function in the lowest sacral segment.[103] Complete injuries often damage the nerve root in the foramen.[49] Function of this root originating from the proximal intact cord can be expected to return within 6 months.[49] The neurological level refers to the most caudal segment of the spinal cord with normal sensory and motor function. The neurological level is recorded separately for the left and right sides of the body. This level must not be preceded by abnormal segments.[103]

With **incomplete lesions** there is partial preservation of sensory and/or motor function below the neurological level and in the lowest sacral segment. Sensation in the anal mucocutaneous junction as well as deep anal sensation must be present for a lesion to be referred to as incomplete.[103]

Spinal shock occurs 30 to 60 minutes after spinal trauma and is characterized by flaccid paralysis and absence of all spinal cord reflex activity below the level of cord lesion.[66] This condition can last for a few hours to several weeks. The completeness of the lesion cannot be determined until spinal shock is resolved.

Clinical syndromes

Some incomplete lesions have a distinct clinical picture with specific signs and symptoms. An understanding of the various syndromes can be helpful to the patient's team in planning the rehabilitation program. Fig. 16-1 depicts the anatomy of the spinal cord.[43,49]

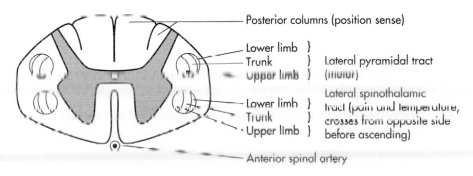

Fig. 16-1. Cross-sectional anatomy of the spinal cord.

Central cord syndrome. Hyperextension injuries usually result in a central cord syndrome.[43] This injury causes bleeding into the central gray matter of the spinal cord, resulting in more impairment of function in the upper extremities than in the lower extremities.[43] The majority of incomplete lesions result in this syndrome.[49] Approximately 77% of patients with central cord syndrome will attain ambulatory function, 53% bowel and bladder control, and 42% hand function.[18]

Anterior spinal artery syndrome. This syndrome is usually caused by flexion injuries in which bone or cartilage spicules compromise the anterior spinal artery.[43] Motor function and pain and temperature sensation are lost bilaterally below the injured segment.[43] The prognosis is extremely poor for return of bowel and bladder function, hand function, and ambulation.[18]

Brown-Sequard syndrome. Occasionally, as a result of penetrating injuries (gunshot or stab wounds), only one half of the spinal cord is damaged. The Brown-Sequard syndrome is characterized by ipsilateral loss of motor function and position sense and contralateral loss of pain sensation several levels below the lesion.[43] The prognosis for recovery is good. Nearly all patients attain some level of ambulatory function, 80% regain hand function, 100% bladder control, and 80% bowel control.[18]

Posterior cord syndrome. Posterior cord syndrome is very rare, resulting from compression by tumor or infarction of the posterior spinal artery. Clinically, proprioception, stereognosis, two-point discrimination and vibration sense are lost below the lesion.[43]

Cauda equina syndrome. Damage to the cauda equina occurs with injuries at the L1 vertebral level and below, resulting in a lower motor neuron lesion, which is usually an incomplete lesion. This lesion results in flaccid paralysis with no spinal reflex activity present.[66,103]

Conus medullaris syndrome. Injury of the sacral cord and lumbar nerve roots within the neural canal results in a clinical picture of lower extremity motor and sensory loss and areflexic bladder and bowel.[103]

ASSOCIATED INJURIES

The incidence of multiple trauma in the patient presenting with a traumatic SCI is 54%.[6] The most frequently associated injury is fracture, occurring in 29.2% of cases.[5] Loss of consciousness was associated with more than one fourth of these injuries.[5] Davidoff and others[34] found incidence of closed head injury (CHI) in 49% of traumatic SCI cases in their sample.[34] Traumatic pneumothorax/hemothorax were reported in 17.8% of these patients.[5] Skull and facial fractures, along with CHI and vertebral artery and esophageal disruptions, are common in cervical injuries.[97] Limb fractures and intrathoracic injuries (rib fractures and hemopneumothorax) are frequent in thoracic injuries, whereas intraabdominal injuries to the liver, spleen, and kidneys are associated with lumbar and cauda equina injuries.[97]

MECHANISM OF INJURY

The majority of SCIs occur as a result of trauma. The degree and type of force that are exerted on the spine at the time of the trauma determine the location and type of damage that occurs.[66] Injuries to the vertebral column can be classified biomechanically as pure flexion or flexion-rotation injuries, hyperextension injuries, and compression injuries.[43] Penetrating injuries to the cord are usually the result of gunshot wounds or knife wounds.[43]

Spinal cord damage also can be caused by nontraumatic mechanisms. Circulatory compromise to the spinal cord resulting in ischemia causes neurological damage at and below the involved cord level. Compression of the cord can be caused by degenerative bone diseases, prolapse of the intervertebral disk into the neural canal, and by various tumors and abscesses of the spinal cord or surrounding tissues. Congenital malformation of the vertebral canal, such as spina bifida, also can damage the spinal cord. Diseases that result in compromise of the spinal cord include Guillain-Barré syndrome, transverse myelitis, and multiple sclerosis. Hysterical paralysis may clinically resemble SCI.

DEMOGRAPHICS

The incidence of traumatic SCI in the United States is approximately 8,000 new cases per year.[6,92,101] Approximately 3,000 new cases of spinal cord impairment secondary to disease and congenital anomalies occur each year.[125] The number of people living in the United States today with SCI is between 180,000 and 225,000.[101] Sixty percent of SCIs occur in persons between 16 and 30 years of age, with a mean age of 30.7 years and the most common age 19 years.[5,40,41] Table 16-1 lists additional demographics.

In 1989, the average length of stay for the acute and rehabilitation phases was 92 days for tetraplegic patients and 75 days for paraplegic patients.[41,101] Average costs for the acute and rehabilitation phases in 1989 were $118,900 for tetraplegic patients and $85,100 for paraplegic patients.[41,101] Obviously, the cost today will exceed those figures. Today, 89% of persons with SCI are discharged to a noninstitutional residence.[5,67] Approximately $8,208 is spent on home modifications.[5,67] After rehabilitation, a person with SCI on average spends $7,866 per year (1988 dollars) for medical services, supplies, etc.[67] These costs increase for higher lesions.[6]

ACUTE MEDICAL MANAGEMENT OF SCI

Acute medical treatment includes (1) pharmacological management to prevent neurological trauma and enhance neural recovery, (2) anatomical realignment and stabilization interventions, and (3) prevention of secondary complications of the SCI.

Pharmacological management

Neurological damage due to SCI may be a result of (1) physical disruption of axons traversing the injury site, (2) local infarction as a result of ischemia or hypoxia, or (3)

Table 16-1. SCI demographics	
Mean age at injury[5,101]	30.7 years
Most common age at injury[5,40,41]	19.0 years
Sex[5]	
Male	82.3%
Female	17.7%
Causes of injury:	
motor vehicle accident	44.8%
falls	21.7%
violent acts	16.0%
sport injuries	13.0%
other	4.5%
Neurological categories at discharge[101]	
Incomplete tetraplegia	31.1%
Complete paraplegia	25.9%
Complete tetraplegia	21.8%
Incomplete paraplegia	20.0%
No deficits	0.9%
Unknown	0.4%
Common injury sites[5]	
C5	15.8%
C4	12.5%
C6	12.5%
T12	7.5%

prevention of impulses by microhemorrhages or edema within the spinal cord at the injury site.[54,55] The initial trauma alone rarely causes anatomical transection of the spinal cord, even when there is a complete loss of sensory and motor function below the level of the injury.[55]

The injury usually causes damage more centrally in the gray matter, with lesser damage occurring to the surrounding white matter.[55] This central contusion is believed to lead to secondary damage 24 to 72 hours after the injury. Investigators believe that secondary injuries to surrounding tissues can be lessened by pharmacological agents, specifically methylprednisolone and monosialotetranexxosylylganglioside (GM-1) ganglioside.

The National Acute SCI Study (NASCIS 2) used high doses of methylprednisolone and showed significant improvements in sensory and motor function 6 months after injury.[19] Young and Flamm[128] showed that methylprednisolone enhances the flow of blood in injured spinal cords, preventing the typical decline in white matter, extracellular calcium levels, and evoked potentials. This acts to prevent progressive posttraumatic ischemia.[54,62,63] Timeliness of administration of this drug is crucial. There was no evidence of improvement in sensory or motor function with methylprednisolone when more than 8 hours elapsed between the time of injury and the initiation of treatment.[19,70] Adverse side effects associated with chronic corticosteroid use are well documented and include gastric ulcer disease, delayed wound healing, hypertension, arrhythmias, electrolyte and endocrine disorders, and alteration in mental status.[95] The complications of high dose, short-term methylprednisolone use do not appear to be as significant as those associated with

chronic administration. The documented adverse effects associated with the protocol include increased wound infection rates and gastrointestinal bleeding.[19]

GM-1 is a complex acidic glycolipid found at high levels in cell membranes in the mammalian central nervous system (CNS). Evidence suggests GM-1 augments neurite growth in vitro, induces regeneration and sprouting of neurons, and restores neuronal function after injury in vivo.[55] The significant improvements in the clients who received GM-1 were manifested in approximately 1 year, with some clinical changes seen as early as 1 day after receiving the drug. Motor function recovery was noted predominantly in the lower extremities. It is thought that neurological return was seen primarily in the lower extremities because GM-1 enhances the function of the surrounding white matter tracks to the lower extremities, but not of the gray matter at the injury site.[54] Individual muscle recoveries were attributed to initially paralyzed muscles that had regained useful motor function as opposed to muscles that had obtained more strength.[54]

Theoretically, it may be more beneficial to combine the administration of these two drugs. Methylprednisolone would allow for initial survival of injured neurons, and GM-1 would enhance recovery in this larger number of surviving neurons.[55] Improvement of as few as one motor level could prove to be functionally relevant to the spinal cord injured individual and may result in the difference between independence and dependence.

Surgical stabilization

One of the first interventions following acute SCI is stabilizing the spine to prevent further cord or nerve root damage. This can be accomplished by several means including skeletal traction, anterior stabilization, posterior stabilization, or external stabilization techniques.

Once paralysis and anesthesia occur, the degree of recovery depends mainly on three factors: the extent of the pathological changes induced by the trauma, the prevention of further trauma during rescue, and the prevention of complications that may further compromise the function of neural tissue. The management of the second and third factors requires specialized expertise.[7]

White and Panjabi[119] define clinical instability as "a loss of the ability of the spine under physiological loads to maintain a relationship between vertebral segments so there is either damage or subsequent irritation of the spinal cord or nerve roots, and there is no development of incapacitating deformity or pain caused by structural changes" (p.85). Clinical evidence of neurological impairment is a strong indication of spinal instability.[52] At the time of injury, paramedics are careful to maintain alignment of the spine if SCI is suspected. In the emergency room, diagnostic studies reveal the severity of the spinal injury as well as the type and degree of the instability. Based on these results, the physician, patient, and family decide on treatment. Indications for surgical intervention include, but are not limited to,

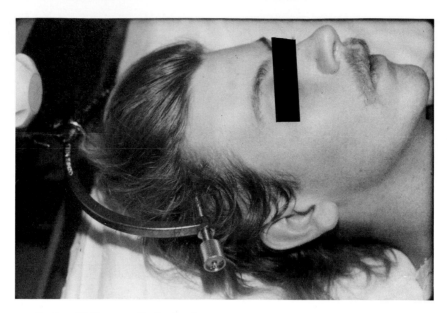

Fig. 16-2. Gardner-Wells tongs. Reduction is accomplished through weights attached to the traction rope. (Courtesy of Dr. H. Herndon Murray, Assistant Medical Director, Shepherd Spinal Center.)

signs of progressive neurological involvement, type and extent of bony lesions, and degree of spinal cord damage.[28]

The purpose of spinal stabilization in the presence of complete SCI is to prevent painful pseudoarthritis or recurrent dislocation. Incomplete SCI is stabilized to decompress and protect the spinal cord from further damage until ligamentous and bony stability is regained.[49] The following discussion includes nonsurgical and surgical interventions.

Cervical spine. Emergency medical technicians use extreme caution to immobilize the injured patient and prevent excessive movement at the unstable spinal site. Spinal alignment can be corrected after the patient is medically stable. If there is compression of neurological tissue, vertebral fracture, or dislocation, reduction must occur to minimize ischemia and edema formation.[52] Reduction is accomplished by cervical traction with the goal of immediate and proper alignment of bone fragments and decompression of the spinal cord until further stabilization.[28,88,124] The most widely used traction is Gardner-Wells tongs (Fig. 16-2), which are inserted into the skull. Weights are added at approximately 5 pounds of traction per level of injury to achieve reduction of the dislocation and to maintain alignment.[88]

While the patient is in traction, a thorough evaluation is performed to assess the extent of the SCI. Certain precautions must be considered during therapy to prevent unnecessary movement at the injury site. The traction rope must be kept in alignment with the long axis of the cervical spine, and the weights must be allowed to hang freely. Cervical rotation must be prevented. In addition, care must be taken to ensure that continued traction is maintained.

When surgical stabilization is indicated, common surgical protocols include posterior and anterior approaches. Unstable compression injuries are usually managed by a posterior procedure except when there is a deficient anterior column. Anterior approaches are used more for decompression of the spinal cord or when more bony support is needed for the anterior column.[52]

One common posterior stabilization procedure, the cervical wiring and fusion (PCWF) (Fig. 16-3), is performed in the following situations: (1) flexion injuries with disruption of the posterior ligament complex, (2) unstable facet dislocation, (3) postlaminectomy, (4) anterior fractures with angulation or translation, and (5) extensive soft tissue damage allowing severe subluxation.[28] Fusion is accomplished through wiring and strips of bone graft harvested from the iliac crest. After this procedure, a hard collar such as a Philadelphia collar (Fig. 16-4) or sterno-occipital-mandibular-immobilizer (SOMI) brace is used until a solid bony fusion has developed. The solid bony fusion usually takes 6 to 8 weeks. Postoperatively, care must be taken to protect the bony fusion.

One disadvantage of the PCWF is that it requires a considerable amount of muscle detachment, which may lead to soft tissue scarring and postsurgical pain. The resultant hypermobility of the joints above and below the fusion may lead to arthritis and increased pain, and in extreme cases, further instability, which a therapist must be aware of in long-term management.[28,49]

Another posterior cervical approach is the insertion of Roy Camille plates commonly used for the middle and lower cervical spine. This procedure is appropriate for fractures of the laminae or spinous process that preclude interspinous wiring and when stabilization of 2 to 3 vertebrae is

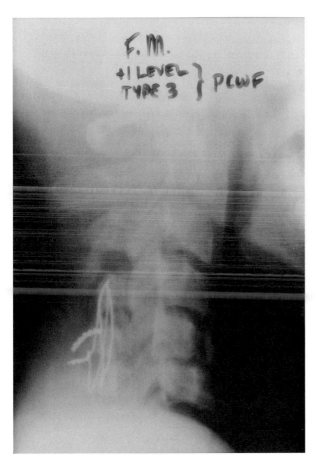

Fig. 16-3. Radiograph of posterior cervical wiring and fusion. (Courtesy of Dr. H. Herndon Murray, Assistant Medical Director, Shepherd Spinal Center.)

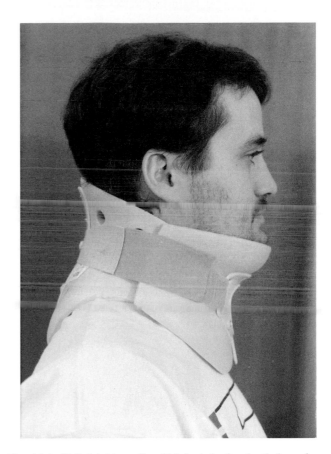

Fig. 16-4. Philadelphia collar. Fabricated of polyethylene foam with rigid anterior and posterior plastic strips. Easily applied via velcro closures. Limits flexion, extension and rotary movements of the cervical spine.

necessary. The presence of osteoarthritis is a contraindication for this procedure. Postoperative care is to wear a cervical collar for 4 to 6 weeks. Anterior fusion is a less commonly used procedure that includes removing the damaged vertebral body, thereby decompressing the spinal canal. A full-thickness iliac crest graft is inserted to replace the resected vertebrae.[28,49] In addition, external stabilization may be indicated for further stabilization.[49] Indications include removal of masses that compress the ventral aspect of the cord, extension injuries in which there is disk disruption, injury to the anterior longitudinal ligament, and previous extensive laminectomy.[28,49]

The advantage of the anterior cervical fusion is that, in conjunction with the halo vest, it provides greater stability with loss kyphotic angulation as compared with the use of the halo vest alone.[49] Disadvantages may include esophageal problems, additional instability, and postoperative subluxation in the presence of posterior longitudinal ligament instability.[28,49] Rehabilitation considerations and postoperative precautions are the same as those described earlier for the PCWF procedure.

Another anterior stabilization procedure is the insertion of ventral plates. Common plating used for this procedure is the use of Arbeitsgemeinshaft für Osteosynthesefragen (AO)

plates. This procedure is contraindicated in the presence of osteoarthritis. Postoperative care is similar to that of the Roy Camille plate.

In situations where surgery is not indicated, an external device can be used. The best available device is halo traction. The halo traction device consists of three parts: the ring, the uprights, and the jacket (Fig. 16-5). The ring fits around the skull, just above the ears. It is held in place by four pins that are inserted into the skull. The uprights are attached to the ring and jacket by bolts. The jacket is usually made of polypropylene and lined with sheepskin. This equipment is left in place for 6 to 12 weeks until bony healing is satisfactory.[90] The advantage of using the halo device is the ability to mobilize the patient as soon as the device has been applied without compromising spinal alignment. This allows the rehabilitation program to commence more rapidly. It also allows for delayed decision making regarding the need for surgery.

The disadvantage of the halo device is that pressure and friction from the vest or jacket may lead to altered skin integrity.[49] Special attention must be taken to ensure that the skin remains intact. Silicone pads may be used over bony prominences to help protect the skin against decubitus ulcers. During more active phases of the rehabilitation

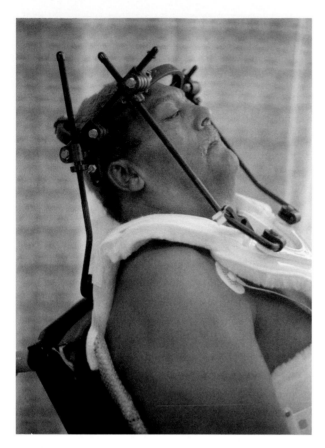

Fig. 16-5. Halo vest. Basic components are the halo ring, distraction rods, and the jacket.

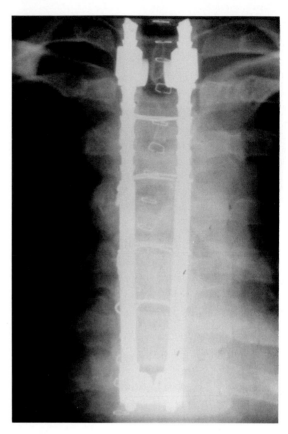

Fig. 16-6. Radiograph of Harrington rod instrumentation. (Courtesy of Dr. H. Herndon Murray, Assistant Medical Director, Shepherd Spinal Center.)

process, the halo device may slow functional progress due to its added weight and its interference with middle to end range of upper extremity movement. In a small percentage of patients, there are complications of dysphagia and temporomandibular joint dysfunction associated with wear of the halo device.[49] Care must be taken not to lift or move the patient by pulling the vest or the upright bars, as this may affect the alignment of the cervical spine. To move the patient, appropriate support must be provided under the vest. The physician should be notified immediately if neck movement is observed.

Thoracolumbar spine. Internal fixation of the thoracolumbar region is necessary when stability and distraction cannot be maintained by other means.[120] The most widely used fixation device for thoracolumbar stabilization is Harrington rod instrumentation and fusion (Fig. 16-6). Whether compressive or distractive forces are indicated, a bony fusion is accomplished through a bone graft taken from the iliac crest.

Postoperatively, an external trunk support is necessary to limit excessive vertebral motion and to maintain proper thoracic and lumbar alignment.[66,120] This may be achieved by a custom thoracolumbosacral orthosis (Fig. 16-7) or by a Jewett brace (Fig. 16-8). Initially, the patient's activity may

be limited to allow for a complete fusion to take place and to minimize the possibility of rod displacement.

A recent advance in spinal stabilization has been the use of transpedicular screws. This method provides a "grip" on the vertebrae that resists loads of any type.[52] The pedicle is the strongest site accessible posteriorly to obtain a three-dimensional fixation which is a safe and strong construct (Fig. 16-9).

Cotrel-Dubousset (CD) instrumentation is another internal fixation procedure used for stabilization of the thoracolumbar spine. The CD instrumentation consists of three implant elements: (1) rods used on either side of the spine that can be contoured, (2) hooks and screws that can be placed in any position or level and apply a distractive or compressive force, and (3) two transverse traction devices that are placed between the horizontal rods. These elements form a stable rectangular construct and provide three-dimensional correction where spinal stability is impaired in both a frontal and sagittal plane.[47,52]

Postoperatively, compression activities should be avoided to prevent bleeding at the site of the hooks.[49] Some physicians require the patient to lie supine for 1 hour after surgery before resuming light activity as tolerated. In some cases, strenuous activities are omitted for 1 year after surgery.[20]

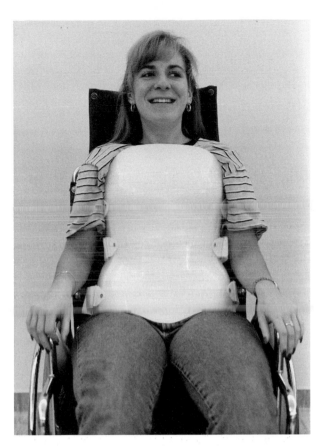

Fig. 16-7. Custom thoracolumbosacral orthosis. A molded plastic body orthosis with soft lining on the interior. Orthosis controls flexion, extension and rotary movements until bony healing occurs.

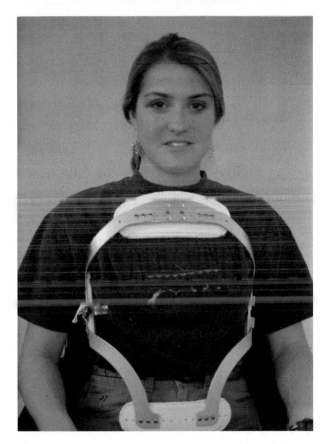

Fig. 16-8. Jewett hyperextension brace. Provides a single three-point force system via sternal pad, suprapubic pad, and thoracolumbar pad. Restricts forward flexion in the thoracolumbar area.

Other options for thoracolumbar stabilization include Jacob distraction rods, Luque rods, Sleflee plates, Weiss springs, and AO internal fixation. Many options must be considered during the decision-making process regarding the optimal operative strategy for the patient with spinal instability.

The goal of the operative procedures at any spinal level discussed is to reverse the deforming forces, to restore proper spinal alignment, and to stabilize the spine.[48] All of these procedures have advantages and disadvantages. The surgeon, patient, and family must be involved in the decision-making process to select the most appropriate method of treatment.

COMPLICATIONS

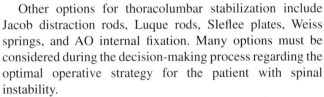

SCI may result in autonomic dysfunction, sensory loss, motor paralysis, and loss of bowel and bladder control, all of which predispose the patient to secondary complications from the time of injury and throughout life. The treating team must be aware of the potential for complications and incorporate appropriate interventions in the treatment program. Additionally, educating the patient in the prevention of

complications is an integral part of the rehabilitation program from admission to postdischarge. This section describes the etiology and incidence of these complications. Refer to the treatment section of this chapter for intervention strategies.

Respiratory complications

Respiratory complications are a common and potentially life-threatening problem related to SCI and may occur acutely or at any time after the initial injury.[9,14,26,39] With inspiratory muscle paralysis, alveolar hypoventilation is imminent and may lead to secondary medical problems. According to the National Data Base, persons diagnosed with complete tetraplegia often developed pneumonia (41.5%), ventilatory failure (40.5%), and atelectasis (41.9%).[3]

Lesions above C4 result in paralysis of inspiratory muscles and will generally require artificial ventilation.[26] The inspiratory muscles are as follows: diaphragm and intercostal muscles (primary), sternocleidomastoids, upper trapezius, scalenes, and the pectoralis major muscles (accessory).[31,80] With diaphragm sparing, patients with C4

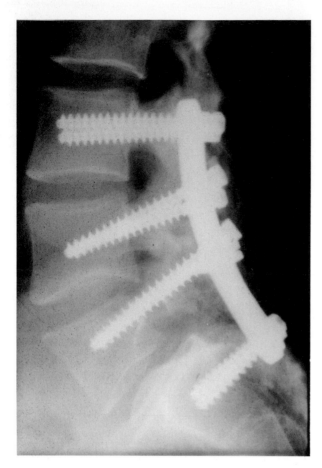

Fig. 16-9. Radiograph of transpedicular screws. (Courtesy of Dr. H. Herndon Murray, Assistant Medical Director, Shepherd Spinal Center.)

tetraplegia may be able to sustain life without artificial means, but may always have marginal ventilatory capacities. C5-T12 lesions result in intercostal paralysis, and patients may demonstrate weakness in the accessory inspiratory muscles as well. Although inspiratory efforts may be reduced, these patients will generally be able to compensate over time. All complete lesions above T10 result in some degree of abdominal muscle paralysis. The abdominal muscles are forceful expiratory muscles, and paralysis reduces cough effectiveness.[35]

General problems for patients with tetraplegia and mid to upper thoracic paraplegia include poor secretion clearance, reduced chest wall mobility, and limited ventilation leading to chronic alveolar hypoventilation.[14,26] The extent of ventilatory impairment is directly proportional to the amount of inspiratory and expiratory muscle involvement.

In addition to direct SCI, patients may sustain injury to the thorax or lung as in a pulmonary contusion. The injury can result in a pneumothorax or hemothorax, altering normal mechanics of ventilation and lung function.[116] If serious enough, a chest tube will be required for management, which

may interfere with access to the chest wall, making treatment more difficult.

DeVivo and others[39] examined the causes of death during the first 12 years after SCI and concluded that pneumonia was the leading cause in tetraplegia. Death within the first year was attributed primarily to pulmonary emboli followed by septicemia and pneumonia. Pulmonary emboli, which interrupt the blood supply to the affected lung, commonly occur from deep vein thrombosis.[52] Any unmanaged alteration in perfusion or ventilation results in ventilatory impairment.[116]

Skin compromise

The incidence of **decubitus ulcers** in the acute and initial rehabilitation phases is between 30% and 56%.[32] A decubitus ulcer can greatly increase length of stay and hospital costs as well as have far reaching consequences for independent functioning. Loss of sensation, immobility, impaired bowel and bladder function, and autonomic disturbances expose the skin to prolonged periods of pressure, shearing, heat, and moisture, all of which predispose the skin to breakdown. When pressure exerted on skin exceeds average arterial capillary pressure, ischemia occurs.[32] If the pressure continues long enough, cellular death and, ultimately, skin breakdown occur.[32] There is a direct relationship between the length of time and amount of pressure required to produce damaging tissue changes. Improper handling of the person with SCI during functional activities such as transfers can cause shearing of the skin. This produces stretching and tearing of the blood vessels that pass between the layers of the skin and the muscle beneath it. Impaired oxygenation and nourishment of the skin may result, leading to breakdown.[49] In the presence of impaired pain perception and proprioception, the individual may be unaware that tissue damage is occurring.

Additional loss of vasomotor tone can result in peripheral edema and poor cellular oxygenation, predisposing the tissues to damage. Many individuals with SCI experience excessive diaphoresis which, combined with incontinence, exposes the skin to extended periods of moisture. In addition, weight loss and anemia, which are common immediately after SCI, increase the likelihood of skin breakdown.[16]

Orthostatic hypotension and edema

Orthostatic hypotension and lower extremity edema occur as a result of loss of sympathetic influences that bring about vasoconstriction.[58] Vasodilation results in hypotension which, combined with the loss of muscle pump action of lower extremity and abdominal muscles, produces venous stasis. Depending on the amount of sympathetic disruption in lesions above the mid-thoracic level and the amount of skeletal muscle paralysis after SCI, there will be varying degrees of edema and problems with orthostatic hypotension.[58]

Deep vein thrombosis and pulmonary embolism

Deep vein thrombosis (DVT) and **pulmonary embolism (PE)** are two serious postinjury complications in SCI. Symptoms of DVT in the patient with sensory loss usually present as noticeable swelling or asymmetry of the involved leg.[71]

The mechanisms important in the formation of venous thromboembolism are venous stasis, activation of blood coagulation, pressure on immobilized lower extremities, and endothelial damage.[58,83,87] During the last 30 years, approximately eight studies have been conducted on the incidence of DVT in acute SCI. The rates of occurrence reported ranged from 12% to 64%.[114] PE occurs in 5% to 15% of patients with the diagnosis of DVT.[52] Incidence was greater in thoracic lesions than in cervical lesions and more prevalent in complete lesions as compared to incomplete lesions.

A drug that is used prophylactically to prevent DVT and PE in the SCI is subcutaneous heparin.[44] Information available to date indicates that heparin decreases but does not eliminate the incidence of DVT and PE.[88] The greatest risk of occurrence of DVT is between 2 to 12 weeks after injury. Prophylactic use of anticoagulant such as coumadin decreases the DVT incidence to 1.3%.[51]

Apneic bradycardia

The first manifestation of autonomic dysfunction is usually apneic bradycardia in response to tracheal suctioning.[17] Restoration of ventilation usually resolves the problem. The exact cause of apneic bradycardia is not well understood, but is believed to be due to sympathetic disruption resulting in vagal dominance in response to noxious stimuli or hypoxia.[17] This condition usually resolves over time.

Autonomic dysreflexia

Autonomic dysreflexia is a massive uncompensated cardiovascular reaction of the sympathetic division of the autonomic nervous system (ANS) to noxious stimuli (usually visceral) below the level of lesion.[49] Vasoconstriction occurs in the vascular beds of the skin and viscera, resulting in an increase in blood pressure.[49] Usually, a sudden rise in blood pressure is sensed by receptors in the aortic arch and carotid sinus, which through the vasomotor center in the brain cause a compensatory vasodilation.[17] Vasodilation occurs only above the level of the lesion, causing flushing of the neck and face and hypertension persists.[17] A sudden rise in blood pressure to extreme levels constitutes an emergency situation which may proceed to subarachnoid hemorrhage.[17] Caregivers must be able to recognize autonomic dysreflexia, understand possible causes, and provide the appropriate response to symptoms.

The most common causes are a distended or irritated bladder, fecal impaction or bowel irritation, decubitus ulcers,

ingrown toenail, burns, stimulation of the genitals, exposure to high temperatures, and constricting garments. Signs and symptoms of the condition are a severe, sudden, pounding headache; hypertension of greater than 40 mm Hg over basal blood pressure; sweating and flushing above the level of lesion; chills without fever (goose bumps); nasal congestion; and penile erection.[17,49] When apparent, removal of noxious stimuli should be the first action taken. The patient should be placed immediately in an upright position to cause postural hypotension to occur. The urinary drainage system should be checked for obstruction, and the patient should be immediately catheterized. Exploration for other causes of noxious stimuli should follow. If these measures do not cause a drop in blood pressure, the physician should be notified immediately.

Thermoregulation

The internal temperature of the body is regulated almost entirely through feedback mechanisms located in the hypothalamus. Heat-sensitive neurons in the hypothalamus send impulses to initiate compensatory reaction either to raise or to lower body temperature along the autonomic pathways to the spinal cord and then through the sympathetic outflow to the skin.[17] Because of the interruption of communication between the ANS temperature control centers in the hypothalamus, there is a disruption of temperature control below the level of lesion.[17] This disruption is manifested by a lack of vasoconstriction, the inability to shiver in cold environments, and the inability to perspire to dissipate heat in warm environments.[17] The higher the lesion, the more severe the problem. The body temperature of the tetraplegic patient is greatly influenced by the temperature of the environment.[17] Individuals with tetraplegia should avoid sudden extremes of temperature. Education regarding seasonal temperature precautions is vital.

Spasticity

Spasticity is the result of an upper motor neuron lesion in which motor neurons below the lesion are released from normal supraspinal descending inhibitory influences. Clinical manifestations of spasticity are a velocity-dependent increase in tonic stretch reflexes (increased resistance to passive stretch), exaggerated deep tendon reflexes, and impaired voluntary control of skeletal muscles.[79,127] Clonus and muscle spasm may also be present.[79]

In the United States, spasticity is a secondary complication in one third of individuals with SCI.[9] Severe spasticity often causes pain, loss of range of motion (ROM), decreased functional independence, increased risk for skin breakdown, difficulty performing routine hygiene, and bowel and bladder dysfunction.[30,49,79] Although spasticity is usually considered a negative side effect of SCI, it may offer several advantages. Spasticity can help to prevent muscle atrophy, improve circulation (thereby decreasing venous stasis), assist with clearing of secretions, and assist with functional tasks.

Standard treatments of spasticity include physical and occupational therapies, oral antispasticity pharmacological agents, motor point blocks, and surgical techniques.[30,72] Various oral pharmacological agents include baclofen (Lioresal), diazepam (Valium), and/or dantrolene (Datrium).[127] Baclofen is the agent most often used. Surgical techniques used to treat spasticity are peripheral neurotomy, posterior rhizotomy, and myelotomy.[79] A relatively new concept in the treatment of spasticity allows for administration of lower doses of baclofen via an indwelling pump into the lumbar subarachnoid space with good results and few side effects.[30,79,87] One of the major drawbacks to this procedure is that it is very costly. Multiple procedures commonly are used by therapists to treat spasticity: slow, prolonged stretching; inhibitive positioning; slow, rotational movements; weight bearing; cryotherapy; inhibitive casting; biofeedback; and pool therapy.

Flaccidity

Lower motor neuron lesions result in flaccid paralysis with no spinal reflex activity below the lesion. This occurs most often at injuries at L1 and below.[43,49] **Flaccidity** can cause the following problems: joint hypermobility or instability, muscle imbalance, muscle atrophy, poor postural control, and dependent edema.

Pain

One third to one half of all individuals with SCI have pain, with 25% of these experiencing severe disabling pain. Pain in SCI may have multiple origins.[84] A variety of pain syndromes are associated with SCI. The times of onset and duration of pain vary from case to case. Radicular pain originating from injury of the neural elements may be described as burning, stabbing, or piercing and usually follows a dermatomal pattern.[49,84] This type of pain is common in cauda equina injuries and other incomplete injuries.[49] Central spinal cord dysesthesia (deafferentation pain) is manifested by poorly localized complaints of constant tingling, numbness, burning, aching, and/or visceral discomfort, which are worsened by activity.[49,84] This is the most common pain syndrome following SCI.[84]

Many persons with SCI experience pain secondary to mechanical trauma that occurred at the time of injury, from surgical procedures, or as a result of improper handling and positioning by caregivers. Trauma to joints, muscles, and soft tissue structures can occur as a result of muscle imbalance. Shoulder pain is common in the initial rehabilitation phase and may be attributed to stretching of structures that shortened during the acute phase of immobilization, muscle imbalance, and the increased use of the shoulder joint in weight-bearing activities. In some individuals with SCI,

shoulder pain increases over time due to the repetitive stresses placed on the shoulder joints.[4,75]

Management of pain post SCI should consist of a team effort to optimize health, including programs for good skin care, bowel and bladder management, maintenance of ROM, proper wheelchair and bed positioning and good nutrition.[10] Relaxation techniques, biofeedback, psychotherapy, physical therapy, antidepressants, anti-inflammatory medications, pain medications, and surgical interventions may be helpful in controlling pain.

Degenerative joint changes

Many mechanical stressors over time cause degenerative joint changes in this population. Muscle imbalance, muscle spasms that may force a joint to the end of its range, flaccidity resulting in unstable joints, performance of repetitive tasks (wheelchair propulsion), improper performance of ROM exercises, and weight-bearing activities using the upper extremities (crutch walking and transfers) all place repetitive stress on joint structures.[6] Painful degenerative shoulders and carpal tunnel syndrome are common problems seen in persons who propel manual wheelchairs, walk with crutches, and perform depression transfers.[4,6,75] The shoulder impairments common to these individuals include bursitis, tendonitis, osteoarthritis, rotator-cuff tears, and impingement syndromes.[4,56]

Some degenerative joint stressors can be decreased by analyzing the performance of functional tasks and modifying them to reduce repetitive motion and weight bearing through the upper extremities. For example, a person with paraplegia could perform a transfer to a tub-seat rather than performing a transfer to the tub bottom. Setting up a lightweight manual wheelchair to maximize the ease of propulsion for the individual can help to minimize stresses on the shoulder.

Urinary tract infection

During the acute and initial rehabilitation phase, 80.4% of patients present with urinary tract infection (UTI).[5] Not surprisingly, UTI continues to be the most frequent complication, ranging from 53% of individuals in the first year after injury to 80% in year 16. Mortality from urinary sepsis has been reduced from 80% in the 1920s to 6% in the 1980s.[5]

Neurological damage to the spinal cord results in bladder voiding dysfunctions (detrusor-sphincter dyssynergias). Upper motor neuron lesions may lead to bladder and sphincter spasticity, voiding dyssynergia, detrusor hypertrophy, and urethral reflux. Lesions at the micturition center cause flaccidity of the bladder and decreased tone of the perineal muscles and sphincters.[86] Some program of catheterization is indicated to drain the bladder (for most patients). Catheterization programs (indwelling, external, or intermittent) all increase exposure of the urinary tract to bacterial infection. Persistent infection can result in nephrolithiasis, hydronephrosis, pyelonephritis, or periurethral abscesses, all of which lead to renal failure.[3]

Most patients with UTI are asymptomatic.[93] General malaise and a slight fever are common and may prevent the individual from participating fully in activities. Chills, a spiking fever, nausea, vomiting, sweating, abdominal discomfort, increased spasticity, increased spontaneous voiding, larger residual volumes, and cloudy malodorous urine may indicate various urinary tract problems including UTI.[3,93] Patients who are symptomatic receive urine cultures and the appropriate antibiotic is prescribed.

UTI can be prevented through a program of appropriate ongoing urological management, patient education, and personal cleanliness. Leg bags, when used, should be emptied as needed to avoid urethral reflux.

Contractures

Contractures occur in 4.5% of patients during the acute and initial rehabilitation phases as a result of spasticity, muscle weakness, muscle imbalance, immobility, and pain. The incidence is higher in complete tetraplegia (8.4%).[5] When contractures are left unmanaged, joint ankylosis may result. Surgical interventions may be indicated including bone resection, capsular releases, and/or tendon lengthening.[118] Following SCI, daily ROM exercises, proper body positioning, and patient education must occur to prevent contractures.

Heterotopic ossification

Heterotopic ossification (HO) is the formation of bone in abnormal anatomical locations. The overall incidence of HO is between 5% and 20%.[122] The etiology of HO is unknown and there is no uniform theory regarding its pathogenesis. Serum alkaline phosphatase levels, however, are significantly increased 6 weeks after injury in individuals presenting with HO.[106,122] The clinical signs of HO are sudden loss of joint range, swelling, local heat, erythema, and nonseptic fever. Vigorous stretching exercises should be avoided to prevent the formation of a pseudoarthrosis.[106] Activities that may traumatize the area should be avoided to reduce the chance of increasing the inflammatory mass. Males develop HO more than twice as often as females.[122] HO occurs more frequently in cervical and mid-thoracic motor complete lesions.[106] Although HO occurs most commonly at the hips, it also forms frequently about the knees.[106] The condition leads to functional restrictions in 3% to 5% of patients.[118] The propensity for development of HO diminishes over time, rarely occurring more than 1 year after injury.[5]

Etidronate disodium (Didronel) may be used prophylactically or in the inflammatory stage to prevent ossification. Surgical intervention is indicated when HO limits joint motion, impairing function or causing abnormal pressure distribution. A wedge resection is made to remove only the amount of bone needed to provide functional joint motion and is more successful if performed on mature bone.[106] Joint manipulation and surgical resection, however, often have poor success.

Osteoporosis

SCI leads to bone demineralization of the entire skeleton except the skull.[53] Many believe that the stimulus for the continual process of bone formation comes from the stress of weight-bearing activities. Bone mass loss continues to progress for approximately 16 months after injury. Homeostasis is reached at two thirds of original bone mass leading to osteoporosis and an increased risk of fractures. After SCI, serum calcium and phosphorus levels rise.[53] This leads to hypercalciuria, predisposing the individual to the formation of bladder and kidney stones.[66]

Controversy abounds regarding the success of treatment in preventing osteoporosis. Standing programs, ambulation with bracing, and electrical stimulation of paralyzed muscles are often performed in hopes of preventing osteoporosis. Overall good health maintenance and good nutrition are important in preventing complications from skeletal changes following SCI.

Spinal deformity

Asymmetrical muscle strength and spasticity, muscle paralysis, poor posture in the wheelchair, loss of mobility, and asymmetrical performance of functional activities predispose the patient to the development of **scoliosis,** lordosis, or **kyphosis.** Spinal deformities occur more commonly in patients with onset of SCI as a child. Spinal deformity may result in impaired respiratory function, abnormal pressure distribution, and decreased function.

Spinal deformity prevention requires the coordinated effort of the treatment team. Spasticity that interferes with good posture must be medically managed. Proper positioning in the bed and wheelchair must be addressed during the acute period and throughout the rehabilitation phase. Therapists must examine the seated posture and performance of functional tasks to avoid repetitive or prolonged asymmetrical posturing. The use of a molded thoracolumbosacral orthosis is indicated to maintain symmetrical trunk alignment in patients with floppy trunks and in growing children. Surgical stabilization of a progressing spinal deformity may be indicated.

Gastrointestinal complications

During the acute phase, disorders of the gastrointestinal tract are caused by a disruption of the nervous system, abdominal trauma, or stress responses of the neuroendocrine system.[98] Acute gastric dilation is usually caused by loss of large amounts of fluid into the stomach. This condition limits diaphragmatic movements and may make ventilation difficult and aspiration more likely to occur. Gastroduodenal ulceration, often referred to as "stress ulceration," has been reported in 22% of patients with SCI. During traumatic SCI, trauma to the viscera may result in gastrointestinal bleeding.[98] These disorders may be life threatening if they are not recognized and treated promptly.[6]

Approximately one third of persons with complete lesions

experience chronic bowel disturbances.[12] Common complications are chronic constipation, fecal impaction, and diarrhea.[12,98] Persons with SCI are also at risk for secondary colonic disorders as a result of prolonged use of bowel management programs.

Management of the bowel after SCI includes dietary management to ensure a high dietary fiber intake, the use of glycerin suppositories and digital stimulation of the rectum to stimulate rectal reflex activity, and manual evacuation.[12] Liquid colace is used with sensory incomplete patients who cannot tolerate manual stimulation. Education is essential for successful bowel management.

Metabolic and endocrine changes

SCI that results in impairment of the ANS and its integration with the brain may result in many changes in the metabolic and endocrine systems.[49] Some of these changes may impair the individual's ability to participate fully in rehabilitation due to fatigue or malaise. Some persons with impaired mobility combined with changes in these systems experience undesirable weight gain.[91] Education in good nutrition, exercise, and weight control is indicated.

REHABILITATION

Banja[11] has defined rehabilitation as a

holistic and integrated program of medical, physical, psychosocial and vocational interventions that empower a disabled person to achieve a personally fulfilling, socially meaningful and functionally effective interaction with the world. Because it seeks to empower, it is a mechanism for a disabled person to reclaim his or her world and a process whose goal is morally congruent with our society's exaltation of "independence" (p. 614-615).

Rehabilitation is a process that extends from the point of admission, well past discharge, to the point of successful reintegration into society. This process involves a continuum of services beginning with the emergency medical system and extending through the acute and rehabilitation hospital stay into a program of lifetime medical care.

Persons with SCI are best treated at tertiary care facilities that include a direct linkage with emergency medical services, full trauma team availability, spine traumatologists, neurourologists, and on-site consultation by the staff of an accredited SCI rehabilitation program. A coordinated system of care shortens hospital stays and improves efficiency of functional gains made during rehabilitation.[6,45,51,68]

The successful rehabilitation process is comprehensive: It includes prevention, early recognition, and inpatient, outpatient, and extended care programs. The comprehensive rehabilitation program for SCI is comprised of several health care professionals including the physicians, occupational therapist, physical therapist, therapeutic recreation specialist, prosthetist-orthotist, nurse, speech pathologist, respiratory therapist, psychologist, social worker, vocational counselor, engineer, and chaplain.[37,42,90]

The coordinated effort of all these professionals is referred to as the team approach. The health care team is defined as a group of health care professionals from different disciplines who share common values and work toward common objectives. Health care professionals agree that health care delivery using the team approach is more effective than fragmented care for patients with long-term disabilities.[37]

Rehabilitation teams may use one of three models: the multidisciplinary model, the interdisciplinary model, or the transdisciplinary model.[37,61] As evidenced by standards set forth by the Joint Commission on Accreditation of Healthcare Facilities (JCAHO) and the Commission on Accreditation for Rehabilitation Facilities (CARF), the interdisciplinary model of team structure is supported in the rehabilitation setting.[2,61,104]

Interdisciplinary refers to activities performed toward a common goal by workers from different disciplines. In this model, the professionals have the added responsibility of a group effort on behalf of the patient. This effort requires the skills necessary for effective group interaction and the knowledge of how to transfer integrated group activities into a result which is greater than the simple sum of the activities of each individual discipline. The group activity of an interdisciplinary program is synergistic, producing more than each could accomplish individually and separately[61] (p. 45).

Phases of rehabilitation

The rehabilitation process may be divided into four or five phases.[36,42] These phases create a framework for visualization of how the person may progress through rehabilitation. The progression of a patient through the rehabilitation process will vary greatly from one individual to another. The SCI patient may move back and forth in the phases as well as have a great deal of overlap between and within the phase framework.

Phase one. Immediately after SCI, there is a loss of function due to neurotrauma and immobilization. The principal emphasis of rehabilitation is to lessen the adverse effects of immobilization. Thus phase one includes all therapeutic intervention during the critical and acute care stages of rehabilitation. This phase may last from a few days to several weeks depending on the severity and level of injury and other associated injuries. Although therapeutic intensity may be limited, patients may begin out-of-bed activities. Goals during this phase may address prevention of secondary complications.

Phase two. This period may be referred to as the early rehabilitation phase. During this time, out-of-bed activities are tolerated for longer periods of time, and the patient begins to work toward specific long-term goals. In accordance with Medicare guidelines for rehabilitation, the patient is able to participate in therapeutic programs a minimum of 3 hours a day.[27] The intensity of therapy may continue to be limited due to unresolved medical issues.

Phase three. This period in rehabilitation is the most active and often the most rewarding. During this period the efforts of weeks and months of work are realized and tangible results can be seen. The SCI person gains varying levels of independence in specific skills and may begin to believe that there is life after SCI. The patient may be taught advanced skills in transferring, wheelchair mobility, gaiting, grooming, and other activities of daily living (ADL). Outings may be scheduled to refine advanced skills and foster community reintegration.

Phase four. This phase largely encompasses activities aimed at a smooth transition to home. Although discharge planning culminates during this phase, it has been ongoing throughout all phases. Discharge planning must be initiated at the time of admission and continue to be integral to treatment planning and goal setting during the entire rehabilitation process.

The following will be completed unless otherwise noted: (1) family training, (2) home modification recommendations, (3) vocational testing/planning (in process), (4) final arrangement for discharge equipment (delivery and fitting), (5) home management, (6) home exercise programs, (7) referrals to outside agencies, and (8) driving evaluation.

Phase five. This phase is comprised of outpatient and other follow-up services, as well as community reintegration. Individuals may return to work or school and resume other family responsibilities. The role of the rehabilitation team is to serve as resources. Refer to section on community reintegration and outpatient services.

Evaluation

A thorough history and evaluation identify the severity and level of neurological injury and is used to establish realistic goals. All areas of the evaluation are outlined below.

History. A thorough review of the medical record before the first contact with the patient is essential. This provides background information and identifies medical precautions necessary to perform a safe and effective evaluation. The history should include personal information, diagnosis, date of onset and cause of injury, pertinent medical/surgical history, nutritional status, and previous rehabilitation. In addition, a social history includes past employment, living situation, marital and family status, and smoking/alcohol status.

Subjective. Any pertinent additions to the history stated by the patient should be described. The patient's statement of goals, problems, and concerns should be included.

Objective. Objective evaluation of the integumentary, neurological, musculoskeletal, and cardiopulmonary systems, as well as functional assessments, are performed.

Skin. Skin breakdown is described in terms of severity, location, width, depth, color, and the presence or absence of odor, drainage, or eschar. Bony prominences that are at high risk to breakdown and the appearance of the skin in relation to turgor and moisture are described. Excessive sweating is

noted due to the increased risk of breakdown in moist areas. The presence of edema and its location with girth measurement are included. Weight shift and turn time schedules, sitting time, cushion type, and skin tolerance for sitting are documented.

Neurological. The patient's sensation is described by dermatome. The recommended tests include (1) sharp-dull discrimination or temperature sensitivity to test the lateral spinothalamic tract, (2) light touch to test the anterior spinothalamic tract, and (3) proprioception or vibration to test the posterior columns of the spinal cord. Sensation is indicated as intact, impaired or absent per dermatome. A dermatomal map is helpful and recommended for ease of documentation. Deep tendon reflexes and cranial nerves are assessed.

Motor. Specific myotomal manual muscle testing is performed, allowing for specific diagnosis of the level and completeness of the injury. Procedures for manual muscle testing are described by Kendall and McCreary[74] and Daniels and Worthingham.[33] A 6-point scale is used:

0 = no visible or palpable contraction is detected
1 = muscle contraction is palpable, but no limb movement is detected
2 = full movement of limb with gravity eliminated
3 = full movement of limb against gravity
4 = full movement with moderate resistance through range
5 = normal strength

Along with the strength of each muscle, the presence, absence, and location of muscle tone should be described. The Modified Ashworth scale is a tool used to describe tone.[73]

Functional mobility and activities of daily living. Functional activities to evaluate include, but are not limited to, bed mobility, transfers, wheelchair mobility, ambulation, dressing, bathing, home management, grooming, bowel and bladder care, and endurance. This section is deferred until the patient is medically and surgically stable.

Range of motion. Available ROM of the upper and lower extremities and the trunk is documented. When indicated, goniometric measurements are included. Specific attention is noted for straight leg raise, ankle dorsiflexion, hip flexion and extension, and all upper extremity mobility. These areas are especially important when performing functional skills such as transfers, dressing, bathing, and ambulation. All postural anomalies are described.

Respiration. All acutely injured patients should be screened for developing ventilatory compromise. Arterial blood gases are noted and the vital capacity measured. The breathing expansion pattern is described, as well as the use of accessory muscles. Artificial breathing devices along with the use of supplemental oxygen are documented. Cough strength and production, the need for assistive coughing and/or suctioning, and the use of an abdominal binder are noted.

Pain. The area and behavior of pain are described. Any devices or modalities used to control pain also should be noted.

Gait. Description of gait includes assistance needed to don/doff any necessary orthotics, ability to assume a standing position, specific gait deviations, and the ability to resume the sitting position. Ambulation on level surfaces, ramps, curbs, stairs, and rough terrain are described. The use of orthotics or assistive devices is documented.

Affect. The patient's appearance and affect are described, along with an appraisal of the patient's ability to actively participate in rehabilitation. The reality of the patient's expectations is assessed.

Equipment. Anticipated equipment needs are described. If the patient already owns equipment, its appropriateness, general condition, need for repairs, rehabilitation technology supplier, funding source, and age of equipment are documented.

Assessment. Goals are described in specific, objective and measurable terms (refer to goal section). Also described are anticipated hindrances to the rehabilitation process. The anticipated length of stay is estimated.

Plan. The treatment plan to achieve both short- and long-term goals is stated, including treatment regimens, frequency, and duration.

American Spinal Injury Association Standards. American Spinal Injury Association (ASIA) standards for assessing and classifying SCI patients are used to facilitate more accurate communication between clinicians and investigators.[103] By systematically examining the dermatomes and myotomes, one can determine the cord segments affected by the SCI. The ASIA neurological examination consists of sensory and motor examinations, which are used to determine the neurological levels, as well as the completeness of the SCI.

The sensory examination consists of testing 28 dermatomes on each side of the body using the modalities of pin prick and light touch. Appreciation of pin prick and light touch at each of the key points is scored on a 3-point scale: 0 = absent, 1 = impaired, and 2 = normal. The scores are added, and total light touch and pin prick scores are assigned. In addition to testing the 28 key points, the external anal sphincter is tested and perceived sensation is graded as a "yes" or "no." The sacral dermatomal information is vital to determine the completeness or incompleteness of the SCI (Fig. 16-10).

The motor examination is completed through testing 10 myotomes on each side of the body. The strength of each muscle is graded, and the scores of the left and right sides of the body are added. Volitional contraction of the anal sphincter also is noted. As with the anal sensory information, the motor information is used to determine if the spinal cord injury is complete or incomplete (Fig. 16-11).

After the completion of the sensory and motor examination, the sensory neurological level, motor neurological level, ASIA impairment scale, and zone of partial preservation are determined. The ASIA impairment scale (modified Frankel and others[50]) is used to describe the completeness of the injury. It is as follows:

A = Complete. No sensory or motor function is preserved in the sacral segment of S4-S5.

B = Incomplete. Sensory but no motor function is preserved below the neurological level and extends through the sacral segments S4-S5.

C = Incomplete. Motor function is preserved below the neurological level, and the majority of key muscles below the neurological level have a muscle grade of less than 3.

D = Incomplete. Motor function is preserved below the neurological level, and the majority of key muscles below the neurological level have a muscle grade greater than or equal to 3.

E = Normal. Sensory and motor function is normal.

Along with the above stated information, the Functional Independence Measure (FIM)[64] is also recommended by ASIA to describe the impact of the SCI on the patient's function. The FIM evaluates different areas of function using a 7-point scale that describes the amount of assistance the patient requires. The evaluation includes areas such as self-care, sphincter control, mobility, locomotion, communication, and social cognition (Fig. 16-12).

Goal setting

Goal setting is a dynamic process that directly follows the evaluation. Evaluation of the patient's baseline status and baseline performance of tasks informs the therapist of factors that limit function. Each rehabilitation problem identified "should be addressed with specific goals to measure enhanced capabilities."[49] The therapist must interpret new information continuously, which leads to ongoing reevaluation and revision of goals.[91] *Goals must always be individualized and should be established in collaboration with the treatment team, the patient, significant others, and with realistic consideration of anticipated needs upon return to the home environment.*

Differing philosophies have been voiced with regard to the responsibility of the rehabilitation team in the careful consideration of appropriate goals and the focus of treatment that follows. One view is that it is the responsibility of the therapist to challenge patients to the maximal level of ability, exposing them to more advanced activities that are beyond their functional ability. This may set the stage for future gains, as patients may learn skills at a later date if the proper foundation has been established.[49] Another view maintains that "in this era of cost consciousness and cost containment, rehabilitation professionals walk a narrow line between training patients to reach their maximum potential for

SENSORY
KEY SENSORY POINTS

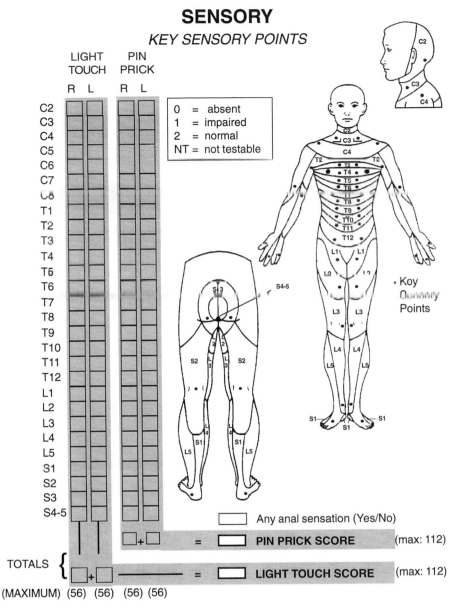

Fig. 16-10. ASIA sensory form. (Courtesy American Spinal Injury Association International, Atlanta, Ga.)

independence and training them to achieve a level of independence which most persons can be expected to continue in their homes and communities (p. 509)."[103] This view differentiates between "the ideal approach and the more realistic, practical approach (p. 509)."[105]

Regardless of how goal setting is approached, goals must not only address functional skills patients require, but also incorporate the long term costs to the musculoskeletal system, and energy conservation techniques that are necessary at times to function successfully.[110,136] Attention must be given to specific limitations or challenges that may result from the discharge disposition. For example, once it is recognized that nursing home placement is likely, the therapeutic goals and treatment program must be structured

for the patient to learn appropriate "techniques to survive and thrive in the facility (p. 832)."[115] These techniques will include assertiveness and care direction.

Factors that must be considered in the goal setting process because they may limit functional outcomes include age, body type, medical problems, additional orthopedic injury, cognitive ability, psychological problems, spasticity, endurance, strength, ROM, funding sources, and motivation. Long term goals for the physical rehabilitation of SCI patients reflect functional outcomes and are based largely on the function of remaining innervated musculature, with consideration for individual limiting factors such as those indicated previously. Short-term goals identify components that interfere with functional ability and are designed to

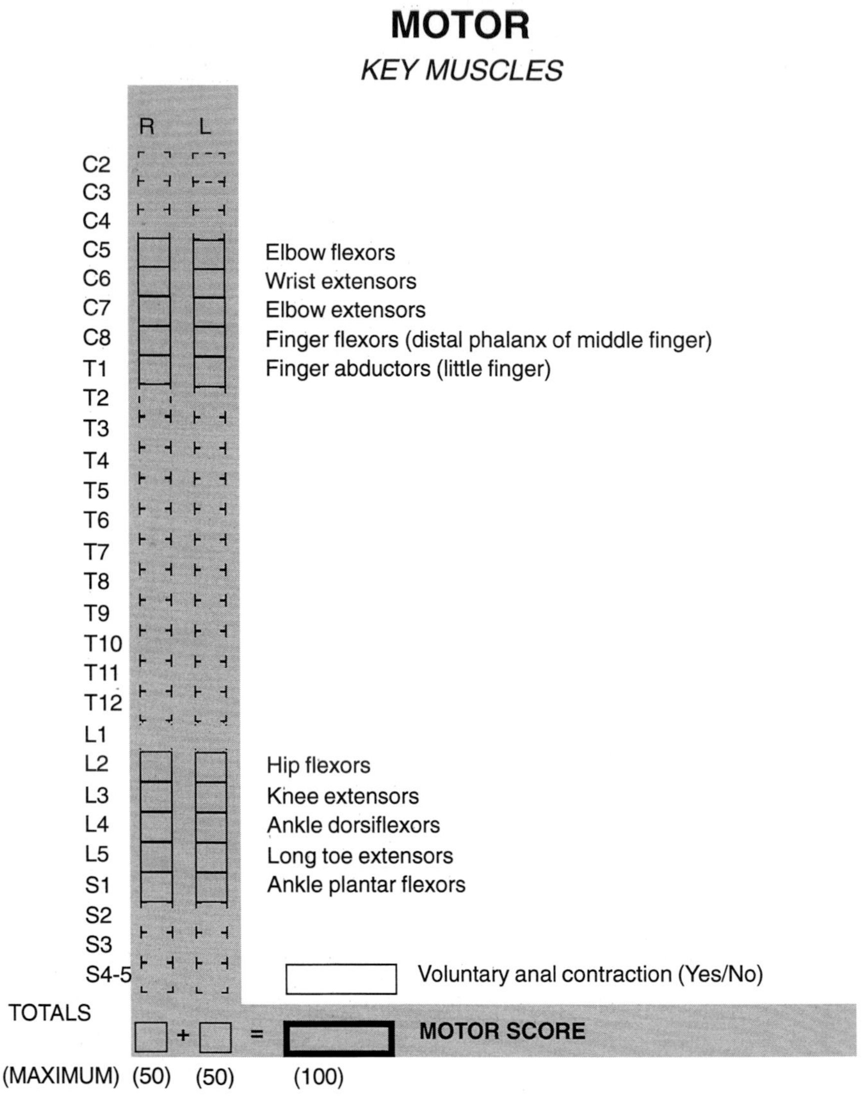

MOTOR
KEY MUSCLES

	R	L	
C2			
C3			
C4			
C5			Elbow flexors
C6			Wrist extensors
C7			Elbow extensors
C8			Finger flexors (distal phalanx of middle finger)
T1			Finger abductors (little finger)
T2			
T3			
T4			
T5			
T6			
T7			
T8			
T9			
T10			
T11			
T12			
L1			
L2			Hip flexors
L3			Knee extensors
L4			Ankle dorsiflexors
L5			Long toe extensors
S1			Ankle plantar flexors
S2			
S3			
S4-5			Voluntary anal contraction (Yes/No)

TOTALS □ + □ = ▭ **MOTOR SCORE**

(MAXIMUM) (50) (50) (100)

Fig. 16-11. ASIA motor form. (Courtesy American Spinal Injury Association International, Atlanta, Ga.)

"address these limiting factors while building component skills"[49] of the desired outcome.

Long-term goals: general outcomes. Before discussing specific long-term goals for patients in relation to the level of injury, it is important to review long-term goals that are appropriate for all rehabilitation patients with SCI. Partial or limited success in attaining these goals directly affects the degree to which more functionally oriented goals are achieved. As these goals are applied to individual patients, objective outcomes should be established (e.g., numbers of hours, degrees of ROM). The following goals are listed without specific objective outcomes.[91]

- Patient will achieve/maintain full ROM in all joints.
- Patient will achieve maximal strength possible in all intact muscle groups.

- Patient will achieve maximal respiratory capacity.
- Patient will tolerate upright sitting without complication.
- Patient will achieve maximal sitting tolerance without skin compromise.
- Patient will have intact skin throughout.
- Patient will attain level of maximum cardiovascular endurance.
- Patient/caregiver are independent with home exercise program for maintaining/increasing strength, ROM, endurance, and respiratory capacity.
- Caregiver will satisfactorily complete training and demonstrate ability to direct and/or perform patient's care as appropriate.
- Patient/caregiver demonstrates appropriate understanding of all equipment operation and maintenance.

L E V E L S	7 Complete Independence (Timely, Safely) 6 Modified Independence (Device)	**No** **Helper**
	Modified Dependence 5 Supervision 4 Minimal Assist (Subject = 75%+) 3 Moderate Assist (Subject = 50%+) **Complete Dependence** 2 Maximal Assist (Subject = 25%+) 1 Total Assist (Subject = 0%+)	**Helper**

Self Care   ADMIT   DISCH
A. Eating
B. Grooming
C. Bathing
D. Dressing-Upper Body
E. Dressing-Lower Body
F. Toileting
Sphincter Control
G. Bladder Management
H. Bowel Management
Mobility
Transfer:
I. Bed, Chair, Wheelchair
J. Toilet
K. Tub, Shower
Locomotion
L. Walk/Wheelchair   W □   W □
                       C □   C □
M. Stairs
Communication
N. Comprehension   A □   A □
                    V □   V □
O. Expression   V □   V □
                    N □   N □
Social Cognition
P. Social Interaction
Q. Problem Solving
R. Memory

Total FIM

NOTE: Leave no blanks; enter 1 if patient not
testable due to risk.

Fig. 16-12. Functional Independence Measure. Guide for the Uniform Data Set for Medical Rehabilitation (Adult FIM^{SM}) Version 4.0 Buffalo, NY 14214: State University of New York at Buffalo, 1993.

- Patient demonstrates ability to direct all care needs.
- All home modification recommendations are issued in a timely manner.
- Appropriate outpatient referrals are completed before discharge.

Long-term goals: functional outcomes. Functional goals are established in the following areas: bed mobility, transfers, weight shifts, wheelchair mobility, wheelchair management, gait, feeding, grooming, dressing, bathing, bowel and bladder management, transportation, communication, skin care/management, and ROM/positioning. Several of these categories of daily living skills are included in

Table 16-2, according to level of SCI. This information must be recognized as general guidelines; variability exists among individuals. These guidelines are most usefully applied to patients with complete SCI. Goal setting for individuals with incomplete SCI is often more challenging given the greater variability of patient presentations and the uncertainty of neurological recovery. As with any patient, ongoing reevaluations provide keys to functional limitations and patient potential and thereby direct the goal setting process.

Short-term goals. Short term goals usually represent components of functional skills and are most often established weekly/biweekly. During the acute phase, short-term goals are established to prepare patients for successful

Table 16-2. Functional outcomes for complete lesions

Functional skills	Level of assistance required (by SCI level groups)			
	High tetraplegia (C1-C5)	Mid-level tetraplegia (C6)	Low tetraplegia (C7-C8)	Paraplegia
Bed mobility • Rolling side to side • Rolling supine/prone • Supine/sitting • Scooting all directions	- Dependent (C1-C4) - Moderate to maximal assistance (C5) - Able to verbally direct all	- Minimal assistance to modified independent with equipment - Able to verbally direct all	- Independent with all	- Independent
Transfers • Bed • Car • Toilet • Bath equipment • Floor • Upright wheelchair	- Dependent (C1-C4) - Maximal assistance with level sliding board transfers (C5) - Able to verbally direct all	- Minimal assistance to modified independent for sliding board transfers - Dependent with wheelchair loading in car - Dependent with floor transfers and uprighting wheelchair - Able to verbally direct all	- Modified independent to independent with level surface transfer (sliding board or depression) - Moderate assistance to modified independent with car transfer - Maximal to moderate assistance with floor transfers and uprighting wheelchair - Able to verbally direct all	- Independent with level surface and care transfers (depression) - Minimal assistance to independent with floor transfer and uprighting wheelchair - Able to verbally direct all
Weight shifts • Pressure relief • Repositioning in wheelchair	- Set-up to modified independent with power recline/tilt weight shift - Dependent with manual recline/tilt/lean weight shift - Able to verbally direct all	- Modified independent with power recline/tilt weight shift - Minimal assistance to modified independent with side to side/forward lean weight shift - Able to verbally direct all	- Modified independent with side to side forward lean, or depression weight shift	- Modified independent with depression weight shift

transition into phase 2 of rehabilitation. Therefore, therapy intervention is focused on minimizing complications, establishing communication, and mobilizing the patient. Beyond the acute phase, short-term goals, as stair-steps toward long-term goal achievement, are useful in assessing whether the treatment program is progressing appropriately. Weekly documentation of short-term goal achievement is necessary. Lack of progress may indicate the need for reconsideration and revision of long-term goals.

Goal revision. The purpose of goal revision is to demonstrate in a timely manner that expectations for

functional skills achievement are continuously being reassessed so that treatment programs are appropriately challenging patients. Goal revision may involve lowering or raising skill expectations or a combination of lowering and raising. Any revision of long-term goals must be discussed with the patient/team and clearly documented.

Goal setting conference. Rehabilitation teams may elect to hold a goal setting conference for each patient during which team members, including the patient, have the opportunity to discuss long-term goals established for the rehabilitation phase. Because this forum may be too

Table 16-2. Functional outcomes for complete lesions—cont'd

	Level of assistance required (by SCI level groups)			
Functional skills	High tetraplegia (C1-C5)	Mid-level tetraplegia (C6)	Low tetraplegia (C7-C8)	Paraplegia
Wheelchair mobility • Smooth surfaces • Up/down ramps • Up/down curbs • Rough terrain • Up/down steps (manual wheelchair only)	- Supervision/ set up to modified independent on smooth, ramp, and rough terrain with power wheelchair - Modified independent with manual wheelchair on smooth surface in forward direction (C5) Maximal assistance to dependent with manual wheelchair in all other situations (C5) - Able to verbally direct all	- Modified independent in smooth, ramp, and rough terrain with power wheelchair - Dependent to maximal assistance up/down curb with power wheelchair Modified independent on smooth surfaces with manual wheelchair - Moderate to minimal assistance on ramps and rough terrain with manual wheelchair - Maximal to moderate assistance up/down curbs with manual wheelchair - Dependent up/down steps with manual wheelchair - Able to verbally direct all	- Modified independent on smooth, ramp, and rough terrain with power wheelchair - Dependent to maximal assistance up/down curb with power wheelchair - Modified independent on smooth surfaces and up/down ramps with manual wheelchair - Minimal assistance to modified independent on rough terrain - Moderate to minimal assistance up/down curbs with manual wheelchair - Dependent to maximal assistance up/down steps with manual wheelchair - Able to verbally direct all	- Minimal assistance to modified independent up/down 6″ curbs with manual wheelchair - Modified independent with descending steps with manual wheelchair - Maximal to minimal assistance to ascend steps with manual wheelchair - Able to verbally direct all
Wheelchair management • Wheel locks • Armrests • Footrests/ legrests • Safety strap(s) • Cushion adjustment • Anti-tip levers • Wheelchair maintenance	- Dependent with all - Able to verbally direct all	- Some assistance required - Able to verbally direct all	- May require assistance with cushion adjustment, anti-tip levers, and wheelchair maintenance - Able to verbally direct all	- Independent with all

Continued.

intimidating or may provide too much information to the patient, individual and ongoing discussions of goals and treatment plans must be shared with the patient. It may be useful to request that the patient sign a statement acknowledging understanding of and agreement to all long-term goals. Interim treatment planning conferences also may be held later in the course of rehabilitation to allow the patient

and the rehabilitation team to evaluate progress, reconsider goals, and determine the focus for the remaining time in formal rehabilitation.

Principles of treatment planning

During rehabilitation, much teaching and learning occur. The health care provider assumes the role of teacher and the

Table 16-2. Functional outcomes for complete lesions—cont'd

Functional skills	Level of assistance required (by SCI level groups)			
	High tetraplegia (C1-C5)	Mid-level tetraplegia (C6)	Low tetraplegia (C7-C8)	Paraplegia
Gait • Don/doff orthoses • Sit · stand • Smooth surfaces • Up/down ramps • Up/down curbs • Up/down steps • Rough terrain • Safe falling acstanding	- Not applicable	- Not applicable	- Not applicable	- Abilities range from: • exercise only with KAFOs* • household ambulation with KAFOs • limited community ambulation with KAFOs or AFOs* • functional community ambulation with or without orthoses
ROM/ Positioning • PROM to trunk, legs, and arms • Pad/position in bed	- Dependent - Able to verbally direct all	- Moderate assistance to modified independent with all - Able to verbally direct all	- Minimal assistance to modified independent with all - Able to verbally direct all	- Independent
Feeding • Drinking • Finger feeding • Utensil feeding	- Dependent (C1-C4) - Minimal assistance with adaptive equipment (C5) - Able to verbally direct all	- Modified independent with adaptive equipment	- Modified independent with adaptive equipment (C7)	- Independent
Grooming • Face • Teeth • Hair • Makeup • Shaving face	- Dependent (C1-C4) - Minimal assistance with adaptive equipment for face, teeth, makeup/ shaving (C5) - Maximal to moderate assistance for hair grooming (C5) - Able to verbally direct all	- Modified independent with adaptive equipment	- Modified independent	- Independent

*KAFO, knee-ankle-foot orthosis; AFO = ankle-foot orthosis.

Table 16-2. Functional outcomes for complete lesions—cont'd

Functional skills	Level of assistance required (by SCI lLevel groups)			
	High tetraplegia (C1-C5)	Mid-level tetraplegia (C6)	Low tetraplegia (C7-C8)	Paraplegia
Dressing • Dressing/ undressing (in bed/ wheelchair) • Upper body/ lower body (in bed/ wheelchair)	- Dependent - Able to verbally direct all	- Modified independent for upper body in bed or wheelchair - Minimal assistance with lower body dressing in bed - Moderate assistance with lower body undressing in bed - Able to verbally direct all	- Modified independent for upper/lower body dressing/undressing in bed - Minimal assistance with lower body dressing/undressing in wheelchair (C7) - Modified independent for upper/lower body dressing/undressing in wheelchair (C8) - Able to verbally direct all	- Modified independent
Bathing • Bathing and drying off • Upper body and lower body	- Dependent - Able to verbally direct all	- Minimal assistance for upper body bathing and drying - Moderate assistance for lower body bathing and drying - Use of shower or tub chair - Able to verbally direct all	- Modified independent with all with shower or tub chair	- Modified independent with all on tub bench or tub bottom cushion
Bowel/bladder programs • Intermittent catheterization • Leg bag care • Condom application • Clean up • In bed/ wheelchair (bladder) • Feminine hygiene • Bowel program	- Dependent - Able to verbally direct all	Bladder: - minimal assistance for male in bed or wheelchair - moderate assistance for female in bed Bowel: - moderate assistance with use of equipment Able to verbally direct all	Bladder: - modified independent for male in bed or wheelchair - modified independent for female in bed; moderate assistance for female in wheelchair Bowel: - minimal assistance to modified independent with use of equipment Able to verbally direct all	Bladder: - modified independent for male and female Bowel: - modified independent for male and female

Continued.

Table 16-2. Functional outcomes for complete lesions—cont'd

Functional skills	Level of assistance required (by SCI level groups)			
	High tetraplegia (C1-C5)	Mid-level tetraplegia (C6)	Low tetraplegia (C7-C8)	Paraplegia
Communication				
• Verbal	- Set-up modified independent using equipment for verbal (C1-C3)	- Independent for verbal	- Independent for verbal	- Independent
• Page turning	- Independent verbal (C4-C5)	- Set-up to modified independent for nonverbal	- Modified independent to independent for nonverbal	
• Keyboard				
• Writing		- Able to verbally direct all		
• Telephone	- Set-up to modified independent with equipment for nonverbal			
	- Able to verbally direct all			
Home management				
• Meal preparation	- Dependent to maximal assistance with meal preparation	- Moderate to minimal assistance with meal preparation	- Minimal assistance to modified independent with meal preparation	- Independent
• Environmental control	- Set-up to modified independent with environmental control unit	- Modified independent with environmental control unit	- Modified independent with environmental control unit	

patient assumes the role of the student. The principles of treatment planning include the following:[91]

- Identify and narrow the problem
- Involve patient in goal setting and treatment planning (this is now a CARF standard)[104]
- Structure the treatment to ensure success
- Organize the treatment in a logical manner to progress smoothly toward the long term goal
- Provide variety in the treatment plan to foster patient participation.

Acute rehabilitation

Acute management of the patient with SCI begins with prevention. Preventing secondary complications speeds entry into the rehabilitation phase and improves the possibility that the patient will become a productive member of society. During the acute phase of rehabilitation, patients are at high risk for decubitus ulcers, joint contractures, DVT, and ventilatory impairment.*

Prevention: decubitus ulcers. Following SCI and during the period of spinal shock, patients may be at greatest risk for developing decubitus ulcers.[85,123] The use of backboards at the emergency scene and during radiographic procedures contributes to potential skin compromise.

---

* References 5, 57, 85, 102, 109, and 123.

Preventive skin care begins with careful inspection. Areas with bony prominences are at greatest risk.[82] Key areas to evaluate include the sacrum, ischii, greater trochanters, heels, malleoli, knees, occiput, scapulae, elbows, and prominent spinous processes. Multiple positions may be used for prevention: prone, supine, right and left sidelying, semiprone, or semisupine.[1,100] Secondary injuries such as fractures and the presence of vital equipment, such as ventilator tubing, chest tubes, and arterial lines, should be considered when choosing positions. Pillows or rectangular foam pads are used to pad around the bony prominence and relieve potential pressure. Padding directly over a prominent area with a firm pillow or pad may only increase pressure. Some patients are not appropriate for rigorous turning schedules (e.g., patients with multiple, unstabilized fractures). Specialty low air loss beds and flotation systems designed to maintain body alignment are also available.[77]

Initially, the patient's position in bed should be changed every 2 to 3 hours[123]; this interval is gradually increased to 6 hours during the rehabilitation phase, depending on the patient's skin tolerance. Once the patient begins out-of-bed activities, even more careful attention to weight-bearing surfaces is recommended. Refer to the seating section of this chapter.

Prevention: joint contractures The development of a contracture may result in postural malalignment or even impede potential function. Daily ROM exercises help prevent contractures.[123] Patients exhibiting spasticity may require more frequent treatments due to an increased risk for contracture development.[123,126] The absence of DVT should be determined, and secondary injuries to an affected limb must be considered when initiating a ROM program.

When planning treatment sessions, the neurological level of the patient and long-term goals should be considered. Although isolated joint ROM should be normal for all patients, allowing adaptive shortening or lengthening of particular muscles may be recommended to enhance the achievement of certain functional skills.[100,117] For example, a patient with mid to low tetraplegia may rely on adaptive shortening of the long finger flexors to replace active grip.[100] As the wrist is extended, the tight two-joint finger flexors passively shorten and create grasp. This is termed *tenodesis* and may assist writing or grooming skills.

Unwanted shortening or lengthening should be prevented. For example a patient with a T-12 lesion may eventually use orthotics to ambulate. However, if the hip flexors are allowed to adaptively shorten which may occur with prolonged sitting in a wheelchair, ambulation will be difficult.

Other considerations specific to SCI patients may include (1) hamstrings should be lengthened to allow 110 degrees to 120 degrees of straight leg raise without overstretching back extensor muscles (the combination of lengthened hamstrings and tight back extensor muscles provides stability for balance in the long sitting position and during transfers) and (2) in the presence of weak or paralysed triceps, adaptive shortening of the elbow flexors impairs transfer skills for the person with mid to low tetraplegia.[49,100] These examples illustrate the importance of muscle length and its effect on function.

Prevention: deep vein thrombosis. As stated earlier, DVT is a common secondary complication. Effective interventions in the treatment of DVT include (1) properly fitted elastic pressure gradient stockings and elastic abdominal binders, (2) early mobilization, (3) positioning to avoid pressure over the large blood vessels, (4) deep breathing exercises, and (5) ensuring adequate hydration.[66,78,114] Intermittent compression garments provide intermittent pressure to the affected extremity, thus attempting to substitute for the loss of muscle pumping action.[78,102,109] Antiembolitic garments, such as Ted hose and Jobst garments, provide a continuous external pressure attempting to prevent venous pooling. These may be especially beneficial when initiating out-of-bed activities.

Prevention: respiratory complications. The acute stage of rehabilitation must focus heavily on preventing pulmonary complications and enhancing available pulmonary function. A patient's ability to breathe must be established before asking the patient to do work.

Vital capacity (VC) is the amount of air that can be moved out of the lung after maximal inspiration.[96,116] It is predicated in normal persons based on age and height, ranging from 4 to 5 liters. The tetraplegic patient may reduce this capacity by 40% or more.[14,26,57,81] Even persons with paraplegia may reduce their VC by 20%.[26,49] The forced expiratory volume in one second (FEV_1) is the amount of air a person can expire during the first second after full inspiration.[57,116] FEV_1 reflects the effectiveness of expiratory efforts and may be used to predict the potential for effective coughing.[116]

The patient must also be able to exchange oxygen (O_2) and carbon dioxide (CO_2) at the alveolar level.[116] This may be impaired in the presence of atelectasis, pneumonia, or pulmonary contusions. Full chest wall mobility must allow adequate inspiratory maneuvers.[26,96] Inspiratory muscle weakness should be evaluated initially.

The therapist should determine which ventilatory muscles are neurologically involved. The primary ventilatory muscle is the diaphragm. The diaphragm is innervated by the phrenic nerve via cervical cord levels 3, 4, and 5 and separates the thoracic and the abdominal cavities. If the diaphragm is weak or paralyzed, its descent will be lessened reducing VC.[26,31,80,89]

Gravity plays a crucial role in the function of the diaphragm.[80] As a person is positioned supine, abdominal contents shift upward and give gentle resistance and support to the muscle. The contents may place a slight stretch on the diaphragm, enabling it to generate a more forceful contraction. If a person is obese or pregnant, this resistance may be too great. Most functionally independent people, however, must attain an upright position.

In normal persons as one moves into an upright position the resting position of the diaphragm drops as the abdominal contents fall.[80] The diaphragm is effectively shortened, which makes generating a strong contraction more difficult. With intact abdominal musculature, however, a counter pressure is produced and adequate intraabdominal pressure is maintained, allowing the diaphragm to perform work.[80] Concomitantly, neural input to the diaphragm also increases in the upright posture, which also counteracts this potentially shortened position.

Conversely, when persons with weakness or paralysis of the abdominal wall sit upright, the ability of the diaphragm to contract effectively may be impaired and reductions in intraabdominal pressure are not accommodated. Abdominal corsets improve diaphragm function in the tetraplegic patient by maintaining normal pressure relationships.[26,29,81,100] If applied appropriately, symptomatic shortness of breath may be reduced.

The intercostal muscles, which are positioned between each rib, are also primary ventilatory muscles.[31,80] The intercostals are innervated by the T1-T12 thoracic nerve roots and may account for 60% of rib cage movement during ventilation.[14] With loss of neural input to the intercostal muscles, the patient will have a reduction in VC.[26]

The loss of intercostal activity may also affect diaphragmatic function. Intact intercostals provide stability of the rib cage.[57] In the presence of weakened or paralyzed intercostal muscles, negative pressure generated by diaphragmatic contraction produces a "sucking in" of the upper chest.[14,26,57,96] This increases the work of breathing for the patient. The therapist should observe the patient closely for evidence of this rib retraction and paradoxical breathing when an increased demand for oxygen is made.[100] If this becomes excessive during functional activities, rest periods should be incorporated and the patient should be monitored for evidence of lowering oxygen levels.

Accessory muscles of ventilation are primarily located in the cervical region.[31] In normal persons, they may be used to augment ventilation when the demand for oxygen increases as during exercise. Accessory muscles also may be recruited to generate an improved cough effort.[123] The most commonly cited accessory muscles are the sternocleidomastoids, the scalenes, the levator scapulae, and the trapezoids.[31,80] The erector spinae group may assist by extending the spine, thus improving the potential depth of inspiration.[49,80]

When working with the tetraplegic patient, training the accessory muscles may be advantageous to augment a weakened diaphragm and paralyzed intercostals.[123] These muscles, however, are only designed to assist ventilation. They are short and less efficient ventilatory muscles and require more oxygen to work in this capacity.[31,80] Consequently, training should proceed carefully so as to avoid fatigue.

Quiet expiration occurs passively through relaxation and recoil of lung tissue.[116] In contrast, forceful expiration and effective coughing are generated by the contraction of the expiratory muscles. The abdominal muscles, including the rectus, the transverse abdominis, and the external and internal obliques, are the primary expiratory muscles.[31,80] The latissimus dorsi, the teres major, and the clavicular portion of the pectoralis major are active during expiration and cough in tetraplegic patients.[35] Maximizing inspiratory efforts enhances cough effectiveness.[89]

Unless the SCI has affected only the lowest sacral and lumbar areas, cough efforts may be hampered because of weak or totally paralyzed abdominal muscles.[26] Loud vocalization and singing also require some active exhalation.[96] Consequently, even lower paraplegic patients may feel some effects of ventilatory impairment.

Ventilatory impairment also occurs when the patient is unable to clear secretions.[26,116] Factors such as artificial ventilation and general anesthesia hamper secretion mobilization. Artificial ventilation is used when the individual can no longer adequately exchange O_2 and CO_2 to sustain life.[116]

With artificial ventilation, patients may require an artificial airway.[15,116] The presence of this airway in the trachea poses an irritant and the patient subsequently produces more secretions.[9] These secretions are most commonly removed by suctioning, which is also an irritant, potentially causing even more secretion production. It is necessary to remove the secretions from the airway, but

caution should be taken so as not to cause undue trauma.

A description of various types and parameters of ventilation is beyond the scope of this chapter. Therapists working with patients requiring artificial ventilation, however, are referred to other publications.[59,116]

Many treatment techniques are available to address problems of ventilatory impairment caused by inspiratory muscle weakness, decreased chest wall mobility, and the inability to clear secretions.[57,89,96,100,117] These techniques include inspiratory muscle training, chest wall mobility exercises, and chest physical therapy.

Inspiratory muscle training

Diaphragm muscle training. The diaphragm should be trained initially in the supine position.[29,96,117] The abdominal excursion produced by diaphragmatic contraction is measured with a soft tape measure using fixed bony landmarks as reference points. The evaluator places the palm of the hand at the xiphoid area and over the lower rib cage, instructing the patient to inspire while appropriate visual and verbal cues are provided. The act of sniffing promotes diaphragm function (Fig. 16-13, *A,B*).

Gentle pressure on inspiration may be used to facilitate a moderately weak diaphragm. Excessive pressure may inhibit diaphragmatic contraction. As the diaphragm begins to strengthen, resistive devices may be used. Inspiratory muscle trainers with adjustable resistance are available. The diaphragm also may be trained using weights on the abdominal wall. Derrickson and others[38] concluded that both inspiratory muscle training devices and abdominal weights were effective in improving ventilatory mechanics. Muscle trainers, however, appear to promote more of an endurance effect than the use of abdominal weights. *The diaphragm is primarily an endurance muscle and should be trained with low resistance and longer treatment sessions as tolerated.*

The next step in inspiratory muscle training is to progress from a supine to a sitting position. An undesired increase of accessory muscle use may be a sign of fatigue.[117] If this occurs, the patient is returned to a more reclined position. Incorrect application of abdominal corsets can interfere with training.

Phrenic nerve pacing may be used to cause the diaphragm to contract and may be indicated when the lesion is at or above the C-3 level.[23,78,112] Electrical stimulation may be applied directly or indirectly through a vein wall or the skin or directly to the phrenic nerve. Family and patients must receive extensive education to learn equipment management and emergency procedure plans in the event of pacer failure.

Accessory muscle training. In the presence of diaphragmatic weakness, accessory muscles are trained to augment ventilation. These muscles may be recruited when the patient is disconnected from the ventilator or to improve inspiratory effort assisting with coughing and vocalization.[35,89] Accessory muscle training begins with the patient in a supine position with a slight stretch on these muscles as tolerated.[117] The stretch is accomplished by shoulder abduction and

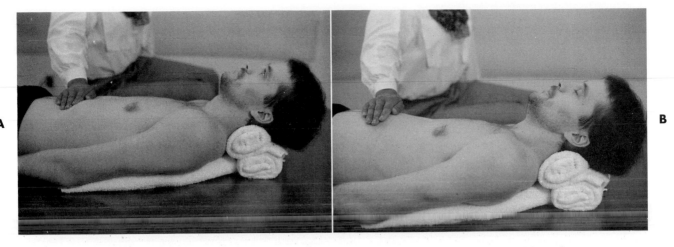

Fig. 16-13. Diaphragm facilitation. **A,** Hand placement and patient positioning to facilitate the diaphragm and inhibit accessory muscle activity. **B,** Firm contact is maintained throughout inspiration. The lower extremities are placed over a pillow in flexion to prevent stretching of the abdominal wall.

external rotation, elbow extension, forearm supination, and neutral alignment of the head and neck. A more challenging position incorporates upper thoracic extension. The therapist's hands are placed directly over the muscle to be facilitated. The patient is instructed to breathe into the upper chest (Fig. 16-14). As the treatment progresses, the diaphragm may be inhibited for short training periods by applying pressure over the abdomen in an upward direction. Care must be taken to avoid excessive pressure preventing occlusion of vital arteries.

When these exercises are effective, they are incorporated into functional activities. For example, using inspiratory maneuvers while working with ROM of the shoulder is an easy way to start. In addition, coordinating inspiratory efforts enhances endurance activities.

Glossopharyngeal breathing. Glossopharyngeal breathing (GPB) is another way of increasing vital capacity in the presence of weak inspiratory muscles.[29,89,96] By moving the jaw forward and upward in a circular opening and closing manner, air is trapped into the buccal cavity. A series of swallowing-like maneuvers forces air into the lungs, increasing the VC. This technique has been reported to increase VC by as much as 1 liter.[117] Although this technique is rarely used to sustain ventilation for long periods of time,[9] it may be used in emergency situations and to enhance cough function. The high tetraplegic patient should attempt to master this skill.

Secretion clearance. Secretions must be moved from the peripheral lung fields to the upper airway for expectoration. Postural drainage, percussion or clapping, and shaking or vibration are used to accomplish this process.[57,89,96] When choosing techniques, one should consider the presence of chest tubes or thoracic trauma. Intracranial pressure also should be monitored if there is a recent head injury.

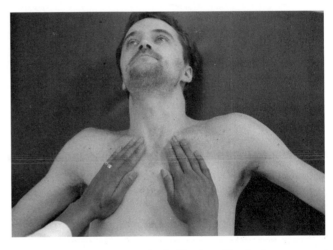

Fig. 16-14. Accessory muscle facilitation. Hand placement and patient positioning.

Quad coughing is a term used to describe assisted coughing for a person unable to generate sufficient effort.[96] The assistant places both hands firmly on the abdominal wall. After a maximal inspiratory effort, the patient coughs and the assistant simply supports the weakened wall. A gentle upward and inward force may be used to increase the intraabdominal pressure yielding a more forceful cough.[96,117] Excessive pressure over the xiphoid process should be avoided to prevent severe injury (Fig. 16-15, *A,B*).

Patients may learn independent quad coughing. In preparation for a cough, the patient positions an arm around the push handles of the wheelchair, which enhances inspiratory effort. The other arm is raised over the head and chest during inspiration. This procedure is followed by a breath hold, then strong trunk flexion and a cough (Fig.

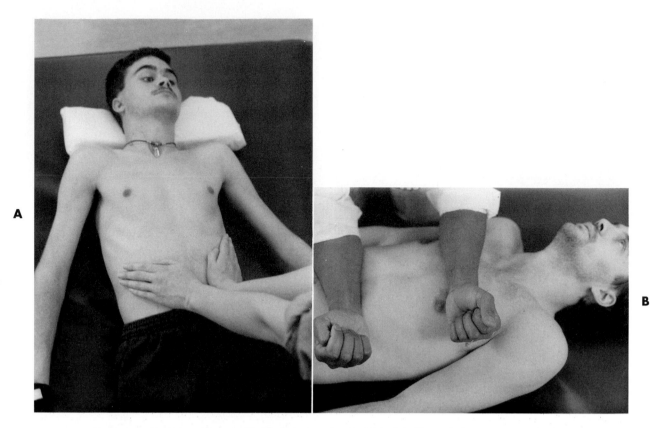

Fig. 16-15. Quad coughing. **A,** Hand placement for the Heimlich-like technique. **B,** Anterior chest wall quad coughing. The inferior forearm supination promotes an upward and inward force during the cough.

16-16 *A,B*).[96] Another technique for independent quad coughing is accomplished by placing the forearms over the abdomen and delivering a manual thrust during cough. This technique, however, is more difficult and may not provide an inspiratory advantage.

Early mobilization. Getting the patient upright as soon as possible promotes self-mobility and begins the transition from phase 1 to phase 2 of the rehabilitation. Beginning upright positioning should be planned carefully. An appropriate seating system for pressure relief and support should be chosen. The possibility of postural hypotension should be considered, and the blood pressure should be monitored when bringing the body upright. As the abdominal wall is not supporting the internal contents, abdominal binders or corsets should be applied to all patients with lesions above T12.[81,89,117] Abdominal binders and antiembolitic garments are used to assist in venous return and in the prevention of orthostatic hypotension. If the patient has a history of vascular insufficiency or prolonged bed rest, wrapping the lower extremities with elastic bandages while applying the greatest pressure distally may be beneficial.

Abdominal binders and corsets are fitted so that the top of the corset lies just over the lower two ribs.[117] They should not be placed too high or allowed to ride up, as may occur in the obese patient, because this may impair ventilation by restricting chest wall excursion. The bottom portion is placed over the anterior iliac spine and figure crest (Fig. 16-17). The corset or binder should be adjusted slightly tighter at the bottom to assist in elevating the abdominal contents.[96,100,117]

Most patients require a reclining wheelchair with elevating footrests when they first get out of bed.[96,100,117] Although the long-term goal may be the use of an upright wheelchair, patients generally do not tolerate full upright position with the initial sitting session. The use of a reclining wheelchair allows progressive acclimation to the upright position.

A weight shift or pressure relief schedule is immediately established. Initially, weight shifts are performed at 30-minute intervals and modified according to skin tolerance.[82] The skin is inspected thoroughly before and immediately after out-of-bed activities. Total sitting time is progressed according to tolerance.

The patient can be transferred via a manual or mechanical lift. Lift systems may be advantageous, as they allow total control of the patient and give the assistant more time to ensure that monitoring devices and lines or tubes attached to the patient remain intact.

The patient is transferred initially to a reclined position and progressed to an upright position as signs and symptoms of medical stability allow. The patient should be monitored for evidence of orthostatic hypotension. Dizziness or

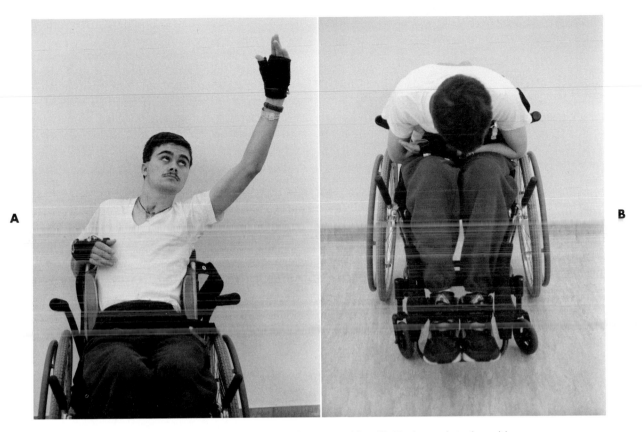

Fig. 16-16. Self quad coughing. **A,** Full inspiratory position. **B,** Expiratory/cough position.

light-headedness are most common. Ringing in the ears and visual changes also may occur. Changes in mental function may indicate more serious hypotension, and the patient should be reclined immediately. Assessing blood pressure before and during activities provides an objective measurement of the patient's status.

Monitoring cardiopulmonary responses, including heart rate and respiratory rate, is also crucial. Devices, such as pulse oximeters, measure the pulse rate and the percentage of oxygen saturation in the distal arterial system. Oxygen saturation refers to the percentage of hemoglobin that is currently carrying oxygen and is thus available to the tissues.[116] The saturation is directly affected by the amount of actual oxygen dissolved in the bloodstream. Generally, a saturation of 92% or greater is recommended in this acutely injured population in the absence of overt premorbid obstructive lung disease. Involving the patient in other activities while working toward upright tolerance helps to encourage active participation in the rehabilitation process from the beginning. Once the patient is able to tolerate upright positioning for at least 3 hours, phase 2 of rehabilitation begins.

Rehabilitation: achieving functional outcomes

The following critical elements are required to achieve functional skills:[7,91]

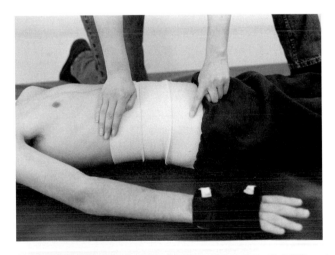

Fig. 16-17. Abdominal binder. Correct placement of ASIS and lower rib cage. Custom corsets may be used if an elastic binder does not provide adequate support to enhance VC.

- Adequate strength
- Adequate ROM
- Stable respiratory system
- Intact skin
- Tolerance for upright sitting
- Adequate cardiovascular endurance

It is important to remember that complications play a significant role in program progression and can affect outcomes and length of stay.

Pressure relief. While the patient is in bed, pressure relief is addressed and appropriate turn times are established and progressed. Pressure relief in the wheelchair is achieved when direct pressure over the bony prominences is relieved or redistributed so as to allow blood flow into the tissue directly under these prominences.

The high tetraplegic patient achieves independent pressure relief in the wheelchair via appropriately prescribed specialty controls. For example a pneumatic control switch may be used to activate the recline mode of a power wheelchair (Fig. 16-18). When the patient is unable to operate a specialty switch, an attendant control is used. When powered options are not feasible due to cognitive deficits, financial limitations, or other reasons, a manual reclining or tilt wheelchair is used (Fig. 16-19). When patients are dependent in performing pressure relief, they are taught to instruct others in this skill. Mid and low level tetraplegic patients are taught to perform a side or forward lean technique for pressure relief (Figs. 16-20, 16-21). The

paraplegic patient is usually taught to perform a push-up (depression) for pressure relief (Fig. 16-22).

Appropriate time to maintain the change in position is usually 60 seconds at intervals of 30 to 60 minutes. The treatment plan should include instructing the client in ways to ensure that the schedule for pressure relief is maintained in all settings. The use of watches, clocks, timers, and attendant care may be necessary.

Mobility

Bed mobility. The components of bed mobility include rolling side to side and supine to prone, coming to sit, and scooting in all directions. Initial training for bed mobility is usually conducted on the mat, as movement on a firm surface is easier and leads to a more successful outcome. The high tetraplegic patient is dependent with these activities and is taught to instruct others.

Bed mobility is a challenging skill to learn for patients with C5, mid, and low level tetraplegia (Fig. 16-23, A-C).[49,91] Due to the functional upper extremity strength of the paraplegic patient, bed mobility skills are often learned in a short time.

Wheelchair transfers. The physical act of moving oneself from one surface to another is described as a transfer. Wheelchair transfers may be accomplished in many different ways. The type of transfer used by a client is determined by the injury level, assistance needed, client preference, and safety of the transfer. When performing transfers, attention must be given to the use of appropriate body mechanics by both the patient and the person assisting.

Dependent transfers may be accomplished with a hydraulic patient lifter, manual pivot, sliding board, or manual lifts,

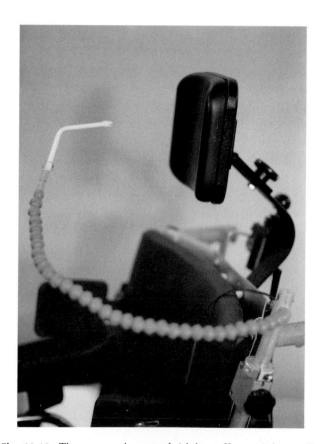

Fig. 16-18. The pneumatic control (sip'n puff straw) is usually ordered on a power reclining wheelchair. The straw is removable and several are supplied with the wheelchair. The straw is attached to a flexible arm so that it is adjustable to different heights and angles to fit the needs of the patient.

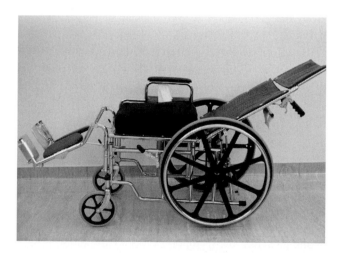

Fig. 16-19. The manual reclining wheelchair is a piece of durable medical equipment which is prescribed on a temporary or a permanent basis. The back of the wheelchair fully reclines and the legrests elevate to allow for effective pressure relief while out of bed. Other features of the wheelchair are desk armrests which may be adjustable in height, removable headrest, and removable legrests. The wheelchair folds and may be transported in the trunk of the car.

which require two or three people. The use of a hydraulic lift may be desirable to decrease wear on the part of the caregiver. On the other hand, the hydraulic lift may not be the method of choice because the lift is bulky, difficult to store, and awkward to transport. Pivot transfers or manual lifts may be taught due to patient or caregiver preference, or when patients are smaller in stature.

Assisted and independent transfers include the use of transfer boards, depression style transfers, and stand pivot transfers. The mechanics of teaching an assisted transfer to a C7 tetraplegic person is depicted in Fig. 16-24 *A-D*. The client is taught to position the wheelchair, position the transfer board, use correct body mechanics to get the best leverage to effect movement in the desired direction, remove the board, and position the body appropriately.[49,91]

Wheelchair transfers are performed to many different surfaces. The training procedure begins with the easiest transfer and progresses to the more difficult transfer. Instructions for wheelchair transfers usually begin on level surfaces and progress to uneven surfaces as individual

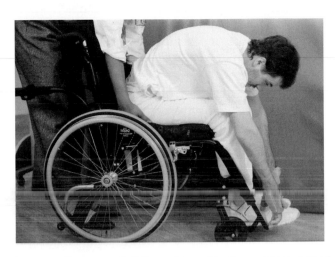

Fig. 16-21. Pressure relief: forward lean. The forward lean method of pressure relief is used for many different injury levels. The subject must have adequate range of motion at the hips and in the lumbosacral spine to allow the ischii to clear the wheelchair cushion at the end range position.

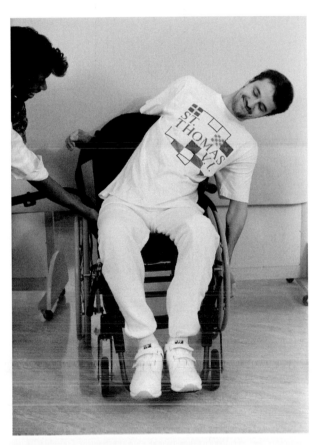

Fig. 16-20. Pressure relief: side lean. The C6/C7 level tetraplegic patient may use a side lean to achieve pressure relief over the ischial tuberosities. The patient hooks one upper extremity around the push handle of the wheelchair on one side and leans away from the hooked upper extremity until the ischium on the hooked side is clear of the wheelchair cushion. The position is maintained for one minute and repeated on the other side.

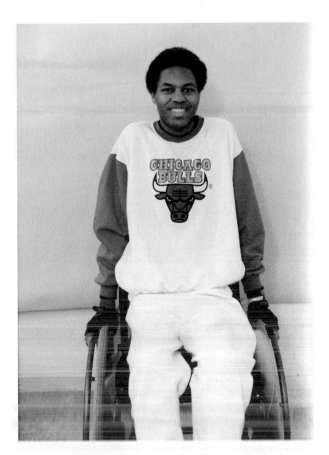

Fig. 16-22. Pressure relief: depression. This method of pressure relief is consistent with a full pushup in the wheelchair. Most paraplegic and some low tetraplegic patients are able to perform this method of pressure relief.

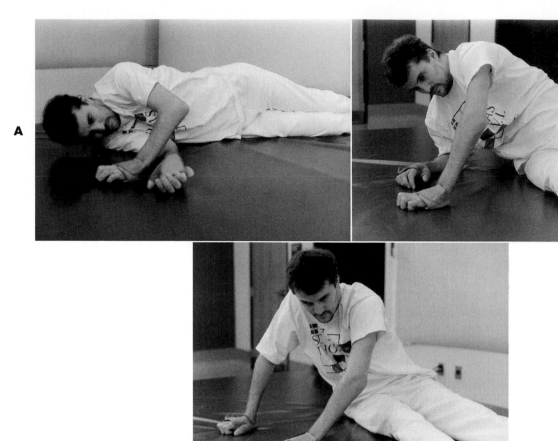

Fig. 16-23. Bed mobility. **A,** After the patient has gained enough strength to effectively roll from supine to sidelying, **B,** he progresses to supporting his weight through the downside elbow and shoulder. **C,** The third step is shifting his upper body weight onto the upper extremity that is top side, and using the head and shoulders to direct the position of the body as he performs a side pushup into the upright sitting position.

strength and skill allow.[49,91] Given these two principles, the list below is an example of how one might proceed with transfer training:

- Mat transfer
- Bed transfer
- Toilet transfer
- Bath transfer
- Car transfer (includes getting wheelchair in/out of car) (Fig. 16-25, *A-E*)
- Floor transfer (Fig. 16-26, *A-E*)
- Other surfaces, e.g., arm chair, sofa, theater seat, pool

Wheelchair mobility skills. Instructions in safe and appropriate use of the wheelchair begin before getting the patient out of bed. The patient is oriented to the wheelchair and its component parts.

Ideally, a power reclining or tilt wheelchair is supplied for high tetraplegic patients to promote maximal independence. A mid to low level tetraplegic patient may be instructed in

the use of both power and manual upright wheelchairs. The paraplegic patient is instructed only in the use of a manual upright wheelchair unless there are extenuating circumstances. For example, a power wheelchair is appropriate for a 50-year-old T12 complete paraplegic patient with severe rheumatoid arthritis.

Both power and manual wheelchair mobility training begins on level surfaces. Training progresses toward more difficult skills as follows:

- Mobility in open areas
- Setup for transfers
- Mobility in tight spaces
- Mobility in crowded areas
- On/off elevators
- Up/down ramps (Fig. 16-27)
- In/out doors
- Wheelies (paraplegic and low level tetraplegic patients, Fig. 16-28)

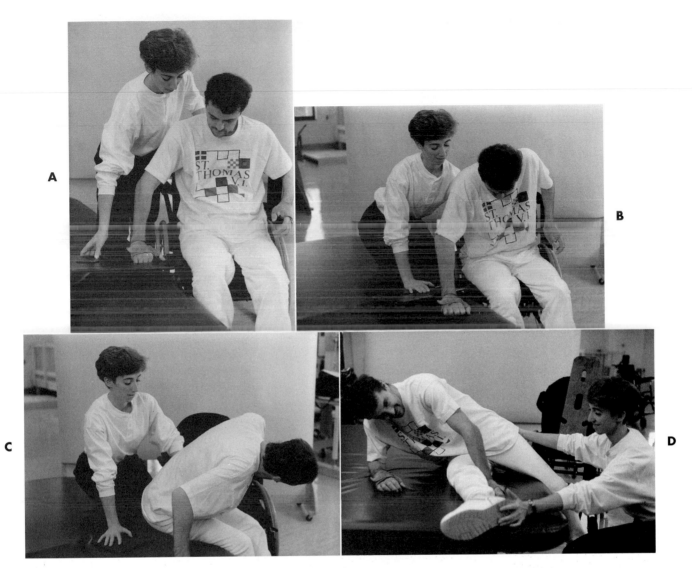

Fig. 16-24. Wheelchair transfer using a transfer board. **A,** The client positions the wheelchair at a 20-30° angle to the surface which he is transferring, and positions the board with assistance. **B,** The client positions the trailing hand close to the trailing hip and the lead hand on the transfer board or on the surface in a diagonal line. **C,** To achieve the appropriate mechanical leverage the client is instructed to twist the upper body and look over the trailing shoulder as he pushes and lifts to effect movement across the board. **D,** When the client has achieved a safe position on the transferring surface, the transfer board is removed and the client is assisted to get his feet onto the surface.

- Negotiation of rough terrains
- Up/down curbs and steps (Figs. 16-29, 16-30).

Wheelies and negotiation of steps is not appropriate for a power wheelchair user. The patient will require varying levels of assistance (Table 16-2) and instruction to reach the desired outcome.[49,51]

Activities of daily living. The scope of ADLs is extensive and may include feeding, grooming, dressing, bathing, transferring, bowel and bladder programs, communications, and home management. Generally, patients with injury levels above C6 who have less than 3/5 strength of the wrist extensors will be dependent or require significant assistance to accomplish ADLs. Specifically, patients with high tetraplegia are able to participate in some feeding and nonverbal communication skills with set-up and appropriate equipment such as electric feeders and computers. These patients, however, are rarely able to effectively participate in skills such as bathing, bowel programs, and home management.

Patients with C6 or lower injuries are capable of achieving higher functional levels of independence. Feeding and grooming skills may be accomplished with modified independence, with equipment ranging from a simple

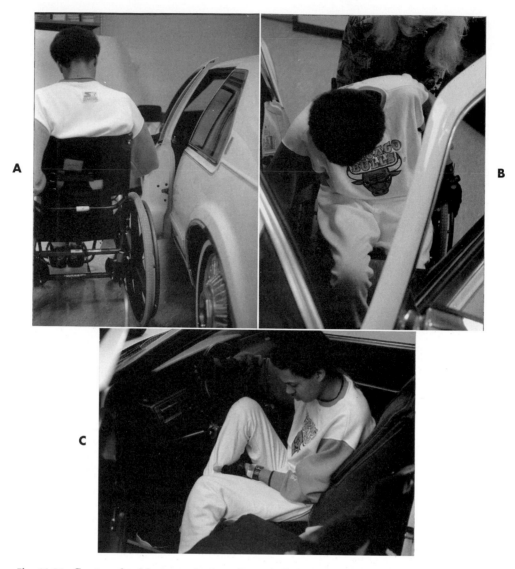

Fig. 16-25. Car transfer. Most paraplegic patients are independent (no equipment needed) in the performance of a car transfer. The client: **A,** approaches the car on the driver's side and opens the door, **B,** positions the wheelchair and does a depression style transfer onto the seat of the car, **C,** positions his lower extremities.

universal cuff adaptation to a customized tenodesis brace. Similarly, upper body dressing is an achievable skill with the use of equipment. More challenging skills for the patient with C6 tetraplegia, who requires greater assistance include lower body dressing, bathing, and bowel/bladder management. Bowel and bladder management in particular requires close coordination of nursing, occupational, and physical therapy professionals.[69,111]

Paraplegic patients, barring unforeseen circumstances, achieve functional independence with most ADLs.

Ambulation. "Will I ever walk again?" is a question often asked during SCI rehabilitation. The team must be empathetic toward and acknowledge the patient's goals for ambulation, and the subject should be discussed openly. The professionals must be careful not to take hope away from the patient. Hope is important to maintain positive survival skills in SCI rehabilitation. Patients who are not candidates for ambulation should receive an explanation of why these goals are not feasible. It is imperative that the rehabilitation team be made aware of all discussions regarding ambulation so that the team may support both the client and the involved team member.

When ambulation is an appropriate goal, the treatment program may be short and relatively uncomplicated for some and laborious for others. Treatment techniques may include therapeutic exercise, biofeedback, neuromuscular stimula-

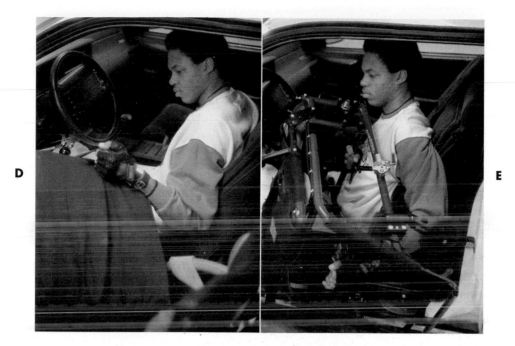

Fig. 16-25, cont'd. D, Prepares to get the cushion and wheelchair into the car. Depending on the make/model of the automobile and the model of the wheelchair (folding vs. rigid), **E,** the wheelchair is placed on the back seat or transferred across the patient and onto the passenger seat. Transferring out of the car is the reverse process beginning with the wheelchair.

tion, balance training, standing, and pregait and gait activities. The therapist must consider the postdischarge environment and include those surfaces in training.

Rehabilitation: measuring functional outcomes

To objectively record progress toward expected outcomes, appropriate measuring tools must be used. Several measuring tools have been tested for reliability and validity in the rehabilitation setting.[13] The following are examples of such tools:

- Barthel Index
- Kenny Self-Care Evaluation
- Katz Index of ADL
- Functional Independence Measure (FIM)[103]
  (Fig. 16-12)

A facility may choose to develop a tool specific to its needs. Refer to Appendix A for an example of a tool developed for use in one of the Model SCI Systems.

Equipment

In SCI rehabilitation, the use of equipment is necessary to achieve the expected outcomes. Therapists work closely with the physician and other team members, including the rehabilitation technology supplier, to determine the most appropriate equipment to meet individual needs. It is important to have access to trial equipment so that the client has the opportunity to practice with equipment similar to that

which is prescribed. The rehabilitation technology supplier should be accessible to the rehabilitation team so that necessary adjustments to the equipment can be made in a timely manner. Additionally, rehabilitation technology suppliers should be knowledgeable and responsible for educating rehabilitation professionals regarding new products. When possible, all equipment should be ordered from a single supplier to reduce confusion when the need for repairs arise. To ensure that the most appropriate piece of equipment is prescribed, the following must be considered: durability, function, transportability, comfort, cost, safety, cosmesis, and acceptance by the user.[91] Generally, the higher the injury level, the more costly the equipment due to the technology involved. Table 16-3 lists equipment according to injury level.

Ideally, equipment should be ordered as soon as possible so that the client can be fitted before discharge. Equipment required by this population is costly, requiring extensive review by third-party payers before funding is approved or denied. Many health care policies do not cover the funding of needed equipment. As a result of these factors, many patients are discharged without the equipment they need. When the patient is discharged without the prescribed equipment, the patient becomes more dependent on others to provide basic needs. Lack of appropriate equipment may result in (1) a feeling of loss of control, (2) contractures and postural deformities, (3) skin breakdown, (4) a loss of skills learned in rehabilitation, and (5) a feeling of poor self-image.

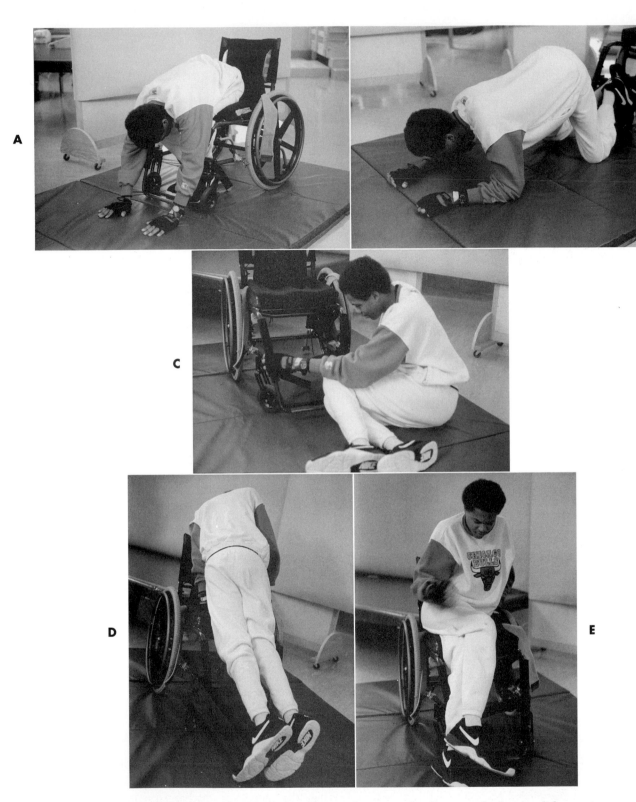

Fig. 16-26. Floor transfer. The independent performance of a floor transfer is a goal for most paraplegic patients. The patient may use different techniques to get onto the floor. **A,** Here the patient positions his feet off the footrest and moves forward onto the front edge of his cushion. **B,** He reaches for the floor with both hands, lowers his knees to the floor and advances his hands forward until his body is clear of the wheelchair. **C,** To get back into the wheelchair he approaches the wheelchair in a forward position and **D,** uses the front frame, seat and/or back of the wheelchair to push himself up into the wheelchair **E,** turning simultaneously to assume the balanced sitting position.

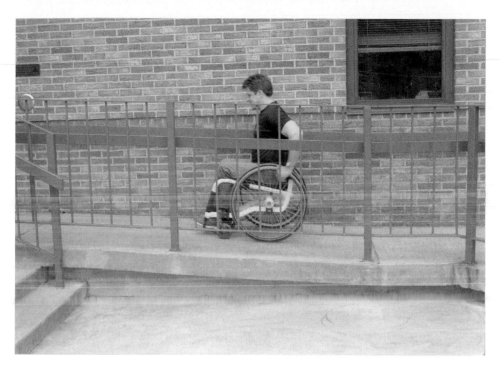

Fig. 16-27. Ascending a ramp. It is necessary to have forward momentum to ascend a ramp efficiently. Forward momentum is achieved when the client leans slightly forward and away from the back of the wheelchair while performing an even pushing stroke for propulsion of the wheelchair. The client must be instructed in safety issues relative to the wheelchair and the percent of incline of the ramp.

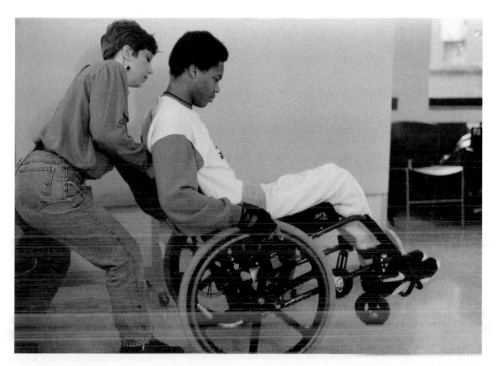

Fig. 16-28. A wheelie is a functional mobility skill which enhances functional independence. The performance of a wheelie is a precursor to negotiating steep ramps, curbs, steps, and rough terrain

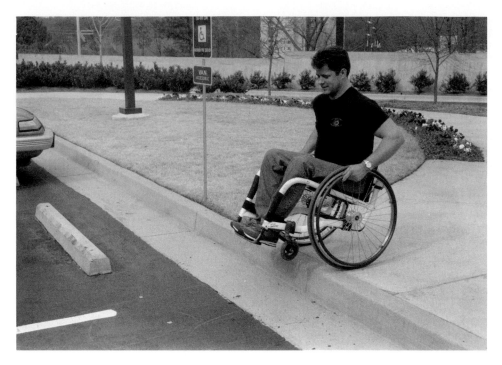

Fig. 16-29. Descending a curb is an advanced wheelchair mobility skill. This T7 paraplegic male assumes the balanced wheelie position and approaches the curb in a forward position. The wheelie position is maintained as he rolls off the curb.

Education

Education of the patient and significant others is an integral part of the rehabilitation process. Formal education includes group and individual instruction and family/caregiver training. Patients and caregivers are taught preventive skin care, bowel and bladder programs, nutritional guidelines, thermoregulation precautions, pulmonary management, cardiopulmonary resuscitation, management of autonomic dysreflexia, equipment management and maintenance, transfer techniques, wheelchair mobility, ambulation, proper body positioning, ROM exercises, and leisure skills. Home programs are taught to maintain or increase strength, endurance, ROM, and function. Energy conservation techniques and proper body mechanics are incorporated in all aspects of training.

Patients are formally tested on their knowledge, and remedial instruction should be provided in deficient areas. During family training, caregivers are formally evaluated on their abilities to safely provide care to the patient. Supervised therapeutic outings and passes allow the patient, caregivers, and the team to identify problem areas and provide additional education in those areas.

Psychosocial issues in SCI rehabilitation

The immediate reaction to the onset of SCI is physical shock accompanied by anxiety, pain, and fear of dying. The response to such an injury varies greatly and depends on the extent of the injury, premorbid activity level, style of coping

with stress, and family and financial resources. There may be great sensory deprivation due to immobilization, neurological impairment, and the monotony of the hospital routine. Several psychological theories have been proposed to describe responses and coping mechanisms.[65] The process of coping with these changes is referred to as adjustment (See Chapter 7).

Rehabilitation personnel are becoming more aware of the need not only to teach functional skills, but also to teach psychosocial and coping skills to the patient and significant others. Education in the following areas facilitates the adjustment process: creative recreation, financial planning, negotiating community barriers, social skills, managing an attendant, creative problem solving, accessing community resources, assertiveness, sexual expression, vocational planning/training, and the use of community transportation. These skills may be introduced in the inpatient rehabilitation setting but will be developed further in the home and community environments. True adjustment and adaptation begin after discharge from rehabilitation.[107,108]

Sexual issues

Altered sexual function is of concern to the SCI population.[130] The injury may result in impairment of erection, ejaculation, orgasm, male fertility, and vaginal lubrication.[46] Table 16-4 lists the relationship of level of spinal injury to sexual function. Formal sexual counseling and education are indicated before discharge from a

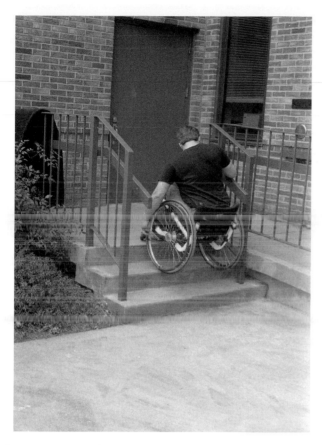

Fig. 16-30. Descending steps using one handrail. This T7 paraplegic person approaches the steps backward, and using the handrail on his right side and the handrim of the wheelchair on the left side lowers himself down three (3) steps. This is one of several methods which may be used to negotiate steps.

Table 16-3. Equipment needs correlated to injury level

Injury level	Equipment	Cost
C1 to C3	Power reclining or tilt wheelchair	$13,000-18,000
	Portable ventilator	7,000-10,000
	Bedside ventilator	7,000-10,000
	Electric hospital bed	1,800-2,200
	Hydraulic patient lifter	1,300
	Reclining shower chair/ stretcher	1,500
	Wheelchair cushion	350-450
	Van modifications	12,000-20,000
	Computer/Access/Printer	4,500
	Environmental control system	2,000
	Communication devices	300-1,500
C4 to C5	Power reclining wheelchair	$10,000-12,000
	Wheelchair cushion	350-450
	Roll-in shower chair	1,300
	Hydraulic patient lifter	1,300
	Electric hospital bed	1,800-2,200
	Van modifications	12,000-20,000
	Computer	4,000
	Environmental control system	1,500
C6 to C7	Power upright wheelchair *or* manual upright wheelchair	$ 6,000-8,000 1,700-2,200
	Roll-in shower chair	1,300
	Wheelchair cushion	350-450
	Electric hospital bed	1,800-2,200
	Van modifications	15,000-25,000
	Hand controls for automobile	495-650
	Hand brace	1,100
C8 to T1	Lightweight manual upright wheelchair	$ 1,700-2,200
	Wheelchair cushion	350-450
	Roll-in shower chair	1,300
	Tub chair/tub bench	600/180
	Raised padded toilet seat	115
	Hand controls for automobile	495-600
T2 to T11	Lightweight upright wheelchair	$ 1,700-2,200
	Wheelchair cushion	350-450
	Tub bench/tub cushion	180/40
	Hand controls for automobile	495-650
	Raised toilet	115
T12-L2	Same as T2 to T11	
	Bilateral knee ankle foot orthoses	$ 3,500-4,000

Based on 1994 Atlanta, Ga retail prices

rehabilitation center. The educational program includes group sessions to address general issues as well as individual sexual function evaluations.[130] Sexual counseling, educational programs, and medical management provide opportunities to address the areas of sexual dysfunction, alternative behaviors, precautions, and other related areas.[46]

Treatment of sexual function is a coordinated effort between the patient, significant other, psychologist, and urologist. Options may include surgical implantation of a penile prosthesis, vacuum erection devices, intracorporeal injection therapy, and the use of lubricants.[99] Refer to Appendix C for additional references regarding sexual function following SCI.

Discharge planning

Discharge planning begins from the time the patient is admitted and continues through the rehabilitation program. It is a continuous process that includes the patient, family, treatment team, and community resources, with the goal being successful community reintegration and a perceived good quality of life. The rehabilitation team must identify the specific needs of the patient and structure the program necessary to enhance the chance of success. Lengths of stay are getting shorter in response to pressure from third-party payers to contain costs. This requires the discharge planning process to be expedited so that procurement of needed equipment, completion of architectural modifications, and referrals to outpatient and community resources occur in a timely manner.

Table 16-4. Relation of level of spinal injury to sexual function

Injury level	Sexual function
Cauda equina/conus	Males: usually no reflex erections rare psychogenic erection ejaculation occasionally occurs Females: vaginal secretions often absent patients generally fertile
Thoracic/cervical	Males: reflex erections predominate (usually short duration) psychogenic erections generally absent ejaculation occasional Females: vaginal secretions present as a part of genital reflex fertility preserved sensation of labor pain absent

Architectural modifications. Architectural barriers in the home, transportation system, work place, or school may prevent access to opportunities. The architectural changes required by the person with SCI for independence in the home and community depend on the degree of impairment, financial resources, and patient/family acceptance of modifications and/or equipment.

Many available resources describe the dimensions of the basic wheelchair and specifications for making homes and facilities accessible to wheelchair users. Refer to Appendix B for resources on architectural modification.

Return to work or school. Successful reintegration after SCI may include returning to work or school. Public school systems have a legal obligation to provide an appropriate school setting for a disabled child. Fewer than 25% of individuals with SCI are employed 5 years after injury.[5,101] Rehabilitation programs must emphasize returning to work throughout the process to improve a patient's successful return to work and facilitate adjustment to SCI.

Many individuals can return to their previous job after SCI.[8,75] The Americans With Disabilities Act (ADA) of 1990, P.L. 101-336, prohibits businesses with 25 or more employees (effective July 26, 1992) and 14 to 24 employees (effective July 26, 1994) from discriminating against "qualified individuals with disabilities" with respect to the terms, conditions, or privileges of employment.[60] Some situations may require modifications to the job site or a change in responsibilities. For those who are unable to perform previous jobs or who were unemployed before injury, many programs exist for training in vocational skills. The Department of Rehabilitation Services (DRS) evaluates clients for skills and functional abilities and provides funding for those qualifying for job training,

job site modification, and the purchase of essential equipment. Services offered by DRS vary from state to state. Each state agency has a list of resources available in the community, such as rehabilitation technology, independent living centers, and job training and placement programs. Individuals should refer to their state DRS for assistance with employment.

Outpatient referral. When patients are unable to reach all of their goals as inpatients, a referral to an outpatient facility with experience in the treatment of SCI is necessary. The need for referral to **outpatient** should be anticipated early in the rehabilitation program so that therapeutic intervention can continue without interruption. An outpatient follow-up appointment should be scheduled before the patient's discharge to reevaluate medical and functional status and make any program changes before complications can occur.

OUTPATIENT SERVICES

Discharge from an **inpatient** rehabilitation program marks only the beginning of the lifelong process of adjustment to disability and community reintegration. Inpatient rehabilitation provides an environment best suited for learning self-care skills, yet "the implications of living in the community with SCI can scarcely be anticipated accurately by the newly injured individual or the able-bodied staff (p. 324)."[65] Comprehensive outpatient services have traditionally been available for routine follow-up assessments, medical care, psychological services, vocational planning/training, and continued therapy services.

Common outpatient therapy treatment programs have included advanced transfer training, advanced wheelchair mobility training, gait training, upgraded ADL training, and upgraded home exercise program instruction. Outpatient therapy, however, is used increasingly for functional training, which traditionally was a part of the inpatient rehabilitation. This is a direct result of cost-containment efforts resulting in shortened length of stays. A direct consequence of this shift results in outpatient treatment of patients who present with more acuity, greater care needs, and fewer skills attained in the inpatient rehabilitation program before entry in the outpatient arena.

The Day Hospital concept has emerged to meet the demand for more cost-saving rehabilitation services. Patients who are medically stable, do not require skilled nursing services during the night, tolerate 3 hours or more of therapy per visit, need a coordinated approach for two or more services, and who have a discharge plan in place are candidates for Day Hospital services.

ADDITIONAL CLINICAL CONSIDERATIONS
Lower extremity orthotic disposition

The philosophy regarding the use of **orthotics** for ambulation for individuals with ASIA impairment scores of A and B varies greatly among rehabilitation centers. Some facilities encourage ambulation for these individuals, whereas others strongly discourage it given that only a small percentage of these clients continue to use orthotics after training has been completed.[21,94]

When the philosophy of the rehabilitation center is to brace the motor complete patient (ASIA impairment A and B), criteria should be established so that both the patient and the professional staff are consistent in the approach to ambulation. This gives the patient specific information and clarifies goals to be attained, ensuring the most positive outcome.

Criteria for ambulation trial may include:

- Expressed desire for ambulation with appropriate goals
- Body weight not to exceed 10% of ideal
- ROM. (hip extension 5 degrees, full knee extension, ankle dorsiflexion 5 to 15 degrees, passive straight leg raise 110 degrees)
- Intact skin
- Stable cardiovascular system
- Controlled spasticity
- Independent function at the wheelchair level

The ambulation trial gives the team and the patient an opportunity to preview what the use of orthotics will be like. If the decision is made to order orthotics, specific goals are set. Goals range from standing and exercise ambulation to community ambulation. Most persons with complete injuries above L2 achieve only exercise ambulation due to the energy necessary for functional ambulation.

According to research performed at Rancho Los Amigos Hospital, the energy cost of ambulation for individuals with complete lesions at T12 or higher is above the anaerobic threshold and cannot be maintained over time. This study also concluded that ambulation for these individuals using a swing through gait pattern is equivalent to "heavy work" or a variety of recreational and sporting activities.[25,94,113] Consequently, it is easy to understand why braces may end up in the closet unused.

The energy cost for ambulation is highest for persons with complete paraplegia who use a swing through gait pattern and lowest for persons who use bilateral ankle-foot orthoses (AFO) or a combination of an AFO and a knee-ankle-foot orthosis (KAFO). Even individuals requiring only bilateral AFOs have a gait efficiency of less than 50% of normal, underscoring the importance of the hip extensor and abductor muscles required for normal ambulation. These muscles are severely or completely paralyzed in this population.

Given intact upper extremities, the energy cost of ambulation is progressively reduced when more residual motor function is present in the lower extremities. Conversely, the person with incomplete tetraplegia has higher energy costs for ambulation despite spared lower extremity function because of upper and lower extremity weakness.[25,94,113]

Levels for ambulation have been classified into four categories:[36]

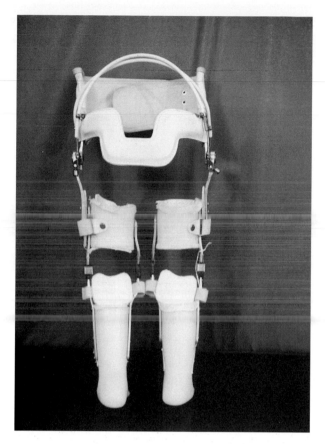

Fig. 16-31. The reciprocating gait orthosis (RGO) while generally used with children is also used with the adult population. Its main components are a molded pelvic band, thoracic extensions, bilateral hip and knee joints, polypropylene posterior thigh shells and AFO sections, and cables connecting the two hip joint mechanisms.

- Standing only
- Exercise—ambulates short distances
- Household—ambulates inside home or work, uses wheelchair much of the time
- Community—independent on all surfaces, does not use the wheelchair

Lower extremity orthotics appropriate for this population are:

- Hip-Knee-Ankle-Foot-Orthosis (HKAFO)
  Reciprocating gait orthosis (RGO), (Fig. 16-31)
  Bilateral KAFOs with pelvic band
- Knee-Ankle-Foot-Orthosis
  Scott-Craig KAFOs, (Fig. 16-32)
  Conventional KAFOs
  Polypropylene KAFOs, (Fig. 16-33)
  New England Rehabilitation KAFOs
- Ankle-Foot-Orthosis
  Conventional AFOs, metal
  Custom polypropylene AFOs, solid ankle, (Fig. 16-34)

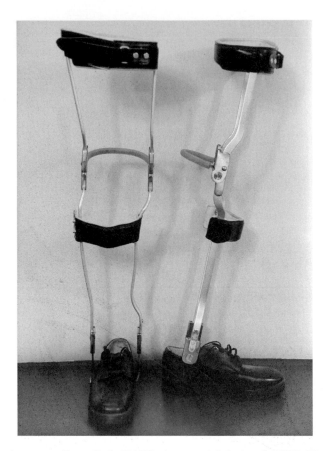

Fig. 16-32. Scott-Craig KAFOs is a special design for SCI. The orthosis consists of double uprights, offset knee joints with pawl locks and bail control, one posterior thigh band, a hinged anterior tibial band, an ankle joint with anterior and posterior adjustable pin stops, a cushion heel, and specially designed longitudinal and transverse foot plates made of steel.

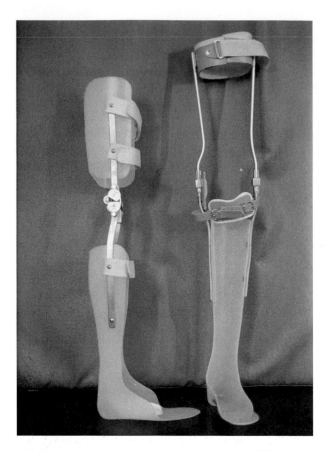

Fig. 16-33. Combination plastic and metal KAFOs.

Custom polypropylene AFOs, articulated ankle, (Fig. 16-35)
University of California Biomechanics Lab (UCBL)

Factors that affect brace selection are cost, experience and bias of the clinician, injury level, residual motor function, and client acceptance. Generally, the HKAFO is used when selected motions of the hip need control, or benefits of the reciprocating gait orthosis are desired, as is the case with the pediatric population. Use of a KAFO is indicated when the quadriceps muscle strength is less than 3/5. AFOs are indicated in the presence of ankle instability and weakness and to prevent hyperextension of the knee joint. Refer to Table 16-5 for correlation of complete injury levels and orthotic disposition.

Orthotic disposition of the incomplete patient is more challenging due to the complexity of problems and varying degrees of impairment. These clients may present with pain, ROM limitations, weakness, and spasticity. These problems sometimes preclude ambulation. Asymmetries such as muscle shortening on the stronger side and lengthening on the weaker side may lead to pelvic obliquity and scoliosis. An orthotic team approach is desirable for all orthotic disposition but is extremely useful and considered a requirement to meet the needs of the incomplete SCI client. Even if orthotic devices enable the patient to become independent, the energy and joint costs on normal joints and muscles over the life expectancy of the individual need to be considered.

Functional electrical stimulation for standing and ambulation

In April 1994 the Food and Drug Administration approved for marketing the first microcomputer-controlled functional neuromuscular stimulation (FNS) device called the Parastep System. The Parastep System comes from the medical engineering sciences known as neuroprosthetics. It is an FNS modality provided as an alternative to traditional bracing and other orthotic approaches to long-term rehabilitation management of SCI.

The Parastep System enables appropriately selected, skeletally mature persons with spinal cord injury (C6-T12) to stand and attain limited ambulation and/or take steps following a prescribed program of physical therapy performed in conjunction with rehabilitation. The Parastep System is noninvasive; it consists of a battery-powered,

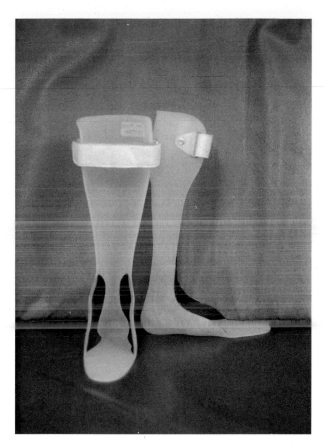

Fig. 16-34. Custom solid ankle AFOs in five degrees dorsiflexion with full footplates.

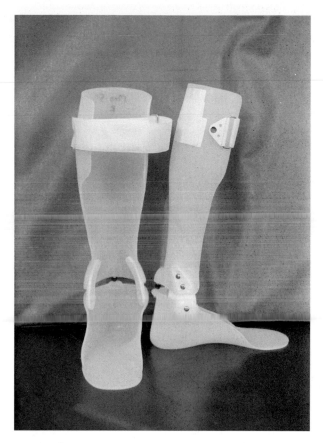

Fig. 16-35. Custom articulated AFOs with adjustable Oklahoma ankle joints.

microcomputer-controlled neuromuscular stimulator and a walker with handgrip-mounted control switches. Unlike other systems, the Parastep System via surface electrodes affords the user the ability to activate his or her own muscles and stand and bear weight on the long bones of the legs.*

Seating principles

Many individuals spend 8 hours or more per day in their wheelchairs after SCI. Consequently, proper seating of these patients may be the most important intervention therapists provide. The seating process should be addressed early in the acute phase, continually throughout the rehabilitation program, and regularly after discharge to help prevent and minimize complications.[49,76] The wheelchair is an integral part of the client's self-image and in many ways will help define personal life-style.[91] Goals for seating the client with SCI are the following:

- Maximize functional independence
- Optimize pressure distribution and relief of pressure

- Optimize comfort
- Enhance the quality of life
- Optimize good postural alignment
- Compensate for fixed deformities
- Maximize ease of transportation of the seating system

The following are basic seating concepts of proper postural alignment:

- Neutral pelvic alignment
- Symmetrical alignment of the trunk and neck
- Neutral head positioning over the pelvis
- Maintenance of a horizontal gaze
- Maintenance of 90 degree angle at the hips, knees, and ankles
- Maintenance of the thighs in neutral abduction
- Neutral shoulder positioning to avoid shoulder elevation, protraction or retraction and to provide adequate upper extremity support[76,129]

Every seating session begins with a thorough evaluation of the client's posture and needs.[76] Trial simulations are essential to determine how the patient will function and maintain posture over time in the seating system. Simulations help to avoid costly mistakes. The patient must be

---

*Habasevich B: Personal communication, Sept 19, 1994. Sigmedics, Inc., One Northfield Plaza, Suite 410, Northfield, IL 60093; telephone (708) 501-3500, fax (708) 501-3404.

Table 16-5. Correlation of complete injury levels and orthotic disposition

Injury level	Muscles present	Orthoses	Goals	Bracing recommended
Above T2	Partial upper extremity function	Standing frames RGOs	Standing ?? Exercise amb.	No
T2 to T6	Complete upper extremity function	Standing frames RGOs KAFOs w/spreader bar	Standing ? Exercise amb.	No
T7 to T10	Partial function of trunk muscles	RGOs KAFOs w/spreader bar	Standing Exercise amb.	No
T11 to T12	Almost complete function of trunk	RGOs KAFOs w/spreader bar	Exercise amb.	Sometimes
L1	Complete trunk function	RGOs KAFOs w/spreader bar	Exercise amb. Sometimes household	Usually
L2	Hip flexors	KAFOs	Exercise amb. Household amb.	Usually
L3	Quadriceps	Combination KAFO/AFO Bil. AFOs	Household amb. Community amb.	Yes
L4 and below	Quadriceps Partial hamstrings Partial ankle Partial hips	AFOs UCBL	Community amb.	Yes

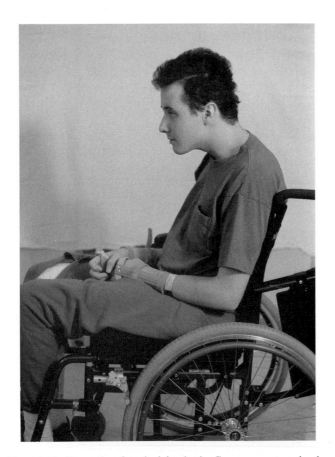

Fig. 16-36. Example of typical kyphotic C-curve posture in the patient with tetraplegia.

involved in the decision-making process to ensure that the seating system will work.

The seating process may be complicated by impaired or loss of sensation and mobility. Great care must be taken to reduce pressure over bony prominences and to distribute pressure over as large an area as possible.[76] Pressure-relieving cushions should be evaluated clinically and with pressure-sensing devices to determine the optimal wheelchair cushion for each individual.[76,129]

Many patients with muscle paralysis of the trunk find that the effects of gravity in a sitting position pull their heads over their laps, resulting in a long kyphosis or a C-curved posture (Fig. 16-36).[129] Two resulting problems are increased weight bearing on the bony sacrum and development of a thoracic kyphosis, leading to neck hyperextension in the effort to maintain a horizontal gaze.[7] Unfortunately, this poor seating posture is quickly learned and difficult to correct.[7] This posture often can be prevented by tilting the wheelchair slightly backwards while maintaining a fixed seat-to-back angle (Fig. 16-37).[76] In that position, the effects of gravity augment sitting balance and facilitate good spinal alignment. The use of a sacral block, a firm wheelchair seat and back, and properly applied seat belts also aid in preventing the C-curved posture.[76]

Asymmetrical muscle strength, asymmetrical spasticity, and power wheelchair propulsion using predominantly one upper extremity often result in poor trunk alignment. The use of lateral trunk supports and lateral thigh bolsters combined, with properly applied seat belts and shoulder harnesses, may aid in maintaining symmetrical trunk posture.

Strong muscle spasms, combined with the effects of gravity, may cause the person with severely impaired mobility to slide down in the wheelchair, resulting in increased pressure on the sacrum and shearing of the skin. For these patients, a wheelchair with a fixed seat-to-back angle that tilts backwards to allow for the performance of pressure relief may help to reduce this problem (Fig. 16-38).

The size, weight, and portability of the seating system affect the individual's life-style. The patient's home or work environment must be evaluated closely for accessibility so that the seating system can be used effectively in those environments. The buildings must be structurally sound and spacious to accommodate heavy power wheelchair systems. The means of transportation of the wheelchair (car versus van) determines whether a fixed or folding wheelchair frame is indicated and possibly whether or not a portable power wheelchair is the best choice.

The wheelchair must be as easy as possible to propel to reduce stress on upper extremity joints. Many manual wheelchairs are lightweight (less than 25 pounds) and have multiple adjustments and choices of tires and casters that make manual wheelchair propulsion more efficient. The correct rear tire size reduces shoulder musculature fatigue. Rear tire size should be selected so that when the wheelchair

user is seated with hands resting on the top of the push rims, there is 60 degrees of elbow flexion and no shoulder elevation.[24] In addition, shifting the distribution of the user's weight back over the rear axle (usually accomplished by moving the rear wheel axle forward) reduces the percentage of weight on the front casters making propulsion more efficient.[24]

Distributing pressure over as large a surface area as possible without endangering function should be considered when taking wheelchair measurements. The width of the seat (wheelchairs are made with the same width seat and back) should be slightly wider than the width of the widest body part. The seat depth should come to within 1 inch of the popliteal fossae. The height of the back should reflect the client's motor function and be no lower than the presence of functional musculature to provide appropriate trunk support. If the back height is too high, it can restrict functional activities such as wheelchair propulsion and wheelies. Tetraplegic patients who use the push handles of the wheelchair to hook while performing functional activities may require custom modification of the wheelchair back (Fig. 16-39).

Finally, the impact of the wheelchair on the individual's self-image must be considered. The entire focus of the

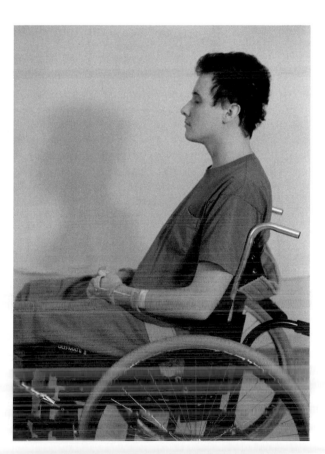

Fig. 16-37. Example of corrected C curve posture.

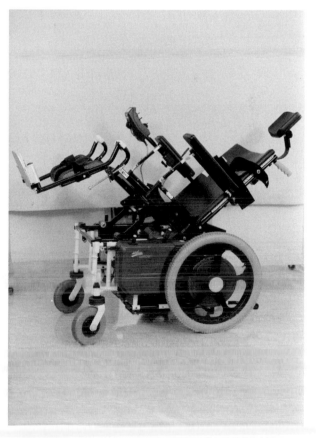

Fig. 16-38. Example of power-tilt-in-space wheelchair.

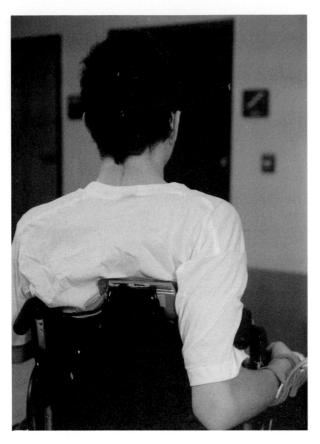

Fig. 16-39. Example of custom modification of a wheelchair back to allow a patient with tetraplegia to hook the push handle with one upper extremity.

rehabilitation process is successful community reintegration. An attractive seating system is an integral tool for the patient's success.

CONCLUSION

Comprehensive treatment of the individual with SCI continues to be a challenge to the rehabilitation team and to society as a whole. Health care reform issues force the rehabilitation team to explore new cost-efficient options to provide quality rehabilitation. New medical interventions improve the prognosis for return of function to a greater extent for the incomplete versus complete lesions. Additionally, the aging of this population presents new problems that require intervention and cause the team to examine past rehabilitation goals and treatment strategies. Passage of the ADA points out that community reintegration of individuals with disabilities is a responsibility of society. These and other issues will present many challenges for individuals with SCI in the future.

CASE 1 ▼ C5-C6 Fracture

The patient, a 24-year-old man, was drag racing on a country road after having consumed several beers. An unrestrained driver, he lost control of his car. The car rolled several times and he was thrown approximately 20 feet from the vehicle. When the emergency medical services arrived at the scene, the patient was unconscious. A cervical collar was applied and he was placed on a spine board for transportation to the closest emergency medical center.

Upon arrival, the patient had regained consciousness, and there was no memory of the accident. The physician ordered radiographs of the spine, skull, and chest. The spine radiographs revealed C5-C6 fracture/subluxation. Chest radiographs demonstrated rib fractures laterally at ribs 4, 5, and 6 on

the left. Skull fractures were ruled out. Physical examination revealed the following: patient awake and alert, absent deep tendon reflexes (indicative of spinal shock), absent sensation below the nipple line, and no volitional movement in the upper or lower extremities except for shoulder shrugs and elbow flexion.

Within 2 hours of the initial injury, methylprednisolone, 30 mg/kg, was administered intravenously. In addition emergency room treatment consisted of starting an intravenous catheter, inserting a Foley catheter, administering oxygen via nasal cannula, and continuing immobilization in the cervical collar. Arrangements were made for transfer to a model spinal cord injury center 20 miles away.

CASE 1 ▼ C5-C6 Fracture—cont'd

Upon admission to the SCI center, the patient was taken to the intensive care unit and evaluated by the attending physician. Confirmation of the previously established C5 motor level was made, and the sensory picture had improved with impaired light touch present in the lower extremities and sacral dermatomes. The diagnosis of C5 tetraplegia with an ASIA impairment of B was given. The patient was immediately placed in cervical traction via Gardner-Wells tongs and was transferred to the computed tomographic (CT) scanner for imaging of the abdomen, cervical spine, and skull. CT of the skull and the abdomen were negative. CT of the cervical spine and the chest confirmed the initial diagnosis of fractures. A decision was made to manage the patient with external fixation using halo traction. The patient was placed on DVT prophylaxis and the methylprednisolone protocol was continued.

Referrals were made to the rehabilitation team including physical therapy, occupational therapy, respiratory therapy, therapeutic recreation, social services, psychological services, speech therapy, and dietary services. Strict turning times, with appropriate padding and positioning, were initiated by the nursing staff to prevent decubitus ulcers, contractures, and pulmonary complications.

All team members made initial contact with the patient within 2 days of admission. The therapy evaluations revealed the following: Functional biceps and wrist extensors bilaterally with absent motor function of all other key muscles of the upper extremity; a strong isometric contraction was noted in the trunk musculature (unable to fully test secondary to the halo vest); hip flexor and extensor muscles were 2/5; knee extensors were 3/5; knee flexors were 1/5; ankle dorsiflexors were 1/5 bilaterally. The motor neurological level was C6 bilaterally, and the ASIA impairment scale had improved to a C.

The patient's vital capacity was 1200 ml, and he complained of left chest wall pain during inspiration. His cough was weak but productive. There was evidence of spasticity with sustained clonus in the right ankle. The Ashworth score was 2 on the left and 3 on the right. Initial treatment consisted of ROM exercises, deep breathing exercises, and a positioning program to prevent adaptive shortening. Out-of-bed orders were received on day 3 and phase 2 began when the patient tolerated 3 hours of therapy daily. Rehabilitation goals were established with the patient and family by all team members.

Through phases 2 and 3 the patient had regained functional strength in the triceps and had weak hand intrinsics. The lower extremities improved to functional strength on the left side; and on the right there was weakness in the gluteal, hip flexor, and ankle musculature. He had normal bowel function. The patient's bladder program was self-voiding; however, he performed intermittent catheterization for residual volume checks using a short opponens brace to assist with a pincer grasp.

The patient was prescribed a rental hemiheight manual wheelchair in seating clinic and was modified independent with propulsion on smooth surfaces and over rough terrain. He was evaluated in brace clinic and began gait training in the parallel bars with the use of a right KAFO. He was independent in all transfers. The patient required minimal assistance in meal preparation and was able to eat using utensils with built up handles. He was able to dress his upper and lower extremities independently using a button hook and zipper pull. He was modified independent in all grooming and bathing skills. A tub bench was necessary during bathing to address balance and endurance deficits, and a long-handled sponge allowed access to hard-to-reach areas. The patient was modified independent in written communication skills with adapted writing equipment (built up pens/pencils or short Wanchik splint). A driving evaluation was completed, and the patient was able to drive with minor modifications. The psychologist counseled the patient and his wife on sexuality and sexual functioning.

The physical therapist completed a home assessment before phase 3. Recommendations were made to accommodate the wheelchair, yet leave flexibility for increased ambulation function. The occupational therapist evaluated the work site to ensure accessibility before the patient returned to work. The social worker contacted the vocational rehabilitation counselor to investigate other work opportunities at the patient's present place of employment. The patient was a car mechanic and would be unable to return to his previous job duties due to hand weakness and an inability to lift heavy objects.

At the time of discharge, the patient and his family understood and appropriately performed his programs. The physical and occupational therapists provided the patient with home exercise programs specific to his strengthening needs. The physical therapist initiated an outpatient referral for gait, balance, and endurance training.

After 6 weeks of outpatient therapy, the patient's endurance and balance had improved, allowing full-time ambulation. The rental wheelchair was discontinued. The patient was discharged from outpatient physical therapy with a revised home exercise program. Physical therapy reassessment and follow-up assessments from all other team members would occur at 8 weeks after discharge from inpatient rehabilitation.

REFERENCES

1. Abruzzesse R: Pressure sores: nursing aspects and prevention. In Lee B and others, editors: *The spinal cord injured patient: comprehensive management,* Philadelphia, 1991, WB Saunders.
2. *Accreditation Manual for Hospitals 1994,* Vol. I standards, 1993 Joint Commission of Accreditation of Health Care Organizations, Oakbrook Terrace, IL.
3. Achong MR: Urinary tract infecions in the patient with a neurogenic bladder. In Bloch R and Basbaum M, editors: *Management of spinal cord injuries,* Baltimore, 1986, Williams & Wilkins.
4. Aljure J, Eltorai I, and Bradley WE: Carpal tunnel syndrome in paraplegic patients, *Paraplegia* 23:182-86, 1985.
5. *Annual reports 9 and 10 for the Model Spinal Cord Injury Care Systems,* The National Spinal Cord Injury Statistical Center, University of Alabama, Birmingham, Ala., 1992.
6. Apple DF and Hudson LM, editors: *Spinal cord injury: the model,* Proceedings of the national consensus conference on catastrophic illness and injury—the spinal cord injury model: lessons learned and new applications, December, 1989, Atlanta, The Georgia Regional Spinal Cord Injury Care System, Shepherd Spinal Center, 1990.
7. Atrice M and others: Acute physical therapy management of individuals with spinal cord injury, *Orthop Clin North Am* 2(1):53-70, 1993.
8. Axelson P and others: *Spinal cord injury: a guide for patient and family,* New York, 1987, Raven Press.
9. Bach JR: New approaches in the rehabilitation of the traumatic high level quadriplegic, *Am J Phys Med Rehabil* 70(1):13-19, 1991.
10. Balazy TE: Clinical management of chronic pain in spinal cord injury, *Clin J Pain* 8(2):102-109, 1992.
11. Banja JD: Rehabilitation and empowerment, *Arch Phys Med Rehabil* 71:614-615, 1990.
12. Banwell JG and others: Management of the neurogenic bowel in patients with spinal cord injury, *Urol Clin North Am* 20(3):517-525, 1993.
13. Barnes ML and others: *Physical therapy,* Philadelphia, 1989, JB Lippincott.
14. Bergofsky EH: Mechanisms for respiratory insufficiency after cervical cord injury: a source of alveolar hypoventilation, *Ann Intern Med* 61(3):435-447, 1964.
15. Biering-Sörensen M and Biering-Sörensen F: Tracheostomy in spinal cord injured: frequency and follow up, *Paraplegia* 30:656-660, 1992.
16. Blissitt PA: Nutrition in acute spinal cord injury, *Crit Care Nurs Clin North Am* 2:375, 1990.
17. Bloch RF: Autonomic dysfunction. In Bloch RF and Basbaum M, editors: *Management of spinal cord injuries,* Baltimore, 1986, Williams & Wilkins.
18. Bosch A and others: Incomplete traumatic quadriplegia: a 10 year review, *JAMA* 216(3):473-478, 1971.
19. Bracken MB: Pharmacological treatment of acute spinal cord injury: current status and future projects, *J Emerg Med* 2:43-48, 1993.
20. Bridwell KH and Dewald RL: *Textbook of spinal surgery,* Philadelphia, 1991, JB Lippincott.
21. Bromley I: Rehabilitation: some thoughts on progress, *Paraplegia* 30:70-72, 1992.
22. Brown DJ: Spinal cord injuries: the last decade and the next, *Paraplegia* 30:77-82, 1992.
23. Brownledd S and Williams S: Physiotherapy in the respiratory care of patients with high spinal injury, *Physiotherapy* 73:3, 1987.
24. Brubaker C: Ergonometric considerations, *JRRD Suppl* 2:37-48, March 1990.
25. Bunch W and others: *Atlas of orthotics: biomechanical principles and application,* ed 2, St Louis, 1985, Mosby.
26. Carter RE: Medical management of pulmonary complications of spinal cord injury, *Adv Neurol* 22:261-269, 1979.
27. CCH Business Law, editors: *Medicare and medicaid guide 1993,* Chicago, 1993, Commerce Clearing House, Inc.
28. Cervical Spine Research Society, ed 2: *The cervical spine,* Philadelphia, 1989, JB Lippincott.
29. Clough P and others: Guidelines for routine respiratory care of patients with spinal cord injury. *Phys Ther* 66(9):1395-1402, 1986.
30. Coffey RJ and others: Intrathecal baclofen for intractable spasticity of spinal origin: results of a long-term multicenter study, *J Neurosurg* 78:226-232, 1993.
31. Crane LD: Functional anatomy and physiology of ventilation. In Zadai CC, editor: *Clinics in physical therapy: pulmonary management in physical therapy,* New York, 1992, Churchill Livingstone.
32. Curry K and Casady L: The relationship between extended periods of immobility and decubitus ulcer formation in the acutely spinal cord injured individual, *J Neurosci Nurs* 24(4):185-189, 1992.
33. Daniels L and Worthingham C: *Muscle testing: techniques of manual examination,* ed 5, Philadelphia, 1986, WB Saunders.
34. Davidoff G and others: Closed head injury in the acute traumatic spinal cord injury: incidence and risk factors, *Arch Phys Med Rehabil* 69(10):869-872, 1988.
35. De Troyer A and Estenne M: Review article: the expiratory muscles in tetraplegia, *Paraplegia* 29:359-363, 1991.
36. Decker M and Hall A: Physical therapy in spinal cord injury. In Bloch RF and Basbaum M, editors: *Management of spinal cord injury,* Baltimore, 1986, Williams & Wilkins.
37. DeLisa JA, Martin GM, and Currie DM: Rehabilitation medicine: past, present, and future. In DeLisa JA, editor: *Rehabilitation medicine: principles and practice,* Philadelphia, 1988, JB Lippincott.
38. Derrickson J and others: A comparison of two breathing exercise programs for patients with quadriplegia, *Phys Ther* 72(11):763-769, 1992.
39. DeVivo MJ, Black KJ, and Stover SL: Causes of death during the first 12 years after spinal cord injury, *Arch Phys Med Rehabil* 74:248-254, 1993.
40. DeVivo MJ and others: Spinal cord injury rehabilitation adds life to years, *West J Med* 154(S):602-606, 1991.
41. DeVivo MJ and others: Trends in spinal cord injury demographics and treatment outcomes between 1973 and 1986, *Arch Phys Med Rehabil* 73:424-430, 1992.
42. Dollfus P: Rehabilitation following injury to the spinal cord, *J Emerg Med* 11:57-61, 1993.
43. Donovan WH and Bedbrook G: Comprehensive management of spinal cord injury, *Clin Symp* 34:2, 1992.
44. Donovan WH and Cutler HW: Traumatic spinal injuries: cervical, thoracic, lumbar. In Hochshuler SH, Cutler HB, Guyer RD, editors: *Rehabilitation of the spine: science and practice,* St Louis, 1993, Mosby.
45. Donovan WH and others: Incidence of medical complications in spinal cord injury: patients in specialized compared with nonspecialized centers, *Paraplegia* 22:282-290, 1984.
46. Ducharme S and others: Sexual functioning: medical and psychological aspects. In DeLisa JA, editor: *Rehabilitation medicine: principles and practice,* Philadelphia, 1988, JB Lippincott.
47. Dunker SB and others: *The unstable spine (thoracic, lumbar and sacral regions),* New York, 1986, Grune and Stratton.
48. Errico TJ and Bauer RD: *Spinal trauma,* Philadelphia, 1991, JB Lippincott.
49. Finkbeiner K and Russo SG, editors: *Physical therapy management of spinal cord injury: accent on independence,* Fisherville, Va, 1990, Woodrow Wilson Rehabilitation Center Project SCIENTIA.
50. Frankel HL and others: Value of postural reduction in the initial management of closed head injuries of the spine with paraplegia and tetraplegia, *Paraplegia* 7.179-192, 1969.

51. Frost FS: Role of rehabilitation after spinal cord injury, *Urol Clin North Am* 20(3):549-559, 1993.

52. Frymoyer JW: *The adult spine-principles and practice,* vol 2, New York, 1983, Raven Press.

53. Garland DE and others: Osteoporosis after spinal cord injury, *J Orthop Res* 10(3):371-378, 1992.

54. Geisler FH: GM-1 ganglioside and motor recovery following human spinal cord injury, *J Emerg Med* 2:49-45, 1993.

55. Geisler FH, Dorsey FC, and Coleman PW: Recovery of motor function after spinal cord injury: a randomized, placebo-controlled trial with GM-1 ganglioside, *N Engl J Med* 324:1829-1838, 1993.

56. Gellman H, Chandler DR, and Petrasek J: Carpal tunnel syndrome in paraplegic patients, *J Bone Joint Surg* 70A:517-519, 1988.

57. Giffin J and Grush K: Spinal cord injury treatment and the anesthesiologist. In Lee B and others, editors: *The spinal cord injured patient: comprehensive management,* Philadelphia, 1991, WB Saunders.

58. Green D and others: Deep vein thrombosis in spinal cord injury: summary and recommendations, *Chest* 102(6):633S-635S, 1992.

59. Grenvik A and others, editors: *Mechanical ventilation and assisted respiration: contemporary management in critical care,* New York, 1991, Churchill Livingstone.

60. Gross GR: What your company could be doing now to implement Title I of the ADA, *Small Business News,* May 1992.

61. *Guide to interdisciplinary practice in rehabilitation settings,* Skokie, Ill, 1992, American Congress of Rehabilitation Medicine.

62. Hall ED: The neuroprotective pharmacology of methylprednisolone: a review article, *J Neurosurg* 56:106-113, 1982.

63. Hall ED, Wolf DL, and Baughler JM: Effects of a single large dose of methylprednisolone sodium succinate on experimental post traumatic spinal cord ischemia-dose response and time-action analysis, *J Neurosurg* 61:124-130, 1984.

64. Hamilton BB and Fuhrer MJ: *Rehabilitation outcomes: analysis and measurement,* Baltimore, 1987, Brooks.

65. Hammell KR: Psychological and sociological theories concerning adjustment to traumatic spinal cord injury: the implication for rehabilitation, *Paraplegia* 30:317-326, 1992.

66. Hanak M and Scott A: *Spinal cord injury: an illustrated guide for healthcare professionals,* New York, 1983, Springer Publishing Co.

67. Harvey C and others: New estimate of the direct costs of traumatic spinal cord injuries: results of a nationwide survey, *Paraplegia* 30:834-850, 1992.

68. Heinemann AW, and others: Functional outcome following spinal cord injury: a comparison of specialized spinal cord injury centers vs general hospital acute care, *Arch Neurol* 46:52-59, 1989.

69. Hill JP: *Spinal cord injury: a guide to functional outcomes in occupational therapy,* Rockville, Md, 1986, Aspen Publishers.

70. Hilton G and Frei J: Methylprednisolone for acute spinal cord injury, *J Neurosci Nurs* 24(4):235-237, 1992.

71. Hull RD: Venous thromboembolism in spinal cord injury patients, *Chest* 102(6):658S-663S, 1992.

72. Katz RT: Management of spasticity, *Am J Phys Med Rehabil* 67(3):108-116, 1988.

73. Katz RT and others: Objective quantification of spastic hypertonia: correlation with clinical findings, *Arch Phys Med Rehabil* 73(4):339-347, 1992.

74. Kendall FP and McCreary EK: *Muscles testing and function,* ed 4, Baltimore, 1993, Williams & Wilkins.

75. Krause JS and Kjorsvig JM: Mortality after spinal cord injury: a four-year prospective study, *Arch Phys Med Rehabil* 73:558-563, 1992.

76. Kreutz DL: Seating and positioning for the newly injured, *Rehab Management* December 1993, pp 67-75.

77. Krouskop T: The role of mattresses and beds in preventing pressure sores. In Lee B and others editors: *The spinal cord injured patient: comprehensive management,* Philadelphia, 1991, WB Saunders.

78. Lee B: Deep vein thrombosis. In Lee B and others, editors: *The spinal cord injured patient: comprehensive management,* Philadelphia, 1991, WB Saunders.

79. Lewis KS and Mueller WM: Intrathecal baclofen for severe spasticity secondary to spinal cord injury, *Ann Pharmacother* 27:767-774, 1993.

80. Luce JM and Culver BH: Respiratory muscle function in health and disease, *Chest* 81(1):82-90, 1982.

81. McCool FD and others: Changes in lung volume and rib cage configuration and abdominal binding in quadriplegia, *J Appl Physiol* 60(4):1198-1202, 1986.

82. Madsen B, Barth P, and Vistnes L: Pressure sores: overview. In Lee B and others, editors: *The spinal cord injured patient: comprehensive management,* Philadelphia, 1991, WB Saunders.

83. Mammen EF: Pathogenesis of venous thrombosis, *Chest* 102(6):640S-644S, 1992.

84. Mariano AJ: Chronic pain and spinal cord injury, *Clin J Pain* 8(2):87-92, 1992.

85. Mawson AR and others: Risk factors for early occurring pressure ulcers following spinal cord injury, *Am J Phys Med Rehabil* 67:123-127, 1988.

86. Menton EB and Tan ES: Bladder training in patients with spinal cord injury, *Urology* 40(5):425-429, 1992.

87. Merli GJ and others: Mechanical plus pharmacological prophylaxis for deep vein thrombosis in acute spinal cord injury, *Paraplegia* 30:558-562, 1992.

88. Meyer RR: *Surgery of spine trauma,* New York, 1989, Churchill Livingstone.

89. Morgan M and Silver J: The respiratory system of the spinal cord patient. In Bloch RF and Basbaum M, editors: *Management of spinal cord injuries,* Baltimore, 1986, Williams & Wilkins.

90. Nickel VL: The rationale and rewards of team care. In Nickel VL and Botte MJ, editors: *Orthopaedic rehabilitation,* ed 2, New York, 1992, Churchill Livingstone.

91. Nixon V: *Spinal cord injury: a guide to functional outcomes in physical therapy management,* Rockville, Md, 1985, Aspen Systems Corp.

92. Parsons KC and Lammertse DP: Rehabilitation in spinal cord disorders: epidemiology, prevention, and system of care of spinal cord disorders, *Arch Phys Med Rehabil* 72:S293-S294, 1991.

93. Perkash I: Long-term urologic management of the patient with spinal cord injury, *Urol Clin North Am* 20(3):423-433, 1993.

94. Perry J: *Gait analysis: normal and pathological function,* Thorofare, NJ, 1992, Slack.

95. *Physician's desk reference,* ed 48, Montrale, NJ, 1994, Medical Economics Data Production Company.

96. Rinehart M and Nawoczenski D: Respiratory Care. In Buchanan L and Nawoczenski D, editors: *Spinal cord injury: concepts and management approaches,* Baltimore, 1987, Williams & Wilkins.

97. Ryan M, Klein S, and Bongard F: Missed injuries associated with spinal cord trauma, *Am Surg* 59:371-374, 1993.

98. Seaton T and Hollingworth R: Gastrointestinal complications in spinal cord injury. In Bloch RF and Basbaum M, editors: *Management of spinal cord injuries,* Baltimore, 1986, Williams & Wilkins.

99. Smith EM and Bodner DR: Sexual dysfunction after spinal cord injury, *Urol Clin North Am* 20(3):535-541, 1993.

100. Somers MF: *Spinal cord injury: functional rehabilitation,* East Norwalk, Conn, 1992, Appleton and Lange.

101. *Spinal cord injury: facts and figures at a glance,* National Spinal Cord Injury Statistical Center, Birmingham, Ala, 1990, University of Alabama.

102. Staas WE and others: Rehabilitation of the spinal cord injured patient. In DeLisa JA, editor: *Rehabilitation medicine: principles and practice,* Philadelphia, 1988, JB Lippincott.

103. *Standards for neurological and functional classification of spinal cord injury,* Ditunno JF, chairman: Chicago, Ill, revised 1992, American Spinal Injury Association.

104. *Standards manual for organizations serving people with disabilities 1993,* Commission on Accreditation of Rehabilitation Facilities, Tucson, Arizona.

105. Stover SL: Functional independence, *Arch Phys Med Rehabil* 70:509, 1989.

106. Stover SL: Heterotopic ossification after spinal cord injury. In Bloch RF and Basbaum M, editors: *Management of spinal cord injuries,* Baltimore, 1986, Williams & Wilkins.

107. Trieschmann RB: Psychosocial research in spinal cord injury: the state of the art, *Paraplegia* 30:58-60, 1992.

108. Trieschmann RB: *Spinal cord injuries: psychological, social and vocational rehabilitation,* ed 2, New York, 1988, Demos Publications.

109. Turpie A: Thrombosis prevention and treatment in spinal cord injured patients. In Bloch RF and Basbaum M, editors: *Management of spinal cord injuries,* Baltimore, 1986, Williams & Wilkins.

110. Umphred DA, editor: *Neurological rehabilitation,* ed 2, St Louis, 1990, Mosby.

111. Vaugeois A: Occupational therapy in the treatment of spinal cord injuries. In Bloch RF and Basbaum M, editors: *Management of spinal cord injuries,* Baltimore, 1986, Williams & Wilkins.

112. Vincken W and Corne L: Improved arterial oxygenation by diaphragmatic pacing in quadriplegia, *Crit Care Med* 15(9):872-873, 1987.

113. Walters RL and Lansford BR: Energy expenditure of normal and pathologic gait: application to orthotic disposition. In Bunch W and others: *Atlas of orthotics: biomechanical principles and application,* ed 2, St Louis, 1986, Mosby.

114. Weingarden SI: Deep vein thrombosis in spinal cord injury: overview of the problem, *Chest* 102(6):636S-639S, 1992.

115. Weingarden SI and Graham P: Young spinal cord injured patients in nursing homes: rehospitalization issues and outcomes, *Paraplegia* 30:828-833, 1992.

116. West JB: *Pulmonary pathophysiology: the essentials,* ed 4, Baltimore, 1992, Williams & Wilkins.

117. Wetzell JL and others: Respiratory rehabilitation of the patient with a spinal cord injury. In Irwin S and Tecklin JS, editors: *Cardiopulmonary physical therapy,* ed 2, St Louis, 1990, Mosby.

118. Wharton GW and Morgan TH: Ankylosis in the paralyzed patient, *J Bone Joint Surg* 52A:105-112, 1970.

119. White III AA and Panjabi MM: *Clinical biomechanics of the spine,* Philadelphia, 1978, JB Lippincott.

120. White AH, Rothman RH, and Ray CD: *Lumbar spine surgery techniques and complications,* St Louis, 1987, Mosby.

121. Whiteneck GG and others: Mortality, morbidity, and psychosocial outcomes of persons spinal cord injured more than 20 years ago, *Paraplegia* 30:617-630, 1992.

122. Wittenberg RH, Peschke U, and Botel U: Heterotopic ossification after spinal cord injury, *J Bone Joint Surg* 74-B(2):215-218, 1992.

123. Yarkony G: Spinal cord injury rehabilitation. In Lee B and others, editors: *The spinal cord injured patient: comprehensive management,* Philadelphia, 1991, WB Saunders.

124. Yashon D: *Spinal Injury,* ed 2, Norwalk, Conn, 1986, Appleton-Century-Crofts.

125. Young JS and Northrup NE: *Statistical information pertaining to some of the most commonly asked questions about SCI* (monograph), Phoenix, Ariz, 1979, National Spinal Cord Injury Data Research Center.

126. Young R and Shahani B: Spasticity in spinal cord injured patients. In Bloch RF and Basbaum M, editors: *Management of spinal cord injuries,* Baltimore, 1986, Williams & Wilkins.

127. Young RR and Delwaide PJ: Drug therapy, spasticity, *New Engl J Med* 304(1):28-33, 1981.

128. Young W and Flamm ES: Effect of high-dose corticosteroid therapy on blood flow, evoked potentials, and extracellular calcium in experimental spinal injury, *J Neurosurg* 57:667-673, 1982.

129. Zarcharkow D: *Wheelchair posture and pressure sores,* Springfield, Ill, 1984, Charles C Thomas.

130. Zigler JE: Rehabilitation of acute spinal cord injury. In Hochschuler SH, Cotler HB, Guyer RD, editors: *Rehabilitation of the spine: science and practice,* St Louis, 1993, Mosby.

APPENDIX A

SHEPHERD SPINAL CENTER
PHYSICAL THERAPY
PROGRESS NOTE: _____

for the week of

_____ _____   ☐ ☐ ☐
Date   Time   Initial Progress D/C

FUNCTIONAL ASSESSMENT

ACT		Current	STG	LTG
	A. BED MOBILITY			
	1. Rolling side to side			
	2. Rolling supine to prone			
	3. Rolling prone to supine			
	4. Coming to sit			
	5. Scooting			
	B. WHEELCHAIR MANAGEMENT			
	Wheelchair type _____			
	1. Brakes			
	2. Arm rests			
	3. Foot rests / Leg rests			
	4. Safety straps			
	5. Adjusts cushion			
	6. Positions self			
	7. Turn Wheelie Bars Up			
	8. Wheelchair Maintenance			
	C. TRANSFERS			
	1. Mat ( )			
	2. Bed ( )			
	3. Car ( )			
	4. Toilet ( )			
	5. Tub ( )			
	6. Floor ( )			
	7. Upright W/C ( )			
	D. WHEELCHAIR MOBILITY			
	Manual Wheelchair			
	1. Smooth surfaces			
	2. Up and down 8 deg. ramps			
	3. Up and down curbs (,6")			
	4. Rough terrain			
	5. Up and down stairs (3)			
	Power Wheelchair			
	6. Smooth surfaces			
	7. Up and down ramps			
	8. Up and down curbs			
	9. Rough terrain			
	E. AMBULATION / GAIT			
	Orthosis/Assistive Device			
	1. don/doff			
	2. sit/stand			
	3. Smooth surfaces			
	4. Up and down 8 deg. ramps			
	5. Up and down curbs (,6")			
	6. Up and down stairs (12-14)			
	7. Rough terrain			
	8. Falling/Standing			
	F. EQUIPMENT (Patient knowledge)			
	1. Name all equipment			
	2. State Vendor/Funding source			

ACT		Current	STG	LTG
	G. SKIN			
	1. Weight Shift, Type ( )			
	2. Rationale - sitting tolerance			
	3. Rationale - shoe tolerance			
	4. Rationale - wheelchair cushion			
	5. Sitting angle (angle/hrs)			
	6. Shoes (# hrs)			
	7. Weight Shift Schedule (min)			
	H. ROM / POSITIONING			
	1. PROM to trunk and BLE			
	2. Rationale for prone			
	3. Rationale for 90/90 hip knee			
	4. Padding and Positioning (bed)			
	5. Prone tolerance (# hrs)			
	I. HOME PROGRAM			

	Initial	Midway	D/C
J. FAMILY TRAINING			

	Yes	N/A	
K. OUTPATIENT REFERRAL			

	Current	Next	LTG
L. HOME MODIFICATIONS			

		Vendor	Current	Next
M. EQUIPMENT				
	1. Power Wheelchair			
	2. Manual Wheelchair			
	3. Hospital Bed			
	4. Cushion			
	5. Patient Lift			
	6. Toilet/Tub			
	7. Orthosis			
	8. Assistive Device			
	9. Other			

N. ADL _____ **MIS (L)** _____ **(R)** _____ **Total** _____

ASIA Impairment _____

Vendor Key:
1. Nat. Seating/Mobility
2. A+ Medical
3. American Rehab
4. Georgia Wheelchair
5. C.H. Martin
6. Atlanta Orthotics
7. Other

Equipment Key: Status
1. Evaluation
2. Rx and LOMN submitted
3. Insurance approved
4. Insurance denied
5. Pending
6. Delivered

ADL Key:
7 – Complete Independence
6 – Modified Independence
5 – Supervision or Setup
4 – Minimal Contact Assistance
3 – Moderate Assistance
2 – Maximal Assistance
1.5 – Verbal Direction
1.0 – Total Assistance

Home Modification Key:
1. Form to family
2. Form returned
3. Recommendations made
4. Other

RELATED SHORT TERM GOALS   LTG Goals Reviewed: Yes ☐ No ☐   Weekly STG met: _____ of _____

Therapeutic pass goal:

Assess:

PLAN:

PT 601 07/90   SIGNATURE _____

APPENDIX B   *ARCHITECTURAL MODIFICATION*

Accessibility in Georgia: A Technical and Policy Guide to Access in Georgia. Designed and developed by Barrier Free Environments, Inc., for the Georgia Council on Developmental Disabilities, 1986, Raleigh, North Carolina.

An Accessible Bathroom. Available from Design Coalition, Inc., 1980, Madison, Wisconsin.

An Accessible Entrance: Ramps. Available from Design Coalition, Inc., 1979, Madison, Wisconsin.

Handbook for Design: Specially Adapted Housing. VA pamphlet 26-13, Department of Veterans Benefits, Veterans Administration, April 1978, Washington, DC.

Harber L and others: *UFAS Retrofit Guide: Accessibility Modifications for Existing Buildings.* Barrier Free Environments Inc., New York, 1993, Van Nostrand Reinhold.

Lebrock C and Behar S: *Beautiful Barrier-Free, A Visual Guide to Accessibility,* New York, 1993, Van Nostrand Reinhold.

Mace RL: *The Accessible Housing Design File.* Barrier Free Environments, Inc., New York, 1991, Van Nostrand Reinhold.

APPENDIX C   *SEXUAL ISSUES*

Althof SE and Levine SB: Clinical approach to the sexuality of patients with spinal cord injury, *Urol Clin North Am* 20(3):527-534, 1993.

Berard EJ: The sexuality of spinal cord injured women physiology and pathophysiology: a review, *Paraplegia* 27(2):99-112, 1989.

Charlifue SW and others: Sexual issues of women with spinal cord injuries, *Paraplegia* 30(3):192-199, 1992.

Drench ME: Impact of altered sexuality and sexual function in spinal cord injury: a review, *Sex Disabil* 10(1):3-14, 1992.

Farrow J: Sexuality counseling with clients who have spinal cord injuries, *Rehabil Couns Bull* 33(3):251-259, 1990.

Kettl P and others: Female sexuality after spinal cord injury, *Sex Disabil* 9(4):287-295, 1991.

Lemon MA: Sexual counseling and spinal cord injury, *Sex Disabil* 11(1):73-97, 1993.

Lloyd LK and Richards JS: Medical and psychological considerations regarding the surgical or pharmacological treatment of impotence in males with spinal cord injury, *J Rehabil Res Dev* 28(1):419-420, 1991.

Nygaard I, Bartscht KD, Cole S: Sexuality and reproduction in spinal cord injured women, *Obstet Gynecol Surv* 45(11):727-732, 1990.

Robbins KH: Traumatic spinal cord injury and its impact upon sexuality, *J Appl Rehabil Couns* 16(1):24-27, 1985.

Sipski ML and Alexander CJ: Sexual activities, response and satisfaction in women pre- and post-spinal cord injury, *Arch Phys Med Rehabil* 74(10):1025-1029, 1993.

Tepper MS: Sexual education in spinal cord injury rehabilitation: current trends and recommendations, *Sex Disabil* 10(1):15-31, 1992.

Trieschmann RB: *Spinal cord injuries: psychological, social, and vocational rehabilitation,* ed 2, New York, 1988, Demos Publications.

White MJ and others: Sexual activities, concerns and interests of men with spinal-cord injury, *Am J Phys Med Rehabil* 71(4):225-231, 1992.

CHAPTER 17

Therapeutic Management of the Client with Inflammatory and Infectious Disorders of the Brain

Rebecca E. Porter

KEY TERMS

brain abscess
meningitis
encephalitis
intervention goals
postural control
hypertonicity
hypotonicity
functional activities

LEARNING OBJECTIVES

After reading this chapter the student/therapist will:
1. Understand the terminology for classifying different types of inflammatory and infectious disorders within the brain.
2. Discuss the range of neurological sequelae that occur.
3. Discuss the components of the comprehensive evaluation process and their interrelationships.
4. Structure the evaluation process to gather the information required to generate an intervention plan.
5. Discuss the general goals of the intervention process.
6. Plan the intervention process to meet the needs of the client.
7. Locate resources (both within this book and in other sources) to assist with ideas for the intervention program.

The diversity of neurological sequelae that may occur after an inflammatory disorder in the brain (brain abscess, encephalitis, or meningitis) provides a range of challenges to the rehabilitation team. The therapist must identify the problems underlying the individual's movement dysfunctions without the template of the cluster of "typical" problems available with some other neurological diagnoses. Each client presents a combination of problems that is unique to that client and that requires the creative design of an intervention program. The following discussion of the therapeutic management of individuals recovering from an inflammatory disorder in the brain focuses on the process of designing an intervention plan to address the specific dysfunctions of the individual client.

AN OVERVIEW OF INFLAMMATORY DISORDERS IN THE BRAIN
Categorization of inflammatory disorders

Inflammatory disorders of the brain can be categorized based on the anatomical location of the inflammatory process and the cause of the infection, as shown below.

A. **Brain abscess**
B. **Meningitis** (leptomeningitis)
   1. Bacterial meningitis
   2. Aseptic meningitis (viral)
C. **Encephalitis**
   1. Acute viral
   2. Parainfectious encephalomyelitis
   3. Acute toxic encephalopathy
   4. Progressive viral encephalitis
   5. "Slow virus" encephalitis

In most individuals the defense mechanisms of the central nervous system (CNS) provide protection from infecting organisms. Compromises of the protective barriers can result in CNS infections as complications of common infections. The response of the CNS to the infection depends on several factors including the type of organism, its route of entry, the CNS location of the infection, and the immunological competence of the individual.[13] CNS infections occur with greater frequency and severity in individuals who are very young or elderly, immunodeficient, or antibody deficient.

The inflammatory process may be a localized, circumscribed collection of pus; may involve primarily the leptomeninges; may involve the brain substance; or may involve both the meninges and the brain substance. The infecting agents may be bacterial, fungal, viral, protozoan, or parasitic. The most common agents producing meningitis are bacterial; the most common agents producing encephalitis are viral. However, bacterial encephalitis and viral meningitis also are disease entities. The following overview of the inflammatory processes within the brain is organized based on the anatomical location of the infection. More comprehensive discussions based on spe-

cific infecting organisms can be found in the references at the end of the chapter.

Brain abscess

Brain abscesses occur when microorganisms reach brain tissue by a penetrating wound to the brain, by extension of local infection such as sinusitis or otitis, or by hematogenous spread from a distant site of infection. The route of infection influences the CNS involved region. A solitary brain abscess in an adjacent lobe tends to occur as an extension of a local infection. Multiple abscesses may originate from the spread of microorganisms through the blood. The introduction of microorganisms by a penetrating trauma may result in an abscess soon after the trauma or several years later. As with the disorders presented in the subsequent discussions, circumstances that result in a compromised immune system (chronic steroid or other immunosuppressive drug administration, administration of cytotoxic chemotherapeutic agents or HIV infection) may predispose the individual to develop opportunistic infections.[6]

While the site and size of the abscess influence the initial symptoms, evidence of increased intracranial pressure is common. Most individuals experience an alteration of consciousness. Focal neurological deficits such as hemiparesis, dysphasia, visual field defects, and ataxia occur in 60% of cases.[6] The most serious manifestations of the abscess relate to the size of the mass rather than the infecting organism.[17] Medical management of the abscess may consist of antibiotic therapy (depending on the infecting agent and size and site of the abscess) or surgical aspiration or excision. Berger and Levy[6] state that permanent neurological deficits occur in half the patients, with 35% of them demonstrating a hemiparesis as a result of parietal lobe involvement.[6] Bharucha and others[7] describe neurological sequelae in 25% to 50% of the survivors, with 30% to 50% having persistent seizures, 15% to 30% with hemiparesis, and 10% to 20% with disorders of speech or language.

Meningitis

Definition. Meningitis (synonymous with leptomeningitis) denotes an infection spread through the cerebrospinal fluid (CSF) with the inflammatory process involving the pia and arachnoid maters, the subarachnoid space, and the adjacent superficial tissues of the brain and spinal cord. Pachymeningitis denotes an inflammatory process involving the dura mater. Meningitis can be caused by a wide variety of organisms, some of which cross the blood-brain barrier and the blood-CSF barrier. The CSF can also become contaminated by a wound that penetrates the meninges as a result of trauma or a medical procedure such as implantation of a ventriculoperitoneal shunt. Once the organism compromises the blood-brain and blood-CSF barriers, the CSF provides an ideal medium for growth. All of the body's typical major defense systems are essentially absent in the normal CSF. The blood-brain barrier may impede the clearance of infecting organisms by leukocytes and interfere with the entry of pharmacological agents. The infecting organism is disseminated throughout the subarachnoid space as the contaminated CSF bathes the brain. Entry into the ventricles occurs either from the choroid plexuses or by reflux through the exit foramen of the fourth ventricle. The spread of the organism via the CSF circulation accounts for the differences in the variety and extent of the neurological sequelae that can result from meningitis.

Bacterial meningitis

Clinical problems. The diagnostic categorization of meningitis depends on the infecting agent (e.g., *Haemophilus influenzae* meningitis, *Streptococcus pneumoniae* meningitis, and viral meningitis) and on the acute or chronic nature of the meningitis (acute, subacute, or chronic meningitis). The term *acute bacterial meningitis* denotes infections produced by any of a wide variety of bacterial organisms. The most common infecting organism producing acute bacterial meningitis varies according to the age of the population. During the neonatal period, infections by gram-negative enterobacilli, especially *Escherichia coli,* and group B streptococci are the most frequently occurring. Typical causative agents in infants and children include *H. influenzae, Neisseria meningitidis,* and *S. pneumoniae.*[1,6] Meningococcal meningitis *(N. meningitidis)* occurs with the greatest frequency in children, adolescents, and young adults.[6,27] Pneumococcal meningitis *(S. pneumoniae)* typically occurs at both ends of the age spectrum or in individuals with predisposing factors such as sickle cell anemia, alcoholism, or diabetes mellitus.[6,27] *Liseria monocytogenes* may be the infecting organism in the immunosuppressed individual.

An example of an organism that uses a typical systemic route of bacterial infection is a *H. influenzae* organism that is a normal flora of the nose and throat. During an upper respiratory tract infection, the organism may gain entry to the blood. The route of transmission of the organism from the blood to the CSF is not well established.

The circulation of CSF spreads the infecting organism through the ventricular system and the subarachnoid spaces. The pia and arachnoid maters become acutely inflamed, and as part of the inflammatory response, a purulent exudate forms in the subarachnoid space. The exudate may undergo organization resulting in an obstruction of the foramen of Monro, the aqueduct of Sylvius, or the exit foramen of the fourth ventricle. The supracortical subarachnoid spaces proximal to the arachnoid villi may be obliterated, resulting in a noncommunicating or obstructive hydrocephalus as a result of the accumulation of CSF. As the CSF accumulates, the intracranial pressure rises. The increased intracranial pressure produces venous obstruction precipitating a further increase in the intracranial pressure. The rise in the CSF pressure compromises the cerebral blood flow, which activates reflex mechanisms to counteract the decreased cerebral blood flow by raising the systemic blood pressure.

An increased systemic blood pressure accompanies increased CSF pressure.

The mechanism producing the headaches that accompany increased intracranial pressure may be the stretching of the meninges and pain fibers associated with blood vessels. Vomiting may occur as a result of stimulation of the medullary emetic centers. Papilledema may occur as pressure occludes the veins returning blood from the retina.

Other routes of bacterial infection may involve a local spread as the result of an infection of the middle ear or mastoid air cells. Meningitis may occur as a complication of a skull fracture, which exposes CNS tissue to the external environment or to the nasal cavity. Fractures of the cribriform plate of the ethmoid bone producing cerebrospinal rhinorrhea provide another route for infection. Meningitis may be a further complication to the clinical problems of the traumatic head injury (see Chapter 14).

Clinical features of acute bacterial meningitis include fever, severe headache, altered consciousness, convulsions (particularly in children), and nuchal rigidity. Nuchal rigidity is indicative of an irritative lesion of the subarachnoid space. Cervical flexion is painful as it stretches the inflamed meninges, nerve roots, and spinal cord. The pain triggers a reflex spasm of the neck extensors to splint the area against further cervical flexion; however, cervical rotation and extension movements remain relatively free.

Several clinical tests are utilized to demonstrate nuchal rigidity. Kernig's test consists of flexion of the cervical area with the client supine. Signs of pain indicate a positive test.[14] Kernig's sign refers to a test performed with the client supine in which the thigh is flexed on the abdomen and the knee extended. This pulls on the sciatic nerve, which pulls on the spinal cord, causing pain in the presence of meningeal irritation. The same results are achieved with passive hip flexion with the knee remaining in extension. This is the same procedure described by Hoppenfeld[14] as the straight leg raising test for determining pathology of the sciatic nerve or tightness of the hamstrings. Passive hip flexion with knee extension can be painful because of meningeal irritation, spinal root impingement, sciatic nerve pathology, or hamstring tightness. Brudzinski's sign refers to the flexion of the hips and knees elicited when cervical flexion (Kernig's test) is performed.[2,6] These signs will not be present in the deeply comatose client who has decreased muscle tone and absence of muscle reflexes. The signs may also be absent in the infant or aged patient.

The diagnosis of bacterial meningitis can be established based on blood cultures and a sample of CSF obtained by a lumbar puncture. Depending on the age of the client and the type of organism involved, blood cultures are positive in 40% to 60% of the cases.[1] Spinal fluid pressure is consistently elevated. The CSF sample in bacterial meningitis typically reveals an increased protein count and a decreased glucose level.

The type and severity of the sequelae of acute bacterial meningitis relate directly to the area affected, the extent of CNS infection, the age and general health of the individual, the level of consciousness at the initiation of pharmacological therapy, and the pathological agent involved. Some of the common CNS complications include subdural effusions, altered levels of consciousness, seizures, involvement of the cranial nerves, and increased intracranial pressure.

Medical management of bacterial meningitis. Medical management of bacterial meningitis consists of the initiation of the antimicrobial regimen appropriate to the infecting organism and procedures to manage the signs and symptoms of meningitis that have been described in the preceding paragraphs. Medical intervention strategies in both these areas change with the development of new pharmacological agents. The reader is encouraged to review recent literature for additional information on current aspects of the medical management of the client with meningitis.

Potential neurological sequelae. Even with optimal antimicrobial therapy, bacterial meningitis continues to have a finite mortality rate, which varies with the infecting organism, age of the individual, and time lapse to initiation of treatment, and the potential for marked neurological morbidity.[1,23] Bacterial meningitis is considered a medical emergency; delays in initiation of antibacterial therapy increase the risk of complications and permanent neurological residua.[2]

Reports of the long-term outcome of individuals with bacterial meningitis indicate that up to 30% of them have long-term neurological sequelae.[1] The neurological sequelae that must be considered by the therapist in developing an intervention plan will differ in each client. The sequelae may be the result of the acute infectious pathological condition, subacute or chronic pathological changes, or late pathological changes. The acute infectious pathological condition could result in sequelae such as inflammatory or vascular involvement of the cranial nerves or thrombosis of the meningeal veins. Subacute or chronic pathological changes include obstructive or communicating hydrocephalus, subdural effusion, and venous or arterial infarction. Late pathological sequelae may develop, such as meningeal fibrosis around the optic nerve or spinal roots or persistent hydrocephalus.

Damage to the cerebral cortex can result in numerous expressions of dysfunction. Motor system dysfunction may be the observable expression of the damage within the CNS, but the location of the damage may include sensory and processing areas as well as those areas typically categorized as belonging to the motor system. Perceptual deficits or regression in cognitive skills may present residual problems. Cranial nerve involvement is most frequently expressed as impairment of ocular mobility or dysfunction of the eighth cranial nerve complex.

Aseptic meningitis. Aseptic meningitis refers to a non-purulent inflammatory process confined to the meninges and choroid plexus usually caused by contamination of the CSF with a viral agent, although other agents can trigger the reactions. The symptoms are similar to acute bacterial meningitis but typically are less severe. Aseptic meningitis of a viral origin is usually benign and self-limiting.[8]

A variety of neurotropic viruses can produce aseptic (viral) meningitis. Common causes are coxsackie B, mumps, echovirus, and lymphocytic choriomeningitis viruses. The primary nonviral agents producing aseptic meningitis are Lyme borreliosis and *Leptospira*.[1] The diagnosis of this type of aseptic meningitis may be established by isolation of the infecting agent within the CSF or by other techniques. Although the glucose level of the CSF in bacterial meningitis is usually depressed, the glucose level in viral meningitis is normal.[1]

Treatment of aseptic meningitis consists of management of symptoms. The condition does not typically produce residual neurological sequelae, and full recovery is anticipated within a few days to a few weeks.

Encephalitis

Clinical problems. Encephalitis refers to a group of diseases characterized by inflammation of the parenchyma of the brain and its surrounding meninges. Although a variety of agents can produce an encephalitis, the term usually denotes a viral invasion of the cells of the brain and spinal cord.

Different cell populations within the CNS vary in their susceptibility to infection by a specific virus.[1] (For example, the viruses responsible for poliomyelitis have a selective affinity for the motor neurons of the brainstem and spinal cord. Viruses such as coxsackie and echovirus typically infect meningeal cells to cause the benign viral meningitis discussed in the previous section.[16]) In acute encephalitis, neurons that are vulnerable to the specific virus are invaded and undergo lysis. Viral encephalitis presents a syndrome of elevated temperature, headache, nuchal rigidity, vomiting, and general malaise (symptoms of aseptic or viral meningitis) with the addition of evidence of more extensive cerebral damage such as coma, cranial nerve palsy, hemiplegia, involuntary movements, or ataxia. The difficulty in differentiating between acute viral meningitis and acute viral encephalitis is reflected in the use of the term *meningoencephalitis* in some cases.

The pathological condition includes destruction or damage to neurons and glial cells resulting from invasion of the cells by the virus, the presence of intranuclear inclusion bodies, edema, and inflammation of the brain and spinal cord. Perivascular cuffing by polymorphonuclear leukocytes and lymphocytes may occur as well as angiitis of small blood vessels. Widespread destruction of the white matter by the inflammatory process and by the thrombosis of the perforating vessels can occur. Increased intracranial pressure, which can result from the cerebral edema and vascular damage, presents the potential for a transtentorial herniation. Residual impairment of neurological functions occurs in

20% to more than 50% of individuals depending on the infecting viral agent.[1]

As the number of individuals who are immunosuppressed as a result of lymphoma, leukemia, organ transplantation, and human immunodeficiency virus infection increases, it is likely that the incidence of encephalitis will increase.

Plum and Posner[20] discuss viral encephalitis in terms of five pathological syndromes. *Acute viral encephalitis* is a primary or exclusively CNS infection. An example would be herpes simplex encephalitis, in which the virus shows a predilection for the gray matter of the temporal lobe, insula, cingulate gyrus, and inferior frontal lobe. *Parainfectious encephalomyelitis* is associated with viral infections such as measles, mumps, or varicella. *Acute toxic encephalopathy* denotes an encephalitis that occurs during the course of a systemic infection with a common virus. The clinical symptoms are produced by the cerebral edema in acute toxic encephalopathy, which results in increased intracranial pressure and the risk of transtentorial herniation. Reye's syndrome is an example. Global neurological signs such as hemiplegia or aphasia are usually present rather than focal signs. The clinical symptoms of the previous three syndromes may be very similar. Specific diagnosis may be established only by biopsy or autopsy.

Progressive viral infections occur from common viruses invading susceptible individuals, such as those who are immunosuppressed or during the perinatal to early childhood period. Slow, progressive destruction of the CNS occurs as in subacute sclerosing panencephalitis. The final category of encephalitis syndromes are *"slow virus" infections* by unconventional agents (the prion diseases)[5,19] that produce progressive dementing diseases such as Creutzfeldt-Jakob disease and kuru.

Medical management of encephalitis. The medical management of virally induced encephalitis has been, and with many infecting agents remains, primarily symptomatic, at times necessitating intensive, aggressive care to sustain life. Pharmacological interventions are available to treat some viral infections, such as herpes encephalitis. The probability of neurological sequelae differs according to the infecting agent. Aggressive management of increased intracranial pressure is required because persistently elevated intracranial pressure is associated with poor outcome.[21] Further information concerning the clinical features, medical management, and potential for neurological sequelae of a specific type of encephalitis should be sought in the literature based on the infecting agent.

Clinical picture of the individual with inflammatory disorders of the brain

An individual with meningitis or encephalitis may demonstrate signs and symptoms similar to generalized brain trauma, tumor disorder, or other identified abnormal neurological state. In the acute phase, the inflammatory process may result in an individual who is in an agitated state, which may range from mild to severe depending both on the client's unique CNS characteristics and on the degree of inflammation. The agitated state may be the result of alterations in the processing of sensory input, with the consequence of inappropriate or augmented responses to sensory input. The client may respond to a normal level of sound as though it were an unbearably loud noise. Dull artificial light may be perceived as extremely bright.

Perceptual and cognitive processes may be affected. Clients may have distortions in their perception of events as well as memory problems. As their memory returns, accuracy of time and events may be distorted leading to frustration and anxiety for both the client and those family and friends who are interacting within the environment.

In addition to alterations in mentation, the individual may demonstrate hypersensitivity or exaggerated emotional responses to seemingly normal interactions. For example, when upset about dropping a spoon on the floor, a client may throw the tray across the table. When another individual was told his girlfriend would be a little late for her afternoon visit, the client became extremely upset and stated his intent to kill himself because his girlfriend did not love him anymore.

Because of the variety of pathological problems following acute inflammation, the client may have residual problems manifested as generalized or focal brain damage. The specifics of these problems cannot be described as a typical clinical picture because they are extremely dependent on the individual client. These variations require the therapist to conduct a thorough evaluation to develop an appropriate individualized intervention program.

EVALUATION PROCEDURES

Just as the medical intervention with clients who have an inflammatory disorder of the CNS is, to a large extent, symptomatic, so is the intervention by therapists. Designing an individualized intervention program based on the client's problems necessitates a comprehensive initial and ongoing evaluation to define the problems and to note changes in them. Although the discussion of evaluation procedures is separated from the discussion of intervention strategies, it must be recognized that the separation is artificial and does not reflect the image of practice. The evaluation process should be considered in relationship to both the long-term assessment of the individual's changes and the short-term within-session and between-session variations. For example, evaluation of the level of consciousness of a client on day one of intervention will provide a starting point for calculation of the distance spanned at the time of discharge. Perhaps more critical to the final outcome is evaluation of the level of consciousness before, during, and after a particular intervention technique to determine its benefit or detriment to the client. The evaluation process is a constant activity intertwined with intervention. The observations and data from the process are periodically recorded to establish the

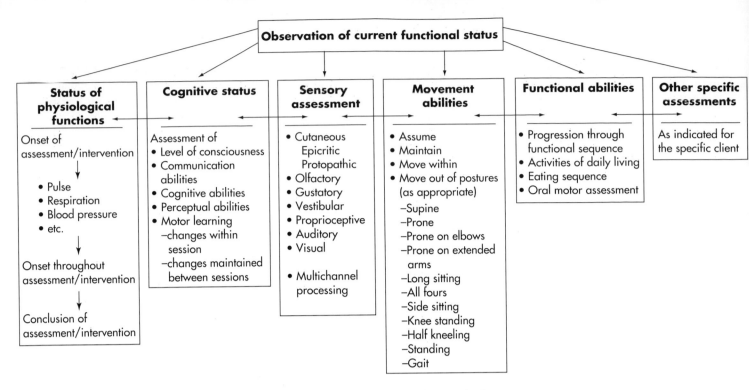

Fig. 17-1. Flow chart of components of the evaluation process.

Observation of current functional status

The evaluation process should be conceptualized as a decision-making tree that requires the therapist to determine actively which components are to be included in a detailed assessment and which can be eliminated or deferred. The first step in this process is the observation of the client's current functional status. If the client is comatose and nonmobile, the focus of the initial session might be an assessment of the stability of physiological functions, level of consciousness, and responses to sensory input. If the client is an outpatient with motor control deficits, the initial session might focus on defining motor abilities and components contributing to movement dysfunctions with a more superficial assessment of physiological functions and level of consciousness. The therapist must be alert to indications of the need for a more detailed evaluation of perceptual and cognitive function (e.g., the client cannot follow two-step commands, indicating the need to assess cognitive skills).

Some of the components discussed in the evaluation process may be assessment skills that are more typically possessed by other professions (e.g., assessment of emotional/psychological status). The inclusion of these items is not meant to suggest that the therapist must complete the formal testing. The items are included to indicate factors that will affect goal setting for the client and that will have an impact on the intervention strategy. Although the therapist may not be the health team member who has primary responsibility for evaluation of these areas, he or she should

course of the disease process and the success of the therapeutic management of the client.

recognize these areas as potential sources of movement dysfunctions.

Observation of the current functional status of the client provides the therapist with an initial overview of the client's assets and deficits. This provides the framework into which the pieces of information from the evaluation of specific aspects of function can be fit. The therapist must not allow assumptions made during the initial observation to bias later observations. The therapist might note that the client is able to roll from the supine to the side-lying position to interact with visitors in the room. When the same activity is not repeated on the mat table in the treatment area, the therapist, knowing the client has the motor skill to roll, might conclude that the client is uncooperative, or apraxic, or has perceptual deficits. The therapist may have failed to consider that the difference between the two situations is the presence or absence of side rails, which may have enabled the client to roll in bed by pulling over to the side-lying position. It is characteristic of human observation skills that we tend to "see" what we expect to see. The therapist must attempt to observe behaviors and note potential explanations for deviations from normal without biasing the results of the subsequent observations.

The following discussion of the specific considerations within the evaluation process does not necessarily represent the temporal sequence to be used during the evaluation process. As different items are discussed, suggestions for potential combinations of items will be made. The sequence of the process is best determined by the interaction of therapist and client. Fig. 17-1 presents the components that should be considered during the evaluation process.

Evaluation of physiological responses to therapeutic activities

It is assumed that the therapist enters the initial interaction with a client after reviewing the available background information. This may provide the therapist with information on the baseline status of the client's vital physiological functions. Any control problems in these areas should be particularly noted. Until the therapist determines that the vital functions such as respiration, heart rate, and blood pressure vary appropriately with the demands of the intervention process, these factors should be monitored. The monitoring process should include consideration of the baseline rate, rate during exercise, and time to return to baseline. The pattern of respiration and changes in that pattern also should be noted.

Clients with depressed levels of consciousness may display temperature regulation dysfunctions. One mechanism for assessing the client's ability to maintain a homeostatic temperature is to review the nursing notes. The events surrounding any periods of diaphoresis should be examined. If no causative factors have been identified, then interventions, which involve thermal agents as discussed in Chapter 6, should be used judiciously.

Evaluation of cognitive status

Because the evaluation process encompasses the stages of recovery from the critical acute phase through discharge from therapy, a range of aspects are included under the evaluation of cognitive status. As indicated previously, the observation of current functional status will direct the therapist toward the appropriate component assessments.

Acute bacterial meningitis and various forms of viral encephalitis may result in changes in the client's level of consciousness. Consciousness is a state of awareness of one's self and one's environment.[20] Coma can be defined as a state in which one does not open the eyes, obey commands, or utter recognizable words.[15] The individual does not respond to external stimuli or to internal needs. The term *vegetative state* is sometimes used to indicate the status of individuals who open their eyes and display a sleepwake cycle but who do not obey commands or utter recognizable words. DeMeyer[11] presents a succinct description of the neuroanatomy of consciousness and the neurological examination of the unconscious patient. Plum and Posner[20] also provide extensive information in this area.

Several scales have been developed to provide objective guidelines to assess alterations in the state of consciousness. Jennett and Teasdale[15] developed the Glasgow Coma Scale, which assesses three independent items—eye opening, motor performance, and verbal performance. The scale yields a figure between 3 (lowest) and 15 (highest) that can be used to indicate changes in the individual's state of consciousness. The evaluation format is simple and the scale demonstrates both interrater and intrarater reliability. The therapist can use assessment tools such as the Glasgow Coma Scale to determine if the intervention program has resulted in any recordable changes in the client's level of consciousness. Ideally, the client will be monitored continuously at consistent intervals to determine changes in status. Any carry-over or delayed effects of the intervention could then be noted. A constant record of the client's level of consciousness might also display a pattern of peak awareness at a particular point in the day. Scheduling an intervention session during the client's peak awareness time may maximize the benefit of the therapy.

In consort with the assessment of the client's state of consciousness is the assessment of his or her ability to communicate—both the expressive and receptive aspects of the process. If a dysfunction is present in the client's ability to communicate, the client should be evaluated by an individual with expertise in this area so that strategies for dealing with the communication deficit can be developed. Evaluation of the movement abilities of the client with communication deficits requires creative planning on the part of the therapist but usually can be accomplished if generalized movement tasks are used. With the client who cannot comprehend a verbal command to roll, the therapist could use an alternate form of communication as discussed in Chapter 26. The therapist could structure the situation to elicit the desired behavior by activities such as placing the client in an uncomfortable position or positioning a desired object so that it can be reached only by rolling.

The emotional and psychological aspects of the client as discussed in Chapter 7 and the cognitive and retention skills of the client should be evaluated informally by the therapist, with referral to appropriate professionals if dysfunction in these areas is suspected. A coordinated team approach is necessary for clients with emotional and psychological, cognitive, perceptual, or communication problems or a combination of these problems. A consistent strategy used by all team members eliminates the necessity of the client to try to cope with different approaches by different people in an area in which he or she already has a deficit. The impact of cognitive deficits on the process of learning motor skills is discussed in the next section on movement assessment. The assessment of the impact of perceptual changes is incorporated within the evaluation of sensory channels.

Evaluation of sensory channels

The evaluation process must include a thorough assessment of the channels for sensory input. Knowledge gained in the assessment of the sensory systems will be utilized in the program-planning process to select the intervention strategies that have the highest probability of success. Although movements can be performed (and in some cases even learned) in the absence of typical sensory feedback, the presence of altered sensory function creates more challenges for both the client/learner and the therapist/teacher. The therapist assesses both the client's ability to perceive the sensory stimulus and the appropriateness of the response to the stimulus. Tactile input could result in an appropriate activation of underlying muscles or a maladaptive increase of muscle activity in a stereotyped distribution.

Variations in the interpretation of sensory input may occur in some clients. Gentle tactile contact may be perceived by the person as a noxious input. Some individuals will have difficulty processing high levels of one type of sensory input (e.g., the noisy clinic area) or multiple simultaneous inputs (e.g., talking to the therapist while walking down a hallway with people moving toward the individual). The therapist should be alert to indications of substitution of sensory feedback channels. The client with impaired proprioception tends to compensate through the use of visual information. Although this compensation may be functional within the constraints of isolated tasks, problems arise when vision is required to monitor other items such as objects in the walking path.

During the evaluation process, the therapist must note the sensory inputs that produce the adaptive behaviors so that they can be utilized as components of the intervention sequence.

The therapist should develop a systematic approach to the initial cursory evaluation of the sensory systems. Deficits identified in the initial evaluation will provide structure for scheduling more comprehensive evaluation of deficits in specific systems. The therapist must also monitor changes in the status of physiological vital functions during sensory input, especially if the client has a history of instability of heart rate, blood pressure, or rate of respiration.

Cutaneous input has several aspects that must be assessed. Some of the inflammatory diseases of the brain may result in cutaneous distributions in which sensation is absent or diminished. These areas should be routinely evaluated for changes in distribution of level of sensation. Tests of light touch, pressure, sharpness, and dullness can be utilized if the client can communicate reliably. A gross assessment of the intactness of the touch system can be made in the noncommunicative client by introducing a mildly adversive (not painful) stimulus, such as a light scratch while monitoring the client for changes in facial expression, posture, or tonus. The possibility of a spinal-level reflex response should be kept in mind when interpreting the results of such a gross assessment.

The olfactory channels are unique among the sensory input routes because the primary olfactory pathway directly synapses with the olfactory cortex within the limbic system before going to the thalamus. Olfactory inputs may provide a mechanism to elicit arousal in an otherwise unresponsive individual. Chapter 6 discusses the procedure for administering olfactory input as a component of evaluation and intervention regimens. Due to the potential hypersensitivity of any or all input systems, it is best to arouse with pleasant odors rather than noxious odors that may elicit a flight-or-fight response.

Gustatory sensory information is not typically an input channel utilized by therapists. In the client who is not receiving any gustatory stimulation because of prolonged tube feeding or in the client who demonstrates dysfunction of the oral musculature, the gustatory avenue of sensory input should not be overlooked. Various tastes can be incorporated in the evaluation of the effects of sensory inputs on clients with depressed levels of consciousness. Gustatory input can be incorporated into an intervention plan with the goal of facilitating movement of the oral and facial musculature. The gustatory/tactile input of a small amount of peanut butter placed on the corner of the client's mouth may elicit tongue protrusion with lateral deviation to remove the morsel. Introduction of a slightly sour taste may facilitate a pucker response of the orbicularis oris. The possibility of achieving desired goals through the inclusion of gustatory input should be considered during the evaluation process.

The complex functions of the vestibular system can be assessed through a variety of avenues. The integrity of the connections underlying a vestibularly induced nystagmus response is assessed by physicians through the caloric test (warm and cold water or air introduced into the ear channel to induce nystagmus). Therapists have used the Ayres Post-Rotatory Nystagmus Test[3,4] and variations of the test to gain information on the postrotatory nystagmus response. Although the postrotatory nystagmus tests provide information on the response of the extraocular muscles to vestibular input, they should not be overinterpreted as yielding insight about the integrity of the vestibular connections underlying postural responses.

Located in the utriculus and sacculus are the maculae, which record changes in the relationship of the head to the pull of gravity (position detectors) and changes in linear acceleration. This end organ is responsible for the tonic labyrinthine reflexes. By manipulating the position of the client's head in relation to the pull of gravity, the therapist can evaluate this aspect of the vestibular system by noting changes in the distribution of muscle activity. The effect of rapid linear accelerations and decelerations can be evaluated as potential activating mechanisms increasing the level of consciousness or level of muscle activity. Slow, rhythmical reversals of linear movements may have a calming effect on the client's behavior or level of muscle activation. Linear movements in all planes and diagonals should be explored.

Assessment of the client's response to proprioceptive input is incorporated within the assessment of the client's movement abilities and is intertwined with the intervention process because a variety of intervention techniques are based on proprioceptive input (Chapter 6). Evaluation of the proprioceptive channels can be conducted through assessment of the client's static position sense and dynamic kinesthesis. These tests allow the therapist to make inferences concerning the client's cognitive abilities to interpret proprioceptive information. Inherent in the successful completion of these tests is the necessity for the client to be able to understand directions and to be able to communicate data to the therapist. Because information input, processing, and output are involved in these tests, failure to comply with the test instructions cannot be definitively attributed to dysfunction of the proprioceptive system. The therapist also should consider information obtained from watching the client move before drawing a conclusion concerning the intactness of the proprioceptive channels. Some of the factors to consider include disregard of an extremity and variations in quality of performance between visually directed and nonvisually directed movements. Although tests of position sense and kinesthetics provide one aspect of the evaluation of the proprioceptive system, the therapist also must be involved constantly in assessing the client's response to the intervention techniques that are part of the treatment plan. This again illustrates the intermingling of assessment and intervention. Intervention places a demand for movement on the client. As the movement occurs, the therapist assesses the quality of the movement. If the quality is not appropriate, the therapist initiates intervention to improve the quality. If the technique does not produce the desired result, a second technique can be tried and the cyclic process continues.

Auditory and visual channels can be grossly assessed by the therapist. More detailed information on the intactness of the sensory channels can be obtained from other health team members. The types of information available from other health team members can vary from the assessment of brainstem evoked potentials in response to auditory and visual inputs in the comatose individual to the identification of visual or auditory acuity deficits. Because the auditory and visual systems provide the therapist with a primary means of communicating with the client and because they can be used to augment performance in the event of deficits in other sensory channels, these systems should be incorporated in the therapist's evaluation process. Simple visual system tests, such as identification of field deficits, assessment of tracking abilities, and a gross evaluation of visual acuity, can be performed quickly. Neurology textbooks can be consulted on the techniques for administering these tests. Simple tests for assessing auditory thresholds can include such techniques as rubbing fingers by the individual's ear, placing a ticking watch to the client's ear, or assessing the presence of a startle response to sounds in the client with altered states of consciousness. Although these quick tests of the visual and auditory systems will not yield quantifiable information, they should provide the therapist with the necessary data to design an intervention plan that accounts for the presence of the deficits or that can use the intact system to compensate for input missing from an impaired system. Refer to Chapter 27 for additional information regarding the visual-perceptual system.

During the evaluation of the client as well as during intervention with the client, the therapist must be aware of the potential to bombard the client with sensory input and overload his or her ability to respond discriminatively to it. If the therapist detects that the client has difficulty in appropriately responding to sensory input, such as the client in a lowered state of consciousness or an agitated state or the

client demonstrating tactile defensiveness, only one type of sensory input should be used during the initial evaluation or intervention sessions. If multiple sensory inputs are used, the positive or negative effects cannot be attributed to a specific input or necessarily to the series of inputs. Evaluation as well as intervention with sensory inputs should proceed in a controlled fashion. Inclusion of additional sensory modalities in the intervention plan should occur systematically.

The individual's response to multichannel sensory conflict input is typically assessed as a component of higher level balance assessment and locomotor abilities. The reader is referred to Chapter 28 for more details on this aspect of the "sensory" assessment. The therapist should apply these concepts during the evaluation of all motor tasks. Consider the following example. A client who relies on visual input to supplement vestibular and somatosensory information is performing the task of sitting on the edge of the mat table. She remains relatively steady until someone walks directly toward her from across the clinic. This change in the environmental context of the performance requires her to assess whether she is moving toward the individual or the individual is moving toward her. Without reliable vestibular and somatosensory check points, the client may activate a postural response to the incorrect assessment. As this example demonstrates, the evaluation of the sensory channels is intertwined with the evaluation of the person's movement abilities.

Evaluation of movement abilities

Assessment of the individual's movement abilities is performed as he or she moves through a sequence of functional postures. The therapist determines the functional postures to be examined for a specific client, ranging from prone and supine (bed mobility activities) through upright ambulation. The assessment focuses on both the quantity and quality of motor performance. The quantity aspect of the movement assessment refers to the number of different functional postures the individual can use. The quality of the movement abilities is assessed within the posture as well as in the process of moving between postures.

A number of additional items relating to the client's movement abilities are assessed during this process. Indications of abnormal ranges of movement of all joints can be obtained. The range may show a limitation of movement or an indication of joint instability. Once the gross deviations are identified, these joints can be examined to determine the source of the problem—joint capsular, ligamentous, bony, skin, or muscular and fascial dysfunction. Conducting the gross assessment of range while the client is moving eliminates the time spent in performing a joint-by-joint goniometric evaluation on articulations with normal excursions.

As the individual is moving (either independently or with the therapist assisting), an assessment of the distribution and fluctuations in muscle activity can be made. The therapist can identify the postures that will be the most conducive to optimal motor performances and those that should be avoided. The therapist can identify the reflexes and reactions influencing each posture. They should be categorized as supporting or interfering with the posture and movement patterns. Assessing the influence of the reflexes and reactions in each of the functional postures provides a more realistic picture of their influence than conducting a reflex inventory test, which considers only one posture. Integration of the tonic reflexes may appear to have occurred in the lower-level postures, while the reflex continues to influence movement at higher-level or more complex postures. Monitoring the influence of the reflexes and reactions as the client progresses through a sequence of postures and movements provides the more comprehensive assessment of the problems to be dealt with in therapy.

Within each posture, the therapist must examine the control the client displays over the posture. Because the assessment takes place as a part of a dynamic sequence, the therapist can assess the client's ability to assume the posture. If the posture cannot be achieved independently, the therapist assesses the factors interfering with achieving the position, the type of assistance necessary to facilitate assumption of the posture, and the effect of the various intervention techniques used to assist the client in achieving the position. Once the client is in the posture, his or her ability to maintain the posture is examined. Factors that interfere with the performance are noted. The client's ability to move within the posture is identified. Movement demands placed on the client should include aspects of both static and dynamic equilibrium. Static equilibrium in the all-fours position could be demonstrated by clients matching the strength of a force attempting to displace them backwards and maintaining the position when the force is suddenly released.

The presence of dynamic equilibrium of the upper torso in the all-fours position could be demonstrated by the client reacting to a quick sideways displacement force administered to the shoulder by crossing one arm over the other to maintain balance. The client also should be able to demonstrate appropriate equilibrium responses to self-imposed perturbations.

The final stage in examining control of a functional posture concerns the ability to move out of the posture. The client should have the ability to move out of the posture to a lower-level posture and to a higher-level posture before mastery of the posture is considered to have been achieved.

As the client is moving through various postures, the function of specific musculature can be examined. Muscle groups should be examined concerning their ability to function in stability (distal segment fixed) situations and in mobility (distal segment free) situations. Because numerous demands are being placed on each muscle group, therapists can assess their ability to perform isometric and isotonic (concentric and eccentric) contractions. Each different posture introduces a new set of variables; therefore the performance of a muscle group must be reexamined as each new movement pattern is performed.

As indicated previously, the evaluation process is not compartmentalized. Many aspects of the client's performance are analyzed simultaneously. When the therapist assists the client in moving to a new posture, an analysis of the influence of facilitation and inhibition techniques is being conducted. The individual's response to these handling techniques cues the therapist in projecting the client's response to an intervention program. The therapist is constantly monitoring the client for changes in physiological functions or changes in the level of consciousness. Anything that results in expressions of pain by the client should be noted. Intervention programs should be a learning experience for clients. If they are attending to pain, they cannot attend to learning. The factor(s) producing the pain should be identified and measures instituted to eliminate the factor(s). If the factors producing the pain cannot be resolved, the intervention program should be designed to avoid triggering the pain. (See Chapter 31 on Pain Management.)

The presence of motor planning dysfunctions can be noted as the client attempts a movement sequence. The therapist may have to cue the client physically to initiate the sequence, which then flows smoothly. The therapist may observe that the client has the correct components to a movement sequence but that the sequence of the components is incorrect. Or the client may demonstrate the ability to produce a movement sequence under one set of conditions but not another. Indications of these types of motor planning problems can be observed during the initial interactions with the client. The therapist also should be aware of any signs of cerebellar dysfunctions (see Chapter 23).

Having observed the client move through a sequence of postures, the therapist will have a baseline knowledge of the client's functional abilities. The details of the client's functional performance are obtained through the assessment of the accomplishment of the activities of daily living (ADL). Whether the assessment of the client's skills in this area is performed by the therapist or other health team member, the results of the assessment are important to add to the database from which the intervention plan will be formulated. Assessment of the client's functional abilities within ADL can provide detailed information on the fine movement skills required of the upper extremity. Evaluation of the performance of these functional tasks provides the therapist with the opportunity to compare the variety of observations, as discussed previously.

Another aspect of the evaluation process that can be integrated in the observations of movement abilities is identification of perceptual deficits. Aspects of the client's motor performance can provide indications for detailed perceptual testing to classify the deficits. This testing should be conducted by the health team member qualified in the area of perceptual testing. During the general evaluation procedures, the therapist can screen the client for signs of perceptual deficits. Clients' abilities to cross their midlines with their upper extremities can be demonstrated in move-

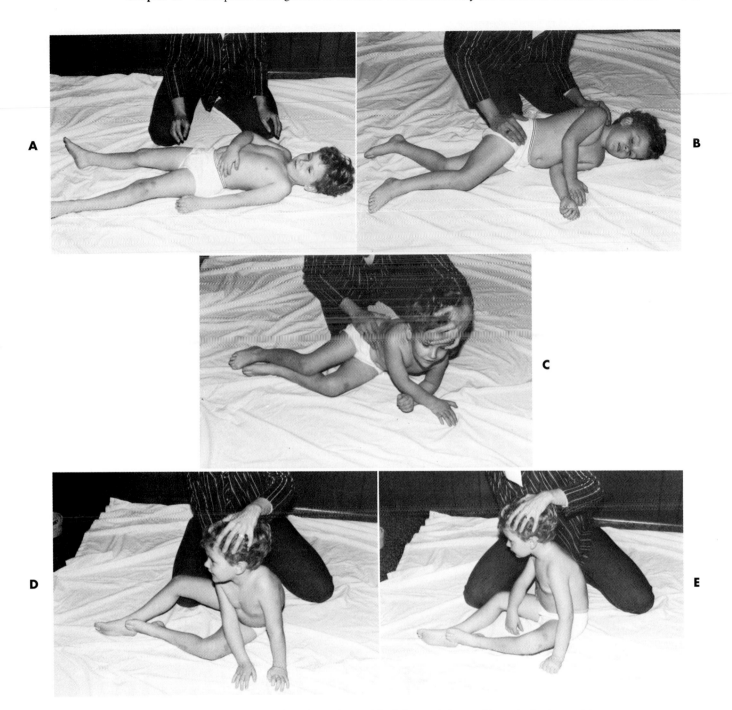

Fig. 17-2. Movement sequence from the supine to side sitting to sitting positions. **A,** Supine position.
B, Handling to side lying. **C,** Handling toward side sitting, arm positions are important. **D,** Side
sitting; note propping patterns with arms. **E,** Handling to symmetrical sitting.

ment sequences such as moving from the supine to the side sitting to the sitting position (Fig. 17-2). The quality of the integration of information from the two sides of the body can be indicated by the symmetry or asymmetry of posture in positions that should be symmetrical. The therapist may suspect that the client has a deficit in body awareness or body image by the poor quality of movement patterns that are within the motor capability of the individual. Spontaneous comments by the client as to how he or she feels when moving ("my leg feels so heavy") also add to the therapist's

assessment of the client's body image. Problems with verticality can be seen with the client who lists to one side when in an upright posture. When the therapist corrects the list to a vertical posture, clients may express that they now feel that they are leaning to one side. Individuals who cannot appropriately relate their positions to the position of objects in their environments may have a figure-ground deficit or a problem with the concept of their position in space. When approaching stairs, these clients may fail to step up or may attempt to step up too soon. These examples should provide an indication of the observations that can indicate the need for detailed perceptual testing. See Chapters 11 and 27 for additional discussion of perceptual deficits.

The preceding aspects of evaluation of movement abilities have focused on facets of motor performance. Within this process, the therapist should intertwine an appraisal of the individual's ability to learn motor tasks (or elements of the task). The therapist attempts to determine whether the client can maintain a change in the ability to perform a movement throughout a therapy session and (ideally) into the next session. The client's ability to capture and integrate changes into the movement repertoire is fundamental to the success of the intervention program. The program can focus on the learning of movement sequences and the generalization of these sequences to movements within other contexts. Individuals with lowered levels of consciousness (typically Rancho Los Amigos Stages 1-3) will be unable to learn or have difficulty learning and generalizing new motor skills. Therapy sessions may be more successful if the focus remains on the performance of motor tasks that were previously "overlearned" and automatic. Although the therapist may be able to manually guide the individual in coming to sitting on the edge of the bed, until the individual demonstrates a higher level of processing, it may be unrealistic to expect that the person will consistently reposition the legs without cuing before attempting the movement sequence.

The general philosophy in the evaluation of the client with neurological deficits as a result of brain inflammation is a whole-part-whole approach. General observations of the client's performance provide a general description of the client's abilities while indicating deficits in his or her performance. The cause(s) of the deficits are explored to provide the pieces of data defining his or her performance. These pieces of data then are arranged within the framework provided by the general observation to define the whole of the client's assets and deficits. As the whole picture is established (with the realization that it will be constantly adjusted), the process of goal setting is initiated. The process presented for refining evaluation data into an intervention plan is applicable whether the client's neurological dysfunction is the result of a bacterial or viral infection, cerebral vascular accident, trauma, or other factors.

GOAL SETTING

Ideally, the process of goal setting for a client is a coordinated effort that involves all members of the health care team, including the client (if feasible) and family. If the therapist is not functioning in a setting where involvement of many disciplines is viable, the therapist can progress through the goal-setting process in the context of his or her role in the client's care.

Having collected data from the evaluation process, the first steps are to establish two lists—one dealing with specific problems the client is encountering and one dealing with his or her assets. Formulating an asset list focuses on the positive data elicited from the evaluation process. Items on the asset list could be observations, such as the client being able to assume the position of prone-on-elbows independently, improved head control in this posture being facilitated by approximation (Chapter 6), and controlled weight shifting being elicited by alternated tapping (Chapter 6). The asset list provides a reference defining the postures and intervention techniques that are effective. This reference is used to develop the **intervention goals** and plan. Formulating and recording a problem list and an asset list can be completed relatively quickly as one gains familiarity with the process. Just as the evaluation process is ongoing, so are the steps involved in goal setting. The asset and problem lists are redefined as the client's status changes.

Having identified assets and problems, the next step is to establish long-term goals. These goals are the general objectives toward which the intervention process is oriented. They identify the end point of the intervention process. The long-term goals are the exit criteria for terminating the intervention. If one of the client's problems was the inappropriate activation of certain muscle groups during attempts to assume and maintain several postures, a long-term goal could be maintenance of appropriate muscle activation while moving between functional postures.

Measurable, objective, short-term goals are established from the long-term goals. The goal should be measurable either in terms of producing a numerical indicator of performance, such as time span, number of repetitions, or distance covered, or in terms of an accurate description of the target motor behavior. The appropriate objective indicator must be carefully selected. Performing a movement more quickly may indicate that the individual is performing it with more normal control and therefore greater ease of movement, or it may indicate that the individual has become more skilled in using an abnormal pattern based on inappropriate muscle activation. If it is not appropriate to write the goal in terms of a numerical indicator, the goal can be written in terms of an observable behavior. The therapist can precisely describe body segment movements based on the component method of movement analysis presented by Van Sant.[24,25] For example, the task of coming to standing from supine can be described in terms of the upper-extremity component, axial component, and lower-extremity component. Formulation of an appropriate short-term goal could specify use of the upper extremities in a push and reach pattern during the task of coming to standing from supine. The short-term goals should be written so that observing the client's behavior will allow the therapist to state whether the criteria of the short-term goal were achieved. Table 17-1 gives an example of some components of short-term goals leading to mastery of functional activities in sitting.

The long-term goals define the client's destination. The short-term goals define the mileposts. The therapist then uses the asset list to design the intervention program, which is the vehicle to get the client to his or her destination. From the asset list, the therapist knows the intervention techniques

Table 17-1. Examples of short-term goals relating to mastery of functional activities in sitting*

Condition variables†		Activity	Criteria
1. When sitting on a mat	a. Using the upper extremities for support	The client will maintain the posture	for ___ seconds.
2. When sitting on the edge of a mat table	b. Using one upper extremity for support c. Without using the upper extremities for support		
3. When sitting in a chair	d. With the therapist displacing the position of the: Pelvis Shoulders Head Lower extremities	The client will make postural adjustments of the head and trunk	appropriate to the degree of displacement.
		The client will bring right foot to left knee (as if to put on a shoe)	without losing balance.

*Long-term goal: The client will master functional activities in sitting. Short-term goals: Select one phrase from each column.
†Therapist needs to consider all aspects of each variable, i.e., 1 a, b, c, d; 2—a, b, c, d; 3—a, b, c, d.

that have the highest probability of success. Adopting this process simplifies the task of outlining the strategy for intervention.

As the therapist considers the appropriate goals for the client, a decision must be made as to whether the format of the intervention will focus on a "training" approach or a "motor learning" approach. During the assessment process, if the therapist concludes that the individual's level of cognitive function precludes the development of insight into movement errors (both the detection and correction of an incorrect performance) or the ability to retain the insight over time, then the therapist should delineate the goals and intervention plan to accommodate this limitation. The "training" approach requires more structure and repetition of activities within that structure. If it is more appropriate to design the intervention plan according to motor learning considerations, the therapist must consider the appropriate schedule and environmental context for the practice, the type and schedule for the feedback provided, and techniques to promote the generalization of the learning beyond the specific practice session. While the goal-setting process results in specification of the outcome objectives for a specific client, the general goals for the intervention process can be delineated to guide the process. As described in the overview of inflammatory disorders at the beginning of this chapter, the extent of the neurological sequelae may range from a single discrete problem to a devastating clinical picture composed of compromised functions in multiple areas. The goals for the intervention process address the problem areas that (1) jeopardize the efficiency and effectiveness of functional activities and (2) are the primary result of compromised neurological function. The listing of goals does not directly include consideration of secondary problems (such as decreases in joint range of motion [ROM], cardiovascular fitness, and endurance). The therapist should

integrate these considerations in the overall assessment of the components of the movement problems.

The goals are written as outcomes of the intervention process and not as goals for a specific client. Because of the broad nature of the goals, other professions also will contribute to the attainment of the goals. The goals of the therapeutic intervention program for clients with inflammatory CNS disorders are as follows:

1. Promotion of optimalization of **postural control** as demonstrated by
   a. the ability to maintain a position against gravity
   b. the ability to automatically adjust before and continuously during movement
2. Promotion of optimalization of selective, voluntary movement patterns within functional activities
3. Enhancement of progression through the sequence of functional activities
4. Fostering integration of sensory input
5. Promotion of optimalization of cognitive and psychosocial responses

Each of these goals is discussed in conjunction with the general therapeutic intervention procedures that can be used to achieve the goal.

GENERAL THERAPEUTIC INTERVENTION PROCEDURES IN RELATION TO INTERVENTION GOALS

Promotion of optimalization of postural control as demonstrated by the ability to maintain a position against gravity and the ability to automatically adjust before and continuously during movement

The intervention goal of promoting optimalization of postural control underlies the ability to make selective, voluntary movement patterns (goal 2) and the ability to progress through the sequence of functional activities (goal 3). Optimization of postural set includes the concepts of decreasing muscle activity that is too high to allow performance of movement sequences, as well as augmenting activation that is too low to support the accomplishment of a movement sequence. The postural set of a client can fluctuate between degrees of **hypertonicity** and **hypotonicity**; the term *optimalization* allows the goal to be stated in a manner that indicates that the optimal postural set for a particular movement is the desired outcome. Intervention techniques to achieve this goal demand that the therapist constantly monitor the client's performance so that appropriate interventions are added when needed and continued only as long as they are needed.

Optimal postural control has been defined by two elements. The client should have the ability to maintain a posture or a position against gravity. Automatic adjustments in the postural set should occur in anticipation of and continuously during movements. Both elements should be performed with minimal physical or cognitive effort on the part of the client.

Readers who are acquainted with the concept of the *normal postural reflex mechanism* introduced by the Bobaths[9] will recognize familiar constructs. This discussion, however, will not incorporate the assumption that dysfunction of postural control is based on problems with specific righting and equilibrium reactions, the presence of associated reactions, the effect of released asymmetrical tonic neck reflex activity, or the effect of released positive supporting reactions.[9] Although one or more of these elements may be present, it will not be assumed to be the causal factor. Clients with neurological sequelae may exhibit "primitive" reflexes—stereotypical motor responses that resemble the reflex responses that are present in the process of normal development but whose influence is suppressed as maturation proceeds. Typically, these motor responses are of a greater magnitude and display less variation than the normal development reflexes.

The utilization of primitive reflexes as part of the intervention techniques for clients who have a limited ability to perform motor responses is controversial. Primitive reflexes can be used to augment a response such as turning the head to the right (asymmetrical tonic neck reflex—ATNR) to augment an extension response of the right upper extremity. The potential problem with this approach is that the client may be learning a behavior that reinforces the limited stereotypical pattern and blocks the process of learning to make appropriate postural adjustments and selective muscle activation.

Primitive reflexes can be useful to elicit a movement response, but should be used only when other tools are not effective. If the movement response is elicited via a primitive reflex, the therapist should immediately attempt to elicit the response without the reflex input. Shaping the sequence in this manner promotes the learning of the desired response and not reinforcement of an undesired stimulus to achieve the response. If the ATNR is used to elicit triceps function, the head then should be returned to the neutral position and function augmented by tapping, vibration, or other proprioceptive inputs. Once the triceps response is achieved with the head in the neutral position, the head should be rotated away from the side of the triceps. This final stage promotes a functional response against the influence of a sensory trigger for the stereotypical pattern.

Basing a decision on the needs of the client, the therapist must decide whether to use these primitive reflexes to augment the initial response despite their potential negative effects. Regardless of this initial decision, the intervention should progress from movement with neutral support from the stereotypical response to movement against the influence of the primitive reflex. As the client progresses to functionally higher level (and more stressful) postures, the influence of primitive reflexes may again be expressed. The process of developing selective control may require repetition in several positions and activities.

The client's ability to demonstrate optimal postural control may be restricted by the presence of hypertonicity or hypotonicity in various muscle groups. These states may be relatively static or may fluctuate with the demands of a particular situation. Inappropriately high levels of muscle activity may be present in a stereotypical muscle distribution in the extremities, whereas the activity of the trunk musculature may be too low to support an antigravity posture. The therapist must design the interventions creatively to meet the shifting responses of the demands of a particular activity.

A saying attributed to the Bobaths is "First make it possible, then make it happen." Although some contend that this philosophy shifts too much of the responsibility away from the client, it also can be interpreted as directing the therapist to create changes in the internal and external environments to afford the person the opportunity to formulate and execute a movement response that otherwise would not be possible. The therapist also must consider structuring the situation so that the client can learn to make the response within a variety of environmental constraints.

Hypertonicity. Inappropriately high levels of activity in a muscle group or groups may limit the client's ability to demonstrate optimal postural control (and optimal selective movements as addressed in the second goal). The therapist can select intervention techniques that are mediated through any of the sensory channels functional for that client. The choice of which channel or combination of channels to use for the input is based on the therapist's initial and continuing evaluation of the client's response to specific types of sensory input (see Chapter 6).

The therapist must address the hypertonicity influencing postural control as a generalized problem before demanding selective voluntary activation of specific muscle groups. Vestibular input that is slow and rhythmical may promote a generalized relaxation of skeletal muscle activity. In some clients, the trunk remains "stiff" in movement sequences in which a segmental response between the upper and lower trunk should occur. Repetitions of rhythmical movements side-lying in which the therapist gently and progressively stretches the client's pelvis in one direction around the body axis while moving the shoulder girdle in the opposite direction and then reverses the movement may effectively alter the biomechanical and neurological contributions to the stiffness (Fig. 17-3).

For some clients, changing the dynamics of a spastic extremity may permit the emergence of more optimal levels of postural control. The appropriately designed ankle-foot orthosis (AFO) may alter the need to rigidly control the position of the pelvis in order to remain upright (Chapter 32). Use of a soft webbing thumb loop to alter the resting position of the first metacarpal may change the overactivity of musculature throughout the upper extremity and allow appropriate adjustment of the shoulder girdle as part of postural responses.

For some of the more involved clients, the therapist may need to use handling techniques to change the alignment relationship of body segments before attempting to elicit automatic postural adjustments. Bobath[9] discusses the use of proximal and distal key points of control to influence the client's distribution of muscle activity. The therapist must remember that the static imposition of control will not help the client learn to move. The therapist imposes control so that the client can move. As the client moves and gains control of the movement, the therapist lessens the amount of control. The therapist's goal should be to remove his or her hands from controlling the client's responses.

Chapter 6 discusses some of the potential combinations of techniques that can produce the desired postural response. The therapist may need to alter the sensory input via several channels before the client will be able to achieve the appropriate postural set. Sensory inputs should be altered systematically until the desired response is achieved. Interventions should be withdrawn systematically to move the client toward responding appropriately and independently to the demands of a situation.

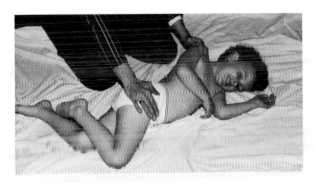

Fig. 17-3. Counterrotation of shoulder girdle backward (retraction) and the pelvis forward. Hand placement of therapist is important so that shoulder and hip movements can occur freely.

If the client is sufficiently alert so that attending to and understanding directions is a possibility, the therapist should direct the person to focus on the sensation of the changes occurring. As the person begins to appreciate the "feel" of what is transpiring, he or she should be asked to assist in maintaining the changes that promote the more skillful movement response. Unless otherwise indicated by the client's status, interventions must actively involve the individual in the process of planning, initiating, completing, and evaluating the movement. Although the therapist may manipulate the environment (internal and external) in which the response is made, the client must be an active participant for learning to occur.

Hypotonicity. Although some clients will demonstrate a pattern of generalized overactivity of the postural muscles of the trunk, many will have difficulty generating sufficient activity in the appropriate groups to sustain a posture or to permit movement in the posture. As presented in Chapter 6, several intervention techniques are available depending on the sensory input channels that are effective. For example, variations in the pressure applied by manual contacts over the contractile portions of muscles provides a means to enhance their activation while the person attempts to maintain a position, prepares for a movement, or executes a movement.

Vestibular input in the presence of generalized hypotonia should be rapid and irregular. The labyrinths should be stimulated by quick stops and starts with changes in direction. The program should include the introduction of movements in all planes. Approximation can be effective in developing appropriate postural activity from a state of either hypertonicity or hypotonicity. Empirically, it seems that more force is applied to increase the postural response than to decrease the response. Approximation appears to elicit a response in all the muscles surrounding a joint as preparation for responding to the demands to the erect posture or the demands of weight bearing. Approximation lends itself to combination with other proprioceptive techniques, such as quick stretch or tapping.

As the therapist applies various techniques in an attempt to elicit a specific response, the therapist must evaluate the desired response in relationship to the environmental context. If the client is sitting on the edge of a mat table, the activity of the trunk musculature will vary depending on whether the feet are flat on the floor, whether the client is engaged in an activity, whether the client is leaning on one arm for support, or whether the client is resting between activities. The client who slouches in sitting when fatigued, bored, or overwhelmed by the sensory input may present a different clinical picture when the appropriate factors are altered.

Promotion of optimalization of selective, voluntary movement patterns within functional activities

The concept of the influence of the environment on the quality of a movement response, discussed in relation to the first goal of the intervention process, is also incorporated in the second goal. Quality, selective, voluntary movement patterns are sought within the framework of functional activities rather than as isolated and abstract movements. Optimalization of the selective movement patterns may require a decrease in the stereotypical linkages of certain muscle groups, an increase in the ability to selectively activate certain muscle groups, the development of the ability to execute the movement in different postures, or a number of other variations.

Performance of functional activities requires that the individual have the capability of performing both mobility and stability patterns with the extremities. Mobility patterns are open kinetic chain movements in which the distal segment is free. These patterns are necessary for placing the extremities (e.g., swing phase of gait or reaching for a doorknob).

Clients who exhibit stereotypical posturing of the upper extremity with a restricted repertoire of available movement patterns require intervention to change the initial position of the extremity before movements are attempted. The influence of the spasticity that interferes with the repositioning of the extremity can be reduced by applying approximation through the long axis of the extremity. Preferably, the therapist's manual contacts for the application of the approximation force are on the weight-bearing surfaces of the hand. If the flexed position of the wrist prohibits application of the force to the heel of the palm, the approximation can be applied gradually through the fisted hand. As the resistance to passive movement diminishes, the wrist can be moved toward the neutral position so that the therapist can then apply the approximation through the heel of the palm (Fig. 17-4). The therapist is moving the extremity toward an alternative resting position so that a new movement sequence can be attempted. It is important to use an intervention technique such as approximation to reduce the level of the spasticity before passive movement is attempted so that a more appropriate position can be assumed without inappropriately stretching the spastic muscles.

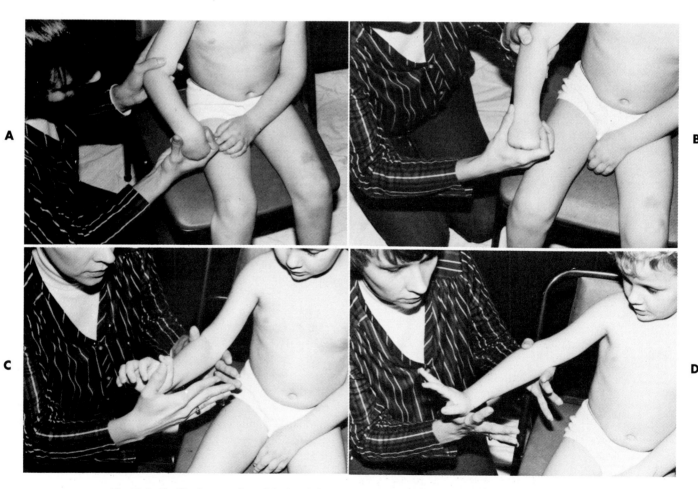

Fig. 17-4. Facilitating opening of the hand. **A,** Fisted hand; stretch to the extensors and approximation through hand, wrist, and elbow is applied. **B,** Approximation is continued; some resistance to the extensors may be applied. **C,** Approximation is applied to the thenar eminence to further facilitate extensor tone. **D,** Full extension is achieved; approximation is maintained.

The client may be asked to assist the therapist with the movement if the person can do so with a minimum of effort. Too often, clients attempt to make a selective movement through a massive effort and overactivation of the muscle groups, which compounds the underlying spasticity. Clients should be encouraged to make easy movements—movements that they are instructed to perform with reduced effort so that they can relearn selective activation of motor units rather than mass firing patterns.

Electrical stimulation can be used as an adjunct to facilitate performance of a particular component of a mobility pattern. The wrist extension component of the proprioceptive neuromuscular facilitation (PNF) pattern of flexion, abduction, and external rotation can be reinforced by using a portable electrical stimulation unit with an adjustable surge duration. The electrical stimulation elicits the correct movement so that the client could learn from the feel of the correct pattern. Adjusting the practice schedule so that the pattern is performed with and without the electrical stimulation support of the movement avoids the potential problem of reliance on the device to produce the movement. Electromyography (EMG) biofeedback can be a useful adjunct to achieve activation of specific muscle groups or to guide the client's attempts to reduce the level of activity of a muscle group (Chapter 30).

Mobility patterns in the upper extremity have as their foundation the freedom of the scapula to appropriately adjust to the position of the humerus. The mobility of the scapula can be addressed through techniques that result in a general decrease in muscle activity (such as neutral warmth) and diagonal movement patterns of the scapula. The scapular stabilizers, such as the rhomboids, trapezius, and serratus anterior, must be capable of allowing appropriate adjustment of the scapula as well as providing the fixation base upon which humeral elevation can occur.

In stability patterns, the distal segment of the extremity is fixed (closed kinetic chain). These patterns are used in the weight-bearing activities of the developmental sequence, such as the stance phase of gait and creeping. The components of the stability patterns are enhanced by proprioceptive input such as approximation. During the performance of both stability and mobility patterns, the therapist should control the situation so that the client learns from the sensation of appropriate movement patterns and not patterns imposed by inappropriate muscle activation.

As the client performs mobility and stability patterns as components of functional activities, all types of muscle contractions should be elicited from each muscle group. If a particular type of contraction poses a problem for a muscle group, the therapist can select an alternate posture in which to build in the ability of the muscle group to perform that type of contraction. For example, if the client has problems with eccentric hamstring control during the swing phase of gait, the pattern can be worked on as a component of the rolling sequence from the supine to the prone position (Fig. 17-5). Once the client gains control of the pattern within one movement context, the therapist must design activities to promote generalization of the pattern to other movement contexts. The client who has difficulty with the cocontraction stability pattern of the upper extremity in the all-fours position may have more success with a forward propping position in sitting, which may allow more control of the amount of weight being supported by the upper extremity. After gaining control in forward propped sitting, attempts can be made to generalize the response to positions such as side sitting and all fours.

Performance of movement patterns should progress toward an ability to easily reverse the direction of the movement. This can be promoted by incorporating rhythmical movements within a posture or between postures as early as possible in the intervention sequence. The end point at which the reversal is required should vary. The client might be asked to move from the sitting position to all fours, and back to sitting; then the client could move from the sitting position to the half-way position to all fours, then reverse to sitting. Incorporating reversal of movement patterns within the intervention program prepares the client to deal with situations that mandate unexpected adjustments in the movement sequence.

Clients who demonstrate problems with the sequencing of movements, such as those with motor dyspraxia, frequently perform better if the movement is performed at a speed that is close to normal. Clients who, previous to the brain infection, had normal movement sequences seem to be able to trigger better movement responses at normal speeds than at slower speeds, which disrupt the normal flow of the movement. In working with clients with sequencing problems, all team members should provide the same, consistent sensory cues to elicit a movement pattern. For example, the therapist may establish a coupling of the verbal cue "roll" with a quick stretch to the ankle dorsiflexors to elicit a rolling pattern. These same cues can be used by other team members to assist the client in changing positions in bed or in performing dressing activities. The consistency of cues may elicit a consistent response from the client. Once the pattern is well established, the intervention program can be designed to include an extinction process for the cues progressing toward the ability of the client to perform the activity in response to the demands of the situation rather than to externally imposed cues.

The flow of a movement pattern may be disrupted by problems categorized as incoordination. The origin of the coordination problems could be dysfunction of the visual-perceptual system (see Chapter 27), or vestibular systems (see Chapters 11 and 28), dyspraxia (see Chapter 11), or dysfunction caused by cerebellar damage (see Chapter 23). If possible, the factors involved in producing a lack of coordination should be identified.

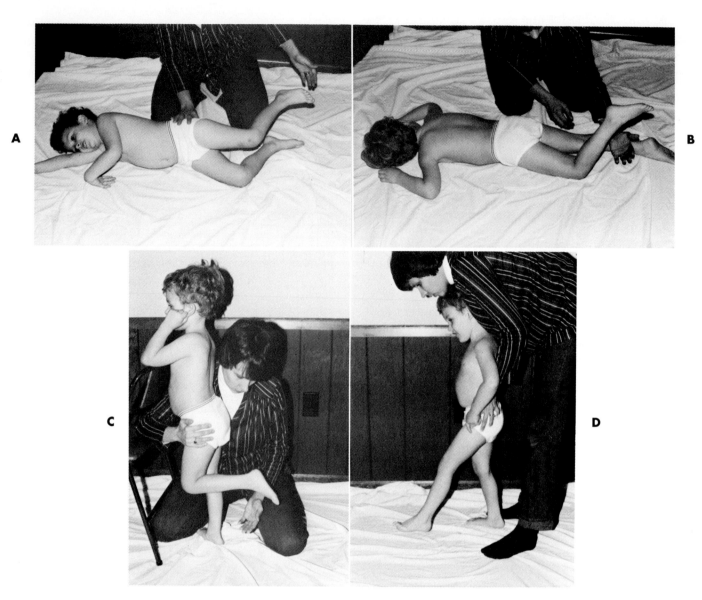

Fig. 17-5. Eliciting eccentric hamstring control within different movement contexts. **A,** Roll from the supine to side-lying position (beginning sequence). **B,** Roll from the side-lying to prone position with controlled lengthening of the hamstrings. **C,** Standing eccentric hamstring contraction. **D,** Controlled hamstring activity during swing phase of gait.

Enhancement of progression through the sequence of functional activities

As the client develops more appropriate postural control and the ability to perform selective movement patterns within functional activities, he or she is developing the basis to progress through a sequence of increasingly challenging **functional activities**. The movement patterns (and the postural control that underlies them) provide the building blocks for mastering an expanding variety of activities.

As the therapist designs the expansion of activities within the intervention program, the demands of each new functional activity and posture must be scrutinized. The client's ability to meet these demands was examined in the evaluation process. The intervention strategy must focus on the quality of the client's ability to assume a posture, maintain the posture, move within the posture (static and dynamic equilibrium responses to both self-generated and external perturbations), and move out of the posture. The therapist will change the sequence of this progression of activities to meet the needs of the client. The client may achieve independence in maintaining a posture while still requiring assistance in assuming the posture.

This progression should be grounded within the context of functionally relevant activities. Unless the individual has difficulty tolerating change, activities should be practiced within different environments to enhance generalization of learning. The creative therapist can design a variety of functionally relevant activities that require similar movement components.

With pediatric clients, the therapist may choose to use the developmental sequence as a model for the functional activities progression. Progression through the developmental sequence should be viewed as a dynamic process so that the intervention incorporates movement both within and between postures.

Samplings of handling techniques that can be adapted to enhance the individual's progression through the sequence of functional activities can be found in the works of Bobath,[9] Carr and Shepherd,[10] Duncan and Badke,[12] Levitt,[18] Sullivan and others,[22] Voss and others,[26] as well as throughout this book. These authors can provide the therapist with ideas for ways to enhance the client's performance within a specific activity.

Fostering integration of sensory input

At the same time that the therapist addresses the previous intervention goals, the goal of fostering integration of sensory input must be considered. Unless the therapist has advanced knowledge of sensory integration theories, this goal may be secondary rather than primary; nevertheless, it cannot be ignored.

The potential for an exaggerated and inappropriate response to sensory input was discussed as part of the clinical picture. Before the therapist expects the client to exhibit adaptive behavior to the potential bombardment of input from combinations of cutaneous, proprioceptive, auditory, and visual input, the therapist must assess the client's ability to respond to multisensory inputs. The ability to respond adaptively progresses from a response to a single sensory system input, to a response to the input in the presence of multiple system input, and then to an adaptive response based on inputs from two or more sources. The therapist must be sure that adding more sensory inputs augments an adaptive response rather than detracts from it. The client may respond to handling techniques providing proprioceptive and cutaneous cues but may demonstrate a deterioration of performance when auditory input is added. When verbal cues are added, the therapist should follow the philosophy that verbal commands should be concise, sparse, and appropriately timed.[26]

All sensory inputs should evoke the correct response on the part of the client rather than cause him or her to sift through the jumble of inputs to recognize the appropriate inputs to which a response should be made. At the highest level, the client will demonstrate cross-modal learning in which input from one sensory system will evoke a response based on input previously obtained via a different system. Recognition of a comb by touch is based on the precept of "combness" usually obtained initially by visual input. If the therapist recognizes the hierarchy in the process of integrating sensory input, intervention situations that require too high a level of performance from the client can be avoided.

The client who can respond adaptively to input from only one source will not be expected to perform in a crowded treatment area that presents extraneous visual and auditory input. The therapist will also recognize the need to include in the intervention plan situations that involve the controlled introduction of sensory inputs so that the client progresses toward the ability to deal with multiple inputs. The reader should explore the writings of Jean Ayres[3,4] to expand these concepts.

Dysfunctions in perceptual integration are addressed as the client moves through functional sequence activities. Although these movement activities would not provide the total program for an individual with a specific perceptual integration dysfunction, goals in this area can be addressed if the therapist is aware of indications of dysfunctions. The therapist must critically observe the performance of a movement sequence to identify substitute actions to compensate for problems such as inability to cross the midline. The therapist must then attempt to redesign the demands of the situation to elicit the desired behavior. The client who moves from the supine to the side sitting to the long sitting positions without the upper extremities crossing the midline could be required to side sit to the left and transfer objects with the right hand from the left side of the body to the right side (Fig. 17-6). The therapist must determine whether the client is truly crossing the midline or rotating the midline of the body to continue to avoid crossing it.

Therapists may be most aware of disturbances in the client's ability to integrate sensory information into an appropriate response when this dysfunction disrupts balance. The ability to maintain and move in upright postures requires successful processing of information from the equilibrial triad—the visual, vestibular, and somatosensory systems. When one component is missing, unreliable, or discrepant with the other two, the person is at risk for loss of balance. During the ongoing evaluation process, the therapist gathers information on the integrity of each system and any evidence of central processing difficulties. Practice of activities to develop postural control, to promote selective movements with functional activities, and to progress further within a sequence of functional activities simultaneously requires practice of the integration of sensory information so that a successful response can be generated.

Clients who are performing at higher levels can be challenged to maintain balance when one element of the equilibrial triad is missing (e.g., vision occluded) or altered (e.g., sitting, standing, or walking on a soft, compliant surface). Successful maintenance of balance outside the protective environment of the therapy clinic requires the ability to switch the primary information source to any one of the three systems. Walking in the dark requires the person to rely on vestibular and somatosensory input. Standing on a moving bus looking out a window requires resolution of the conflict between visual input (the external world is moving), vestibular input (you are moving), and somatosensory input

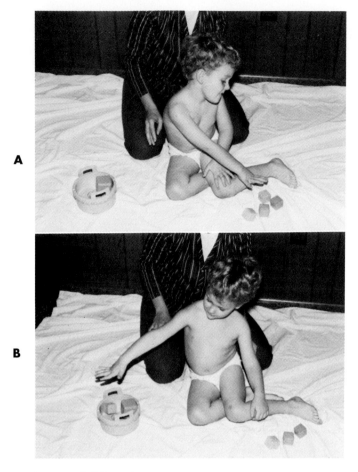

Fig. 17-6. Child crossing midline of body when transferring objects from left to right. **A,** Beginning active on contralateral side. **B,** Ending sequence by crossing midline and placing objects on ipsilateral side.

(you are stationary). Movement experiences within the therapy program should foster practice of this sensory integration process (see Chapter 28).

Promotion of optimalization of cognitive and psychosocial responses

In addition to attending to the factors directly related to motor performance, the therapist also must attend to the client's psychosocial and cognitive responses. Although the therapist does not have primary responsibility in this area, a goal of the intervention process should be to promote optimalization of psychosocial and cognitive responses.

Particularly in the agitated state that may be a component of the response to the inflammatory process, the client may demonstrate exaggerated and inappropriate emotional responses to events. Dealing with these emotional fluctuations can become a major determinant in goal attainment in the other areas. Maintaining a positive, nonthreatening interaction allows the client to use the therapist as a reference for judging the appropriateness of emotional responses.

If the client's state of agitation is interfering with the

intervention program, the therapist may alter the program to include sensory inputs that have a calming effect. Cutaneous inputs, such as wrapping the person in a cotton sheet blanket, or vestibular inputs, such as rhythmical repetitive rocking, can be productive. Auditory and visual input should be controlled to avoid overloading sensory processing mechanisms.

In Chapter 7 Burton discusses the psychosocial adjustment that occurs in the process of recovering from a neurological disability. The therapist must be aware of how the client's regression in affective and cognitive domains affects the intervention process. The therapist should seek assistance from the health care team members responsible for intervention in these areas to deal with the client constructively. The therapist must remember that both the family members and the client are in the process of adjusting to the client's changed and, it is hoped, changing status. Family members may be an asset or a liability to the client's recovery process. During the therapist's interactions with the family members in activities such as instructions in the client's home program, the therapist should be prepared to deal with expressions of the individual's difficulty in adjusting to the situation. The therapist also should be prepared to assist family members in identifying appropriate sources to help them deal with their problems.

Changes in mentation, perception of events, and memory losses present challenges to both the client and the therapist. Repetition in the recounting of past events may help reorder past knowledge. Use of brief verbal or visual cues may assist the client in recalling safety instructions or the components of the exercise program. The therapist should try to generate a nonstressful environment when working on these deficits so that attention and recall are not overshadowed by emotional pressure.

As the therapist works with the client on an intervention program, situations arise that require problem solving to determine a way to accomplish a task. If the task is to accomplish an independent transfer from a wheelchair into a bathtub, decisions must be made concerning the sequence of movements. Therapists can approach this situation in two ways. They can instruct clients step-by-step in what to do, or they can involve clients to the extent possible in the process of deciding what to do. If the therapist instructs the client step-by-step, the client may master the task but may not be able to perform it under different conditions. If the therapist involves the client in the decision-making process, the client may be learning not only how to accomplish the specific task, but also how to accomplish the task under varied conditions. The intervention process should lead to the ability to respond to the demands of a situation, and involvement of clients in the problem-solving process helps prepare them for independence. The therapist must structure the client's role in decision making to the level of the client's ability to participate so that the experience is not frustrating. Although the client's participation may initially increase the time required to complete a task, it promotes skills that may lead more quickly to independence of function.

INTERACTION WITH OTHER PROFESSIONALS

The therapist needs to design an intervention program that is articulated with that of other members of the health care team. The recovery process of the client should be facilitated by a care plan in which each team member reinforces the goals of the other team members. The care of the person must be a collaborative effort. Each client deserves an intervention process that considers him or her as a whole person, not as a set of fragmented problems.

SUMMARY

This chapter has presented a brief discussion of the pathology and medical management of various inflammatory processes that affect the brain. The process of assessment, the role of assessment in designing an intervention program, the goals of the intervention process, and means to meet those goals were presented to assist the reader in more effective management of these clients.

While the problem-solving process presented in this chapter for assessment, goal identification, and treatment planning is not limited to clients with inflammatory supraspinal disorders, its application in the presence of typical neurological sequelae has been described. When dealing with inflammatory disorders of the brain, the variability of neurological sequelae is examined based on the anatomical location of the inflammatory process and the cause of the infection.

Although the neurological disorders discussed in this chapter are life threatening and may be fatal, many clients recover and return to their previous life-styles. Clients will vary within the spectrum of minimal to severe involvement and specific to generalized CNS dysfunction and will demonstrate little to full recovery after the acute distress. Prognosis for recovery depends on the type of infecting organism and the extent of involvement. The therapist must remain flexible and willing to adjust every aspect of therapeutic intervention to meet the specific needs of each client.

REFERENCES

1. Adams RD and Victor M: *Principles of neurology,* ed 5, New York, 1993, McGraw-Hill.
2. Adams RD and Victor M: *Principles of neurology—companion handbook,* ed 5, New York, 1994, McGraw Hill.
3. Ayres JA: *Sensory integration and learning disorder,* Los Angeles, 1972, Western Psychological Services.
4. Ayres JA: *Southern California postrotatory nystagmus test,* Los Angeles, 1975, Western Psychological Services.
5. Baringer JR: Viral infections. In Asbury AK, McKhann GM, McDonald WI, editors: *Diseases of the nervous system: clinical neurobiology,* vol II, Philadelphia, 1992, WB Saunders.
6. Berger J and Levy RM: Infections of the nervous system. In Grotta JC, editor: *Management of the acutely ill neurological patient,* New York, 1993, Churchill Livingstone.
7. Bharucha NE, Bhabha SK, and Bharucha EP: Bacterial infections. In Bradley WG and others, editors: *Neurology in clinical practice,* Boston, 1991, Butterworth-Heinemann.
8. Bharucha NE, Bhabha SK, and Bharucha EP: Viral infections. In Bradley WG and others, editors: *Neurology in clinical practice,* Boston, 1991, Butterworth-Heinemann.
9. Bobath B: *Adult hemiplegia: evaluation and treatment,* ed 3, London, 1990, William Heinemann Medical Books.
10. Carr JH and Shepherd RB: *Movement science—foundations for physical therapy in rehabilitation,* Rockville, Md, 1987, Aspen Publishers.
11. DeMeyer W: *Technique of the neurological examination,* ed 4, New York, 1994, McGraw-Hill.
12. Duncan PW and Badke MB: *Stroke rehabilitation—the recovery of motor control,* St Louis, 1987, Mosby.
13. Griffin DE and Johnson RT: Host responses to infection of the nervous system. In Asbury AK, McKhann GM, McDonald WI, editors: *Diseases of the nervous system: clinical neurobiology,* vol II, Philadelphia, 1992, WB Saunders.
14. Hoppenfeld S: *Physical examination of the spine and extremities,* New York, 1976, Appleton-Century-Crofts.
15. Jennett B and Teasdale G: *Management of head injuries,* Philadelphia, 1981, FA Davis.
16. Johnson RT: Neurovirology. In *Encyclopedia of neuroscience,* vol II, Boston, 1987, Birkhäuser.
17. Kirkpatrick JB: Neurological infections due to bacteria, fungi, and parasites. In Davis RL and Robertson DM: *Textbook of neuropathology,* ed 2, Baltimore, 1991, Williams & Wilkins.
18. Levitt S: *Treatment of cerebral palsy and motor delay,* ed 2, London, 1982, Blackwell Scientific.
19. Pendlebury WW: Central nervous system diseases caused by unconventional transmissible agents and chronic viral infections. In Bradley WG and others, editors: *Neurology in clinical practice,* Boston, 1989, Butterworth-Heinemann.
20. Plum F and Posner JB: *The diagnosis of stupor and coma,* ed 3, Philadelphia, 1980, FA Davis.
21. Schooley RT: Encephalitis. In Roper AH, editor: *Neurological and neurosurgical intensive care,* ed 3, New York, 1993, Raven Press.
22. Sullivan PE and Markos PD: *Clinical decision making in therapeutic exercise,* Norwalk, Conn, 1995, Appleton and Lange.
23. Tunkel AR and Scheld WM: Bacterial infections in adults. In Asbury AK, McKhann GM, McDonald WI, editors: *Diseases of the nervous system: clinical neurobiology,* vol II, Philadelphia, 1992, WB Saunders.
24. VanSant AF: Analysis of movement dysfunction: usefulness of a component approach. In *Proceedings of the 13th Annual Eugene Michels Researchers' Forum,* Alexandria Va, 1993, Section on Research American Physical Therapy Association.
25. VanSant AF: Rising from a supine position to erect stance—description of adult movement and a developmental hypothesis, *Phys Ther* 68(2):185-192, 1988.
26. Voss DE, Ionta MK, and Myers BJ: *Proprioceptive neuromuscular facilitation,* ed 3, Philadelphia, 1985, Harper & Row.
27. Weinstein L: Meningitis, pyogenic. In *Encyclopedia of neuroscience,* vol II, Boston, 1987, Birkhäuser.

CHAPTER 18

The Role of Rehabilitation after Human Immunodeficiency Virus (HIV) Infection

Laura LeCocq, Johnny Bonck, and Anne MacRae

OUTLINE

KEY TERMS

AIDS

HIV

LEARNING OBJECTIVES

After reading this chapter the student/therapist will:

1. Have a greater understanding of human immune function, particularly acquired immunity.
2. Be familiar with neuropathology associated with HIV infection.
3. Be knowledgeable about systemic and opportunistic infections that accompany HIV infection.
4. Have an increased awareness of the psychopathology of HIV.
5. Be aware of side effects related to medical treatment for primary HIV infection and secondary opportunistic infections.
6. Consider comprehensive neuromuscular and psychological evaluation and treatment needs of HIV infected individuals.
7. Practice universal precautions with all patients.

IDENTIFICATION OF THE CLINICAL PROBLEM

First reported in 1981, acquired immunodeficiency syndrome (**AIDS**) was deemed an epidemic in 1985. The vast array of physical and psychological dysfunction associated with AIDS, as well as the social and political implications of the disease, will continue to have a profound impact on all rehabilitation professionals.

The nomenclature and the acronyms developed for the study of AIDS can be confusing. Furthermore, the clinical and pathological information about this disease is constantly increasing. Certainly our understanding of the disease process will change between the writing and publication of this book. Changes in terminology reflect this evolution of clinical knowledge. The definitions used throughout this chapter reflect current use.

The virus thought to be responsible for the transmission of AIDS was identified as **HIV** (human immunodeficiency virus) in July 1986 at the International Conference on AIDS in Paris. A second virus, HIV-2, was identified in western Africa. This second subtype, less widely distributed, has since been established in Europe and in South, Central, and North America. Both HIV-1 and HIV-2 have resulted in AIDS, but evidence suggests that HIV-2 may be less virulent than HIV-1. In addition to these subtypes, several strains of HIV-1 have been identified. Different strains reflect variations in cellular affinities and resistance to medications.

During the early attempts to understand the natural history of HIV infection, the term AIDS-related complex (ARC) was used to describe a host of immunodeficiency-related illnesses that did not fit the formal diagnostic criteria for AIDS. It was speculated that milder forms of the illness might be present that were chronic but nonprogressive. The evidence has not supported this theory, however, and the term ARC is now seldom used.

In 1993 the Centers for Disease Control (CDC) revised its definition of AIDS and classification system of HIV infection. To reflect current scientific knowledge, the new system elucidates the importance of helper-T (CD4+) cell counts as indicators for pharmacological disease management. The changed definition of AIDS now includes those with HIV infection and CD4+ counts below 200/mm^3, regardless of the status of concomitant disorders. In addition, three clinical conditions—pulmonary tuberculosis, recurrent pneumonia, and invasive cervical cancer—were added to the existing list of 20 AIDS-defining diseases.[7] It is hoped that these changes will allow greater accuracy in accounting for HIV-related immunosuppression. The entire spectrum of illness from seroconversion to full-blown AIDS can be covered by the term *HIV infection.*

Epidemiology

Discussion of the epidemiology of HIV infection is multifaceted. Both reported and estimated figures must be examined. There is a wide discrepancy between reported (611,589) and estimated (2.5 million) global AIDS cases. Africa has 34.5% of reported AIDS cases, but 71% of estimated global incidence. The United States reported 39.5% of diagnosed cases, but is estimated to support 13% of the global cases.[62] Such differences are attributed to data gathering practices. Given the extended time between initial HIV infection and the development of AIDS, estimated figures provide the most accurate account of the pandemic.

A further distinction must be made between infection with HIV and the development of AIDS. Statistically, HIV infection is not equivalent to having AIDS. According to the

World Health Organization (WHO),[63] approximately 13 million individuals have been infected since the beginning of the HIV pandemic. In the United States, 1 million estimated HIV infections translate into 1 infection per 250 people.[8] As of December 1992, the African countries of Burundi, Congo, Malawi, Uganda, and Zimbabwe and the Caribbean regions of the Bahamas and Bermuda reported the highest rates of AIDS. Currently, the majority of new infections are appearing in sub-Saharan Africa and Southeast Asia.[63]

Women are the fastest growing HIV infected population. With more than 3 million women infected worldwide, AIDS has become the leading cause of death for women aged 20 to 40 in metropolises of sub-Saharan Africa, Western Europe and the Americas.[22,58] In the United States, women currently represent 15% of all AIDS cases.[7] African-American and Latin-American women who comprised 14% of the total population are disproportionately affected with 72% of the female AIDS cases.

Globally, heterosexual transmission is responsible for 71% of HIV infections. Among women in the United States, however, intravenous drug use is largely responsible—50% by direct intravenous drug use and 21% by sexual contact with an intravenous drug user.[59]

Most asymptomatic pregnant women are diagnosed seropositive after the birth of an ill child.[12] The rate of infection for the children of HIV infected women in the United States is approximately 33%—between 1,500 and 2,000 infants annually.[56]

Nearly 5,000 cases of AIDS among children in the United States have been reported by the CDC.[7] About 90% of these result from maternal-infant transmission. Disease progression is much swifter in children. The majority of perinatally infected infants exhibit symptoms of advanced infection by age 18 months.[12] This quicker progression is the result of immunological immaturity.[1,12]

Global projections for the year 2000 estimate the number of individuals infected with HIV at 30 to 40 million. The majority of these will be in developing countries. Tragically, at least 10 million AIDS orphans under the age of 10 will most acutely feel these losses.[62]

Normal immunity

The immune system is complex and dynamic, comprising a multitude of components and subsystems, all of which interact continuously. The normal immune system has two main components or lines of defense against illness (Fig. 18-1). The first is the innate, or inborn, component that includes the skin, the cilia and mucosal linings of the respiratory and digestive systems, the gastric fluids and enzymes of the stomach, and the phagocytic phase-cells. This innate component of the immune system keeps pathogens out of the body by creating barriers against them, by ejecting them, or by enveloping them and eliminating them. The second, acquired component of the immune system, develops defenses against specific pathogens, starts

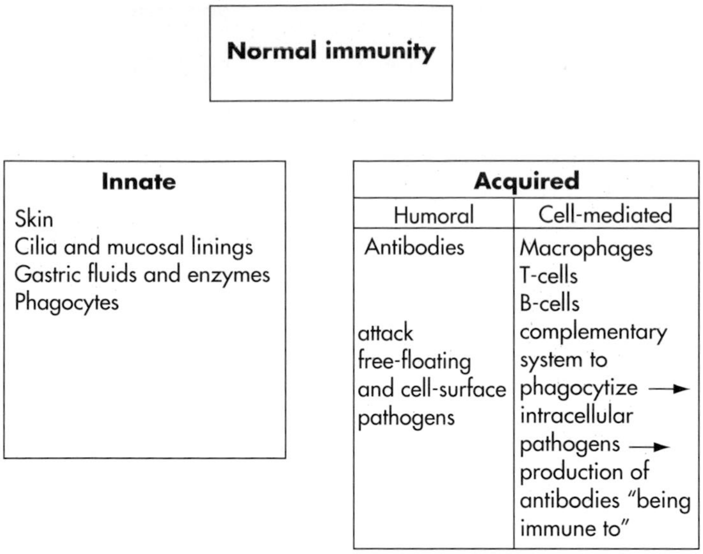

Fig. 18-1. Main components of immunity.

in utero, and continues throughout life. It is the second, acquired (or antibody) immunity that is most pertinent to understanding HIV and its progression.

Acquired immunity

Acquired immunity is divided into humoral and cell-mediated responses. Humoral immunity depends on the production of antibodies. This response is effective for dispatching free-floating or cell-surface pathogens. The cell-mediated response is required to destroy infected cells, those with intracellular pathogens. Cell-mediated immunity is essential for destroying pathogens responsible for the opportunistic infections and neoplasms that are associated with AIDS.[10,11]

For the study of HIV pathology, it is important to consider three types of immune system cells: macrophages, T lymphocytes (T cells), and B lymphocytes (B cells). Macrophages originate in the bone marrow, then migrate to the organs in the lymphatic system. Macrophages recognize, then phagocytize, antigens—substances deemed foreign to the body. All but a fragment of the antigen is digested by the macrophage. This remaining portion protrudes from the cellular surface, where it is recognized by T and B cells.[40]

Both of the lymphocytes originate in the bone marrow. Their differentiation into T and B cells depends on where they develop immunocompetence. T cells migrate to the thymus to perform this task. B cells complete it before leaving the bone marrow. T cells then travel to lymph nodes, the spleen, and connective tissue, where they wait to phagocytize the antigens in the manner previously described. B cells function in the same way against free-floating blood-borne pathogens.[40]

There are at least eight types of T cells with varying functions. Two relevant types are helper T cells (CD4+) and suppressor T cells (CD8). These cells are regulatory and

complementary. Upon recognition of an antigen, CD4+ cells chemically stimulate production and activation of other lymphocytes to destroy the foreign material. When the action of the T and B cells is sufficient, CD8 cells stop this action, thus preventing destruction of noninfected cells.

In the process of identifying and destroying these antigens, the acquired immune system also retains a memory of the antigen, which allows it to respond more rapidly and effectively to the pathogen if it is reintroduced into the body. Herein lies the pertinence of vaccination and the phenomenon of "being immune to" an illness.[40]

PATHOGENESIS OF AIDS

HIV belongs to a class of viruses known as retroviruses, which carry their genetic material in the form of RNA rather than DNA. HIV primarily infects the mononuclear cells, especially CD4+ and macrophages, but B cells also are infected.[35] HIV binds to the receptor sites on the surface of the lymphocytes, eventually fusing, then entering the cells. Reverse transcriptase released from the HIV allows a DNA copy of the virus to be made within the host cell, which can then become integrated into the host cell genome. The lymphocyte becomes a "virus factory" as replicated virions bud out of the cell to infect others.

Within days of HIV infection, lymph nodes become sites of rampant viral replication, during which the individual remains asymptomatic. This time of seroconversion usually occurs within 3 months, but can take 12 months. On retrospect, many people describe nonspecific and self-limited flulike symptoms: fever, diarrhea, myalgias, and fatigue. An asymptomatic period follows in which the individual tests seropositive. The interim stages of HIV infection are marked by generalized swelling of the lymph nodes followed by an extended period when the infected person will not necessarily develop further symptoms, but laboratory tests will reveal immune dysfunction, particularly a decline in CD4+ cells. This clinical latency spans up to 7 years in children and 14 years in adults.[33,38,52] The relatively recent development of this pandemic affords little information on longer survival.

Neuropathology

HIV affects every division of the human nervous system (see the box). Early in the investigation of HIV, devastating effects on the central nervous system (CNS) became evident. The mechanism by which HIV infects the CNS is unclear. Isolated HIV seems unable to cross the blood-brain barrier, but infected macrophages and T cells do. It may also be that infected capillary endothelial cells of the brain infect glial cells lining the blood-brain barrier. This process causes a breakdown of the barrier, allowing even greater passage of infected macrophages and T cells.[35]

Once inside the CNS, HIV can be isolated from glial cells and neurons. It is possible that infected CNS cells produce toxic biochemicals that result in neuropathology. The virus

Neuropathology of HIV

Central Nervous System

Mechanism of CNS infection unclear, but HIV seems unable to cross blood-brain barrier alone. Probably crosses in macrophages and T cells. Most directly affects subcortical structures (basal ganglia, thalamus, brainstem).

AIDS dementia complex (ADC), a subcortical dementia, is different from cortical dementia such as Alzheimer's disease.

Estimated 70% of infected → cognitive, motor, and behavioral constellation that is ADC.

Peripheral Nervous System

Sensory—In early and middle stages, largely involves distal lower extremities; paresthesia, and decreased temperature sensitivity. In advanced stages, decreased ankle and knee reflexes, temperature and vibration sensitivity and proprioception, hyperesthesia.

Motor Most closely resembles Guillain-Barré syndrome (progressive muscle weakness → paralysis, decreased deep tendon reflexes) → splints, ankle-foot orthosis may prevent deformities.

Autonomic Nervous System

Arrhythymias—especially tachycardia.

Abnormal blood pressure—orthostasis and with isometric exercises.

Autonomic nervous system involvement has been associated with dementia, myelopathy and peripheral sensory neuropathies.

Table 18-1. Neurological disorders associated wth AIDS

Agent classification	Organism/disease
Primary viral	HIV/ADC, encephalopathy, atypical aseptic meningitis, vacuolar myelopathy, peripheral neuropathy
Secondary viral	Cytomegalovirus/meningoencephalitis, retinitis, peripheral neuropathies
Secondary viral	Herpes simplex I and II; herpes varicella zoster/encephalitis, retinitis, peripheral neuropathies
Secondary viral	Papovavirus/progressive multifocal leukoencephalopathy
Protozoan	*Toxoplasma gondii*/toxoplasmosis
Fungal	*Cryptococcus neoformans*/cryptococcal meningitis
Fungal	*Candida albicans*/intracerebral candidiasis
Fungal	*Aspergillus fumigatus*/meningitis, encephalitis and/or abscess
Fungal	*Coccidioides immitis*/meningitis
Bacterial	*Mycobacterium avium-intracellulare*/encephalitis, meningitis, cranial and/or peripheral neuropathies
Bacterial	*Mycobacterium tuberculosis hominis*/meningitis and/or mass lesion
Neoplastic	Primary CNS lymphomas Metastatic systemic lymphoma
Iatrogenic	Extrapyramidal motor symptoms Acute myelopathies Neuropathies

primarily alters the subcortical structures, specifically the basal ganglia, thalamus, and brainstem.[36] Biological variation between HIV isolates in blood and in neural tissue implies the existence of a neurotropic strain. It may be that ". . . a viral strain in the same host can evolve differently in the brain and the blood, and can be distinguished by molecular as well as biological features" (p.227).[35]

Peripheral neuropathy that accompanies HIV infection is both sensory and motor in nature. Mild sensory involvement manifests in early and middle stages of disease. They most frequently involve the feet, causing paresthesia and decreased temperature sensitivity. In advanced stages of disease, the involvement is bilateral. Diminished ankle and knee reflexes, sensation (temperature and vibration), and proprioception complicate hyperesthesia. In some cases, ambulation is precluded by pain from hypersensitivity to touch. Motoric peripheral neuropathy mimics clinical presentation of Guillain-Barré syndrome. Microscopic analysis of cerebrospinal fluid (CSF) is necessary to distinguish the disorders.[4]

Autonomic nervous system (ANS) dysfunction has been associated with HIV infection. In one study, individuals with the greatest ANS involvement also had dementia, myelopathy, and sensory peripheral neuropathy. Variations in heart rate, including resting tachycardia, were common. Abnormal blood pressure readings were identified in response to isometric exercise and positional changes (sit to stand and tilting).[19]

It is not possible in this context to discuss the neuropathology of each of the many secondary infections and neoplasms of HIV illness. It is important to realize, however, that the clinical manifestations of these pathological processes overlap with one another, as well as with the signs and symptoms of primary HIV infection of the CNS; lesions of the CNS can be the site of more than one opportunistic disease process simultaneously. Table 18-1 lists a wide variety of organisms and/or conditions responsible for the neurological manifestations associated with HIV infection. These include primary and secondary viral, protozoan, fungal, and mycobacterium infections, as well as neoplasms and iatrogenic conditions. In addition, neurological disorders can result from the breakdown of tissue seen with neoplasia and resulting cerebrovascular infarction, hemorrhage, or vasculitis.

Systemic manifestations

Although the clinical course of HIV infection can vary greatly among individuals, researchers and practitioners

560

have begun to track the overall course of the disease. A progressive and highly variable pattern of clinical manifestations of the pathological process has emerged.[25,37,41]

When the immune system can no longer protect the body from recrudescent (already existing in the body) or ubiquitous (commonly found in the environment) pathogens, a variety of systemic diseases develop. The following is a brief explanation of the most common complications of HIV infection.

Pneumocystis carinii pneumonia (PCP) is the most common opportunistic infection among HIV infected individuals. Recent evidence indicates that the PCP-causing organism is usually acquired in childhood and that between 65% and 85% of healthy adults possess PCP antibodies. Reactivation of latent infection is responsible for the recurrent fever, dyspnea, and hypoxia that characterize PCP.[3,28]

Candida albicans is also found in healthy individuals. Unchecked proliferation of these organisms secondary to immunocompromise results in yeast infections of mucosal tissue—oral, esophageal, and vaginal.

Cryptococcus neoformans is also a yeast. This organism, however, manifests primarily in the CNS in the form of meningitis or abscesses. Signs and symptoms of cryptococcosis include headache, altered mental states, nausea, vertigo, somnolence, seizures, and coma. Cryptosporidiosis infects the gastrointestinal (GI) tract and causes chronic diarrhea and malabsorption. Both of these factors contribute to the wasting syndrome that characterizes HIV infection.[32,48]

Involuntary loss of more than 10% of baseline body weight and chronic diarrhea or unexplained weakness and fever constitute HIV wasting syndrome.[6] Retrospective demographic research in the United States found that 17.8% of individuals with AIDS experienced wasting syndrome.[45] The ensuing malnutrition contributes to further immunosuppression.[24]

Roughly 30% to 40% of healthy adults have contracted *Toxoplasma gondii,* the organism responsible for toxoplasmosis.[43,61] Unchecked by the immune system, toxoplasmosis results in CNS dysfunction, namely, altered cognition, headache, focal neurological deficits, encephalitis, and seizures.

The cytomegalovirus (CMV) can effect the GI and respiratory tracts, but primarily targets optic structures. CMV infection also appears to be latent. Between 40% and 100% of healthy adults possess CMV antibodies.[34] Predominant consequences of HIV/CMV coinfection are unilateral or bilateral deficits in visual acuity, visual field cuts, and blindness.

Mycobacterial infections in HIV-infected individuals usually present as either *Mycobacterium avium-intracellulare* complex (MAC) or *Mycobacterium tuberculosis* (TB). Currently, WHO estimates HIV/TB coinfection at 4.4 million worldwide.[62] HIV is the primary cause for the resurgence of

TB in the United States. Steadily increasing incidence of infection by *Mycobacterium tuberculosis* is likely the result of two factors: better medical management of HIV as a whole and the development of multidrug resistant strains of TB.

MAC tends to present late in the course of HIV infection. Estimates of incidence in persons with AIDS (PWAs) range from 18% to 56%. Autopsy findings indicate that the prevalence of MAC is underestimated.[44] Initial infection involves the GI and pulmonary tracts and eventually disseminates throughout the body. This disorder probably is not due to latent reactivation of the organism, but rather from primary infection by ingestion or inhalation.[27] Signs and symptoms of MAC infection include pneumonia, fever, weight loss, malaise, sweats, anorexia, abdominal pain, and diarrhea.

By contrast, TB is usually identified early in the course of HIV infection. Latent *Mycobacterium tuberculosis* reactivation appears to be responsible for 90% of the resultant disease among immunocompromised people.[27] Large outbreaks in hospitals and residential care centers for PWAs, however, have been reported, indicating susceptibility to primary infection.[13,15]

As in many other infections, initial signs and symptoms of TB include fever, weight loss, malaise, cough, lymph node tenderness, and night sweats. Pulmonary involvement constitutes between 75% and 100% of TB infection in HIV patients, but extrapulmonary infection, especially lymph nodes and bone marrow, occur in up to 60% of these individuals as well.[2,27,28,50] Other less common areas of infection include the CNS, cardiac, and mucosal tissues.

Mycobacterium tuberculosis is communicable, preventable, and treatable. Tuberculin skin testing should be available and routinely offered to individuals at HIV testing sites. Highest risk individuals for concomitant HIV and TB infections include the homeless, intravenous drug users, and prisoners.[2,50] The risk of infection to health care personnel as well as to the general public is a concern. Isolation rooms that provide negative pressure, nonrecirculated ventilation, and specific air filters and air exchange rates offer the best protection to health care providers exposed to TB-infected individuals. Properly fitted face masks that filter droplet nuclei should be worn. Monitoring of personnel who work with these populations will identify the need for necessary preventive therapy.[2]

AIDS-Kaposi's sarcoma (AIDS-KS) is the most frequently identified neoplasm among HIV infected people. This vascular neoplasm afflicts about 20% of seropositive gay men. Interestingly, AIDS-KS is less common among intravenous drug users and rare in women and children. T-cell count is not a valuable prognosticator for development of KS.[28] The disorder presents as cutaneous purple nodular lesions, or as rife visceral lesions. AIDS-KS has been intimately associated with the lymphatic system, specifically deficient lymphatic transport, nodal dysfunction, and tumors, which contribute to lymphedema that clinicians observe as swollen extremities.[60]

HIV appears to have a quicker, more severe course in women. Median survival times for women, once diagnosed with AIDS, is 7 months and for men, 24 months. What remains unclear is whether this difference is biological or a result of socioeconomic circumstances that delay diagnosis or limit access to health care.

Both sexes are susceptible to the same opportunistic infections and malignancies, but their patterns differ. Women are more likely to contract PCP, toxoplasmosis, and *Candida* infections, but less likely than men to develop AIDS-KS. Infected women have higher incidence with persistent recurrence of cervical dysplasias, human papillomavirus, herpes simplex virus, and pelvic inflammatory disease than noninfected women.

Infected children often present with chronic diarrhea and a failure to thrive—likely complications of oral and GI infections. Adenopathy is common and salivary gland enlargement occurs more frequently than in adults. Otitis media and measles, despite immunization, are also more frequent complications of children.[12,59]

Children are susceptible to disorders seen in adults—herpes virus, pneumonia, toxoplasmosis, meningitis, and encephalitis. Additional neurological manifestations in children include cerebral atrophy, ataxia, rigidity, hyperreflexia, and the inability to achieve or sustain developmental milestones.[12]

AIDS-Related psychopathology

Psychiatric manifestations of HIV infection seem to have gone underreported or underdiagnosed. Careful consideration of psychological function is warranted during clinical encounters with HIV-infected persons. AIDS-related psychopathologies mimic many previously described consequences of primary HIV infection, opportunistic infections, and medicinal side effects. These psychiatric complications can be affective or organic in nature. Indicators include disturbances in sleep and appetite patterns, diminished memory and energy, psychomotor retardation, withdrawal, apathy, and emotional lability. Anxiety disorders (particularly posttraumatic stress disorder), adjustment reactions, reactive and endogenous depressions, and obsessive disorders frequently result.[18,26,47]

Using the American Psychiatric Association's standard for diagnosis of mental disorders (DSM-III-R), one study found Axis I disorders (excluding substance abuse) in 61.9% of the subjects.[54] Reported incidence of mood disorders among PWAs approaches 83%.[49] Indeed the virus' affinity with subcortical structures of the CNS that regulate affect and mood support research indicating a prevalence of manic episodes that is 10 times higher than that of the general population.[39] Manic syndrome has been identified at all stages of the disease process: initial HIV seropositivity, AIDS, and in response to azidothymidine (AZT) therapy.[14,20,53] When associated with HIV, mania appears to be secondary to structural CNS changes.[16,29] Described manic episodes generally respond well to psychiatric medications and may not recur.[5,20,42,46] The onset of manic syndrome is an ominous marker in the course of HIV. Nearly one fourth of the patients reviewed in one study died within 6 months.[16]

Analyses of new onset psychosis among HIV-infected individuals yielded the following information. Psychotic episodes are preceded by a period (days to months) of affective and behavioral changes.[21] Admitting diagnoses to psychiatric units included "undifferentiated schizophrenia, schizophreniform disorder, reactive psychosis, atypical psychosis, depression with psychotic features and mania." Some psychiatric diagnoses were revised during the course of hospitalization to "AIDS encephalitis, cryptococcal meningitis, or 'organic psychosis.'"[23] Eighty-seven percent of the subjects in one study displayed delusions, usually persecutory, grandiose, or somatic in nature. Affective disturbances were present in 81% of the subjects. Hallucinations and thought process disorders were each prominent in 61%. Several subjects received the diagnosis of AIDS during their psychiatric hospitalization.[23]

More than 70% of all PWAs experience the progressive subcortical dementia that constitutes AIDS dementia complex (ADC).[37] Since the identification of AIDS, the constellation of cognitive, motor, and behavioral symptoms of ADC also has been referred to as HIV encephalopathy or encephalitis, HIV dementia, and most recently HIV associated cognitive/motor deficit, AIDS-related dementia, and HIV-related organic brain syndrome.[16,47,51] ADC is characterized by a subtle onset of forgetfulness, distractibility, slowing of mentation, apathy, and isolation. The subcortical changes inherent in ADC allow the individual to be aware of these progressive deficits, creating the potential for affective complications.

Motoric manifestations of ADC include gait disturbances, intention tremor, and abnormal release of reflexes. Frequent concomitant vacuolar myelopathy and peripheral neuropathies complicate the course of ADC. Vacuolar myelopathy, the result of swollen myelin sheaths, manifests as hypertonicity of both lower extremities, including plantar flexion. Accompanied by ataxia, the result is a rigid, wide gait and difficulty walking heel-to-toe.[4]

Differentiation between psychiatric and physiological manifestations is complicated. Psychiatric and organic disorders are initially indistinguishable on the basis of behavior, and they may exist concurrently. Furthermore, other primary disease processes and medicinal reactions imitate psychopathologies. Differentiation is nonetheless essential, for many disorders respond well to established therapies, both psychological and pharmacological, once differential diagnoses are established. Awareness of the intricate interplay of all factors is essential for competent rehabilitative efforts for those infected with HIV.

MEDICAL MANAGEMENT
Cell counts and prophylaxis

Pharmacological interventions to combat the opportunistic infections of HIV are beyond the scope of this chapter, but a simplified summary of clinical information is pertinent. Medical management of HIV infection is most often guided by the CD4+ cell count. Controversy is emerging regarding the use of CD8 cell counts as more valuable indicators of prophylactic agent administration.[10] Currently, CD4+ cell directives are as follows: CD4+ counts above 500/mm^3 usually indicate no need for antiretroviral therapy, as individuals are generally asymptomatic. CD4+ counts between 200/mm^3 and 500/mm^3 indicate the need for antiretroviral therapy. Those with CD4+ cell counts below 200/mm^3 direct preventive PCP and toxoplasmosis measures. Those with counts below 100/mm^3 may also receive prophylactic agents against the above as well as CMV, MAC, and fungal infections such as cryptococcus and candidiasis.[11] Table 18-2 provides a summary of common pharmacological agents prescribed to combat opportunistic infections and, most pertinent to rehabilitation, their potential side effects.

Now that a viral etiology has been established with some certainty, researchers are concentrating on developing effective antiretrovirals and safe vaccines. Currently, three antiretroviral drugs have been approved by the Food and Drug Administration (FDA) to combat HIV infection. They are zidovudine (AZT), didanosine (ddl), and dideoxcytidine (ddC) (see the box).

AZT

AZT is the most well-studied and often-used antiretroviral to combat HIV. It has shown efficacy at inhibiting both HIV-1 and HIV-2.[37] AZT is often begun when CD4+ cell counts are between 200/mm^3 and 500/mm^3. Its use appears to delay the progression of symptomatic illness. When CD4+ counts are below 200/mm^3, AZT is dispensed to decrease incidence and severity of opportunistic infections. Patients have reported increased energy, appetite, and weight gain. Improved cognition with AZT use has been noted in those with AIDS dementia complex.[28]

Resistance to AZT develops in some patients. This phenomenon appears to be a function of time, stage of disease at initiation of therapy, and viral strain. Toxic but reversible side effects of the drug include bone marrow suppression, anemia, leukopenia, nausea, abdominal pain, and headache. Use of AZT for more than 1 year has contributed to myowasting, weakness, fever, seizures, confusion, and esophageal ulcerations in some patients.

ddl

ddl is recommended for those who are intolerant of or failing AZT treatment. A small number of ddl users have reported clinical improvements—primarily weight gain and

---

Antiretroviral medications

Zidovudine (AZT)

Often begun when CD4+ counts between 200/mm^3 and 500 mm^3. Delays progression, below 200 mm^3, used to decrease frequency of opportunistic infections (OIs). Resistance develops. Toxic -- bone marrow suppression, anemia, leukopenia, nausea, abdominal pain, headache. Use > 1 year → muscle wasting, fever, seizures, confusion, esophageal ulcers.

Didanosine (ddl)

Indicated when AZT intolerant, less effective and less toxic. Reversible toxicity (diarrhea, pancreatitis, hepatitis, seizures, cardiomyopathy, peripheral neuropathies).

Dideoxycytodine (ddC)

Least used; severe peripheral neuropathies, rashes, fever, malaise, oral ulcers. Most effective pharmacotherapy is combination of these drugs and ddl is only one of these with FDA approval for combination with AZT.

---

improved cognition. ddl is less toxic than AZT to bone marrow. Signs and symptoms of ddl's reversible toxicity include diarrhea, pancreatitis, hepatitis, seizures, cardiomyopathy, and peripheral neuropathy.[28,57]

ddC

High doses of ddC have demonstrated some clinical improvement—weight gain and CD4+ counts—but with severe peripheral neuropathy. Other toxic effects are rashes, malaise, fever, and oral ulcers. Preliminary investigations reveal that a combination of drugs may be more effective than monotherapy. ddC is, to date, the only FDA-approved agent for use in combination with AZT.[28,57]

Vaccines

Vaccination is likely the best hope of controlling disease progression. The first human immunizations with potential AIDS vaccine took place in 1986 in healthy seropositive volunteers in France and Zaire. Low levels of both humoral and cell-mediated immune responses resulted. One conclusion of this study is that booster vaccinations could be effective.[30]

Genetic mutation of the virus further complicates attempts to disable it. It is thought that genetically similar but distinguishable strains of HIV can exist in one individual. Further, AZT-resistant strains of HIV have been identified.[55]

Another difficulty with vaccination development is a lack of animal models. Chimpanzees replicate simian immune deficiency virus (SIV), a similar but not identical disease. Furthermore, an average of 12 years and $231 million is required for a new drug to gain FDA approval. Many major pharmaceutical companies seem wary of the immense research expenses and potential liability risks linked to

Table 18-2. Common disorders related to HIV: medications and side effects

Disorder	Medication	Side effects
PCP	Trimethoprim-Sulfamethaxazole	blood cell destruction (WBCs and platelets), nausea, vomiting, orthostasis, allergic skin reaction: rash, fever, hives
	Pentamadine (inhaled)	bronchospasm, cough, conjunctivitis
	Pentamadine (IV)	hypoglycemia, hyperglycemia, hypotension, nausea, vomiting, arrhythmias, vertigo, fever, pancreatitis, acute renal failure
Toxoplasmosis	Pyrimethamine and Sulfadiazine	bone marrow suppression (RBCs, WBCs, platelets), anorexia, abdominal cramps, vomiting, photosensitivity, urticaria
	Pyrimethamine and Clindamycin	nausea, vomiting, abdominal pain, diarrhea, rash
	Pyrimethamine and Clarithromycin	hearing loss
		elevated liver enzymes
Meningitis	Amphotericin	renal toxicity, anemia, thrombophlebitis, flulike symptoms (fever, chills, nausea and vomiting [n&v], headache [h/a], myalgia)
	Flucytosine	renal toxicity, n&v, abdominal pain, bone marrow suppression
CMV	Ganciclovir	blood cell destruction, mental status changes
	Foscarnet	nephrotoxicity with incontinence, electrolyte abnormalities
	Acyclovir	rash, blood cell destruction, renal deficiencies, lethargy, tremors, confusion
Candidiasis	Nystatin	altered taste
	Ketoconazole	n&v, abdominal pain, vertigo, somnolence
	Amphotericin	renal toxicity, thrombophlebitis, anemia, flulike symptoms
Mycobacterium TB	Isoniazid	hepatic toxicity, peripheral neuropathy, vertigo, lupus, muscle twitch, convulsion
	Pyrazinamide	hepatic damage, joint pain, increased uric acid
	Streptomycin	ototoxicity, nephrotoxicity
	Rifampin	flulike symptoms, GI intolerance, hepatitis
	Ethambutol	blurred vision, red/green color blindness
MAI	Rifampin	see above
	Ethambutol	see above
	Clofazimine	GI intolerance, increased skin pigmentation (red-brown to black)
	Amikacin	ototoxicity, nephrotoxicity
	Ethionamide	GI intolerance, peripheral neuropathy, orthostasis, psychiatric symptoms, liver toxicity, poor diabetic control
	Cycloserine	convulsions, psychosis, h/a, somnolence
MAC	Rifabutin	altered taste
Herpes (simplex and zoster)	Acyclovir	rash, blood cell destruction, renal deficiencies, lethargy, tremors, confusion
AIDS-KS	Radiation/Chemotherapy	n&v, weight loss, hair loss, lethargy
Cryptococcal Meningitis	Amphotericin B/flucytosine	blood cell destruction, liver malfunction, anemia, chills, rigors (sudden chill->high temp->hot, diaphoresis)

vaccine development. The result is that smaller biotechnology companies with fewer resources are assailing the complicated problems of HIV infection.[81] It is estimated that a vaccine will not be readily available for another 5 to 10 years. This vaccine will ideally induce both humoral and cellular immune responses and have no toxic effects. It will protect against initial infection and retard disease onset in infected individuals.

REHABILITATIVE RAMIFICATIONS

The evaluation procedures for HIV illness are broadly outlined below. Of course, each case varies and the evaluation process is individualized according to the specific needs of the client (see the box on p. 564)

What is the relationship of the person with HIV infection to the environment, both at present and in the future? The rehabilitation therapist should keep this question in mind throughout the evaluation process. In this context, the term *environment* is meant to include not only the physical aspects of surroundings, but also the psychological and emotional climate in which the individual functions.

The evaluation process has a different focus for different stages of the disease. If the client is in the early stages of the disease, the therapist should determine whether he or she is still managing in accustomed life roles. Important issues might include new or adapted vocational and leisure skills. During later stages, the focus may change to more basic daily functional concerns. The therapist must remember, however, that the client may place more importance on participation in avocational interest than on independent self-care. This choice is not only valid, but must be respected and supported by health care professionals. Another crucial determination to be made during the evaluative process is whether the person is to be discharged to home or some other supervised setting. In either case, what kind of community-based support networks are available to the individual?

Astute evaluative questions about the psychosocial status of the client include the following:

1. Does the client's perception of his or her status and prognosis agree with that of the treatment team?
2. What is the client's predominant coping style?
3. Who are the client's caregivers? Social support system?

The support system can be a critical issue for many people with HIV infection who are part of the high-risk groups of homosexual and bisexual men and intravenous drug users. Many of these people have traditional networks of family, spouse, and friends; a significant number have equally strong nontraditional support systems. Some will be lacking in the kinds of support needed to cope with the devastating effects of the disease.

It is possible to use models developed for oncology and progressive neurological disorders, such as amyotrophic lateral sclerosis, for HIV neurological rehabilitation. How-

---

Evaluation procedures for HIV illness

A. Baseline data (premorbid functional level)
   1. Accustomed life roles
B. Stage in disease process
C. Psychosocial issues
   1. Coping mechanisms
   2. Social support system
D. Cognitive/perceptual status
   1. Reality orientation
   2. Memory
   3. Organizational skills
   4. Visual perception
   5. Motor planning
   6. Safety awareness
   7. Judgment
E. Communication
   1. Oral language
   2. Written language
F. Sensory/motor status
   1. Balance
   2. Gait
   3. Coordination
   4. Sensation/pain
   5. Muscle tone
   6. Strength
G. Activities of daily living (ADLs)
   1. Grooming/hygiene
   2. Feeding
   3. Bathing
   4. Dressing
   5. Housework
   6. Community management
   7. Other self-care regimens (i.e., medications)
   8. Avocational interests
   9. Activity tolerance

Neuromuscular rehabilitation treatment procedures for HIV infection

A. Psychosocial intervention
   1. Facilitation of the expression of grief
   2. Validation and education of caregivers
B. Cognitive/perceptual intervention
   1. Rehabilitation
   2. Maintenance
   3. Compensation (including communication)
C. Sensory/motor intervention
   1. Sensory stimulation
   2. Maintenance of strength, range of motion, and endurance
   3. Tone normalization
   4. Functional mobilities (including ambulation equipment)
D. Pain control
   1. Psychological modalities
   2. Behavioral modalities
   3. Physical modalities
E. ADL training
   1. Leisure or avocational skill development
   2. Community management skills
   3. Transfer training
   4. Recommendations for adaptive equipment
   5. Self-care retraining
   6. Energy conservation
   7. Work simplification
F. Continuity of care
   1. Discharge planning
   2. Community linkages

ever, dramatic functional fluctuations that characterize HIV and secondary infections must be understood.

The neurorehabilitation evaluation of HIV infection should include standard cognitive, perceptual, and motor components of function. The idiosyncratic nature of the disease may necessitate more detailed evaluation of these specific areas. Recommended cognitive and perceptual evaluations are both formal and observational. Safety, judgment, and money management need to be assessed. In addition to the organicity of ADC, evaluation of the systemic complications of HIV is necessary for optimal rehabilitative planning and treatment team efficacy.

The ADL evaluation is best made within the context of the immediate and projected life roles of the individual. Maximal independent functioning is the goal of rehabilitation, whatever the stage of illness. If the person is at home or is being discharged to home, a crucial component of the ADL examination is the assessment of community management skills. Consider access to transportation, socialization opportunities, shopping, banking, ability to negotiate health care and insurance systems, and community involvement. Many people with HIV infection and their caregivers have little experience with disability because of their age or social status. This combined with the stressors of illness can create unrealistic expectations and unnecessary frustrations.

Treatment process

The neuromuscular rehabilitation treatment procedures for HIV infection are outlined in the box on p. 564. The box below provides an overview of treatment techniques for opportunistic infections.

Cognitive deficits in attention, concentration, and memory require consistency, structure, and environmental cues to minimize confusion. Safety and judgment deficits can be countered by environmental adaptations. Lethargic clients benefit from sensory enhancement. Maintenance of endurance and strength, passive and active range of motion (ROM) are important components of any motor function treatment plan. Neuromuscular facilitation and inhibition, positioning, and splinting are feasible modalities to normalize tone as needed. Gait training, the use of ambulatory aids, training in motor planning, and balance and endurance exercises may be appropriate.

In addition to techniques and modalities, active listening, empathy, and unconditional positive regard are important aspects of one's therapeutic use of self. The clinician must "bracket" or set aside personal biases and beliefs to accurately hear the perspective of the individual client. The use of expressive modalities facilitates the development of coping skills while providing appropriate exploration and release of powerful emotions. Human touch can counter the

---

Most common opportunistic infections and rehabilitation interventions

Pneumocystic carinii **pneumonia (PCP)**—most common OI. Infectious agent unclear but probable latent infection; 65% to 85% healthy adults possess PCP antibodies. Fever, dyspnea and hypoxia → diaphragmatic breathing, energy conservation.*

Candida albicans—present in healthy people, immunocompromise → yeast infections of oral, esophageal and vaginal mucosal tissues → teach good oral care with soft brush, bland diet, salt water rinses.

Cryptococcus neoformans—also a yeast, but manifests in CNS as abcesses and meningitis. Headache, altered mental states, nausea, vertigo, somnolence, seizures and coma → pain management, safety and gait training, cognitive and sensory stimulation.

Cryptosporidiosis infects GI tract → chronic diarrhea and malabsorption, contributes to wasting syndrome → nutritional and hydration strategies

Wasting syndrome—involuntary loss of 10% of baseline body weight, weakness, chronic diarrhea and unexplained fever. Nutrition, hydration, energy conservation.

Toxoplasmosis—affects CNS of 30% to 40%; headache, altered cognition, encephalitis, seizures, local deficits → imposed structure, concrete tasks, pain management.

Cytomegalovirus (CMV)—Present in 40% to 100% of healthy adults. Can effect GI and respiratory tracts, but most often in optic structures → unilateral or bilateral decreased visual acuity, field cuts and blindness → compensatory skills, safety tasks and mobilities, home evaluation, supportive service referrals.

Mycobacterial infections—Two are most pertinent—MAC and TB. MAC affects 18% to 56%, but autopsies reveal this is a low estimate. *Not* latent, but primary infection. Appears late in infection, begins in GI or pulmonary tracts, then disseminates. Pneumonia, fever, weight loss, malaise, sweats, anorexia, abdominal pain, diarrhea. TB appears early, latent reactivation in 90% of HIV infected. Pulmonary TB estimates 75% to 100% in HIV infected with this bacteria. Also infects lymph nodes and bone marrow in 60% of these. Also infects CNS, cardiac, and mucosal tissues. Fever, weight loss, malaise, cough, lymph node tenderness and night sweats → energy conservation, nutrition and hydration, caregiver and patient education in safe management of infection. Is communicable; wear a mask, follow respiratory isolation protocol.

AIDS-Kaposi's sarcoma (AIDS-KS) Most frequent neoplasm and most frequent in gay men, rare in women and intravenous drug users. Purple skin or visceral lesions. Associated with deficient lymphatic transport, nodal tumors and lymphedema → swollen, painful lower extremeties. Nutrition, pain management, task simplification, mobility and ADL training.

*Underlined components identify potential treatment procedures recommended for the specific problem.

powerful and isolating effect of fear of contagion. Rehabilitation therapists can demonstrate and educate caregivers about the safety and benefit of touch.

Pain management is best approached with a behavioral and a physical approach. Pain reduction is achieved through training in breathing techniques, visualization, progressive muscle relaxation, autogenics, music, meditation, and engagement in meaningful activities. Transcutaneous electric nerve stimulation (TENS), ultrasound, and massage are also therapeutic tools (See Chapters 30 and 31.)

The process of grieving is often mistakenly associated solely with the death of another. It is a natural reaction to loss, including the loss of one's own health and diminished independence. Loss of abstract human qualities, such as perceived attractiveness and productivity, results in grief. Such emotions are often difficult for a client to articulate. It is the therapist's responsibility to be sensitive to the client's individualized grief pattern.

Placement issues accompany discharge planning from acute health care facilities. The rehabilitation professional is often called on to make recommendations regarding the level of assistance the client will need. All of the previously discussed areas of cognitive/perceptual, sensory/motor, and ADL management combined with available psychosocial and practical support influence these recommendations. Options include a return to independent living, assisted independent living by a loved one, home with supportive services (often supplied by community based AIDS organizations), home with hospital-based home care, hospice, or extended care facility.

IMPLICATIONS FOR THE HEALTH CARE PROFESSIONAL

Any discussion of the clinical manifestations of HIV infection must include important emotional considerations regarding the high morbidity of the disease and the attitudes of persons with the disease and health professionals. Fear of infection is a valid concern for the health care worker. It should be addressed with accurate information about risk factors and methods of transmission. Although HIV has been isolated from nearly all body fluids, the only documented mechanisms of transmission are (1) sexual contact, (2) parenteral contact with blood or blood products, and (3) perinatal infection from an infected mother to her offspring. The virus is fragile, begins to weaken immediately upon exposure to air, and is destroyed by household bleach. Very specific and invasive acts need to be performed to acquire HIV.

The association of HIV with the high-risk groups of homosexual men and intravenous drug users and the high mortality rate of the disease caused an inordinate fear response in many health care workers in the early years of the epidemic. The actual danger of infection of HIV to a health care worker is very low. To date the CDC reports 33

Universal blood and body fluid precautions

1. Routinely use barrier precautions to prevent skin and mucous membrane contact with blood or body fluids when such exposures are anticipated. Wear gloves when touching patient body fluids, mucous membranes, non-intact skin, or items soiled by body fluids. Wear masks and protective eye wear to protect mucous membranes when you anticipate exposure to droplets of body fluids. Wear a gown if you anticipate splashes of body fluids. Change these items (gloves, masks, eye wear, and gowns) between each patient.

2. Wash your hands immediately after removing gloves. Wash your skin surfaces immediately and thoroughly if you contact body fluids.

3. If you have an occasion to handle a needle, *do not* recap, bend, or separate it. Place it and all other sharps in the red plastic "sharps" container. Disposal into trash containers and plastic biohazard bags has resulted in punctures of housekeeping personnel.

4. Transmission of HIV via saliva is undocumented, but if called on to perform CPR, use a mouthpiece or resuscitation bag.

5. If you have weeping dermatitis or other skin lesions, refrain from direct patient care until you are healed. Cover all minor breaks in the skin (hangnails, cuts, etc.).

6. Pregnancy does not appear to increase susceptibility to HIV infection, but if infection does occur, the child has a 33% chance of being infected. Therefore strict adherence to these precautions is required.

---

documented occupational transmissions to health care workers, primarily (75%) among nurses and housekeeping staff.[9] Partly in response to this statistic, the health care industry and governmental regulating agencies have recommended new standards of infection control. Universal precautions and body substance isolation (see the box) eliminate the need for the health care worker to determine which clients or which body substances are dangerous.

Precautions must be taken with all clients whenever there is any possibility of exposure to body fluids. For rehabilitation therapists, this means gloves and gowns are used in handling clients who are incontinent or who have open lesions or wounds with which the therapist will come into contact. Gloves are necessary for feeding training or oral-bulbar facilitation if the therapist puts a hand in the client's mouth. Handwashing is indicated even with the use of latex gloves. Gloves are especially important if there is a lesion or dermatitis on the therapist's hands. These precautions protect both clients and health care workers.

The opportunistic infections described are predominantly latent and proliferate because of the immunocompromised state of the individual. Although the majority of TB in PWAs is also latent, health care workers present during cough-inducing procedures for patients with TB should don face masks to filter droplets. Finally, therapists, even pregnant ones, do not need to avoid or be prevented from treating HIV-infected clients, as long as infection control procedures are followed.

The sociocultural background of many clients with HIV illness may be foreign to the therapist. This is usually an issue in theory more than in practice. The competent and caring health care worker responds to individuals, putting aside personal moral, political, and cultural viewpoints to focus on the needs that result from illness.

SUMMARY

AIDS is the end-stage of a disease process of pandemic proportions that is predicted to kill millions of people worldwide before effective medical interventions are available. Research and resultant treatments are extending lives so that more people require rehabilitative services that maximize function and quality of life.

HIV infection is caused by a retrovirus that attacks the humoral and cellular immune system and the CNS. Acquisition of the virus is limited to risky sexual behaviors, sharing of needles by intravenous drug users, and lateral infection from mother to infant. Infrequent exceptions to these modes of transmission include: (1) occupational infections to health care workers (in the United States, 33 documented and 69 possible transmissions)[9] and (2) blood product infection, a rare occurrence since blood screening began in 1985. Practice of universal precautions minimizes the risk to health care workers.

After infection, nonspecific "flulike" symptoms signal seroconversion of the blood to antibody positive. This period normally takes approximately 6 weeks. An asymptomatic period follows during which disruption of immune function or CNS involvement is demonstrated only in laboratory tests or pathological studies. HIV infection and resultant immunocompromise produce CNS dysfunction, psychiatric complications, deadly opportunistic infections, and neoplasms.

Medical management has focused on the treatment of the secondary illnesses and on palliative care. The 12 years since identification of the virus is remarkable for a lack of effective antiretroviral therapies.

Neuromuscular rehabilitation evaluation and treatment for HIV infection are similar to those of other progressive neuromuscular disorders. The final stage of the syndrome, AIDS, can be addressed as are other wasting diseases such as cancer, but with an emphasis on cognitive and perceptual function. Neurotropic qualities of the virus result in a high incidence of AIDS dementia complex.

Rehabilitation treatment focuses on specific dysfunctions and psychosocial ramifications of infection. Compensation, mobility, ADL retraining, pain control, and community management skills constitute a well-developed treatment plan.

The epidemic is a major challenge on a personal as well as a professional level because of the natural fear of contagion. The illness originally appeared in subcultures that are often disenfranchised. Social, racial, and economic status and controversial behaviors contribute to prejudice, fear, and limited access to health care. Rehabilitation professionals have responded significantly to this challenge. Continued advocacy and compassion combined with professional enlightenment will, in a small way, alter the course of the disease.

CASE STUDIES

Three case studies are presented to help the reader understand and identify various stages of this clinical problem and how each stage may require a different therapeutic focus.

CASE 1   ▼   Early Stage

Ruby is a 23-year-old African American/Hispanic woman. She has a history of intravenous drug use and learned of her HIV status at the time of her AIDS diagnosis—9 months ago. At that time Ruby was also diagnosed with *Pneumocystis carinii* pneumonia and pulmonary tuberculosis. Ruby is without an address or a job. She lives on the streets with other addicts or in transient hotels. Her social contacts revolve around obtaining and using drugs. She is not part of the welfare system.

Ruby was admitted to the acute psychiatric unit of a hospital after a hotel resident telephoned the police to report a woman was running through the halls, pounding on doors, shouting and threatening to "get those children!"

Ruby's agitation and delusions responded well to neuroleptics. During her hospitalization, Ruby received methadone to counter narcotic withdrawal symptoms. An abscess on her left anterior deltoid was present upon admission. Pain caused decreased left shoulder strength to poor (3/5), as opposed to normal (5/5) in her right shoulder.

Rehabilitation focused on left upper extremity ROM, one-handed ADLs, dressing changes, and HIV prevention (needle sterilization). She was discharged with a limited supply of medication and a referral to community mental health services at the end of the week for follow-up medication and monitoring. Ruby was issued a voucher for a city-paid transient hotel, but she did not stay. Most patients report feeling unsafe in them. Ruby returned twice for outpatient therapy to maintain her left shoulder ROM.

John is a 51-year-old white man who tested HIV positive in 1987. He received a diagnosis of AIDS in 1992 after his initial (and ongoing) struggle with cytomegalovirus retinitis. Additional significant medical history includes two bouts of *Pneumocystis carinii* pneumonia and a left cerebrovascular accident with mild residual right-sided weakness. This hospitalization also identified the presence of toxoplasmosis.

John has worked as a front office manager for a large hotel chain for 13 years. He transferred to his newest position in a large city 5 years ago. This job demanded that he often work more than 50 hours a week. Accrued vacation time has helped John combat illness while maintaining his job. His supervisors and co-workers are aware of and generally supportive of his condition. In the last 10 months John has been delegating more duties to his assistant to limit his work to between 30 and 40 hours a week. Four weeks before this hospitalization, John took a medical leave of absence from work.

John was admitted to the hospital after having fallen (with loss of consciousness) to the floor of his apartment, where he lay for 24 hours. He was severely dehydrated and confused. John lives with a roommate who is not a significant other, but is willing to assist in home management for both of them.

However, the roommate is uncomfortable with providing more personal assistance for John.

Rehabilitation services found John to have poor static and dynamic balance with decreased insight, safety, and judgment about his status. Although he was able to identify some of his limitations, he was unable to exercise problem-solving skills to ameliorate them. For example, after repeatedly falling to the side while attempting to don his sock, John's solution was to state, "I have lousy balance." John was unable to demonstrate independent management of his 11 different medications, or to sequence a 5-step simple meal preparation process, despite written instructions. John insisted on his capacity for independent self-care despite such problems. Physical therapy was able to improve John's ambulation from the level of moderate assist to contact guard with a front-wheeled walker. Occupational therapy was able to adapt John's home environment by rearranging furniture and installing assistive equipment that increased John's safety. Visual cues and structured routines were incorporated into his environment to compensate for cognitive deficits. Rehabilitation team collaboration resulted in John's return to home with 24-hour light supervision that included his roommate in the evenings. Referrals were made to existing community services for daily meal delivery.

Lorenzo is a 37-year-old man born in Ecuador. He has lived in the United States for 25 years. He has been married for 10 years. Lorenzo and his wife have a 9-year-old daughter. Lorenzo is an associate professor of history at a university. He is currently on sabbatical. He tested positive for HIV in 1987 and was diagnosed with AIDS in 1991. Lorenzo's wife and daughter know of his AIDS diagnosis and are supportive of all medical interventions on his behalf. Lorenzo's wife reports a negative HIV test. The family fears discrimination and reprisal based on his HIV status. Consequently, none of his co-workers and few (3) friends know. Lorenzo's wife is his primary caregiver.

Lorenzo has experienced relatively few opportunistic infections associated with HIV infection. In 1993 he was diagnosed with AIDS-Kaposi's sarcoma, AIDS wasting syndrome, and anemia. Cachexia, generalized weakness, and frequent headaches have been tolerated by Lorenzo since that time. Lorenzo described a marked decrease in strength with more severe headaches in the last 3 weeks.

This hospitalization resulted from acute left-sided neurological dysfunction. He fell twice, without loss of consciousness or seizure, on the day before admission. Upon examination, Lorenzo reported anorexia, insomnia, dizziness, and left-sided sensory and motor impairment. Both right extremities were within normal limits for sensorimotor function. Severe pain in both left extremities precluded active or passive ROM. Moderate spasticity and hyperreflexia were noted in both left extremities. Muscle strength in these were poor (2/5)—he was unable to move them against gravity. Left elbow flexor and heel cord contractures were present. Decreased

left-sided coordination and numbness also were present. Sensation was intact for light touch, vibration, and proprioception. Lorenzo was alert and oriented X4. No changes in mentation were reported by either Lorenzo or his wife, except for an ongoing depressed mood without suicidal ideation. During this hospitalization, some days he was somnolent and lethargic, responding with one word answers. On other days he easily engaged in conversation and self-care. The diagnosis yielded by this hospitalization was acute bacterial meningitis. A persistent cough throughout his 3-week stay resulted in a diagnosis of *Pneumocystis carinii* pneumonia. His CD4+ cell count was 38.

The physical therapist was unable to complete her examination because of severe pain and hyperesthesia. The necessity for physical therapy to touch and urge patient movement, along with Lorenzo's poor prognosis, resulted in discontinued physical therapy in this case. The occupational therapist found Lorenzo to be bedridden and to require set-up and moderate assistance to perform bed-level ADLs. Yet Lorenzo expressed motivation to maintain independence. Interventions included a multidisciplinary team approach to provide comfort care for Lorenzo, emotional support for his family members, and community service connections. After family meetings with all disciplines, discharge plans were made for home-based hospice care, rather than extended care facility placement. Rehabilitation considerations were for quality of life issues; equipment needs; nonpharmaceutical pain control through relaxation training; and the use of meaningful activities, energy conservation training, environmental adaptations, and caregiver training.

ACKNOWLEDGMENT

The authors wish to thank Mark Holodniy, MD, Director of AIDS Clinic and Acting Chief of Infectious Diseases, Palo Alto Veterans Administration, Palo Alto, California, for his assistance in the preparation of this manuscript.

REFERENCES

1. Ammann A: Immunopathogenesis of pediatric acquired immunodeficiency syndrome, *J Perinatol* 8(2):154, 1988.
2. Barnes PF and others: Tuberculosis in patients with human immunodeficiency virus infection, *N Engl J Med* 324(23):1644, 1991.
3. Bernard EM and others: Pneumocystis, *Med Clin North Am* 76(1):107, 1992.
4. Brew JB and Currie JN: HIV related neurological disease, *Med J Aust* 158(2):104, 1993.
5. Buhrich N, Cooper DA, and Freed E: HIV infection associated with symptoms indistinguishable from functional psychosis, *Br J Psychiatry* 152.649, 1988.
6. Centers for Disease Control: Revision of the CDC surveillance case definition for acquired immunodeficiency syndrome. *MMWR* (suppl 2S), 1987.
7. Centers for Disease Control: Projections of the number of persons diagnosed with AIDS and the number of immunosuppressed HIV-infected persons—United States, 1992-1994, *MMWR* 41(RR-18), 1992.
8. Centers for Disease Control: *The scope of the HIV/AIDS epidemic in the United States,* Atlanta, 1993, CDC.
9. Centers for Disease Control: *US AIDS cases reported through December 1992, HIV/AIDS Surveillance Report,* Atlanta, 1993, CDC.
10. Clericic M and Shearer GM: A TH 1 → TH 2 Switch is a critical step in the etiology of HIV infection, *Immunol Today* (14)3:107, 1993.
11. Cohen C and Silenzio VMB: Current guidelines for preventing opportunistic infections in HIV disease, *Drug Therapy* 38, 1993.
12. Czarniecki L and Dillman P: Pediatric HIV/AIDS, *Crit Care Nurs Clin North Am* 4(3):447, 1992.
13. Daley CL and others: A prospective study of the risk of tuberculosis with accelerated progression among persons infected with the human immunodeficiency virus, *N Engl J Med* 326:231, 1992.
14. Dauncey K: Mania in early stages of AIDS, *Br J Psychiatry* 152:716, 1988.
15. Di Perri G and others: Nosocomial epidemic of active tuberculosis among HIV-infected patients, *Lancet* 2:1502, 1989.
16. El-Mallakh RS: Mania in AIDS: clinical significance and theoretical considerations, *Int J Psychiatry* 21(4):383, 1991.
17. Ellerbrock F and others: Epidemiology of women with AIDS in the United States, 1981 through 1990, *JAMA* 265:2974, 1991.
18. Fernandez F: Neuropsychiatric syndromes and their treatment in HIV infection. In *A psychiatrist's guide to AIDS and HIV disease,* Washington DC, 1990, American Psychiatric Association.
19. Freeman R and others: Autonomic function and human immunodeficiency virus infection, *Neurology* 40:575, 1990.
20. Gabel RH and others: AIDS presenting as mania, *Compr Psychiatry* 27(3):251, 1986.
21. Halstead S and others: Psychosis associated with HIV infection, *J Br Psychiatry* 153:618, 1988.
22. Hankins CA and Handley MA: HIV disease and AIDS in women: current knowledge and a research agenda, *J Acquir Immune Defic Syndr* 5:957, 1992.
23. Harris MJ and others: New-onset psychosis in HIV-infected patients, *J Clin Psychiatry* 52(9):369, 1991.
24. Hellerstein MK and others: Current approach to the treatment of human immunodeficiency virus—associated weight loss: pathophysiologic considerations and emerging management strategies, *Semin Oncol* 17(6) (suppl 9):17, 1990.
25. Hopp JW and Rogers EA: AIDS and the allied health professions, Philadelphia, 1989, FA Davis.
26. Jacobsberg LB and Perry S: Psychiatric disturbances, *Med Clin North Am* 76(1):99, 1992.
27. Kerlikowske KM and Katz MH: *Mycbacterium avium* complex and *Mycobacterium* tuberculosis in patients infected with the human immunodeficiency virus, *West J Med* 157(2):44, 1992.
28. Kessler HA and others: AIDS Part II, *Dis Mon* 38(10):691, 1992.
29. Kieburtz K and others: Manic syndrome in AIDS, *Am J Psychiatry* 148(8):1068, 1991.
30. Koff WC: The prospects for AIDS vaccines, *Hosp Pract* 99, 1991.
31. Koff WC and Glass MJ: Future directions in HIV vaccine development, *AIDS Res Hum Retroviruses* 8(8):1313, 1992.
32. Kotler DP: Gastrointestinal manifestations of HIV infection and AIDS. In DeVita VT, Hellman S, Rosenberg SA, editors: *AIDS: etiology, diagnosis, treatment and prevention,* ed 3, Philadelphia, 1992, JB Lippincott.
33. Krasinski K, Borkowsky W, and Holzman RS: Prognosis of human immunodeficiency virus infection in children and adolescents, *Pediat Infect Dis J* 8:216, 1989.
34. Krech U: Complement-fixing antibodies against cytomegalovirus in different parts of the world. *Bull World Health Organ* 49.103, 1973.
35. Levy JA: Pathogenesis of human immunodeficiency virus infection, *Microbiol Rev* 57(1):183, 1993.
36. Levy RM, Bredesen DE, and Rosenblum ML: Neurological complications of HIV infection, *Am Family Phys* 40(2):517, 1990.
37. Libman H: Pathogenesis, natural history, and classification of HIV Infection, *Crit Care Clin* 9(1):13, 1993.
38. Lifson AR and others: Long-term human immunodeficiency virus infection in asymptomatic homosexual and bisexual men with normal CD4+ lymphocyte counts: immunologic and virologic characteristics, *J Infect Dis* 163:959, 1991.
39. Lyketsos CG and others: Manic syndrome early and late in the course of HIV, *Am J Psychiatry* 150:326. 1993.
40. Marieb EN: *Human anatomy and physiology,* Redwood City, Calif, 1989, Benjamin/Cummings.
41. Markowitz JC and Perry SW: Effects of human immunodeficiency virus on the central nervous system. In Yudofsky SC and Hales RE, editors: *The American Psychiatric Press Textbook of Neuropsychiatry,* ed 2, Washington DC, 1992, American Psychiatric Association.
42. Maxwell S and others: Manic syndrome associated with zidovudine treatment, *JAMA* 259(23):3406, 1988.
43. McCabe RE and others: Clinical spectrum in 107 cases of toxoplasmic lymphadenopathy, *Rev Infect Dis* 157:1, 1987.
44. Mehta JB and Morris F: Impact of HIV infection on mycobacterial disease, *Am Family Phys* 45(5):2203, 1992.
45. Nahlen BL and others: HIV wasting syndrome in the United States, *AIDS* 7:183, 1993.
46. O'Dowd MA and McKegney KP: Manic syndrome associated with zidovudine, *JAMA* 260(24):3587, 1988.
47. Ostrow DG: *Psychiatric aspects of human immunodeficiency virus infection,* Kalamazoo, MN, 1990, Upjohn Pharmaceuticals.
48. Patterson BK, Ehrenpreis ED, and Yokoo H: Focal enterocyte vacuolization: a new microscopic finding in the acquired immune deficiency syndrome, *Am J Clin Pathol* 99:24, 1993.
49. Perry SW and Tross S: Psychiatric problems of AIDS inpatients at a New York hospital: preliminary report, *Public Health Rep* 99:20, 1984.
50. Pitchenik AE and Fertel D: Tuberculosis and nontuberculous mycobacterial disease, *Med Clin North Am* 76(1):121, 1992.
51. Report of a working group of the American Academy of Neurology AIDS Task Force: Nomenclature and research case definitions for neurologic manifestations of human immunodeficiency virus type 1 (HIV 1) infection, *Neurology* 41:778, 1991.
52. Rutherford GW, Lifson AR, and Hessol NA: Course of HIV-1 infection in a cohort of homosexual and bisexual men: an 11 year follow-up study, *Br Med J* 301:1183, 1990.

53. Schmidt U and Miller D: Two cases of hypomania in AIDS, *Br J Psychiatry* 152:839, 1988.

54. Snyder S and others: Prevalence of mental disorders in newly admitted medical inpatients with AIDS, *Psychosomatics* 33(2):166, 1992.

55. Stine GJ: *Acquired immune deficiency syndrome: biological, medical, social and legal issues,* Englewood Cliffs, NJ, 1993, Prentice-Hall.

56. Tinkle MB, Amaya MA, and Tamayo OW: Part1. Epidemiology, pathogenesis, and natural history, *J Obstet Gynecol Neonatal Nurs* 21(2):86, 1992.

57. Torres RA, Franke-Ruta G, and Barr M: Future therapies in the management of critically ill AIDS patients, *Crit Care Clin* 9(1):153, 1993.

58. Williams AB: The epidemiology, clinical manifestations and health-maintenance needs of women infected with HIV, *Nurse Pract* 17(5):27, 1992.

59. Williams AB: Women in the HIV epidemic, *Crit Care Nurs Clin North Am* 4(3):437, 1992.

60. Witte MH, Witte DL, and Way MF: AIDS, Kaposi's sarcoma and the lymphatic system: update and reflections, *Lymphology* 23:73, 1990.

61. Wong B and others: Central-nervous-system toxoplasmosis in homosexual men and parenteral drug abusers, *Ann Intern Med* 100(36):36, 1984.

62. World Health Organization: *The current global situation of the HIV/AIDS pandemic,* Geneva, January 4, 1993.

63. World Health Organization: World Health Organization Global AIDS Statistics, *AIDS Care* 5(1):125, 1993.

CHAPTER 19

Poliomyelitis and the Postpolio Syndrome

Laura K. Smith and Marsha Mabry

KEY TERMS

poliomyelitis	management
postpolio sequella	postpoliomyelitis
postpolio syndrome (PPS)	postpolio muscular atrophy

LEARNING OBJECTIVES

After reading this chapter the student/therapist will:

1. Describe the pathological lesion occurring in poliomyelitis.
2. List three physiological processes that are the basis for recovery of muscle strength following the acute phase of poliomyelitis.
3. List five symptoms commonly seen in people who have postpolio syndrome.
4. Describe the difference between fatigue in postpolio syndrome and normal fatigue.
5. Describe the most likely etiology of new muscle weakness in postpolio syndrome.
6. State the goal for clinical management of the postpolio syndrome.
7. State four musculoskeletal objectives designed to achieve this goal.
8. Explain why energy conservation techniques play such an important role in the management of postpolio syndrome.
9. State why exercises designed to strengthen polio-involved muscles can cause further weakness and pain.
10. Describe three common styles used by people with postpolio to cope with their impairments.

OVERVIEW

Poliomyelitis or infantile paralysis is an endemic disease of humans first recorded in paralytic form in 1300 BC.[81] It is an acute infectious disease caused by an enteric virus with worldwide distribution. Transmission is by human contact, and most of the people ingest the virus. Few persons, however, develop the paralytic form because they have developed immunity from breast-feeding, subclinical infections, clinical infections without paralysis, and now vac-

cines. In the paralytic form, the virus selectively attacks the motor neuron cell bodies with resulting flaccid muscle paresis or paralysis.

As sanitation levels increased in industrialized countries in the first half of this century and formula-feeding was advocated, acute poliomyelitis escalated to epidemic proportions. Frightening epidemics swept across North America and Europe from 1910 to 1959. In 1921 New York City recorded 9,000 cases with 2,000 deaths. Franklin Roosevelt contracted poliomyelitis at this time. In 1937, when he was President of the United States, he founded the March of Dimes (The National Foundation for Infantile Paralysis). An unprecedented outpouring of public funds occurred to provide treatment, research, and professional education. The results were spectacular. In just 20 years the "War on Polio" was won with the introduction of the inactivated vaccine (Salk, 1955) and the live attenuated oral vaccine (Sabin, 1960). Polio was promptly forgotten as medicine and rehabilitation turned attention to other pressing disabilities. The March of Dimes changed focus to birth defects, and the surviving polio victims went on with their lives to compensate, compete, and become productive citizens.

Acute poliomyelitis and its sequelae, however, did not stop but rather continued on in its many phases. Currently there are an estimated 250,000 to 300,000 postpolio individuals in the United States. These people have all of the diseases and injuries found in an adult population. Evaluation and treatment are complicated by the previous paresis and by the poor or altered response to medical, surgical, and rehabilitation procedures. Over 25% of the postpolio individuals are experiencing new symptoms of fatigue, weakness, pain, and decreased functional ability of the postpolio syndrome.[34] Although the virus is still prevalent within industrialized countries, infection is prevented by immunization. There are 10 or more new cases of acute poliomyelitis per year in the United States, mostly vaccine related. The World Health Organization (WHO) has calculated that there is an average of 275,000 new cases per year in developing countries.[93]

IDENTIFICATION OF THE CLINICAL PROBLEM: PATHOLOGY

In most instances the widely prevalent polio viruses are destroyed in the stomach or excreted via the intestinal tract without clinical infection, or they may enter the bloodstream and produce a flulike infection with recovery and development of immunity. If the virus crosses the blood-brain barrier, it attacks almost all of the motor nerve cells in the brain, brainstem, and spinal cord. Symptoms during this 2-week febrile illness include headache, sore throat, elevated temperature, severe meningismus, severe muscle pain to touch and stretch, and flaccid muscle paresis or paralysis (signs and symptoms of severe life-threatening poliomyelitis are outlined by Spencer[81,82]). Many motor neurons fought off the virus and recovered, but many were destroyed. Bodian[12] in animal studies found only 4% of the anterior horn cells histologically normal at 2 to 6 days from onset, but by 14 days the neurons were either destroyed or of normal appearance.

Following the febrile illness a motor neuron with its 5 to 1,500 muscle fibers could be unaffected, recovered, or destroyed with resulting denervation of the muscle fibers (Fig. 19-1). The 100 to 1,000 motor neurons to a particular muscle might be unaffected or recovered, all of the motor neurons to a muscle could be destroyed, or the muscle could be partially denervated with combinations of recovered and destroyed motor neurons. Diagnostic EMG at this time would show fibrillation potentials indicating recent denervation of muscle fibers.

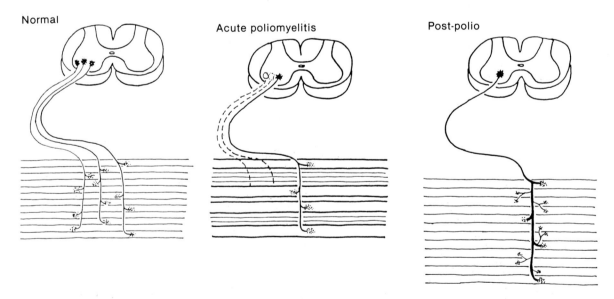

Fig. 19-1. Schematic representation of motor units to a muscle. *Normal* represents the 100 to 1000 motor neurons of a muscle and the 5 to 1500 muscle fibers each axon innervates. *Acute poliomyelitis* depicts viral destruction of some of the anterior horn cells with atrophy of denervated muscle fibers. *Postpolio* represents axon sprouting by recovered nerve cells with reinnervation of the orphaned muscle fibers and subsequent hypertrophy.

Physiological processes of recovery of muscle strength

In convalescent poliomyelitis, muscle strength in partially denervated muscles increases to a maximum over a 2-year period, with 50% of the muscle strength recovery occurring in the first 3 months after onset and 75% in the first 6 months (Fig. 19-2). The rate and magnitude of the recovery, however, can be compromised by injudicious treatment, activity, and excessive exercise.[9,45,81,82]

Muscle strength recovery and increase in functional ability occur by several physiological processes. Recovered neurons develop terminal axon sprouts to reinnervate orphaned muscle fibers.[32,85,92] (Fig. 19-1). It is estimated that a single motor neuron can reinnervate up to five times its normal complement of muscle fibers. Electromyographically the action potentials of the single motor units are polyphasic with large amplitudes and are called giant motor units. The innervated muscle fibers can be hypertrophied by exercise and activity during the rehabilitation phase. This has been referred to as denervation hypertrophy. The third process provides an increase in functional ability and an

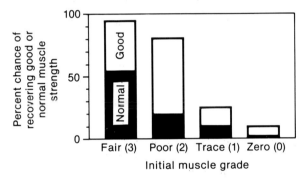

Percent chance of severely involved muscles recovering to "good" or "normal" eventual strength:

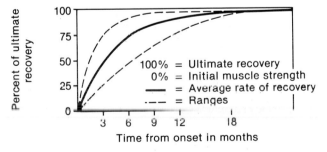

Rate of muscle recovery irrespective of the initial or final strength:

Fig. 19-2. The rate and extent of increase in manual muscle test scores in postacute poliomyelitis. Muscles showing some strength on initial examination will increase in strength unless they are overworked, in which case they may plateau or lose strength. The grade of Normal (5) is a clinical definition and not an indication of fullness strength. This grade can be recorded with loss of 60% of the anterior horn cells to a muscle.[39] (Adapted from Spencer, WA: *Treatment of acute poliomyelitis,* Springfield, Ill, 1956, Charles C Thomas, with permission).

apparent increase of strength by neuromuscular learning whereby practice of an exercise or an activity leads to increased skill and performance without necessarily increasing muscle strength.[74] The fourth process is the increased recruitment of the giant motor units with use of the muscle at high levels of its capacity.

Such extensive compensatory physiological processes mask the profound neurological deficits caused by the disease. This was demonstrated by Sharrard,[76] who counted the number of anterior horn cells in the spinal cords of postpolio individuals who died from other causes. He compared the percentage of cells present with previous muscle test grades. Muscles graded 5 (N) could have lost up to 60% of their anterior horn cells; muscles previously graded 4 (G) had lost 60% to 90% of their motor neurons; and muscles of grades 3, 2, and 1 (F, P, T) lost 90% to 98%.

Functional compensation

The body possesses a number of compensatory mechanisms to maintain function in the presence of residual paralysis (Fig. 19-3). These compensations include use of weak muscles at high levels of their capacity, substitution of strong muscles with increased energy expenditure for the task, and use of ligaments for stability with resulting hypermobility. Many convalescent polio clients in the early epidemics were encouraged to exercise for years and to use heroic compensatory methods for function. In the long term, however, such overcompensation leads to microtrauma of ligaments and joint structures and exhaustion of neuromuscular units.

The postpolio syndrome (PPS)

The late effects of poliomyelitis have been recorded in the literature since 1875 by various authors.* These new problems occur at an average of 35 years after the acute onset, and thus it was not until the 1980s that the large number of survivors from the great epidemics of 1940 to 1957 made an impact on the medical system.[56] The **postpolio sequella** is a combination of neurological, musculoskeletal, and psychosocial manifestations. The most common physical problems are profound fatigue, pain, and new weakness with decreased function, safety, and quality of life (Table 19-1). Other physical problems include muscle fasciculations and cramps,[25] hypoventilation, swallowing difficulties, and sleep disturbances.

The etiology of the new weakness and atrophy is unknown because few autopsy studies have been made. Several causes have been proposed and are reviewed in detail by Jubelt and Cashman.[42] There is little current evidence to implicate reactivation of the polio virus or an autoimmune response. Normal aging, with loss of neurons occurring after age 60,[86] may be a factor in the older

* References 3, 9, 17, 33, 36, 44, and 67.

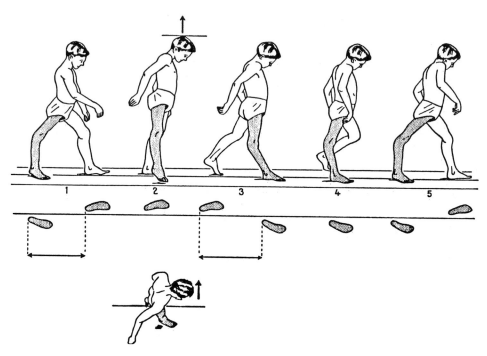

Fig. 19-3. The functional compensations of a boy with paralysis of the right lower extremity show increased energy expenditure and progressive ligamentous laxity. (Adapted from Ducroquet R and others: *Walking and limping—a study of normal and pathological walking,* Philadelphia, 1968, JB Lippincott Co, with permission of the copyright holder.)

Table 19-1. Most common new health problems in 132 confirmed postpolio individuals with a diagnosis of postpolio syndrome

	N	%
Health problems		
Fatigue	117	89
Muscle pain	93	71
Joint pain	93	71
Weakness		
Previously affected muscles	91	69
Previously unaffected muscles	66	50
Cold intolerance	38	29
Atrophy	37	28
ADL problems		
Walking	84	64
Climbing stairs	80	61
Dressing	23	17

Adapted with permission from Halstead L and Wiechers D, editors: *Research and clinical aspects of the late effects of poliomyelitis,* White Plains, NY, 1987, March of Dimes, p 17.

postpolio individuals because the loss of a few neurons from an already markedly depleted neuronal pool could result in a significant decrease in strength. It has been suggested that the neurons that showed histological recovery from the virus may not have been physiologically normal and may be subject to premature aging and failure.[44,52]

Most of the evidence as to the cause of **postpolio syndrome (PPS)** points to an increased metabolic demand on the giant motor units, with pruning of the axon sprouts to reduce the number of muscle fibers innervated by the motor nerve cell (Fig. 19-4). The sprouting and pruning process has evidently been going on since the convalescent stage of polio as a mechanism to maintain as many denervated fibers as possible. In time there is more pruning than sprouting, with downsizing of the number of fibers in the motor units leading to muscle weakness and fatigue.* Some muscle biopsies are suggestive of new denervation of muscle fibers.[19,20] A similar process of axon sprouting and pruning has been found in normal aging.[84]

A second area of dysfunction in the giant motor units is at the neuromuscular junction. Single-fiber electromyographic (EMG) studies show instability or failure of transmission of the nerve impulse at the axon terminal. This problem may be the cause of fatigue and decreased endurance.[53,70,71,92]

MANAGEMENT: EVALUATION, GOAL SETTING, AND TREATMENT
Acute and convalescent polio

Treatment in all of the stages of poliomyelitis is complex because the disease produces a spotty and asymmetrical paralysis, with no two clients alike. Treatment needs differ

* References 11, 33, 53, 54, 70, 71, and 92.

according to the stage of the disease, age of the person, time from onset, severity of involvement, amount of recovery, presence of joint hypermobility or hypomobility, previous treatment, and level of activity. Effective treatment is based on pathology and is individualized by evaluation of the person. During the febrile illness the goal of treatment is to preserve and protect life and physiological functions. Rest and anticipatory medical and nursing care are obligatory. Physical measures other than positioning to relieve pain and pain-free passive range of motion (ROM) are contraindicated. In the convalescent phase the goal is to develop useful function compatible with the patient's residual capacity. Physical and occupational therapy predominate with emphasis on pain relief, exercise, and independent function, with major modifications for those with respiratory muscle paralysis. The following references provide details of the principles and methods of treatment of acute and convalescent poliomyelitis.[39,45,81,82]

Postpolio evaluation

The manifestations of the late effects of polio are non-specific and similar to symptoms of many other conditions. A comprehensive interdisciplinary evaluation is essential to (1) confirm the original diagnosis of poliomyelitis because approximately 10% to 15% of people who thought or were told they had polio did not,[33,81] (2) identify all other physical-psychosocial health problems that may occur in the age ranges of 20 to 90 years, and (3) establish current diagnoses. The differential diagnosis of PPS is made by exclusion.[34,35,56]

Physical therapy evaluation in PPS differs markedly from that needed in the postacute and convalescent stages, where definitive manual muscle testing and goniometry form the basis of the treatment plan. In PPS selective gross group testing is sufficient to provide information to help in the diagnosis of polio and direction of treatment needs. Time need not be spent searching for nonfunctional contractions (P+ to T or 2+ to 1) or to belabor the narrow range of grades from N- to P+ (5- to 2+), because these grades vary markedly with previous activity. Comparisons with old muscle tests are interesting but are reliable only when the ability of the examiners and the criteria used for each muscle are known. Major aspects of the physical therapy evaluation include the following:

1. History and analysis of physical activity by type, time, and intensity in the home, at work, in travel, in community activities, in avocations, and in recreation and exercise
2. Detailed evaluation of habitual sleeping, sitting, standing, and walking postures
3. Modified spinal and upper lower quarter evaluations according to problems presented
4. Evaluation of current orthoses and needs for orthotic interventions

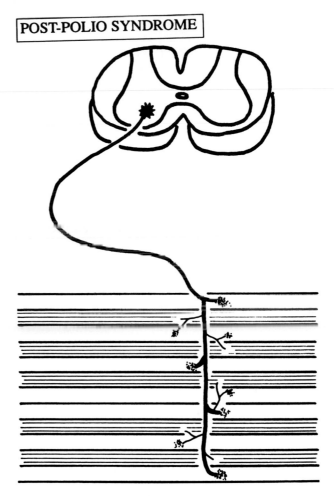

POST-POLIO SYNDROME

Fig. 19-4. Schematic representation of pruning back of axon sprouts in postpolio syndrome resulting in reduced numbers of muscle fibers per motor unit and atrophy of the orphaned muscle fibers.

Management of postpolio syndrome

The general goal at this stage is to provide the person with principles and methods for self-**management** of his or her body. The most important aspect of the program is patient and family education regarding the pathology caused by acute poliomyelitis, the processes of recovery, and the effects of long-term compensation. Specific musculoskeletal objectives are to:

1. Alleviate and prevent the causes of pain
2. Decrease the abnormally high work load of muscles relative to their limited capacity
3. Correct and minimize postural and gait deviations mechanically
4. Maintain and increase function, safety, and the quality of life

Pain

Muscle pain. Pain was found to be the predominant problem of reporting **postpoliomyelitis** individuals, with an incidence of 85% in those walking without orthotic assistance and 100% in those using crutches or manual wheelchairs for locomotion.[79] The types and causes of pain are multiple. One type of pain is diffuse and generalized and often described as "bone pain" or "like having the flu." This pain occurs both in known weak muscles and particularly in extremities that have been thought to be normal. Most people report that this type of pain is not affected by medications or physical modalities and that it is increased by physical activity and decreased by rest. The pain or fatigue is unusual because it usually does not occur at the time of the activity but rather 1 or 2 days later. Treatment should be directed to nonfatiguing functional activities, energy conservation techniques,[95] more frequent rest periods, and pacing of activities by interspersing rest periods or change of activity.[4]

Examples of some of the life-style changes that are recommended include avoiding stairs, low chairs, and deep knee bends and encouraging use of elevators, elevated chairs, bathtub bench or shower stool, reserved parking, and weight control. Recommendations for the neck and upper extremities include seating and workstation corrections, support of books and newspapers for reading, use of rolling carts for carrying, telephone headsets, and computer wrist rests. Decreasing workloads on the muscles may require eliminating unessential walking, using an orthosis or a personal mobility vehicle (motorized cart or chair), avoiding strengthening and aerobic exercises, and in some cases disability retirement.

Recovery from the diffuse muscle pain takes many months and depends on the severity, length of time present, and the client's compliance with treatment recommendations. Peach and Olejnik[62] found that muscle pain was resolved in 28% and improved in 72% of people who complied with recommendations. In those who were noncompliant, muscle pain was improved in 14%, unchanged in 57%, and increased in 29%.

Joint pain. Joint pain is more localized than muscle pain and is caused primarily by long-term microtrauma from abnormal biomechanical forces, as well as by injuries from falls. Joint pain may accompany PPS, but joint pain by itself is usually a repetitive injury and not a symptom of PPS. Common conditions include osteoarthritis,[91] sacroiliitis, trochanteric bursitis, ligamentous laxity of the knee and ankle, patellar-femoral tracking problems, shoulder impingements, lateral epicondylitis (humerus), and carpal tunnel syndrome. Neck, shoulder, and back pain radiating to the hip and leg were reported by over 65% of postpolio individuals.[79] This pain should not be unexpected because the incidence of major postural abnormalities and gait deviations is also high as shown in Table 19-2. Treatment is complicated by the presence of osteoporosis, lack of compensatory substitutions to rest the injured part, and often poor response to exercise.

Local pain and dysfunction can be treated as athletic

Table 19-2. Major postural abnormalities in sitting, standing, and walking in 111 confirmed postpolio clinic clients

Posture (N)	Abnormal deviation	No.	Percent
Sitting (N = 111)	Absent lumbar curve	64	54
	Forward head (loss of cervical curve)	50	45
	Uneven pelvic base*	29	26
	Structural scoliosis	38	34
Standing (N = 76)	Absent lumbar curve	52	68
	Uneven pelvic base*	40	53
	Weight bearing on stronger leg	29	38
Walking (N = 76)	Abnormal gait deviations	76	100
	Major lateral trunk oscillations	33	43
	Obvious forward lean	40	53

Adapted from Smith L and McDermott K: Pain in post-poliomyelitis: addressing causes versus effects. In Halstead L and Wiechers D, editors: *Research and clinical aspects of the late effects of poliomyelitis,* White Plains, NY, 1987, March of Dimes (with permission).
*Pelvic asymmetry was ½ inch or more.

injuries from overuse, but require major modifications and careful monitoring of performance, pain, and fatigue. Many joint pain problems can be relieved and controlled by a home program such as methods to rest the injured part, mechanical postural corrections, cold packs, nonsteroidal antiinflammatory drugs (NSAIDs), orthotics, and ROM exercises. Successful treatment of joint pain, however, requires identification and elimination of the cause of the pain. These goals frequently are difficult to achieve because the person with postpolio may not have the strength in other parts of the body to compensate and carry out an essential function, or the person may be unable or unwilling to make necessary life-style changes. Most clients can benefit from a short course of outpatient therapy to specifically address inhibiting muscle spasm, stretching fascia and muscles, decreasing edema and increasing nutrition in joint structures, mobilizing or stabilizing joints, and reeducating muscles to properly stabilize joints in activity. This program should include assisting the client in carrying out the home program and life-style changes and the development of an ongoing program of appropriate exercises. This program should include relaxation, meditation, self-mobilization, underwater exercises, or body awareness techniques such as the Feldenkrais method.[72] Many clients have had courses of heat treatments or a series of unattended modalities and although they felt better during the treatment, they either did not improve or got worse.

Other types of pain. Many persons who had poliomyelitis underwent extensive orthopedic surgery, and some are experiencing pain or hypersensitivities at these sites. Hypersensitivities can be decreased and even eliminated with desensitization exercises if the client is willing to devote the necessary time. The most frequent sites of pain at old surgical sites are in (1) the trunk from surgery for scoliosis and (2) the foot near subtalar arthrodeses, or in hypermobility of the transverse tarsal joint due to fusion of all the ankle joints. In most instances, stabilization of the ankle and foot in a custom-made ankle-foot orthosis (AFO) and use of a rocker-bottom shoe has relieved the pain and permitted weight bearing and walking. Custom-made corsets and trunk supports in chairs have helped some people control the pain at previous surgical sites in the trunk. A few clients find transcutaneous electrical nerve stimulation (TENS) helpful and continue to use it to control pain (see Chapters 30 and 31). Most individuals, however, stop using these devices because masking the pain permits them to physically overdo, which leads to further injury to their bodies. Temporary alleviation of pain is not particularly difficult, but correction of the causes and teaching the client to control and prevent pain is indeed a challenge.

Abnormal fatigue. Abnormal fatigue is reported by almost 90% of the postpolio clients as a new problem (see Table 19-1). This is a profound fatigue that may not seem to be related to a particular activity, and recovery does not occur with usual rest periods. In one study, postpolio subjects described their fatigue as increasing loss of strength during exercise, increasing weakness, and heavy sensation of muscles. These were significantly different descriptors than those used by a nonpolio control group.[10] This fatigue also has been described as a sudden and total wipe out and in a few instances may include headaches and sweating suggestive of autonomic nervous system overload.[78] Often the fatigue occurs at the same time each day, usually in the early afternoon. This fatigue causes people to decrease activities and permit their world to become smaller. These individuals may develop excuses to avoid participation in social activities, shopping, family outings, and vacations. As the fatigue becomes worse the person is tired all the time and gets up in the morning fatigued and worn out. Many individuals go into a cycle of getting up to go to work, coming home to go to bed, getting up to go to work, and spending weekends in bed.

Abnormal fatigue is treated similarly to muscle pain and new muscle weakness through decreasing the workload on the muscles by using nonfatiguing functional activities, energy conservation techniques, breaking activities up into parts with frequent rest periods,[1] and by daily rest periods including a nap if possible.[95] The client needs help in relaxation or meditation exercises and in gaining permission to rest. Sometimes short-term sick leave (weeks to months) with appropriate decrease in activity can relieve the fatigue, and work can be resumed with modifications. In severe fatigue problems, disability retirement is needed.

Recovery from this type of fatigue takes 3 to 12 months, depending on the severity of the problem and compliance with recommendations. Peach and Olejnik[62] found on re-

evaluation that fatigue was resolved or improved in the group who complied and unchanged or increased in the group who did not.

New muscle weakness. New muscle weakness occurs in extremities known to have polio involvement and frighteningly in stronger extremities not thought by the client to have been affected. Weakness is primarily noticed in repetitive and stabilizing contractions rather than with single maximum efforts. The problem may be in decreased ability of the muscles to recover rapidly after contracting. Recovery of quadriceps muscle strength after fatiguing exercise was significantly less in symptomatic postpolio subjects compared to nonsymptomatic and control subjects.[69] Decreases in strength do not usually show up on the manual muscle test because it is a single effort maximum contraction, a large range of force is represented in grades 4 and 5, and few examiners are now tested for reliability.[40] In a 1 year follow-up using quantitative muscle force testing no differences were found in muscle strength, work capacity, endurance capacity, or recovery from fatigue of the quadriceps in either nonsymptomatic or symptomatic groups with postpolio.[2] Nevertheless, there is at best a slow decline in functional ability, which clients describe as loss of strength.

Other signs relating to new muscle involvement include fasciculations, muscle cramps, atrophy, and elevation of muscle enzymes in the blood. Fasciculations are seen in muscles at rest and during contraction, and they tend to persist even when muscle pain and fatigue have been resolved. Muscle cramps are commonly found in fatigued muscles and are alleviated by decreased activity. New **postpolio muscular atrophy** of muscles is sometimes reported and is most noticeable when it occurs in the gastrocnemius or the anterior tibialis. Elevation of muscle enzymes, indicative of muscle damage, has been found in people with postpolio and has been related to the intensity of work.[61,89,90]

Overuse of muscles for their limited capacity has long been associated with these new problems.[9,61,66] New weakness and atrophy have been attributed to metabolic overload of the giant motor units, with more pruning of muscle fibers than axon sprouting.[88,92] Muscle overload occurs from use of muscles at high levels of their capacity for a long period. To perform the same activity with weak muscles, the muscles need to contract at a higher percentage of their capacity than is normally required. For example in walking, muscles in postpolio subjects may contract at both higher intensities and for prolonged or even continuous periods in the gait cycle.[66] Energy expenditure for the task is increased, and the prolonged contractions keep the capillaries compressed to limit needed muscle nutrition. Fasciculations are often observed using nearly maximum voluntary contractions to perform a daily activity. Like elite athletes, the muscles of people with postpolio cannot continue to maintain these high levels indefinitely.

To determine whether the cause of the new weakness is

overuse or possibly disuse, a detailed assessment is required of home, work, recreational, and community activities.[95] If the client is merely asked what his or her activity level is, the answer will usually be something like, "I don't do anything anymore." This response leads the investigator to assume that weakness is from disuse. With specific questioning, one usually finds that the client is doing an extraordinary amount of physical activity. There are few "couch potatoes" in this group. What the client means by not doing anything is relative to the previous higher level of activity. It is important to establish a total picture of the client's activities in sitting, standing, walking, lifting, carrying, climbing stairs, using a telephone or a computer, as well as activities such as cooking, vacuuming, mowing the lawn, playing tennis, singing in a choir, or taking care of grandchildren.

The goal of treatment of overuse weakness is to slow the rate of progression by decreasing the workload on the muscle. This may include life-style changes with use of nonfatiguing functional activities, energy conservation techniques, pacing of activities with frequent rest periods, weight control or reduction, orthoses, and motorized assistance.

Generalized weakness from disuse is seen in clients who have had infections, fractures, surgery, and other illness requiring bed rest or immobilization. Treatment requires a modified conditioning program with careful monitoring of response (see **Exercise** p. 581).

Environmental cold intolerance. The involved extremities in people with postpolio are frequently abnormally cold. This condition is due to sympathetic nerve cell involvement leading to decreased vasoconstriction and venoconstriction with heat loss to the environment. This problem may become worse with PPS, and most people have learned to control the heat loss with clothing.

Cold intolerance can cause a problem with the use of cold in the treatment of injuries. Most people with postpolio do not want to use local cold on any part of the body. They use heating pads and hot water, which feels good at the time but may perpetuate or increase the edema, inflammation, and pain. Local cold is often more effective and is well tolerated by most people with postpolio. Successful application requires more client education about the use of cold and demonstration of the effects.

Sleep disturbances. Sleep disturbances have been found in over 50% of reporting postpolio individuals.[28] These disturbances may be caused by pain, stress, underventilation, or obstructive apnea.[5,38,77] The role of the therapist is primarily in the area of pain. A history of pain or numbness that is worse at night or on rising points to sleeping surfaces that are too firm or sleeping with joints in closed packed positions—usually the neck and shoulders. These problems are correctable with foam mattress covers or waterbeds, cervical pillows, and modification of sleeping postures.

Life-threatening conditions. Life-threatening conditions such as hypoventilation, dysphagia, and cardiopulmo-nary insufficiency require management by medical specialists.[5,6,80,81] These problems occur in people with previous bulbar poliomyelitis who may or may not be using ventilatory assistance and in those with severe kyphosis or scoliosis. The role of the therapist is to modify activities and teach glossopharyngeal breathing, manually assisted coughing, or bronchial drainage as indicated.[18,24] If trunk supports are considered, vital capacity should be checked with and without an abdominal binder to determine the effect on breathing.

Decreasing the work load of muscles

Energy conservation techniques. Energy conservation techniques provide the easiest way to decrease the work of muscles without loss of function. An occupational therapy program to assist the person in analysis of all activity by type, time, distance, and intensity is valuable. Such an inventory forms the basis for setting priorities and determining where and how individuals wish to use their limited neuromuscular capacity.[95] Questions to be addressed include the following:

1. Can one trip do for two or three?
2. Can the activity be performed in a less strenuous way, such as by sitting or using a rolling basket?
3. Are there easier ways to perform the activity with modern comforts and technology, including motorization and electronics?
4. Can the activity be broken up into parts with change of activity or rest?
5. Are there other people who can perform some of the physical aspects of the activity?

Weight reduction. Weight reduction is the single most effective way to decrease the muscle workload, but it is one of the most difficult. Weight loss is slow without exercise, but it can be accomplished. Weight control needs to be incorporated as a permanent modification of nutritional habits rather than achieved in a short-term diet. Dietetic counseling and support groups are important components of this difficult life-style modification.

Locomotion. Assymetrical or abnormal gait patterns, crutch walking, or propelling manual wheelchairs for several decades are frequently the major sources of the pain, weakness, and fatigue in people with PPS. For example, the incidence of pain in a group of 114 confirmed postpolio patients increased from 84% in those who were ambulatory without orthotics to 100% for those who used crutches or wheelchairs for locomotion.[79] The high prevalence of osteoarthritis in patients with PPS was documented in the hand and wrist by radiography.[91] Over twice the number of postpolio subjects had osteoarthritis of the wrist or hand than would be expected in a normal population of the same age. The risk factor was significantly increased with lower extremity muscle paralysis and use of assistive devices.[91] Despite severe difficulties with locomotion, changes or modifications are hard for polio survivors to consider. As locomotion becomes more arduous or painful, many begin to limit outside activities rather than modify individual methods of locomotion. They find more and more reasons to avoid activities at work, with the family, and in the community. Resistance to life-style changes is common in the postpolio population and leads to needless suffering and functional decline.[62]

Prevention of this spiraling disability and restoration of lost function requires marked decrease in the amount of walking or propelling a chair and a change to methods of locomotion that do not cause pain, weakness, and fatigue. Those who have been walking without assistive devices or with inadequate assistance may need to use a cane, forearm crutches, trunk support, shoe corrections, or new orthoses. Clients who have been walking for years with crutches with or without orthoses develop shoulder, elbow, and wrist injuries, as well as new muscle weakness, muscle pain, and fatigue. They need to use personal mobility vehicles (motorized carts) for distance locomotion or as their primary form of locomotion, with walking reserved for transfers and short distances only. Lightweight manual wheelchairs only perpetuate the problems and create new ones. Those propelling manual wheelchairs develop shoulder, elbow, wrist, and hand injuries. These people need to obtain electric wheelchairs or motorized carts if suitable. Manual wheelchairs at best only postpone problems.

Increased use of motorized vehicles for locomotion should be considered by almost all individuals with PPS to decrease unessential loads on muscles. Some require only occasional use of these vehicles, such as in airports, grocery stores, convention centers, and theme parks. All-terrain vehicles (ATVs), riding lawn mowers, tractors, and golf carts can be used to permit continuing participation in farm, ranch, seashore, hunting, camping, fishing, and other outdoor activities. Some people need motorized locomotion only at work, home, or in the community, whereas others may use motorization as their primary form of locomotion. To transport the motorized carts and electric wheelchairs, hoists or ramps are required to place the vehicles into and out of autos, trucks, or vans.

The purposes of the changes in methods of locomotion are to increase safety and prevent costly falls, reduce energy expenditure and decrease fatigue, prevent further injury and pain, and most important to increase function and quality of life. Those who do make these difficult changes in their methods of locomotion seem to undergo a metamorphosis from pain and dysfunction to renewed activity and increased function. They enthusiastically state that they wished they had made these changes earlier.

Correction of posture and gait deviations. In addition to sitting in poorly supporting chairs, sofas, auto seats, and wheelchairs, the postpolio individual may have trunk muscle paresis or asymmetries of the pelvic base and may spend up to 16 hours per day in the seated position. The typical posture is slumped hanging on posterior vertebral ligaments with loss of lumbar and cervical curves. Neck, shoulder, and back pain are common. Mechanical restoration of the lumbar curve in all seating at home, during meals, at work, in automobiles, in wheelchairs, at church, in meetings, and at social events can correct the problem. This can be accomplished by use of properly fitted clerical chairs, ergonometric chairs, anterior tilt seats, gluteal pads, and the many types of lumbar rolls, back supports, and seating systems.

Persons with abdominal muscle paralysis benefit from custom-made thoracolumbar corsets, with the posterior rigid stays bent to produce a normal standing lumbar curve. Paretic or paralyzed neck muscles can be rested and supported by soft foam collars or the more supportive microcellular neck collars.

People with severe trunk muscle paralysis or scoliosis with or without spinal fusion often support their trunk or relieve pain by pushing down with their hands or elbows on chairs, tables, and on their hips (Fig. 19-5). In time such self-traction results in pain and weakness in their arms. Chair inserts and fixed supports as well as custom-made corsets, back braces, and molded body jackets should be considered. The rigid trunk supports, however, take away mobility used for function. Usually they can be worn for part of the day in activities where trunk mobility is not essential.

Orthotics. Unlike most rehabilitation clients, people with postpolio have strong and usually negative feelings about orthotics. Most individuals long ago discarded their braces and have relied on body compensations for walking (see Fig. 19-3). If an orthosis was essential for walking it has become

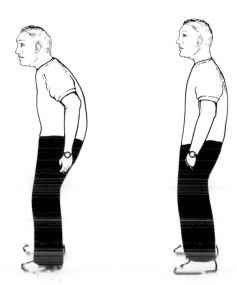

Fig. 19-5. Polio paralysis of the erector spinae (and abdominal) muscles with inability to sit or stand erect. Erect posture is frequently achieved by casual appearing activities such as pushing down on the body and chairs.

a part of the body image, and the client does not want any changes. Some have already tried plastic orthoses and found them painful and of no use. Thus it is difficult to get the person with PPS to consider orthoses or an orthotic change.

To gain the client's respect, the therapist must respect the client's knowledge of how his or her extremities function and give each individual specific useful reasons to use the orthoses. Some of these reasons include preventing falls and potential fractures, limiting joint motion and preventing pain, restoring weight bearing on the weak leg and decreasing the work of the strong leg in standing, gaining erect posture and decreasing back pain, and decreasing energy expenditure and fatigue.

In some cases both the upper (talo-crural) and the lower (subtalar) ankle joints were fused surgically. To walk, the subject places abnormal forces on the posterior structures of the knee and/or the transverse tarsal joint. In time hypermobility and pain occur in these areas. Motion for walking can be restored by wearing rocker bottom shoes. Pain in the transverse tarsal joint can be decreased by stabilizing the ankle and foot in an AFO. Pain at the knee may require a Knee-Ankle-Foot Orthosis (KAFO).

AFOs are needed for dorsiflexor weakness resulting in drop-foot or slap-foot, for plantar flexor weakness with absent heel rise, and for mediolateral instability. The reason that people with postpolio have so much difficulty with plastic AFOs is that they are usually made in 5 to 10 degrees of dorsiflexion and are then placed in a shoe with a slight positive heel, increasing the angle of the posterior shell to the floor. In standing and walking this causes a knee flexion torque, with buckling of the knee if the quadriceps muscle is weak. Pain occurs because the client tries to straighten the knee by pushing back against the posterior shell of the AFO. If this is the problem, AFOs should be made in slight plantar flexion so that the tibia is perpendicular to the floor in the shoes the client is going to wear. This is the normal position of the ankle for toe and heel clearance.[60] In case of a plantar flexion contracture, more plantar flexion is required in the AFO. Most jointed AFOs are of limited value because they are heavier and bulkier, require a larger shoe than those with metal joints, and do not control the ankle. The advantage of jointed AFOs is their ability to adjust to find the best angle in function.

The floor reaction AFO prohibits all ankle motion and can place forces to control the knee.[50,73,94] The orthosis prevents drop foot, promotes heel rise, provides an extension torque on the proximal tibia to supplement weak quadriceps muscles, and can limit hyperextension of the knee. This orthosis requires precision in fabrication to have the knee extension torque occur only when the tibia is perpendicular to the floor in the gait cycle. When this orthosis is used with rocker bottom shoes to give back motion, a person with a flail foot can walk with a normal gait pattern. Subjects with ligamentous laxity of the knee, excessive tibial torsion, or

paralysis of the quadriceps muscles are poor candidates for this type of AFO.

Heel lifts, shoe inserts, molded foot orthoses, and some normal footwear can provide a number of unobtrusive corrections. Positive heel shoes with a broad base, such as cowboy boots, stacked or Cuban heels, or the Swedish clog,[64] decrease the amount of dorsiflexion and plantar flexion motion and work needed in the gait cycle. Rocker bottom soles provide mechanical heel rise to assist the calf muscles and are available commercially or can be added to shoes. Work boots, dress boots, or basketball shoes may provide needed ankle stability.

People with unilateral lower-extremity paralysis or pain stand with weight on the stronger limb, which must perform continuous, high-level isometric contractions (Fig. 19-6). Unloading the stronger leg requires restoration of weight bearing on the more involved leg using a KAFO or, in some instances, an AFO which prevents advance of the tibia in the stance phase.[50,73,79,94]

Fifty percent of ambulatory postpolio individuals walk with an obvious forward lean. This posture requires continuous contraction of the erector spinae muscles and leads to back pain, often radiating to the hip and leg. The forward lean posture is found in people with quadriceps muscle paresis and in those with ankle weakness. Those with quadriceps weakness must move the center of gravity of the

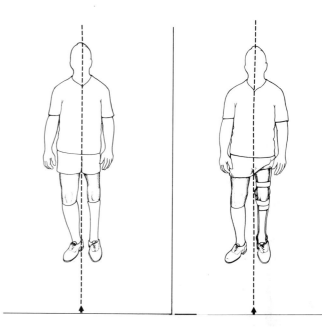

Fig. 19-6. This man has paralysis of the left lower extremity with severe fatigue, low-back pain, pain and weakness in the right lower extremity, and decreased function. He can be seen to bear weight and stand on the right leg. Application of a left KAFO with a free knee joint (with a drop lock for use in prolonged standing and walking on rough terrain) and a limited motion ankle joint unloaded his right leg and permitted him to walk in an erect posture. His pain disappeared and he has regained function at work and in social activities.

body anterior to the knee axis to lock the knee and prevent knee flexion in stance. This posterior force also produces ligamentous instability and genu recurvatum (see Fig. 19-3). In some instances light-weight athletic knee braces allowing 10 to 15 degrees of hyperextension provide adequate control. More often a KAFO with an offset knee joint allowing necessary hyperextension is required.[15,63,65] People with dorsiflexor muscle paralysis or ankle instabilities walk in the forward lean posture to watch the floor and foot placement to avoid tripping and falling. Athletic ankle supports or boots may be sufficient to control some ankle instabilities. Molded and posted plastic AFOs with or without ankle joints are needed for more control. Flexible plastic AFOs and the dynamic spring dorsiflexion assists correct simple drop foot.[79] Once the need to walk in a forward-leaning posture is removed, the person can walk upright, and back pain may disappear in a few days.

Walking with lateral trunk shift in the stance phase (gluteus medius gait) produces abnormal forces and joint dysfunction from the spine to the foot (Fig. 19-7). These forces can be reduced by use of a forearm crutch or cane.

People who are long-term crutch walkers with or without orthoses and those whose walking is slow, precarious, or labored should be guided to consider use of motorized vehicles as their primary form of locomotion. Orthotic corrections or applications may be indicated to improve transfers and short-distance walking.

Exercise. With the onset of new problems of weakness and fatigue, most people with PPS have been directed or are self-directed to engage in strengthening, aerobic, or sports

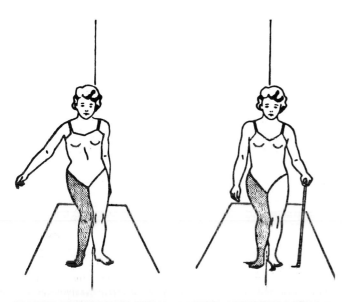

Fig. 19-7. Lateral trunk shift in a postpolio individual to illustrate abnormal forces occurring in the back, knee, and ankle with resulting joint dysfunction and pain. Prevention of these abnormal forces and some correction can be provided by use of a cane or forearm crutch. (Adapted from Ducroquet and others. *Walking and limping—a study of normal and pathological walking,* Philadelphia, 1968, JB Lippincott Co.)

exercise programs. Instead of correcting problems, these activities produce an increase in fatigue, muscle weakness, and pain.[3,10,61] Exercise may cause increased problems because it is applied to motor units that are working at high levels of capacity and that may be in a state of decompensation. The initial objective of treatment is to reduce the load on the muscles, eliminate the pain and fatigue, and build a reserve capacity. Most clients with PPS are willing to stop exercise as part of life-style changes, at least on a trial basis. Later exercise can be evaluated for purpose, magnitude of energy expenditure relative to total energy expenditure, and the risk/benefit ratio to present and future muscle performance.

Exercises for stretching fascia and muscles, mobilizing joints, reeducating muscles to stabilize joints in activity, increasing joint nutrition, and decreasing edema are frequently used in therapy for the treatment of pain and injuries. For clients with PPS these exercises can be used safely with modification and careful monitoring. A beginning rule of thumb is for the therapist to estimate the intensity that the subject can tolerate and then apply one half, reduce the estimated repetitions to one half, and double the time of estimated rest periods. If fatigue does not last longer than 30 minutes or appear in the next 2 days and if pain does not increase, the program can be continued and gradually increased. Increased fatigue or pain is an indication for reevaluation of the exercise (and any other activities that the person may have engaged in) with consideration of decreasing the amount of exercise or activity.

The same modifications can be used in reconditioning exercises. Weakness of disuse may occur with fractures, illness, or surgery. If a preillness manual muscle test is not available, it is important to recreate with the client a gross picture of preillness muscle function. Individuals with PPS can relate what and to what extent they could move previously, if the right questions are asked. It is important to obtain this information to avoid extensive efforts to try to strengthen muscles that are below functional strength and to identify new peripheral nerve lesions that may have occurred.

Many clients with PPS have excessive muscle tension (especially around the head and neck) and an inability to relax or to maximize rest periods. Initially, they may need treatment to alleviate pain, regain motion, and develop a home exercise program. Ongoing valuable exercise programs are relaxation exercises, imagery, Feldenkrais body awareness techniques,[72] beginning yoga (avoiding all difficult exercises), and nonresistive underwater exercise.

Many recreational and sporting activities have important family and social purposes. These activities should be evaluated with the client for possible modifications that would reduce strenuous aspects but retain the client's ability to participate in the activity. Motorized carts, ATVs, golf carts, snowmobiles, or trucks permit continued participation in outdoor activities such as camping, birding, fishing, playing golf, winter recreation, scouting, or coaching youth activities. Horseback riding can be continued if mounting and dismounting platforms are available. Those who enjoy the water should avoid competitive lap swimming but can participate in easy recreational and family fun activities. A few golfers are able to continue their sport in a modified manner, using a golf cart, longer clubs, graphite shafts, and learning to swing the club using momentum rather than brute force. One mother hired a teenager to pick up toys, push swings, serve refreshments, and take children to the bathroom on the days when neighborhood friends came to play. This approach allowed the mother to be sedentary but interact with the children.

Individuals with postpolio are exercise-oriented from their early association of exercise and muscle strength recovery. Most of them again request exercises to make their muscles stronger, to lose weight, and to improve cardiorespiratory fitness. Unfortunately for the person with postpolio, these types of exercises need to be strenuous or of long duration to be effective. Exercise should be evaluated by the therapist in relation to the client's total activity and the risk/benefit ratio. Those who have asymptomatic postpolio (and are in good health) should respond well to appropriate exercise programs. True gains in muscle strength will be limited because most people with postpolio long ago achieved their maximum strength limits. Clients should know the signs of PPS and should exercise in moderation. Those who have PPS with muscle pain and fatigue are already getting too much exercise in their daily activities. These people need to further modify their life-styles and avoid placing additional loads on decompensated muscles. When the muscle pain and fatigue are eliminated and a reserve capacity has been developed, additional activities and exercise can be considered. Most people will opt to increase nonfatiguing functional activities or social recreation rather than exercise in and of itself.

The box lists the general guidelines for activity and exercise given to clients with postpolio and PPS. Spencer and Jackson's caution in the 1950s regarding treatment of the person with poliomyelitis remains an important guideline today: "The patient's capacity to do work must always continue to exceed the demands placed upon him."[82]

Exercise studies. A few exercise studies using quantitative measurements have been done with subjects with postpolio. Aerobic testing using modified protocols to reduce fatigue has been used on the treadmill,[21] bicycle ergometer,[41] and arm ergometer.[46] There were no cardiorespiratory training effects in the first study, probably due to the low intensity of the exercise, but the duration and distance of walking increased.[21] The two ergometry studies showed an increase in maximum oxygen consumption of 15% and 19%, which is a training effect comparable to normal values for age. There were, however, no changes in blood pressure or heart rate, particularly the expected decrease in resting heart rate that occurs with aerobic training.[21,41,44] Although the

Postpoliomyelitis*

General guidelines for physical activity and exercise

- Obtain a complete medical examination. The symptoms of the late effect of polio are similar and may be combined with the symptoms of other conditions. Self-diagnosis is dangerous.
- Preserve and protect your limited muscle and joint capacities. Post-polio problems are caused by long-term overuse at high levels of capacity.
- Control and reduce body weight by permanent modification of nutritional habits without use of exercise.
- Make a detailed diary of your activities in type, time, and amount over days and averaged for a week or months. Analyze, set priorities, and use methods to conserve energy.
- Maintain function by doing things the easy way. Take advantage of modern comforts and technology including motorization and electronics.
- Correct injury producing abnormal postures in sleeping, SITTING, standing, and working using mechanical supports and assists.
- Break up activities into parts with rest periods or change of activity. Incorporate frequent rest periods or a nap as needed.
- Learn techniques of relaxation or imagery to maximize rest periods.
- Avoid unessential physical activity such as walking, bicycling, or swimming laps and aerobic, "toning", body building or strengthening exercises.
- Preserve muscle capacity for important function, work, family, and social activities.
- LISTEN TO YOUR BODY! Build a reserve capacity and avoid facing every posture and activity with exhaustion or pain in muscles or joints.

*Printed with permission of the Institute for Rehabilitation and Research Postpolio Clinic, Houston, Tex.

intensity of the exercise protocols had to be reduced for some of the subjects, none had to terminate the exercise because of overuse symptoms, nor did these symptoms occur at the end of the studies. A problem in evaluating these studies is that it is not always clear whether the postpolio study subjects were asymptomatic, symptomatic (PPS), or mixed.

Isokinetic and isometric dynamometers have been used to record maximum muscle forces (or torques) in postpolio subjects before and after resistive exercise programs designed to increase muscle strength. Two of the studies were of single cases[31,57] and two had 12 and 17 subjects.[23,27] Both of the multisubject studies tested the quadriceps femoris. Einarsson and Grimby[23] reported an average gain of 29% in isometric strength and 24% in isokinetic strength over a period of 6 weeks. The same type of muscle contractions, however, were used for testing and training. Fillyaw and others[27] reported a strength gain of 8% over a 2-year period. An isometric contraction was used for testing and concentric-eccentric contractions for the exercise. These results do not compare to the strength gains of 100% and higher made by normal subjects undergoing training, but rather compare to serial testing when no exercise is done.[58,59] For example Munin and others[58] measured the affected and nonaffected quadriceps muscle every 6 months over 3 years to document muscle weakness in persons with PPS. They reported increases in muscle strength up to 25%. In older persons without polio, test performance gains of the quadriceps increased an average of 174% in 90-year-old subjects[26] and 107% in 60- to 72-year-old men.[30] In these two studies thigh muscle area (as documented by computed tomography [CT] scan) increased by 9% and 11%, respectively, indicating an increase in muscle bulk.

Because there are neural adaptations specific to the type of muscle contraction used for measurement and training, it is difficult to determine the differences in true increases in strength from the ability to increase a specific test performance. Another term for this phenomenon or increase in performance is *motor learning*. The theory states that the subject learns to perform the measurement or the exercise better without true gains in strength. This happens even with an apparently simple weekly maximum isometric contraction.[74] Evidence of this phenomenon can be seen when improvements are made in the opposite untrained muscle group (transfer of training), when the apparent strength gains are maintained for months after cessation of the training, and when there are no increases in the size of the muscle. The greatest increases in test performance occur when the muscle contraction is the same for both the test and the training. Smaller increases are seen when the measurement and training muscle contractions are different and when measures to decrease the effect of motor learning have been used.

The neural adaptation specific to the type of measurement or training is illustrated in the following study on older men.[30] Multiple tests to assess strength were performed. The training program required lifting and lowering 80% of the weight of one repetition maximum (1 RM), which was assessed weekly. After 12 weeks, there were average increases in quadriceps muscle strength of 104% for the 1 RM, 7% for maximum isometric, 8% for maximum isokinetic at 60 degrees/second, and 10% for isokinetic at 240 degrees/second. In addition there was an increase in cross-sectional area of the quadriceps of 10%, and muscle biopsy showed approximately 30% increase in muscle fiber size.[30] This study illustrates some of the complexities in designing or evaluating studies that attempt to measure changes in muscle strength.

Psychosocial considerations

The psychosocial issues confronting persons with PPS often are more disruptive than the physical problems.* To better understand this condition it is helpful to know about

---

*References 29, 33, 43, 47, 48, and 87.

the background of those with postpolio and a few of the myths that helped to shape their lives.

During the polio epidemics of the 1940s and 1950s, fear of the disease was rampant. Parents kept children out of public swimming pools in the summer, away from movies, and from congregating in groups. If children did get polio, many parents suffered guilt feelings, which often were expressed later by encouraging the child to high levels of physical achievement. Approval and perks were gained by activities such as walking farther or faster and keeping up with or exceeding the performance of siblings and friends. The best treatment available was provided to all polio victims by the March of Dimes. To receive this treatment, polio patients were hospitalized for months at a time away from their families, friends, and communities. Many of the patients were children who felt abandoned, afraid, and totally dependent on strangers for their care and nurturing. The polio patient was expected to be a "good patient" and to "work hard." Indeed, they did work hard to reeducate weakened muscles and compensate for lost function.[14,16,34,75] Later in the recovery process, parents made the decisions for children to undergo multiple surgical procedures so that the heavy braces could be eliminated and the children would look "normal and fit in." One can understand why clients react so negatively to the suggestion of orthotics.

One of the myths that flourished in the polio years was "don't wallow in self-pity." Courage, determination, and cheerfulness were attributes to be prized. The myth gained strength when polio patients' levels of disability were compared—"Look at him. He can't move. You should be grateful. It could be much worse!" The children were often shamed into silence and learned not to express feelings about their disability.

Coping styles. Those with postpolio developed several styles to cope with their disability. Maynard and Roller[55] described coping styles according to severity of muscular involvement. *Passers* are those with little or no obvious physical involvement. They are able to hide atrophy with clothing, and they avoid activities that reveal the weakness. Many invested much energy in projecting normality to others and were so adept at denial that they disconnected themselves from the polio experience. Often spouses do not know of the history of polio. This group can develop the most severe cases of PPS. They do not identify with others with postpolio and they are difficult to help. *Minimizers* are those with obvious physical involvement such as a limp, an atrophied extremity, or use of an assistive device. They usually have pushed themselves to function at a normal or supernormal level. Physical imperfections have been ignored by tuning out pain and discomfort brought about by their high levels of activity. They suffer tremendous pain before they will acknowledge the late effects of polio. *Identifiers* are the most severely impaired of the postpolio groups. They usually require wheelchairs for mobility and many have respiratory involvement. Attaining independence in self-care activities required great effort and persistence. Identifiers integrated their disability into their self-image and have led active, productive lives. They are often involved in disabled rights and independent living movements.

The majority of polio survivors were adept at disguising their impairments and achieved high levels of productivity, enabling them to disappear into society.[87] The rate at which these individuals have been educated, employed, and married indicates that their success at living "normal" lives. However, they have pushed themselves and lived with internal and external stresses similar to those persons with Type A behavior.[14] Many polio survivors may have compensated for underlying low self-esteem and fear of losing control of their lives by exhibiting this excessive drive.

Response to new diagnosis. When the client seeks help for new problems, the encounters with the medical community can be frustrating. Most health professionals are unfamiliar with the late effects of polio and as a consequence, the procedure for arriving at a diagnosis of PPS can take time and involve a series of physician consultations.[7,14,16,37] Publicity by support groups has helped refer clients to postpolio clinics or to specialists who have knowledge of PPS.[68]

The response to the diagnosis of PPS can vary from relief to despair. Relief occurs in those who have been searching for a diagnosis and those who have been told their symptoms were psychosomatic. Despair occurs as the treatment program of life-style changes is described. Most of the clients are distressed when diagnosed with PPS and are resistant to making changes in their lives. They have worked hard to accomplish their goals and are at the peak of their careers. They distrust the medical community because they are presented with management suggestions that are opposed to the ones they followed to recovery decades ago. They are being told that "use it or lose it" and "no pain, no gain" does not apply to them. Clients wonder whether the shift in philosophy is valid. They are disillusioned because their former medical heroes/heroines did not foresee their future problems.

The individual's feeling of pride and accomplishment about the initial recovery is often diminished, and he or she experiences a feeling of failure. These individuals fear the future for themselves and their loved ones. Some will not be able to hide physical problems and will have to admit their disability. They are anxious about the prospects of changing roles with their families, friends, and co-workers.[7,16,55] Many postpolio clients experience the reemergence of repressed feelings. It is as if they are reliving the initial illness. The defenses and coping strategies they used successfully for so many years have broken down and they experience overwhelming anxieties and conflicts.[7]

Most people who had polio never grieved their physical losses. They were sick for 2 weeks, and the following months

and years were focused on muscle strength gains and improvements in function. There was no time for sadness and mourning necessary for emotional healing. To gain acceptance of their changing situation, these people need to grieve their physical losses both old and new.* Tate and others[83] reported an association of feelings of depression with severity of physical symptoms in individuals with PPS who lacked appropriate coping behaviors. Some clients suffer from clinical depression and need treatment. Most clients could benefit from individual, group, or family psychotherapy during this period of emotional turmoil.

Compliance. A few clients readily accept suggestions for life-style changes and start making these changes immediately; a few clients refuse to consider any life-style modifications. Most clients, however, make needed changes but require support, patience, and time for processing and decision making.

Physical and occupational therapists can help clients in many ways to function while living with purpose and quality of life. First, it is important to respect their knowledge of their body and how it functions. Many of these people still remember the anatomical names of their muscles. They have developed their own unique methods of handling, transferring, walking, and performing activities. Attempts to "correct" their performance or do it another way can be disastrous and have resulted in unnecessary fractures. It is extremely important to follow the client's directions for transfers and other functional activities. Another important help is to allow the client to vent feelings about the new challenges, their past high levels of physical achievement, and their previous treatment.

Compliance of the postpolio client is markedly improved by the therapist's ability to provoke or alleviate pain in the initial evaluation and to suggest management strategies that are accepted as normal. Use of cold packs and lumbar pillows to relieve pain during the initial visit can markedly promote compliance. Recommendations for cervical pillows, ergonometric chairs, computer wrist rests, or water beds help pave the way for more emotionally charged suggestions such as orthoses, decreasing ambulation, or motorized carts. Therapists can be a source of information about postpolio support groups.[68] People in these groups have faced their losses and many have adopted new coping skills. The support groups eagerly share knowledge about every facet of living with PPS, and many of the members can be positive role models for the newly diagnosed individual.

Therapists can make recommendations in a way that helps clients view compliance as life enhancing and empowering and not as capitulation and failure. Polio survivors should be reassured that the resilience and ingenuity that helped them live successfully for so many decades will also enable them to face this new challenge.

---

* References 7, 8, 13, 37, 49, and 51.

J.R. had normal muscle strength in his arms and trunk, major weakness in his left leg, and what he considered a normal right leg. His complaint was of pain and weakness in his strong right leg and low back pain. It was noted that he shifted to the right when standing and bore almost all his weight on the right extremity. All of the muscles in this extremity were in a constant state of contraction. He accepted a left KAFO and all of his pain was eliminated. He also decreased his weight by 20 pounds.

W.N. has almost total body paralysis and is ventilatory dependent. She has a few muscles active at a fair or less value in her left hand and she uses an electronic feeder to move her shoulder and elbow, which allows her to operate a computer and phone. She has been employed full-time as a department head in a hospital for 30 years. She is now having pain and increased weakness in the muscles of her left hand. Evaluation showed that she used these muscles extensively for gestures as she talked. She was advised to avoid contracting these muscles except when needed to operate her computer, write, or eat. She did so and the symptoms disappeared.

M.B. has generalized muscle weakness in her legs and walks with a drop foot gait. Her major complaint was low back pain. Evaluation of her gait showed that she walked with a forward lean to watch the floor. AFOs were recommended. With these she was able to walk in an erect position and her back pain was eliminated.

J.S. is a 45-year-old teacher with paraplegic type involvement. He walked with long leg braces and crutches for over 30 years. About a year ago his right shoulder became painful with weight bearing, and in a few months the left shoulder also became painful. He was advised to use a motorized cart as his primary form of locomotion. He continued to walk with braces and crutches, and his physician recommended physical therapy for treatment of shoulder pain. His shoulder pain increased. When seen in Postpolio Clinic he had bicepital tendonitis and painful arcs with shoulder flexion. He was advised to use a motorized cart for his primary form of locomotion and to obtain a van and a lift to place him and the cart into the van. He was advised to apply to agencies for financial help to supplement his resources for needed equipment. Physical therapy treatment was recommended to relieve and control shoulder pain. He followed these recommendations with total relief of pain. He is now independent in his community and particularly enjoys going to malls, theme parks, and sporting events with his family. He regrets that he did not accept motorized locomotion sooner.

J.W. is a 40-year-old single mother of two children. She self reported a history of drug abuse. Her primary involvement from polio was in the right lower extremity. She walked with a marked lateral trunk shift (gluteus medius gait) on stance phase and drop foot in the swing phase. She had acute pain in the hips, radiating posteriorly to the knee and more severe on the right. The pain was worse in the morning and decreased as the day progressed. It was exacerbated by sitting, standing, and walking. She moved constantly from one position to another. The sacroiliac joints were acutely painful to palpation. Compression of the ilia relieved the pain. She was advised to have outpatient therapy for treatment of sacroiliitis, but because of financial and transportation problems, she requested alternatives. She was advised to obtain a sacroiliac belt, cane for use in the left hand, cold packs to apply to her sacroiliac joints six to eight times a day, and a right AFO. She was advised to correct her sitting posture with lumbar supports and a well-fitted clerical chair with arms to stretch her piriformis muscles, and to use nonsteroidal antiinflammatory medication. This regimen was quite rigorous to undertake without assistance, but she was able to comply with all the recommendations and her pain was virtually eliminated. Perhaps the most important aspect of the program is that she gained control of the pain and it has now become insignificant.

CASE EXAMPLES

People with PPS usually have multiple problems and require multiple modifications and life-style changes to relieve or eliminate the fatigue, pain, and rate of progression of muscle weakness. Case histories are long and complex. To reduce the complexity in the above case examples, single problems and their solutions are presented.

CONCLUSION

The understanding of (1) polio and acute treatment of this disease and (2) PPS and its management is still evolving. The therapist needs to update his or her understanding to provide the best treatment solutions for each individual.

REFERENCES

1. Agre JC and Rodriquez AA: Neuromuscular function in polio survivors, *Orthopedics* 14:1343-1347, 1991.
2. Agre JC and Rodriquez AA: Neuromuscular function in polio survivors at one-year follow up, *Arch Phys Med Rehabil* 72:7-10, 1991.
3. Agre JC, Rodriquez AA, and Tafel JA: Late effects of polio: critical review of the literature on neuromuscular function, *Arch Phys Med Rehabil* 72:923-931, 1991.
4. Agre JC and Rodriquez AA: Intermittent isometric activity: its effect on muscle fatigue in postpolio subjects, *Arch Phys Med Rehabil* 72:971-975, 1991.
5. Bach J and others: Mouth intermittent positive pressure ventilation in the management of postpolio respiratory insufficiency, *Chest* 91:859, 1987.
6. Bach JR and Alba AS: Pulmonary dysfunction and sleep disordered breathing as post-polio sequelae: evaluation and management, *Orthopedics* 14:1329-1337, 1991.
7. Backman ME: The post polio patient: psychological issues, *J Rehabil* 53 4:23-26, 1987.
8. Beisser A: *Flying without wings*, New York, 1990, Bantam Ed.
9. Bennett RL and Knowlton GC: Overwork weakness in partially denervated skeletal muscle, *Clin Orthop* 12.22, 1958.
10. Borlly MH, Strauser WW, and Hall KM: Fatigue in postpolio syndrome, *Arch Phys Med Rehabil* 72:115-118, 1991.
11. Birk TJ: Poliomyelitis and the post-polio syndrome: exercise capacities and adaptation—current research, future directions, and widespread applicability, *Med Sci Sports Exerc* 25:466-472, 1993.

12. Bodian D: The virus, the nerve cell, and paralysis, *Bull Johns Hopkins Hosp* 83:1, 1948.

13. Bozworth-Campbell A: *Life is goodbye, life is hello,* ed 2, Minneapolis, 1986, CompCare.

14. Bruno RL and Frick NM: The psychology of polio as prelude to post polio syndrome: behavior modification and psychotherapy. *Orthopedics* 14 (11):1185-1193, 1991.

15. Clark D, Perry J, and Lunsford T: Case studies—orthotic management of the adult post polio patient, *Orthop Prosthet* 40:43, 1986.

16. Conrady L and others: Psychological characteristics of polio survivors: a preliminary report, *Arch Phys Med Rehabil:* 1 70:458-463, 1989.

17. Cornill L: Sur un cas de paralysie generale spinale anterieure subaipue, suivi d'autopsie, *Gaz Med* (Paris) 4:127, 1875.

18. Dail C: Clinical aspects of glossopharyngeal breathing: report of its use by 100 post-polio patients, *JAMA* 158:445, 1955.

19. Dalakas MC and others: Late effects of poliomyelitis muscular atrophy: clinical, virologic and immunologic studies, *Rev Infect Dis* 6(suppl):S562, 1984.

20. Dalakas MC and others: A long term follow-up study of patients with post-poliomyelitis neuromuscular symptoms, *N Engl J Med* 314:959, 1986.

21. Dean E and Ross J: Effect of modified aerobic training on movement energetics in polio survivors, *Orthopedics* 14:1243-1246, 1991.

22. Ducroquet R, Ducroquet J, and Ducroquet P: *Walking and limping—a study of normal and pathological walking,* Philadelphia, 1968, JB Lippincott Co.

23. Einarsson G and Grimby G: Strengthening exercise program in post-polio subjects. In Halstead L and Wiechers D, editors: *Research and clinical aspects of the late effects of poliomyelitis,* White Plains NY, 1987, March of Dimes Birth Defects Series 23:4.

24. Fergelson C: Glossopharyngeal breathing as an aid to the coughing mechanism in patients with chronic poliomyelitis in a respirator, *N Engl J Med* 254:611, 1956.

25. Fetell MR and others: A benign motor neuron disorder: delayed cramps and fasciculations after poliomyelitis or myelitis, *Ann Neurol* 11:423, 1982.

26. Fiatarone MA and others: High-intensity strength training in nonagenarians, *JAMA* 263:3029-3034, 1990.

27. Fillyaw MJ and others: The effects of long-term non-fatiguing resistance exercise in subjects with post-polio syndrome, *Orthopedics* 14:1253-1256, 1991.

28. Fisher A: Sleep-disordered breathing as a late effect of poliomyelitis. In Halstead L and Wiechers D, editors: *Research and clinical aspects of the late effects of poliomyelitis,* White Plains, NY, 1987, March of Dimes Birth Defects Series 23:4.

29. Frick N: Post-polio sequelae and the psychology of second disability, *Orthopedics* 8:851, 1985.

30. Frontera WR and others: Strength conditioning in older men: skeletal muscle hypertrophy and improved function, *J Appl Physiol* 64:1038-1044, 1988.

31. Gross MT and Schuch CP: Exercise programs for patients with post-polio syndrome: a case report, *Phys Ther* 69:72-76, 1989.

32. Halstead L and Wiechers D, editors: *Late effects of poliomyelitis,* Miami, 1985, Symposia Foundation.

33. Halstead L and Wiechers D, editors: *Research and clinical aspects of the late effects of poliomyelitis,* White Plains, NY, 1987, March of Dimes Birth Defects Series 23:4.

34. Halstead L: The residual of polio in the aged, *Top Geriatric Rehabil* 3(4): 9-26, 1988.

35. Halstead L: Assessment and differential diagnosis for post-polio syndrome. *Orthopedics* 14(11):1209-1217, 1991.

36. Hamilton EA, Nichols PIR, and Tair GBW: Late onset of respiratory insufficiency after poliomyelitis; a preliminary communication, *Ann Physiol Med* 10:223, 1970.

37. Hanson B: *Picking up the pieces: healing ourselves after personal loss,* Dallas, 1990, Taylor.

38. Hill R and others: Sleep apnea syndrome after poliomyelitis, *Am Rev Resp Dis* 127:129, 1983.

39. Huckstep RL: *Poliomyelitis: a guide for developing countries including appliances and rehabilitation of the disabled,* New York, 1975, Churchill Livingstone.

40. Iddings DM, Smith LK, and Spencer WA: Muscle testing. Part 2. Reliability in clinical use, *Phys Ther Rev* 41:249-256, 1961.

41. Jones DR and others: Cardiorespiratory responses to aerobic training by patients with postpoliomyelitis sequelae, *JAMA* 261:3255-3259, 1989.

42. Jubelt B and Cashman N: Neurological manifestation of the post-polio syndrome, *Crit Rev Neurobiol* 3:199, 1987.

43. Kaufert J and Kaufert PA: Aging and respiratory polio, *Rehabil Digest* 13:15, 1982.

44. Kayser-Gatchalian MC: Late muscular atrophy after poliomyelitis, *Eur Neurol* 10:371, 1973.

45. Kendall H and Kendall F: Orthopedic and physical therapy objectives in poliomyelitis treatment, *Physiother Rev* 27:2, 1947.

46. Kriz JL and others: Cardiorespiratory responses to upper extremity aerobic training by postpolio subjects, *Arch Phys Med Rehabil* 73:49-54, 1992.

47. Laurie G and Raymond J, editors: *Proceedings of Rehabilitation Gazette's Second International Post-Polio Conference and Symposium on Living Independently with a Severe Disability,* St Louis, 1984, Gazette International Networking Institute.

48. Laurie G and Raymond J, editors: *Proceedings of Gazette International Networking Institute's Third Internation Polio and Independent Living Conference, St Louis,* 1986, Gazette International Networking Institute.

49. Leech P and Singer Z: *Acknowledgement: opening to grief of unacceptable loss,* Taytonville, Calif., 1988, Wintercreek Publications.

50. Lehmann J and others: Ankle-foot orthoses: effect on abnormalities in tibial nerve paralysis, *Arch Phys Med Rehabil* 66:212, 1985.

51. LeMaistre J: *Beyond rage: the emotional impact of chronic physical illness,* Oak Park, 1985, Alpine Guild.

52. McComas A, Upton A, and Sica R: Motor neuron disease and aging, *Lancet* 2:1474, 1973.

53. Martinez A, Ferrer M, and Conde M: Electrophysiological features in patients with non-progressive and late progressive weakness after paralytic poliomyelitis: conventional EMG automatic analysis of the electromyogram and single fiber electromyography study, *EMG Clin Neurophysical* 24:469, 1984.

54. Martinez A, Perez M, and Ferrer M: Chronic partial denervation is more widespread than is suspected clinically in paralytic poliomyelitis—an electrophysiological study, *Eur Neurol* 22:314, 1983.

55. Maynard FM and Roller S: Recognizing typical coping styles of polio survivors can improve re-rehabilitation, *AM J Phys Med Rehabil* 70(2): 70-72, 1991.

56. Maynard F: Post-polio sequelae—differential diagnosis and management, *Orthopedics* 8:857, 1985.

57. Milner-Brown HS: Muscle strengthening in a post-polio subject through a high-resistance weight-training program, *Arch Phys Med Rehabil* 74:1165-1167, 1993.

58. Munin MC and others: Postpoliomyelitis muscle weakness: a prospective study of quadriceps muscle strength, *Arch Phys Med Rehabil* 72:729-733, 1991.

59. Munsat TL and Andres P: Preliminary observations on long-term muscle force changes in the post-polio syndrome. In Halstead LS and Wiechers DO, editors: *Birth Defects: Original Article Series.* 23:329-334, 1987.

60. Murray MP, Drought AB, and Kory BC: Walking patterns of normal men, *J Bone Joint Surg [Am]* 46:335, 1964.

61. Peach PE: Overwork weakness with evidence of muscle damage in a patient with residual paralysis from polio, *Arch Phys Med Rehabil* 71:248-250, 1990.

62. Peach P and Olejnik S: Effect of treatment and non-compliance on post-polio sequelae, *Orthopedics* 14:1199-1203, 1991.

63. Perry J and Hislop H, editors: *Principles of lower extremity bracing,* Washington, DC, 1967, American Physical Therapy Association.

64. Perry J, Gromley J, and Lunsford T: Rocker shoe as a walking aid in multiple sclerosis, *Arch Phys Med Rehabil* 62:59, 1981.

65. Perry J and Fleming C: Polio: long-term problems, *Orthopedics* 8:877, 1985.

66. Perry J, Barnes G, and Gronley JK: The postpolio syndrome: an overuse phenomena, *Clin Orthop* 233-145-162, 1988.

67. Potts CS: A case of progressive muscular atrophy occurring in a man who had acute poliomyelitis nineteen years previously, *Univ Pennsylvania Med Bull* 16:31, 1903.

68. *Post-Polio Directory—1993,* St Louis, 1993, International Polio Network.

69. Rodriguez AA and Agre JC: Electrophysiological study of the quadriceps muscles during fatiguing exercise and recovery: a comparison of symptomatic and asymptomatic postpolio patients and controls, *Arch Phys Med Rehabil* 72:993-997, 1991.

70. Rosenheimer J: Effects of chronic stress and exercise on age-related changes in end-plate architecture, *J Neurophysiol* 53:1582, 1985.

71. Rosenheimer J and Smith D: Differential changes in the end-plate architecture of functionally diverse muscles during aging, *J Neurophysiol* 53:1567, 1985.

72. Ruth S and Kegerreis S: Facilitating cervical flexion using a Feldenkrais method: awareness through movement, *J Orthop Sports Phys Ther* 16:25-29, 1992.

73. Saltiel J: A one piece laminated knee locking short leg brace, *Orthop Prosthet* 23:68, 1969.

74. Schenck J and Forward E: Quantitative strength changes with test repetitions, *Phys Ther* 45:562, 1965.

75. Scheer J and Luborsky ML: The cultural context of polio biographies, *Orthopedics* 14 (11):1173, 1181, 1991.

76. Sharrard WJW: The distribution of permanent paralysis in the lower limb in poliomyelitis, *J Bone Joint Surg* 37(B):540, 1955.

77. Sleeper G, Kignman P, and Armeni M: Nasal continuous positive pressure for at-home treatment of sleep apnea, *Respir Care* 30:90, 1985.

78. Smith E, Rosenblatt P, and Limauro A: The role of the sympathetic nervous system in acute poliomyelitis, *J Pediatr* 34:1, 1949.

79. Smith L and McDermott K: Pain in post-poliomelitis: addressing causes versus effects. In Halstead L and Wiechers D, editors: *Research and clinical aspects of the late effects of poliomyelitis,* White Plains, NY, 1987, March of Dimes Birth Defect Series 23:4.

80. Spencer GT: Respiratory insufficiency in scoliosis: clinical management and home care. In Zorab PA, editor: *Scoliosis,* London, 1977, Academic Press.

81. Spencer WA: *Treatment of acute poliomyelitis,* Springfield, Ill, 1956, Charles C Thomas.

82. Spencer WA and Jackson RB: Poliomyelitis, acute. In Conn HF, editor: *Current Therapy.* Philadelphia, 1957, WB Saunders.

83. Tate DG and others: Prevalence and associated features of depression and psychological distress in polio survivors, *Arch Phys Med Rehabil* 74:1056-1060, 1993.

84. Thompson LV: Effects of age and training on skeletal muscle physiology and performance, *Phys Ther* 74:71-81, 1994.

85. Thompson W and Jansen JKS: The extent of sprouting of remaining motor units in partly denervated immature and adult rat soleus muscle, *Neuroscience* 2:523, 1977.

86. Tomlinson BE and Irving D: The numbers of limb motor neurons in the human lumbosacral cord throughout life, *J Neurol Sci* 34:213, 1977.

87. Trieschmann R: *Aging with a disability,* New York, 1987, Demos Publications.

88. Trojan DA, Gendron D, and Cashman N: Electrophysiology and electrodiagnosis of the post-polio motor unit, *Orthopedics* 14:1333-1361, 1991.

89. Waring WP, Davidoff G, and Werner R: Serum creatine kinase in the post-polio population, *Am J Phys Med Rehabil* 68:86-90, 1989.

90. Waring WP and McLaurin TM: Correlation of creatine kinase and gait measurement in the postpolio population: a corrected version, *Arch Phys Med Rehabil* 73:447-450, 1992.

91. Werner RA, Waring W, and Maynard F: Osteoarthritis of the hand and wrist in the post poliomyelitis population, *Arch Phys Med Rehabil* 73:1069-1072, 1992.

92. Wiechers D and Hubbel S: Late changes in the motor unit after acute poliomyelitis, *Muscle Nerve* 4:524, 1981.

93. World Health Organization: Poliomyelitis in 1985. Part I, *Weekly Epidemiological Record* 62:273, 1987.

94. Yang C and others: Floor reaction orthosis: clinical experience, *Orthop Prosthet* 40:33, 1986.

95. Young G: Energy conservation, occupational therapy, and the treatment of post-polio sequelae, *Orthopedics* 14:1233-1239, 1991.

ADDITIONAL READINGS

Krauss P and Goldfischer M: *Why me? coping with grief, loss, and change,* New York, 1988, Bantam.

Carter NB: *Of myths and chicken feet: a polio survivor looks at survival,* Omaha, 1992, NPSA Press.

CHAPTER 20

Multiple Sclerosis

Debra Frankel

KEY TERMS

multiple sclerosis (MS)	myelin basic protein
myelin	Betaseron
demyelination	autoimmune disease
exacerbations and	Copolymer (COP I)
remissions	oral tolerance
relapse and remission	oligodendrocyte

LEARNING OBJECTIVES

After reading this chapter the student/therapist will:
1. Describe the medical basis of multiple sclerosis including epidemiology, etiology, signs and symptoms, diagnosis and course.
2. Describe current research strategies and findings.
3. Describe the medical management of the MS patient.
4. Identify the unique psychosocial and neuropsychological effects of MS.
5. Identify appropriate rehabilitation goals, formulate a rehabilitation plan, and develop rehabilitation strategies to maximize function and quality of life.

BACKGROUND

Multiple sclerosis (MS) is one of the most common neurological diseases of young adults. It was first recorded in 1822 by Sir Augustus D'Este, who apparently had the disease and documented in his diary a 25-year search for a cure.[6]

In 1838, Robert Carswell, a British medical illustrator, made drawings of a brainstem and spinal cord, showing patchy, hardened, and discolored tissue he had seen during an autopsy, and in 1842, Jean Cruveilhier, a French physician, observed similar patchy areas that he called "islands of sclerosis" on an autopsy of a paralyzed woman.[6]

It was not until 1868, however, that Jean Martin Charcot formally identified and described MS. He called the disease "sclerose en plaques," describing the hardened patchlike areas found (on autopsy) disseminated throughout the central nervous system (CNS) of individuals with the disease.[6]

In the normal human nervous system, impulses in many nerve fibers travel in excess of 200 mph. This remarkable velocity is achieved, to a large extent, by the insulation property of **myelin,** a complex of lipoprotein layers formed early in development by oligodendroglia in the CNS, which sheaths the axons.

MS is characterized by inflammatory lesions (plaques)—distinct areas of myelin loss scattered throughout the CNS, primarily in the white matter (Fig. 20-1). These plaques of **demyelination** are accompanied by inflammation (or the accumulation of white blood cells and fluid around blood vessels that lie within the CNS). Cell bodies and axons are, for the most part, spared; however, axons may be destroyed when fibrous gliosis (scarring) occurs—thus the observation of sclerotic plaques by medical historians. Because of destruction of myelin, neurotransmission is disrupted.

MS involves demyelination in the CNS only. CNS demyelination also occurs as a predominant finding in several other less common disorders, including acute disseminated encephalomyelitis, optic neuromyelitis, and diffuse cerebral sclerosis.

AN OVERVIEW OF MULTIPLE SCLEROSIS
Epidemiology

MS is generally diagnosed between the ages of 15 and 50 years, with the majority of people in their 30s at the time of diagnosis. It appears more predominantly in women with a ratio of almost 2:1. MS is rare in some races, e.g., African Blacks and Eskimos, and is most predominant in whites.

A number of studies have established geographical patterns of MS prevalence. MS appears more prominently in areas of the world farther from the equator (Fig. 20-2). A related observation is that the location where a person spends the first 15 years of life determines a greater or lesser likelihood of developing MS as opposed to where they live at the time of diagnosis. A person born in the north who moves to the south after age 15 brings with him or her the higher risk of a northerner.[1] The prevalence rate of MS in the northern United States is over 100/100,000, whereas in the southern United States, it is about 30/100,000.[1]

Data collected from incidence in the Faroe, Orkney, and Shetland Islands (in the Northern Atlantic) indicated a rise in recorded cases of MS for a 15- to 25-year period around World War II followed by a drop to prewar rates.[17] This rise and fall suggests that a viral agent may have been introduced by troops who occupied the islands during the war.

Also relevant to the epidemiological picture of MS is genetics. Family studies show a major genetic influence on susceptibility to MS. Five percent of people with MS have a sibling with MS, and about 15% have a close relative with the disease. The mode of inheritance and number of genes involved have not been determined, and it is clear from twin concordance data, that an environmental trigger must also be at play.[13] Epidemiological studies have helped to identify MS as a disease that most probably has an environmental trigger and that occurs in genetically susceptible individuals.

Etiology

It is probable that myelin damage is mediated by the immune system. It appears that in genetically susceptible individuals there is an abnormality in the way in which the immune response is regulated and controlled that results in a widespread attack on the individual's own neural tissue—that is, an autoimmune response. A specific antigen has not yet been identified.

It is theorized that a virus is responsible. However, it is believed to be a ubiquitous virus that infects a large number of people with only a few of the infected developing the secondary process (MS) or an unusual virus with a low rate of infection but a high rate of clinical expression.[5]

Signs and symptoms

Functional and clinical deficits correlate with localized areas of demyelination in the CNS. Because of the great variability of the anatomical location and time sequence of lesions in clients with MS, the clinical manifestations of the disease vary among individuals. Symptoms may develop quickly, within hours, or slowly over several days or weeks. Most commonly, symptoms develop within 6 to 15 hours, although rapidity of onset and appearance of symptoms depend on the locus and size of the underlying lesion. The most common symptoms are motor weakness, paresthesia, unsteady gait, double vision, and micturition disorder (see the box on p. 592 for a summary). Other types of onset, such as hemiplegia, trigeminal neuralgia, and facial palsy, are less common. In many individuals a history of vague functional impairment precedes definite symptoms, and in some definite neurological signs do not confirm initial complaints.

The subject of cognitive and affective changes that are mediated by the MS disease process has recently been addressed in a formalized way. It has been concluded that 50% to 65% of people with MS show evidence of some cognitive impairment. The majority of these individuals have mild impairment, with approximately 10% to 20% showing significant dysfunction. Research does not support the notion that the occurrence of cognitive symptoms is related to severity of physical symptoms or to duration of the disease.[21,22] Specifically, cognitive functions that seem most often affected are short-term memory, conceptual reasoning, and problem solving. Verbal fluency and speed of information processing are sometimes affected. It is rare to see widespread deterioration of intellectual function in MS.[21,28]

Depression appears more common in those with MS than in the general population or those with other medical conditions.[15,16] This finding probably results from a complex interaction of variables including the pathophysiology of the disease, the unique stressors that characterize MS, and the individual's particular circumstances.

A wide variety of symptoms are associated with the disease and should be understood by a therapist dealing with these problems (see the box on p. 592 for a summary of the most common signs and symptoms of MS).

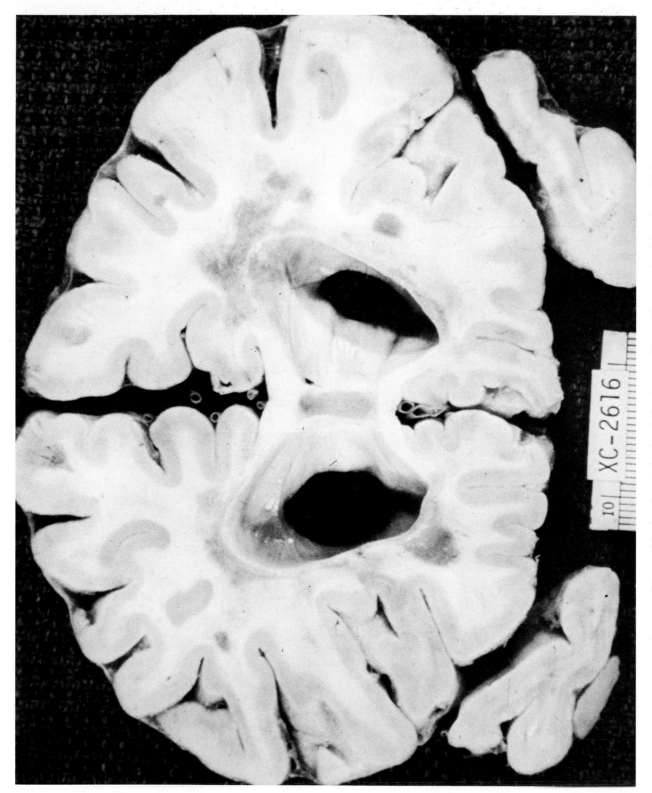

Fig. 20-1. Photo of brain slice indicating MS plaques. (From *Therapeutic claims in multiple sclerosis*, published under the auspices of the International Federation of Multiple Sclerosis Societies, 1982; photo, courtesy Cedric Raine M.D., Albert Einstein College of Medicine, Yeshiva University, New York.)

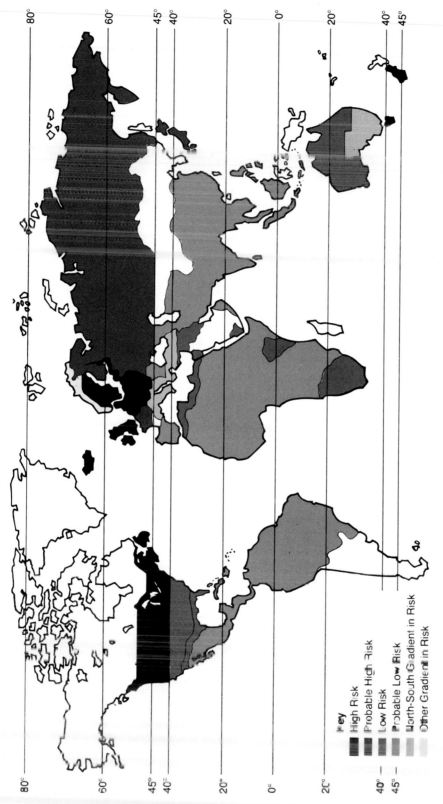

Fig. 20-2. World map indicating MS incidence. (Modified by National Institute of Neurological and Communicative Disorders and Stroke: Multiple sclerosis: hope through research, Nos 79-75, Washington, DC, 1981, National Institutes of Health; from McAlpine D and others: *Multiple sclerosis, a reappraisal*, Edinburgh, 1965, E & S Livingstone, Ltd.)

Key
High Risk
Probable High Risk
Low Risk
Probable Low Risk
North-South Gradient in Risk
Other Gradient in Risk

Summary of common signs and symptoms

Motor symptoms

Spasticity and reflex spasms
Weakness
Contractures
Gait disturbance
Fatigue
Cerebellar and bulbar symptoms
- Resultant swallowing/respiratory difficulties
- Nystagmus
- Intention tremor

Sensory symptoms

Numbness
Pain (most often of musculoskeletal origin)
Paresthesia
Dysesthesia
Distortion of superficial sensation

Visual symptoms

Diminished acuity
Double vision
Scotoma
Ocular pain

Bladder/bowel symptoms

Urgency
Frequency
Incontinence
Urinary retention
Constipation

Sexual symptoms

Impotence
Diminished genital sensation
Diminished genital lubrication

Cognitive and emotional symptoms

Depression
Lability
Disorders of judgment
Agnosia
Memory disturbance
Diminished conceptual thinking
Decreased attention and concentration
Dysphasia

Course and prognosis

The clinical course of MS can be divided roughly into three patterns. One is the classic pattern, characterized by **exacerbations and remissions.** It features sudden onset or reappearance of symptoms that indicate the development of a fresh lesion or extension of an old one. This is followed by partial or total disappearance of the symptom or symptoms. In benign cases (which may account for 20% of the total MS population) this pattern may recur throughout life with little or no residual disability. Mild cases may be evidenced by deficits that accumulate over the series of exacerbations but are not severe enough to interfere with near-normal functioning. Moderate cases carry a more severe degree of residual deficit, which subsequently may become progressive, resulting in significant disability.

The second pattern, progressive MS, is characterized by slow or rapid worsening of disability from the onset, without delineated periods of **relapse and remission.** Existing deficits may increase in severity, and new symptoms occur as the disease progresses. For the most part, progression is slow; however, in a small number of cases the disease fulminates, progressing rapidly over a few years, leading to severe disability or death.

The third pattern consists of a combination of the first two. It starts with a classic relapsing/remitting course but becomes progressive, with limited remissions.

Overall prognosis is variable and the course of the disease quite unpredictable (Fig. 20-3). Although there have been efforts to identify prognostic guidelines, these guidelines have not proved reliable.

Various factors have been associated with exacerbations or temporary worsening. These include excessive fatigue, trauma, and rise in body temperature because of fever, hot bath or shower, or hot weather conditions. However, no specific cause-effect relationship has been identified. For the most part, the course of MS remains unpredictable.

Diagnosis

The diagnosis of MS is largely clinical. The basic diagnostic criteria are (1) evidence of multiple lesions in the CNS and (2) evidence (clinical or paraclinical) of at least two distinct episodes of neurological disturbance in an individual between the ages of 10 and 59 years.[20] Paraclinical evidence may include neuroimaging with magnetic resonance imaging (MRI) or computed tomography (CT) scanning, evoked potentials or cerebrospinal fluid (CSF) analysis (see the box on p. 593).

MRI is currently the preferred method to detect MS lesions. Use of MRI has hastened the diagnosis in many cases; however, MS cannot be diagnosed solely on the basis of this test. About 5% of people confirmed to have MS based on other criteria show no lesions on an MRI scan. Conversely, many other diseases may cause lesions that appear on the MRI, and many healthy individuals also may exhibit unidentified bright spots on MRI.[20]

Evoked potentials may include visual evoked potentials (VEP), brainstem auditory evoked potentials (BAEP), and somatosensory evoked potentials (SSEP). These tests, which measure nerve conduction along visual, auditory, and sensory pathways, often provide evidence of altered nerve conduction that may not be apparent on neurological examination. (see Chapter 29).

CSF examination is not routine in diagnosing MS but may provide additional clues in complicated cases. Elevated

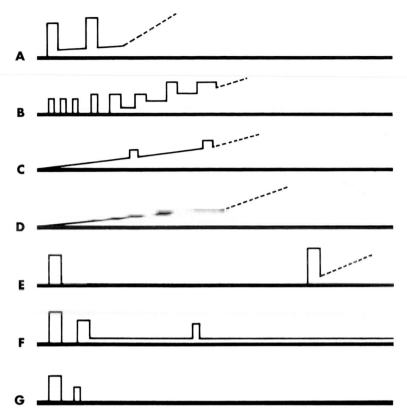

Fig. 20-3. Course of MS. **A,** Severe relapses, increasing disability and early death. **B,** Many short attacks, tending to increase in duration and severity. **C,** Slow progression from onset, superimposed relapses, and increasing disability. **D,** Slow progression from onset without relapses. **E,** Abrupt onset with good remission followed by long latent phase. **F,** Relapses of diminishing frequency and severity; slight residual disability only. **G,** Abrupt onset; few if any relapses after first year; no residual disability. (From McAlpine D and others: *Multiple sclerosis: a reappraisal,* Edinburgh, 1965, E & S Livingstone, Ltd.)

Diagnostic guidelines for multiple sclerosis

Definite MS

1. Two attacks and clinical evidence of two separate lesions
2. Two attacks, clinical evidence of one and paraclinical evidence of another separate lesion

Probable MS

1. Two attacks and clinical evidence of one lesion
2. One attack and clinical evidence of two lesions
3. One attack, clinical evidence of one lesion, paraclinical evidence for another separate lesion

From Poser C and others: *The diagnosis of multiple sclerosis,* New York, 1984, Thieme-Stratton.

---

gamma globulin is found in many cases of MS, and about one fourth of persons with active MS may show white blood cells in the CSF.[14] Analysis also may show fragments of myelin or **myelin basic protein** in individuals with acute episodes.

Psychosocial considerations

The personality of the individual along with the family and community environment before the development of any physical disability crucially affect the response to illness. The nature of the disability itself will also, obviously, determine the response.

MS is a demanding disease emotionally. Its impact is strong and is felt by all members of the family. Grief and anxiety accompany the diagnosis and may fluctuate with the disease and the individual's particular circumstances.

Several clinical aspects of MS influence the emotional impact of the disease:

1. **Ambiguity of diagnosis:** Although MRI and increased knowledge about MS have hastened the diagnostic process, there is often a period of ambiguity during which the individual is experiencing symptoms without a clear explanation. During this time, individuals may harbor fantasies of life-threatening or debilitating illness or may not be taken seriously by physicians or friends. Once a confirmed diagnosis of MS is made, some individuals report feeling relief to

have an explanation, even though the implications of the diagnosis remain ambiguous.

2. **Unpredictability of the course:** The course of MS is uncertain. The disease remains benign for some but may be severely disabling for others. An individual may be symptom-free for months or years and then unexpectedly experience an exacerbation. Symptoms may even vary from morning to evening of the same day. This unpredictability and the accompanying sense of loss of control can frequently cause depression, anxiety, and fear. Planning for the future becomes difficult and has an impact on family, work, and social interactions and activities.

3. **Covert symptoms:** Many symptoms of MS, including fatigue, double vision, bladder dysfunction, and paresthesias, are not visible to others yet can be very disabling and disturbing to the individual. Many people find that they are misunderstood, seen as lazy or lacking initiative (when they are actually fatigued), and find it difficult to explain the effect of these hidden symptoms to others. Some struggle with the decision to disclose their diagnosis to employers or friends. They fear job discrimination or alienating friends, but find that MS is a stressful and disturbing secret to keep.

Certainly, the stress of MS is in many ways like the stress of any kind of serious illness. A profound sense of fear, vulnerability, and exhausting self-concern underlies the coping process. The loss of a sense of control over one's body and life-style may precipitate an ongoing grieving process and a search to make some sense and give meaning to an otherwise confusing and purposeless event.

MEDICAL MANAGEMENT

Major treatment measures focus on easing of symptoms and attempting to maximize health, minimize associated complications, and lessen the severity or length of an exacerbation. Overall nursing and medical management calls for principles that will effect maximal health in general. These include ensuring adequate nutrition, encouraging balanced rest and exercise, avoiding exposure to infections, and—certainly of importance—preventing complications secondary to reduced activity (Fig. 20-4). It is also important to facilitate coping resources and to minimize family problems and individual anxiety and depression. Specifically, the following medical treatments can be beneficial:

1. **Acute exacerbations:** Natural improvement of acute exacerbations generally occurs within 4 to 12 weeks. The degree of improvement varies, although the reasons for this are not entirely understood, but probably have to do with reduction in inflammation.[26] For acute exacerbations of MS drugs having major antiinflammatory effect are used including: adrenocorticotropic hormone (ACTH) and synthetic adrenal steroids such as prednisone, methylprednisolone,

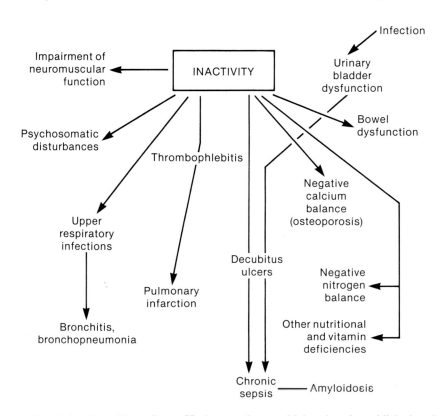

Fig. 20-4. Inactivity chart. (From Bauer H: A manual on multiple sclerosis, published under the auspices of the International Federation of Multiple Sclerosis Societies, 1977.)

betamethasone, and dexamethasone (see Chapter 33). Although these agents are used widely in acute attacks of MS, there is little evidence that they alter the extent of residual disability or the overall course of the disease.[5,8,24,26]

2. In 1993, the FDA approved the first drug in 25 years to be licensed to treat MS. Beta interferon IB **(Betaseron)** was found in clinical trials to reduce the number and severity of exacerbations in individuals with relapsing/remitting MS.[17] Administered by injection every other day, this medication will soon also be tested in chronic progressive patients. Immunosuppressive drugs such as azathioprine (Immuran) and cyclophosphamide (Cytoxan) have been tried to reduce worsening, but they have toxic side effects and their efficacy is controversial.[5,24]

3. **Spasticity:** Baclofen (Lioresal) is the most commonly used medication to control spasticity in MS. Side effects such as increased weakness, lethargy, and fatigue may occur with baclofen. The surgical implantation of a baclofen pump, which administers baclofen intrathecally, has been beneficial to many people with severe spasticity. The pump is implanted beneath the skin, usually on the lower abdomen, and the rate of drug delivery can be adjusted to meet individual need.[26]

   Sodium dantrolene (Dantrium) also may be helpful, although it may induce weakness even at low doses. Diazepam (Valium) is also used, most frequently for spasms that occur at night. Cyclobenzaprine HCl (Flexoril) is sometimes prescribed for back spasms and also may have an overall antispasticity effect. With all these medications, a tolerance may occur over time, rendering them less effective. Carbamepazine (Tegretol) is generally used to control tonic or paroxysmal spasms, and cortisone may also decrease overall spasticity but long-term use is not advocated.[24]

   Phenol blocks or tendon release surgical procedures may be required if severe spasticity interferes with personal hygiene and other activities of daily living, although a combination of exercise, stretching, and medication can usually avoid these measures.[6]

   Severe tremor is sometimes treated with isonicotonic acid hydrazide (INH) or clonazepam (Clonopin) with inconstant results.[24,30]

4. **Fatigue:** Amantadine (Symmetrel) may be effective in managing MS fatigue, as are some stimulants such as pemoline (Cylert) and methylphenidate (Ritalin). These stimulants may cause sleeplessness or other side effects and must be monitored carefully. Principles of energy conservation along with drug therapy can help minimize fatigue. The experimental use of 4-aminopyridine, a nerve conduction enhancer, has shown improvement in fatigue, spasticity, and other symptoms in some patients.[24]

5. **Bladder:** Urinary frequency and urgency may be reduced by smooth muscle relaxants or nerve blockers such as propantheline (Pro-banthine) and oxybutynin (Ditropan), Cystospaz, Urispas, and Ornade. Urinary retention is frequently treated with bethanechol (Urecholine) or phenoxybenzamine (Dibenzyline). Crede technique and intermittent catheterization are used with the bladder that does not empty sufficiently. If a bladder problem cannot be solved with medication or intermittent catheterization, continuous catheterization using a Foley catheter may be necessary.[4,24]

   Bladder infections, secondary to urinary retention, are treated with an antibiotic specific to the bacteria present. Prevention of infection is the best approach.

6. **Bowel:** Absence of good bowel control may lead to constipation or incontinence. Bulk formers such as hydrophilic colloid (Metamucil) or stool softeners such as Colace may be recommended. Laxatives such as Milk of Magnesia or Doxidan may be prescribed if expelling stool is the cause of the constipation. Rectal stimulants may also be effective such as glycerine or Ducoax suppositories. Frequent use of enemas should be avoided. A bowel program including dietary and drug regimens can usually control the constipation and incontinence of MS.

7. **Pain:** Trigemninal neuralgia, occasionally seen in MS, may be effectively treated with carbamepazine (Tegretol) but can cause sleepiness. Phenytoin (Dilantin) is also used for pain as is baclofen. The use of transcutaneous nerve stimulation (TENS) over the area of pain may also bring relief. Some tricyclic antidepressant drugs (e.g., amitryptiline) may be helpful in some cases.

8. **Sexual dysfunction:** In impotent men, penile implants or injections into the penis can produce erections. In women, artificial lubricants or other mechanical aids may facilitate orgasm. Urological and psychological counseling for the couple is recommended.

9. **Psychological and cognitive disturbances:** Neuropsychological testing can assist in determining the degree of cognitive and affective impairment. When reactive depression complicates MS, standard antidepressant therapy is often effective. Antidepressant medication is less effective in cases where cognitive abnormality is the underlying cause. Counseling can improve understanding and provide coping mechanisms, and rehabilitative efforts by neuropsychologists and occupational therapists may help to compensate for these problems.

In considering any therapy or treatment, one must keep in mind that a large percentage of persons with MS show improvement at various times during their illness regardless of treatment. Recent research regarding the placebo effect and the "mind-body" effect is further evidence that improvement is not always a direct result of treatment procedures themselves.

RESEARCH CONSIDERATIONS

MS is still a disease of unknown cause. It is generally accepted that MS occurs in genetically susceptible individuals. It is suspected that a viral infection is involved as well, yet efforts to culture a specific virus have not been successful, nor have efforts to transmit a virus to other mammals. The most widely accepted theory of the etiology of MS is that MS is an **autoimmune disease** of the CNS, triggered by an environmental agent in genetically susceptible individuals, which causes inflammation and ultimately destruction of myelin.

The search for the cause and cure of MS is the focus of efforts in the United States by both the National Multiple Sclerosis Society and the US Federal National Institutes of Health. Internationally, work is being conducted in academic and scientific institutions worldwide. The International Federation of MS Societies works to coordinate these efforts and to facilitate communication among investigators. Research efforts focus generally on four biomedical areas: immunology, genetics, virology, and biology of glial cells.

Immunology: Immune-modifying strategies have received considerable attention over the last several years. Global immunosuppressant therapies including cyclophosphamide, cyclosporine, azathioprine, methotrexate, total lymphoid irradiation, and plasmapheresis have undergone numerous clinical trials. The drawback to these global methods is that they leave the body open to serious infection, and their impact on the progression of MS is not conclusive. New mechanisms that target specific T cells such as monoclonal antibodies and synthetic peptides may be safer and have had some early success in blocking T-cell function in experimental allergic encephalomyelitis (EAE), the animal model of MS. Efforts to enhance immunological tolerance to myelin or its antigens include injecting **Copolymer (COP I),** a synthetic peptide similar to myelin components, and the use of **oral tolerance** therapy,[30] another new area of investigation in which the natural immunological functions in the digestive tract are manipulated to block the autoimmune response. Clinical trials with COP I hold promise for reducing the exacerbation rate with few side effects.[29] The use of interferon to induce immulological changes has proved successful in the development of interferon beta 1B (Betaseron) as a licensed treatment for relapsing-remitting MS.[17]

Genetics: A combination of several genes that determine immune function and control will probably be implicated in MS susceptibility. Efforts to identify these genes is underway using families in which there are multiple cases of MS along with molecular genetic technology.

Virology: Dozens of viruses have been proposed as the trigger of MS, yet none has been shown to have a cause-and-effect relationship to the disease. Many researchers suspect that a single virus does not cause MS but that the problem lies in the way a genetically susceptible individual handles common viral infection in general.

Glial biology: The study of **oligodendrocytes,** the glial cells that make and maintain myelin, offers the best hope for recovery of function. It is thought that astrocytes, another glial cell, produce toxic substances that damage myelin and create the nerve tissue lesions typical of MS. Efforts to transplant oligodendrocytes in mice and to manipulate the immune system to accelerate remyelination are showing promise in improving function.

EVALUATION

The clinician must consider various factors when evaluating the individual with MS. Subjective perceptions of problems by the individual and family members are of great importance. Functional assessment at times may not correlate with clinical measure—that is, MS lesions may be functionally silent in some cases; yet in others, significant functional impairment may result from apparently minimal clinical disease activity. The individual with MS must be evaluated at intervals during the fluctuating course of the disease. Additionally, factors that influence performance such as heat and time of day (fatigue factor) must be considered when the client is evaluated.

An assessment profile must be developed before establishing treatment goals. Such a profile should include assessment of:

- Strength
- Tone
- Range of Motion
- Balance
- Coordination
- Ambulation
- Fatigue/Endurance
- Cardiovascular and respiratory status
- Bed mobility/transfers
- Bowel/bladder/sexual impairment
- Swallowing/speech impairment
- Visual status
- Sensory impairment
- Activities of daily living independence
- Cognition/perception
- Vocational and avocational status
- Psychosocial status (including family adjustment)
- Physical environment/Community resources
- Medical stability

Each patient serves as his or her own baseline because the course of MS and severity of symptoms are so variable.

A standardized profile such as the Functional Independence Measure (FIM) is sometimes used in MS assessment. This tool, available from Uniform Data Systems for Medical

Rehabilitation,* documents the severity of patient disability and outcomes of medical rehabilitation. It helps to develop a patient profile, can be compared to previous assessments, helps to develop functional goals, and is available as a software product.

The Kurtzke Disability Status Scale (DSS)[10] is the standardized assessment of MS disability used widely by MS clinicians and researchers to quantify the degree of disability and provide a common language to describe patient status. This Neurological Assessment uses measures from an assessment of Functional Systems (FS) (See the Kurtzke Disability Scale in the box on p. 598) including pyramidal, cerebellar, brainstem, sensory, bowel and bladder, optic, cerebral, and other functions. The patient's grade on the Kurtzke DSS scale (For specific scoring of the disability scale, see the box on p. 599) is frequently used to measure the effectiveness of a particular treatment or as a criteria for participation in a clinical trial. An expanded scoring system to quantify disability status was developed in 1985 by the International Federation of Multiple Sclerosis Societies and is called the Minimal Record of Disability (MRD), which can be obtained from the National Multiple Sclerosis Society. In addition to the Kurtzke FS and DSS it includes demographic and socioeconomic information, activities of daily living (ADL) status, and environmental information. The MRD can be obtained directly from the National Multiple Sclerosis Society.† Because it is specifically designed for the person with MS, this useful tool provides a comprehensive, standardized profile that can assist the health care team in planning the management of these individuals.

Additional efforts by the Rehabilitation Subcommittee of the Consortium of MS Centers‡ to identify uniform assessment tools may also lead to additional resources for establishing a standardized patient profile.

SETTING GOALS

A statement from *A Manual on Multiple Sclerosis*[2] summarizes important guidelines in setting goals:

In every rehabilitation program, the patient must be treated as a whole, the best physical and psychological condition under the circumstances must be achieved, complications eliminated as far as possible and realistic motivations exploited. This can only be accomplished by the well-coordinated teamwork of doctors, nurses, physiotherapists, occupational therapists, clinical psychologists, social workers, the patient and his family and friends, and organizations with a genuine interest and sense of responsibility for him (p. 34).

The ideal rehabilitation model acknowledges the client's responsibility and resources. It recognizes both the client's

---

* 232 Parker Hall, SUNY South Campus, 3435 Main St., Buffalo, NY 14214.
† 733 Third Ave., New York, NY 10017.
‡ c/o Bernard Gimble M.S. Center, Holy Name Hospital, 718 Teaneck Rd., Teaneck, NJ 07666.

and family members' priorities and values; it considers not only the home environment but community resources, medical issues, history of the disease, and the cognitive and affective status of the individual.

To date there is no evidence that rehabilitation efforts have an influence on the principal pathological process in MS. Therefore the overriding principle in setting rehabilitation goals is to maximize independence, self-determination, and quality of life within the context of the individual's life-style and abilities (see the box on p. 599).

Often, for more stable or clear-cut disabilities, goals are set according to a functional skill such as ambulatory or wheelchair level. This may not be appropriate for clients with MS. A large number may be ambulatory for short distances but require a wheelchair for more demanding tasks. Additionally, for periods of exacerbation, training in wheelchair mobility may be a temporary yet important necessity. The variations in MS confirm the need for ongoing reestablishment of goals in response to therapy and to changes in the client's condition, home environment, and the family situation.

REHABILITATION MANAGEMENT
Overview

Involvement in a rehabilitation program may take several forms. From a practical point of view, fiscal considerations may dictate the frequency and duration of therapy visits as well as location, that is, whether the care is administered at home or on an inpatient or outpatient basis. Unfortunately, the availability of third-party payment for therapy is often conditional, with many individuals ineligible for reimbursement, particularly for maintenance and preventive therapies.

The place at which treatment is provided can often dictate the form it takes. An inpatient setting, for example, provides an opportunity for intensive therapies, a therapeutic community, multidisciplinary support, a comprehensive treatment environment, and easy availability of equipment and modalities. It is also important to realize that such a setting requires learning skills outside of the home environment, transferring those skills after discharge, and adjusting psychologically to the home setting, where the client has the opportunity and responsibility to carry out his or her program.

Home-based treatment, as an alternative, provides a familiar environment; however, availability of equipment or modalities may be limited. The treatment environment selected needs to be based on the client's needs, the availability of resources, and cost.

Treatment focuses on helping the patient achieve optimal functional independence and is best carried out by an interdisciplinary team. Members of the team include the physician, occupational therapist, physical therapist, speech therapist, nurse, dietitian, social worker, recreation therapist, and of course the patient and his or her family. Not all members will be involved at all times, and financial realities

Kurtzke Disability Scale (FS)

1. Pyramidal functions
   0 = Normal
   1 = Abnormal signs without disability
   2 = Minimal disability
   3 = Mild or moderate paraparesis or hemiparesis; severe monoparesis
   4 = Marked paraparesis or hemiparesis; moderate quadriparesis; or monoplegia
   5 = Paraplegia, hemiplegia, or marked quadriparesis
   6 = Quadriplegia
   V = Unknown
2. Cerebeller functions
   0 = Normal
   1 = Abnormal signs without disability
   2 = Mild ataxia
   3 = Moderate truncal or limb ataxia
   4 = Severe ataxia all limbs
   5 = Unable to perform coordinated movements due to ataxia
   V = Unknown
   X is used after 0-3 when weakness of grade 3 or more interferes with testing.
3. Brainstem functions
   0 = Normal
   1 = Signs only
   2 = Moderate nystagmus or other mild disability
   3 = Severe nystagmus, marked extraocular weakness or moderate disability of other cranial nerves
   4 = Marked dysarthria or other marked disability
   5 = Inability to swallow or speak
   V = Unknown
4. Sensory functions
   0 = Normal
   1 = Vibration or figure-writing decrease only
   2 = Mild decrease in touch or pain; moderate decrease in position, vibration, or discrimination
   3 = Marked hyposensitivity (not complete)
   4 = Analgesia or anesthesia to groin; hemianesthesia or hemianalgesia
   5 = Analgesia and anesthesia to neck
   V = Unknown

5. Bowel and bladder functions
   0 = Normal
   1 = Mild hesitancy, urgency or retention
   2 = Moderate hesitancy, urgency, retention, or rate urinary incontinence
   3 = Frequent incontinence
   4 = In need of almost constant catheterization but with intact bladder sensation; severe bowel retention and/or incontinence
   5 = Lack of sensation and control of bowel and bladder function
   V = Unknown
6. Visual functions
   0 = Normal
   1 = Scotoma with visual acuity (corrected) better than 20/30
   2 = Worse eye with scotoma with maximal visual acuity (corrected) of 20/30 to 20/59
   3 = Worse eye with large scotoma, or moderate decrease in fields, but with maximal visual acuity (corrected) of 20/60 to 20/99
   4 = Worse eye with marked decrease of fields and maximal visual acuity (corrected) of 20/100 to 20/200; grade 3 plus maximal acuity of better eye 20/60 or less
   5 = Grade 4 plus maximal visual acuity of better eye 20/60 or less
   V = Unknown
   X is added to grade 0-6 for presence of temporal pallor.
7. Mental functions
   0 = Normal
   1 = Mood alteration only
   2 = Mild decrease mentation
   3 = Moderate decrease mentation
   4 = Marked decrease in mentation (chronic brain syndrome, moderate)
   5 = Dementia; or chronic brain syndrome, severe, incompetent
   V = Unknown
8. Other functions
   0 = None
   1 = Any other findings (specify)
   V = Unknown

Kurtzke JF: *Neurology* 11(8):688, 1961.

may prohibit involvement of all team members; however, the team approach is the most comprehensive approach to management. The team uses a variety of methods to reduce disability and improve the quality of life for a person with MS: physical treatment, education, environmental changes, compensation with adaptive equipment, and counseling. Table 20-1 indicates how the interdisciplinary team might collaborate on many common MS problems.[13]

General problem areas

The following problem areas are often evaluated and treated by the physical therapist, frequently in collaboration with other team members.

Fatigue. Fatigue is the most common MS symptom and can cause significant disability, even in those with few other symptoms. As an invisible symptom, fatigue is frequently misunderstood by friends, family, or employers. MS fatigue is described as nerve fiber fatigue and results when the body requires more energy for nerve impulses to travel along demyelinated fibers. Rise in body temperature, even body temperature fluctuations during the course of the day, also may affect nerve conduction velocity, resulting in fatigue. Additionally, fatigue may result as stronger muscle groups compensate for weaker groups or from using walking aids that require greater energy expenditure. Using energy conservation techniques and planning exercise and activities

Specific scoring of the disability scale: Kurtzke Scale (DSS)

0 = Normal neurological examination (all grade 0 in functional groups).
1 = No disability, minimal signs (Babinski, minimal finger-to-nose ataxia, diminished vibration sense) (grade 1 in functional groups).
2 = Minimal disability—slight weakness or stiffness, mild disturbance of gait, or mild visuomotor disturbance (1 or 2 functional grade 2).
3 = Moderate disability—monoparesis, mild hemiparesis, moderate ataxia, disturbing sensory loss, or prominent urinary or eye symptoms, or combinations of lesser dysfunctions (1 or 2 functional grade 3 or several grade 2).
4 = Relatively severe disability not preventing ability to work or carry on normal activities of living, excluding sexual function. This includes the ability to be up and about 12 hours a day (1 functional grade 4 or several grade 3 or less).
5 = Disability severe enough to preclude working, with maximal motor function walking unaided up to several blocks (1 functional grade 5 alone, or combination of lesser).
6 = Assistance (canes, crutches, braces) required for walking (1 functional grade 6 alone or combination of lesser).
7 = Restricted to wheelchair—able to wheel self and enter and leave chair alone (combinations with at least 1 above functional grade 4).
8 = Restricted to bed but with effective use of arms (combinations usually junctional grade 4 or above in several functional groups).
9 = Totally helpless bed patient (combinations usually functional grade 4 or above in most functional groups).
10 = Death due to multiple sclerosis.

Kurtzke JF: *Neurology* 11(8):688, 1961.

Aspects of quality of life

Psychophysiological equilibrium

Understanding of the disease, the symptoms, and how to manage them
Understanding of limitations and strengths; functioning up to but respecting limits
Maintenance of function with minimum effort and maximum safety (balancing rest and activity appropriately)
Functional improvement despite persistent neurological signs
Return to preexacerbation physical status
Altering environment to support independence, diminish disability
Wellness life-style
Mastery over potential uncertainty and loss of control

Interrelatedness

Realistic expectations for patient and family
Preservation of family unit
Learning new ways to fulfill family/friendship roles
Knowing and practicing how to be realistically independent—not being a burden—but also being able to communicate when and how help is needed
Avoiding social isolation
Knowing and appropriately using community resources

Productivity

Developing alternative plans to already established vocational goals (job, education, other training)
Establishing a productive life (paid or volunteer)

Creativity

Developing problem-solving skills
Developing avocational interests
Reaching important life goals; focusing on remaining possibilities
Developing an enjoyable, personally meaningful life (MS not being the focus of one's life)

Adapted from Maloney FP and others: *Interdisciplinary rehabilitation of multiple sclerosis and neuromuscular disorders*, Philadelphia, 1985, JB Lippincott.

at times of higher energy during the course of the day may compensate for fatigues. Adapting the work environment for energy conservation often allows the MS patient to continue employment. In addition exercise to increase general endurance, cardiovascular health, and overall conditioning may address this symptom.

Weakness. Decreased strength results from several causes: upper motor neuron weakness, fatigue, disuse, or overriding spasticity in an antagonistic muscle. To enhance function in weak muscles active assistive exercise, active and/or resistive exercise should be incorporated into a daily program. Proprioceptive neuromuscular facilitation techniques (PNF) may increase the benefit of assisted, active and resisted exercise. Although strengthening exercises will not alter the disease process, compensatory strengthening of nonaffected muscle groups, preventing weakness secondary to disuse and strengthening agonist muscles to overcome spasticity in antagonistic muscle groups may improve function.

If compensatory strengthening proves to be limited in improving mobility, bracing may be effective in reducing gait abnormalities and improve the individual's ability to function with less effort. Ankle foot orthoses (AFOs) are used to stabilize the ankle and compensate for foot drop and are commonly used for MS gait problems. Other orthotics also may compensate for weakness in both upper and lower extremities. See the box on p. 602 for general principles of a strengthening program.

Spasticity. In managing spasticity, the therapist should consider reflex dominance, hypertonicity, and abnormal movement. A stretching routine may be beneficial and should allow for slow elongation of the muscle through relaxation. The application of cold has been useful in some cases in reducing hypertonicity as have other inhibitory relaxation

Table 20-1. Examples of team interaction on common MS problems

Problem	Goals	Team*	Plan
Weakness	Strengthen disuse component Maintain fitness	MD/nurse/OT/PT†	Strengthening exercises, substitution, compensation, protective splints
Spasticity	Normalize tone without causing loss of support	MD/nurse/OT/PT	Medication, stretching, positioning, cold bath or spray, movement techniques, motor point block
Incoordination/tremor/ impaired balance	Improve balance and control	MD/nurse/OT/PT	Medication, coordination/balance exercises, joint approximation, adaptive equipment, extremity weights, compensatory techniques, air splints, weighted canes/crutches, gait training
Impaired sensation	Enhance sensory awareness Teach precautions	MD/nurse/OT/PT	Education, visual compensation, developmental sequence exercises, joint approximation, tapping, brushing, weights
Pain	Decrease source of pain Decrease perception of pain	Biofeedback†/ counselor/MD/ nurse/OT/PT	Medication, improve posture, transcutaneous nerve stimulation, increase activity, stress management, muscle relaxation, diminish pain behavior
Visual impairment	Improve vision Compensate for loss	Blind services/MD/ nurse/OT/PT/ ophthalmologist	Medication for acute optic neuritis, patch for double vision, compensatory techniques, talking books, home visit
Fatigue	Increase and conserve available energy	Biofeedback/ counselor/MD/ nurse/OT/PT	Teach energy conservation, treat depression, improve endurance, efficient compensatory techniques and equipment, stress management, have patient keep record of activities and readjustment, rest periods at onset of fatigue
Memory/cognitive impairment	Identify Compensate	Counselor/MD/OT/ speech†/ neuropsychologist	Evaluation, educate patient and family, teach compensatory techniques, alteration of home environment
Ambulation/transfers	Safe and efficient mobility	Nurse/OT/PT	Decrease spasticity, strengthen and improve balance, improve trunk stability, gait training, gaiting aids, practice on ward, evaluate environment (hospital, home, work) for safety, accessibility, wheelchair evaluation, training
Activities of daily living/community skills	Efficient and safe self-care Energy conservation Access to community	Driver education/ nurse/OT/PT/ recreation†	Transfers, balance, bed mobility, home equipment, new skills, adaptive equipment, energy conservation, and practice on ward, at home and on supervised recreational outing

From Maloney FP and others: *Interdisciplinary rehabilitation of multiple sclerosis and neuromuscular disorders,* Philadelphia, 1985, JB Lippincott.
*Team members are listed in alphabetical order.
†MD, physician; OT, occupational therapist; PT, physical therapist; speech, speech/language pathologist; biofeedback, biofeedback technician; recreation, recreation therapist.

techniques including joint approximation, slow rolling from supine to side, slow rocking, slow stoking of the paravertebral muscles and pressure on the tendinous insertion of the spastic muscle (see Chapter 6).

Reflex-inhibiting movement patterns and positioning (side-lying) may inhibit abnormal postural reflex mechanisms (e.g., asymmetrical tonic neck reflex or tonic labrynthine reflex and abnormal movements). Additionally, the use of functional exercise and weight bearing performed in various spatial positions may be helpful in normalizing movement. Daily active and passive range of motion (ROM) exercises will help maintain joint range. Training in self-ROM and encouragement of participation in functional tasks will aid in the prevention of contractures. Severe ROM limitations may require surgical intervention such as myotenotomy. Medications, as discussed earlier, may augment physical treatment. (For additional information refer to Chapter 33.)

Problems With Balance and Coordination. (see Chapter 28). Cerebellar problems are common in MS and difficult to manage. Ataxia, incoordination, dysmetria, and tremor that becomes exaggerated with movement may be present in both the extremities and trunk. Treatment sequences in functional activities may help improve balance in various positions. Progress is made from a wide to narrow base of support, from static to dynamic activities, and from a low to a high center of gravity. Additionally, strengthening the fixation musculature, using visual cues, and biofeedback may improve balance and lessen tremor. For the most part, however, treatment is compensatory. Use of adaptive equipment in ADLs, weighted cuffs to reduce tremor, or weighted canes to reduce ataxia may prove useful. These weighted cuffs may increase the imbalance and once removed exaggerate the problem. The use of elastic tubing or band such as Theraband, which also gives resistance but incorporates compression versus distraction, also will reduce

Table 20-1. Examples of team interaction on common MS problems—cont'd

Problem	Goals	Team*	Plan
Bowel dysfunction	Regularity without constipation, diarrhea, incontinence	Dietitian/MD/nurse/OT/PT	Diet, decrease constipating medications, manage bladder program, sitting balance, transfers, hand function, increase daily activity
Bladder dysfunction	Freedom from incontinence and infection	MD/urologist/nurse/OT/PT	Evaluation, medication, teach bladder program, sitting/standing balance, transfers, hand function, treat infections
Sexual dysfunction	Compensation/education	Counselor/MD/urologist/OT/PT	Evaluation, education, mobility, balance, decrease spasticity, contractures, hand function, bowel and bladder control, compensatory techniques, prosthesis, support, self-image
Dysarthria	Improve communication Maintain functional communication Compensation Energy conservation	Nurse/OT/PT/speech	Retraining, teach others to listen, abdominal breathing exercises, oral exercises, decrease spasticity, practice on ward, communication boards, hand function for boards
Dysphagia	Nutrition Safety Energy conservation	Dietician/MD/nurse/OT/speech	Diet, patient and family training and education, evaluation of alternative routes of nutrition if needed
Adjustment/motivation	Facilitate adjustment Appropriate independence/dependence Prevent isolation Stress management	Biofeedback/counselor/MD/nurse/OT/PT/recreation/speech	Supportive counseling, alternative goals, success at valued tasks, improved ability to communicate, antidepressant medication, biofeedback/relaxation, positive social/recreational experiences
Medical complication: decubitus ulcer	Prevent/treat	Dietician/MD/nurse/OT/PT	Evaluate, educate patient and family, strengthen and position, decrease spasticity, improve nutrition, protective equipment, correct contractures
Medical complication: contractures	Prevent/decrease	MD/nurse/OT/PT/surgeon	Stretching, positioning, educate patient and family, equipment, strengthen, surgical release
Medical complication: nutrition	Maximize nutrition Avoid fads	Dietician/MD/nurse/OT/PT	Evaluate, educate, train in swallowing, body position, hand control, treat depression, proper diet
Medical complication: respiratory problems	Improve breath control Avoid respiratory illness	MD/nurse/PT	Breathing exercises, improve posture, increase activity, medical care if needed
Vocation Family adjustment Avocation Home-making	Best and most interesting job and recreation available Strengthen family Mobilize community resources	Counselor/MD/nurse/OT/PT/recreation/speech/vocation counselor	Physical skills, motivation, help to overcome environmental barriers, build bridges to community resources, counseling

the ataxia without exaggerating the problem when they are removed. Tremors of the head and neck may be controlled with a collar or brace. Increased fatigue related to the extra weight may contraindicate their use. Drug treatment, as discussed earlier, may augment compensatory training techniques. In extreme cases, thalamic surgery or stimulation has been tried. The risks of such a procedure, however, outweigh the benefits in most cases.[26]

Sensory dysfunction. Impaired sensation is frequently a problem in MS. Treatment is aimed at compensating for the loss, maximizing safety, and increasing awareness of the distribution of sensory impairment. Inability to perceive temperature or pain must be attended to by training in visual compensation and safety techniques. Routine skin inspection, particularly where there is significant immobility, should be taught, appropriate wheelchair cushioning or mattresses provided, and pressure relief techniques taught.

Dysphagia and dysarthria. Fatigue, weakness, tremors, incoordination, and abnormal tone may contribute to imprecise articulation, vocal harshness, slurring, changes in rate of speech, hypernasality, and other problems in oral communication. After evaluation, speech therapy generally focuses on compensating for dysfunction. Specific techniques of speech therapy include using pauses to improve speech that is slurred, rapid, and run together; exaggerating articulation; reducing phrase length; increasing voice volume; using oral exercise to maximize ROM and strength of oral musculature; and using augmentative communication devices including writing, computer driven systems, communication boards, and pointing. Those who have motor difficulties, however, may be limited in the use of some of these methods.

Treatment for dysphagia focuses on body positioning (to prevent aspiration), style of eating "think swallow" (a

General principles of a strengthening program

Following are common principles to remember while implementing a strengthening program.

1. Unaffected muscle groups should be maximally strengthened to allow maximal use of compensation techniques that involve unaffected limbs.
2. Use adaptive devices, i.e., canes and crutches, to allow the patient to remain ambulatory longer and maintain functional strength levels as long as possible.
3. Strengthening exercises must be safe and efficacious. Therapists must teach the patient a judicious balance between rest and exercise.
4. The patient should progress through the strengthening program very slowly. For example, if s/he is starting at 8-10 repetition (reps) of each exercise, s/he can increase 1-2 reps every 2-3 weeks, to 20-25 reps. One- to two-pound weights may then be added and the reps decreased to 8-10, with the progression starting over. This slow increase in progression accompanied by good compliance will lead to successful strengthening. A cool atmosphere allows for more efficient exercise, as MS patients are often highly sensitive to heat.
5. Home programs for these exercises are essential; the effectiveness of any exercise program depends on its being carried out on an ongoing basis.
6. Prior to strengthening, stretching exercises should be performed to decrease spasticity, increase flexibility, and increase blood flow to the area.
7. To improve functional strength, exercises should be performed at submaximal resistance with frequent repetitions.
8. Emphasis should be placed on proximal strengthening in order to decrease energy consumption during functional activities.
9. Large fluid movements to enhance coordination should be used.
10. If a patient has difficulty initiating movement, try starting with large body/trunk movements, then moving from proximal to distal.
11. Light weights may help stabilization if a patient has significant tremors.
12. Combining strengthening exercises with aerobic, balance, and/or spasticity-reducing exercises whenever possible will maximize benefits within the patient's exercise tolerance.
13. Avoid excessive fatigue of a muscle: 1-5-minute rest periods throughout the exercise session will facilitate recovery of neurotransmission.
14. Set realistic goals and expectations with the patient. Be creative, realistic, and simplistic. The more enjoyable the exercises, the better the compliance.

From Schapiro R: *Multiple sclerosis: a rehabilitation approach to management,* New York, 1991, Demos Publications.

conscious swallow as opposed to relying on reflexive swallowing), and food and liquid selection (semisoft, moist foods and thick liquids with progression to more challenging foods). Because fatigue can exacerbate swallowing problems, larger meals taken earlier in the day followed by smaller meals later, may be easier to handle. Placement of feeding tubes may be required if a practical degree of swallowing cannot be achieved.

Ambulation/mobility. Gait in MS patients is influenced by weakness, spasticity, impaired sensation and proprioception, problems with balance, fatigue, visual problems, and incoordination. In addressing ambulation, trunk control and balance should be addressed first, followed by normalization of tone and maximizing flexibility and ROM. Gait is often more functional when strength can be improved in the trunk and extremities. Some patients also may require a graduated sitting tolerance program, tilt-table routine, and graduated standing tolerance schedule before specific gait training. Using visual and tactile cues may help compensate for sensory and proprioceptive loss. Prescription of specific ambulation aids can improve safety, decrease energy expenditure, and improve endurance. Upper extremity strength and motor control, cognitive status, and emotional response to using the device must be considered in prescription. Bracing to improve ambulation should follow these guidelines outlined in the box on p. 603.[23]

In wheelchair prescription, the goal is proper positioning to be sure the pelvis, spinal column, and limbs are in correct alignment and the patient is secure in the chair. Seating may be modified by the use of foam inserts, clamp-on side supports, and customized contour seating systems. Footrests should be adjusted so that the thighs are parallel to the floor. A seat belt should be used for safety. Functional training should include propulsion, retropulsion, and maneuvering in narrow areas and on various terrains. Manipulation of arm rests, leg rests, foot rests, brakes, and other wheelchair accessories must be included in wheelchair mobility training. A reclining chair may be most effective for those with head, neck, and trunk instability. Electric wheelchairs may be necessary when fatigue, weakness, or tremors make independent propulsion of a manual chair impossible. Three-wheel scooters are used frequently by people with MS with adequate trunk stability and upper extremity function. The three-wheeler also offers greater ease of dismantling and loading into a car than a traditional electric wheelchair. Cushion prescription to minimize skin breakdown and discomfort should be made with regard to the patient's risk for developing these problems.

Cognitive dysfunction. Cognitive problems in MS result from demyelination in the cerebral tracts that connect with primary sensory areas, motor, speech and integration areas of the cerebrum. This results in poor recognition of deficits as well as an inability to store and retrieve new information, a combination that may present a major impediment to rehabilitation.[23]

Bracing

The most common braces used to brace the lower extremities in MS are standard polypropylene AFOs and those with an articulated joint. The following guidelines may be helpful.

A standard AFO is indicated if the patient exhibits
1. Consistent foot drop or toe drag
2. Poor knee control (especially hyperextension)
3. Weakness of grade 2 or 3 at the ankle with dorsi-flexion testing
4. Minimal-to-moderate spasticity
5. Poor endurance in gait
6. Poor proprioception and sensory sense

The advantages of an AFO are that it
1. Saves energy during gait because the patient does not work as hard to clear his/her toes during the swing through phase of the gait
2. Improves foot drop or toe drag during the swing phase of gait
3. Improves general safety during walking by avoiding many falls due to the toe drag
4. Provides more knee control during mid-stance phase of gait by avoiding hyperextension of the knee
5. Provides greater ankle stability
6. Improves the overall gait pattern
7. Provides better cosmesis for the patient

The advantages of the AFO with an articulating joint are
1. All of the above listed for the standard AFO.
2. It allows some mobility at the ankle joint. This permits a more natural movement at the ankle during gait, which looks more normal. It allows the patient to drive while wearing the brace, and allows more freedom for squatting down in order to reach objects on the floor.

3. It provides a plantar flexion stop to prevent the foot from further plantar flexion during swing phase of gait.
4. It still allows for dorsiflexion assist, and can be set up to 5 degrees of dorsiflexion to clear the foot during the swing through phase.

Relative contraindications for these types of braces are
1. Moderate or severe spasticity in the lower extremities
2. Severe foot edema
3. Severe weakness (muscles grades 2 or less) at the hips

A double upright metal brace can provide some of the same advantages listed above, and usually provides more adjustments for the ankle and the knee. However, this brace is usually not the preferred choice due to its weight and poorer cosmetic appearance.

The polypropylene AFOs may be set in a few degrees of dorsiflexion to provide better knee control. If hyperextension is severe, a Swedish hyperextension knee cage may be useful. In some people this device may be quite helpful, but it is decidedly more bulky and often moves down the leg, which decreases its effectiveness. Custom bracing of the knee can be the answer to this problem, as effective orthotics may make up for instability of the joints, tendons, and ligaments. This usually requires the skills of a trained orthotist and is a topic beyond the scope of this book.

Some therapists have found rocker clog shoes to be of some help for those few people who need to have the plantar flexed position neutralized while the curved forefoot sole will initiate knee flexion. A skilled therapist should determine if this situation is present before purchase of this device is recommended.

For additional information on bracing refer to Chapter 32.

From Schapiro R: *Multiple sclerosis: a rehabilitation approach to management* p. 52, New York, 1991, Demos Publications.

Rehabilitation strategies focus mostly on compensatory strategies, for instance using a memory book, tape recorder, timers or alarms, or "ticker files." In therapy deficits in judgment, logical analysis, reasoning, and self-monitoring may require the use of clear, written, sequenced steps for exercises or adapted methods of performing ADL, transfers, and ambulation. The therapist should be aware that what may appear to be low motivation or poor follow-through in therapy, may be the presence of cognitive deficits.

It is important to remember that people with MS are not monolithic, nor is there an "MS personality." In addition the relationships among age, severity of disability, and duration of illness are not good predictors of cognitive or affective changes.

Given this information, many with MS would derive benefit from a neuropsychological evaluation. Such an evaluation could be helpful in several ways: The person with MS as well as family members can gain a better understanding of the nature and extent of the illness; the evaluation can identify impaired and intact functions; the evaluation may

assist the person in developing realistic vocational and other life goals; the results can clarify misconceptions on the part of others who may incorrectly attribute cognitive problems to uncooperative or oppositional behavior; and the results can suggest compensatory techniques.

General conditioning and fitness. A reduction in physical activity because of MS limitations may result in a general reduction in fitness. This reduction is characterized by (1) increased neuromuscular tension, (2) increased pulse rate at rest, (3) decreased adrenocortical reserve, (4) decreased muscular strength, (5) decreased vital capacity at rest, (6) decreased maximal vital capacity, (7) increased fatigue, (8) increased anxiety, and (9) increased depression.[23]

A physical conditioning program will not necessarily have an impact on the course of MS. It is likely, however, that enhanced overall health and fitness can improve a sense of well-being and reduce the other secondary effects of inactivity. With attention to raising body temperature, incoordination, cycles of fatigue, and safety, a conditioning program geared to the individual can offer a sense of control over some aspects of health and improve the quality of life. Aerobic exercise such as swimming, walking, stationary bikes, and rowers may be appropriate. Swimming and other water exercise can be ideal for those with MS, especially if water temperature can be maintained to avoid overheating. All patients should have a cardiovascular examination by a physician before starting an aerobic program.

Activities of daily living

Functional improvement or maintenance of functional independence is the overall goal of the rehabilitation program. Carry-over of therapeutic exercise, mat exercises, and ambulation training to ADL tasks are vital. In addition, specific training in techniques of dressing, bathing, toileting, personal hygiene, feeding, and bed mobility can improve or maintain independence in ADL. Adaptive equipment can be used to conserve energy and compensate for weakness and incoordination. For example, weighted silverware and plate guards can compensate for tremor and incoordination in self-feeding. Button hooks, reachers, stocking aids, and Velcro may improve independence in dressing. Transfer training should be incorporated into functional activities. The use of sliding board, hydraulic lift, or assistance from another individual must be geared to the client's ability and priorities regarding expenditure of energy.

Adapted tools for communication skills (i.e., writing or typing), such as built-up pencils, typing shield, or universal cuffs, may assist written communication. Homemaking tasks and child care from a wheelchair level, ambulatory-assisted level, or ambulatory level can be practiced with the aid of assistive devices and energy conservation techniques.

Driving often presents problems for the individual with MS. Diplopia or blurred vision, decreased coordination, weakness, and spasticity may interfere with safe driving or require the use of hand controls or adapted van. Perceptual and cognitive considerations must be made in a predriving evaluation or in driver training.

Persons with MS, whether they are experiencing mild or severe symptoms, may have job and career concerns. Individuals engaged in heavy physical labor may not be able to continue. Persons who are unable to stand for long periods or walk long distances and those who fatigue easily or have visual or coordination problems may need to make adjustments at the work site or build flexibility into their career plan. Although some persons with MS may be severely disabled, significant areas of good functioning often remain as well as periods of disease stability. Attention to these periods in prevocational and vocational counseling is, of course, important. Psychological adjustment, as well as cognitive and perceptual status, also influence career planning and vocational goal setting. The passage of the Americans with Disabilities Act (ADA) in 1990 has improved access and opportunity in both employment and social life.

PSYCHOSOCIAL ISSUES

In regard to psychosocial functioning, many families cope well with MS and find that, along with the problems, MS has brought about useful changes. It is important to recognize, however, that the family feels the pain of this disease, too. Family members may wonder how much to help the person with MS; they may feel burdened with his or her dependence; and they may be worried about the future, concerned about financial pressures, and exhausted by the care requirements of their family member. Sexual dysfunction, which is often not addressed by caregivers, may also have a significant impact on family functioning. This aspect of daily living merits attention, counseling, and practical information, all of which should be made available to families.

The meaning of illness or disability in a family relates to culture, religion, and personal values and beliefs. For some, illness means weakness, imperfection, and asexuality and is a result of sin or wrongdoing. For others, illness may be seen as a learning opportunity or an enriching experience—a challenge to confront or a catalyst to making one more compassionate and aware of what is really important in life. We also are influenced strongly by the viewpoints of our friends, family, medical caregivers, and rehabilitation team members. Personal awareness of attitudes and beliefs about disability is important to examine because therapists sometimes communicate these beliefs in subtle ways to their clients.

Helping families cope with MS also may involve an examination of their premorbid patterns of dealing with stress, conflict, and tragedy. Often, MS magnifies preexisting problems and tensions so that families who present "MS-generated" problems may have had these problems before the diagnosis was made.

The relationship among attitude, psyche, and physical wellness or disease is well documented.[3,23] Although stress cannot be implicated in causing exacerbations per se, the ability to manage stress can positively influence overall health and well-being. To treat the body without adequate consideration of the accompanying psychological and emotional issues would be a great injustice.

SUMMARY

MS is a chronic and usually progressive disease of the CNS, characterized by disseminated patches of demyelination in the brain and spinal cord, resulting in multiple and varied neurological symptoms and signs. Destruction of myelin, accompanied by edema and inflammation and followed by tissue scarring, appears to be the underlying cause that impedes or prevents neurotransmission.

The clinical diagnosis of MS depends on evidence of two or more distinct CNS lesions, of symptoms and signs that have appeared in distinct episodes or have progressed over time, and the exclusion of other neurological explanations.

Laboratory and electrophysiological tests provide support of a clinical diagnosis; however, at the present time no test is pathognomonic for MS.

The course of the disease is characterized by an unpredictable series of exacerbations and remissions in some cases, progressive disability over time in other cases, or a combination of the two, often accompanied by periods of disease stability.

The etiology of MS appears to be an autoimmune process in which myelin is destroyed. The trigger of this abnormal immune response is unknown, although a viral cause is under investigation.

Treatment of MS is primarily symptomatic. Immunosuppressive, antiviral, and antiinflammatory agents have shown some therapeutic benefit, particularly beta interferon, which was approved by the FDA in 1993. Several other agents are being investigated. Rehabilitative measures, including physical, occupational, and speech therapy, do not appear to alter the underlying pathology of the disease. Therefore the overriding principle in setting rehabilitation goals for a person with MS is to maximize functional independence, minimize complications and problems secondary to decreased mobility, and compensate for loss of function. Psychosocial adjustment, vocational disposition, and family issues merit significant attention by the treatment team, because MS generates tremendous need in these areas.

REFERENCES

1. Alter M and others: Migration and risk of multiple sclerosis, *Neurology* 28:1089, 1978.
2. Bauer H: *A manual on multiple sclerosis,* Vienna, 1977, International Federation of Multiple Sclerosis Societies.
3. Benson H: *The mind/body effect,* New York, 1979, Simon & Schuster.
4. Catanzaro M: Nursing car of the person with MS, *Am J Nurs* 80(2):286, 1980.
5. Cook S: *Handbook of multiple sclerosis,* New York, 1990, Marcel Dekker.
6. Dean G: The multiple sclerosis problem, *Sci Am* 223(1):40, 1970.
7. Dimitrijevuc MR and Sherwood AM: Spasticity—medical and surgical treatment, *Neurology,* 30(7pt2):19, 1980.
8. Ellison GW and Myers LW: Immunosuppressive drugs in multiple sclerosis:pro and con, *Neurology* 30(7 pt2):28, 1980.
9. Johnson KP: Cerebrospinal fluid and blood assays of diagnostic usefulness in multiple sclerosis, *Neurology* 30(2):107, 1980.
10. Kurtzke JF: On the evaluation of disability in multiple sclerosis, *Neurology* 11(8):686, 1961.
11. Kurtzke JF and Hyllested K: Multiple sclerosis in the Faroe Islands. 1. Clinical and epidemiological features, *Ann Neurol* 5:6, 1979.
12. Lisak RP: Multiple sclerosis: evidence for immunopathogenesis, *Neurology* 30(2):99, 1980.
13. Maloney FP and others: *Interdisciplinary rehabilitation of multiple sclerosis and other neuromuscular* disorders, Philadelphia, 1985, JB Lippincott.
14. McAlpine D and others: *Multiple sclerosis: a reappraisal,* Edinburgh, 1965, E&S Livingstone.
15. Minden SL and others: Depression in multiple sclerosis, *Gen Hosp Psychiatry* 9:426, 1987.
16. Minden SL and Schiffer R: Affective disorders in multiple sclerosis, *Arch Neurol* 47:98, 1990.
17. Paty DW and others: Interferon beta-Ih is effective in relapsing-remitting multiple sclerosis, *Neurology* 43:655, 1993.
18. Pelettier KL: *Mind as healer, mind as slayer,* New York, 1977, Dell.
19. Percy AK and others: MS in Rochester, Minn: a 60 year appraisal, *Arch Neurol* 25.105, 1971.
20. Poser C and others: *The diagnosis of multiple sclerosis,* New York, 1984, Thieme-Stratton.
21. Rao SM: Neuropsychology of multiple sclerosis: a critical review, *J Clin Exp Neuropsychol* 8(5):503, 1986.
22. Rao SM and others: Cognitive dysfunction in multiple sclerosis, *Arch Neurol* 41:685, 1991.
23. Schapiro R: *Multiple sclerosis: a rehabilitation approach to management,* New York, 1991, Demos Publications.
24. Schapiro R: *Symptom management in multiple sclerosis,* New York, 1987, Demos Publications.
25. Schiffer RB and Slater RJ: Neuropsychiatric features of multiple sclerosis: recognition and management, *Semin Neurol* 5(2): 127, 1985.
26. Sibley W: *Therapeutic claims in multiple sclerosis,* New York, 1992, Demos Publications.
27. Slater RJ and others: *Minimal record of disability for multiple sclerosis,* New York, 1985, National Multiple Sclerosis Society.
28. Surridge D: Psychiatric aspects of multiple sclerosis, *Br J Psychol* 115:5245, 1969.
29. Waksman BH and others: *Research on multiple sclerosis,* 3rd ed, New York, 1987, Demos Publications.
30. Weiner H and others, Double blind trial of oral tolerization with myelin antigens in multiple sclerosis, *Science* 259:1321-1324, 1993.
31. Williams A and others: An investigation of multiple sclerosis in twins, *Neurology* 30:1139, 1980.

CHAPTER 21

Basal Ganglia Disorders

Metabolic, hereditary, and genetic disorders in adults

Marsha E. Melnick

LEARNING OBJECTIVES

After reading this chapter the student/therapist will:
1. Describe the circuitry of the basal ganglia.
2. Relate the anatomy and physiology of the basal ganglia to its role(s) in sensorimotor and cognitive processes.
3. Utilize the information on the anatomy, physiology, and pharmacology to explain the signs and symptoms seen in the classic disease states of Parkinson's disease and Huntington's disease.
4. Develop an evaluation plan for patients with diseases of the basal ganglia.
5. Develop a treatment plan for these patients with the rationale for intervention methods.
6. Describe the effects of alcoholism on the peripheral and central nervous system.
7. Integrate the information in this chapter with the information provided in Section I of this book to develop treatment plans for patients with metabolic and/or toxic disorders.

KEY TERMS

Huntington's chorea
alcoholism
Parkinson's disease

basal ganglia
physical therapy
exercise

This chapter considers the metabolic, hereditary, and genetic disorders that typically have their onset in adulthood, including **Huntington's chorea,** Wilson's disease, **alcoholism,** heavy metal poisoning, and drug intoxication. Because of the wide variety of diseases with a wide variety of causes, the concentration here is on understanding the clinical problems and commonalities that exist within this grouping. The predominant area of the brain affected by these disorders is the basal ganglia. For this reason **Parkinson's disease,** a degenerative disease of the **basal ganglia,** is also included. Therefore the first part of this chapter is devoted to the diseases of these structures, and the second part incorporates diseases of other areas of the brain. The reader should also review other chapters of the book that discuss in particular cerebellar dysfunction and hemiplegia.

THE BASAL GANGLIA

The most commonly seen disorders affecting the basal ganglia include Parkinson's disease, Huntington's chorea, Wilson's disease, and the drug-induced dyskinesias. All involve changes in muscle tone, a decrease in movement coordination, and the presence of extraneous movement. Taken together, these disorders affect approximately 450,000 people.[7]

To understand how one interrelated area of the brain can account for such a wide variety of symptoms, it is first necessary to understand the anatomy, physiology, and pharmacology of these structures.

Anatomy

The basal ganglia are comprised of three nuclei located at the base of the cerebral cortex—hence their name. These

nuclei are the caudate nucleus, the putamen, and the globus pallidus. Two brainstem nuclei, the substantia nigra and the subthalamic nucleus, are included as part of the basal ganglia because they have a close functional relationship to the forebrain nuclei. Some authors include the amygdala, the claustrum, and the red nucleus as part of the basal ganglia. Functionally, the amygdala and claustrum are not part of this system despite their anatomical location, and the red nucleus has not been shown to be anatomically connected with the other nuclei of the basal ganglia. Therefore these structures are not included in this portion of the chapter. (The anatomical location of the various parts of the basal ganglia is shown in Fig 21-1.)

The varying terminology associated with this brain region can be confusing. Based on their location and shape, the putamen and globus pallidus together have been referred to as the lentiform (lens-shaped) nucleus. However, embryologically, anatomically, and functionally the caudate nucleus and the putamen are similar, and many recent texts and articles refer to the caudate and putamen together as the

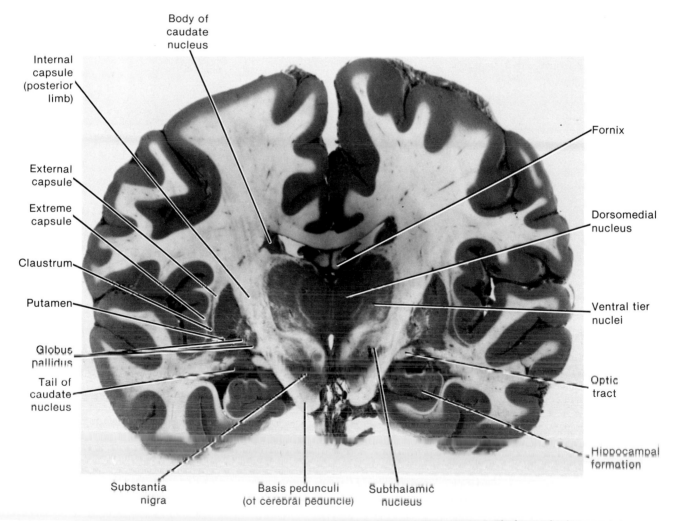

Fig. 21-1. Anatomical location of various parts of the basal ganglia (From Nolte J: *The human brain: an introduction to its anatomy,* St. Louis, 1981, Mosby.)

neostriatum—a term derived from *striate* and used to denote pathways from and to the caudate and putamen. Further, the term *corpus striatum* refers to the caudate, putamen, and globus pallidus. The various connections and interconnections of this system are discussed on the basis of these definitions.

The basal ganglia may contain two functional but interacting units. The dorsal portion of the system, or dorsal striatum, is the functional sensorimotor unit. The ventral portion, or ventral striatum, is related to motivation and therefore is closely related to the limbic system.[76] This chapter concentrates on the dorsal striatum, but the reader should examine Chapter 5 for a full appreciation and understanding of the limbic system.

Afferent pathways. Functionally, the basal ganglia can be divided into an afferent portion and an efferent portion (Fig. 21-2). The afferent structures are the caudate and putamen. They receive input from the entire cerebral cortex, the intralaminar thalamic nuclei, and the centromedian-parafascicular complex of the thalamus, as well as from the substantia nigra and the dorsal raphe nucleus. The projections from the cortex are systematically arranged so that the frontal cortex projects to the head of the caudate and putamen and the visual cortex projects to the tail. In addition, the prefrontal cortex projects mainly to the caudate, whereas the sensorimotor cortex projects mainly to the putamen.[107] Those projections from the cortical regions, which represent the proximal musculature, and those from the premotor regions may be bilateral.[91,106] These very close and very profuse connections between the cortex and the basal ganglia

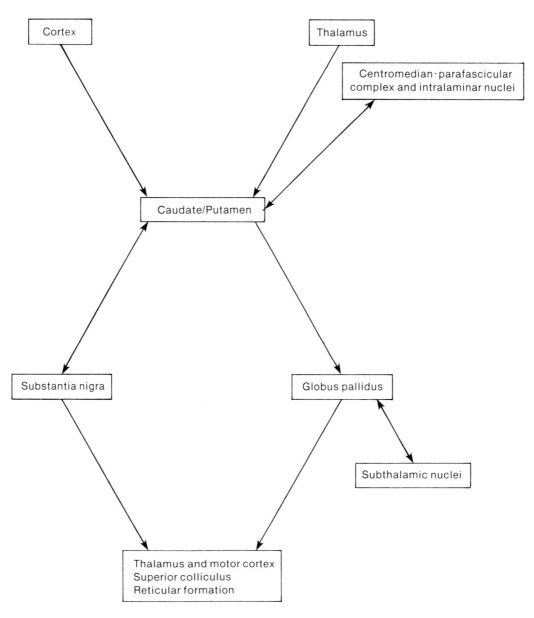

Fig. 21-2. Afferent and efferent portions of the basal ganglia.

are suggestive of a close interfunctional relationship between the cortex and the neostriatum. The projections from the thalamus to the caudate-putamen are also somatotopically arranged. The heaviest projections are from the centromedian nucleus, which also receives massive input from the motor cortex.[91,107]

The somatotopic arrangement of the cortico-striatal-thalamic-cortical pathways are maintained throughout the loop. This finding has led to an important functional hypothesis that the basal ganglia form parallel pathways subserving specific sensorimotor and associative functions.[4] The putamen is linked to the sensorimotor functions and the caudate to the associative functions.

As our knowledge of the circuitry of the basal ganglia has advanced, so has the knowledge regarding the microscopic structure. The caudate-putamen looks somewhat homogeneous because of the predominance of one cell type. Careful analysis using precise staining methods have demonstrated the appearance of patches within these nuclei. Input can be segregated depending on whether the patches are innervated or the areas around the patches (matrix) are innervated.[68] The intrinsic structure of the caudate-putamen also suggests that at least nigral input occurs in a way that could immediately modulate the input coming from the cortex.[176]

Efferent pathways. The input that has been processed in the caudate-putamen is then sent to the globus pallidus (pallidum) and substantia nigra (nigra), which comprise the efferent portion of the basal ganglia. The globus pallidus and substantia nigra are each divided into two regions. The globus pallidus has an external and an internal region; the substantia nigra consists of the dorsal pars compacta and the ventral pars reticulata. Embryologically and microscopically, the internal segment of the globus pallidus and the pars reticulata of the substantia nigra are very similar. These two regions are the primary efferent structures for the basal ganglia. The projections from the caudate and putamen to the pallidum and nigra maintain the somatotopic arrangement. The caudate projects primarily to the rostral and dorsal third of the pallidum and the anterior portion of the substantia nigra. The putamen projects to the caudal and ventral portions of the pallidum and the caudal nigra.[33,55] Evidence suggests that the projection from the caudate and putamen are separate in the pallidum and nigra.[91] From these structures the information is transmitted to the thalamus and then to the cortex. The pallidum projects to the lateral portions of the ventrolateral and ventroanterior nuclei of the thalamus. The nigra projects to the medial portions of these nuclei. The superior colliculus, the pedunculopontine nucleus (PPN), and other less defined brainstem structures (perhaps the reticular formation) also receive pallidal and nigral output. All output of the basal ganglia has then been processed through the globus pallidus and/or the substantia nigra before proceeding to other areas of the brain (see Fig 21-2).

Pathways to the motor system. Information processed

in the basal ganglia can influence the motor system in several ways, but no direct pathway to the alpha or gamma motor neurons exists. This first route is the projection to the ventroanterior and ventrolateral nuclei of the thalamus, which then projects to the motor and premotor cortex. Another pathway is through the superior colliculus and then to the tectospinal tract. There are also pathways from the globus pallidus and substantia nigra that terminate in areas of the reticular formation (e.g., the pedunculopontine nucleus) and then through the reticulospinal pathways. Anatomically therefore the basal ganglia are in good position to affect the motor system.

The circuitry of the basal ganglia comprise two loops.[3] This is shown for the sensorimotor system in Figure 21-3. The direct loop is the loop that begins in the cortex and projects to the putamen and then directly to the globus pallidus, internal segment, and on to the thalamus. The indirect pathway adds the subthalamic nucleus between the

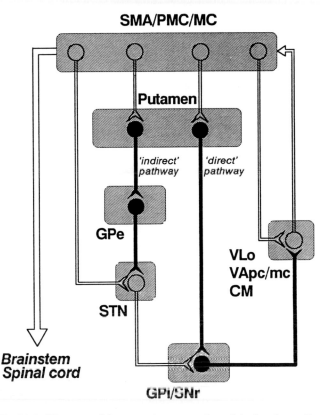

Fig. 21-3. Diagram of the sensorimotor portion of the basal ganglia depicting the "direct" and "indirect" pathways. Darkened circles represent inhibitory neurons; open circles, excitatory neurons. Abbreviations: SMA, supplementary motor cortex; PMC, premotor cortex; MC, motor cortex; GPe, globus pallidus external segment; GPi, globus pallidus internal segment; STN, subthalamic nucleus; VLo, ventral lateralis pars oralis nucleus of the thalamus; VApc/mc, ventral anterior pars parvocellularis and pars magnocellularis of the thalamus; CM, centromedian nucleus of the thalamus; SNr, pars reticularis of the substantia nigra. (From Alexander GE and Crutcher MD: *Trends in Neuroscience* 13:266-271, 1990. Reprinted with permission.)

globus pallidus, external segment, and the thalamus. The subthalamic nuclei also receive direct input from the premotor and motor cortex as well as from the pallidum.[73,141] The darkened neurons represent inhibitory connections, and the open neurons represent excitatory connections. In general, the direct pathway, via disinhibition, activates the thalamocortical pathway; the indirect pathway inhibits the thalamocortical system. The role of these loops in normal and diseased states will become clearer as we discuss the physiology and pharmacology of the basal ganglia.

In summary, input from the motor cortex, all other areas of the cortex, parts of the thalamus, and the substantia nigra enter the basal ganglia through the caudate and putamen. Here they are processed and sent on to the globus pallidus and substantia nigra. The appropriate "gain" of the system is adjusted, and the information is sent to the muscles by way of the thalamus and motor cortex, the superior colliculus, or the reticular formation.

Physiology

The understanding of the physiology of the interactions among areas of the basal ganglia has greatly increased in the last decade. Initially, the prevalent view was that the basal ganglia exerted an inhibitory influence on the motor system. An early study by Mettler and others[135] demonstrated an inhibition of cortically evoked movements following caudate stimulation. More recent studies show both excitatory and inhibitory influences.

The caudate and putamen are composed of neurons that fire very slowly, whereas the neurons in the globus pallidus fire tonically at fairly high rates. (The spontaneous activity of the caudate and putamen is therefore low, whereas that of the globus pallidus is high.) The low firing rates of neostriatal neurons are partially a result of the nature of thalamic synaptic inputs.[29]

Stimulation of the cortex, thalamus, and substantia nigra almost always produces excitatory postsynaptic potentials (EPSP) followed by longer inhibitory postsynaptic potentials (IPSP)—EPSP-IPSP sequence. Further, input from the cortex seems to have priority over input from the thalamus and substantia nigra.[85] The data provide evidence that the cortex is instrumental in regulating the responsiveness of caudate neurons.[113-115]

Cortical recruiting responses have been demonstrated following caudate, putamen, and pallidal stimulation,[27,28,45] especially over the area of the motor cortex. This led Dieckmann and Sasaki[45] to conclude that the neostriatum and pallidum have an important functional role in controlling the activity level of the cerebral cortex. The cortical response from caudate stimulation is a long-term hyperpolarization. Hull and co-workers[83] hypothesized that this hyperpolarization served to "enhance the magnitude of subsequent excitatory inputs" (p. 97), that is, the caudate would affect the bias of cortical neurons. They also suggested that a long-lasting hyperpolarization might be a useful model for the "timing and sequencing of behavioral responses in the presence of relatively constant stimulus inputs as for example, in a delayed response situation" (p. 175).[84]

The physiology of the direct and indirect pathways also tends to support a role for the basal ganglia in modifying input to the cortex. The neurons of the efferent portion of the basal ganglia respond with either phasic increases or phasic decreases in activity which in turn will affect the activity in the thalamus and hence the cortex. A decrease in activity of the internal segment of the globus pallidus removes inhibition to the thalamus and thus enables cortical activation. It is not yet known whether the two pathways are activated concurrently or whether different activities activate the two pathways separately. In the former possibility, the indirect pathway is seen as a "break" on ongoing activity; if the latter, the indirect pathway would act to decrease all other patterns in a form of lateral inhibition.[3] In both cases, the basal ganglia would have a role in cortical activation and modulation. In fact, the current view in relationship to disease processes is that an underactive direct pathway and/or an overactive indirect pathway would lead to decreased activation of the cortex and hence bradykinesia and akinesia, whereas, an overactive direct pathway and/or underactive indirect pathway would lead to the presence of extraneous movements.[2,70]

Relationship of the basal ganglia to movement and posture

Functionally, what might be happening in these anatomical and physiological connections? Researchers and clinicians have been attempting to answer this question for several centuries. Lesion experiments, single unit recording in awake, behaving animals, and careful observations of the sequelae of human disease processes have provided some answers.

Automatic movement. Based on the anatomical knowledge of this time, Willis in 1664 wrote that "the corpus striatum represents an exchange between brain stem and cortex" (p. 7).[199] He therefore suggested that this structure "receives the notion of spontaneous localized movements in ascending tracts. . . . Conversely, from here tendencies are dispatched to enact notions without reflection [automatic movements] over descending pathways" (p. 7).[199] Magendie in 1841 demonstrated that removal of the striatum bilaterally produced compulsive movements. He described the response of acaudate rabbits as follows: "The animal runs forward as if under an irresistible impulse. . . . One may say that the animal believes it is hunted and hears the barking of the dogs running in its footsteps" (p. 8).[124] Removal of only one striatum produced no visible effect. Studies by Nothnagel[147] demonstrated that destruction of the globus pallidus produced a twisting of the spine with the convexity toward the side of the lesion. Lesions of the nigra tended to produce immobility. With the advent of the use of electrical stimulation in the late nineteenth century, further information on the function of the basal ganglia was gathered. Stimulation of the caudate nucleus did not (and does not) produce movement of muscles or limbs as did stimulation of the motor cortex. However, total body patterns and postures were usually evoked.

Ferrier[58] was the first to describe the results of stimulation of the caudate nucleus. He noted that there was an increase of flexion of the head and trunk, that the limbs remained in a flexed position, and that the facial muscles also went into tonic contraction. Ferrier concluded that "in the corpus striatum there would thus appear to be an integration of the various centers which are differentiated in the cortex."[58] From these early experiments came the idea that the basal ganglia are involved not only in sensorimotor integration but in initiation of movements and postural and movement programming. (Recent experimental evidence continues to support the concept that the basal ganglia are involved in the preparatory stages but not in the excitation of movement.)

Motor problems in animals. Contemporary experiments concerning lesions show a wide variety of motor problems in a variety of animals. Hypokinesia following the occurrence of lesions in the basal ganglia is one frequent result. Stern[182] observed that bilateral lesions of the substantia nigra produced poverty of movement and a tendency to assume fixed postures. Monkeys with large lesions in the basal ganglia assume a "somersault" position; that is, the animal is flexed so that the head rests on the floor while the animal is standing.[48] Cooling of the putamen and the pallidum in the monkey produces a slowing of movements as well as the tendency toward flexed postures.[74] In one experiment electromyogram (EMG) recordings of the biceps and triceps of monkeys demonstrated an increase in cocontraction of these muscles.[79] Although movement is still possible, it must be made with an abnormal starting position and a delay in appropriate activation of the prime movers.

Movement initiation and preparation. The hypothesis that the basal ganglia are involved in movement initiation and preparation also receives support from human experiments. Kornhuber[102] observed, while recording from the scalp in humans, a slow negative potential bilaterally just before movement. This "Bereitschafts-potential" or "readiness potential" was not present in individuals with Parkinson's disease. Kornhuber hypothesized that the generator for this readiness potential was not in the motor cortex but rather in subcortical structures and, further, that there were two types of movement generators: one for ramp function, or "voluntary speed smooth movement," and another for ballistic, or fast, movement. Ramp movements require integration among the parts of the body for control of constant speed and fluidity of movement. Based on his observations that the signs of lesions in the basal ganglia produced a deficiency in the voluntary production of smooth movements and that lesions of the motor cortex did not, Kornhuber concluded that the generator for ramp move-

ments in the extremities, trunk, and head was the basal ganglia.

A more precise investigation into how movements were programmed and initiated used the technique of single unit recording in awake, performing animals: Evarts[54] in the motor cortex, Delong[46] in the basal ganglia, Thach[189,190] in the cerebellum, and Massion and Smith[128] and Strick[184] in the ventroanterior-ventrolateral nuclei of the thalamus. All these researchers found that units in these areas alter their activity before changes in the EMG activity of the muscles performing the task; that is, before arrival of sensory feedback information from the muscles, joints, and skin could modify the centrally generated movement program. These changes in neuronal activity occurred 50 to 200 msec before the EMG activity changes, and there was enough overlap of the onset of these changes so that no clear answer established which of these areas gave the command to move. However, these results do indicate that all of these brain sites are involved in movement generation. Delong's experiments showed that some units in the basal ganglia changed their activity preferentially with performance of slow (ramp) movements and that units in the cortex, cerebellum, and some pallidal units showed activity changes in both ramp and ballistic movements,[46] in partial agreement with Kornhuber's hypothesis. Experiments using cooling procedures demonstrated that cooling the ventrolateral nucleus,[20] the cerebellum, or basal ganglia[25,80] produced a delay in the onset of the movement but also a slowing in the velocity of the movement itself, again indicating that these structures are involved in the initiation phase of the movement.

Neafsey and others[142,143] and Melnick and co-workers[132] presented further evidence for the involvement of the globus pallidus, ventroanterior-ventrolateral nuclei, and motor cortex in the preparation of movement. Of the units recorded in the globus pallidus, ventroanterior-ventrolateral nuclei, and medial precruciate cortex of the cat, 30% to 70% changed their firing pattern more than 250 msec before changes in EMG activity. Neafsey hypothesized that these early unit activity changes were the "neural correlate of the state of set" (p. 712), or readiness that exists as a preparatory adjustment for performing a task, as proposed by Woodworth and Schlosberg.[202] Buchwald and others[28] have defined this preparatory activity as "response set," which entails "the ability to initiate and carry out smoothly and in proper sequence a set of movements that comprise a defined response" (p. 175).[29] Denny-Brown,[48] in studying the effects of lesions of the basal ganglia on movement, has also suggested that the basal ganglia participate in the "activating set." He defined this set as the preparation of the mechanism preparatory to a motor performance oriented to the environment."[49] The difficulty in parkinsonism of initiating movements or in changing from one movement to another is an example of a disruption in this "response set" process.

Postural adjustments. The involvement of the basal

ganglia in the initiation of movement may include a role in directing the postural adjustments necessary before distal movement can take place. In fact, in addition to the assumption of flexed, fixed postures, other postural abnormalities have been observed following lesions of the basal ganglia. In an experiment by Winkelmuller and Nitsch,[201] rats with bilateral lesions of the substantia nigra were unable to balance skillfully or correct imbalance by quick movements or by shifting their weight. Cats with lesions of one caudate nucleus who had been trained to alternate bar presses have been shown to have similar deficits in postural adjustments. The normal animal keeps the body in a central position and moves only its paws in these alternating movements. The animals with lesions had to move the entire body back and forth between the bars to perform the task.[149]

Similar postural deficiencies have been observed in monkeys with lesions of various parts of the basal ganglia. These deficiencies led Denny-Brown and Yanagesawa[49] to conclude that the basal ganglia "must be concerned in the elaboration of specialized motor reactions to the environment by modification of the labyrinthine and body-contact righting reactions." Similarly, Potegal[160] observed that animals with lesions in the anterior caudate were unable to guide their behavior by taking their own body position into account. He referred to this deficit as a breakdown in "egocentric localization." Similarly studies of human disease processes support the hypothesis that the basal ganglia have a role in the postural mechanisms active before movement. Martin,[127] in his extensive studies of individuals with Parkinson's disease, found that these patients, in addition to their akinesia, demonstrated severe disturbances in posture. He noted that especially when vision was occluded these persons were unable to make the normal postural shifts involved in equilibrium reactions.

Despite the preceding discussion regarding the role of the basal ganglia in postural mechanisms, the data are inconclusive. The early unit activity changes seen in the basal ganglia are not related in a simple fashion to early EMG activity in the proximal and axial muscles. Neither Melnick and others[132] nor Neafsey and co-workers[142,143] found early EMG changes in the proximal muscles that correlated with changes in basal ganglia neuronal activity changes. It is possible that the basal ganglia are involved in biasing and setting the gamma motorneuron system in preparation for extrafusal muscle contraction. The lack of early EMG activity is not inconsistent with a theory of biasing spinal reflex mechanisms to enhance or inhibit the eventual firing of alpha motor neurons of specific muscles.[64] Perhaps the central nervous system (CNS) prepares the muscles for a certain amount of postural tone; if this tone is already present, then no activity changes occur in the muscles. Changes in neuronal activity in preparation for movement would therefore occur with no corresponding change in the EMG activity. Kubota and Hamada[104] reported gradual changes in pyramidal tract neuronal activity up to 1 second

before movement without any visible changes in the posture of the monkey or any changes in EMG activity. They interpreted their finding as also indicating a preparatory state for voluntary movement. This early neuronal activity might also be preparing neurons in the reticulospinal, tectospinal, and corticospinal pathways so that when movement is required, the alpha motor neuron will be more ready or less ready to fire and therefore the movement will occur with the appropriate speed and coordination. This would be similar to the theory of long-term biasing of the cortex discussed earlier. Stimulation of the caudate nucleus or globus pallidus can modify alpha and gamma motor responses evoked by motor cortex or pyramidal tract stimulation.[67,144] Delong and Strick[47] interpreted the changes in basal ganglionic activity preceding movement to be a facilitory discharge to "establish the climate for the performance rather than the detailed pattern of the movement" (p. 334).

Perceptual and cognitive functions. The basal ganglia's function is not solely in the initiation and control of movement and posture. Several studies demonstrate that the basal ganglia are involved in aspects of sensory integration. Lidsky and others[118] found that neurons in the basal ganglia were related to the reward properties and particularly to the sensation of perioral stimulation. Their work and the work of Schneider and colleagues[168] demonstrated that the basal ganglia were involved in modulating reflex responses about the face. Hore and others[79,80] and Brooks,[25] recording from the striatum during cooling, found that the animals had the greatest difficulty with performance of learned movements in the absence of vision. The studies of Crutcher and DeLong[41] found that movement related cells in the putamen were also sensitive to proprioceptive input. Schneider and others[169] found that animals made parkinsonian by a neurotoxin had deficits in operantly conditioned behavior. They suggested that the decrease in performance was due to a "defect in the linkage" between a stimulus and the motor output centers.

There is also evidence to show that the basal ganglia are involved in perceptual and cognitive functions. Following lesions of the basal ganglia, deficits appear in the performance of a variety of alternation tasks in rodents, carnivores, primates, and humans (see Teuber[188] for a review). One reason for these deficits is the animal's tendency toward perseveration of a previously reinforced cue. In learning a delayed spatial alternation task, the animal must learn the temporal sequence (i.e., the alternation of position) and must be able to remember the location and consequences of its last response.[121] Stimulation of the caudate nucleus immediately following movement to the goal prevents the acquisition of this task and also disrupts performance of the task once it is learned, but it does not affect motor ability. Livesey and Rankine-Wilson[121] therefore concluded that interference in caudate functioning at this time selectively disrupted the registration of information generated internally. Frontal cortical lesions also produce deficits in delayed spatial response tasks, but the cortex and the neostriatum appear to mediate separate aspects of delayed response behavior.[50,121,194]

Further support for differences between the cortex and caudate in these tasks comes from experiments involving lesions of these areas in neonatal primates and cats. Kling and Tucker[97] found that early combined lesions of the frontal cortex and caudate nucleus had "devastating" effects on early survival, on somatomotor function, and on the ability to perform delayed-response tasks. Lesions of the frontal cortex alone, occurring at the same period in development, did not show these effects.Tucker and Kling[192] concluded that subcortical structures were more important in control of movement in the neonate and also for the retention of certain cognitive functions if the animal had sustained early brain injury. Goldman[66] obtained similar results in early lesions of the cortex or caudate nucleus. She suggested that the caudate nucleus might be responsible for mediating delayed-response performance in both normal monkeys and those with cortical lesions at early ages. She also hypothesized that the caudate "does not take over functions of the dorsolateral cortex in a compensatory sense, by assuming functions it would not normally have, but is simply the structure primarily responsible for mediating spatial-mnemonic abilities in monkeys under 2 years of age" (p. 409). Olmstead and Villablanca,[149] however, found that cats with lesions of the caudate nucleus made early in life were not as impaired on tasks such as alternating bar pressing and reversal of a spatial discrimination task as cats who sustained this lesion later in life. The kittens used in the experiment showed fewer perseveration tendencies than the adult animals. Deficits have been found in tasks other than delayed-response tasks in animals with basal ganglia lesions. Animals show difficulties in performance of *go-no go* tasks because of a difficulty in suppressing a response to the *no-go* cue.[16]

Humans with basal ganglia disease also show problems in perceptual abilities. Bowen[24] found that these individuals exhibited deficits in a variety of tasks involving perception of interpersonal and intrapersonal space. In pursuit-tracking tests individuals with Parkinson's disease had particular difficulties in correcting errors, which is consistent with Teuber's view that "the basal ganglia may play a role in the regulation of 'corollary' discharges, that is, in presetting of the motor system by sensory stimuli" (p. 164).[188] If the motor system is inflexibly set, corrections can be made only by a complete reprogramming. Further, Bowen noted differential responses when individuals with Parkinson's disease were categorized according to the side of their major neurological symptoms. She suggested that hemispheric specialization in humans may be affected by basal ganglia lesions.[24] It is interesting to note that children with learning disabilities frequently display deficits in the postural mechanisms thought to be mediated by the basal ganglia.[7]

Further evidence that the basal ganglia participate in the performance of delayed-response tasks is found in the results of single unit recording studies. Units in the frontal cortex

change their activity during the delay period in these types of tasks.[61,105] Soltysik and others[178] found neuronal activity changes related to at least one epoch of the delayed-response paradigm in 60% of the units recorded from the globus pallidus, putamen, and caudate. In particular, they found a high percentage of these units responded during the delay period, which would be expected if these structures play a role in the regulation of this task. They stated: "If we consider the delay period to represent a maintaining of a response set, and the pre-response epoch to be a preparatory period enabling the specific response, then neurons of both the pallidum and caudate appear to be associated in significant numbers with this behavior" (p. 75).[178]

Based on the literature indicating involvement of the basal ganglia in these complex behaviors, Buchwald and others[29] have hypothesized that the basal ganglia are involved in "cognitive set" as well as "response set." They defined "cognitive set" as "the ability to discriminate a situational context and make an appropriate response to a given signal" (p. 175). The term *cognitive* was used for "situations where information has to be transferred across some period of time before a response is initiated" (p. 177). They further suggested that the basal ganglia were more involved in complex tasks than in simpler behaviors. Animal experiments seem to indicate that complex learned responses are the ones most affected by basal ganglia lesions.[47,127]

The ability to perform cognitive activities involves integrating sensory information and, based on this information, making an appropriate response. The basal ganglia seem to have a sensory integrative function as evidenced by experiments that show a multisensory and heterotopic convergence of somatic, visual, auditory, and vestibular stimuli.[103,129,139,163] Segundo and Machne[170] observed unitary discharges of the basal ganglia to both somatic and vestibular stimuli. They hypothesized that the function of the basal ganglia was not in a subjective recognition of the stimuli but rather in the regulation of posture and movements of the body in space and in the production of complex motor acts (see Potegal and others[161] for a similar hypothesis).

For movements to be properly controlled and properly sequenced, the two sides of the body need to be well integrated. Some anatomical evidence suggests some means of bilateral control for the basal ganglia. A lesion of one caudate nucleus or nigrostriatal pathway produces a change in the unit activity of the remaining caudate.[113,115] Studies of the dopaminergic pathway also indicate interactions between the two sides of the body.[119] For this reason one may find deficits in function even on the "uninvolved" side of an individual with disease of the basal ganglia. It is also possible that diseases of the basal ganglia may go unnoticed until damage is found bilaterally.

It is hoped that this summary of experimental results on the function of the basal ganglia illustrates several points. Despite many years of research an exact and precise role for these structures remains to be discovered. It does appear, however, that at least in some general way the basal ganglia are involved in the processes of movement related to preparing the organism for future motion. This may include preparing the cortex for approximate time activation, "setting" the postural reflexes or the gamma motor neuron system, and perhaps organizing sensory input to produce a motor response in an appropriate environmental context. The various parts of the basal ganglia may subserve different aspects of movement, which might account for the differences between an individual with Parkinson's disease and one with Huntington's disease. In a clinical assessment one must carefully examine the loss of automatic postural adaptations appropriate for the task at hand. It is hoped that the day approaches when it will no longer be necessary to say, "The exact nature and function of the large mass of basal grey matter known as the corpus striatum have hitherto constituted, it is no exaggeration to say, one of the unsolved problems of neurology" (p. 428).[200] The therapist's job will certainly be easier. Until then it is crucial that clinicians carefully observe all aspects of movement and postural tone during treatment. For additional information refer to Chapter 5.

Neurotransmitters

Before a detailed analysis of the diseases of the basal ganglia can be considered, a brief description of the neurotransmitters of this region is necessary. The primary diseases discussed in this chapter indicate a deficit in specific neurotransmitters. The pharmacological treatment of Parkinson's disease and, in the future, perhaps of Huntington's disease is based on these neurochemical deficits. The basal ganglia possess high concentrations of many of the suspected neurotransmitters: dopamine (DA), acetylcholine (ACh), gamma-aminobutyric acid (GABA), substance P, and the enkephalins and endorphins. This discussion, however, includes only the first three neurotransmitters. A diagram of the basal ganglia pathways, which includes the neurotransmitters, is shown in Fig. 21-4.

DA is the major neurotransmitter of the nigrostriatal pathway. It is produced in the pars compacta of the substantia nigra. The axon terminals of these dopaminergic neurons are located in the caudate nucleus. For years a battle raged as to whether DA was excitatory or inhibitory. At present there is evidence that DA is both excitatory and inhibitory.[33] Dopamine appears to be excitatory to the neurons in the direct pathway (GABA/substance P neurons) and inhibitory to the neurons in the indirect pathway (GABA/enkephalin neurons).[152] This dual effect means that a loss of DA will lead to a loss of excitation in the direct pathway and an excess of excitation of the indirect pathway leading to a powerful decrease in activation of the thalamocortical pathway.

There are now five DA receptors; however, their chemical interactions permit the continued usage of D_1 and D_2 receptor classes.[6] Many new drugs will influence only one

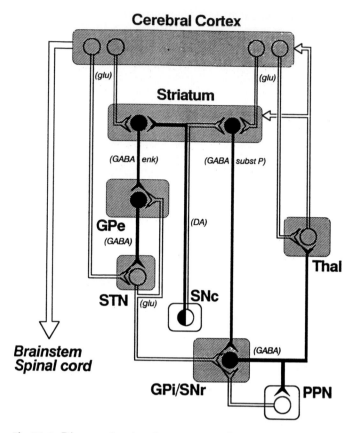

Fig. 21-4. Diagram showing the neurotransmitters of the direct and indirect pathways of the basal ganglia. Darkened circles represent inhibitory neurons; open circles, excitatory neurons. Abbreviations: glu, glutamate; GABA, gamma-aminobutyric acid; enk, enkephalin; subst P, substance P; DA, dopamine; Thal, thalamus; GPe, globus pallidus external segment; GPi, globus pallidus internal segment; STN, subthalamic nucleus; SNr, pars reticularis of the substantia nigra; PPN, pedunculopontine nucleus. (From: Alexander GE and Crutcher MD: *Trends in Neuroscience* 13:266-271, 1990. Reprinted with permission.)

of these receptors. Recent experiments have been trying to determine which behaviors are mediated by which DA receptor in the hope that this research may lead to more effective drug treatment with fewer side effects. All dopamine receptor agonists useful in treating Parkinson's disease are D_2 receptor agonists. The exact role of D_1 receptors is still under investigation.

Because various drugs and chemicals can act as agonists (similar to) and antagonists (block the action of) of DA, they are used in treating disease involving the basal ganglia. Agonists include amantadine, apomorphine, and a class of drugs called the ergot alkaloids (e.g., bromocriptine). Amphetamine, which prevents the reuptake of DA, can enhance the effect of any DA present in the system. Antagonists include haloperidol and other antipsychotic drugs of the phenothiazine class. With time these drugs may deplete the basal ganglia of DA and thus cause Parkinson's disease or tardive dyskinesia. The DA agonists and antagonists will be discussed further in the treatment of Parkinson's disease and the occurrence of drug-induced dyskinesia.

ACh is believed to be the neurotransmitter of the small interneurons of the caudate and putamen. It is presumed to inhibit the action of DA in this region and classically must be "in balance" with DA (and GABA). Dopaminergic axon terminals are found on cholinergic neurons. Substances that increase dopaminergic activity decrease release of ACh and vice versa.[145] The antagonists of ACh, such as belladonna alkaloids and atropine-like drugs, were one of the first class of drugs used in the treatment of Parkinson's disease.

GABA is an inhibitory neurotransmitter that is found throughout the brain. In the basal ganglia it is synthesized in the caudate nucleus and transmitted to the globus pallidus and substantia nigra.[163] GABA in the basal ganglia may permit movement to occur by allowing a distribution of neuronal firing. It also may provide a means of feedback inhibition in the efferent parts of the basal ganglia so that the program of activity is not repeated unless needed (see reference 163 for a summation of the role of GABA). Individuals with Huntington's disease have a deficiency of this chemical. Although agonists of GABA exist (e.g., muscimol and imidazole-acetic acid), a successful drug for the treatment of Huntington's disease has not yet been found. This may be a result of either the ubiquitous nature of GABA or the very complex circuitry and interrelationships that exist among GABA, ACh, and DA.

In addition to the transmitters discussed, there may be cotransmitters in the basal ganglia. Two such cotransmitters are cholecystokinin and neurotensin. The interactions of these cotransmitters may alter the sensitivity of DA receptors. Fuxe and others[62] suggest that the interactions of cotransmitters may alter the "set point" of transmission in synapses. They may therefore be important in one of the side effects of DA therapy, supersensitivity.

SPECIFIC CLINICAL PROBLEMS ARISING FROM BASAL GANGLIA DYSFUNCTION
Parkinson's disease

Parkinson's disease, first described by Parkinson in 1817, is a disease characterized by rigidity, bradykinesia (slow movement), micrography, masked facies, postural abnormalities, and a resting tremor.[7] As might be suspected from the review of functional physiology of the basal ganglia, the postural abnormalities include an assumption of a flexed posture, a lack of equilibrium reactions, especially of the labyrinthine equilibrium reactions, and a decrease in trunk rotation.

The pathology of Parkinson's disease consists of a decrease in the DA stores of the substantia nigra with a consequent depigmentation of this structure and the presence of Lewy bodies (intracellular inclusions). It is DA that gives the substantia nigra its coloration (and hence its name); therefore the lighter the nigra the greater the DA loss. It has been proposed that Parkinson's disease is an abnormal

acceleration of the aging process.[130] DA shows an increase in concentration very early in life, followed by a rapid decrease from 5 to 20 years of age and a slow continuous loss between ages 20 to 80. Carlsson[33] proposed that while a loss of or damage to the DA neurons early in life (because of, for example, infection or toxicity) may be insufficient to precipitate Parkinson's disease, the additional loss of neurons with the natural physiological aging process may add cumulatively to that early loss, and the signs of Parkinson's disease are seen when some critical level is reached. Indeed the average age of onset for Parkinson's disease is 35 to 60 years. The disease affects men slightly more than women.

The etiology of Parkinson's disease remains unknown. Calne[36] suggests that, like pneumonia, Parkinson's disease may have several causes. A slow viral process or long-term effects of early infection were implicated in post-encephalitis-parkinsonism. There is evidence that environmental factors are involved in the etiology and that the interaction of environment and aging lead to a critical decrease in DA. Several investigators have found a link between growing up in a rural area and Parkinson's disease; the important factors include pesticide use, insecticide use, and well water.[12,31,100,162] Genetics may also be a factor in Parkinson's disease. Although twin studies indicate that there may not be a single gene involved in Parkinson's disease, as in Huntington's disease, a family history is an important risk factor.[31] Hubble and others[82] also found that a history of depression was a risk factor for Parkinson's disease. The accumulation of free radicals, cell death from toxins to excitatory neurons, and dysfunction of nigral mitochondria have been implicated from studies of a known neurotoxin (discussed later in this chapter); however, this has not been proven in idiopathic Parkinson's disease.

In view of possible treatment effects for parkinsonism, it is interesting that a study by Sasco and others[166] found an inverse relationship, albeit small, between participation in exercise or sports and later development of parkinsonism. Most researchers agree that the etiology is an interaction of toxic exposure, genetics, and aging. The loss of DA from the SN leads to alterations in both the direct and indirect pathways of the basal ganglia and a decrease in excitatory thalamic input to the cortex and the symptomatology of Parkinson's disease.

Symptoms

Bradykinesia and akinesia. Bradykinesia (a decrease in motion) and akinesia (a lack of motion) are characterized by an inability to initiate and perform purposeful movements. They are also associated with a tendency to assume and maintain fixed postures. All aspects of movement are affected, including initiation, alteration in direction, and the ability to stop a movement once it is begun. Spontaneous or associated movements, such as swinging of the arms in gait or smiling at a funny story, are also affected. Bradykinesia is hypothesized to be the result of a decrease in activation of the supplemary motor cortex, premotor cortex, and motor cortex.[156] The resting level of activity in these areas of the cortex may be decreased so that a greater amount of excitatory input from other areas of the brain would be necessary before movement patterns could be activated. In the individual with Parkinson's disease, an increase in cortically initiated movement even for such "subcortical" activities as walking supports this hypothesis. These automatic activities are now cortically controlled, and each individual aspect seems to be separately programmed. Associated movements in the trunk and other extremities are not automatic activity. This means that great energy must be expended whenever movement is begun.

Bradykinesia and akinesia affect performance of all types of movements; however, complex movements are more involved than simple movements.[18,19,26,193] This fact was demonstrated in a study showing that the readiness potential preceding gait was more abnormal than the same potential preceding simple ankle dorsiflexion performed in an open kinetic chain.[193] Additionally, patients with parkinsonism have increased difficulty performing simultaneous or sequential tasks, over and above that seen with simple tasks. Parkinsonian patients must complete one movement before they can begin to perform the next, whereas control subjects are able to integrate to movements more smoothly in sequence. This deficit has been shown in a variety of tasks from performing an elbow movement and grip to tracing a moving line on a video screen. The parkinsonian patient behaves as if one motor program must be completely played out before the next one begins, and there is no advance planning for the next movement while the present movement is in progress.[18,19,26,138,153] Further, sequential movements become more impaired as more movements are strung together; for example, a square is disproportionately slower to draw than a triangle; a pentagon, more difficult than a square.[1,18] These results indicate that parkinsonian patients have difficulty with transitions between movements. Transitional difficulties are more impaired in tasks requiring a series of different movements than tasks requiring a series of repetitive movements. (This fact is important when planning a comprehensive treatment program.)

Results of reaction time experiments are controversial. Some studies find that simple reaction time tasks (the direction and extent of movement are known) are more impaired than choice reaction time tasks (direction and/or extent of movement are not known),[70] others find that choice tasks are more impaired than simple,[26] still others find that they are equally impaired.[88] These conflicting views may be hard to reconcile in the evaluation and treatment process; however, the task differences may be indicative of task-dependent impairments. Differences in results may involve differences in subject familiarity with the task, whether there is a warning cue, whether the cues involve many sensory systems, and whether the movement sequence must be represented internally. Those authors that find simple

reaction time tasks less impaired suggest that parkinsonian patients can use prior information to preplan movement[203]; those that find choice reaction time tasks more impaired suggest that parkinsonian patients are able to select the correct movement, but have difficulty in initiation only. There does seem to be agreement that programming of movements in parkinsonism is definitely task dependent and that familiarity with the task and the use of multisensory systems improve performance.

It is important to remember that bradykinesia is *not* caused by rigidity or an inability to relax. This was demonstrated in an EMG analysis of voluntary movements of persons with Parkinson's disease.[71] Although the pattern of EMG agonist-antagonists burst is correct, these bursts are not large enough, resulting in an inability to generate muscle force rapidly enough. Even in slow, smooth movements, however, these individuals demonstrated alternating bursts in the flexor and extensor muscle groups. This type of pattern is expected in rapid movements that require the immediate activation of the antagonist to halt the motion, but it would interfere with slow, smooth, continuous motion. Other experimenters[69,136] found an alteration in the recruitment order of single motor units. Milner-Brown and others[136] hypothesized that recruitment of the first motor units participating in the initiation of movement involved a pathway from the substantia nigra to the caudate, then through loops to the thalamus and motor cortex, and on down by way of the pyramidal system. Once initiated, smooth movement can continue only with a continuous firing of agonist motor units, along with recruitment of more motor units or the ability to increase firing rates. In individuals with Parkinson's disease, there was a delay in recruitment, pauses in the motor unit once it was recruited, and inability to increase firing rates. These persons therefore would have a delay in activation of muscles and an inability to properly sustain muscle contraction for movement.

Rigidity. The rigidity of Parkinson's disease may be characterized as either "lead pipe" or "cogwheel." The cogwheel type of rigidity is a combination of lead-pipe rigidity with tremor. In rigidity there is an increased resistance to movement throughout the entire range in both directions without the classic clasp-knife reflex so characteristic of spasticity. Procaine injections can decrease the rigidity without affecting the decrease of spontaneous movements, confirming that rigidity is not the same phenomenon as bradykinesia.[159,197]

Rigidity is not due to an increase in gamma motor neuron activity, a decrease in recurrent inhibition, or a generalized excitability in the motor system.[112] Long latency reflexes are enhanced in parkinsonism, and the increase in long latency reflexes approximates the observable increase in muscle tone.

Tatton and others[186] found differences in certain cortical long-loop reflexes in normal and drug-induced parkinsonian monkeys, which led them to speculate that the "reflex gain" of the CNS may lose its ability to adjust to changing environmental situations. That is, in normal persons the descending input that would establish the appropriate level of excitability of the alpha and gamma motor neurons for writing is different from that necessary to lift a heavy object; in individuals with Parkinson's disease it would be at the same level. (The descending input for excitability of the motor neurons to the commands "push" or "pull" would also be the same in the parkinsonian person.) In other words, for the normal person the command to "push" in response to an external perturbation would increase the excitability of the triceps motor neuronal pool; the command to "pull" would decrease triceps excitability. In the individual with Parkinson's disease, the excitability of the triceps motor neuronal pool would be the same to both commands, and therefore the response to either would be delayed. It is possible that the basal ganglia help to modulate the gain of proprioceptive feedback occurring through the motor cortex. Disease in these structures might then limit the range of this modulation so that all inputs are treated the same, and the whole system is adjusted at a higher level of activity. This means that the person with parkinsonism may have the perception of moving farther than he or she is actually moving.

Some studies have shown a decrease in interneuronal circuitry, which accompanies a quicker recovery of reflexes. This might account for some of the earlier literature that reported an increase in alpha or gamma motorneuron activity or an altered response in H-reflex activity.[15] Hallett[70] has suggested that increased reflex responsiveness may be the result of "release" of the pedunculopontine nucleus from globus pallidus inhibition.

An important aspect of rigidity is that it might increase energy expenditure.[126] This would increase the patient's perception of effort on movement and may be related to feelings of fatigue.[59]

Tremor. The tremor observed in Parkinson's disease is present at rest, it usually disappears or decreases with movement, and it has a regular rhythm of about 4 to 7 beats per second. The EMG tracing of a person with such a tremor shows rhythmical, alternating bursting of antagonistic muscles. Tremor can be produced as an isolated finding in experimental animals that have lesions in various parts of the brainstem or that have been treated with drugs, especially DA antagonists. DA depletion, however, is not the sole cause of tremor. It appears that efferent pathways, especially from the basal ganglia to the thalamus, must be intact because lesions of these fibers decrease or abolish the tremor.[158] Poirier and others[158] proposed that tremor results from a combined lesion of the basal ganglia and cerebellar nucleus pathways. Because both the basal ganglia and the cerebellum project to the thalamus, a lesion of the thalamus can abolish the tremor regardless of the specific pathway(s).

Postural instability is a serious problem in parkinsonism that leads to increased episodes of falling and the sequelae of falls. Koller and others[99] found that over one third of all patients with parkinsonism fall and that over 10% fall more than once a week. They also found that the likelihood of falling increased as the length of duration of disease increased. Drug treatment is not usually effective in reducing the incidence of falls.

One explanation for postural instability is ineffective sensory processing. Martin,[127] for example, found that labyrinthine equilibrium reactions were delayed in parkinsonian patients. Studies of the vestibular system itself, however, have shown that this system functions normally. Pastor and others[154] studied central vestibular processing in parkinsonian patients and found that the vestibular system responds normally and that patients can integrate vestibular input with the input from other sensory systems. This group hypothesized that the parkinsonian patients had an inability to adequately compensate for baseline instability. This theory is in partial agreement with studies by Beckley and others[17] demonstrating that parkinsonian patients were unable to adjust the size of long latency reflex responses to the degree of perturbation. Glatt and others[68] found that parkinsonian patients did not demonstrate anticipatory postural reactions and, in fact, behaved exactly as a rigid body with joints. Horak and others[78] reported similar findings and found defects in strategy selection; parkinsonian patients chose neither a pure hip strategy nor a pure ankle strategy but mixed the two in an inappropriate and maladaptive response. Taken together, it appears that postural instability results from the interaction of akinesia, bradykinesia, and rigidity, with some disturbance in central sensory processing.

Gait. Another characteristic of Parkinson's disease is the presence of a festinating gait. This is a gait characterized by a progressive increase in speed and shortening of stride as if the individual is trying to catch up with his or her center of gravity. Forward festination is called propulsion; backward festination is known as retropulsion. The festinating gait may be caused by the decreased equilibrium responses. If walking is a series of controlled falls and if normal responses to falling are delayed or not strong enough, then the individual will either fall completely or continue to take short, runninglike steps. The abnormal motor unit firing seen with bradykinesia may also be the cause of ever-shortening steps. If the motor unit cannot build up a high enough frequency or if it pauses in the middle of the movement, then the full range of the movement would decrease; in walking this would lead to shorter steps. Festination may be similar to the description of a rabbit running as if chased by dogs. In this regard then it could be similar to what Villablanca and Marcus call "obstinate progression."[191] Cats with lesions of the basal ganglia will fixate on a singular sensory object and follow it continuously even if they bump into the wall. If a new, more potent stimulus is presented, the animal will refocus its attention or at least halt the activity. A client walking with a festinating gait can be made to alter this gait pattern by introducing a potent new stimulus (e.g., a loud clap), which is similar to the cat displaying "obstinate progression."

The gait of a person with Parkinson's disease shows other abnormalities besides festination. Typically, there is a loss in the heel-toe progression of the normal gait cycle. Instead there is a flat-footed or, with progression, a toe-heel sequence. It is as if the Parkinsonian patient has lost the adult gait pattern and is using a more primitive pattern. The flat-footed gait decreases the ability to step over obstacles or to walk on carpeted surfaces.

Attentional and cognitive deficits. Especially in recent years, researchers have tried to address the cognitive and perceptual deficits of patients with Parkinson's disease. Whereas the movement deficits are hypothesized to be due to a decrease in putamenal excitation of the cortex, the learning and perceptual deficits are hypothesized to be due to a decrease in cortical excitation from the caudate nucleus.[153] The deficits are of frontal lobe function and include an inability to shift attention, an inability to quickly access "working memory," and difficulty with visuospatial perception and discrimination. Research attention has focused on the specific deficits of parkinsonian patients compared with patients with Alzheimer's disease, patients with frontal lobe damage, and those with temporal lobe damage. There appears to be an increase in these perceptual deficits with progression of the disease process. In general, patients have difficulty in shifting attention to a previously irrelevant stimulus,[150] learning when selective attention is necessary,[150,180] or selecting the correct motor response based on the sensory stimuli.[169]

Learning deficits also have been found in patients with parkinsonism; procedural learning has been particularly implicated. Procedural learning is learning that occurs with practice or, as defined by Saint-Cyr and others,[165] "the ability gradually to acquire a motor skill or even a cognitive routine through repeated exposure to a specific activity constrained by invariant rules." In their tests, parkinsonian patients did very poorly on tests of procedural learning, but their declarative learning was within normal limits. Pacual-Leone and colleagues[153] studied procedural learning in more detail. They found that parkinsonian patients could acquire procedural learning but needed more practice than controls subjects. They also found that the ability to translate procedural knowledge to declarative knowledge was more efficient if it occurred through visual input only rather than visuomotor practice. Visual input alone is better than the combination of visual input with a motor task.

Stages of the disease. Parkinson's disease is a progressive disorder. Usually the initial symptom is a resting tremor or micrography (bradykinesia of the upper extremity) unilaterally. With time rigidity and bradykinesia are seen and postural alterations begin to occur. This commonly starts with an increase in neck, trunk, and hip flexion, which, accompanied by a decrease in righting and equilibrium responses, leads to a decreasing ability to balance.

While these postural changes are occurring, there is also an increase in rigidity, which is most apparent in the trunk and proximal musculature. Trunk rotation is severely decreased. There is no arm swing in gait and no spontaneous facial expression, and movement becomes more and more difficult to initiate. Movement is usually produced with great concentration and is perhaps cortically generated, therefore bypassing the damaged basal ganglia pathways. This great concentration then makes movement tiring, which also heightens the debilitating effects of the disease.

Eventually the individual becomes wheelchair bound and dependent. In the late and severe stages of the disease, especially without therapeutic attention to movement, the client may become bedridden and may demonstrate a fixed trunk-flexion contracture no matter what position the person is placed in. This posture has been called the "phantom pillow" syndrome because, even when lying supine, the person's head is flexed as if on a pillow.

Throughout this progressive deterioration of movement, there is also a decrease in higher-level sensory processing. This is especially evident in the performance of spatial tasks,[13,24] for example, following a map. The difficulty occurs because these individuals cannot orient their own body in space with reference to the map; they display a loss of egocentric localization. In addition, they can perform only one task at a time. Despite these changes there is no conclusive evidence of a loss in cognitive abilities.[24] Reports of dementia range from 30% to 93% of Parkinson's disease patients.[87] It is generally thought that the appearance of dementia in parkinsonian patients is a result of the presence of extranigral and/or cortical changes similar to those seen in Alzheimer's disease. Frequently, the amount of dementia is related to the age of the patient, and these patients may represent a subset of Parkinson's disease. The presence of dementia with Parkinson's disease may indicate involvement of acetylcholine and/or the noradrenergic mesolimbic system. In this case, treatment with anticholinergic drugs may increase a tendency toward dementia, especially in older patients. Sometimes cognitive deficits are inferred because of spatial problems, sensory processing problems, and a masked face.

The most serious complication of Parkinson's disease is bronchopneumonia. Decreased activity in general, along with decreased chest expansion, may be contributing factors. The mortality rate is greater than in the general population, and death is usually from pneumonia.

Pharmacological considerations and medical management. The knowledge that the symptoms of Parkinson's disease are caused by a decrease in DA led to the pharmacological management of this disease. DA itself does not cross the blood-brain barrier, but levo-dihydroxy-phenylalanine (L-dopa), a precursor of DA, does. This led to the use of L-dopa in treatment in the late 1960s.[40,81,122] Because L-dopa can be changed to DA in the body before ever reaching the brain, it is now usually given with an inhibitor of aromatic amino acid decarboxylation (carbidopa). These inhibitors do not enter the brain readily; thus at the dosages used, their actions are limited to peripheral tissue. This then allows more of the L-dopa to enter the brain and undergo decarboxylation where it will do the most good. Further, the decarboxylase inhibitor allows a reduction in dosage of L-dopa itself, which helps decrease the cardiac and gastrointestinal side effects it causes through the increase in DA in the peripheral organs.

Amantadine is another drug that has been effective in treatment of Parkinson's disease. Although the mechanism of action of this antiviral medication is unknown, it is thought to include a facilitation of release of catecholamine (of which DA is one) from stores in the neuron that are readily releasable. It is often administered in combination with L-dopa.

Treatment of Parkinson's disease with L-dopa in these various combinations is extremely helpful in reducing bradykinesia and rigidity. It is less effective in reducing tremor. Because Parkinson's disease involves the nigral neurons, the receptors and the neurons in the striatum (which are postsynaptic to DA neurons) remain intact and initially are somewhat responsive to DA.[58] With time, however, the receptors appear to lose their sensitivity, and the prolonged effectiveness (10 years or more) of L-dopa therapy is questionable.[90,125,131] A further complication of L-dopa therapy is the development of involuntary movements (dyskinesias) and the "on-off" phenomenon—a short-duration response resulting in sudden improvement of symptoms followed by a rapid decline in symptomatic relief and perhaps the appearance of dyskinesias. With time the "on" effect becomes of shorter and shorter duration.[90] The effectiveness of L-dopa does not appear to be closely correlated with the stage of the disease.

The use of L-dopa alone or in combination with carbidopa has not provided a cure or even prevented the degeneration of Parkinson's disease. Therefore many new drugs are being tested and tried. As scientists learn more about the dopamine receptors and their role in motor control, more effective medications may be found. Some of these "newer" drugs include bromocriptine and pergolide, both D_2 receptor agonists. Low doses of bromocriptine seem to decrease the wearing off phenomenon of L-dopa and may also decrease the dyskinesia.[32] However, the side effects include hallucinations, nausea, and vomiting. Pergolide also appears to be effective in treatment; however, double-blind studies seem to indicate recovery in placebo as well.[90] It is quite likely that newer D_1 and/or D_2-D_1 agonists will be developed.

Another approach to pharmacological treatment of Parkinson's disease developed from research on a designer drug that contained the neurotoxin 1-methyl-4-phenyl-1,2,3,6-tetrahydropyridine (MPTP). It was found that the conversion of MPTP to the active neurotoxin MPP+ could

be prevented by monamine oxidase inhibitors such as deprenyl and pargyline.[75] Deprenyl is now used before the initiation of, or in conjunction with, L-dopa/carbidopa. Although its mechanism of action is still not fully understood, it may act as a neuroprotective agent.[37,101] Other catechol-O-methyltransferase (COMT) inhibitors (e.g., entacapone) are under investigation. Future pharmacological interventions may include a variety of neurotrophic factors and possible neuroprotective factors.[89]

Stereotaxic surgery is an old technique[90] that has made a comeback based on the new knowledge of basal ganglia connectivity and improvements in the instrumentation. Lesions are made in specific areas of the globus pallidus and, in nonhuman primates, in the subthalamic nucleus. Following the appearance of these lesions, which are small in size and restricted to the posteroventral region of the globus pallidus, there is improvement in the rigidity, bradykinesia, and akinesia. Patients demonstrate associated reactions spontaneously. In many cases the dyskinesias also improve. The surgical treatment resurgence is new and must be tested over time.

Another possibility is fetal transplantation of the substantia nigra. Studies of this technique are presently under investigation.

Evaluation of the client with Parkinson's disease. Evaluation of the client with Parkinson's disease should focus on the degree of rigidity and bradykinesia and how much these symptoms interfere with activities of daily living. These evaluations should of course be as objective as possible, and one method is the rating scale developed by Webster (1968) and shown in Fig. 21-5.[77] This type of scale also allows assessing the progression of the disease. The Hoehn and Yahr Scale[77] is used as a descriptor for the patients's level of involvement. Unilateral involvement places the patient at stage I. Early bilateral involvement with full independent activities of daily living (ADL) ability and no postural instability is stage II. In stage II most patients first encounter physical therapy. In stage III, the patient has postural instability. In stage IV, although the patient is still ambulating independently, most activities require some assistance. In stage V, the patient is confined to a wheelchair or to bed. The most prevalent and most comprehensive evaluation is the Unified Parkinson's Disease Rating Scale (UPDRS), which evaluates cognitive and emotional status, ADL ability, and motor function. This scale is helpful, but is not as objective or as useful in planning a **physical therapy** plan of treatment.

In assessing function of the client with Parkinson's disease, the therapist must note not only that an activity can be accomplished but also how long it takes to perform a task. Gait can be assessed by general pattern and also by speed and distance. Forward and backward walking as well as braiding should be evaluated. (Similarly, the time it takes to go from sitting to standing, standing to sitting, and supine lying to sitting and back again should be recorded.) Handwriting

PARKINSON'S DISEASE PATIENT EVALUATION

Select the appropriate rating for each symptom and mark it in the space provided
in the right-hand column.

BRADYKINESIA
OF HANDS—
INCLUDING
HANDWRITING
0   No involvement
1   Detectable slowing of the supination-pronation rate evidenced by be-
    ginning difficulty in handling tools, buttoning clothes, and with
    handwriting
2   Moderate slowing of supination-pronation rate, one or both sides,
    evidenced by moderate impairment of hand function. Handwriting
    is greatly impaired, micrographia present
3   Severe slowing of supination-pronation rate. Unable to write or
    button clothes. Marked difficulty in handling utensils

RIGIDITY
0   Nondetectable
1   Detectable rigidity in neck and shoulders. Activation phenomenon is
    present. One or both arms show mild, negative, resting rigidity
2   Moderate rigidity in neck and shoulders. Resting rigidity is positive
    when patient not on medication
3   Severe rigidity in neck and shoulders. Resting rigidity cannot be
    reversed by medication
                                                                        ____

POSTURE
0   Normal posture. Head flexed forward less than 4 inches
1   Beginning poker spine. Head flexed forward up to 5 inches
2   Beginning arm flexion. Head flexed forward up to 6 inches. One or
    both arms raised but still below waist
3   Onset of simian posture. Head flexed forward more than 6 inches.
    One or both hands elevated above the waist. Sharp flexion of
    hand, beginning interphalangeal extension. Beginning flexion
    of knees
                                                                        ____

UPPER
EXTREMITY
SWING
0   Swings both arms well
1   One arm definitely decreased in amount of swing
2   One arm fails to swing
3   Both arms fail to swing
                                                                        ____

GAIT
0   Steps out well with 18-30 inch stride. Turns about effortlessly
1   Gait shortened to 12-18 inch stride. Beginning to strike one heel.
    Turn around time slowing. Requires several steps
2   Stride moderately shortened now 6-12 inches. Both heels beginning
    to strike floor forcefully
3   Onset of shuffling gait, steps less than 3 inches. Occasional stut-
    tering-type of blocking gait. Walks on toes turns around very
    slowly
                                                                        ____

TREMOR
0   No detectable tremor found
1   Less than 1 inch of peak-to-peak tremor movement observed in limbs
    or head at rest or in either hand while walking or during finger
    to nose testing
2   Maximum tremor envelope fails to exceed 4 inches. Tremor is severe
    but not constant and patient retains some control of hands
3   Tremor envelope exceeds 4 inches. Tremor is constant and severe.
    Patient cannot get free of tremor while awake unless it is a
    pure cerebellar type. Writing and feeding self are impossible
                                                                        ____

FACIES
0   Normal. Full animation. No stare
1   Detectable immobility. Mouth remains closed. Beginning features of
    anxiety or depression
2   Moderate immobility. Emotion breaks through at markedly increased
    threshold. Lips parted some of the time. Moderate appearance of
    anxiety or depression. Drooling may be present
3   Frozen facies. Mouth open ¼ inch or more. Drooling may be severe
                                                                        ____

SEBORRHEA
0   None
1   Increased perspiration, secretion remaining thin
2   Obvious oiliness present. Secretion much thicker
3   Marked seborrhea, entire face and head covered by thick secretion
                                                                        ____

SPEECH
0   Clear, loud, resonant, easily understood
1   Beginning of hoarseness with loss of inflection and resonance. Good
    volume and still easily understood
2   Moderate hoarseness and weakness. Constant monotone, unvaried pitch.
    Beginning of dysarthria, hesitancy, stuttering; difficult to
    understand
3   Marked harshness and weakness. Very difficult to hear and to under-
    stand
                                                                        ____

SELF-CARE
0   No impairment
1   Still provides full self-care but rate of dressing definitely im-
    peded. Able to live alone and often still employable
2   Requires help in certain critical areas, such as turning in bed, ris-
    ing from chairs, etc. Very slow in performing most activities but
    manages by taking much time
3   Continuously disabled. Unable to dress, feed self, or walk alone
                                                                        ____

                                                           TOTAL   ____

OVERALL DISABILITY (total value of):
1-10, Early illness; 11-20, moderate disability; 21-30, severe or advanced disease.

Fig. 21-5. Parkinson's disease patient evaluation form. (From Endo Laboratories, Inc, Garden City,
NY. Copyright 1979.)

should be periodically sampled. Additionally, active and passive range of movement should be measured.

A careful analysis of equilibrium is imperative for the parkinsonian client. This must include assessment with and *without* vision and the differences in the two recorded. The author's own investigation also highlights the importance of assessing tandem walking, especially in the early stages of the disease. This may be the first sign of equilibrium impairment.

Another aspect of assessment would include the detailed observation of associated postural movements. For example in rising from a chair, does the patient move forward in the chair, place the feet underneath the knees, and lean forward before rising? At present a complete and easy-to-use form for evaluation does not exist for Parkinson's disease. The evaluation format should also include the performance of simultaneous and sequential tasks.

An assessment of chest expansion and vital capacity should also be included in the evaluation. This is important because of the complication of pneumonia.

General treatment goals and rationale. As with all treatment, the general goals will be related to the findings on evaluation of each client. In general, goals include increasing movement as well as range of motion, maintaining or improving chest expansion, improving equilibrium reactions, and maintaining functional abilities. Increased movement may in fact modify the progression of the disease and prevent contractures.[53] It may further help to retard dementia. Although L-dopa decreases the bradykinesia, it alone will not be effective in increasing movement, and therefore aggressive intervention in the early stages is necessary. Increasing trunk rotation goes hand in hand with increasing range of movement and motion in general. The longer clients are kept mobile, the less likely they are to develop pneumonia and maintain independence in ADL.

Treatment procedures. The person with parkinsonism must be encouraged to move throughout a full range of motion early in the disease process to prevent changes in the properties of muscle itself. In these patients the contractile elements of flexors become shortened and those of the extensor surface become lengthened.[167] This enhances the development of the flexed posture traditionally seen. To increase movement there must be a decrease in rigidity. Many relaxation techniques appear to be effective, including gentle, slow rocking, rotation of the extremities and trunk, and even the use of yoga. With the parkinsonian client success in relaxation may be better achieved in the sitting position because rigidity may increase in the supine position.[10] Further, because the proximal muscles are often more involved than the distal muscles, relaxation may be easier to achieve by following a distal to proximal progression. The inverted position may be used with care. Initially, this position facilitates some relaxation (increase in parasympathetic tone) and then increases trunk extension, which is important for the parkinsonian client.

Once a decrease in rigidity is achieved through relaxation, movement must be initiated. For the client with Parkinson's disease, this movement should be large and through the entire range. As with relaxation techniques it may be easier to start with distal motions first and gradually increase the movement, bringing in proximal and trunk muscles. Sitting is a good position from which to begin, starting perhaps with swinging of the arms in ever-increasing amplitude. Because bilateral symmetrical patterns are easier than reciprocal patterns, they should be used first. To add trunk rotation (which will also help decrease the proximal rigidity)[22] proprioceptive neuomuscular facilitation (PNF) patterns and rhythmical initiation might be used.[98] Additionally, neurodevelopmental treatment (NDT) and mobilization techniques may be useful to increase scapular and pelvic mobility.

The use of rhythm and auditory cues facilitates movement. Rhythm, especially as in a march, seems to enable the client to move continuously with alternating flexion and extension without becoming fixated. Clapping or music enhances this effect. At present no explanation can be given for this phenomenon, but perhaps it diminishes cortical initiation and abnormal EMG activity (which was discussed earlier). Movement is thus accomplished in a more automatic, nonfragmented manner.

As the client's movement increases, bilateral activities can be replaced with reciprocal patterns. Use of functional types of activities is likewise important. In gait activities large steps with large arm swings should be encouraged. Additionally, changes in direction, changes in movement patterns, and stopping and starting activities should be stressed.

Equilibrium reactions in all planes of movement and under different control should be encouraged. Rhythmical stabilization may be used *if* the use of resistance does not lead to an increase in truncal rigidity. The timing of the resistance must be very gradual, allowing the client time to develop force in one set of muscles before increasing resistance and then switching directions. This alters the context of the environment and allows the client to practice a variety of variations of the original plan. If proper time is not allowed, the therapist may reinforce the already inefficient, ineffective patterns of motor activity. (See Chapters 6, 9, 14, 17, 23, and 24 for other procedures.) Further, there may be a relationship between longevity and physical activity and some evidence to indicate that **exercise** may alter the magnitude of free radicals and other compounds linked to aging and to parkinsonism. Immunological function may also be improved with exercise. (See the article by Sasco and others[166] linking a lack of exercise with development of parkinsonism.) Exercise is most beneficial when it is begun early in the disease process. All research on the effects of exercise programs in parkinsonism indicate this point. Hurwitz[86] found that patients who were still independently mobile at home and in the community benefitted the most from a home program. Schenkman and Butler[167] also indicated that patients in the earlier stages of the disease had the best potential for improvement. If patients practice regular physical exercise in conjunction with disease-specific exercises, the ill effects of inactivity will not potentiate the effects of the disease process itself. Although most patients with parkinsonism can achieve an adequate exercise level, many had fitness levels that were poor or very poor.[126]

While working on upper-extremity activities, chest expansion may be increased as arm swings increase. The clinician may also have the client shout—again, especially with some kind of rhythmical chant, even a simple "left, right" while walking. If needed, specific breathing exercises can be incorporated.

In addition to treatment in the therapy department, the parkinsonian client also should be given a home program, which is necessary to encourage making moderate, consistent exercise a part of the normal day. Fatigue should be avoided and the exercise graded to the individual's capability. The therapist should keep in mind that learned skills such as various sports are sometimes less affected than automatic movements,[55] perhaps because these skills may rely on cortical involvement.

Physical or occupational therapy in the treatment of Parkinson's disease can be quite effective whether or not the client is taking medication. Physical therapy is suggested in most brochures and books[53] for parkinsonian individuals and their families. However, little has been published on effective therapeutic procedures for the individual with Parkinson's disease.[9] One recent report by Palmer and others[151] utilized precise, quantitative measures to assess motor signs, grip strength, coordination, and speed as well as measurements of the long latency stretch reflex following two exercise programs in Parkinson's patients. These two programs were the United Parkinson Foundation program and karate training. Their results indicated improvement over 12 weeks in gait, grip strength, and coordination of fine motor control tasks but no change in a decline in movements requiring speed. The patients all felt an increase in general well-being. The results of this careful study indicate that more research and careful documentation of exercise programs are needed.

Physical activity and movement appear to increase quality of life by decreasing the depression and lack of initiative that occur in Parkinson's disease. Group classes can serve as an extra support system for Parkinson's patients and their spouses.[63,151] A carefully structured low-impact aerobics program appears to be beneficial to patients even with long-standing disease (Melnick and others, unpublished results). One program begins with seated activities for upper extremities (Fig. 21-6, A) and then combination movements for warm-up (Fig. 21-6, B). The participants then progress to standing and marching activities that incorporate coordinated movements of arms and legs as well as balance and trunk rotation (Fig. 21-7). All movements are performed to

music similar to that used in aerobics classes in any gym or health spa. Heart rate should be monitored periodically. Many Parkinson's disease associations also have audio tapes for exercises (e.g., United Parkinson's Foundation).

Ballroom dancing is also an excellent form of therapy for Parkinson's patients, as it promotes rhythmical movement, rotation, balance, and coordination. The waltz or fox trot is a good beginning dance as it is easy and somewhat slow (Fig. 21-8). The mambo promotes separation of the pelvis from the trunk and increases coordination. A modified Charleston can be used to increase one-legged balance, as can modified tap dancing. The use of dance also facilitates changing direction.

Some of the group activities and possible exercises are depicted in Figs. 21-6 to 21-9. Data are presently being gathered on functional changes and ROM changes in patients participating in a weekly program of aerobics.

Aerobic exercises, especially those that incorporate context-dependent responses and a varied environment, ameliorate many of the dysfunctions associated with parkinsonism. Examples of these activities are presented in the box on p. 625. (Aerobic exercises that are not as effective in requiring context-dependent responses are presented in the box on p. 625.) Research has shown the importance of adjusting the response to the specific task and has also demonstrated the importance of practice for the parkinsonian patient.[38,187] The principles of motor learning are of paramount importance in the treatment program of these patients. Random practice may enable the patient to learn the correct schema by which to regulate the extent, speed, and direction of the movement. Random practice also may be important in facilitating the ability of the patient to shift attention and to learn to access "working memory." The parkinsonian patient may benefit from visual instruction and mental rehearsal *before* performing the movement.[164,181] The research on sensory systems in Parkinson's disease indicates that effectiveness of the use of multisensory cuing. Finally, the role of aerobic fitness itself may be a factor in reducing dysfunction.[134] Aerobic exercise may improve pulmonary function in parkinsonian patients because these functions appear to suffer from deficiencies in rapid force generation of the respiratory muscles,[43] similar to limb musculature.

Patients frequently ask about the timing of medication and exercise. For any form of exercise in parkinsonism to be effective, movement must be possible, especially movement through the full arc of the joint. It seems plausible therefore that exercise should be performed during the "on" period. On the other hand, perhaps there would be a more long-lasting effect if the parkinsonian patient tried to exercise without medication. The question of the effects of exercise on dopamine agonist absorption were recently investigated by Carter and others.[35] They concluded that the effect was variable from patient to patient; however, the response of each patient was consistent. It should be noted, however, that

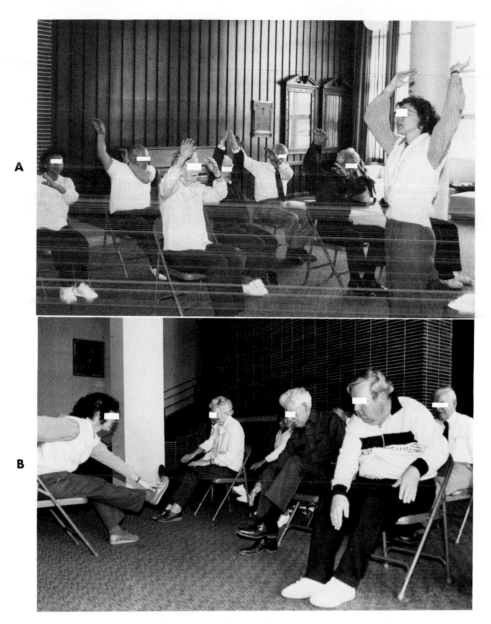

Fig. 21-6. Seated aerobics or warm-up exercises. **A**, Clients are utilizing bilateral upper extremity patterns to facilitate trunk rotation. Instruction was to let the head follow the hands. **B**, This exercise encourages trunk rotation, large movements, and coordination of the upper and lower extremities. Clients are to reach with the arms and touch the opposite foot. This coordination is very difficult in Parkinson's disease, and initially many clients could not move the arms and legs at the same time.

none of the patients exercised vigorously, which may have skewed the results. Nevertheless, this study supports the concept that the patient needs to be "in tune" with his or her own response and adjust medications and exercise to a schedule accordingly. Patients appear able to integrate their exercise and medication schedule well.

The use of assistive devices in gait for the Parkinson's patients is an area with no clear-cut guidelines. Because coordination of upper and lower extremities is often difficult, the ability to use a cane or walker is often lacking. The

patient may drag the cane or carry the walker. Walkers with wheels seem to increase the festinating gait, and the patient may just fall over the walker. For those patients with a tendency to fall backwards, an assistive device may simply be something to carry backwards with them. Therefore the reason for using the assistive device must be carefully assessed. Walkers or canes can be helpful for the person with postural instability and the ability to walk with a heel-toe gait. The height of walker or cane should be adjusted carefully to promote extension and avoid an increase in trunk

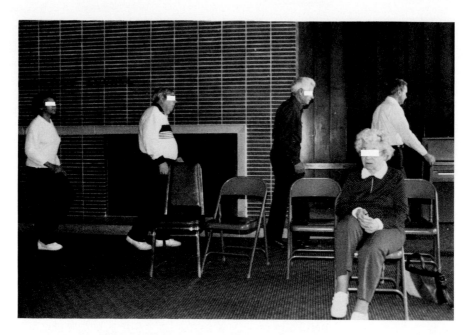

Fig. 21-7. Initial warm-up in standing. Clients are to walk with the head up, back as straight as possible, and take large steps. When the group began, walking was the major aerobic activity and used to increase endurance and encourage movement. Nonambulatory patients march in place in the chair.

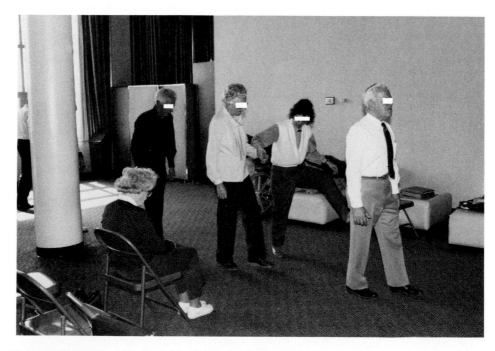

Fig. 21-8. Walking in a "waltz rhythm" (slow, quick, quick) emphasizes a big step for the slow step. Notice lack of automatic arm swing. Also notice flexed posture of seated patient during rest period.

flexion. Dunne and others[52] described a cane that could present a visual cue for the patient who has freezing episodes. I have found it especially useful for patients who fall because of freezing. A survey by Mutch and colleagues[140] in Ireland found that nearly half of the patients responding used some type of assistive device. These devices were used for reaching, ADLs, and walking. Parkinson's patients may also benefit from assistive devices for eating and/or writing. For a few patients small cuff weights may decrease tremor when walking; however, for many patients cuff weights only exacerbate the tremor.

Bed mobility is another important consideration for

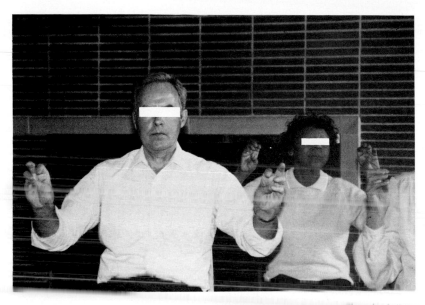

Fig. 21-9. Cool-down period allows time to work on fine finger movements. Thumb abduction with rounded fingers and various rhythm is used to increase coordination. Notice "masked face."

Examples of exercise regimens that promote context-dependent responses

1. Walking outdoors
2. Karate and other martial arts
3. Dancing (all forms)
4. All ball sports
5. Cross-country and downhill skiing
6. Well-structured, low-impact aerobics classes

This list is an example of activities; it should not be considered all inclusive.

Exercise regimens that promote fitness and increase in ROM but no context-dependent responses

1. Walking on treadmill
2. Stationary bicycle
3. Strengthening machines and free weights (with low weights or low resistance)
4. Step exercises and stair climbers
5. Rowing machines
6. Swimming laps

This list is an example of activities; it should not be considered all inclusive.

Parkinson's patients. A firm bed may make getting in and out of bed easier. Most patients report that satin sheets with silk or satin pajamas make moving in bed far easier. This is true in both the early and later stages of the disease. Beds with a head that can be raised electrically may be helpful as the disease progresses, but while sleeping the patient should lower the head as close to horizontal as possible. If getting up from a chair becomes too difficult, chairs with seats that lift up have been used effectively.

As Parkinson's disease progresses the patient may experience difficulty in swallowing and even in chewing. Therapy for oral-motor control should be initiated, and a dietitian consult may be necessary to ensure adequate nutrition.

A dietitian may also be beneficial in guiding the patient's protein intake. High protein may reduce the responsiveness of the patient to dopamine replacement therapy.[148] Regulating the amount and timing of protein ingestion can improve the efficacy of drug treatment in some patients.

Finally, Parkinson's disease is a progressive, degenerative disease. Therapy and exercise may modify the progression but cannot halt or reverse it. Quality of life throughout the course of the disease may be enhanced, however, and the therapist can assist the client and family in coping with the constraints of this disease. (See Case 1 on p. 626 and Case 2 on p. 627.)

Huntington's disease

Huntington's disease (formerly Huntington's chorea) is another degenerative disease of the basal ganglia. This disease gets its name from the family of physicians who described its pattern of inheritance. Huntington's disease is inherited as an autosomal dominant trait and affects approximately 6.5/100,000 people.[55]

Symptoms. Some of the signs and symptoms of Huntington's disease are similar to Parkinson's disease: abnormalities in postural reactions, trunk rotation, distribution of tone, and extraneous movements. Individuals with Huntington's disease, however, are at the other end of the spectrum;

CASE 1 ▼ Ms. T

Ms. T is a 55-year-old woman who was diagnosed with Parkinson's disease 1 year ago. The disease began in her left arm and leg when she noticed increasing stiffness and difficulty moving. She complains of some instability in walking and recently has developed a slight resting tremor in the left hand. On initial evaluation she had full active and passive ROM in all extremities, neck, and trunk. There is a mild resting tremor present in the left hand. There is mild cogwheel rigidity in the left upper and lower rigidity; there is some intermittent resistance to passive movement in the right upper extremity as well. Strength is grossly within normal limits throughout. Sensation is intact throughout. Equilibrium reactions are delayed, but the patient demonstrates an ankle strategy on a flat surface and a hip strategy when standing on the balance beam; there is no mixing of the synergies and her balance responses are appropriate to the degree of displacement.

The patient is able to stand in the Sharpened Romberg position for 30 seconds with the eyes open and 20 seconds with the eyes closed. She can stand on the right leg for 30 seconds with the eyes open and 15 seconds with the eyes closed; she can stand on the left leg for 15 seconds with the eyes open and 10 seconds with the eyes closed. When walking, she has a heel-toe sequence, shortened stride length, and normal stride width. There is no arm swing on the left and a diminished arm swing on the right. There is no trunk rotation and very slight trunk flexion throughout the gait cycle. Speed is within normal limits for a 25-foot walk. The patient is able to turn freely. She has recently begun to suffer from a foot dystonia, which is worse with fatigue. It has interfered with her daily walking program and her tennis, an activity she enjoys with her husband twice a week. Her only medications is deprenyl.

This patient is in Hoehn and Yahr stage I, with some beginning of bilateral symptoms and progression to stage II. She is young, employed full-time and has been involved in regular exercise for the past 10 years. Her complaints are of stiffness, slowed movements, and foot dystonia. Because her symptoms are mild at present and she has good balance in standing and walking, this patient should be encouraged to continue exercising regularly. She should try to maintain her tennis, as this requires complex, sequential, context-dependent movements. Although tennis involves motor responses to external cues, it does necessitate rapid force generation and anticipatory movements. This should encourage continued motor learning. Additionally, she should be encouraged to continue walking out of doors and practice alternating speed of walking. The dystonia is more difficult to resolve. It may be tied to medication and differing medication schemes are now being tried. She is also on a program of stretching and strengthening of the ankle as well as a sensory stimulation program for the feet. Foam between the toes has helped to decrease dystonia early in the day.

Ms. T has also been informed about the importance of maintaining chest expansion and monitoring her breathing. This will be important as the disease progresses. She attends a support group for young parkinsonian patients to increase her awareness of the disease, new treatments, and support. As the disease progresses, she will need a home program appropriate for her symptoms. The home program will be reassessed every 3 to 6 months.

---

rather than a paucity of movement, they exhibit too much movement, which is evident in the trunk and face in addition to the extremities. The gait takes on an ataxic, dancing appearance (in fact, chorea means *to dance*), and fine movements become clumsy and slowed. As with the parkinsonian individual there is a decrease in associated movements (e.g., arm swing). The extraneous movements are of the choreoathetoid type, consisting of "single, isolated muscle action, producing a short, rapid uncoordinated jerk of the trunk, limb or face" (p. 312).[83] Usually, however, these occur in successive movements so that the entire picture is one of complex movement patterns. It is as if the "movement generator" aspects of the basal ganglia are continuously active, as would fit the hypothesis of a disruption in the indirect pathway. As the disease progresses, the choreic movements may give way to akinesia and rigidity.

In addition to the involvement of the motor systems, the individual with Huntington's also shows signs of dementia and emotional disorders that become worse as the disease progresses. The client may show lack of judgment and loss of memory, a deterioration in speech and writing (i.e., severe decrease in ability to communicate), depression, hostility, and feelings of incompetence. There is a decrease in IQ with performance measures decreasing more rapidly than verbal levels. There is also evidence of ideomotor apraxia, especially as the disease progresses.[172] Suicide is fairly common.

Huntington's disease is usually manifested after the age of 30, although childhood forms appear rarely. Death from this disease occurs about 15 years after the onset of symptoms.

The movement disorders of Huntington's disease are presumed to be related to degeneration of the striatal neurons, specifically the enkephalinergic neurons.[183] The dementia is associated with cortical destruction. Recently, the locus of the gene for Huntington's disease has been found. It is located on the short arm of chromosone 4. The gene itself has now been isolated, and a marker for the gene has been detected.[72] If the family pedigree is known and the chromosomes of the parents can be obtained, it is now possible to detect presymptomatically which offspring have the faulty chromosome.

Although this may be a great step forward, genetic testing is still fraught with ethical considerations. At present,

---

CASE 2 ▼ Mr. R

Mr. R is a 68-year-old man with a 7-year history of Parkinson's disease. He now falls two to three times a day, has difficulty eating, and has noticed weakness in his right hand. He would like to return to full activity including golf twice a week, swimming, and skiing. On evaluation he has moderate rigidity in all extremities; the right side is worse than the left. It is most marked in the right wrist, forearm, and hand. Shoulder flexion and abduction lack 15 degrees bilaterally. He has a 15-degree knee flexion contracture on the right; all other joints in the lower extremity have range within functional limits. Strength is a grossly 4 - 4+ throughout including grip strength. Sensation is within normal limits throughout. Static and dynamic sitting balance is good.

The patient sits with a posterior pelvic tilt, rounded shoulders, and flexed neck. On rising to a standing position, he does move forward in the chair which positions his feet under his knees. He does not lean forward as he stands. He momentarily loses his balance upon rising from a chair. Static standing balance is fair, dynamic balance is fair. When pushed on the sternum, he takes one to two steps backward, even to a gentle push. When pushed from behind he takes several steps forward. He lost his balance and required assistance when trying to catch a large ball thrown to the side. His gait pattern is typical of a parkinsonian patient. There is a shortened step and a flat-footed foot contact. He complains of festination and of freezing, but neither were observed during the evaluation. He turns "en bloc." There is no arm swing and no trunk rotation.

He walks slowly and was unable to increase his speed measurably in a 25-foot walk. He is taking 1-dopa/carbidopa and deprenyl. He has tried another D_2-agonist but experienced hallucinations. He was able to ski until last winter. At that time, he found that he could not stand up once he fell down, and sometimes he fell without realizing that he was falling. He stated that he "did not think it was safe to ski." He also no longer swims because he has difficulty breathing in the pool and coordinating his breathing with the strokes. He does not play golf because it takes him so long.

This patient needs to be encouraged to continue both to exercise and to socialize while exercising. He has been encouraged to resume golf at times when his club is less crowded. Additionally, he has been given a home program consisting of activities performed in the seated and standing positions, which encourage trunk rotation and large movements and are coordinated with good breathing practices. He has been given some balance exercises that challenge his equilibrium in a safe environment. His home program will be monitored every 3 months because of the distance he must travel to come to the clinic. His wife was instructed to exercise with her husband and to exercise to music with him. He was referred to the speech pathologist for a swallowing evaluation and he was given a joint program for his speech and breathing. He is able to play golf once a week; he is not yet ready to resume swimming or skiing.

---

although testing is available it is not widely used. Further, testing for Huntington's disease is typically only available to those over the age of 18. Despite these problems, localizing the portion of the chromosome involved means that ultimately the gene product will be identified, and this will perhaps lead to improved means of treatment.

The exact mechanisms for the production of choreoathetoid movements are unknown. Because these extraneous movements are part of a person's normal repertoire of movement patterns, it is possible that they are "released" at inappropriate times and without any modulation. A postmortem examination showed a decrease in GABA which was greater in the GPe than the GPi. This agrees with the previously described current model.[183] Recent use of position emission tomography (PET) scans demonstrates loss of ACh and GABA neurons. A pattern therefore may be released before it is necessary, and inappropriate portions of pattern cannot be inhibited. Petajan and others[157] also found motor unit activity indicative of bradykinesia. Recordings of single motor units in the muscles indicates that persons with Huntington's disease have a loss of control evidenced by an inability to recruit single motor units.[157] As the efforts at control increased, these individuals demonstrated an overflow of motor unit activity that resulted in full choreiform movements. Those in the earlier stages of the disease demonstrated what the experimenters termed "microcho-

rea," small ballistic activations of motor units.[157] As in Parkinson's disease, difficulty occurs in modulating motor neuron excitability. Another finding in this experiment revealed motor unit activity indicative of bradykinesia. Yanagasawa[204] used surface EMG recordings to classify involuntary muscle contractions in Huntington's disease patients with varying movement disorders from chorea to rigidity. He found brief, reciprocal, irregular contractions in those patients with classical chorea and tonic nonreciprocal contractions in those patients with rigidity. Presence of athetosis or dystonia was associated with slow, reciprocal contractions. During sustained contractions EMG activity demonstrated brief, irregular cessation of activity in the choreic patients. Thus patients with Huntington's disease have interruption of normal motor function at rest and during sustained activity (e.g., stabilizing contractions).

The abnormal postural reactions of the person with Huntington's disease may occur from a misinterpretation of sensory input, especially vestibular and proprioceptive (similar to the parkinsonian syndrome). However, the dementia of Huntington's disease precludes further testing. Although it appears as if the thalamus also plays a role in the movement disorders of Huntington's disease, the specifics are unknown at present.[49,156]

Stages of the disease. Huntington's disease is a progressive disorder. The initial symptoms are most often complaints of incoordination, clumsiness, or jerkiness. A classic test for eliciting choreiform movements in this early stage is a simple grip test. The client grips the examiner's hand and maintains that grip for a few seconds. The person with Huntington's disease will display what is descriptively called the "milkmaid's sign"; there will be alternate increases and decreases in the grip, perhaps the equivalent of the EMG abnormalities seen during sustained contractions. Facial grimacing or the inability to perform complex facial movements also may be present very early.

In many cases the dementia and psychological symptoms of Huntington's disease occur after the onset of the neurological signs. In those cases where very subtle personality changes occur first, the diagnosis may be more difficult. Such persons may appear forgetful or unable to manage appointments and financial affairs. They may be thought to have early senility, or they may show signs of severe depression or schizophrenia.

With time, the combination of the psychological and neurological problems causes the individual to lose all ability to work and perform ADL. This person eventually can be cared for only in an extended care facility. By this time the choreiform movements have given way to rigidity, and the patient is bedridden. Fig. 21-10 shows the stages of Huntington's disease according to Shoulson and Fahn.[173]

Pharmacological considerations and medical management. The great advances in pharmacological management of Parkinson's disease have led to a great deal of research to find appropriate drugs for the management of Huntington's disease. At present, however, there is no fully effective medication for this disease.

The symptoms of Huntington's disease indicate an increase in dopaminergic effect. At autopsy there is a decrease in the number of intrinsic neurons of the striatum that contain the neurotransmitter GABA or ACh. Biochemical studies reveal a definite decrease in GABA concentration in addition to a decrease in ACh concentration in the basal ganglia. Therefore drug therapy depends on those drugs that are cholinergic or GABA-containing agonists and those that act as DA antagonists. To date the DA antagonists have been more effective in ameliorating neurological symptoms.

In general, pharmacological treatment is not started until the choreiform movements interfere with function[72] because these drugs have side effects that may be worse than the chorea (see the section on tardive dyskinesia). Perphenazine, haloperidol (Haldol), and reserpine are still the most commonly used medications. The first two block the DA receptors themselves; reserpine depletes DA stores in the brain. Side effects include depression, drowsiness, a parkinsonian type of syndrome, or sometimes dyskinesia. Drugs such as choline, which would increase ACh concentrations, have produced only transient improvement.[185] There have been many efforts to find a GABA agonist that would reduce the symptoms of Huntington's disease, but these have so far been unsuccessful.[21,175] The problem with finding a medi-

cation to increase GABA is that such a drug will probably cause inhibition throughout the brain, not just in the basal ganglia. Thus the individual's level of alertness and ability to function might be reduced—something the person with Huntington's disease can ill afford.[21]

Because management of the dementia and personality problems is not satisfactory with any present drug therapy, it becomes more difficult than the choreiform problem. Cortical degeneration is most certainly involved, but disruption of the heavy corticostriate projections also may be a factor in the progression of this disease. Although alterations in DA have been implicated in psychotic problems such as schizophrenia, the role of the basal ganglia in thought processes is, at best, little understood. In the words of Woody Guthrie:

> There's just not no hope
> Nor not no treatment known
> to cure me of my dizzy
> called Chorea.[74]

At present the best hope for the person with Huntington's disease lies in a better understanding of the genetic mechanisms causing destruction of the GABA-containing cells in the striatum and cortical destruction. In the meantime correct and early diagnosis is important in providing the proper early intervention, which must include counseling.[95] The Committee for the Control of Huntington's Disease has set up several research centers, including a brain and tissue bank, in an effort to facilitate research into the causes of the disease.

Evaluation of the client with Huntington's disease. In evaluating a person with Huntington's disease, one must assess the degree of functional ability and how the chorea interferes with function. Which extremities, including the face, are involved? Does the client have any cortical control of the chorea or any means of allaying these extraneous movements? What exacerbates the symptoms? What lessens them? At present no rating scale exists other than the capacity to perform ADL (see Fig. 21-10). A standard ADL form with space to write in how the client performs these activities or why she or he cannot perform them would be helpful.

In addition, posture and equilibrium reactions should be tested. What associated reactions, if any, are present? In assessing posture, care should be taken to observe the posture of the extremities in addition to the trunk, head, and neck. Dystonic posturing should be carefully noted, especially if the client is taking medication. Any changes should be reported to the physician.

A gross assessment of strength should be made with particular attention paid to the ability to stabilize the trunk and proximal joints. To reduce the effects of rigidity, ROM becomes important as the disease progresses.

In the assessment of the client with Huntington's disease, the stage of psychological involvement and mental state

Stage	Engagement in occupation	Score	Capacity to handle financial affairs	Score	Capacity to manage domestic responsibility	Score	Capacity to perform activities of daily living	Score	Care can be provided at	Score
Stage 1	Usual level	3	Full	3	Full	2	Full	3	Home	2
Stage 2	Lower level	2	Requires slight help	2	Full	2	Full	3	Home	2
Stage 3	Marginal	1	Requires major help	1	Impaired	1	Mildly impaired	2	Home	2
Stage 4	Unable	0	Unable	0	Unable	0	Moderately impaired	1	Home or extended care facility	1
Stage 5	Unable	0	Unable	0	Unable	0	Severely impaired	0	Total care facility only	0

From Shoulson and Fahn (1979).

Fig. 21-10. Functional stages of Huntington's disease. (From Shoulson I and Fahn S: Neurology 29:_, 1979.)

must be reliably assessed both during evaluation and treatment. Computed tomography (CT) data will give some clues to the amount of cortical and basal ganglia degeneration, which can assist in determining possible cortical functioning.

General treatment goals and rationale. Maintaining the optimal quality of life is the most important goal for treatment of persons with Huntington's disease and their families. This will include maintenance of functional skills and advice to the family on adaptive equipment. Techniques that reduce tone may also reduce choreiform movements. Increasing stability about the shoulders, trunk, neck, and hips will help maintain function. Again, it must be reiterated that the evaluation results will dictate treatment procedures.

Treatment procedures. The Commission on the Control of Huntington's Disease[174] stated that these individuals are underserved by physical and occupational therapy. Peacock[155] surveyed physical therapists in one state. Of the 585 therapists who responded, only 15.5% had worked with at least one patient with Huntington's disease; 6.2% had worked with more than one patient, thus confirming the underutilization of physical and occupational therapy today. Hayden[74] and Peacock[155] suggest that therapy can improve the quality of life. Yet there are few articles on treatment procedures. Theories as to which techniques may prove most beneficial are offered here with the warning that to date none have been documented. (See also Chapter 6 for specific treatment techniques.)

The treatment of the person with Huntington's disease has some parallels with the treatment of cerebral palsy athetosis. These techniques, however, must be adapted to the adult. Of critical importance are the techniques for improving coactivation and trunk stability. The use of the pivot-prone and withdrawal patterns of Rood are helpful, and their benefit may be increased with the use of Theraband. Neck cocontraction and trunk stability may improve or at least maintain oral functions. Additionally, the techniques of rhythmical stabilization in all positions as well as heavy work patterns of Rood should be helpful.[98] Yet plans practiced out of context may not carry over in the functional plans; thus the reader is recommended to practice coactivation in functional patterns during activities if at all possible.

Relaxation aids reduction of extraneous movements. In the early stages methods that require active participation of the client, such as biofeedback and traditional relaxation exercises, may be included. As dementia becomes more apparent, more passive techniques such as slow rocking and neutral warmth must be used. These techniques are also helpful in reducing the choreiform movements of the mouth and tongue, which may prove useful for the dentist and those responsible for proper nutrition of the client. In most cases of Huntington's disease, the individual is quite thin (almost emaciated) and begins to age rapidly as the disease progresses. The extraneous movements, especially as they become more severe, increase metabolic demands, and nutrition therefore becomes increasingly important. Attention therefore must be paid to head, neck, and oral-motor control. Increased pressure on the lips may aid in lip closure and facilitate swallowing. Special straws with a mouthpiece similar to a pacifier therefore may be useful. A dietitian should be consulted for assistance in teaching the family how to prepare balanced and appetizing meals and snacks that are still easy to swallow.

The degree of dementia influences the treatment. Conscious efforts to control extraneous movements will be more difficult as cognitive function decreases. Further, new memories and new patterns of movements will be difficult to establish. The therapist therefore must use techniques that require subcortical control and must keep in mind that the client can sometimes remember old, normal patterns of movement.

Peacock's study[155] suggests that group programs including strength, flexibility, balance, coordination, and breathing exercises may be very successful, especially in the early stages of the disease. No amount of physical or occupational therapy, however, can prevent neuronal cell loss. Because Huntington's disease is a progressive, degenerative disease, the client will get worse. Eventually, goals must be aimed at preventing total immobility and assisting caretakers in transfer techniques and advising them in the use of adaptive equipment. One aspect of treatment that cannot be measured but is important in the author's view is the degree of hope offered just by the fact that a health professional is providing ongoing care. This may lessen the client's degree of despair and depression and may help maintain quality of life.

Wilson's disease

Wilson's disease, or hepatolenticular degeneration, is a disease caused by faulty copper metabolism. The toxic effects of copper lead to degeneration of the liver and the basal ganglia, hence the name. Wilson's disease, inherited as an autosomal recessive trait, affects a very small percentage of the population.

In Wilson's disease there is an increase in the amount of copper absorbed from the intestinal tract, a subsequent elevation in the amount of copper in the blood serum, and an increase in the amount of copper deposited in tissue.[198] There is a concomitant reduction in ceruloplasmin. The increase in tissue copper may interfere with various enzyme systems of particular cells. The connection of copper with DA metabolism may account for the basal ganglia involvement.

Neuronal degeneration is present in the globus pallidus and putamen and to a lesser extent in the caudate nucleus. There also may be atrophy in the gray matter of the cortex and the dentate nucleus of the cerebellum.

Symptoms. The deposition of the excess copper in the cornea results in the classic diagnostic sign of Wilson's disease, the Kayser-Fleischer ring—a brownish-green or brownish-red colored ring found in the sclerocorneal junction.

Based on constellations of the signs and symptoms, there are several forms of Wilson's disease. One type entails only liver involvement and no neurological signs. A dystonic form is most common in those with an onset of the disease after the age of 20. The individual shows the same abnormal positioning of the limbs and trunk that characterizes the dystonia, rigidity, and bradykinesia seen in Parkinson's disease. Associated reactions and facial expressions are absent. There is a festinating gait and flexed posture. There may be a tremor of the hand, head, and body.

If the onset of the disease occurs before age 20, the appearance of choreoathetoid movements of the face and upper extremities is usually present. The gait resembles that of the individual with Huntington's disease. This early onset form is accompanied by a very rapid deterioration.

Common to all forms of Wilson's disease that involve brain structures is difficulty in speaking and swallowing, incoordination, and personality changes. The personality changes are the first signs of the disease, especially emotional lability and impaired judgment. If the disease progresses, there is increased dementia, increased cirrhosis of the liver, and progressive decrease in motor function.

The term *dystonia* is used for involuntary movements with a sustained contraction at the end of the movement.[55] Usually these movements involve a twisting of the extremity. If the contraction at the end of the movement is prolonged, the term *dystonic posture* is used. A very peculiar aspect of dystonia is that it can be decreased with proprioceptive or tactile input.[55] Dystonia is usually seen with widespread involvement of the basal ganglia and intralaminar nuclei of the thalamus.[156] The cerebellum also may be involved.[39]

Dystonia, like bradykinesia and choreoathetosis, belongs on a continuum of the extraneous movements present with basal ganglia involvement. The movement patterns are total and involve rotation of the limb. As in the other diseases of the basal ganglia discussed so far, there is also a decrease in the normal associated movements. As Wilson's disease progresses, the classic abnormal posture of increased flexion occurs, along with rigidity and, if severe enough, the total inability to move. As with other diseases of the basal ganglia, there appears to be an imbalance or abnormal response in the neurotransmitters; however, the precise imbalance is not yet known.

Stages of the disease. The first symptom of Wilson's disease is usually a change in the individual's personality. Either when this becomes severe enough or when the movement disorder appears, a diagnosis can be made by the presence of the Kayser-Fleischer ring or by an analysis of copper metabolism. Because Wilson's disease is now treatable by chemical means, the full progression of this disease is usually not seen. If left untreated, the dystonia

becomes worse and the person becomes more rigid. Additionally, muscle weakness can occur and progress, seizures may develop, and the dementia and personality disorder also become worse.

Medical management. Because the signs and symptoms of Wilson's disease are caused by an increased absorption of copper, treatment consists of drugs that will inhibit this absorption. Concomitantly, copper intake in the diet should be restricted. Penicillamine is the drug of choice, usually in combination with vitamin B_6.[55] There are some side effects of penicillamine, but these appear to be infrequent. If the copper imbalance is treated, the neurological signs do not progress.

Evaluation and treatment intervention. Because Wilson's disease is fully treatable and can be diagnosed early, it is possible that it will not concern the therapist. If the client is referred for therapy, treatment techniques should be wholly based on symptomatology. Evaluation is similar to that of the parkinsonian or Huntington's person. It consists of describing the type of extraneous movement present, when it is present, and factors that influence the degree of dystonia. Ease of movement also should be assessed, and it may be timed as for the parkinsonian client. Additionally, range of movement and strength should be evaluated, especially if the disease is progressing.

Treatment will then be designed to alleviate the problems. Extraneous movements may be reduced by any technique that will reduce tone. Positioning is important. If bradykinesia is the major sign, then treatment would be similar to that used in Parkinson's disease; if trunk stability is poor, the therapist proceeds as in Huntington's disease. The client with Wilson's disease has knowledge of what normal movement feels like and usually has good cognitive abilities at the time treatment is started. Because of the emotional liability, which is one of the first symptoms in this disease, the treatment session should be well planned and quite structured.

Tardive dyskinesia

Tardive dyskinesia is a drug-induced disorder and thus will be used to indicate the problems that can arise from drug intoxication. In particular this section concentrates on the problems associated with drugs that affect DA metabolism, including amphetamine, haloperidol, and classes of drugs used in treatment of psychotic disorders: the phenothiazines, butyrophenones, and thioxanthenes. As the use and misuse of drugs becomes more common, these types of disorders may become more frequent. (Refer to Chapter 33 for additional information.)

The use of phenothiazines (one of the neuroleptics) has become a very effective and common treatment for schizophrenia. This treatment protocol has enabled many schizophrenics to leave the mental institution. These drugs are DA antagonists and thus decrease the amount of DA in the brain.

The exact site of the brain involved in schizophrenia itself is not within the scope of this chapter, but the neurological signs that occur will be discussed. As might be expected, they involve structures within the basal ganglia. Tardive dyskinesia is a gradual disease that occurs after long-term drug treatment. The most typical involvement is of the mouth, tongue, and muscles of mastication; therefore tardive dyskinesia may be called orofacial or buccolingual-masticatory (BLM) dyskinesia.

Symptoms. Dyskinesia is defined as an inability to perform voluntary movement.[94] In practical terms, however, dyskinesia is usually a series of rhythmical extraneous movements. In tardive dyskinesia this typically begins with, or may be confined to, the region of the face. These extraneous movements may include choreoathetoid or dystonic movements. Because of abnormality in basal ganglia function, there are also accompanying abnormalities in postural tone and postural adjustments. Instead of the typical flexed posture of Parkinson's disease, clients with tardive dyskinesia show extension of the trunk with increased lordosis and neck flexion.[123] This description of the disease is rather broad, but the problems of drug-induced movement disorders are varied. They may take the form of drug-induced Parkinson's disease or dystonia. In tardive dyskinesia, akinesia and rigidity similar to that seen in parkinsonism may exist simultaneously with the choreoathetoid-like movements. The key factor in tardive dyskinesia is its slow onset after the ingestion of neuroleptic medications.

Etiology. Although many people take neuroleptic medication, only a small percentage acquire tardive dyskinesia. Many factors may predispose an individual to movement disorders. One of these is age.[177] This might be expected because of the influence of aging processes on the concentration of DA. Sex may also be a factor. Women are more at risk for tardive dyskinesia.[123] The fact that sex can affect DA levels is supported in studies of animals with brain lesions. In one study, female rats had a lower concentration of DA after early brain lesion than did their male litter mates.[171] The absolute amount of neuroleptic ingested may also be a factor, but to date definitive studies have not been completed. So far it appears that the length of time the individual takes medication is not a strong predisposing factor. As the biological abnormalities of schizophrenia become better understood, further understanding of the causes of tardive dyskinesia also may be elucidated. It is hypothesized that the development of tardive dyskinesia is caused by supersensitivity.[8,94] With the use of drugs that deplete the brain of DA, the brain becomes more sensitive to it. And, in fact, in humans the withdrawal of neuroleptics tends to heighten the disease; essentially, withdrawal of the DA antagonist means that far more DA is able to act on these already sensitive terminals.[8,30,94]

Because of the effectiveness of long-term treatment for schizophrenia provided by neuropletics, research into the underlying cause and therefore treatment of the major side effect, the motor disorders, has greatly increased. But as with Parkinson's disease and Huntington's disease, animal models are difficult to produce. For one thing, the normal function of the basal ganglia in movement is obscure. However, experimental evidence indicates that the basal ganglia are involved in movements about the face, especially the mouth, and buccolingual dyskinesia is the most frequently encountered symptom in tardive dyskinesia.[119,120,121] Lidsky and others[118] hypothesized that sensory input about the face was involved in the high number of globus pallidus units responsive to licking. Further experiments showed that basal ganglia stimulation could alter the threshold of mouth reflexes.[108] The response of basal ganglia neurons to sensory input shows increasing localization of response with age; the region about the mouth becomes increasingly sensitive.[168] Further research along these lines, both in normal animals and those with lesions, may answer the question of what is happening at a neuronal level. This would facilitate drug and physical therapy intervention.

Pharmacological and medical management. One serious problem of tardive dyskinesia is that it is often irreversible. The withdrawal of medication, in fact, may increase the movement disorders. Or it may be that recovery takes even more time than the time required for the onset of the disease. It is a strange fact that sometimes the drug that caused the disease may be the drug that reduces the symptoms; that is, increasing the dose may lessen the movement disorder. This might be expected if supersensitivity to DA is involved. But again, with time the increased dose will also cause a reappearance of the symptoms.

The use of other drugs in conjunction with the neuroleptics has been tried in various animal models of the disease. As might be expected, anticholinergic drugs (which would worsen an imbalance between DA and ACh) worsen the dyskinesia. Lithium has been successful in one animal model of dyskinesia.[94] Some neuroleptic drugs seem to have less effect on movement than others; however, the side effects of one such drug, chlorpromazine, are life threatening. More research is needed into both the mechanisms of schizophrenia and the mechanisms for the production of the abnormal movements.

Evaluation and treatment intervention. The effectiveness of therapy intervention in drug-induced dyskinesia is, as yet, not completely known. However, since the neuroleptics do provide an effective long-term treatment of schizophrenia, therapists need to become aware of the problem and offer some assistance. Early drug holidays (time without use of drugs) may be of value in treatment of tardive dyskinesia, and therefore early awareness of incipient changes in motor function may be of value. Assessment of patients receiving drug therapy could perhaps begin before treatment and then at prescribed intervals. The knowledge that postural adjustments are abnormal in most basal ganglia diseases means that analysis of posture statically and in motion might provide early clues of development of movement disorders.

The same would be true for equilibrium reactions and changes in tone with changes in position. Once movement disorders appear, an assessment of when and where the extraneous movements occur is important. Refer to Chapter 28 for test of balance.

General treatment is similar to that used in Huntington's disease; oral treatment corresponds to that for the athetotic child with cerebral palsy. If a hyperreactivity to sensory stimulus exists, then oral desensitization may be of value.

Ameliorating the oral grimacing, of course, would be helpful for the schizophrenic person who is trying to return to society. The effectiveness of physical and occupational therapy treatment cannot be assessed until therapists become involved with these clients and record their results. In cases in which the parkinsonian-like symptoms are stronger than the dyskinetic movements, treatment would follow the plan for the individual with Parkinson's disease.

Other considerations

Other drugs besides neuroleptics may also produce movement disorders. Amphetamine, for example, has been shown to cause long-term changes in brain function even from very small doses.[116,117,195] Adults who were hyperactive children sometimes show a decrease in the readiness potential.[23] Further research is under way to determine the role that medications, such as methylphenidate (Ritalin), used in treating hyperactive children might play in causing movement disorders. The problem of drug-induced movement disorders may become an ever-increasing one for the therapist.

In 1982 several young people were treated for rigidity and "catatonia" after the use of what they thought was heroin. Careful examination of these patients revealed that they had parkinsonian-like symptoms.[42,109] The chemical responsible for the symptomatology was 1-methyl-4-phenyl-1,2,3,6-tetrahydropyridine (MPTP), a meperidine analog that was an impurity in the designer heroin. This discovery has enabled research in animals and clinical studies in humans. Although there are some differences among idiopathic Parkinson's disease, MPTP-induced Parkinson's disease, and MPTP-induced parkinsonism, there are important similarities: MPTP selectively damages DA cells in the substantia nigra; L-dopa is effective in alleviating the symptoms, and the symptoms seen are irreversible and progressive. In animal studies, age does affect the degree of damage,[133,196] and in humans, some of those who used the drug MPTP are now beginning to show symptoms of parkinsonism.[110] This delay in appearance of symptoms fits a model of Parkinson's disease that suggests that an initial insult to the DA system may not result in disease until a critical level is reached. The critical level of DA depletion may occur with age because of a gradual loss of DA in the aging process. The real importance of the discovery of MPTP-induced parkinsonism is that it may enable better understanding of the pathogenesis and, in turn, of the treatment of the disease. One hypoth-esized cause of Parkinson's disease implicated environmental toxins (because some herbicides such as paraquot resemble the chemical structure of MPTP) and the involvement of superoxide free radical.[14,37,101] Epidemiology studies are now underway to investigate Parkinson's disease in areas known for high herbicide usage, and alpha tocopheral is under investigation as a protective agent.

METABOLIC DISEASES AFFECTING OTHER REGIONS OF THE BRAIN

All alterations of metabolism, if allowed to continue, will affect nervous system function. This includes alterations in sodium, water, sugar, and hormonal balance. Table 21-1 lists metabolic diseases that often have neurological sequelae. Proper treatment is usually medical management of the imbalance. Physical therapeutic intervention, if necessary, should address specific neurological symptoms. (See other chapters that discuss these individual problems.)

Ingestion of or exposure to heavy metals may also lead to CNS disease. Table 21-2 describes the sequelae of these problems.

One metabolic problem, however, warrants in-depth consideration: drug-induced neurological disorders that arise from over ingesting alcohol. Movement disorders involve the effects of alcohol on the CNS and the effects of nutritional deficiency that are part of the alcoholic syndrome.

Alcoholism

Alcohol, as a drug, has a direct effect on the nervous system. Additionally, the chronic effects of alcohol include vitamin and general nutritional deficiency. Alcohol has a high caloric value and therefore the chronic alcoholic tends to decrease food intake: the classic "drinking lunch or dinner." Thus acute intoxication, while not producing nutritional deficiency, contributes to it.

Signs and symptoms of acute alcohol intoxication. Most people are well aware of the symptoms of acute alcohol intoxication, perhaps through personal experience. Initially, alcohol produces relaxation and a loss of inhibitions. This is followed by a loss of judgment and coordination. If alcohol ingestion continues, a stuporous stage may be reached: The person "passes out" and awakens the next morning with a hangover. Drinking water and eating tend to alleviate the sick feeling, and the neurological signs are reversible at this stage. However, overly large volumes of alcohol can lead to coma and death. The symptoms of acute intoxication result from the direct effect of alcohol on the excitability of neurons, that is, inhibitory neurons become less excitable. Alcohol causes a decrease in membrane excitability. The cortex is usually affected first, and this effect descends the neuraxis. Coma is an indication of medullary involvement.

The individual with signs of acute intoxication will rarely, if ever, be seen in the clinic. The person with chronic alcohol intoxication, however, often will show neurological complications. The most prevalent problems involve cortical

Table 21-1. Neurological complications of metabolic disorders

Metabolic problem	Treatment	Neurological complication
Decreased sodium (too much H_2O)	Restricted water intake	Muscle twitching, seizures, coma
Increased sodium	Rehydration, *slowly*	Cerebral edema, muscle rigidity, decerebrate rigidity
Decreased potassium (hypokalemia) often caused by aldosteronism	Restoration of calcium levels after assessing primary cause	Changes in resting potential of neuron; hyperpolarization; muscle weakness and fatigue with eventual total paralysis
Magnesium imbalance	Improved diet, intravenous magnesium	Mental confusion, muscle twitching, myoclonus, tachycardia, hyperreflexia, extraneous movements, seizures
Diabetes mellitus	Proper control of diabetes	Peripheral neuropathy, pseudotabes, possible seizures and coma
Hypoglycemia	Treatment of primary cause; diet adjustment	Anoxia of the brain, seizures, mental confusion
Hyperthyroidism	Thyroid-blocking agents; intravenous fluids, hydrocortisone and propranolol if patient in thyroid crisis	Hyperkinesia, irritability, nervousness, emotional lability, symmetrical peripheral neuropathy
Hypothyroidism	Thyroid supplement	Sluggishness, mental and motor retardation, muscle weakness, sometimes muscle pain
Hypercalcemia	Treatment of primary cause, which is often hyperparathyroidism, vitamin D malignancy (therefore surgical removal)	Headache, weakness, fatigue, proximal neuropathy, rigidity, tremor, disorientation
Hypocalcemia	Intravenous administration of calcium (possible medical emergency)	Hyperexcitability of the peripheral and central nervous systems, which can lead to tetany and convulsions

Table 21-2. Neurological complications of heavy metal poisoning

Type of metal	Treatment	Neurological complication
Lead Source: lead paint, industrial (fumes of molten lead)	Elimination of source, reduction of fluids, intravenous urea or mannitol, use of chelating agents	Interstitial edema and hemorrhage (especially in cerebellum) in acute poisoning; all levels of CNS affected in chronic poisoning In children: seizures, mental retardation, behavior problems, and hyperactivity In adults: spasticity, rigidity, dementia, personality changes Peripheral neuropathy may occur in adults and children
Arsenic Source: paint and insecticides	Removal of source, gastric lavage, intravenous fluids, and maintenance of electrolyte balance; penicillamine used in acute poisoning	Demyelinization of peripheral nerves in all extremities
Manganese Source: industrial if manganese dust is not removed; symptoms appear 2 to 25 years after exposure	L-dopa	Neuronal loss in basal ganglia, substantia nigra, and cerebellum Initially psychiatric disturbances, including nervousness, irritability, and a tendency toward compulsive acts Later, muscular weakness and parkinsonian-like symptoms
Mercury Rare but may affect farmers and dental office workers	Penicillamine; function returns only with physical, occupational, and speech therapy	Loss of neurons, especially in cerebellum; also in cortex near calcarine fissure Alternating periods of confusion, drowsiness, and stupor with restlessness and excitability Ataxia, dysarthria, visual deterioration

function, cerebellar function, and peripheral neuropathies. The cortical and cerebellar problems involve the combination of alcohol effects and nutritional deficiency; peripheral neuropathies are believed to be a result of nutritional deficiencies.[93] Because large neurons are more difficult to excite, it is possible that the large neurons of the cortex and cerebellum are more easily affected by decreases in excitability. The cerebellum and frontal lobes of the cerebral cortex are more sensitive to the deleterious effects of alcohol. The nutritional deficits further exacerbate these problems as the lack of food causes a decrease in glucose available for brain metabolism. Vitamin deficiency, especially of the B vitamins, is a further cause of the symptomatology seen.

In addition to the effects of chronic alcohol on the adult, alcohol can also be devastating to an unborn child. Because alcohol crosses the placenta, the developing brain with its high metabolic rate may be affected even in the absence of symptoms in the mother. Binge drinking by the mother can be as detrimental as abuse. This has become a great enough problem with enough similarities among affected infants that fetal alcohol syndrome is a recognizable disease at birth. In addition to a low birth weight and irritability, distinct facial anomalies also are associated with this disease. A long-term evaluation of these children will provide information on other neurological problems that may become more evident as the child ages. Animal research indicates that brain maldevelopment, and delays in reflex and motor development are not reversible.[146] One of the areas showing a decrease in size is the frontal cortex.[146] (See Chapters 8, 9, and 10 for further information on pediatric problems.)

Signs and symptoms of chronic alcoholism. The individual suffering from chronic alcoholism can have neurological and psychological impairment. Neurological symptoms include ataxia (especially in the trunk and lower limbs), incoordination, and peripheral neuropathy. Seizures also may be a complication. The ataxia that occurs is the classic staggering, wide-based gait depicted on every television program showing an alcoholic. The person cannot perform a tandem gait (walking forward in heel-to-toe fashion on a straight line) and has difficulty maintaining an upright posture with the feet together. If weakness because of neuropathy is present, the ataxia, of course, is worsened. Vestibular deficits also are present and persist even after periods of abstinence. Abstinent alcoholics showed performance deficits on all sensory organization tests during dynamic posturography; these deficits reached statistical significance for those conditions that entailed proprioceptive conflict.[111]

The psychological problems also are probably fairly well known. These include delirium tremens (DTs), dementia, and the Wernicke-Korsakoff syndrome. DTs are most frequently seen in any withdrawal from alcohol. This is when the alcoholic sees the "pink elephants." The individual is restless, irritable, disoriented, and often hallucinates when awake; speech may be unintelligible. Temperature is elevated, and the person is dehydrated. DTs are probably

caused by a type of rebound phenomenon: The depressed neuronal firing is freed from the alcohol and neurons are overly irritable. Deep tendon reflexes are also hyperactive.

Wernicke-Korsakoff syndrome (hyphenated because the two syndromes are usually seen together) is caused by frontal lobe involvement complicated by vitamin B_1 deficiency. In Korsakoff's syndrome there is a loss of memory, especially short-term and recent memory. The individual then tends to make up answers and may "remember" the physician or even the therapist as someone she or he met in a bar; a simple breakfast just completed may become a banquet feast. These confabulations are a classic sign of the chronic alcoholic. They are probably an attempt to function without recent memory. Wernicke's syndrome includes ataxia (already described), disorientation, dementia, and ophthalmoplegia. The eye problems include nystagmus followed by lateral rectus weakness and double vision.

The peripheral neuropathies exacerbate all of these problems. The muscles are tender to touch, and there may be a burning sensation in the hands and feet, which intensifies the irritability of DTs. Muscle weakness will increase the apparent ataxia, and decreased sensation causes a further loss of proprioceptive cues the individual might otherwise use.

Pharmacological considerations and medical management. The biggest factor in treatment is, of course, withdrawal from alcohol. Librium, which is synonymous with chlorpromazine and chlordiazepoxide, is used to keep the individual sedated and to reduce DTs. At the same time, the electrolyte and water balance of the body must be restored. Because alcohol usually causes dehydration, the body's fluids must be replaced, but refurnishing necessary electrolytes also requires attention. In addition, nutrition is important because the nutritional deficiencies are as harmful as the effects of alcohol itself. Large supplements of B complex vitamins should be added to the diet.

If the individual has been hospitalized fairly early, abstains from alcohol, and controls the diet, some of the symptoms of the disease can be reversed. This is especially true of the eye involvement and of much of the ataxia. Permanent memory deficits, however, often occur; the longer the alcoholism, the worse the memory. The neuropathies, if they recover, recover very slowly. Both the myelin sheath and the axon have been damaged. In long-standing alcoholism the nerve roots also become involved, lessening the chances for regeneration and recovery. The best cure therefore is prevention.

Evaluation. Before proceeding with a neurological evaluation, the therapist needs to assess the client's mental status. Is there any short-term retention? Can the individual's perception of sensation be trusted as accurate? If the client cannot perform a task, is it because he or she did not understand the instructions or has forgotten them? All commands should be single commands and kept as short as possible. Because weakness and loss of sensation, especially proprioception, can produce signs similar to ataxia, it is a good idea to evaluate peripheral nerve function first. Nerve conduction tests are useful evaluation tools for the alcoholic patient. The faster myelinated nerves are the most sensitive to alcohol.[60] (Refer to Chapters 29 and 30 for additional information.)

In assessing the degree of cerebellar involvement, static posture and movement need to be evaluated. This includes the ability to stand upright with the feet together, the width between the legs in standing or walking, and the presence or absence of equilibrium reactions. Sometimes there is a delay in equilibrium reactions that needs to be recorded. Persistent involvement of the vestibular system means that tests of vestibular function including vestibular-ocular reflex (VOR), optokinetic nystagmus (OKN), and balance should be performed.

Treatment considerations. Chapter 23 on cerebellar disease deals with actual treatment methodologies; however, treatment of the alcoholic adds a few problems that may not be encountered in these other disease entities. The first problem encountered is one of setting goals because the client may not be sufficiently mentally alert to participate in goal setting. Second, the degree of recovery is impossible to know; the therapist should strive for as much recovery as possible. Of course, the achievement of whatever goals are established depends on abstinence from alcohol.

In treatment of alcoholism, the mental status is a crucial problem. If dementia is present, the client will not be able to use higher-level thought processes or achieve cortical control over movement. Therefore techniques that require attention or learning may have very limited success. In addition, carry-over from one session to the next will be hampered because the client may have no recollection of the previous treatment or even of the therapist. The lack of attention and memory also means that, just as in evaluation, all commands must be brief and simple. The treatment session should be well structured so that the client's thoughts are not allowed to wander. Sometimes it may also be advisable to adjust the length of treatment to the individual's tolerance. The addition of both physical and occupational therapy may produce a more holistic treatment approach.

There is another consideration in the treatment of the alcoholic, and this is the effect of exercise on physical well-being in general. Even without neurological signs, alcoholic individuals may benefit from a carefully monitored program of physical activity—carefully monitored because this client may be in a debilitated condition with generalized weakness and even respiratory problems. A study in Japan has shown that physical exercise can help the alcoholic's general rehabilitation progress.[191] As in all diseases discussed so far, the exact treatment procedures depend on the results of the evaluation. Documentation of the effects of therapy should be clear and, whenever possible, quantifiable.

SUMMARY

This chapter has focused on the pathophysiology, evaluation, and treatment of genetic, hereditary, and metabolic diseases affecting adults. In all of these diseases the therapist is an important (though sometimes underused) part of the rehabilitation team. A knowledge of the possible mechanisms involved in the production of the varying movement disorders may make the appropriate evaluation and subsequent treatment more meaningful. Even with degenerative, progressive disorders the therapist plays an important role in maintaining quality of life and assists the client and family in coping with the disease. Throughout this chapter the importance of documentation and publication has been stressed. Both will assist in the development of improved therapeutic techniques and also may help researchers in planning and interpreting appropriate experimental studies.

REFERENCES

1. Agostino R and others: Sequential arm movements in patients with Parkinson's disease, Huntington's disease and dystonia, *Brain* 115:1481, 1992.
2. Albin RL and others: The functional anatomy of basal ganglia disorders, *Trends Neurosci* 12:366, 1989.
3. Alexander GE and Crutcher MD: Functional architecture of basal ganglia circuits:neural substrates of parallel processing, *Trends Neurosci* 13:266, 1990.
4. Alexander GE and others: Basal ganglia-thalamocortical circuits: parallel substrates for motor, oculomotor, "prefrontal" and "limbic" functions, *Prog Brain Res* 85:119, 1990.
5. Amato G and others: The role of internal pallidal segment on the initiation of a goal directed movement, *Neurosci Lett* 9:159, 1978.
6. Ariano MA and others: D2 dopamine receptor distribution in the rodent CNS using antipeptide antisera, *Brain Res* 609:71, 1993.
7. Ayres AJ: *Sensory integration and learning disorders,* Los Angeles, 1972, Western Psychological Services.
8. Baldessarini RJ and Tarsy D: Dopamine and the pathophysiology of dyskinesias induced by antipsychotic drugs, *Annu Rev Neurosci* 3:23, 1980.
9. Ball J: Demonstration of the traditional approach in the treatment of a patient with parkinsonism, *Am J Phys Med* 46:1034, 1967.
10. Ball J: Personal communication, 1983.
11. Banks MA: Physiotherapy benefits patients with Parkinson's disease, *Clin Rehabil* 3:11, 1989.
12. Barbeau A and others: Ecogenetics of Parkinson's disease: prevalence and environmental aspects in rural areas, *Can J Neurol Sci* 14:36, 1987.
13. Barbeau A: Parkinson's disease: etiologic considerations. In Yahr MD, editor: *The basal ganglia,* New York, 1976, Raven Press.
14. Barbeau A and others: Ecogenetics of Parkinson's disease: prevalence and environmental aspects in rural areas, *Can J Neurol Sci* 14:36, 1987.
15. Bathien N and Rondot P: Reciprocal continuous inhibition in rigidity of parkinsonism, *J Neurol Neurosurg Psychiatry* 40:20, 1977.
16. Battig K and others: Comparison of the effects of frontal and caudate lesions on discrimination learning in monkeys, *J Comp Physiol Psychol* 55:458, 1962.
17. Beckley DJ and others: Impaired scaling of long latency postural reflexes in patients with Parkinson's disease, *Electroencephalogr Clin Neurophysiol* 83:22, 1993.
18. Benecke R and others: Disturbance of sequential movements in patients with Parkinson's disease, *Brain* 101:361, 1987.
19. Benecke R and others: Performance of simultaneous movements in patients with Parkinson's disease, *Brain* 109:739, 1986.
20. Benita M and others: Effects of ventrolateral thalamic nucleus cooling on initiation of forelimb ballistic flexion movements by conditioned cats, *Exp Brain Res* 34:435, 1979.

21. Bird ED: Biochemical studies on γ-aminobutyric acid metabolism in Huntington's chorea. In Bradford HF and Marsden CD, editors: *Biochemistry and neurology,* London, 1976, Academic Press.

22. Bobath B: *Adult hemiplegia: evaluation and treatment,* London, 1976, William Heinemann Medical Books.

23. Boop R and others: Methylphenidate (MPH): absence of readiness potential in patients with Parkinson's disease and in patients following long-term MPH treatment, *Neurosci Abst* 7:779, 1981.

24. Bowen FP: Behavioral alterations in patients with basal ganglia lesions. In Yahr MD, editor: *The basal ganglia,* New York, 1976, Raven Press.

25. Brooks VB: Roles of cerebellum and basal ganglia in initiation and control of movements, *Can J Neurol Sci* 2.265, 1975.

26. Brown RG and others: Response choice in Parkinson's disease: the effects of uncertainty and stimulus—response compatibility, *Brain* 116:869, 1993.

27. Buchwald NA and others: The "caudate-spindle." III. Inhibition by high frequency stimulation of subcortical structures, *Electroencephalogr Clin Neurophysiol* 13:525, 1961.

28. Buchwald NA and others: The "caudate-spindle." IV. A behavioral index of caudate-induced inhibition, *Electroencephalogr Clin Neurophysiol* 13.536, 1961.

29. Buchwald NA and others: The basal ganglia and the regulation of response and cognitive sets. In Brazier MAB, editor: *Growth and development of the brain,* New York, 1975, Raven Press.

30. Burt DR and others: Antischizophrenic drugs: chronic treatment elevates dopamine receptor binding in brain, *Science* 196:326, 1977.

31. Butterfield PG and others: Environmental antecedents of young-onset Parkinson's disease, *Neurology* 43:1150, 1993.

32. Calne DB and others: Bromocriptine in parkinsonism, *Br Med J* 4:442, 1974.

33. Carlsson A: Some aspects of dopamine in the basal ganglia. In Yahr MD, editor: *The basal ganglia,* New York, 1976, Raven Press.

34. Carpenter MB: Anatomy of the basal ganglia and related nuclei: a review. In Yahr MD, editor: *The basal ganglia,* New York, 1976, Raven Press.

35. Carter JH and others: The effect of exercise on levodopa absorption, *Neurology* 39 (Suppl 1):320, 1989.

36. Calne DB: Is idiopathic parkinsoniam the consequence of an event or a process? *Neurology* 44:5, 1994.

37. Cohen G and Heikkila RE: The generation of hydrogen peroxide, superoxide radical and the hydroxyl radical by 6-hydroxy dopamine, dialuric acid and related aytotoxic agents, *J Biol Chem* 249:2447, 1974.

38. Conner NP and Abbs JH: Task-dependent variations in Parkinsonian motor impairments, *Brain* 114:321, 1991.

39. Cooper IS: *Involuntary movement disorders,* New York, 1969, Paul B Hoeber.

40. Cotzias GC and others: Modification of parkinsonism: chronic treatment with L-dopa, *N Engl J Med* 280:337, 1969.

41. Crutcher MD and DeLong MR: Single cell studies of the primate putamen. II. Relations to direction of movement and pattern of muscular activity, *Exp Brain Res* 53:244, 1984.

42. Davis CG and others: Chronic parkinsonism secondary to intravenous injection of meperidine, *Psychiatry Res* 1:249, 1979.

43. deBruin PFC and others: Effects of treatment on airway dynamics and respiratory muscle strength in Parkinson's disease, *Am Rev Respir Dis* 148.1576, 1993.

44. Diamond SG and Markham CH: One year trial of pergolide as an adjunct to sinemet in the treatment of Parkinson's disease, *Adv Neurol* 40:537, 1984.

45. Dieckmann G and Sasaki K: Recruiting responses in the cerebral cortex produced by putamen and pallidum stimulation, *Exp Brain Res* 10:236, 1970.

46. DeLong MR: Activity of basal ganglia neurons during movement, *Brain Res* 40:127, 1972.

47. DeLong MR and Strick P: Relation of basal ganglia, cerebellum and motor cortex units to ramp and ballistic limb movements, *Brain Res* 71:327, 1974.

48. Denny-Brown D: *The basal ganglia and their relation to disorders of movement,* Liverpool, UK, 1962, Liverpool University Press.

49. Denny-Brown D and Yanagesawa N: The role of the basal ganglia in the initiation of movement. In Yahr MD, editor: *The basal ganglia,* New York, 1976, Raven Press.

50. Divac I: Neostriatum and functions of perfrontal cortex, *Acta Neurobiol Exp* 32:461, 1972.

51. Dom R and others: Neuropathology of Huntington's chorea, *Neurology* 26:64, 1976.

52. Dunne JW and others: Parkinsonism: upturned walking stick as an aid to locomotion, *Arch Phys Med Rehabil* 68.380, 1987.

53. Duvoisin RC: *Parkinson's disease: a guide for patient and family,* New York, 1978, Raven Press.

54. Evarts EV: Pyramidal tract activity associated with a conditioned hand movement in the monkey, *J Neurophysiol* 29:1011, 1966.

55. Fahn S: The extrapyramidal disorders. In Wyngaarden JB and Smith LH, editors: *Cecil's textbook of medicine,* ed 16, Philadelphia, 1982, WB Saunders.

56. Fahn S and Elton RL: Unified Parkinson's disease rating scale. In Fahn S and others, editors: *Recent developments in Parkinson's disease,* vol 2, NJ, 1987, MacMillan Healthcare Information.

57. Feltz P: γ-Aminobutyric acid and a caudato-nigral inhibition, *Can J Physiol Pharmacol* 49:1113, 1971.

58. Ferrier D: *The functions of the brain,* London, 1876, Smith, Elder.

59. Friedman J and Friedman H: Fatigue in Parkinson's disease, *Neurology* 43:2016, 1993.

60. Fujimura and others: Assessment of the distribution of nerve conduction velocities in alcoholics, *Environ Res* 61:317, 1993.

61. Fuster JM and Alexander GE: Neuron activity related to short-term memory, *Science* 173:652, 1971.

62. Fuxe K and others: Heterogeneities in the dopamine neuron systems and dopamine cotransmission in the basal ganglia and the relevance of receptor-receptor interactions. In Fahn S and others, editors: *Recent developments in Parkinson's disease,* New York, 1986, Raven Press.

63. Gauthier L and others: The benefits of group occupational therapy for patients with Parkinson's disease, *Am J Occup Ther* 41:360, 1987.

64. Gelfand IM and others: Some problems in the analysis of movements. In Gelfand VS and others, editors: *Models of the structural-functional organization of certain biological systems,* Cambridge, 1971, The MIT Press.

65. Glatt S and others: *Anticipatory and feedback postural responses in perturbation in Parkinson's disease,* Phoenix, 1989, Society for Neuroscience Abstract.

66. Goldman PS: The role of experience in recovery of function following orbital prefrontal lesions in infant monkeys, *Neuropsychologia* 14:401, 1976.

67. Granit R and Kaada BR: Influence of stimulation of central nervous structures on muscle spindles in cat, *Acta Physiol Scand* 27:130, 1952.

68. Graybiel AM: Functions of the nigrostriatal system, *Clin Neurosci* 1:12, 1993.

69. Grimby L and Hannerz J: Disturbances in the voluntary recruitment order of anterior tibial motor units in bradykinesia of parkinsonism, *J Neurol Neurosurg Psychiatry* 37:47, 1974.

70. Hallett M: Physiology of basal ganglia disorders: an overview, *Can J Neurol Sci* 20.177, 1993.

71. Hallett M and others: Analysis of stereotyped voluntary movements at the elbow in patients with Parkinson's disease, *J Neurol Neurosurg Psychiatry* 40:1129, 1977.

72. Harper PS: Localization of the gene for Huntington's chorea, *Trends Neurosci* 7:1, 1984.

73. Hartmann-von Monakow K and others: Projections of the precentral motor cortex and other cortical areas of the frontal lobe to the

subthalamic nucleus in the monkey, *Exp Brain Res* 33:395, 1978.

74. Hayden MR: *Huntington's chorea,* Berlin, 1981, Springer-Verlag.

75. Heikkila RE and others: Protection against the dopaminergic neurotoxicity of MPTP by monoamine oxidase inhibitors, *Nature* 311:467, 1984.

76. Heimer L: *The human brain and spinal cord: functional neuroanatomy and dissection guide,* New York, 1983, Springer-Verlag.

77. Hoehn MM and Yahr MD: Parkinsonism: onset, progression and mortality, *Neurology* 17:427, 1967.

78. Horak FB and others: Postural instability in Parkinson's disease: motor coordination and sensory organization, Anaheim, 1984, Society for Neuroscience Abstract.

79. Hore J and Vilis T: Arm movement performance during reversible basal ganglia lesions in the monkey, *Exp Brain Res* 39:217, 1980.

80. Hore J and others: Basal ganglia cooling disables learned arm movements of monkeys in the absence of visual guidance, *Science* 195:584, 1977.

81. Hornykiewicz O: The mechanisms of action of L-dopa in Parkinson's disease, *Life Sci* 15:1249, 1974.

82. Hubble JP and others: Risk factors for Parkinson's disease, *Neurology* 43:1693, 1993.

83. Hull CD and others: Intracellular responses in caudate and cortical neurons. In Crane G and Gardener R, editors: *Psychotropic drugs and dysfunctions of the basal ganglia,* Washington, DC, 1969, US Public Health Service.

84. Hull CD and others: Intracellular responses of caudate neurons to brainstem stimulation, *Brain Res* 22:163, 1970.

85. Hull CD and others: Intracellular responses of caudate neurons to temporally and spatially combined stimuli, *Exp Neurol* 38:324, 1973.

86. Hurwitz A: The benefit of a home program exercise regimen for ambulatory Parkinson's disease patients, *J Neuro Nurs* 21:180, 1989.

87. Jellinger K: Pathology of parkinsonism. In Fahr S and others, editors: *Recent developments in Parkinson's disease,* New York, 1986, Raven Press.

88. Jordan N and others: Cognitive components of reaction time in Parkinson's disease, *J Neurol Neurosurg Psychiatry* 55:658, 1992.

89. Kaakkola S and others: Effect of entacapone, a COMT inhibitor, on clinical disability and levodopa metabolism in parkinsonian patients, *Neurology* 44:77, 1994.

90. Kelly PJ and Gillingham FJ: The long-term results of stereotaxic surgery and L-dopa therapy in patients with Parkinson's disease: a 10-year follow-up study, *J Neurosurg* 53:332, 1980.

91. Kemp JM and Powell TPS: The connexions of the striatum and globus pallidus: synthesis and speculation, *Phil Trans R Soc Lond* (Biol) 262:441, 1971.

92. Kim R and others: Projections of globus pallidus and adjacent structures: an autoradiographic study in the monkey, *J Comp Neurol* 169:263, 1976.

93. Kissin B and Begleiter H, editors: *The biology of alcoholism,* vol 5, New York, 1977, Plenum Publishing Corp.

94. Klawans HL: Therapeutic approaches to neuroleptic induced tardive dyskinesia, *Res Publ Assoc Res Nerv Ment Dis* 55:447, 1976.

95. Klawans HL and others: Presymptomatic and early detection in Huntington's disease, *Ann Neurol* 8:343, 1980.

96. Klawans HL Jr and Weiner W: The effect of δ-amphetamine of choreiform disorders, *Neurology* 24:312, 1974.

97. Kling A and Tucker TJ: Effects of combined lesions of frontal granular cortex and caudate nucleus in the neonatal monkey, *Brain Res* 6:428, 1967.

98. Knott M and Voss D: *Proprioceptive neuromuscular facilitation patterns and techniques,* ed 2, New York, 1968, Harper & Row.

99. Koller WC and others: Falls and Parkinson's disease, *Clin Neuropharmacol* 12:98, 1989.

100. Koller W and others: Environmental risk factors in Parkinson's disease, *Neurology* 40:1218, 1990.

101. Kopin IJ and others: Mechanisms of neurotoxicity of MPTP. In Fahr S and others, editors: *Recent developments in Parkinson's disease,* New York, 1986, Raven Press.

102. Kornhuber HH: Motor functions of cerebellum and basal ganglia: the cerebellocortical saccadic (ballistic) clock, the cerebellonuclear hold regulator, and the basal ganglia ramp (voluntary speed smooth movement) generator, *Kybernetik* 8:157, 1971.

103. Krauthamer GM and Albe-Fessard D: Electrophysiological studies of the basal ganglia and striopallidal inhibition of non-specific afferent activity, *Neuropsychologia* 2:73, 1964.

104. Kubota K and Hamada I: Preparatory activity of monkey pyramidal tract neurons related to quick movement onset during visual tracking performance, *Brain Res* 168:435, 1979.

105. Kubota K and Niki H: Prefrontal cortical unit activity and delayed alteration performance in monkeys, *J Neurophysiol* 34:337, 1971.

106. Kunzle H: Bilateral projections from precentral motor cortex to the putamen and other parts of the basal ganglia: an autoradiographic study in Macaca fascicularis, *Brain Res* 88:195, 1976.

107. Kunzle H: Projections from the primary somatosensory cortex to basal ganglia and thalamus in the monkey, *Exp Brain Res* 30:481, 1977.

108. Labuszewski T and Lidsky TI: Basal ganglia influences on brain stem trigeminal neurons, *Exp Neurol* 65:471, 1979.

109. Langston JW and others: Chronic parkinsonism in humans due to a product of meperidine analog synthesis, *Science* 219:979, 1983.

110. Langston JW: MPTP neurotoxicity: an overview and characterization of phrases of toxicity, *Life Sci* 36:201, 1985.

111. Ledin T and Odkvist LM: Abstinent chronic alcoholics investigated by dynamic posturography, occular smooth pursuit and visual suppression, *Acta Otolaryngol* 111:646, 1991.

112. Lelli S and others: Spinal cord inhibitory mechanisms in Parkinson's disease, *Neurology* 41:553, 1991.

113. Levine MS and others: Pallidal and entopeduncular intracellular responses to striatal, cortical, thalamic and sensory inputs, *Exp Neurol* 44:448, 1974.

114. Levine MS and others: The spontaneous firing patterns of forebrain neurons. II. Effects of unilateral caudate nuclear ablation, *Brain Res* 78:411, 1974.

115. Levine MS and others: The spontaneous firing pattern of forebrain neurons. III. Prevention of induced asymmetries in caudate neuronal firing rates by unilateral thalamic lesions, *Brain Res* 131:215, 1977.

116. Levine MS and others: Long-term decreases in spontaneous firing of caudate neurons induced by amphetamine in cats, *Brain Res* 194:263, 1980.

117. Levine MS and others: Long-term behavioral and neurophysiological effects of neonatal δ-amphetamine administration in kittens, *Neurosci Abst* 8:965, 1982.

118. Lidsky TI and others: Pallidal and entopeduncular single unit activity in cats during drinking, *Electroencephalogr Clin Neurophysiol* 39(1):79, 1975.

119. Lidsky TI and others: The effects of stimulation of trigeminal sensory afferents upon caudate units in cats, *Brain Res Bull* 4:9, 1979.

120. Lidsky TI and others: Trigeminal influences on entopeduncular units, *Brain Res* 141:227, 1978.

121. Livesey PJ and Rankine-Wilson J: Delayed alternation learning under electrical (blocking) stimulation of the caudate nucleus in the cat, *J Comp Physiol Psychol* 88:342, 1975.

122. Lloyd KG and others: The neurochemistry of Parkinson's disease: effect of L-dopa therapy, *J Pharmacol Exp Ther* 195:453, 1975.

123. MacKay AVP: Clinical controversies in tardive dyskinesia. In Marsden CD and Fahn S, editors: *Movement disorders,* Boston, 1981, Butterworth.

124. Magendie M: *Fonctions et maladies du système nerveux,* Paris, 1841, Lecapalin. (Translated in *Assoc Res Nerv Ment Dis* 21:8, 1940.)

125. Markham CH and Diamond SG: Evidence to support early levodopa therapy in Parkinson disease, *Neurology* 31:125, 1981.

126. Markus HS and others: Raised resting energy expenditure in Parkinson's disease and its relationship to muscle rigidity, *Clin Sci* 83:199, 1992.

127. Martin JP: *The basal ganglia and posture,* London, 1967, Pitman Books, Ltd.

128. Massion J and Smith AM: Activity of ventrolateral thalamic neurons related to posture and movement during contact placing responses in the cat, *Brain Res* 61:400, 1973.

129. Matsunami K and Cohen B: Afferent modulation of unit activity in globus pallidus and caudate neurons and changes induced by vestibular nucleus and pyramidal tract stimulation, *Brain Res* 91:140, 1975.

130. McGeer PL and others: Aging and extrapyramidal function, *Arch Neurol* 34:33, 1977.

131. Melmon KL and Morrelli HF: *Clinical pharmacology: basic principles in therapeutics,* ed 2, New York, 1978, Macmillan.

132. Melnick M and others: Activity of forebrain neurons during alternating movement in cats, *Electroencephalogr Clin Neurophysiol* 57:57, 1984.

133. Melnick ME and others: Comparison of behavioral effects of MPTP in young adult and year old rats. In Markey SP and others, editors: *MPTP, a neurotoxin producing a Parkinsonian syndrome,* Orlando, Fla, 1986, Academic Press.

134. Melnick ME and Palmer G: Physical therapy. In Koller WC and Paulson G, editors: *Therapy of Parkinson's disease.* New York, 1990, Marcel Dekker.

135. Mettler FA and others: The extrapyramidal system, *Arch Neurol Psychiatry* 41:984, 1939.

136. Milner-Brown HS and others: Electrical properties of motor units in Parkinsonism and a possible relationship with bradykinesia, *J Neurol Neurosurg Psychiatry* 42:35, 1979.

137. Montgomery EB and others: Motor initiation versus execution in normal and Parkinson's disease subjects, *Neurology,* 41:1469, 1991.

138. Montgomery EB and others: Reaction time and movement velocity abnormalities in Parkinson's disease under different task conditions, *Neurology* 41:1476, 1991.

139. Muskens L: The central connection of the vestibular nuclei with the corpus striatum and their significance for ocular movements and for locomotion, *Brain* 45:452, 1922.

140. Mutch WJ and others: A pilot study of patient rated disability and the need for aids in Parkinson's disease, *Clin Rehabil* 3:151, 1989.

141. Nauta HJW and Cole M: Efferent projections of the subthalamic nucleus: an autoradiographic study in monkey and cat, *J Comp Neurol* 180:1, 1978.

142. Neafsey EJ and others: Preparation for movement in the cat. I. Unit activity in the cerebral cortex, *Electroenchephalogr Clin Neurophysiol* 44:706, 1978.

143. Neafsey EJ and others: Preparation for movement in the cat. II. Unit activity in the basal ganglia and thalamus, *Electroencephalogr Clin Neurophysiol* 44:714, 1978.

144. Newton RA and Price DD: Modulation of cortical and pyramidal tract induced motor responses by electrical stimulation of the basal ganglia, *Brain Res* 85:403, 1975.

145. Nieoullon A and others: Interdependence of the nigrostriatal dopaminergic systems on the two sides of the brain in the cat, *Science* 198:416, 1977.

146. Norton S and others: Early motor development and cerebral cortical morphology in rats exposed prenatally to alcohol, *Alcoholism* 12:130, 1988.

147. Nothnagel H: Experimentalle Untersuchungen uber die Funktion des Gehirns, *Virchows Arch* 57:184, 1873. (Translated in *Assoc Res Nerv Ment Dis* 21:8, 1940.)

148. Nutt JG and others: The "on-off" phenomenon in Parkinson's disease: relation to levodopa absorption and transport, *N Engl J Med* 310:483, 1984.

149. Olmstead CE and Villablanca JR: Effects of caudate nuclei or frontal cortical ablations in kittens: bar pressing performance, *Exp Neurol* 63:244, 1979.

150. Owen AM and others: Contrasting mechanisms of impaired attentional set-shifting in patients with frontal lobe damage or Parkinson's disease, *Brain* 116:1159, 1993.

151. Palmer SS and others: Exercise therapy for Parkinson's disease, *Arch Phys Med Rehabil* 67:741, 1986.

152. Pan HS and Walters JR: Unilateral lesion of the nigrostriatal pathway decreases the firing rate and alters the firing pattern of the globus pallidus neurons in the rat. *Synapse* 2:650, 1988.

153. Pascual-Leone A and others: Procedural learning in Parkinson's disease and cerebellar degeneration, *Ann Neurol* 34:594, 1993.

154. Pastor MA and others: Vestibular induced postural responses in Parkinson's disease, *Brain* 116:1177, 1993.

155. Peacock IW: A physical therapy program for Huntington's disease patients, *Clin Management* 7:22, 1987.

156. Pechadre JC and others: Parkinsonian akinesia, rigidity and tremor in the monkey, *J Neurol Sci* 28:147, 1976.

157. Petajan JH and others: Motor unit control in Huntington's disease: a possible presymptomatic test. In Chase TN and others, editors: *Advances in neurology,* vol 23, New York, 1979, Raven Press.

158. Poirier LJ and others: Striatonigral lesions and movement disorders in monkeys, *Adv Neurol* 10:5, 1975.

159. Pollock LJ and Davis L: Muscle tone in parkinsonian states, *Arch Neurol Psychiatry* 23:303, 1930.

160. Potegal M: The caudate nucleus egocentric localization system, *Acta Neurobiol Exp* 32:479, 1972.

161. Potegal M and others: Vestibular input to the caudate nucleus, *Exp Neurol* 32:448, 1971.

162. Rajput AH and others: Geography, drinking well water chemistry, pesticides and herbicides and the etiology of Parkinson's disease, *Can J Neurol Sci* 14:414, 1987.

163. Roberts E: Some thoughts about GABA and the basal ganglia. In Yahr MD, editor: *The basal ganglia,* New York, 1976, Raven Press.

164. Robertson C and Flowers KA: Motor set in Parkinson's disease, *J Neurol Neurosurg Psychiatry* 53:583, 1990.

165. Saint-Cyr JA and others: Procedural learning and neostriatal dysfunction in man, *Brain* 111:941, 1988

166. Sasco AJ and others: The role of physical exercise in the occurrence of Parkinson's disease, *Arch Neurol* 49:360, 1992.

167. Schenkman M and Butler RB: A model for multisystem evaluation treatment of individuals with Parkinson's disease: rationale and case studies, *Phys Ther* 69:932, 1989.

168. Schneider JS and Lidsky TI: Processing of somatosensory information in striatum of behaving cats, *J Neurophysiol* 45:841, 1981.

169. Schneider JS and others: Deficits in operant behavior in monkeys treated with MPTP, *Brain* 111:1265, 1988.

170. Segundo JP and Machne X: Unitary responses to afferent volleys in lenticular nucleus and claustrum, *J Neurophysiol* 19:325, 1956.

171. Shellenberger MK: Persistent alteration of rat brain monoamine levels by carbon monoxide exposure: sex differences and behavioral correlation, *Neurotoxicology* 2:431, 1981.

172. Shelton PA and Knopman DS: Ideomotor apraxia in Huntington's disease, *Arch Neurol* 48:35, 1991.

173. Shoulson I and Fahn S: Huntington's disease: clinical care and evaluation, *Neurology* 29:1, 1979.

174. Shoulson I and others: Clinical care of the patient and family with Huntington's disease. In Commission for the control of Huntington's disease and its consequences, vol 1, National Institute of Health, Washington, DC, 1977.

175. Shoulson I and others: Huntington's disease: treatment with muscimol, a GABA- mimetic drug, *Trans Am Neurol Assoc* 102:124, 1977.

176. Smith AD and Bolam JP: The neural network of the basal ganglia as

revealed by the study of synaptic connections of identified neurones, *Trends Neurosci* 13:259, 1990.

177. Smith JM and Baldessarini RJ: Changes in prevalence, severity and recovery in tardive dyskinesia with age, *Arch Gen Psychiatry* 37:1368, 1980.

178. Soltysik S and others: Single unit activity in basal ganglia of monkeys during performance of a delayed response task, *Electroencephalogr Clin Neurophysiol* 39:65, 1975.

179. Sotrel A and others: Evidence for neruonal degeneration and dendritic plasticity in cortical pyramidal neurons of Huntington's disease: a quantitative Golgi study, *Neurology* 43:2088, 1993.

180. Stam CJ and others: Disturbed frontal regulation of attention in Parkinson's disease, *Brain* 116:1139, 1993.

181. Stelmach GE and others: Movement preparation in Parkinson's disease: the use of advanced information, *Brain* 109:1179, 1986.

182. Stern G: The effect of lesions in the substantia nigra, *Brain* 89:449, 1966.

183. Storey E and Beal MF. Neurochemical substrates of rigidity and chorea in Huntington's disease, *Brain* 116:1201-1222, 1993.

184. Strick PL: Anatomical analysis of ventrolateral thalamic input to primate motor cortex, *J Neurophysiol* 39:1020, 1976.

185. Tarsy D and others: Physostigmine in choreiform movement disorders, *Neurology* 24:28, 1974.

186. Tatton WG and others: Altered motor cortical activity in extrapyramidal rigidity. In Poirier LJ and others, editors: *Advances in neurology,* vol 24, New York, 1979, Raven Press.

187. Teasdale N and others: Temporal movement control in patients with Parkinson's disease, *J Neurol Neurosurg Psychiatry* 53:862, 1990.

188. Teuber HL: Complex functions of basal ganglia. In Yahr MD, editor: *The basal ganglia,* New York, 1976, Raven Press.

189. Thach WT: Discharge of cerebellar neurons related to two maintained postures and two prompt movements. I. Nuclear cell output, *J Neurophysiol* 33:527, 1970.

190. Thach WT: Discharge of cerebellar neurons related to two maintained postures and two prompt movements. II. Purkinje cell output and input, *J Neurophysiol* 33:537, 1970.

191. Tsukue I and Shohoji T: Movement therapy for alcoholic patients, *J Stud Alcohol* 42:144, 1981.

192. Tucker TJ and Kling A: Differential effects of early and late lesions of frontal granular cortex in the monkey, *Brain Res* 5:377, 1967.

193. Vidailhet M and others: The bereitschafts potential preceding simple foot movement and initiation of gait in Parkinson's disease, *Neurology* 43:1784, 1993.

194. Villablanca JR and Marcus R: Effects of caudate nuclei removal in cats: comparison with effects of frontal cortex ablation. In Buchwald NA and Brazier MAM, editors: *Brain mechanisms in mental retardation,* New York, 1975, Academic Press.

195. Wagner GC and others: Long-lasting depletions of striatal dopamine and loss of dopamine uptake sites following repeated administration of methamphetamine, *Brain Res* 181:151, 1980.

196. Wagner GC and Jarvis MF: Age-dependent effects of MPTP. In Markey SP and others, editors: *MPTP: a neurotoxin producing a Parkinsonian syndrome,* Orlando, Fla, 1986, Academic Press.

197. Walshe FMR: Nature of musculature rigidity of paralysis agitans and its relationship to tremor, *Brain* 47:159, 1924.

198. Walshe JM: Wilson's disease: the presenting symptoms, *Arch Dis Child* 37:253, 1962.

199. Willis T: Cerebri anatomic cui accessit nervorum descriptio et usus, 1664. (Translated in *Assoc Res Nerv Ment Dis* 21:8, 1940.

200. Wilson SAK: An experimental research into the anatomy and physiology of the corpus striatum, *Brain* 36:427, 1914.

201. Winkelmuller W and Nitsch FM: Quantitative registration of motor disorders following bilateral lesions of S.N. in the rat, *Appl Neurophysiol* 38:291, 1975.

202. Woodworth RS and Schlosberg H: *Experimental psychology,* New York, 1961, Holt, Rinehart & Winston.

203. Worringham CJ and Stelmach GE: Practice effects on the preprogramming of discrete movements in Parkinson's disease, *J Neurol Neurosurg Psychiatry.*

204. Yanagasawa N: The spectrum of motor disorders in Huntington's disease, *Clin Neurol Neurosurg* 94 Suppl: S182, 1992.

Brain Tumors

Gertrude Freeman

KEY TERMS

classification
clinical malignancy
radiation
chemotherapy

Karnofsky Scale of
  Performance Status (KPS)
Dietz classification
hope

LEARNING OBJECTIVES

After reading this chapter the student/therapist will:

1. Become familiar with the classification of brain tumors.
2. Gain an awareness of the most common symptoms that may occur depending on the site and extent of tumor involvement.
3. Value the importance of other history and a thorough neurological examination when evaluating a patient suspected of having a brain tumor.
4. Become familiar with the most common procedures for the diagnosis of a brain tumor.
5. Become familiar with the side effects of the medical and surgical management of a brain tumor and how they may affect the therapy program.
6. Become familiar with the functional evaluation scales frequently used by other oncology team members.
7. Develop an appreciation for the importance of including all systems in an evaluation of a patient following diagnosis of a brain tumor.
8. Develop an awareness of the need to apply the principles of motor learning to the management of patients following treatment for a brain tumor.
9. Appreciate the role of the therapist when interacting with patients who are in a deteriorating condition.

Rehabilitation is the restoration or improvement of the physical function of a patient, which has been impaired by accidents, disease, or its treatment. Among the patients who may benefit from the rehabilitative services of the physical therapist are those with a brain tumor.[77] Until recently, most people could not see any rationale for applying the benefits of rehabilitation to a group of patients who, if not cured, were likely to die within a relatively short time. Today, however, many people are cured of tumors, whereas others live with chronic illness that is interspersed with remissions. Unfortunately, these patients are often left with severe functional problems. The therapist can make a significant contribution toward improving the quality of life remaining to such patients.[25,41,42,43,53]

The management of a patient with a tumor is much like that of any patient with a chronic neurological condition (i.e., patients with problems resulting from vascular insult or trauma).[22,78] In patients with other conditions, however, the disease process usually has been arrested before rehabilitative measures are initiated, enabling the therapist to make certain assumptions about the patient's future and to plan a rehabilitative strategy. Absolute goals can be formulated in the secure knowledge that the rehabilitative program will not be complicated by a deteriorating physical condition. This may not be true of the patient with a brain tumor, although the rehabilitative plan may have essentially the same goals. As with any patient, the therapist must be flexible, adjusting expectations as the patient's physical status changes in the course of the disease.[53]

The multifaceted team approach, using the combined skills of all its members, has been successful in the rehabilitation of chronic neuromuscular disability and can be profitably applied to managing the patient with a brain tumor. Rehabilitation results can be predicted with greater certainty when the natural history of the primary tumor, the therapeutic medical-surgical approach and its complications, and the patient's current clinical status are taken into consideration. It is essential for the therapist to work closely with the entire medical team to determine appropriate care.[26] Therapists must be sensitive to the patient's physical and psychological needs and adjust rehabilitation goals and methods accordingly. To be a respected member of the oncology team, a therapist must have a knowledge of tumor management, as well as management of the particular neurological deficit.[53]

AN OVERVIEW OF BRAIN TUMORS
History

The microscopic characteristics of brain tumors were first recognized during the last half of the nineteenth century. However, an orderly scheme of **classification** based on cell morphology was not established until 1926 when Bailey and Cushing published a monograph in which tumors were named according to the histological resemblance between their cells and cells of normal development.

More recently, there has been a trend toward simplification so that a diagnosis with prognostic implication can be made. Two grading systems that may be used are the classifications of Kernahan and Ringretz. In the classification of Kernohan and others, the name of the tumor is based on cells present in the adult brain combined with a malignancy grading of I to IV (IV being the most malignant) The Ringretz scale is a similar three-grade system. Grades III and IV on the Kernohan scale have been combined into Ringretz grade III.[1,5,40,41]

Realizing the need for a universal classification of central nervous system (CNS) tumors, the World Health Organization (WHO) established a center for this purpose in 1970. In the resulting 1979 publication, *Histological Typing of CNS Tumors*, tumors were named according to microscopic characteristics. The WHO classification has been used successfully since its publication. As our understanding of tumor cells increases, the present classification will continue to change.[54,80]

Etiology and incidence

Brain tumors are a health problem for all age groups, and data suggest that their incidence is increasing. The estimated number of primary CNS tumors in the United States for 1993 is 17,500. Estimated deaths for the same period are 12,100. Approximately 80,000 to 100,000 metastatic tumors occur annually.[46] The statistics for brain tumors, however, show great variation and in some cases may be artificial. The development of noninvasive diagnostic procedures, improved medical care for the elderly, and the availability and quality of medical services in the more developed countries may account for the increased incidence in some categories.[46,57,62]

The majority of brain tumors occur in two age ranges: childhood (3 to 12 years) and later life (50 to 70 years). In adults, brain tumors occur in white Americans more than black Americans and slightly more often in men than women. Men have a higher incidence of malignant glioma and neuroma, whereas women have a higher incidence of meningoma and pituitary adenoma.[31,51,58]

In children, primary brain tumors are the second most common form of cancer; however, the presence of malignancy is lower than in adults. Pediatric tumors are also quite different in histology and behavior from those of adult tumors. Nearly two thirds of pediatric CNS lesions are infratentorial, whereas an equivalent proportion of adult tumors are supratentorial.[31,40,68]

Little is known about the etiology of brain tumors. Certain tumors appear to be congenital; others may be related to hereditary factors, but the evidence is weak.[58,79] For many years a history of head trauma was considered a risk factor for glial tumors; however, recent studies have theorized that the trauma aggravates an already present tumor.[49,69] Studies of exposure to environmental agents are currently of interest; chemicals and medications are among those most suspected. In a study of nonoccupational risk factors, no association was determined between brain tumors and exposure to pets, irradiation to the head, or family history of CNS malignancies.[68] Other studies have examined the relationship of brain tumors with electrical occupations and ionizing radiation. The evidence of electromagnetic field radiation, resulting in brain cancer is strongly suggestive although not yet conclusive.[8]

Some studies have shown that ionizing radiation *may* be an important risk factor for meningioma, whereas others accept it as a well-established fact. Regarding family clustering of brain tumors, reports suggest that the mortality rate from cerebral glioma may be four times higher in relatives of patients with tumors than in the general population.[50,68]

Further research to identify etiological risk factors is of

critical importance. Identification of factors that could be modified might lead to a decrease in the future incidence of brain tumors.[50]

Classification of tumors

Therapists who treat patients with brain tumors must have a knowledge of tumor classification. Understanding the clinical behavior of a brain tumor depends on an accurate classification of the cell of origin and on the degree of aggressiveness of the cells.

The brain tumor classification of Kernohan and Sayre, along with the percentage of occurrence, is presented in Table 22-1. Characteristics of the most common brain tumors are described in the following paragraphs, and biological and histological malignancy is discussed.[14,41] Most primary intracranial tumors fit into one of two histological categories. The first category represents tumors of the primary supporting elements (gliomas). The second category concerns the usually benign tumors of the covering of the dura of the brain (meningiomas).[17,63]

Tumors may be further classed as primary, originating from cells found within the brain, or secondary (metastatic), originating from structures outside the brain. As seen in Table 22-1 the common primary tumors include the glial series, meningiomas, pituitary tumors, and neurilemomas. For discussion the varieties of gliomas are considered as pure entities; however, a mixture of glial elements is commonly present. The prognosis of these mixed tumors is determined by their most malignant component.[50,70]

Gliomas vary in their biological and growth characteristics; some are benign and slow growing, whereas others are highly malignant. Although they may occur at any age, they are generally tumors of the young adult. Gliomas produce symptoms that are focal in nature as a result of local infiltration, destruction, or pressure on the brain; they rarely metastasize.[14,15,41,51,70]

Astrocytomas, the most common glioma, may occur throughout the brain, but most are supratentorial and primarily involve the cerebral hemispheres. They range from the benign slow-growing variety to the highly malignant glioblastoma multiforme. The peak incidence of cerebral astrocytomas occurs during the third and fourth decades, with the frontal lobes the most common site of origin. The cerebellar astrocytoma is the most common infratentorial tumor of children.[26,79]

Glioblastoma Multiforme (GMA) grade III and IV, the most common intracranial neoplasm of the adult, occurs most often in the 45- to 55-year-age group. It may be found in any area of the brain but occurs most frequently in one frontal lobe and may spread via the corpus callosum to the opposite side. Males are affected twice as frequently as females. Life expectancy after diagnosis of GM-A Grade III or IV is usually about 12 to 18 months.[41]

Medulloblastoma is the second most common posterior

Table 22-1. Incidence of intracranial tumors at all ages and in children younger than 15 years of age*

Tumor	All ages (%)	Children (%)
Glioma	45	70
Astrocytoma	15	30
Glioblastoma	15	5
Oligodendroglioma	8	1
Medulloblastoma	4	20
Ependymoma	4	10
Meningioma	15	1
Neurinoma	6	<0.5
Pituitary adenoma	6	1
Metastases	5–20	<0.5
Craniopharyngioma	3	10
Choroid plexus papilloma	0.5	3
Pinealoma	1	2
Hemangioma	3	1
Epidermoid	2	0.5
Dermoids–teratoma	<0.5	3
Sarcoma	2	4
Optic glioma	1	4

From Evans RG: In Morantz RA and Walsh JW, editors: *Brain tumors: a comprehensive text,* New York, 1994, Marcel Dekker.

fossa tumors of children. These highly malignant tumors usually develop in the vermis of the cerebellum during the first two decades of life. The presence of a tumor close to the fourth ventricle results in the early development of hydrocephalus.[59,69]

The *oligodendrogliomas* are found in proximity to neurons made up of cells involved in the process of myelination. These tumors occur in adults, most often during the fifth and sixth decades, and are located predominantly in the frontal and parietal lobes of the cerebral hemispheres. Oligodendrogliomas diffusely infiltrate in a nondestructive manner and can achieve great size before they are symptomatic. Patients often survive with this type of tumor for 15 to 20 years.

Ependymoma, a type of nonastrocytic glioma, is most common in childhood and adolescence. It is derived from the lining of the walls of the ventricular system and spinal canal. Those found in the parietal occipital region show a tendency to malignancy, whereas those in the spinal cord are relatively benign.[15,41]

The *meningioma* is the most important tumor of the meningeal group. The majority of these tumors are benign, encapsulated, and slow growing. They are common in the fifth and sixth decades and are more frequent in women by a ratio of approximately 2:1.[11] In the very young and elderly the sex distribution is even. Because meningiomas are slow-growing tumors that compress the underlying structures rather than infiltrating adjacent tissue, abnormal signs and symptoms may be overlooked and the diagnosis missed completely.*

Pituitary adenomas are tumors derived from cells of the anterior portion of the pituitary gland. They are usually found in middle-aged or older individuals. The clinical signs and symptoms are caused by the secretion of hormones through compression of the normally functioning pituitary.[26,41,59]

Neurilemomas (neurinoma, schwannoma) are slow-growing, benign tumors that originate from Schwann cells. The most common is a tumor on the vestibular portion of the VIII cranial nerve. Treatment consists of surgical removal, which results in facial paralysis and deafness.[11,26,41,59]

Metastases to the brain constitute a major problem in the management of patients with malignancies. The number has risen over the years, and currently between 20% and 40% of the general cancer population develop metastases. As people in general live longer and other therapies are more successful in controlling disease outside the CNS, it is likely that the incidence will continue to increase. Because of its ability to retard metastases in other sites, the use of multiagent chemotherapy has also contributed to this trend. The lesions that most commonly give rise to metastases to the brain are carcinomas of the lung and breast. The incidence of the lung as a source of metastasis is approximately 50%,[46] paralleling the frequency of the primary tumors (Table 22-2). Thus the combination of an increasing incidence of lung cancer, with its predilection for brain metastases, and patients developing metastases while on systemic chemotherapy has led to a large influx of this disease.

Metastatic brain tumors are most frequently reported between the fourth and seventh decade. About half appear on computed tomography (CT) scan to be single lesions. The occurrence may be at a late stage in the metastatic process or the first sign of a previously unrecognized primary tumor. The great majority of metastases reach the CNS through the arterial system.

The frontal lobe of the cerebrum is the most common site for metastatic disease. Other frequent sites are temporal, parietal, and occipital lobes. Cerebellar metastases are infrequent and those to the brain stem are the most rare.[40,41,46,73]

The use of the word *benign* in the classification of brain tumors can be misleading. When a neoplasm is designated as benign, one assumes that a complete cure is possible; conversely, a malignant tumor indicates a poor prognosis. This distinction is made on the basis of histological examination and is termed *cytological malignancy*. In assessing the malignant potential of a brain tumor, we must also consider biological malignancy, which is the likelihood that a tumor will kill the patient. Most cytologically malignant brain tumors are also biologically malignant.

* References 11, 26, 41, 46, 50, and 59.

Table 22-2. Metastatic brain tumors*— distribution by primary cancer

Primary cancer	Percentage of brain metastases
Pulmonary	50
Breast	15
Gastrointestinal	8
Genitourinary	6
Melanoma	6
Unknown primary	10
Other	5

From Laws ER and Thaper K: *Brain Tumors: A Cancer Journal for Clinicians* 1993: 43: 263-71.
*Annual US incidence: 80,000 to 100,000 cases

Irrespective of the histological malignancy of the tumor, its unimpeded growth as a space-occupying and expanding lesion within the confines of the skull inevitably leads to death, which, by definition, is equated to **clinical malignancy.** Various other factors, including the brain's exquisite sensitivity to increased internal pressure, tumor volume, surrounding brain edema, or ventricular obstruction dictate that certain cytologically benign tumors are biologically malignant and inevitably fatal.[14,40,41,57] Many current difficulties in the classification of tumors arise from our incomplete knowledge of their nature and should dissipate as our understanding of the embryology of tumor cells increases.

Signs and symptoms

The progression and type of neurological symptoms depend on the site, growth rate, and type of brain tumor. Neurological deficits are generally thought to be the result of two factors: focal disturbances caused by a tumor and increased intercranial pressure. Focal disturbances are a result of direct invasion or infiltration, causing destruction of neural tissue, and of compression of the brain. Compression also may result in necrosis as a result of alteration in circulation.[31,41,59] The increased intracranial pressure may be a result of several factors: an increase in the mass within the skull, edema formation around the tumor, and alteration in cerebrospinal fluid (CSF) circulation. By the time increased pressure appears, a significant tumor mass or corresponding amount of cerebral edema is present. The symptoms of increased pressure include lethargy, drowsiness, irritability, and difficulty with ambulation. It is not surprising therefore that these symptoms reflect an unfavorable prognostic value.[5,26,41,59]

The most frequent signs and symptoms of tumors are headache, vomiting, and papilledema, which are seen during the course of illness in approximately 70% of brain tumor patients. Headache is the most common presenting symptom occurring in approximately 65% of cases.[46] It may be in a generalized area, or there may be regional correlation, in

Table 22-3. Correlation between clinical symptoms and common neuroanatomical location of tumor sites

Symptoms	Frontal lobe	Parietal lobe	Temporal lobe	Occipital lobe	Lateral and third ventricle	Fourth ventricle	Cerebellum	Midbrain	Brainstem	Cerebellopontine angle	Pineal	Pituitary	Pons	Posterior fossa
Headache				X	X	X		X			X	X		X
Nausea and vomiting				X	X	X		X			X	X		X
Vertigo				X						X	X			X
Light-headedness														
Convulsions														
Personality changes	X													
Papilledema	X		X											
Cranial nerve palsies										X				
Loss of social and sexual inhibitions or apathy/lethargy	X													
Astereognosis		X												
Nystagmus		X					X	X					X	
Contralateral hemiparesis														
Interruptions of consciousness				X										
Visual and auditory hallucination														
Contralateral hemianopsia		X	X	X										
Aphasia		X	X											
Sensory loss		X				X								
Motor loss						X	X	X	X					
Ataxia							X	X			X			
Hearing loss	X													
Alexia				X										
Homonymous hemianopsia		X		X										

which case it has a localizing value. The headache associated with brain tumor is caused by irritation, traction, or compression on pain-sensitive structures including blood vessels, venous sinuses, and cranial nerves. The pain may be described as deep, aching, steady, dull, or severe. It is most severe in the morning, gradually decreasing during the day because of the increased CSF drainage in the erect versus the recumbent position. Vomiting related to increased intracranial pressure and brainstem compression occurs in approximately 10% of the cases as a result[46] of stimulation of the emetic center in the medulla. It occurs most frequently in children, is most likely to occur in the morning, is unrelated to meals, may be unaccompanied by other symptoms, and may be projectile in nature. Papilledema is caused by venous stasis, which leads to engorgement and swelling of the optic disc. In association with the papilledema, disturbances in vision such as decreased visual acuity, diplopia, and deficits in the visual fields—occurs in approximately 30% of cases.[31,41,46]

Other symptoms common in adults with brain tumors are seizure activity and personality changes in about 15% of cases.[46] Seizures, as a manifestation of altered neuronal excitability, are related to compression invasion or alteration

in blood supply. They are present in about 30% of cases and may take the form of a generalized grand mal type or a focal Jacksonian seizure (which can be helpful in localization).[46] Often the first seizure is a momentary loss of alertness or concentration and may be ignored by the patient. It is of interest that the presence of a seizure as an early presenting symptom has a positive correlation in prognosis.[26,31,41]

Encroachment on highly specialized cerebral tissue produces specific neurological deficits, depending on the area and extent of involvement (Table 22-3). The most common frontal lobe symptoms involve higher-level reasoning and judgment skills and may manifest themselves as inappropriate behavior, inability to concentrate, or indifference (see Chapter 5). Other frontal lobe symptoms involve hemiparesis, caused by pressure on the neighboring precentral cortex and pathways and unsteadiness in gait, often imitating cerebellar ataxia (patients with frontal ataxia tend to fall backward). When the dominant frontal lobe is affected, aphasia and apraxia may be evident.

Lesions in the parietal lobe pose particular problems. Removal of significant portions of this area produce major, and often disabling, deficits. The left parietal lobe controls speech as well as sensory and motor functions in right-handed patients. The right parietal lobe, which has control of the left side of the body, is concerned with complex cognitive functions (concepts of space, music, and other abstractions) and sensory-motor control.

Visual loss in the upper quadrant of the eye opposite the lesion, which may progress to a complete hemianopsia and psychomotor seizures (which are described as visual, auditory, or olfactory hallucinations), are two common symptoms that occur with temporal lobe involvement. Varying degrees of receptive aphasia, beginning with difficulty in naming objects, occur when the involvement is in the dominant hemisphere. Facial weakness may result from pressure in the frontal cortex, and total destruction of the temporal lobe will result in mental changes such as irritability, depression, poor judgment, and childish behavior.

Tumors of the occipital lobe occur less frequently than tumors of the previously mentioned lobes. Symptoms include convulsive seizures preceded by an aura. When the occipital cortex is involved, contralateral homonymous hemianopsia, visual agnosia, difficulty in judging distances, and the tendency to get lost in familiar surroundings may occur.

Cerebellar tumors cause early papilledema and may produce a headache at the base of the skull. Lesions of the cerebellum produce a variety of movement disorders, depending on the location of the tumor. Ataxia often suggests a midline cerebellar lesion. Dysmetria and dysdiadochokinesia reflect cerebellar hemisphere deficits, usually of ipsilateral representation. Symptoms that are less obvious than movement disorders, but equally characteristic of a cerebellar tumor, are hypotonia and scanning speech—a tendency to speak with a staccato rhythm, pronouncing each syllable rather than the word (see Chapter 23).

Cerebral tumors manifest their effects through increased intracranial pressure, causing specific cranial nerve compression, such as optic nerve compression resulting in blindness or ocular motor nerve damage resulting in ocular motility defects. Increased pressure also can cause clinical symptoms indirectly with ventricular compression or blockage resulting in hydrocephalus. Another major area is pituitary dysfunction with all of its ramifications of changes in body function, hypopituitarism, giantism, acromegaly, and Cushing's syndrome, depending on the type of tumor and its location.[31,40,41,59]

Tumors of the hypothalamus can affect fat and carbohydrate metabolism, water balance, sleep patterns, appetite, and sexual behavior.[31,40,41,59,79]

Diagnosis

Evaluation: History and neurological examination. The history of a patient suspected of having a brain tumor is a crucial part of the evaluation, because a presumptive diagnosis can be made from the symptoms of headache, evidence of seizure, or indications of a progressive loss of function. The neurological examination enables one to determine the current overall neurological status of the patient and can be helpful in localizing the lesion and predicting outcome. Patients with the poorest level of neurological function have the worst prognosis, regardless of therapy.

The neurological evaluation of a patient suspected of having a brain tumor must encompass the following areas: intellectual, cranial nerve, motor, sensory, reflex, and coordination functions. The most crucial of these areas is intellectual orientation to person, place, and time. The more subtle evaluation of intellectual function involves speech, memory, arithmetic, verbal skills, and association. In general, intellectual functions can be associated with anatomical areas; for example, speech is involved with temporal and parietal areas, especially left parietotemporal (in right-handed patients), memory is frontal and temporal, and mathematical skills are parietal. Association functions are primarily frontal and temporal in location.

Visual field and cranial nerve deficiencies can be very important in diagnosis. Expanding tumors frequently affect cranial nerves III, IV, and VI; and similar dysfunction may be produced by the compression and stretching of the cranial nerves. Visual deficits involve the entire visual pathway from occipital lobe to optic nerve. Motor functions involve pathways from the contralateral parietal motor area through the midbrain and brainstem; lesions at any point in the course of these tracts can result in weakness. Cerebral lesions affecting motor function tend to produce a spastic paralysis with distal parts and fine motor functions first to be affected.

Sensory functions follow a complex pathway from the sensory areas of the contralateral parietal lobes by way of the midbrain, thalamus, and medulla to the cord. Brain tumors of the parietal lobes often produce sensory loss in distal parts earlier than distal parts, and testing for reactions to a pin, temperature, or vibration, as well as for tactile discrimination are all effective.

Reflexes are hyperactive with intracranial mass lesions, becoming hypoactive in the terminal phases. Careful determination of the amplitude of the reflex responses on a numerical scale is helpful. Tumors in the cerebellar area result in transient symptoms of incoordination and are frequently observable for only short intervals.[40,41]

Diagnostic studies. When the history and neurological examination are suggestive of a brain tumor, definitive diagnostic studies are of value to substantiate the suspected diagnosis. Due to the recent advances in neuroimaging techniques, these diagnostic studies are currently reported to be nearly 100% accurate.[79] In the earlier part of this century, skull radiographs, lumbar puncture with cerebral spinal fluid examination, electroencephalography, pneumoencephalography, and ventriculography were relied on for diagnosis of a brain tumor.[46] Currently, in most instances, CT scan and magnetic resonance imaging (MRI) have replaced these tests as the primary diagnostic tools for detection of brain tumors.

During a CT scan as radioactive beams pass through the head, images are generated based on the amount of radiation absorbed. A CT scan provides a 360-degree view of the brain, with tomographic cuts at 1-degree intervals.[3,79]

Development of this technology has permitted the size and density of the tumor to be visualized and its precise location calculated in three-dimensional space. The associated displacement of other intracranial structures and the surrounding areas of ischemia also can be seen. Introduction of a contrast agent may enhance the clarity of the images. The contrast agent also assists to further characterize the tumor, distinguish edema, and differentiate radiation-induced changes from residual or recurrent tumor.[1,9,70,79]

The MRI may be the most precise type of imaging available for diagnosis of brain tumor. Like CT, MRI is a noninvasive computer-based imaging modality that depicts anatomical sections in tomographical slices of varying thickness. The MRI's image production, based on magnetic fields and radio frequency pulses, is superior to CT as a diagnostic tool. Its clear, detailed images have the capability to detect small neoplasms and oxygen-deprived or necrotic tissue. In addition to offering excellent anatomical detail, the MRI also allows for a physiological assessment of the tumor and surrounding area.[3,9,46,70,79]

In some instances the results of the CT scan and MRI can be misleading. The contrast agent does not cross the blood-brain barrier, therefore the tumor masses visualized correspond to the regions of the brain with a disrupted barrier. The malignant cells that have infiltrated into an area of brain in which the barrier is intact may not be visualized.[48]

Position-emission tomography (PET) also provides further insight into brain tumors. PET scanning augments CT scan and MRI. It provides information regarding brain metabolism and regional blood flow and, based on oxygen utilization, is able to assist in prognosis.[65] It is hoped that the newer techniques may aid in differential diagnosis, thus allowing for more precise treatment decisions.

Medical and surgical management

Once the presence of a brain tumor has been positively established, an appropriate therapeutic plan must be selected. The goal is to improve the patient's quality of life and survival time by decreasing the size of the tumor mass. The three most common methods for treatment of brain tumors are surgery, **radiation,** and **chemotherapy.** These modalities can be used alone or in any combination.[12,31,79]

In most instances surgery is the last step in a positive diagnosis of a brain tumor. The surgical procedure can be one of three types: biopsy, partial, or radical resection. The selection depends on the location of the tumor, the purpose of the surgery, and the neurological status of the patient.[1,46]

Biopsy is the removal of sufficient tissue to establish the diagnosis without removing a significant portion of the tumor. Biopsy is indicated for individuals who have deep seated lesions, debilitated patients, or others who are poor surgical risks. A biopsy can be performed by open craniotomy or by CT-guided stereotactic methods. Stereotactic methods allow needle biopsies to be safely obtained in virtually any area of the brain. The major drawback of a needle biopsy is in the sampling. The biopsy may reveal a low grade tumor when in fact the major portion of the tumor is a higher grade. Open resection increases the accuracy of tissue samples because the tumor can be visualized.[1,77,79]

The general procedures for the major operative approaches are similar; the major differences occur during the surgery and vary according to the specific situation. Surgery usually is a combination of diagnostic biopsy and cytoreductive surgery.[1,11,75,77,79]

Many brain tumors cannot be removed completely. The tumor may not have a clear demarcation, or it may be in a strategic location or involved with vital areas of function. In these instances a partial tumor resection that is as extensive as possible improves survival rate. The resection also increases the benefit of radiation and chemotherapy by removing the tumor's hypoxic tumor core.[1,41,46]

Progress in localizing tumors and neuroimaging technology has greatly increased the anatomical information available to neurosurgeons. This information, along with the development of instrumentation such as the laser and the operating microscope, has allowed aggressive resection to become a viable procedure.[1,3,46,75]

Computer-assisted stereotactic resection is a relatively new procedure. It provides the surgeon with precise feedback on tumor margins, limits procedure-induced edema, and by decreasing exposure and manipulation minimizes injury to the normal brain.

Additional advantages of stereotactic resection are the potentially decreased costs of hospitalization and early discharge. Long-term results do not indicate that individuals receiving this procedure have a better prognosis than those treated with conventional surgery; however, with further development it may become the choice for removal of intracranial tumors.[1,3,46]

Ventilation, intracranial pressure measurements, and blood pressure status are carefully monitored following surgery; and cerebral edema is controlled by continued fluid restriction and corticosteroids. Changes in neurological status can be anticipated on the second to fourth day after the operation because of evolving cerebral edema. Because these patients are dehydrated and are usually in one position for a long time, they are prime candidates for thrombophlebitis and pulmonary embolism. The use of anticoagulants is contraindicated postoperatively because of risk of intracranial bleeding. Therefore elevation, bed rest, and elastic stockings are extremely important during the immediate postoperative period. During this time positioning, range of motion, and other activities that affect intracranial pressure cannot be avoided; however, these activities should be spread throughout the day.[41,76]

Surgery followed by radiation and/or chemotherapy may

be the most common approach to primary brain tumors. Radiation is planned for tumors that are surgically inaccessible or for remnants of a tumor that could not be removed completely. Tumor cells are more radiosensitive than nontumor cells. Therefore the objective is to destroy tumor cells without injury to the normal cells. Radiation has the advantage of treating locally a small, defined, nonmetastasizing tumor. Radiotherapy has its limitations because there is a maximal tolerated dose that normal brain tissue can accept without the adverse effect of radiation necrosis.[1,31,46,75,79]

The treatment dose for the tumor depends on several variables including histological type, radio responsiveness, location, and level of tolerance. Many patients improve remarkably after partial surgical resection and radiation. If radiation is not preceded by surgery, radiation, accompanied by large doses of corticosteroids, can temporarily reverse and control symptoms of increased intracranial pressure. Several approaches are currently undergoing investigation in an attempt to sensitize the tumor and to improve the efficiency of irradiation for patients with malignant tumors.[31,79]

One problem receiving attention is the radioresistance of the hypoxic tumor cells. Well-oxygenated tissues are approximately three times more sensitive to radiation than anoxic tissues. To address this problem attempts have been made to develop chemicals to sensitize the cells and to deliver increased oxygen to the tumor via a hyperbaric system. Because heat has the ability to alter the sensitivity of resistant cells, another possibility may be the use of hyperthermia along with radiation therapy.[21,39,79]

Interstitial implantation of radioactive sources (brachytherapy) has become an alternative delivery system. Brachytherapy enables sources of radiation to be accurately placed directly adjacent to the tumor. This strategy allows high doses of radiation to be delivered, with significantly lower doses delivered to the surrounding tissue. Brachytherapy may offer an additional option in the management of metastatic lesions.[1,72,75,79]

Stereotactic radiosurgery is a relatively new treatment modality that uses stereotactically directed beams of ionizing radiation to destroy small intracranial lesions. This very intense radiation can destroy tumor cells as compared to radiotherapy, which aims to supress tumor growth. The gamma knife and the linear accelerator are two types of units in current use. Radiosurgery is a safe and effective procedure, especially for patients who are not surgical candidates or have inoperable tumors.*

Due to the impressive advances made with chemotherapy outside the CNS, attention has focused on its use with CNS malignancies. Studies reported modest improvement when chemotherapy was included with surgery and radiation as part of the overall therapeutic plan.[41,51,76,77]

Multiple chemotherapeutic agents are available. CNUs (Nitrosoureas Carmustine BCNU or Lomustine CCNU) have been the most widely accepted because they are lipid-soluble agents with the ability to cross the blood-brain barrier.[41,75,76,77] The mode of action of CNU agents is to destroy the cell by interfering with DNA during cell division. CNUs may be applied alone or in combination with another chemotherapeutic agent. The appropriate combination of drugs and their sequencing may improve the response through synergistic activity.[51,79]

Chemotherapy can be applied regionally or systemically. This type of therapy almost always exhibits its primary toxicity in organs other than the brain; therefore the systemic side effects limit the systemic therapy.[41,51,79] Approaches to decrease the side effects have included combining the use of BCNU with bone marrow to combat the effects of bone marrow suppression or bone marrow transplant in order to obtain dose intensification.[13,79] External variables that can influence the effect of chemotherapy include type and location of the tumor, the patient's neurological status and body tolerance, and the stage of the disease.

Variables within the tumor cells can have implications for the timing of chemotherapy treatments. Changes in the characteristics of the cells can vary the response to therapy, or a cell that is sensitive to chemotherapy may be replaced by a drug-resistant cell in a short period of time.[51]

Future advances in chemotherapy of CNS tumors are likely to include the development of drugs with greater specificity and a diminished toxicity for normal organs. Intraarterial therapy, intrathecal injection, and other methods of drug delivery are under investigation. Biological agents that modify the characteristics of tumor cells and methods for disruption of the blood-brain barrier are also being studied. The suggestion that heat alters cell membrane permeability has led to the speculation that it may enhance the uptake of chemotherapeutic agents.[13,41] Most of the results of recent chemotherapy studies, however, show no real hope, and there is need for further research.[13]

Although early attempts at immunotherapy for brain tumors were disappointing, newer methods including interferon therapy and targeted therapy using monoclonal antibodies have emerged as promising areas of investigation. Researchers in this area suggest that the knowledge of the entire concept of immune response must be increased before it can be applied to brain tumors.[13,34,46,75]

Management of a metastatic tumor differs from primary tumor management. In most cases, radiotherapy is the principal and often the sole treatment, although surgery may be considered for the young patient who has a solitary metastasis in a silent area, with the primary tumor a site other than the lung. The surgical techniques are essentially the same as those for primary tumors except that resection of surrounding normal brain, such as lobectomy, is rarely indicated. Certain medical approaches, such as the use of corticosteroids for management of the increased intracranial

*References 1, 3, 23, 52, 55, and 79.

pressure, can often preclude the need for acute surgical intervention. Such surgery may be done on an elective basis later in the course of care. Recent research indicates that the recurrence of metastasis in the CNS is far lower following surgery combined with radiation than with radiation alone, suggesting that patients who might benefit from such prolonged suppression of symptoms should have surgery. The future of the treatment of human CNS neoplasms offers a tremendous challenge to all of those concerned with the treatment of these patients.[22]

REHABILITATION
Overview

Rehabilitation is an important component in the management of patients with brain tumors, and it is becoming more valuable as new technology lengthens the patient's life after diagnosis. The tumor makes its presence known through its symptoms—the functional limitations it imposes on the patient's activities and the pain it produces. The rehabilitation plan is essentially the same as that used in the management of other chronic CNS disabilities. The multifaceted team approach, successfully used in the rehabilitation of patients with other disabilities, can be used with equal facility for patients with brain tumors. The patient must be a participant in the therapeutic plan. The physical therapist who interacts with the patient at the level of symptom management generally focuses his or her attention on the functional consequences of the disease. However, patients with brain tumors present problems and opportunities different from those of patients with other diagnoses. When developing a rehabilitation program for these patients, the therapist must consider the prognosis, the highly emotional impact of the disease, the consequences of immobilization, and the effect of therapeutic interventions on both the physical and emotional responses of the patient. In some patients, hemiparesis and aphasia can clear dramatically, whereas the resolution of symptoms following a vascular occlusion is slow. Unfortunately, the therapists' evaluations must frequently culminate in program changes to accommodate increasing disability; initial efforts directed at ambulatory self-care may be reoriented to wheelchair, then assisted self-care, and finally to supportive, total bed care.*

Interest in neurooncology continues. Scientific advances continue to be coupled with technological advances, and this combination will inevitably lead to a better outcome for individuals with brain tumors.[46]

Evaluation

The patient with a brain tumor typically presents to physical therapy with problems of hemiplegia similar to those that occur as a result of CNS damage due to vascular or traumatic insult.[63] For a detailed description of the definitive evaluation technique refer to Chapter 24.

---

* References 18, 24, 27, 28, 43, 45, and 53.

The clinical label of hemiplegia may not be sufficient to explain all the problems encountered by these patients. The tumor may have infiltrated to multiple areas of the brain; therefore numerous deficits may be exhibited. The site and characteristics of the tumor dictate what other difficulties must be considered.[12,18,46,56] A thorough evaluation of all systems is required to identify adequately the problems to be addressed for successful rehabilitation.[12,18,45,56] Careful observation of performance in functional tasks provides documentation of the psychomotor and musculoskeletal systems. Evaluation of the sensory system may identify deficits, as well as the components that will be most useful in providing feedback.[25,40] Pain, fatigue associated with a limited cardiopulmonary reserve, and weakness as a side effect of tumor treatment are additional areas to assess before activity levels are established.[12,18,47]

The clinical picture for this patient is a changing one; the therapist is dealing with a progressive disease that demands attentive ongoing evaluation. Pain during assistive joint range of motion (ROM) may be the first indicator of a metastasis or pathological fracture, and progressive weakness may be the initial sign of increasing intracranial pressure.[45]

Functional assessment. The functional assessment is the most important evaluation to consider when developing a treatment plan. The degree of functional difficulty, factors that are preventing performance of the activity, and the level of energy expenditure involved must be noted. In addition to providing a system of analyzing the deficits and formulating a problem list, the assessment can assist in determining clinical care outcomes by comparing measures of function before and after treatment.[4,27]

The Functional Independence Measure (FIM), one example of a functional assessment, identifies basic problems and provides a method for measuring progress. This instrument, which is intended to measure disability regardless of underlying pathology, has been used successfully for patients with brain tumors (Table 22-4).[56,63] (Refer to Chapter 16 for FIM assessment.)

Other evaluation scales. The therapist must be aware of the functional evaluation scales that are frequently used by other oncology team members for monitoring treatment. The **Karnofsky Scale of Performance Status (KPS)**[36] is widely used in clinical research and treatment decisions (Table 22-5). During early cancer therapy, radiologists recognized the need to clinically evaluate the chemotherapeutic agents. Four general criteria were suggested: subjective improvement, objective improvement, performance status, and length of remission or prolongation of life. The KPS was the first evaluation scale in which performance status was included. An individual's performance status was rated on a numerical scale from 0 to 100, representing ability to perform normal activity and the patient's need for assistance (Table 22-5). The KPS has been used in randomized trials of chemotherapeutic agents, in evaluating an individual's

Table 22-4. An integrated functional assessment of cancer patients using the Karnofsky Performance Scale (KPS) and the Functional Independence Measure (FIM)

General category*	Probable FIM scores (KPS)	Useful rehabilitation treatment modalities				
		Physiatry consult	PT	OT	Speech	Nursing
A†	126 (100)... No deficits	No	No	No	No	No
	126 (90)... No deficits	Yes	Yes	Yes	Yes	Yes
	120-126 (80) .... May have minimal loss of function in mobility, continence, memory	Yes	Yes	Yes	Yes	Yes
B‡	115-120 (70) .... Increasing loss of function may require supervision	Yes	Yes	Yes	Yes	Yes
	90-115 (60) .... May require minimal assistance from others	Yes	Yes	Yes	Yes	Yes
	70-90 (50) .... Regularly requires moderate assistance with self-care	Yes	Yes	Yes	Yes	Yes
C§‖	60-70 (40) .... Needs maximum assistance for all activities of daily living	Yes	Yes	Yes	Yes	Yes
	40-60 (30)	Yes	Yes	Yes	Yes	Yes
	18-45 (20)	Yes	No	No	No	No
	18 (10)...	No	No	No	No	No
	0 (0)..	No	No	No	No	No

From: O'Toole DM and Golden AM: *West J Med* 155: 387, 1991.
OT = occupational therapy, PT = physical therapy
*See Table 1 for a description of each category and the index scores.
†Corresponds to Dietz stage I, preventive.
‡Corresponds to Dietz stage II or III, restorative or supportive.
§Corresponds to Dietz stage III or IV, supportive or palliative.
‖One role of rehabilitation is to educate family members in providing safe and effective assistance with self-care activities.

Table 22-5. Karnofsky performance status scale

Condition	Performance status %	Comments
A. Able to carry on normal activity and to work. No special care is needed.	100	Normal. No complaints. No evidence of disease.
	90	Able to carry on normal activity. Minor signs or symptoms of disease.
	80	Normal activity with effort. Some signs or symptoms of disease.
B. Unable to work. Able to live at home, care for most personal needs. A varying degree of assistance is needed.	70	Care of self. Unable to carry on normal activity or to do active work.
	60	Requires occasional assistance, but is able to care for most of personal needs.
	50	Requires considerable assistance and frequent medical care.
C. Unable to care for self. Requires equivalent of institutional or hospital care. Disease may be progressing rapidly.	40	Disabled. Requires special care and assistance.
	30	Severely disabled. Hospitalization is indicated although death not imminent.
	20	Very sick. Hospitalization necessary. Active supportive treatment necessary.
	10	Moribund. Fatal processes progressing rapidly.
	0	Dead.

From Karnofsky DA and Burchenal JH: In Macleod CM, editor: *Evaluation of chemotherapeutic agents,* New York, 1949, Columbia University Press.

response to treatment, and in evaluating the impact of therapeutic agents on the patient's quality of life. Because of the relationship between KPS and prognosis, physicians also use the performance status as a guide to treatment plans.

A physician who routinely assesses the KPS may identify specific areas of difficulty indicating a need to make referrals for rehabilitation services. These early referrals may lead to a better quality of life and care for patients with advancing tumors.[10,36,56,71]

To increase physician's awareness of the potential of the KPS in selecting patients appropriate for rehabilitation, one group of rehabilitation specialists identified similarities and showed a correlation between their functional measure and the Karnofsky scale (see Table 21-3). By developing further use of the KPS in this way, the scale may become a measure of life rather than its more common use as a measure of time to death.[56]

Other measurements of functional ability that are used in the field of oncology are the needs assessment of Lehman and others and the Long Range Evaluation System developed by Carl V. Granger. In 1978, Lehman and others[47] reported that a significant number of cancer patients they reviewed had functional disabilities that could be improved by rehabilitation techniques. Problems that contributed to the functional disabilities included pain, generalized weakness, and psychological problems. Primary barriers to rehabilitation were failure to identify functional problems and unfamiliarity with the value of rehabilitation. As a result of the chart review, they defined a needs assessment system, followed by the development of a model of care.[12,29,47,66] The Long Range Evaluation System (LRES) is a functional assessment system designed, tested, and used in a variety of clinical settings. It is a measurement tool for describing areas of service need, severity of handicap, and change in individuals over time. The data collection forms are descriptive checklists prepared for computer entry with allowance for descriptions. Scores are generated incorporating modified versions of the Barthel Index, a measure of independence in self-care and mobility, and the Pulses Profile, a measure of independence in personal care. For examples of the Barthel Index, refer to the index on evaluations for specific locations of specific tests. The level of social support is measured by the ESCROW scale profile. It is postulated that the physically disabled person with a marginal level of independence is more likely to have potential for independent living if social supports are high as represented by high ESCROW scale.[47] The LRES was structured so that it measures change over time. Through periodic assessments the rehabilitation program can be adapted to the patient's needs in either a stable or progressive clinical situation. The utilization of this instrument for many years has permitted validation of interrater reliability, making it a well-established test.[12,77]

Rehabilitation plan

It is difficult to predict the response to treatment or the life expectancy of an individual with a brain tumor. Therefore no patient should be denied the benefits of rehabilitation even though the prognosis may be uncertain. The rehabilitation plan should be developed based on the diagnosis, the effects of treatment, the definitive evaluation, and the Deitz oncology classification.[56,63]

In carrying out the rehabilitation plan, therapists use their skills as they would with any other similarly disabled patient. Realistic goals must be established. In addition, a program to achieve the goals, subject to adaptation to accommodate the patient's response to treatment and the course of the disease, must be initiated as early as possible.[45,53]

Dietz classification. At the Sloan-Kettering Cancer Center, the late J. H. Dietz, Jr. pioneered the establishment of standards of care based on which adaptation may be necessary to meet the patient's physical and personal needs. The Dietz classification, based on four phases of care (preventive, restorative, supportive, and palliative), is widely accepted. Through the use of this classification, the appropriate rehabilitation stage of the disease can be delineated and realistic goals set. Specific rehabilitation goals and a plan of care are established depending on individual need within each classification.

The majority of patients fall into the category of preventive rehabilitation, which seeks to apply appropriate interventions at an early stage to prevent or retard the development or reduce the impact of a potential disability. Patient education should be a significant part of preventive rehabilitation. The patient in the restoration phase can be expected to return to the premorbid status. This stage is intended to maximize the patient's ability within the residual disability. The focus of therapy within this stage is defined as the process of evaluating the patient's condition and setting specific treatment goals to assist the restoration of function. Supportive rehabilitation seeks to increase self-care skills and mobility using quick, effective methods. Patients in this phase may remain active with known residual tumor and possibly a slowly progressive disability. These patients require the most rehabilitation. Because the patients can be easily overlooked, reasonable and realistic goals may not be fully achieved. During the palliative stage increasing disability and decreasing functional capacity reflect the rapid progression of the tumor. Appropriate measures set in parameters of short-term goals can reduce complications, increase comfort or independence, and provide emotional support to patients during the terminal stage.*

Complications and side effects

Although the traditional goals of neurorehabilitation apply, the length of the immobilization period and the side

---

* References 12, 31, 33, 43, 53, and 63.

effects of treatment are somewhat unique in tumor patients. For the patient with a brain tumor, there is often a prolonged period of inactivity. This period may actually precede the diagnosis of the tumor or be a consequence of the medical/surgical care.

Although the control of the tumor usually causes a temporary improvement in activity, the complications of muscle weakness and the other effects of inactivity can deter this improvement. Because of the loss of the gravitational stimulus and the diminished stress of exercise, prolonged bed rest may make the marginally independent patient require total care. These deconditioning effects may be more pronounced in patients whose systems have been subjected to chemotherapy.

With bed rest, changes in blood volume and viscosity result in an increased risk of thrombophlebitis and pulmonary embolism. Reduction in plasma volume can be limited by exercises with, isotonic being more effective than isometric. If a patient receives chemotherapy, the inability of the circulatory system to adapt to the upright position after a period of forced bed rest may occur sooner than with other types of patients. Early intervention of physical therapy in the form of positioning and carefully graded exercise helps to diminish the adverse effects of immobilization.[12,16,18]

Along with preventing the complications of immobilization, an enriched environment including sound, color, and motion should be created for patients with a brain tumor.

It is equally important to include a variety of individuals in the therapeutic environment. Implementing a program for volunteers is an excellent means to accomplish this goal.

Recent trends in treatment have resulted in intensive combinations of treatment modalities as well as patient multidrug chemotherapy protocols. As a result, more complications occur now than in the past, when treatment was simpler but less effective in reducing tumor mass. The patient and family usually benefit from knowing the potential psychological and neurological effects of chemotherapy and radiation. To hide the facts from the patient may cause unnecessary distress. Considering the relationship therapists build with their patients, they are often the ones the patients question. It is important that the therapist have a knowledge of the side effects of treatment and be aware of signs and symptoms that may develop.[2,12,18,22]

The patient's ability to respond to rehabilitation measures may fluctuate during radiation and chemotherapy. Although the long-term effects of these therapies may be a "cure" or rapid improvement, during intensive treatment the patient may exhibit a transient decline in neurological or hematological conditions. Complications of tumor treatment, which should be anticipated in planning a rehabilitation program, include the toxic effect to the patient's gastrointestinal tract and hematopoietic system. In the case of the gastrointestinal tract, complications may include anorexia, difficulty in swallowing, nausea, and irritation of the gut lining. These problems may result in decreased caloric intake and markedly reduced tolerance for activity. Tumor therapy may also result in decreases in platelet as well as white cell production. Decreased platelet counts may increase the potential for bleeding episodes (bruising), whereas decreased white counts herald the increased susceptibility to infections. These complications may require a reduction in activity for a limited time or a more complicated response, such as the use of reverse barrier precautions to reduce the risk of infection.[12,31]

Treatment

Appropriate goal setting: adaptive or functional program. Use of the terms *adaptive* or *functional* discourages the misconceptions and unrealistic expectations by the patient of being restored to a former level of function. Their use creates an environment that permits the patient to adjust according to his or her needs or to develop better tolerance for a progressive disease. The long-term goal of rehabilitation for a patient with a brain tumor is to achieve an independent or maximal level of function in the patient's own environment despite the possibility of residual disability.[12,18,19,20]

The key to achieving this goal is the identification of functional problems. Success of a home program can depend on the patient's ability to transfer and ambulate. Too often when a patient is discharged from an acute care setting, the importance of these activities may be overlooked.[56] Problems should be identified early and every effort made to implement the patient's rehabilitation along with other types of intervention.[63] The patient must not be made to wait until all therapeutic treatment for the tumor has been completed because adaptive measures first introduced at that point may well be too little and come too late. Short-term goals for patients in the restorative and supportive phases include managing the problems that are resulting in functional limitations and mastering the appropriate functional tasks. For the treatment program to be successful, the patient must regain active control and assume the role of initiator in performing tasks. Incorporating the principles that affect performance into an interdisciplinary treatment plan will ensure the best result. Considering the possibility of a deteriorating condition, it is especially important to integrate problem-solving experiences into the treatment plan.

Cognitive deficits may be a problem for an individual following treatment for a brain tumor. It may take greater effort by the therapist to ensure that the patient is assuming an active role in the treatment session. Special efforts must be made to ensure that the activity is meaningful and the patient is aware of what he or she is trying to achieve. The level of the activity must provide both a challenge and some measure of success.

The timing of treatment sessions may affect the patient's ability to be actively involved. The therapist must take into account the effects of medications and other treatments the patient is receiving and schedule the therapy sessions when the patient is most alert and best able to participate.

Damage from a tumor can also disturb the normal feedback mechanisms that play an essential role in motor learning. The therapist must be aware of the methods of feedback that the patient is best able to process and use these methods as guides. For example, if movement errors are the result of problems with the internal mechanisms, it may be valuable to introduce external feedback such as through the auditory or visual systems.[44]

For patients to adapt to changes in their physical condition or a changing environment, a treatment program also should provide the patient with every opportunity to vary movement patterns. The patient who has the ability to appropriately alter functional activities will have a better chance for success.[*]

Obstacles to the successful attainment of functional goals may be lack of initiation and perceptual problems. Patients who lack the ability to initiate movement are often incorrectly described as obstinate, uncooperative, unmotivated, or depressed. Conversely, because some tumor patients have normal verbal skills, their impulsiveness and perceptual problems may be overlooked and their rehabilitation potential overestimated. They are at high risk for accidents and need a fixed routine and predictable environment.[18,47]

Despite rehabilitation efforts most patients with brain tumors will have residual impairments. For those with significant problems, too much stress must not be placed on independence. The use of compensatory strategies and/or assistive devices may be preferable to increase safety and efficiency and allow for an earlier discharge. For patients who achieve independence, the continuum of rehabilitative care may involve evaluating the work place and the community. Compensatory strategies and appropriate modifications may allow these patients to safely return to work or favorite leisure activities.[38] An individually planned comprehensive rehabilitation program including efforts to mobilize family and community resources usually yields the best results.[63]

Hospice

A nontraditional role therapists might assume when treating patients with a brain tumor is that of a hospice team member. Referral to a hospice program is appropriate when the patient's tumor is unresponsive to therapy and a "cure" or long-term remission is no longer possible. In medieval Europe, the word "hospice" was used to describe a place of shelter and comfort for travelers who were ill or suffering from wounds. Today hospice is the name given to a new health care movement in which the emphasis is placed on

control of physical symptoms. These facilities assist both the patient and his or her family to live life fully before death. Because one person cannot fully meet the needs of the terminally ill, the hospice program is organized on the basis of the interdisciplinary team. The patient is the central figure in this team.

The therapist, like other members of the team, provides palliative care, including positioning for comfort, applying modalities to alleviate pain, and maintaining functional range of motion. An equally important area of involvement for the physical therapist is adapting the activities of daily living to accommodate the capabilities of the patient and family. It is important to use techniques of energy conservation and to identify equipment that will enable the patient to maintain his or her independence or ease the family's burden of care. Although the physical therapist often will provide "hands-on" treatment for the hospice patient, more prevalent roles are those of counselor, educator, and facilitator. With proper background in the psychological implications of terminal illness and the hospice philosophy of care, the physical therapist is well equipped to provide valuable assistance.[37,64,74]

PSYCHOSOCIAL PROBLEMS

Therapists develop a special supportive relationship with their patients. They are usually one of the few consistent providers of care in the acute setting and often continue to see the patient after discharge. This strong interpersonal relationship is a key to successful rehabilitation. When a therapist allows this bond to develop, he or she must be committed to continuing the relationship with a patient who potentially may die.[12,17,25,30]

Hope forms the basis for a positive attitude and is an essential element for living with a brain tumor. The physical therapist can enable realistic hope by focusing on short-term goals. Achieving these goals can bring a purpose to the patient's existence and incorporating humor into the treatment plan can further develop an awareness of life.[32,67]

When the tumor has progressed to the stage where the only purpose of treatment is to slow its progression, physical therapy can continue to guide the patient focusing on maintenance of comfort and reduction of pain awareness. A patient's primary need at this time is to know he or she will not be abandoned.

Another key role is that of being an active listener to the patient and the family. Particularly important is the skill of listening without expressing pessimism and, conversely, not giving false hope.[22] The physical therapist can also be a support to family and friends by encouraging active participation in the treatment plan.

The more common treatment focus in therapy is centered toward recovery, and it is natural for the therapist to feel a sense of frustration and depression when evidence of recurrence of the disease is identified. Treatment becomes a

CASE 1 ▼ **Brain Tumor Patient Problem**

Mr. W. is a 46-year-old accountant who was moderately active and in good health until 4 weeks ago when he began to notice difficulty speaking and experiencing severe generalized headaches in the mornings. Aspirin did not provide any significant relief. He made an appointment to see his local medical doctor (LMD) but before then was brought to the emergency room by ambulance after sustaining a grand mal seizure at work. Based on a history and neurological examination he was admitted and further neurological tests were performed. MRI showed evidence of a left frontal-parietal lobe tumor. Open biopsy confirmed the diagnosis of an astrocytoma and a partial resection was carried out.

At this time Mr. W. is 1-week postop and you have received a physical therapy consult. Radiation therapy was started yesterday. Chemotherapy is under consideration for a later date. During a bedside evaluation you have determined that Mr. W. is alert and oriented. He shows evidence of a moderate expressive aphasia and a mild apraxia. He seems depressed and indifferent regarding his therapy. It appears that he is somewhat impulsive and has a problem following complex directions. He states his right forearm and hand feel numb. A specific sensory evaluation was not performed at this time.

Examination reveals generalized right-sided weakness. His right lower extremity grades 3+ at the hip and knee with a 2+ grade at the ankle. The right upper extremity graded 2+ to 3 throughout with greater weakness distally. There is evidence of mild extensor tone in the lower extremity and a + supporting reaction was elicited. He is independent in coming to sitting and performs a standing pivot transfer by the use of his left side. His sitting and standing balance are asymmetrical. Mr. W. stated that he feels unsteady when standing and that he has not attempted to walk since his surgery.

---

personal as well as a professional challenge, and the success in meeting this challenge depends on the personality of the individual and the existence of support systems. The therapist must develop insight to his or her own feelings and attitudes toward cancer and its disabling effects, dying, and death. Therapists who have not resolved their own feelings may find themselves avoiding the patient by spending less time with the patient, avoiding eye contact, or limiting touch. These behaviors may reinforce the feelings of loneliness and isolation.

Members of the oncology team can be an excellent support system, encouraging the members to express their attitudes and feelings and helping them to strike an emotional balance between aloofness and overinvolvement.[3,22,25,26,30]

Patients and family members may experience a number of reactions when evidence of recurrence or progression of the disease is identified. There is the inevitable realization that a cure is less likely now. The therapist who has not taken the opportunity to evaluate and address the psychosocial status of the patient and family will find obstacles in treatment and education.[22]

SUMMARY

Rehabilitation is a vital component of the treatment plan for patients with brain tumors. The first step in developing an appropriate plan is to identify what functional limitations will result from the tumor or the treatment procedures. These areas then become the focal point for rehabilitation. The ultimate goal is to improve the quality of survival so that patients will be able to lead lives as independent and productive as possible regardless of life expectancy. Even in instances where the patient's life expectancy is limited, efforts toward maintaining function at maximum potential may produce results that transcend economic return.[18,20]

REFERENCES

1. Adams BA, Clancey JK, and Eddy M: Malignant glioma: current treatment perspectives, *J Neurosci Nurs* 23:9-15, 1991.
2. Amato CA: Malignant glioma: coping with a devastating illness, *J Neurosci Nurs* 23:20-23, 1991.
3. Arbour RB: Stereotactic localization and resection of intracranial tumors, *J Neurosci Nurs* 25:14-21, 1993.
4. Balridge RB: Functional assessment of measurements, *Neurology Report* 17:3-10, 1993.
5. Barnard RO: Pathological classification of tumors of the central nervous system. In Walker MD and Thomas GT, editors: *Biology of brain tumor,* Boston, 1986, Martinus Nijoff.
6. Barnes ML and others: Principles of motor learning. In *Reflex and vestibular aspects of motor control, motor development and motor learning,* Atlanta, 1990, Strokesville Publishing.
7. Barton L and Black K: Setting functional outcomes for inpatient rehabilitation: a justification for motor learning treatment strategies. Proceedings of the forum on efficacy of physical therapy treatment for patients with brain injury, Neurology section of the American Physical Therapy Association. Alexandria, Va, (1990).
8. Bates MN: Extremely low frequency electromagnetic fields and cancer: the epidemiologic evidence, *Environ Health Perspect* 95:147-156, 1991.
9. Batnitzky S and Eckard DA: The radiology of brain tumors: general consideration and neoplasms. In Morantz RA and Walsh JW, editors: *Brain tumors: a comprehensive text,* New York, 1994, Marcel Dekker.
10. Cammack JM: Interdisciplinary care of the patient with cancer in a community hospital, *Clinical Management PT,* 2:7, 1982.
11. Chang Y and Horoupian DS: Pathology of benign brain tumors. In Morantz RA and Walsh JW, editors: *Brain tumors: a comprehensive text,* New York, 1994, Marcel Dekker.
12. Charrette EE and O'Toole DM: Cancer rehabilitation. In Higby DJ, editor: *Issues in supportive cancer care,* Boston, 1986, Martinus Nijhoff.
13. Chatel M, Lebrun C, and Frenay M: Chemotherapy and immunotherapy in adult malignant gliomas, *Curr Opinion Oncol* 5:464-473, 1993.

14. Clark RL and Howe CD: *Cancer patient care at M.D. Anderson hospital and tumor institute,* Chicago, 1976, Year Book Medical Publishers.
15. Coons SW and Johnson PC: Pathology of primary intracranial malignant neoplasms. In Morantz RA and Walsh JW, editors: *Brain tumors: a comprehensive text,* New York, 1994, Marcel Dekker.
16. Dean E: Bedrest and deconditioning, *Neurology Report* 1993; 17:6.
17. DeGroot J and Chusid JG: *Correlative neuroanatomy,* San Mateo, 1988, Appleton & Lange.
18. DeLisa JA and others: Rehabilitation of the cancer patient. In DeVita V and others, editors: *Cancer: principles and practice of oncology,* Philadelphia, 1985, JB Lippincott.
19. Dietz JH: Adaptive rehabilitation in cancer: a program to improve quality of survival, *Post Grad Med* 68.145, 1980.
20. Dietz JH: *Rehabilitation oncology,* New York, 1981, John Wiley & Sons.
21. Edwards DK, Stupperich TK, and Welsh DM: Hyperthermia treatment for malignant brain tumors: nursing management during therapy, *J Neurosci Nurs* 23:34-38, 1991.
22. Ethrington MF: Physical therapy management. *Clin Manage Phys Ther* 7.12, 1987.
23. Evans RG: The role of radiation therapy in the treatment of brain tumors in children. In Morantz RA and Walsh JW, editors: *Brain tumors: a comprehensive text,* New York, 1994, Marcel Dekker.
24. Fink DJ: Cancer rehabilitation the team approach. In McKenna RJ and Murphy GP, editor: *Fundamental of surgical oncology,* New York, 1986, Macmillian.
25. Flomenhoff D: Understanding and helping people who have cancer, *Phys Ther* 64:1232, 1984.
26. Gilroy J and Holliday PL: *Basic neurology,* New York, 1982, Macmillian.
27. Granger CV and Seltzer GB: *Primary care of the functionally disabled: assessment and management,* Philadelphia, 1987, JB Lippincott.
28. Gunn AE and others: Physical rehabilitation. In Gunn AE, editor: *Cancer rehabilitation,* New York, 1984, Raven Press.
29. Harvey RF and others: Cancer rehabilitation an analysis of 36 program approaches, *JAMA* 247:2127, 1982.
30. Hersch SP: Psychological aspects of patients with cancer. In De Vita VT and others, editors: *Cancer: principles and practice on oncology,* Philadelphia, 1985, JB Lippincott.
31. Hickey J: *The clinical practice of neurological and neurosurgical nursing,* ed 2, Philadelphia, 1992, JB Lippincott.
32. Hickey SS: Enabling hope, *Cancer Nursing* 9:133-137, 1986.
33. Hinterbuchner C: Rehabilitation of physical disability in cancer, *NY State J Med* 78:1066, 1978.
34. Holladay FP, Griffitt WE, and Wood GW: Immunology and immunotherapy of brain tumors. In Morantz RA and Walsh JW, editors: *Brain tumors: a comprehensive text,* New York, 1994, Marcel Dekker.
35. Horak FB: Assumptions underlying motor control for neurologic rehabilitation. In *II STEP conference,* Norman Okla, 1991, Foundation for Physical Therapy.
36. Karnofsky DA and Burchenal JH: The clinical evaluation of chemotherapeutic agents in cancer. In Macleod C, editor: *Evaluation of chemotherapeutic agents,* New York, 1949, Columbia Union Press.
37. Katterhagen JG: Specialized care of the terminally ill patient. In De Vita VT and others, editor: *Cancer; principles and practice of oncology,* Philadelphia, 1985, JB Lippincott.
38. Klarßßn CF and Frank JM: Rehabilitation of physically disabled dentists. a model for a vocationally specific rehabilitation program, *Arch Phys Med Rehabil* 75:332-333, 1991.
39. Kimler BF: Radiotherapy of brain tumors: basic principles. In Morantz RA and Walsh JW, editors, *Brain tumors: a comprehensive text,* New York, 1994, Marcel Dekker.
40. Hornblith DL: Neoplasms of the central nervous system. In De Vita VT and others, editors: *Cancer; principles and practice of oncology,* Philadelphia, 1985, JB Lippincott.
41. Kornblith PL and others: *Neurologic oncology,* Philadelphia, 1987, JB Lippincott.
42. Kottke FJ, Stillwell K, and Lehman J: *Krusen's handbook of physical medicine and rehabilitation,* ed 3, Philadelphia, 1982, WB Saunders.
43. Kudsk EG and Hoffman GS: Rehabilitation of the cancer patient, *Primary Care* 14:381, 1987.
44. Kwolek A and Pop T: Use of biological vicarious biofeedback in the rehabilitation of patients with brain damage, *Neurol Neurochir Pol* 1:321-327, 1992.
45. LaBan MM and Merscharert SR: Cancer therapy an emmerging role for physical medicine and rehabilitation, *Ariz Med* 37:483, 1980.
46. Laws ER and Thaper K: Brain tumors, *A Cancer Journal for Clinicians,* 43:263-271, 1993.
47. Lehman JF and others: Cancer rehabilitation: assessment of need, development, and evaluation of model of care, *Arch Phys Med Rehabil* 59:410, 1978.
48. Lesser GJ and Grossman SA: The chemotherapy of adult primary brain tumors, *Cancer Treat Rev* 19:261-281, 1993.
49. Lewis A: Documentation of movement patterns used in the performance of functional tasks, *Neurology Report,* 14:13, 1990.
50. Longsuethr W and others: Epidemiology of intracranial meningioma, *Cancer* 72:639-648, 1993.
51. Lord J and Coleman EA: Chemotherapy for glioblastoma multiforme, *J Neurosci Nurs* 23:68-70, 1991.
52. Lunsford LD, Kondziolka B and Flickinger JC: Stereotactic radiosurgery: current spectrum and results, *Clin Neurosurg* 38:151-159, 1992.
53. McLaughlin WJ and Holz S: Cancer rehabilitation—an integrated support system, *Clin Manage Phys Ther* 5:9, 1985.
54. Mennel H: Grading of intracranial tumors following the WHO classification, *Neurosurg Rev* 14:249-260, 1991.
55. Neatherlin JS and Brent VA: The gamma knife: implications for nursing practice and patient education, *J Neurosci Nurs* 23:71-74, 1991.
56. O'Toole DM and Golden AM: Evaluating cancer patients for rehabilitation potential, *West J Med* 155:384-387, 1991.
57. Poulson S: Neurosurgical nursing care. In Tiffany R, editor: *Cancer nursing: surgical,* London, 1980, Farber and Farber.
58. Prados MD and Wilson CB: Neoplasms of the central nervous system. In Hollond, J and others, editors: *Cancer medicine,* Philadelphia, 1993, Lea & Febiger.
59. Price SA and Wilson LM: *Pathophysiology: clinical concepts of disease processes,* ed 2, New York, 1982, McGraw Hill.
60. Quinn L: Principles of motor learning. In *Clinical management in physical therapy,* vol 7, pp 6-11, 1987.
61. Quinn L: *Motor learning considerations in treating neurologically impaired patients.* Proceedings of the forum on efficacy, Arlington, Va, 1990. Neurology section of the American Physical Therapy Association.
62. Radhakrishnan K, Bohnen NI, and Kurland LT: Epidemiology of brain tumors. In Morantz RA and Walsh JW, editors: *Brain tumors: a comprehensive text,* New York, 1994, Marcel Dekker.
63. Ragnarsson KT: Principles of cancer rehabilitation medicine. In Hollond J and others, editors: *Cancer Medicine,* Philadelphia, 1993, Lea & Febiger.
64. Reuss R: One physical therapists's personal account, *Clin Manage Phys Ther* 4:28, 1984.
65. Rominski FB, Riu G, and Songer MI: Central nervous system tumors. In Baib BD and others, editors: *Cancer nursing: a comprehensive textbook,* Philadelphia, 1991, WB Saunders.
66. Romsaas EP and McCormick JM: Assessment and resource utilization for cancer patients, *Arch Phys Med Rehabil* 67:459, 1986.
67. Schein JC: Getting back, *PT, Today,* 1(6):12-15, 1993.
68. Schiffer D: Pathology and neuroepidemiology of the brain and nervous system, *Curr Opin Oncol* 3:449-458, 1991.
69. Schmidek HH: Molecular genetic events in some primary human brain

tumors. In Morantz RA and Walsh JW, editors: *Brain tumors: a comprehensive text,* New York, 1994, Marcel Dekker.

70. Schwartz RB and Mantello MT: Primary brain tumors in adults. *Semin Ultrasound CT MR* 13:449-472, 1992.

71. Shag CC: Karnofsky performance status revisited. *J Clin Oncol* 2:187, 1984.

72. Sneed PK and Gutin PH: Interstitial radiation therapy of brain tumors. In Morantz RA and Walsh JW, editors: *Brain tumors: a comprehensive text,* New York, 1994, Marcel Dekker.

73. Tikhtman AJ and Patchell RA: Brain metastases. In Morantz RA and Walsh JW, editors: *Brain tumors: a comprehensive text,* New York, 1994, Marcel Dekker.

74. Toot J: Physical therapy and hospice: concept and practice, *Phys Ther,* 64:655, 1984.

75. Ushio Y: Treatment of gliomas in adults, *Curr Opin Oncol* 3:467-475, 1991.

76. Wegmann JA: Central nervous system cancers. In Groenwald SL and others, editors: *Cancer nursing principles and practice,* Boston, 1993, Jones and Bartlett Publishers.

77. Welch WC and Kornblith PL: Chemotherapy of brain tumors: fundamental principles. In Morantz RA and Walsh JW, editors: In *Brain tumors: a comprehensive text,* New York, 1994, Marcel Dekker.

78. Wellisch DK and Cohen RS: Psycholsocial aspects of cancer. In Haskel C, editor: *Cancer treatment,* Philadelphia, 1985, WB Saunders.

79. Willis D: Intracranial astrocytoma: pathology, diagnosis and clinical presentation, *J Neurosci Nurs* 23:7-11, 1991.

80. Zulch KJ: *Histological typing of tumors of the central nervous system,* Geneva, 1979, World Health Organization.

CHAPTER 23

Cerebellar Dysfunction

Nancy I. Urbscheit and Barbara S. Oremland

KEY TERMS

cerebellum
motor control
movement disorder

LEARNING OBJECTIVES

After reading this chapter the student/therapist will:
1. Understand the function and normal physiology of the cerebellum.
2. Identify the symptoms of cerebellar disorders.
3. Explain the physiology responsible for the clinical presentation of patients with cerebellar disorders.
4. Understand the relationship between the cerebellum and other parts of the brain and how the important feedback loops affect movement.
5. Select an appropriate treatment technique for the patient with a cerebellar disorder.

Receipt of a referral of a client with cerebellar dysfunction can be a frustrating event for a therapist. The first problem facing the therapist is the proper recognition and evaluation of motor problems peculiar to cerebellar disease. Second, a treatment program with known beneficial effects for the improvement of the motor deficits must be implemented. In solving these two problems a therapist can run into difficulty for a number of reasons. Although therapists typically learn a list of signs and symptoms accompanying cerebellar disease, they are not taught precise methods of examination and quantification of these symptoms. In addition, the relative significance and progression of each symptom have not been clearly defined. Last, and perhaps most serious of all, is the limited knowledge of the mechanisms underlying each motor symptom in cerebellar disease. This lack of awareness is the most serious limitation because it hampers development of effective treatment programs.

Therapists are not the only individuals struggling to understand the intricacies of cerebellar function. In this century scientists have generated tremendous volumes of literature on the anatomy and discharge characteristics of neurons of the **cerebellum,** yet much of this material does not readily explain normal or pathological **motor control** by the cerebellum. For example, the anatomy, synaptic interaction, and discharge behavior of neurons of the cerebellar cortex have been defined in detail. However, the link between the behavior of this complex sheath of neurons and normal coordination of movement remains obscure. In attempting to resolve the mystery of the cerebellum, scientists repeatedly have turned to the classic studies of cerebellar dysfunction by

Holmes.[48-53] With relatively simple tools, Holmes carefully observed and evaluated the motor problems of soldiers who had sustained cerebellar wounds in World War I. From this data he offered definitions and proposed theories of cerebellar functions that have centralized the focus for both the inquisitive investigator and the clinician.

Although the observations of Holmes cannot be completely explained, new insight into cerebellar function has been developed since Holmes' work was done. Other studies on humans and animals have revealed additional physical characteristics of the motor problems, the association of the lesion to the symptom, and the prognosis of the problem. Refer to Chapter 4 on motor control for additional information on cerebellar function.

IDENTIFICATION OF MOVEMENT DISORDERS ASSOCIATED WITH CEREBELLAR LESIONS
Hypotonicity

Hypotonicity is a typical symptom of a cerebellar lesion.* Hypotonicity occurs ipsilaterally to the lesions that are restricted to the lateral cerebellum but may be bilateral or contralateral to lesions in the intermediate area of the cerebellum. If cerebellar hypotonicity is present bilaterally, the intensity is greater in the involved limbs than with unilateral hypotonicity. All muscles of the involved extremities are affected, but those muscles that move proximal joints are involved most significantly. In adult monkeys with acute cerebellar lesions, hypotonicity dissipates with time, resulting in minimal deficit after several months.[7]

Hypotonicity can be detected in a variety of ways.[4,41,49] The muscles of an involved limb have a reduced firmness or turgor to palpation. Upon passive shaking, the limb will move through a greater arc of motion than does a normal limb. In the case of unilateral lesions, hypotonicity may result in a wider, flatter barefoot print on the ipsilateral side. When the client attempts to maintain a hypotonic extremity against gravity, the extremity will tend to drop slowly. Also if a client is distracted while holding an object in his hand, the object may drop from his grasp. In addition, if an extremity is passively supported and the support withdrawn unexpectedly, the extremity will tend to fall heavily. The client's posture may also be poorly maintained or asymmetrical as a result of hypotonicity.

Although deep tendon reflexes may be subnormal, this symptom does not necessarily accompany hypotonicity.[4] Even though the amplitude of the deep tendon reflexes may be normal, the limb may briefly oscillate back and forth after tendon tap (Fig. 23-1). This phenomenon has been called a pendular deep tendon reflex. Pendular deep tendon reflexes are typically associated with hypotonicity.

Holmes compared the myogram of the knee jerk in hypotonic men with cerebellar damage to that of normal men.[49] The myogram of the normal knee jerk response displays two peaks of tension (Fig. 23-2, A). The initial peak

* References 5, 6, 30, 35, 49, and 53.

is evoked by the tendon tap and is responsible for the brisk twitch of knee extension. The second contractile response is presumed to be caused by another stretch reflex of the quadriceps femoris muscle evoked by the descent of the leg. The descent of the leg is actually slowed by the second contractile response. In the myogram of the knee jerk of a client with a cerebellar lesion, only the early tension peak appears (Fig. 23-2, B). The second response, which would brake the return of the limb, is not present, and the limb falls heavily. Thus, during a knee jerk, the leg behaves as a pendulum that falls by its own weight and oscillates momentarily because of momentum.

A client with hypotonicity may be unable to fixate a limb posturally. This problem can lead to incoordination during voluntary movement. For example, flexion and extension of the elbow in an unsupported position can be very erratic in a hypotonic client, yet the same movement can become very smooth and controlled when the arm is supported on a table.[50] Also, a hypotonic client may be unable to flex one finger and hold the other in extension.[50] This may at first be considered incoordination but is really caused by lack of stability induced by hypotonicity.

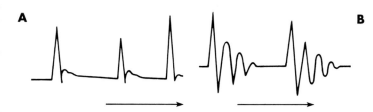

Fig. 23-1. Tracings of the excursion of the leg during a knee-jerk response in a normal person, **A,** and a person with cerebellar hypotonicity. **B,** Direction of arrows indicate progression of record in time. Note pendular response of a person with cerebellar damage. (From Holmes G: *Lancet* 1:1181, 1922.)

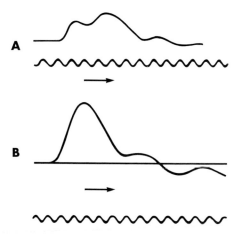

Fig. 23-2. Myogram of quadriceps muscle on normal knee-jerk response, **A,** and that evoked from a person with cerebellar lesion. **B,** Time indicated below each trace by vibrations of tuning fork at 25 Hz. Note absence of second peak of tension in response of person with cerebellar disease. (From Holmes G: *Lancet* 1:1181, 1922.)

Several mechanisms have been suggested for the appearance of cerebellar hypotonicity. Hypotonicity can occur in primates and humans who have isolated lesions in the lateral region of the hemispheres of the cerebellum.* Dow and Moruzzi[30] noted in primates that hypotonicity after cerebellectomy (total removal of the cerebellum) is very similar to that appearing after medullary pyramidotomy (section of the corticospinal tract at the pyramids), and they assumed a common mechanism. The cortex of the lateral region of the cerebellar hemispheres or neocerebellum sends fibers to the dentate nucleus of the cerebellum, which in turn sends fibers to the ventral lateral nucleus of the thalamus via the superior cerebellar peduncle. The fibers from the ventral lateral nucleus of the thalamus terminate in the motor cortex. This pathway produces a facilitation of neurons of the motor cortex.[71,72,95,97] If this facilitation to the motor cortex is lost, the ability of the motor cortex to facilitate spinal motor neurons via the corticospinal tract will be reduced.

By recording the discharge of muscle spindle afferent fibers in response to stretch, gamma motor neuron discharge has been found to decrease after pyramidotomy, motor cortex ablation, and cerebellectomy in monkeys.[37-39] Following acute cerebellectomy in the monkey, Ia afferent fiber discharge decreases in response to both static and dynamic stretch (Fig. 23-3). Recovery of a relatively normal pattern of discharge is evident 56 days after the lesioning, which supports the observation that hypotonicity can improve after acute injury of the cerebellum. Interestingly, the discharge of secondary afferent fibers from the muscle spindles is not significantly influenced by cerebellectomy.[37]

The cerebellum can facilitate lower motor neurons not only through the corticospinal system but also via the vestibulospinal, rubrospinal, and reticulospinal pathways (see Chapters 3, 4, and 6). The activity of these latter spinal pathways is influenced by the medial and intermediate regions of the cerebellum. In a study of clients with cerebellar tumors, Amici and others[4] noted a high incidence of hypotonicity with tumors located in the medial or intermediate regions of the cerebellum. Presumably, the facilitatory influence of the vestibulospinal, rubrospinal, and reticulospinal systems on alpha and gamma motor neurons is depressed by such tumors.

Asthenia

A lesion of the cerebellum can produce the condition of asthenia, or generalized weakness. Holmes noted that, in people with traumatic unilateral injury to the cerebellum, muscle strength on the involved side of the body may be reduced by 50% when compared to the normal limb.[10] Posture also may be poorly maintained in the client displaying asthenia. The clients complain of a sense of heaviness, excessive effort for simple tasks, and early onset of fatigue.[53] Asthenia is not as common as other symptoms accompanying cerebellar lesions. Amici and others[4] noted

that the symptom occurred in only 10% of their clients with cerebellar tumors. Likewise, Gilman and others[41] noted it in only two of 162 clients with cerebellar lesions caused by a variety of problems.

The mechanism underlying asthenia is not clear. Hagbarth and others[45] performed an experiment that offered a possible model for cerebellar asthenia. They infiltrated lidocaine about the median nerve in normal subjects, producing weakness in the hand. Lidocaine blocks conduction in thin nerve fibers, including gamma motor neurons. During voluntary contraction both alpha and gamma motor neurons to a muscle are normally coactivated. If the gamma motor neurons are blocked by lidocaine, an excitatory input to alpha motor neurons from muscle spindles will be reduced. Without the excitatory input from muscle spindles, the supraspinal drive to alpha motor neurons may have to increase to produce the voluntary movement. The normal perception of heaviness or force of effort is thought to be related to intensity of supraspinal signals required to produce the movement.[78] Thus any increase in the supraspinal drive to produce voluntary movement will be perceived as increased effort and fatigue, which is a common complaint in asthenic clients.

A decrease in fusimotor activity is known to occur in cerebellar lesions and also has been suggested as the mechanism for hypotonicity. Hypotonicity and asthenia, however, do not necessarily accompany one another. This suggests that although the conditions may share similar features, the mechanisms for them may not be identical.

Bremer[9] theorized that asthenia is caused by a loss of cerebellar facilitation to the motor cortex, which in turn could reduce the activity of spinal motor neurons during voluntary movement. A loss of facilitation of the cortex also has been suggested as a mechanism underlying hypotonicity. If loss of facilitation of the cerebral cortex is responsible for asthenia and hypotonicity, perhaps the areas of the cortex that are affected in asthenia and hypotonicity are not identical. Future research is required to untangle the similarities and differences of these two symptoms of cerebellar dysfunction.

Ataxia

Ataxia is a general term used to describe the lack of coordination displayed by individuals with cerebellar lesions; however, the phenomenon of ataxia includes many distinctive traits, all of which need not be present in order for a person to be described as ataxic. Therefore so that all the dimensions of ataxia may be covered, the phenomenon is described by body regions with the distinctions of ataxia associated with each.

Trunk and extremities
Disturbances of posture and balance. Lesions of the neocerebellum cause only slight postural instability, whereas lesions of the vestibulocerebellum cause an extreme instability of stance.[28] Acute or longstanding lesions of the cerebellum that affect one side of the body can result in

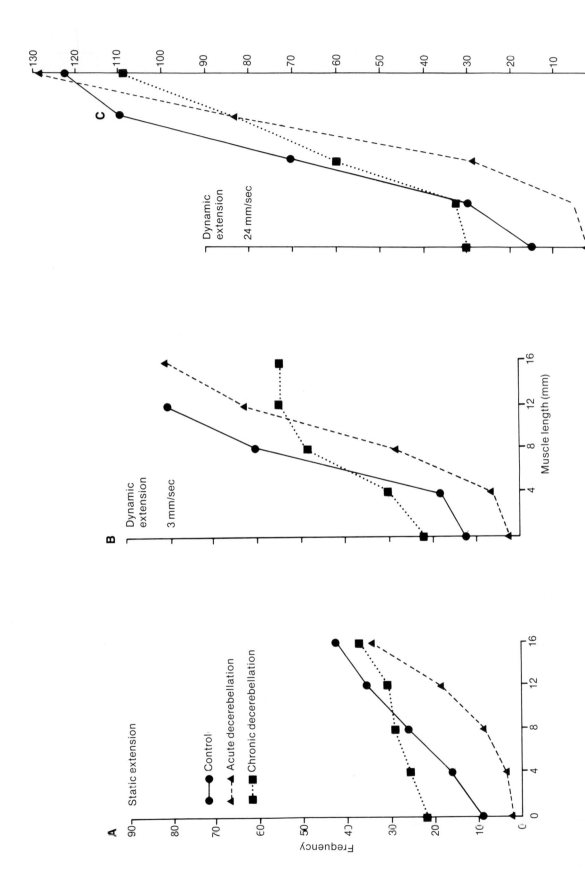

Fig. 23-3. Mean frequency of discharge of Ia afferent fibers from muscle spindles of the gastrocnemius muscle in monkeys: control (*solid lines*), 5 to 6 days decerebellate (*interrupted lines*), and 56 days after decerebellation (*dotted lines*). Responses to static stretch are represented in **A**, and responses to dynamic stretch at rates of 3 mm/sec and 24 mm/sec are represented in **B** and **C** respectively. (From Gilman S: *Brain*, 92:629, 1969.)

lateral curvature of the spine.[51] Individuals with bilateral involvement of the cerebellum may assume extreme slouching and leaning positions when seated if support is not provided.[51] When standing, individuals have a tendency to spread their feet apart and use their arms for balance. Some clients fall to one side consistently. Opening or closing the eyes appears to have no significant effect on the ability to maintain standing balance.[48,53,85] Lateral deviation of the head can occur, but this is not a common symptom.[4,41]

Posture may be distorted by changes in proprioceptive control loops that operate via the cerebellum. There are several areas of the cerebellum that may contain these loops. The dorsal spinocerebellar tract, the ventral spinocerebellar tract, and the spinoolivary tract carry proprioceptive information from the spinal cord to the midline cerebellum or vermis. The output of the vermis is to either the Deiter's nucleus (lateral vestibular nucleus) or to the fastigial nucleus of the cerebellum. Both these nuclei can affect the excitability of the alpha and gamma motor neurons: the fastigial nucleus via the reticulospinal tract and Deiter's nucleus via the vestibulospinal tracts. Through these feedback loops the cerebellum can provide a corrective output for disruptions of body posture. Ablation or stimulation of the medial zone of the cerebellum in monkeys leads to disruption of equilibrium of the body.[17]

The intermediate region of the cerebellum also receives proprioceptive input from the spinal cord. The cortex of the intermediate region of the cerebellum has output to the interpositus nucleus in monkeys and cats and, in humans, to the globose and emboliform nuclei. These nuclei affect posture by connections with the motor cortex and red nucleus. Postural control exerted by such a feedback system appears to be associated with voluntary movements of the ipsilateral limb rather than with basic equilibrium of the entire body because electrical stimulation or ablation of the intermediate region of the cerebellum evokes postural changes only in the ipsilateral limbs.[6,17]

Lesions of the cerebellum might disrupt body posture by means other than loss of proprioceptive control loops operating via the cerebellum. The cerebellum normally has the ability to adjust the gain or sensitivity of proprioceptive reflexes that operate over segmental or suprasegmental paths. If this gain modulation is altered by cerebellar disease, the automatic postural adjustments may become distorted. An example of this has already been mentioned in relation to hypotonicity: Decreased fusimotor activity (which decreases the sensitivity of the stretch reflexes) appears to be related to the inability of the person to support himself or herself adequately against gravity.

Patients with late cerebellar atrophy, which often includes the anterior lobe, almost never fall, even though they have severe disturbances in stance and gait.[28] The absence of falling appears to be due to intact intersegmental movements between the head, trunk, and legs. According to Dichgans and Mauritz,[28] these patients "show exag-

gerated intersegmental reactions. Since trunk and leg movements are roughly 180 degrees out of phase, a backward movement of the legs is compensated for by a forward inclination of the trunk (p. 634)."[28]

Nashner[85] noted that clients with cerebellar disease lacked the ability to adapt long-loop stretch reflexes in situations in which normal individuals could do so. A long-loop stretch reflex is evoked by stretch and has a latency of approximately 120 msec for the lower extremity. The pathway is presumably supraspinal, but the exact location is not clear. The reflex can be demonstrated in the medial gastrocnemius muscle of normal individuals when they stand on a platform that suddenly shifts backwards. The gastrocnemius muscle undergoes a long latency stretch reflex, which reduces the sway of the body in this situation (Fig. 23-4, *A*). After repeated trials, the long latency stretch reflex increases in amplitude. The reflex also occurs when the platform directly dorsiflexes the ankle; however, the reflex in this situation produces postural instability. After repeated trials the reflex disappears in normal individuals when the ankle is dorsiflexed by the platform (Fig. 23-4, *B*). Thus in normal people the long-loop stretch reflexes can be modified to fit the external circumstances. The medial gastrocnemius muscle of clients with cerebellar lesions also displays the long-loop stretch reflex under the above conditions. The amplitude of the reflex, however, does not change with repeated trials with either type of stretch. These experiments suggest that the normal cerebellum is involved in the adaptation of postural reflexes to external conditions.

Another disturbance of posture that clients often display is postural or static tremor. The client's body may oscillate back and forth while standing, or a limb may oscillate up and down when the person attempts to hold it against the force of gravity. For example a tremor may appear in an abducted arm but will disappear if support is provided at the axilla. The frequency of this oscillation is typically about 3 Hz, and both antagonistic muscles about a joint participate.[29,49,103] Although disturbances of balance and body position are common symptoms, postural tremor is an infrequent symptom, occurring in 9% (14 of 162 patients) studied by Gilman and others[41] and in 13.1% of patients studied by Amici and others.[4]

The mechanisms underlying postural tremor are far from clear. Mechanisms for postural tremor and intention tremor (tremor during a movement) may not be identical. For example administration of L-dopa will relieve postural tremor but not intention tremor.[42] Also, the two tremors are not always coincident, postural tremor being much less common than intention tremor.[4,41]

The postural tremor of cerebellar disease also displays differences from the typical resting tremor of parkinsonism. The tremor of parkinsonism has a higher frequency and can persist even when the subject is supine and relaxed.[66] The involvement of distal musculature is more prevalent in parkinsonism tremor than in cerebellar postural tremor.

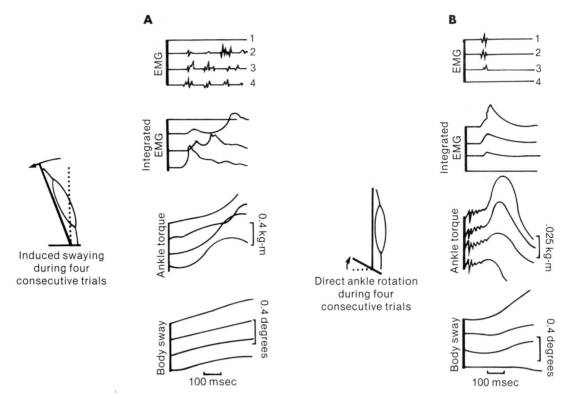

Fig. 23-4. A, Long-loop reflex of the medial gastrocnemius muscle in a normal subject induced by unexpected anterior sway of body. Note that the reflex increased in amplitude with each consecutive trial. **B,** Long-loop reflex of the medial gastrocnemius muscle in a normal subject induced by unexpected dorsiflexion of ankles. Note that amplitude of reflex decreases with each consecutive trial. (From Nashner LM: *Exp Brain Res* 26:65, 1976.)

Although there are differences between the postural tremor of cerebellar disease and the resting tremor of parkinsonism (see Chapter 21), there are some similarities in that administration of L-dopa or stereotaxic lesions of the ventral lateral nucleus of the thalamus relieves both tremors.[24,42] In addition, the transection of the rubro-olivo-cerebello-rubral pathway in the monkey will lead to postural tremor if there is a concomitant depletion of dopamine in the animal's brain.[67]

The resting tremor of parkinsonism appears to be induced by a rhythmically discharging center in the brain. Neurons in the ventral lateral nucleus of the thalamus and the motor cortex discharge rhythmically with the tremor in clients with Parkinson's disease. Although no one has recorded such activity in clients with postural tremor, a rhythmically discharging center in the thalamus might generate postural tremor, suggesting the importance of cerebellothalamocortical connections for normal posture and movement.[84]

Another possible mechanism for cerebellar postural tremor could be disruption of proprioceptive feedback loops. If the body shifts position, proprioceptors signal this change, and via a suprasegmental or long-loop pathway involving the cerebellum or another region in the brain, an automatic postural correction is made. When the limbs of a normal person shift because of gravity, sensory input leads to a motor output that returns the limb automatically to the desired position. The motor output occurs in time to prevent a noticeable disruption of position. An oscillation can occur in this feedback system if there is a delay in the processing of sensory input or motor output because of a lesion. Thus clinically we see the limb tremor in a client with a cerebellar lesion when the client attempts to hold it steady against gravity.

Evidence for the actual delay of a long-loop reflex has been found in a variety of studies on clients with cerebellar disease. Marsden and others[76] noted that tonically contracting thumb flexors in normal individuals will undergo an initial segmental reflex with a latency of 25 msec in response to abrupt stretch, followed by two later reflexes with latencies of 42 and 55 msec, respectively. These latter two are considered to operate over a suprasegmental path. In these experiments clients with cerebellar disease display the early reflex at the same latency as normal people; however, only one late response occurs with a very long latency of 80 msec.

Rather than using the physical stimulus of stretch to activate muscle spindle afferents, Mauritz and others[77] electrically stimulated the tibial nerve to excite muscle spindle afferent fibers. Using this technique to evoke segmental and suprasegmental stretch reflexes, they found that persons with postural tremor had delayed long-loop reflexes. Postural tremor was also produced by this stimulation technique in persons with incipient degenerative cerebellar disease.

Postural tremor also may be explained by another hypothesis. Sensory feedback systems, which operate over supraspinal as well as spinal pathways, all oscillate even in a normal person. For example, the spinal stretch reflex pathway oscillates at 8 to 12 Hz, the corticospinal pathway has an oscillation of 3 to 5 Hz, and the transcerebellar pathway has an oscillation of 4 to 6 Hz. In spite of these potentially oscillating circuits, a normal person displays no visually obvious tremor because none of the feedback pathways operate in isolation from the others. By acting together these multiple pathways effectively dampen one another's oscillation so that little oscillation is actually expressed. If one of these multiple reflex pathways is absent or delayed, however, a noticeable oscillation of the body or limbs may occur. If the transcerebellar reflex path is absent, the spinal reflex path is ineffective in dampening the low frequency oscillation (3 to 5 Hz) induced by the corticospinal pathway.[105] Thus the body will tend to oscillate at the low frequency—that of postural tremor.

Clients with postural tremor display the tremor only when attempting to hold a fixed position, not necessarily all the time. Any limb displays a mechanical oscillation, similar to that of a metal spring or tuning fork when perturbed. When a limb or joint changes in stiffness, as from relaxation to an attempt at stabilization against gravity, its properties of mechanical oscillation also change. The mechanical oscillations of a stabilized limb may actually reinforce the low-frequency oscillation of the limb in a client with cerebellar disease and lead to a noticeable postural tremor, but not necessarily a movement tremor.

Dysmetria. People with cerebellar lesions often have difficulty placing their limbs correctly during voluntary motion. They typically overestimate or underestimate the range of movement needed. If normal individuals, with eyes closed, flex their shoulders to 90 degrees and then bring their arms quickly over their heads without hesitation, they can accurately reposition their arms to 90 degrees of flexion. People with cerebellar damage usually cannot return their arms to the original position without noticeable error. People with cerebellar damage may also display intention tremor, in which a hand oscillates back and forth as they try to touch their nose or the heel oscillates as they attempt to slide it down the opposite shin. The tremor has a frequency of 3 to 5 Hz and is typically enhanced during the termination of a goal-directed movement.[50]

Holmes[53] suggested that dysmetria results from errors in the level and rate of force production. He demonstrated this by having a client with a left cerebellar lesion press his right and left arms against springs of equal strength.

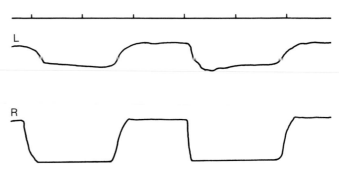

Fig. 23-5. Tracings on a slowly rotating drum of simultaneous depression of the right and left arms against springs of equal tension, from a man with a lesion of the left side of the cerebellum. The tracings show delay in starting and slowness in effecting the movements, reduced and irregular exertion of power, and slowness in relaxation on the affected side. Time in seconds. (From Holmes G: *Brain* 62:10, 1939.)

Because of the ipsilateral cerebellar involvement, the tension developed by the left arm displayed a slow onset, reduced intensity, and a slow release compared to that of the right arm (Fig. 23-5). Holmes noted another error in the rate of force production, which he labeled as the rebound phenomenon.[49] If a restraining force is suddenly removed from an isometrically contracting limb in a normal person, the limb will not change position. In contrast, the limb of a person with a cerebellar lesion will move abruptly as if still opposing the resistance.

Recent studies have extended the observations of Holmes on the deficits of force production that accompany cerebellar lesions. If a normal subject performs a ballistic motion (high speed), the antagonist and agonist display a consistent triphasic pattern of activity (Fig. 23-6, *A*). The agonist undergoes an initial burst of activity, then the antagonist undergoes a burst, followed by a second burst from the agonist.[46,76] The first burst from the agonist has a consistent duration of 50 to 110 msec. The antagonist muscle burst displays a consistent duration of 40 to 100 msec. The duration of the second agonist muscle burst varies. The amplitude of the first agonist burst is related to the distance moved. The amplitude of the antagonistic muscle burst is not related to the amplitude of the movement or forces of deceleration but probably does assist in checking the movement. The amplitude of the second agonist burst varies with accuracy of movements and might serve as a means of correction.

Ballistic movements are assumed to be centrally programmed, the timing and amplitude of the activity being automatically organized by the brain. A neural program that requires sensory input to adjust for peripheral conditions, as evidenced by inaccurate ballistic movements in deafferented humans.[11] The cerebellum may be an important part of this neural program because clients with cerebellar lesions lose the ability to perform normal ballistic motions. Although the triphasic pattern of antagonistic muscles still exists, the

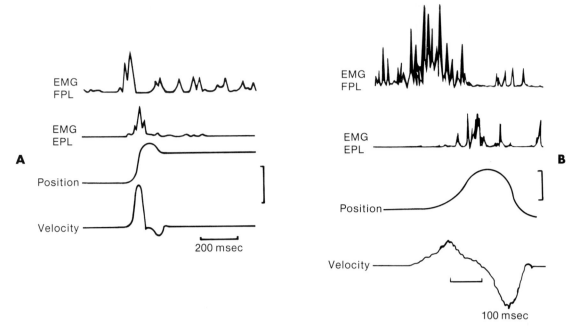

Fig. 23-6. A, Fast ballistic movements in normal man. Subject flexed distal joint of thumb through 20 degrees. Records are from top down, rectified EMG of flexor pollicis longus *(FPL),* rectified EMG of extensor pollicis longus *(EPL),* position, and velocity. Calibration is 200 msec and 20 μV, 27 degrees or 336 degrees/second. **B,** Fast thumb flexion from a 62-year-old man with unilateral cerebellar ataxia resulting from stroke. Records from top down are ordered as in **A.** Calibration is 100 msec and 100 μV, 25 degrees and 313 degrees/sec. Note the slower movement, inability to hold final position, and very prolonged bursts of activity in the agonist and antagonist muscle. (From Marsden CD and others: *Physiological aspects of clinical neurology,* Oxford, 1977, Blackwell Scientific Publications, Ltd. Edited by CF Rose.)

duration of the bursts is prolonged; thus the total motion has a longer duration and will obviously be dysmetric (see Fig. 23-6, *B).*[47] Clinical examples of this would be the overshoot when a client attempts to reach for something quickly or is unable to walk briskly and control the position of his or her feet.

Hallett and others[46,47] noted another abnormality in the activity of antagonist muscles of subjects with cerebellar lesions. If normal subjects isometrically extend their elbows against a resistance and then are unexpectedly told to flex their elbows very fast, the discharge of the triceps muscle will cease before the onset of the biceps activity. The triceps does not cease activity so abruptly in subjects with cerebellar lesions. In fact, the triceps may continuously discharge during the biceps activity. Such abnormal coactivation of the antagonists could contribute to dysmetria. This would lead to a delay in reversing any resistive movement, producing an overshoot and very imprecise alternating movement against resistance.

Other investigators utilizing normal and cerebellar-lesioned monkeys have examined aspects of cerebellar function related to the symptoms of dysmetria. In these studies the lateral and intermediate zones of the cerebellum and the associated deep cerebellar nuclei appear to control

the onset, rate, and ultimate level of force produced by muscle contraction. Discharge of neurons of the dentate nucleus has been observed to precede that of the motor cortex by 15 msec in monkeys trained to move in response to a light.[111] This suggests that the dentate nucleus acts as a trigger for the motor cortex during voluntary movement. Discharge of the dentate nucleus also appears to be tightly related to properties of intended movements as well as properties of ongoing movement.[10] Discharge of the interpositus nucleus is strongly related to properties of ongoing movement rather than those of intended movement.[10,107,111]

As might be expected, lesions of the dentate nucleus or interpositus nucleus in animals result in dysmetria. Specific, but temporary, lesions have been placed in the deep cerebellar nuclei in monkeys by use of a cooling probe. For example, during ipsilateral cooling of the dentate nucleus, the initiation of arm movements of two monkeys trained to respond immediately to a visual signal was delayed by 0.05 to 0.15 seconds.[80] Onset of movement-related discharge of neurons in the precentral motor cortex also was delayed by 0.05 to 0.15 seconds during dentate cooling. This suggests that disruption of the function of the dentate nucleus interferes with the trigger for the motor cortex during initiation of movement. Thus a client with a cerebellar lesion affecting the dentate nucleus might experience a delay in the initiation of movement and difficulty in movements that require bursts of speed.

Conrad and Brooks[21] also temporarily cooled the dentate nucleus in monkeys. The animals had been trained to perform fast alternating flexion and extension of the ipsilateral elbow. Range of movement was limited by mechanical stops at the end of flexion and extension. During the cooling, termination of the agonistic activity was delayed, but velocity or acceleration of motion was unaffected. For slower movements in which the spatial dimension of the movement was learned but not mechanically stopped, dentate cooling produced an overshoot or hypermetria, increased velocity, and acceleration of motion.[12]

Dentate dysfunction also influences oscillations that accompany voluntary movement. Normal movement is accompanied by very low amplitude oscillations, which are presumably the result of oscillating activity in long-loop feedback pathways. In monkeys performing a self-paced tracking task, dentate cooling causes a shift in the predominant peak of the power spectra of limb oscillation from 6 to 3 to 5 Hz.[23] As mentioned before, intention tremor in clients with cerebellar disease also has a frequency of 3 to 5 Hz. Thus damage of the dentate nucleus could be involved in the generation of intention tremor. The slower oscillation of intention tremor might result from the time-consuming relay of sensory input to the motor cortex needed to modulate movement when the cerebellum no longer functions effectively.[3,79,115,116] Thus a client with intention tremor may have trouble performing tasks requiring precision of limb placement and steadiness, such as drinking from a cup, placing a key in the door, or putting on makeup.

Lesions of the interpositus nucleus in animals also can be responsible for dysmetria. Monkeys trained to perform a self-paced tracking task with the forearm displayed hypometria and decreased velocity of motion after local cooling of the interpositus nucleus. Thus very circumscribed lesions of the cerebellum may cause different characteristics of dysmetria.[112] Specific research on human subjects is not available, but the assumption is that lesions similar to those studied in the monkeys will cause similar symptoms in humans.

According to Brown and others,[14] the cerebellum has a coordinative role during oculomanual tracking tasks. When there is a lesion in the cerebellum the patient takes longer to initiate purposeful limb movements on the affected side. When only the eyes are required to track a target, saccadic onset times are the same as those of normal individuals. When initiation of eye and arm movements is coupled in the cerebellar patient, however, the initiation times are significantly prolonged, not unlike in patients with parkinsonism. The cerebellum may be the center linking oculomotor and limb motor systems during a task requiring coordination of eye and limb movement.

Disturbances of gait. Perhaps the most striking clinical feature of cerebellar dysfunction is the staggering gait, which resembles that of someone who is very intoxicated. Arm swing is typically gone. The individual cannot walk a straight line without lurching, step length is uneven, and the feet may be too close or too far apart or lifted without a regular rhythm or height. The gait pattern becomes even more distorted by walking heel to toe, walking in a small circle, or walking backward.

Gait disturbances are very common in cerebellar damage. Gilman and others[41] noted that 100 of 162 clients with cerebellar lesions displayed the phenomenon. Amici and others[4] found ataxic gait the most frequent symptom in their clients with cerebellar tumors.

Although a disturbance of gait is considered a general manifestation of ataxia, gait can be the only feature of movement that is distorted. Gait is typically altered without changes in limb movement, muscle tone, or equilibrium with late atrophy of the cerebellum or chronic severe alcoholism.[70,114] Both of these conditions selectively involve the cortex of the anterior lobe of the cerebellum.

The cerebellum has been theorized to play a significant role in the generation of the pattern of locomotion. Activity of descending tracts during locomotion in cats is in phase with the gait cycle (Fig. 23-7). The rubrospinal pathway discharges in rhythm with the swing phase; the reticulospinal and vestibulospinal tracts discharge in rhythm with stance.[90] After cerebellectomy, rhythmical discharge disappears (Fig. 23-7) in the descending tracts. Thus the cerebellum's control of gait extends beyond the integration of sensory input and correcting for errors in movement. In humans the clinical problem might be observed as a total disruption of the rhythm of gait: the stance and swing phase are totally irregular in duration, and the client cannot adjust for deviations in the surface on which he or she walks.

Gait disturbances also can occur in combination with other problems in cerebellar lesions. Gait disruption can be a result of errors in rate and absolute level of force of muscle contraction and can accompany dysmetria of isolated movement. Cerebellar lesions that affect posture also will influence the person's ability to walk.

Movement decomposition. A client with a cerebellar lesion may perform a movement in a distinct sequence of steps rather than in one smooth pattern. For example, if a supine client is asked to place a heel on the opposite knee, he or she may first raise the extended leg, then flex the knee, and last lower the heel to knee. Such a movement abnormality is called decomposition.[50] Based on such observations, Holmes theorized that the cerebellum functions to sequence and time simple movements into one smooth, complex act. In the absence of this function, the movement becomes separated into individual components.

Dysfunction of the dentate nucleus has been implicated in decomposition because temporary cooling of this area will produce this disturbance in monkeys.[21]

Dysdiadochokinesia. Many clients with cerebellar le-

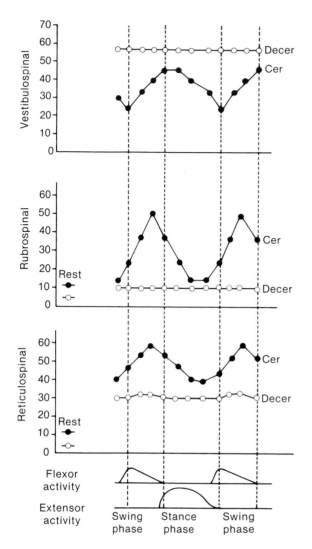

Fig. 23-7. Activity of descending tracts during locomotion. Mean values of the discharge rate of neurons of the vestibulospinal, rubrospinal, and reticulospinal tracts are plotted as a function of the hind limb position (ipsilateral for vestibulospinal and reticulospinal tracts; contralateral for rubrospinal tract). Curves obtained in cats with the cerebellum intact *(CER)* and those who have been decerebellated *(DECER)* are presented. A mean value of the resting discharge rate is also presented *(REST)*. Flexor and extensor activity is shown schematically. (From Orlovsky GN and Shik ML: Control of locomotion: a neurophysiological analysis of the cat locomotor system. In Porter R, editor: *International review of physiology, neurophysiology* II, vol 10, Baltimore, 1976, University Park Press.)

sions are unable to perform rapidly alternating movements. This deficit can be demonstrated by having clients rapidly supinate and pronate their forearm or rapidly tap their hand on their knee. Compared to that of a normal person, the movement appears slow and quickly loses range and rhythm.

Holmes[48] attributed dysdiadochokinesia to an inability to stop ongoing movement rather than to a reduced velocity of motion. Use of electromyography (EMG) has revealed discrete, nonoverlapping bursts of antagonistic muscle activity during rapid, alternating movements in normal people.[110] In people with cerebellar lesions, however, antagonistic muscle activity typically overlaps, resulting in a braking action for movement, such that activities like brushing one's teeth or stirring food will become ineffective.

Dysdiadochokinesia is related to dysmetria in that both result from the inappropriate timing of muscle activity. The inability to stop a goal-directed movement in one direction will be displayed as hypermetria, whereas the attempt to abruptly reverse the direction of movement will reveal dysdiadochokinesia.

In monkeys trained to perform rapid, rhythmical flexion and extension of the elbow, dentate cooling increased the duration of agonistic activity up to 0.1 to 0.2 seconds.[21] The onset of activity of the antagonist was delayed and often overlapped the activity of the agonist. No change in actual movement velocity was noted. Control of reciprocal motion by the cerebellum is also revealed by the observation that discharge of Purkinje cells in the intermediate zone of the cerebellum is related to reciprocal action of muscles. During cocontraction these same Purkinje cells become inhibited.[104] If the cerebellum is damaged, such neural discharge patterns may not occur.

Speech. Speech is a complex motor function that, as might be expected, is disturbed by cerebellar lesions. A client's grammar or word selection is not altered, but the melodic quality of speech is changed. The resultant disturbance is labeled dysarthria. Lechtenberg and Gilman[69] noted that 19% of 162 clients with various cerebellar lesions developed dysarthria, and Amici and colleagues[4] found dysarthria in 8.5% of a large population of clients with cerebellar tumors.

Scanning speech is a typical example of cerebellar dysarthria. Words or syllables are pronounced slowly, accents are misplaced, and pauses may be inappropriately short or long.[20] Clients also may display explosive speech or staccato speech.[125] The voice can become invariant in pitch and loudness, tremulous, nasal, or very soft.[13,49,51]

Attempts to localize areas of speech function in the cerebellum have revealed a relatively high incidence of dysarthria in clients with damage in the left cerebellar hemisphere.[69] The left cerebellar hemisphere is influenced by the right (nondominant) cerebral hemisphere, which has among its functions perception of melodies, tone, and rhythm.[91,100] If the left cerebellum plays a role in the melodic production of speech, input from the nondominant cerebral hemisphere seems appropriate in the context of this task.

Mechanisms responsible for dysarthria are most likely similar to those producing dysmetria of the limbs. For example, inability of muscles of the larynx to initiate or stop contractions quickly or hypotonicity of the larynx could produce a slurring in the pronunciation of consonants and vowels, slow speech, prolonged pauses, or uneven stress on syllables.[13,62] Hypotonicity of the larynx may also be responsible for the inability to increase loudness or vary pitch of the voice.

Eye movement. Although physical therapists are not expected to treat deviations of eye movement, they will see a relatively high frequency of such problems in clients with cerebellar lesions. An awareness of the variety of problems and the underlying mechanisms should be helpful in interacting with a client who displays such phenomena.

Just like posture of the limbs, the *resting position of the eyes* is affected by cerebellar dysfunction. After an acute lesion of a cerebellar hemisphere, both eyes deviate toward the contralateral side.[33,86]

Voluntary movement of the eyes is also affected by cerebellar lesions. A relatively common disturbance in eye movement is gaze-evoked nystagmus.[5] As the eyes are voluntarily moved to gaze at an object in the periphery, they move quickly in the intended direction and then drift involuntarily to neutral. The sequence is repeated as long as the effort is sustained to keep the gaze deviated toward the periphery. Clients with cerebellar atrophy may display a permanent gaze-evoked nystagmus bilaterally, whereas those with an acute unilateral lesion may display nystagmus temporarily to the ipsilateral side.[59] A rebound nystagmus often appears if gaze deviation is maintained 20 seconds or longer. The nystagmus then occurs briefly in a direction opposite to the prior gaze when the eyes are voluntarily returned to neutral.[54]

The inability of the eyes to move accurately toward an object in the periphery of vision is referred to as ocular dysmetria. When a normal person directs gaze toward an object in the periphery, the eyes move in a rapid step called a saccade. The amplitude of the saccade must be very accurate to place the intended image on the fovea of the retina. After cerebellar damage the saccadic movement of the eyes can become too large or too small, and corrective saccades will have to be made, resulting in ocular dysmetria.[64,93,99] Ocular dysmetria is related to the initial position of the eyes, such that hypermetria occurs when the eyes are eccentric to the target and hypometria occurs when the eyes move from neutral to a peripheral target.

Ocular dysmetria also can occur with pursuit movements of the eyes. When a normal person follows a slowly moving object, the eyes move in a smooth, continuous fashion but will stop abruptly if the object stops moving. However, if a client with cerebellar dysfunction visually pursues an object, the eyes may move only in saccades and will continue to move after the object stops.[18,19,117]

In the degenerative disease ataxia telangiectasia, clients are typically unable to initiate conjugate eye movement and accomplish lateral gaze by vigorous head movements.[5] Normal subjects can shift their eyes 30 degrees without accompanying head motion, but clients with cerebellar dysfunction typically move their heads within the first 30 degrees of eye movement.[102]

Reflex movements, as well as voluntary movements of the eyes, are also distorted by cerebellar lesions. The vestibular system influences the discharge of motor neurons of the extraocular muscles to appropriately regulate the velocity of eye movement with that of head movement. If such a reflex did not occur, the image on the retina would tend to shift with head movement and vision would be distorted. The effectiveness of the reflex can be demonstrated by watching a fixed object at arm's length while shaking the head. The visual image of the object remains clear because the eyes are held steady within the moving head. This response is called the vestibuloocular reflex. The sensitivity of the vestibuloocular reflex can be calculated by a ratio of eye velocity to head velocity. Although the sensitivity of the reflex is not universally altered in clients with cerebellar lesions, in such problems as the Arnold-Chiari syndrome and spinocerebellar degeneration, the ratio can exceed that of normal individuals.[122,123]

The amplitude of the vestibuloocular reflex will adapt to changes in internal or external conditions. For example, unilateral damage to the vestibular apparatus results in spontaneous nystagmus toward the damaged side, which typically disappears in a few weeks.[81] If normal subjects are asked to fix their eyes on a target attached to a rotating chair in which they are sitting, the vestibuloocular reflex nearly disappears.[122] These adaptations are possible only if the cerebellum is intact.

When a normal person watches stripes on a revolving drum moving horizontally or vertically, nystagmus develops in which the eyes snap quickly (fast phase) in the direction opposite to that of the revolving drum. The eyes then drift back slowly (slow phase) and the sequence is repeated. This phenomenon is called optokinetic nystagmus. In acute lesions of the cerebellum, the amplitude of the optokinetic nystagmus is often decreased, whereas in chronic problems, the amplitude of both phases or just one of the phases of optokinetic nystagmus is often increased.[41]

As might be expected, some clients with cerebellar lesions complain of visual defects. These defects include blurred vision, diplopia, loss of perspective, and difficulty seeing when their body is in motion.[121,122]

The *mechanisms* by which the cerebellum influences eye movement are not completely clear. Presumably, lesions of different areas of the cerebellum affect different aspects of eye movement because a client may have distortion of one type of eye movement but not another. However, the diagnostic value of eye movements for cerebellar disease is limited because brainstem lesions can produce identical symptoms.

Gaze-evoked nystagmus has been explained by the loss of a holding function provided by the cerebellum. When the eyes are held steady at the end of a normal saccade, the discharge of motor neurons innervating the extraocular muscles is proportional to the position of the eyes in the head. However, the sensory systems that influence eye position transmit signals of velocity. For example, the semicircular canals detect velocity of head movement and the retina detects the velocity of the image moving across it. These signals must undergo a "mathematical" integration to code position rather than velocity. This process of neurointegration does not appear to occur in the cerebellum and is believed to occur in the brainstem;[15] however, the cerebellum is essential for the normal integration of the velocity signals. If the cerebellum is damaged, the integration undergoes a rapid decay, which is reflected in the poor maintenance of eye position. Thus the cerebellum is necessary to sustain or boost the output of the brainstem integrator of sensory signals influencing eye position.[124] The appearance of gaze-evoked nystagmus does not correlate with a specific cerebellar lesion in humans, although nystagmus occurring with downward gaze is particularly common in clients with the Arnold-Chiari malformation.[121] In addition, removal of the flocculus and paraflocculus in monkeys leads to a serious defect in the ability to sustain gaze in any direction.[124]

The ability of the eye to keep a smooth visual pursuit of a slowly moving target also appears to be related to the ability to keep gaze fixated on a still object. During normal smooth pursuit, the motor neurons to the extraocular muscles discharge at a rate proportional to eye movements. The sensory feedback from pursuit movement of the eyes codes target velocity rather than the position of the eyes. Thus velocity signals influencing smooth pursuit movements must be integrated to create a usable command for eye position. This neurointegration also presumably occurs in the brainstem. The control of the sensitivity of the integrator, however, is believed to be a function of the cerebellum. The flocculus and the paraflocculus are, again, presumed to be involved in this function because damage in these areas disrupts smooth pursuit movements.

Neurons that discharge before a saccade have been located in the thalamus, cerebellum, vestibular nuclei, superior colliculus, pontine reticular formation, and mesencephalic aqueductal gray matter. However, the area of the brain that appears primarily responsible for the generation of the saccades is the pontine paramedian reticular formation because specific lesions at this region will produce permanent loss of saccadic eye movement.[123] Damage to this region disrupts the rapid phases of both vestibular and optokinetic nystagmus. Although the cerebellum does not initiate saccades, it does influence their accuracy. To initiate saccades, the neurons in the pontine reticular formation send a burst of activity to the motor neurons of the extraocular muscles. This burst is believed to code the difference in the visual target position and the actual eye position at the start of the saccade. Thus for this burst to move the eye to the exact location needed, the pontine reticular formation must have accurate estimates of the starting position of the eye as well as any other short-term or long-term changes in the eye and its muscles because of fatigue, injury, or aging. The

cerebellum appears to provide this feedback to the saccadic pulse generator in the brainstem.[89]

Distortions of optokinetic nystagmus may be a result of disruption in the cerebellar systems, which control either smooth pursuit or saccadic movement of the eyes. For example, a client may display a loss of smooth pursuit movement and a disturbance of the slow phase of optokinetic nystagmus. Presumably, the cerebellar mechanisms responsible for these two features of eye movement are the same. Similarly, saccadic eye movement may be distorted as well as the fast phase of optokinetic nystagmus.

Cerebellar dysfunction in other movement disorder syndromes. Dr. Walter J. Olson, Jr., Director of the Movement Disorders Clinic at the University of Louisville, is investigating new evidence that pathology of the cerebellum must be considered when evaluating a patient with a movement disorder associated traditionally with basal ganglia involvement.[88] Because of developments in technology that allow clear and precise imaging of the cerebellum, patients with parkinsonism and Huntington's disease have documented involvement with the cerebellum as well. As seen in Fig. 23-8, *A,* which represents a magnetic resonance imaging (MRI) film, a normal cerebellum is indicated by the arrow denoting the solid white area in the cerebellum. Fig. 23-8, *B* presents a patient with spinocerebellar atrophy in the cerebellum, noted by the arrow. A branching effect with some darkness in the cerebellum, which is the atrophy, can be seen. A patient with Huntington's disease is seen in Fig. 23-8, *C.* A traditional basal ganglia disorder is shown, as well as some atrophy in the cerebellum, as denoted by the branching or dark areas within the cerebellum. It is not unusual for a patient with multiple infarcts in the cerebral cortex to have cerebellar atrophy, which results in the pathological movement of ataxia.[88]

Olson explains that some of the earliest signs in Huntington's disease are abnormal saccades, which are clearly associated with cerebellar dysfunction. The loss of balance posteriorly, which is common in patients with parkinsonism, is also characteristic of a patient with a cerebellar lesion. Olson has also observed that the patient with early parkinsonism often displays a postural tremor and an intention tremor, similar to that present in patients with early cerebellar degeneration. If the patient with early cerebellar degeneration is given L-dopa, he or she often improves. Positron emission tomography (PET) and MRI have contributed greatly to revealing the role of the cerebellum in a variety of movement disorders. Technology is confirming the theory that many movement disorders are an aggregate of symptoms associated with lesions in both the basal ganglia and cerebellum.[88,94]

Theories of cerebellar function in coordination. Understanding the contribution of the cerebellum to movement has come a long way from the original concept in 1839 that its only function was to maintain sexual potency.[34] Although

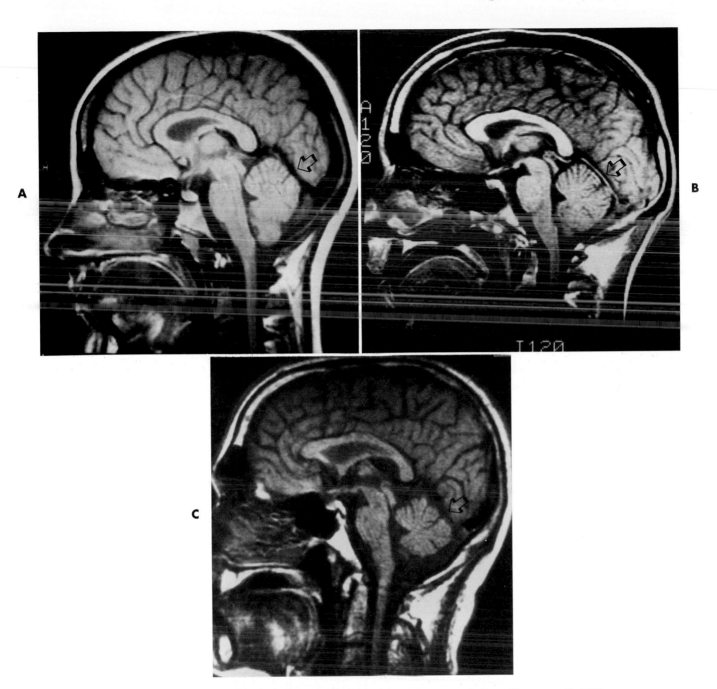

Fig. 23-8. **A,** MRI of normal cerebellum. Note full solid white area as indicated by arrow. **B,** MRI of spinocerebellar atrophy. Note dark and branching areas of cerebellum as indicated by arrow, which denotes atrophy. **C,** MRI of Huntington's disease. Note dark and branching areas of cerebellum, which indicates atrophy.

studies of the normal function and consequences of lesions of the cerebellum strongly suggest that the cerebellum controls the onset, level, and rate of force production by muscles, there are only theories to explain how this is accomplished. One theory suggests that the cerebellum acts essentially as a comparator between sensory input and motor output.[31,32,96] The cerebellum is the recipient of a tremen-

dous sensory input, including that from muscle spindles, Golgi tendon organs, cutaneous receptors, joint receptors, and the vestibular apparatus. The cerebellum also receives motor output from the motor cortex. Presumably, the cerebellum "compares" the voluntary command for movement with the sensory signals produced by the evolving movement. If the motor commands and evolving sensory signals are not appropriately matched, the cerebellum will provide corrective feedback to motor pathways capable of influencing the movement.[32]

A second theory of function of the cerebellum suggests that it acts as a compensator, instead of a comparator. Rather than providing corrections to ongoing voluntary movement, the cerebellum is assumed to perform predictive compensatory modification of reflexes in preparation for movement.[73] The success of voluntary movement depends largely on the stability and adjustment of many different reflexes. For example if the stretch reflexes of a limb are too sensitive, a high-speed movement may be impossible because of evoked stretch reflexes. Thus muscle spindle activity will have to be reduced before and during such movement. This reduction can be produced by inhibition of gamma motor neurons or interneurons in the stretch reflex pathway. In other circumstances the sensitivity of muscle spindles may have to be increased before movement. The cerebellum may be the initiator of such compensatory modification of the stretch reflex as well as many other reflexes.

The cerebellum also has been theorized to learn effective motor behavior. Ito[56] proposed that the cerebellum acts as an adaptive feedforward control system, which programs or models voluntary movement skills based on a memory of previous sensory input and motor output. According to this theory, learned movement is controlled by an internal model stored in or triggered by the cerebellum. If the cerebellum is damaged, the learned motor programs cannot be utilized. Movement will then be guided by long delay sensory feedback loops through the cerebrum, just as in learning a new skill, and incoordination will result.

If the cerebellum learns or memorizes movements, are programs retained for complex movements, such as a serve in tennis, or for simple qualities of movements? Brooks[10] suggested that the lateral and intermediate cerebellum act to sequence simple movements that make up complex actions. The cerebellum may thus learn small, simple programs, which are then triggered in the order needed to produce the complex motion.

Although no one knows where and how learning in the cerebellum may take place, several ideas have been proposed that put heavy emphasis on the role of the inferior olivary nucleus.[2,75] The neurons of the inferior olive have a $1:1$ relationship with Purkinje cells via the climbing fibers. Each olivary neuron is presumed to be activated by the cerebral cortex during a demand for an elemental or simple movement. The Purkinje cell activated by a particular inferior olivary neuron can then initiate this movement. The discharge of Purkinje cells is also affected by input from the mossy fibers, which reflects the sensory context in which the elemental movement is demanded. Possibly, the climbing fiber input potentiates the mossy fiber input so that mossy fiber input to the Purkinje cell may be able to evoke an elemental movement from the Purkinje cell in the absence of input from the cortex.

The cerebellum also participates in motor imagery (MI) also known as mental practice. According to Ryding and others[98] MI is a pure mental activity, requiring no muscle involvement and the same amount of time as the actual motor performance. They observed that the area of the brain showing the most activity during MI is the cerebellum, particularly the dentate nucleus and the cerebellar hemispheres. Patients who show damage in the lateral region of the cerebellar hemispheres have a reduced or absent capacity for anticipatory cues when performing a pretrained motor task.[68]

There is other evidence that the role of the cerebellum is not purely motor. Roland[94] explains that the posterior lobule of the cerebellum participates in pure cognitive activities such as thinking and verbal encoding.

Akshoomoff and Courchesne[1] believe the cerebellum can affect voluntary control of a specific cognitive operation such as rapid and accurate shifts of attention. Patients with damage in this area, such as those with autism, astrocytoma, and idiopathic cerebellar atrophy, showed a deficit in shifting attention from one sensory domain to another, where no motor action was involved. The implication is that the neocerebellar action for cognitive processes does not necessarily depend on the motor control system. In essence, Akshoomoff believes that possibly the neocerebellum "helps us to effortlessly shift from one domain of thought to another (p. 737)."[1]

No one is certain whether the cerebellum functions in all three of these capacities or predominantly in just one. If the cerebellum does perform all three of the described functions, different lesions may disturb one function more than another. Recognition of these theories and the consequences of their disruption may help a therapist more carefully examine a client and plan a therapeutic program. For example, if the cerebellum no longer functions as a comparator, movement will obviously be dysmetric. This individual will need time-consuming practice, but in selected activities that will be most useful for him or her and not in all movements. Even though the cerebellum may not automatically correct movement errors, the client may consciously be able to correct movement with practice or the remaining CNS may be able to assume a role of automatic correction.

If the cerebellar function of a reflex compensator is lost, the client may display abnormal muscle tone, inappropriate postural adjustment, and loss of associated limb movements, as well as being dysmetric. The therapist may need to evoke reflexes during an activity that would assist the postural stability and progression of movement. The presumption, again, is that the client can consciously learn to control the activity or that another part of the nervous system can begin to make the reflex adjustment automatically.

The concept of learning by the cerebellum is especially

important for therapists to consider. If clients have lost "learned motor programs" controlled by the cerebellum, they will obviously by dysmetric. Therapy for any neurologically involved client is offered with the hope that a long-term modification of motor behavior will take place. However, if the cerebellum is the primary area where adaptive movement can be "learned," the client may never receive much benefit from therapy. Currently, no studies quantify the ability of clients with cerebellar lesions to learn new motor skills or relearn lost skills with training. Obviously, such work would be a valuable guide to therapists in providing activities that can achieve better motor performance. Therapists, however, need to recognize that even though the best therapeutic program possible is offered, the motor learning capabilities of some clients with a cerebellar lesion may be very limited and gains achieved slowly at best.

The role of the cerebellum has been reviewed in terms of its control of normal movement and what happens when the cerebellum is damaged. The cerebellum also may play a role in the rate of recovery from lesions elsewhere in the brain. Boyeson and others[8] suggested that hemiparesis in rats produced by sensorimotor cortex injury could be compensated for by cerebellar activity. This compensation appears dependent on the noradrenergic axonal branching of the locus coeruleus to the cerebellum. The locus coeruleus projects to the ipsilateral sensorimotor cortex and the contralateral cerebellum. Damage to the branches of the sensorimotor cortex may produce compensatory arborization and/or receptor hypersensitivity in the contralateral cerebellum. If the locus coeruleus is damaged the recovery of function after sensorimotor cortex injury is slowed, but enhancement of the action of the locus coeruleus facilitates recovery.

RECOVERY FROM CEREBELLAR LESIONS

After a brain lesion there is always some level of spontaneous recovery of compensation; the level depends on the severity of the lesion and its location. For cerebrovascular accidents and head trauma, therapists do have some published guidelines for recovery patterns to which they can refer; however, such information has not been well documented for cerebellar lesions. For this reason, this chapter cannot provide a complete description of recovery patterns following cerebellar damage. However, it is hoped that the information presented will provide therapists with some clarifying expectation for their clients.

Various investigators have attempted to study the recovery patterns following cerebellar damage with animal models. Poirier and others[92] observed the motor behavior of monkeys for up to 1 year after various surgical lesions had been placed in the cerebellum. The most severe problems resulted from total cerebellectomy and included truncal ataxia, dysmetria of the limbs, hypotonicity, and postural

tremor. These problems decreased in severity over the first 4 weeks after surgery, but improvement then reached a plateau. The animal was still severely compromised, dysmetria and postural tremor being the least obvious of the above symptoms.

Goldberger and Growdon[43] bilaterally lesioned the dentate and interpositus nucleus in monkeys. The animals displayed gross oscillations of the limbs at a frequency of 2 per second, hypermetria of the limb, and primitive movement locomotion during the first 2 weeks. As the animals improved over the next 50 weeks, the limbs developed a smaller and faster amplitude tremor of 6 to 8 Hz and a marked improvement in gait and accuracy of movement of the extremities. In contrast, if only one cerebellar hemisphere is damaged with no nuclear involvement in a primate, the animal displays ipsilateral dysmetria, postural tremor, and awkward leaping gait for the first 1 to 2 weeks and becomes essentially normal over the next 2 months. If the midline structure of the cerebellum is involved, the animal's chief problem is truncal ataxia, which improves over the first 3 to 5 months but never disappears. Thus from animal work it appears that recovery is very poor from a total cerebellectomy; a bilateral lesion is more devastating than a unilateral lesion; damage to the deep cerebellar nuclei is more serious than that to the cortex; and spontaneous compensation will be complete within 6 months to a year.

Although one cannot assume that humans will respond to acute cerebellar injury exactly as primates do, the information provided by animal work does indeed provide a general framework for humans. A feature of cerebellar lesions that cannot be readily studied in animals is the effect of a degenerative disease or an expanding tumor. If a client develops a degenerative cerebellar disease or a tumor, the developing symptoms are generally milder than those produced by the same damage occurring acutely. Thus compensation appears to be concurrent with a steadily progressing lesion.

If compensation for a cerebellar lesion is possible, what other neurological structures are necessary for the compensation to take place? If the cerebellum is not totally destroyed, some available adaptation for the movement distortions may occur because of the remainder of the cerebellum. Evidence for this is the observation that compensation for a cerebellar lesion will be disrupted by a second lesion in which deficits are more serious than those that have occurred if the second lesion had been produced alone.[4] The motor cortex is also considered to be an essential structure upon which compensation for a cerebellar lesion depends.[19]

EVALUATION AND GOALS

As for any neurologically involved client, the primary goal of therapy is to make the client as functional as possible under conditions of maximum safety, reasonable energy cost

Assessment of movement disorders

Hypotonicity

Specific tests
1. Muscle palpation
2. Deep tendon reflexes
3. Passive shaking of limbs
4. Wet footprint
5. Hold object while conversing
6. Voluntary flexion and extension of knee or elbow supported and unsupported
7. Flex one finger only

Observation
1. Resting posture

Positive
1. Reduced firmness
2. Pendular
3. Limbs move through greater arc of motion than does normal limb
4. Print broader on involved side
5. Drops object when distracted
6. Ataxic when unsupported; controlled when supported
7. All fingers flex

1. Slack, asymmetrical

Asthenia

Specific tests
1. Maintain arm(s) in 90-degree position of flexion or abduction
2. Maximal resisted muscle contraction for major muscle groups
3. Repeat submaximal muscle contractions, such as rising on toes, push-ups, squeezing tennis ball

Observation
1. Everyday activities

Positive
1. Arm(s) tire quickly
2. Weaker on involved side or unable to work against resistance, which is normal for size and age
3. Tires quickly

1. Tires easily, complains of heaviness

Balance and postural control

Specific test
1. Hold limb against pull of gravity
2. Nudge client unexpectedly when sitting or standing
3. Stand on one foot or walk backward

Observation
1. Standing posture

Positive
1. Postural tremor
2. Loses balance easily
3. Loses balance easily

1. Feet apart, trunk flexed slightly, needs to hold for stability, postural tremor of legs

to the client, and cosmesis. In deciding how to achieve this goal, a therapist has to decide what basic functions the client cannot achieve and specific reasons why. Evaluation of a client with a cerebellar lesion therefore should include an initial determination of basic functional capabilities such as:

1. Bed mobility and posture
2. Ability to sit up from a reclining position
3. Maintenance of sitting posture
4. Ability to stand up from a sitting position
5. Maintenance of standing posture
6. Ambulation
7. Ability to dress, groom, and eat

No special tests are needed to isolate these abilities other than observing the client's attempts at each. Description of performance can include assistance needed, level of effort involved, time to complete the activity, potential hazards to the client, and unusual accompanying movements or noticeable features unique to that client.

Once an assessment of basic fundamental capabilities of clients has been completed, therapists should determine why their clients display the difficulties observed by looking

carefully for the movement disorders associated with cerebellar lesions (described at the beginning of the chapter). A list of each movement disorder, a description of specific tests, and simple observations needed to determine the presence of each disturbance are presented in the box. Both sides of the body need to be examined even if a unilateral cerebellar lesion has been diagnosed. Although therapists are not expected to provide detailed evaluations of eye movement or speech, brief notations of obvious distortions may help clarify the total problem facing the client. If the client has multiple sites of brain involvement, the symptoms caused by cerebellar damage may be masked by spasticity or sensory loss, and tests for these features will need to be added.

The cerebellar movement disorders the client displays will help the therapist decide why any of the basic functions cannot be performed. The therapist can then select the therapeutic activities that would best correct the movement disorder and hence improve the client's functional behavior. For example if an individual is hypotonic, his or her resting posture while reclining, sitting, and standing will be changed. The treatment for such a client would need to

Assessment of movement disorders—cont'd

Dysmetria

Specific test
1. Flex arms to 90-degree position, quickly elevate overhead and then return to 90-degree position
2. Put peg in a hole, trace circle with pencil, trace circle on floor with big toe, slide heal down shin slowly, place feet on markers when walking
3. Therapist resists client's elbow flexion and releases unexpectedly
4. Voluntarily flex and extend knee or elbow in supported and unsupported position
5. Submaximal isometric effort against force transducer
6. Electromyogram of antagonistic pair of muscles during ballistic contraction

Posture
1. Not able to resume 90-degree position without initial error
2. Intention tremor, undershoots or overshoots target
3. Arm rebounds
4. Limb ataxic whether supported or not
5. Onset and release of force of involved limb delayed
6. Duration of triphasic pattern longer than 300 msec

Gait disturbance

Specific test
1. March to cadence
2. Walk on heels or toes
3. Walk clockwise and counterclockwise
4. Walk on uneven ground

Observation
1. Typical gait pattern

Positive
1. Unable to follow rhythm
2. Loses balance and rhythm
3. Stumbles in one direction
4. Cannot compensate and stumbles

1. Slow, stumbles easily, not rhythmical, step length and height irregular

Dysdiadochokinesia

Specific test
1. Tap hand on knee or toes on floor
2. Walk as fast as possible

Observation
1. Activities of daily living

Positive
1. Rapidly loses rhythm and range
2. Gait becomes very impaired only when fast

1. Unable to brush teeth, stir food, shake salt shaker

Movement decomposition

Specific test
1. Supine client touches heel to opposite knee

Observation
1. Typical movement

Positive
1. Movement broken up into separate phases, does not flow

1. Activity appears as if in slow motion, mechanical like a puppet

include activities that enhance tone of antigravity muscles. If asthenia exists, postural stability and ambulation will be affected. Resistive exercises to antigravity muscles may improve such a client's posture and endurance in ambulation. If a client does not display hypotonicity or asthenia but still has poor postural stability, dysmetria may be the major problem. In this situation the client needs many sessions of practice in the precise posturing of the trunk, upper extremities, or legs in an attempt to make posture an automatic function or, second best, a consciously controlled function. If a client displays gait disturbances but does not have dysmetria, hypotonicity, or asthenia, the cerebellar motor program for gait may have been selectively disturbed and attention in therapy will need to be directed only toward gait. However, if dysmetria of isolated movements in the

limbs is present as well as gait abnormalities, selected coordination exercises for the extremities as well as gait training should be implemented. Inability to dress, feed, or groom oneself effectively may be caused by hypotonicity, dysmetria, or asthenia but may also be specifically caused by movement decomposition or dysdiadochokinesia. The predominant distortion will need to become the focus of treatment.

TREATMENT

The program described in this section is for the client with a relatively severe, but stabilized, lesion of the cerebellum, such as might be produced by trauma, cerebrovascular accident, or a tumor that has been surgically removed. Many parts of the program, however, could be used to help maintain function of the client with degenerative cerebellar disease. The reader should be aware that success of any of the following activities has not been well documented. Thus they are to be taken only as ideas for obtaining selective goals. Several goals toward which a therapist can work with a client having a cerebellar lesion are (1) postural stability, (2) functional gait, and (3) accuracy of limb movement.

Head and trunk control

A client with postural instability needs to be assisted sequentially to each level of independently maintained posture. Thus a client is a candidate for sitting only when there is sufficient head and trunk control and a candidate for standing only when sitting balance can be maintained. If clients have inadequate head control, they can be treated in the prone position while propped on elbows with pillow under chest or by being placed on a wedge bolster. If clients are not comfortable in the prone position, treatment can be performed with them seated with hips tucked back in a chair, feet flat on the floor, and elbows supported by a lap table or pillow. The goal is to have clients lift the head and hold it steady. This position is the same as that which a baby first learns in control of the head. It can be promoted by brushing of neck and upper back, 3 to 5 seconds of ice to the neck extensors, stretch to the neck extensors followed by heavy resistance to extensors to maintain extension in the shortened range, and downward compression on the shoulders.[106] To progressively promote trunk control, less support to the elbows from the pillows and bolsters should be offered. The client in the prone position should attempt to prop on both elbows and progress to the use of just one elbow for support to promote weight shift at the shoulders (refer to Figs. 6-10 and 6-11 for additional information on head control treatment).

Biofeedback might be tried in an attempt to promote upright head position in the severely involved client. For example, the client could wear a helmet that provides a visual and auditory clue when the vertical position of the head is not maintained.[119]

Sitting balance

When clients can hold their heads up and have developed some trunk control, they need to be offered progressive challenges to sitting balance. This can be accomplished by treating the client in a chair without arms or a back, depending on the individual's performance. If available, a safer and more versatile place to treat a client is on the edge of a mat table. To promote trunk stability the therapist applies joint approximation at the client's hips or shoulders. To help a client sustain contraction of the trunk muscles, rhythmical stabilization for trunk rotation may be utilized. In this situation rhythmical stabilization is provided not to increase strength but to give clients the sensation of stability, which they can then attempt alone. If clients cannot sustain an isometric contraction of the trunk muscles, a pattern of slow-reversal-hold over a steadily decreasing range of trunk rotation might be attempted instead.[63] Therapists can also help clients control balance by joining hands with them and having them meet a gentle resistance through their extended arms.

Clients next need to practice weight shift in all directions while sitting. This can first be practiced with clients using both hands for support, progressing to no support from their hands. Clients also should try to sustain balance with the arms overhead and the trunk rotated because this position will be used in activities of daily living. Although not essential, clients can be provided with practice in maintaining different sitting positions (Fig. 23-9). (Refer to Chapters 13 and 16 for additional information.)

Rising from supine or prone position to sitting

At the same time the client is developing control of sitting balance, work on safe and efficient ways of moving from the supine or prone position to sitting will be necessary. Work

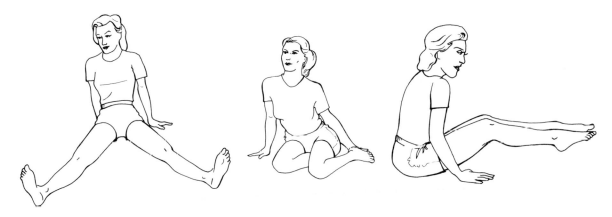

Fig. 23-9. Alternate positions in sitting to attempt with the client with a cerebellar lesion to promote control of posture and balance.

toward this goal also can be performed on a mat table. The procedure used will depend on the client's weight, side of involvement, and underlying muscle strength. A very heavy or weak individual may need first to roll to one side and push up from the side-lying posture. The client should first lie near the edge of the table with knees bent and feet flat on the table. As the knees drop passively to the side, the trunk should rotate as well. If clients still have difficulty getting to side lying, their efforts can be strengthened by the therapist's providing gentle resistance in the side-lying position to flexion, adduction, external rotation of the shoulder, and trunk rotation (Fig. 23-10). As clients become stronger, the resistance can be applied when they are between the side-lying and supine positions. When clients can achieve a side-lying position alone, they can proceed to drop their legs off the edge of the table and push up with their arms to a sitting position. Ideally, clients should be taught to roll in both directions, but for practical purposes emphasis may need to be placed on one direction only. If clients have primary involvement on one side, they may find it easier to roll toward that side. However, this may create difficulty when they attempt to push up to sitting with the involved arm. Under these circumstances the therapist will have to decide the direction easiest for the client to roll and sit.

A more natural method of rising from the supine position is to rely primarily on the action of the abdominal muscles. For stability, a client can drop one leg off the edge of the table, placing the foot on the floor if possible. The client can then rise to a sitting position using the abdominal and iliopsoas muscles. A weak or heavy client can use this method if a side rail is provided for a pull. The difficulty with external aids for clients with dysmetria is that the inaccuracy of reach may disrupt the ongoing flow of movement or actually be a hazard. If time allows, the client should practice assuming the sitting position from prone. Clients can push up on their arms and rotate their bodies backward onto their hips (Fig. 23-11). Clients also can push up on their hands and knees and drop onto a hip; however, this requires better control of balance.

Independent transfers

If clients develop adequate sitting balance but are not considered safe candidates for ambulation, they should be taught as many independent transfers as possible. A sliding transfer from a wheelchair to another chair or bed will be the safest. A trapeze over a bed or bars in the bath may increase the level of independence if the accuracy of limb movements allows such activity.

Preparing for ambulation

If the goal is to progress clients toward ambulation, a series of preliminary activities would be beneficial before they attempt to stand. The stability at the hip needed for standing can be developed by working initially in the

crawling or kneeling position on a mat table. This allows the person to practice weight shifting through the hips without the harmful consequences of falling from standing. The client who is preparing to ambulate should be able to assume a quadriped position from sitting on the mat. If not, the therapist can help the client achieve this position from the prone position (Fig. 23-12). From hands and knees clients can, using the assistance of a therapist or stall bars, work their way up to a kneeling position or sit back on their heels and then straighten the trunk and legs.

If a person cannot easily practice crawling or kneeling activities because of age or other problems, standing activities will have to be started without this preliminary practice. If a client has been in a wheelchair, the therapist should prepare the person's cardiovascular system for being upright by placing him or her on a tilt table. Standing

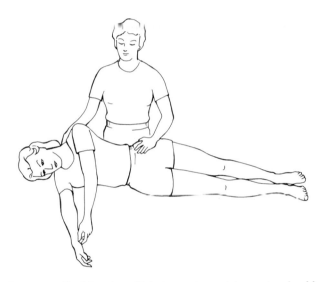

Fig. 23-10. Position in which to apply resistance to shoulder flexion, adduction, external rotation, and trunk rotation to promote rolling from supine to side-lying.

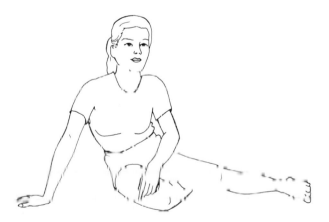

Fig. 23-11. Client pushing up from prone position and rotating back onto hips to sit up.

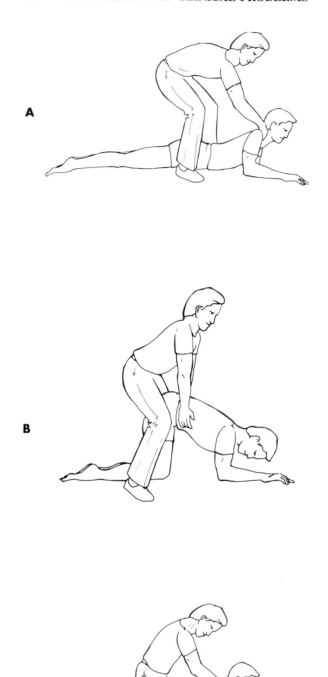

Fig. 23-12. Method to assist a client from prone to quadruped position. **A,** While lifting shoulders to prop client on forearms, therapist directs client to lift head. **B,** Therapist lifts client's pelvis to bring him up on knees. **C,** While lifting client's shoulders to place weight on hands, therapist directs client to lift head.

activities should be started in the parallel bars. Clients may not be able to assume a standing position without help. When standing up from sitting, clients need to remember to slide forward in the chair and flex their trunks considerably, placing the center of gravity over their feet. The trunk and legs should be extended only after gaining balance on the feet. This may be the most difficult step for an ataxic individual, who will either lean too far forward or extend the trunk too early and drop back into the chair. Another method a client may use to come to standing is to pull up on the stall bars from a kneeling position. However, this is less practical and will be useful only if the client should end up on the floor. Whatever the method used to come to standing, it will require much repetition by the client and verbal feedback from the therapist. In addition to verbal feedback, viewing a videotape may help a client recognize and correct mistakes.

Once upright, the person should practice balancing, which can be reinforced by approximation through the hips and shoulders. Tremor can be reduced by ankle weights or a weighted belt. Rhythmical stabilization applied to rotation of the trunk may also be valuable in gaining stability. Biofeedback from a force platform may also help the person control the center of gravity. It is hoped that the client can learn to come to standing and maintain standing without pulling on the bars; however, for some people this will be impossible. Those individuals who rely on the bars will not become independent ambulators but may, with the assistance of another person, be able to get up and walk. Once standing and stable, the client needs to practice alternate lifting of the feet. These activities can be practiced in rhythm with music to promote skill. A mirror also will be valuable at this time.

Ambulation

When the person begins to walk in the bars, he or she will need precise verbal feedback as to step length, body rotation, accessory movements, and trunk position. As in the initial learning of a sport, the therapist will need to isolate one problem at a time and provide practice. When the person is ready to walk outside of the bars, a decision will need to be made about an ambulatory aid. Aids may be necessary but also may be an obstacle because clients will now need to control position and movement of the device as well as themselves. Although a walker is typically the most stable, it can be so only when all legs are placed down together and at a correct distance from the body. Accuracy of placement may be facilitated by weighting the legs of the device. Also a piece of tape placed from side to side, midway across the walker, will help keep the client from walking too far into the walker and falling backwards. Crutches or canes may be used but require reciprocal movement of the arms and legs with appropriate timing and placement; this too can be very hard or impossible for some clients. The person may actually do better by using tall poles for support rather than the typical cane or crutches. Therapists can measure clients' progress in ambulation by the number of times they lose their balance in a treatment session, frequency of a specific error, the distance ambulated, or the level of assistance needed (see Chapters 14 and 28 for additional suggestions).

Activities for temporary reduction of dysmetria

Clients with cerebellar lesions will be frustrated in many activities by the presence of dysmetria. A therapist attempting to modify this impairment needs to recognize that no therapeutic procedure will totally eliminate dysmetria; however, before clients practice specific functional activities, the therapist can have them perform activities that will temporarily decrease dysmetria. For example, use of proprioceptive neuromuscular facilitation (PNF) patterns of rhythmical stabilization or slow-reversal-hold for the lower extremities will allow clients to ambulate with better control.[60,61] Similarly, functional tasks involving the arms can be preceded by PNF patterns for the arms.[83] Frenkel's exercises can also be used to modify dysmetria of the lower extremities.[65] These exercises can be performed in the supine, sitting, or standing positions. Each activity is to be performed slowly, with the client watching the extremity very carefully. When the client has gained reasonable control of one activity, he or she should proceed to the next.

Although Frenkel's exercises are classically described for the leg (see the box), they can be modified for the arm. For example, the client can first practice flexing and extending the elbow horizontally, supported on a sliding board, then move the arm without support to place the hand on the opposite elbow, next slide the hand down and up the forearm, and, finally, place the hand in the therapist's moving hand. Whether using Frenkel's exercises or PNF patterns to improve coordination, these activities should not comprise the entire therapy session but should be used to prime the client to practice a subsequent functional activity. Another procedure that can reduce dysmetria of an extremity is to place weights on the extremity.[82] The weights required vary from client to client. The greater the movement error, the heavier the weight needed; however, if the weight is too heavy, dysmetria will become worse.

The use of EMG or goniometrical biofeedback also may assist the client in receiving training in very specific acts. For example, brushing the teeth may be impossible because the toothbrush misses the mouth or hits the teeth and once inside the mouth does not effectively clean the teeth. EMG feedback from the deltoids, biceps, wrist flexors, and extensors or goniometrical position of the shoulder and elbow may be relayed to clients as they try to learn a pattern that works for them or to duplicate the pattern of signals produced by normal individuals when brushing their teeth.

CEREBELLAR STIMULATION

Results of physiological studies of the function of the cerebellum have led to the use of electrical stimulation of the cerebellum in treatment of various neurological disorders. Electrical stimulation of the cerebellum in cats disrupts

seizure activity induced by electrical stimulation of the pericruciate cortex and the hippocampus.[22,57,58] Based on such observations, cerebellar stimulation has been tried for treatment of severe epilepsy uncontrolled by medication. The results of the treatment have been controversial. Cooper and others[25] reported substantial reduction of seizure frequency in 18 of 32 individuals receiving chronic cerebellar stimulation. Gilman and others[40] also reported favorable results in a study of seven clients with epilepsy. However, Van Buren and others,[113] who performed a double blind cross-over study in five people with epilepsy, were unable to demonstrate objective improvement in the character or frequency of the clients' seizures.

Spasticity in experimental animals can be reduced by electrical stimulation of the anterior lobe of the cerebellum.[70,101] Such findings led to the attempt to reduce involuntary movement disorders in humans by chronic cerebellar stimulation. The results of these efforts also have been controversial. Cooper and others[26] implanted stimulating electrodes over the anterior lobe of the cerebellum of 141 clients with cerebral palsy having severe spasticity and athetosis. In 124 of these individuals who were followed for 1 year after surgery, spasticity was considered improved in 41% and athetosis improved in 24%. Other studies using clients with a variety of movement disorders also have

---

Frenkel exercises

Supine

1. Flex and extend one leg, heel sliding down a straight line on table.
2. Abduct and adduct hip smoothly with knee bent, heel on table.
3. Abduct and adduct leg with knee and hip extended, leg sliding on table.
4. Flex and extend hip and knee with heel off table.
5. Place one heel on knee of opposite leg and slide heel smoothly down shin toward ankle and back to knee.
6. Flex and extend both legs together, heels sliding on table.
7. Flex one leg while extending other leg.
8. Flex and extend one leg while abducting and adducting other leg.

Sitting

1. Place foot in therapist's hand, which will change position on each trial.
2. Raise leg and put foot on traced footprint on floor.
3. Sit steady for a few minutes.
4. Rise and sit with knees together.

Standing

1. Place foot forward and backward on a straight line.
2. Walk along a winding strip.
3. Walk between two parallel lines.
4. Walk, placing each foot in a tracing on floor.

reported significant reduction in spasticity and improvement in the quality of voluntary movement.[108,120] However, double blind studies have not been positive for the effects of chronic cerebellar stimulation.[36,118] In these studies neither professional evaluators nor the clients themselves could tell when the stimulator was turned on.

Another problem with cerebellar stimulation has been to develop electrodes and methods of placement that do not induce damage yet provide adequate current on a long-term basis. Significant damage to the stimulating site and encapsulation of electrodes with connective tissue have been reported, but it is not known if this situation is a universal problem.[27,109] On the basis of the above uncertainties with chronic electrical stimulation of the cerebellum, the approach must still be considered experimental and a last resort for intractable epilepsy, severe spasticity, or other involuntary movement disorders.[57]

REFERENCES

1. Akshoomoff NA and Courchesne E: A new role for the cerebellum cognitive operations, *Behav Neurosci* 106:731, 1992.
2. Albus JS: A theory of cerebellar function, *Math Biosci* 10:25, 1971.
3. Allen GI and Tsukahara N: Cerebrocerebellar communications systems, *Physiol Rev* 54:957, 1974.
4. Amici R and others: *Cerebellar tumors: clinical analysis and physiopathologic correlations,* New York, 1976, S Karger.
5. Baloh RW and others: Vestibulo-ocular function in patients with cerebellar atrophy, *Neurology* 25:160, 1975.
6. Botterell EH and Fulton JF: Functional localization in the cerebellum of primates. II. Lesions of the midline structures (vermis) and deep nuclei, *J Comp Neurol* 69:47, 1938.
7. Botterell EH and Fulton JF: Functional localization in the cerebellum of primates. III. Lesions of the hemispheres (neocerebellum), *J Comp Neurol* 69:63, 1938.
8. Boyeson MG and others: Unilateral locus coeruleus lesions facilitate motor recovery from cortical injury through supersensitivity mechanisms, *Pharmacol Biochem Behav* 44:297, 1993.
9. Bremer F: Le cervelet. In Roger GH and Binet L: *Traité de physiologie normale et pathologique,* vol 10, Paris, 1935, Masson.
10. Brooks VB: Control of intended limb movement by the lateral and intermediate cerebellum. In Asanuma H and Wilson VJ: *Integration in the human nervous system,* New York, 1979, Igaku Shoin.
11. Brooks VB: Motor programs revisited. In Talbott RE and Humphrey DR: *Posture and movement,* New York, 1979, Raven Press.
12. Brooks VB and others: Effects of cooling dentate nucleus on tracking task performance in monkeys, *J Neurophysiol* 36:974, 1973.
13. Brown J and others: Ataxic dysarthria, *Int J Neurol* 7:302, 1970.
14. Brown SH and others: Role of the cerebellum in visuomotor coordination, *Exp Brain Res* 94:478, 1993.
15. Carpenter RHS: *Movement of the eyes,* London, 1977, Pion, Ltd.
16. Carrea RME and Mettler FA: Physiologic consequences following extensive removals of the cerebellar cortex and deep cerebellar nuclei and effect of secondary cerebral ablations in the primate, *J Comp Neurol* 87:169, 1947.
17. Chambers WW and Sprague JM: Functional localization in the cerebellum. I. Organization in longitudinal corticonuclear zones and their contribution to the control of posture, both extrapyramidal and pyramidal, *J Comp Neurol* 103:105, 1955.
18. Chase RA and others: Modification of intention tremor in man, *Nature* 206:485, 1965.
19. Cogan DG: Ocular dysmetria: flutter like oscillations of the eyes and opsoclonus, *Arch Ophthalmol* 51:318, 1954.
20. Cole M: Dysprody due to posterior fossa lesions, *Trans Am Neurol Assoc* 96:151, 1971.
21. Conrad B and Brooks VB: Effects of dentate cooling on rapid alternating arm movements, *J Neurophysiol* 37:792, 1974.
22. Cooke PM and Snider RS: Some cerebellar influences on electrically induced cerebral seizures, *Epilepsia* 4:19, 1955.
23. Cooke JD and Thomas JS: Forearm oscillation during cooling of the dentate nucleus in the monkey, *Can J Physiol Pharmacol* 54:430, 1976.
24. Cooper IS: *Involuntary movement disorders,* New York, 1969, Harper & Row.
25. Cooper IS and others: A long-term follow up study of cerebellar stimulation for the control of epilepsy. In Cooper IS: *Cerebellar stimulation in man,* New York, 1978, Raven Press.
26. Cooper IS and others: A long-term follow-up of chronic cerebellar stimulation for cerebral palsy. In Cooper IS: *Cerebellar stimulation in man,* New York, 1978, Raven Press.
27. Dauth GW and others: Long-term surface stimulation of the cerebellum in monkey. I. Light microscopic, electrophysiologic and clinical observation, *Surg Neurol* 7:377, 1977.
28. Dichgans J and Mauritz K: Patterns and mechanisms of postural instability in patients with cerebellar lesions, *Adv Neurol* 39:633, 1983.
29. Dichgans J and others: Postural sway in normals and atactic patients, analysis of the stabilizing and destabilizing effects of vision, *Agressologie* 176:15, 1976.
30. Dow RS and Moruzzi G: *The physiology and pathology of the cerebellum,* Minneapolis, 1958, University of Minnesota Press.
31. Eccles JC: Long-loop reflexes from the spinal cord to the brain stem and cerebellum, *Atti Accad Med Lomb* 21:1, 1966.
32. Eccles JC: The dynamic loop hypothesis of movement control. In Leibovic KN, editor: *Information processing in the nervous system,* New York, 1969, Springer.
33. Fisher CN and others: Acute hypertensive cerebellar hemorrhage: diagnosis and surgical treatment, *J Nerv Ment Dis* 140:38, 1965.
34. Fisher JD: Contributions illustrative of the functions of the cerebellum, *Am J Med Sci* 23:352, 1839.
35. Fulton JF and Dow RS: The cerebellum: a summary of functional localization, *Yale J Biol Med* 10:89, 1937.
36. Gahn NH and others: Chronic cerebellar stimulation for cerebral palsy: a double blind study, *Neurology* 31:87, 1981.
37. Gilman S : The mechanism of cerebellar hypotonia: an experimental study in the monkey, *Brain* 92:621, 1969
38. Gilman S and others: Effects of medullary pyramidotomy in the monkey. II. Abnormalities of spindle afferent response, *Brain* 94:515, 1971.
39. Gilman S and others: Spinal mechanisms underlying the effects of unilateral ablation of areas 4 and 6 in monkeys, *Brain* 97:49, 1974.
40. Gilman S and others: Clinical, morphological, biochemical, and physiological effects of cerebellar stimulation. In Hambrecht FT and Reswick FB: *Functional electrical stimulation,* New York, 1977, Marcel Dekker.
41. Gilman S and others: *Disorders of the cerebellum,* Philadelphia, 1981, FA Davis.
42. Goldberger ME and Growden JH: Tremor at rest following cerebellar lesions in monkeys: effect of L-dopa administration, *Brain Res* 27:183, 1971.
43. Goldberger ME and Growdon JH: Pattern of recovery following cerebellar deep nuclear lesions in monkeys, *Exp Neurol* 39:307, 1973.
44. Growden JH and others: An experimental study of cerebellar dyskinesia in the rhesus monkey, *Brain* 90:603, 1967.
45. Hagbarth KE and others: The effect of gamma fiber block on afferent muscle nerve activity during voluntary contractions, *Acta Physiol Scand* 79:27A, 1970.
46. Hallett M and others: EMG analysis of stereotyped movements in man, *J Neurol Neurosurg Psychiatry* 38:1154, 1975.

47. Hallett M and others: EMG analysis of patients with cerebellar deficits, *J Neurol Neurosurg Psychiatry* 38:1163, 1975.

48. Holmes G: The symptoms of acute cerebellar injuries due to gunshot injuries, *Brain* 40:461, 1921.

49. Holmes G: The Croonian lectures on the clinical symptoms of cerebellar diseases and their interpretation, *Lancet* 1:1177, 1922.

50. Holmes G: The Croonian lectures on the clinical symptoms of cerebellar diseases and their interpretation, *Lancet* 1:1231, 1922.

51. Holmes G: The Croonian lectures on the clinical symptoms of cerebellar diseases and their interpretation, *Lancet* 2:59, 1922.

52. Holmes G: The Croonian lectures on the clinical symptoms of cerebellar diseases and their interpretation, *Lancet* 2:111, 1922.

53. Holmes G: The cerebellum of man, *Brain* 62:1, 1939.

54. Hood JD and others: Rebound nystagmus, *Brain* 96:507, 1973.

55. Horvath FE and others: Effects of cooling the dentate nucleus in alternating bar pressing performance in monkey, *Int J Neurol* 7:252, 1970.

56. Ito M: Neurophysiological aspects of the cerebellar motor control system, *Int J Neurol* 1:162, 1970.

57. Ivan LP and Ventureyra ECG: Chronic cerebellar stimulation in cerebral palsy, *Appl Neurophysiol* 45:51, 1982.

58. Iwata K and Snider RS: Cerebello-hippocampal influences on the electroencephalogram, *Electroencephalogr Clin Neurophysiol* 11:439, 1959.

59. Jung R and Kornhuber HH: Results of electronystagmography in man: the value of optokinetic vestibular, and spontaneous nystagmus for neurologic diagnosis and research. In Bender MB: *The oculomotor system,* New York, 1964, Harper & Row.

60. Kabat H: Studies on neuromuscular dysfunction. XII. Rhythmic stabilization: a new and more effective technique for treatment of paralysis through a cerebellar mechanism, *Permanente Found M Bull* 8:9, 1950.

61. Kabat H: Analysis and therapy of cerebellar ataxia and asynergia, *Arch Neurol Psychiatry* 74:375, 1955.

62. Kent R and Netsell R: A case study of an ataxic dysarthric: cineradiography and spectrographic observations, *J Speech Hear Disord* 40:115, 1975.

63. Knott M and Voss DE: *Preprioceptive neuro-muscular facilitation,* ed 2, New York, 1968, Harper & Row.

64. Kornhuber HH: Neurologie de kleinherns, *Zbl ges Neurol Psychiat* 191:13, 1968.

65. Krusen FH and others: *Handbook of physical medicine and rehabilitation,* ed 2, Philadelphia, 1971, WB Saunders.

66. Lamarre Y and others: Central mechanisms of tremor in some feline and primate models, *J Can Neurol Sci* 2:227, 1975.

67. Larochelle L and others: The rubro-olivo-cerebello nubral loop and postural tremor in the monkey, *J Neurol Sci* 11:53, 1970.

68. Lectenberg R: Ataxia and other cerebellar syndromes. In Jankovic J and Eduardo T, editors: *Parkinson's disease and movement disorders,* Baltimore, 1993, Williams & Wilkins.

69. Lechtenberg R and Gilman S: Speech disorders in cerebellar disease, *Ann Neurol* 3:285, 1978.

70. Lowenthal M and Horsley V: On the relations between the cerebellar and other centers (namely cerebral and spinal) with reference to the action of antagonistic muscles, *Proc R Soc Lond* 61:20, 1897.

71. Luciani L: *Il cervelletto: nuovi studi di fisiologia normale e patologica,* Florence, 1891, Le Monnier.

72. Luciani L: De l'influence qu'exercent les mutilations cérébelleuses sur l'excitabilité de l'écorce cérébrale et sur les réflexes spinaux, *Arch Ital Biol* 21:190, 1894.

73. MacKay WA and Murphy JT: Cerebellar modulation of reflex gain, *Prog Neurobiol* 13:361, 1979.

74. Marie P and others: De l'atrophie cérébelleuse tardive à prédominance corticale, *Rev Neurol* (Paris) 38:849, 1082, 1922.

75. Marr D: A theory of the cerebellar cortex, *J Physiol* 202:437, 1969.

76. Marsden CD and others: Disorders of movement in cerebellar disease in man. In Rose CF, editor: *Physiological aspects of clinical neurology,* Oxford, 1977, Blackwell Scientific Publications.

77. Mauritz KH and others: Delayed and enhanced long latency reflexes as the possible cause of postural tremor in late cerebellar atrophy, *Brain* 104:97, 1981.

78. McCloskey DI: Kinesthetic sensibility, *Physiol Rev* 58:763, 1978.

79. Meyer-Lohmann J and others: Effects of dentate cooling on precentral unit activity following torque pulse injections into elbow movements, *Brain Res* 94:237, 1975.

80. Meyer-Lohmann J and others: Cerebellar participation in generation of prompt arm movements, *J Neurophysiol* 38:871, 1977.

81. Miles FA and Fuller JH: Adaptive plasticity in the vestibulo-ocular responses of the rhesus monkey, *Brain Res* 8:512, 1974.

82. Morgan MH: Ataxia and weights, *Physiotherapy* 61:332, 1975.

83. Nakamura R and Taniguchi R: Kinesiological analysis and physical therapy of cerebellar ataxia. In Sobue I: *Spinocerebellar degenerations,* Baltimore, 1978, University Park Press.

84. Narabayashi H: Involuntary movements and cerebellar pathology. In Massion J and Sasaki K: *Cerebro-cerebellar interactions,* Amsterdam, 1979, Elsevier/North Holland Biomedical Press.

85. Nashner LM: Adapting reflexes controlling human posture, *Exp Brain Res* 26:59, 1976.

86. Nashold BS and others: Ocular reactions in man from deep cerebellar stimulation and lesions, *Arch Ophthalmol* 81:538, 1969.

87. Nyberg-Hansen R and Horn J: Functional aspects of cerebellar signs in clinical neurology, *Acta Neurol Scand* 48(suppl 51):219, 1972.

88. Olson Jr WJ: Personal communication, 1994.

89. Optican LM and Robinson DA: Cerebellar-dependent adaptive control of primate saccadic system, *J Neurophysiol* 44:1058, 1980.

90. Orlovsky GN and Shik ML: Control of locomotion: a neurophysiological analysis of the cat locomotor system. In Porter R, editor: *International review of physiology neurophysiology* II. vol 10, Baltimore, 1976, University Park Press.

91. Oscar-Barman M and others: Dichotic ear-order effects with nonverbal stimuli, *Cortex* 10:270, 1974.

92. Poirier LJ and others: Physiopathology of the cerebellum in the monkey. II. Motor disturbances associated with partial and complete destruction of cerebellar structures, *J Neurol Sci* 22:491, 1974.

93. Ritchie L: Effect of cerebellar lesions on saccadic eye movements, *J Neurophysiol* 39:1246-1256, 1976.

94. Roland PE: Partition of the human cerebellum in sensory-motor activities, learning and cognition, *Can J Neurol Sci* 20(suppl 3):S75, 1993.

95. Rossi G: Sugli effetti consequenti alla stimolazione contemporanea della corteccia cerebrale e di quella cerebellare, *Arch Fisiol* 10:389, 1912.

96. Ruch TC: Motor systems. In Stevens SS, editor: *Handbook of experimental psychology,* New York, 1951, John Wiley & Sons.

97. Russell JSR: Experimental research into the functions of the cerebellum, *Philos Trans R Soc Lond* 185:819, 1894.

98. Ryding E and others: Motor imagery activates the cerebellum regionally. A SPECT rCBF study with 99mTc-HMPAO, *Cogn Brain Res* 1:94, 1993.

99. Selhorst JB and others: Disorders in cerebellar ocular motor control I. Saccadic overshoot dysmetria, *Brain* 99:497, 1976.

100. Shankweiler D: Effects of temporal lobe damage on perception of dichotically presented melodies, *J Comp Physiol Psychol* 62:115, 1966.

101. Sherrington CS: Double (antidrome) conduction in the central nervous system, *Proc R Soc Lond* 61:243, 1897.

102. Shimizu N and others: Eye-head co-ordination in patients with parkinsonism and cerebellar ataxia, *J Neurol Neurosurg Psychiatry* 44:509, 1981.

103. Silfverskjold BP: A 3 sec leg tremor in a cerebellar syndrome, *Acta Neurol Scand* 55:385, 1977.

104. Smith AM and Bourbonnais D: Neuronal activity in cerebellar cortex related to control of prehensile force, *J Neurophysiol* 45:286, 1981.

105. Stein RB and Oguztoreli MN: Reflex involvement in the generation and control of tremor and clonus. In Desmedt JE, editor: Physiological tremor, pathological tremor and clonus, *Prog Clin Neurophysiol* (Basel) 5:28, 1978.

106. Stockmeyer S: An interpretation of the approach of Rood to the treatment of neuromuscular dysfunction, *Am J Phys Med* 46:900, 1967.

107. Strick PL: Cerebellar involvement in "volitional" muscle response to load changes, *Prog Clin Neurophysiol* 4:85, 1978.

108. Sukoff MH and Ragatz RE: Cerebellar stimulation for chronic extensor-flexor rigidity and opisthotonus secondary to hypoxia, *J Neurosurg* 53:391, 1980.

109. Tennyson VM and others: Long-term surface stimulation of the cerebellum in the monkey. II. Electron microscopic and biochemical observations, *Surg Neurol* 8:17, 1977.

110. Terzuolo TA and Viviani P: Parameters of motion and EMG activities during some simple motor tasks in normal subjects and cerebellar patients. In Cooper IS and others, editors: *The cerebellum, epilepsy and behavior,* New York, 1973, Plenum Press.

111. Thach WT: Correlation of neural discharge with pattern and force of muscular activity, joint position, and direction of the intended movement in motor cortex and cerebellum, *J Neurophysiol* 41:654, 1978.

112. Uno M and others: Effects of cooling the interposed nuclei on tracking-task performance in monkeys, *J Neurophysiol* 36:996, 1973.

113. Van Buren and others: Preliminary evaluation of cerebellar stimulation and other biologic criteria in the treatment of epilepsy, *J Neurosurg* 48:407, 1978.

114. Victor M and others: A restricted form of cerebellar cortical degeneration occurring in alcoholic patients, *AMA Arch Neurol* 1:579, 1959.

115. Vilas T and Hore J: Effects of changes in mechanical state of limb on cerebellar intention tremor, *J Neurophysiol* 40:1214, 1977.

116. Vilas T and others: Dual nature of the precentral responses to limb perturbations revealed by cerebellar cooling, *Brain Res* 117:336, 1976.

117. von Noorden GK and Preziosi TJ: Eye movement recordings in neurological disorders, *Arch Ophthalmol* 76:162, 1966.

118. Whittaker CK: Cerebellar stimulation for cerebral palsy, *J Neurosurg* 52:653, 1980.

119. Woolridge CP and Russell G: Head position training with the cerebral palsied child: an application of biofeedback techniques, *Milbank Mem Fund Q* 57:407, 1976.

120. Wong PKH and others: Cerebellar stimulation in the management of cerebral palsy: clinical and physiological studies, *Neurosurgery* 5:217, 1979.

121. Zee DS and others: The mechanism of downbeat nystagmus, *Arch Neurol* 30:227, 1974.

122. Zee DS and others: Ocular motor abnormalities in hereditary ataxia, *Brain* 99:207, 1976.

123. Zee DS and others: Slow saccades in spinocerebellar degeneration, *Arch Neurol* 33:243, 1976.

124. Zee DS and others: Effects of ablation of flocculus and paraflocculus on eye movements in primate, *J Neurophysiol* 46:878, 1981.

125. Zentay PJ: Motor disorders of the nervous system and their significance for speech. I. Cerebral and cerebellar dysarthrias, *Laryngoscope* 47:147, 1937.

CHAPTER 24

Hemiplegia

Susan D. Ryerson

KEY TERMS

hemiplegia	embolism
thrombosis	hypertonicity
hemorrhage	postural instability
transient ischemic attack (TIA)	

LEARNING OBJECTIVES

After reading this chapter the student/therapist will:

1. Identify the various types of causes of neurovascular diseases.
2. Identify the typical patterns of motor activity seen after a vascular insult.
3. Identify the stages of recovery of motor function observed in clients who have had a neurovascular insult.
4. Analyze musculoskeletal and central pattern generator or motor control problems.
5. Identify various treatment procedures and understand how they affect motor performance.

OVERVIEW

The treatment of **hemiplegia** is controversial. Various treatment methods have been devised and advocated. This chapter reviews the problems and management of hemiplegia and uses normal movement as a base on which appropriate techniques of facilitation and reeducation can be chosen to allow the person with hemiplegia to return to life with the highest quality of function.

Definition

Hemiplegia, a paralysis of one side of the body, is the classic sign of neurovascular disease of the brain. It is one of many manifestations of neurovascular disease, and it occurs with strokes involving the cerebral hemisphere or brainstem. A stroke, or cerebrovascular accident (CVA), results in a sudden, specific neurological deficit. It is the suddenness of this neurological deficit—seconds, minutes, hours, or a few days—that characterizes the disorder as vascular. Although hemiplegia may be the most obvious sign of a CVA and a major concern of therapists, other symptoms are equally disabling, including sensory dysfunction, aphasia or dysarthria, visual field defects, and mental and intellectual impairment. The specific combination of these neurovascular deficits enables a physician to detect both the location and the size of the defect. Cerebrovascular accidents can be classified according to pathological type—**thrombosis,** embolus, or **hemorrhage**—or by temporal factors—completed, in-evolution, or **transient ischemic attacks (TIA).**

Epidemiology

Although the incidence of cerebrovascular disease has been decreasing for the last 25 years, stroke is still the third most common cause of death in the United States.[1] The incidence of stroke rises rapidly with increasing age; in the 80- to 90-year-old age group, the mortality rates approach the corresponding incidence rates. In the United States, the incidence of stroke is greater in males than in females, and it is greater in the blacks than in whites.[66] Cerebral infarction (thrombosis or **embolism**) is the most common form of stroke, accounting for 70% of all strokes. Hemorrhages account for another 20%, and 10% remain unspecified. An idea of the prevalence of stroke can be gained by looking at the results of a study of three states: Of every 100 persons who survive a stroke, 10 return to work without impairment, 40 have mild residual disability, 40 are disabled and require special services, and 10 need institutional care.[65]

The three most commonly recognized risk factors for cerebrovascular disease are hypertension, diabetes mellitis, and heart disease. The most important of these factors is hypertension.[55] Systolic and/or diastolic blood pressure, pulse pressure, and variability of pressure are all good predictors of stroke for all age groups.

Clinically evident diabetes is also significantly related to stroke. Interestingly, the risk of stroke for a diabetic client is not related to the treatment or nontreatment of the disease.

Heart disease, especially electrocardiogram (ECG) abnormalities and heart enlargement, also increases the chance of a completed stroke. Cardiac and cerebrovascular disease are concomitant lesions. See Irwin and Tecklin: *Cardiopulmonary Physical Therapy* for more information.

Risk factors that have been correlated to stroke include increased blood fat levels, obesity, and cigarette smoking. Because high blood pressure is the greatest risk factor for stroke, human characteristics and behavior that increase one's blood pressure will increase the risk of stroke.

Ostfeld[55] noted that mortality rates for stroke have declined, slowly at first (from 1900 to 1950), then more quickly (from 1950 to 1970), and with a sharp drop noted around 1974. Experts have speculated that the greater use of hypertensive drugs in the 1960s and 1970s started this decline, and the creation of screening and treatment referral centers for high blood pressure may account for the marked decline in the late 1970s. Although approximately 100,000 people die from cerebrovascular disease each year, an additional 1 million people survive strokes but are left disabled.

Outcome

The long-term follow-up on the Framingham study revealed that long-term stroke survivors, especially those with only one episode, had a good chance for full functional recovery.[28] For those people left with severe neurological and functional deficits, studies have demonstrated that rehabilitation is effective and that it can improve functional ability.[20,40,69] It has been demonstrated that age is not a factor in determining the outcome of the rehabilitation process.[2] Presently, it is thought that all clients should be given an opportunity to participate in the rehabilitation process unless it is medically contraindicated.[40]

Prediction of ultimate functional outcome has been hampered by the inaccuracy of commonly used predictors (medical items, income level, intelligence, functional level). Computed tomography (CT) scanning and regional cerebral blood flow (rCBF) studies are presently being studied for their potential use as predictors of functional recovery following stroke.[45,61]

Pathoneurological and pathophysiological aspects

Classification. The pathological processes that result from a cerebrovascular accident can be divided into three groups—thrombotic changes, embolic changes, and hemorrhagic changes.

Thrombotic infarction. Atherosclerotic plaques and hypertension interact to produce cerebrovascular infarcts.[1] These plaques form at branchings and curves of the arteries. Plaques usually form in front of the first major branching of the cerebral arteries. These lesions can be present for 30 years or more and may never become symptomatic. Intermittent blockage may procede to permanent damage. The process by which a thrombus occludes an artery requires several hours and explains the division between stroke-in-evolution and completed stroke.

TIAs are an indication of the presence of thrombotic disease and are the result of transient ischemia. Although the cause of TIAs has not been definitively established, cerebral vasospasm or transient systemic arterial hypotension are thought to be responsible factors.

Embolic infarction. The embolus that causes the stroke may come from the heart, from an internal carotid artery thrombosis, or from an atheromatous plaque of the carotid sinus. It is usually a sign of cardiac disease. The infarction may be of pale, hemorrhagic, or mixed type. The branches of the middle cerebral artery are infarcted most commonly as a result of its direct continuation from the internal carotid artery. Collateral blood supply is not established with embolic infarctions as a result of the speed of obstruction formation, so there is less survival of tissue distal to the area of embolic infarct than with thrombotic infarct.[1]

Hemorrhage. The most common intracranial hemorrhages causing stroke are hypertensive, ruptured saccular aneurysm, and atrioventricular (AV) malformation. Massive hemorrhage frequently results from hypertensive cardiac-renal disease and causes bleeding into the brain tissue in an oval or round mass that displaces midline structures. The exact mechanism of hemorrhage is not known. This mass of extravasated blood decreases in size over 6 to 8 months.

Saccular, or berry, aneurysms are thought to be the result of defects in the media and elastica that develop over years. This muscular defect plus overstretching of the internal elastic membrane from blood pressure causes the aneurysm to develop. Saccular aneurysms are found at branchings of major cerebral arteries, especially the anterior portion of the circle of Willis. Averaging 8 to 10 mm in diameter and variable in form, these aneurysms rupture at their dome. Saccular aneurysms are rare in childhood.

AV malformations are developmental abnormalities that result in a spaghetti-like mass of dilated arteriovenous fistulas varying in size from a few millimeters in diameter to huge masses located within the brain tissue. Some of these blood vessels have extremely thin, abnormally structured walls. Although the abnormality is present from birth, symptoms usually develop between the ages of 10 and 35. The hemorrhage of an AV malformation presents a pathological picture similar to the saccular aneurysm. The larger AV malformations frequently occur in the posterior half of the cerebral hemisphere.[1]

Clinical findings. The focal neurological deficit resulting from a stroke, whether embolis, thrombus, or hemorrhage, is a reflection of the size and location of the lesion and the amount of collateral blood flow. Unilateral neurological deficits result from interruption of the carotid vascular system, and bilateral neurological deficits result from interruption of the vascular supply to the basilar system. Clinical syndromes resulting from occlusion or hemorrhage in the cerebral circulation vary from partial to complete. Signs of hemorrhage may be more variable as a result of the effect of extension to surrounding brain tissue and the possible rise in intracranial pressure. Table 24-1 summarizes the clinical symptoms and the anatomical structures involved according to specific arterial involvement.

The frequencies of the three types of cerebrovascular disease—thrombotic, embolism, and hemorrhage—vary according to whether they were taken from a clinical study or from an autopsy study, but their frequency ranks in the order presented in this section (National Stroke Survey[75]). The clinical symptoms and laboratory findings for each type have been condensed in Table 24-2.

Movement disturbances. Hemiplegia, the motor dysfunction of stroke, is one of the most obvious clinical signs of the disease. Although the site and size of the cerebral vascular lesion initially determine the degree of motor function, the concomitant presence of sensory impairment adds to and compounds the problem of motor dysfunction. Although theories of generator control systems and efferent drive have explained how purposeful movements can occur without "input" from integrated sensory systems, movement is refined, coordinated, and adapted through the interaction of exteroceptive and kinesthetic messages.

After the onset of CVA with hemiplegia, a state of low tone or flaccidity exists. The length of this state of flaccidity may be short or last for weeks or months.

This state is followed by the development of patterns of returning muscle function, compensations due to weakness, loss of control, or poor balance and patterns of increased tone. The rate at which these patterns of muscle function return is dictated by the site and severity of the lesion and by the focus of the rehabilitation process. Early return of movement is seen in the shoulder and pelvic girdle elevators (upper trapezius, levator scapulae, quadratus lumborum, latissimus dorsi).[13,43] Distal return often is available early in recovery and is used by the client to reinforce weak proximal musculature. As the client begins to function, in the presence of incomplete or unbalanced muscle return and control, other problems will emerge: inefficient patterns of movement, improper initiation patterns, poor joint alignment, and reflexive responses to stress. This results in stereotypical movement patterns such as the following:

1. Use of unilateral paracervical muscles of the neck results in ipsilateral flexion (the ear approximates the affected shoulder) and contralateral rotation (turning the face away from the affected side) (Fig. 24-1).
2. Use of shoulder elevators on a downwardly rotated scapula slowly changes the position of the scapula from one of depression on the thorax to elevation on the thorax and contributes to shoulder subluxation.
3. Use of pelvic hikers to initiate swing phase of gait prevents the emergence of lower trunk and pelvic rotation.

The development of abnormal movement patterns occurs not only in the arm and leg, but also in the musculature of the head, neck, and trunk. The trunk is the critical site for the development of abnormal movement patterns because trunk movements form the basis for postural control of movement. This is the same phenomenon displayed in children with

Table 24-1. Clinical symptoms of vascular lesions

Vessel	Clinical symptoms	Structures involved
Middle cerebral artery	Contralateral paralysis and sensory deficit	Somatic motor area
	Motor speech impairment	Broca's area (dominant hemisphere)
	"Central" aphasia, anomia, jargon speech	Parietooccipital cortex (dominant hemisphere)
	Unilateral neglect, apraxia, impaired ability to judge distance	Parietal lobe (nondominant hemisphere)
	Homonomous hemianopsia	Optic radiation deep to second temporal convolution
	Loss of conjugate gaze to opposite side	Frontal controversive field
	Avoidance reactio of opposite limbs	Parietal lobe
	Pure motor hemiplegia	Upper portion of posterior limb of internal capsule
	Limb-kinetic apraxia	Premotor or parietal cortex
Anterior cerebral artery	Paralysis—lower extremity	Motor area—leg
	Paresis in opposite arm	Arm area of cortex
	Cortical sensory loss	Sensory area
	Urinary incontinence	Posteromedial aspect of superior frontal gyrus
		Medial surface of posterior frontal lobe
	Contralateral grasp reflex, sucking reflex	Uncertain
	Lack of spontaniety motor inaction, echolalia	Uncertain
	Perservation and amnesia	
Posterior cerebral artery		
Peripheral area	Homonomous hemianopsia	Calcarine cortex or optic radiation
	Bilateral homonomous hemianopsia, cortical blindness, inability to perceive objects not centrally located, occular apraxia	Bilateral occipital lobe
	Memory defect	Inferomedial portions of temporal lobe
	Topographic disorientation	Nondominant calcarine and lingual gyri
Central area	Thalamic syndrome	Posteroventral nucleus ophthalmus
	Weber's syndrome	Cranial nerve III and cerebral peduncle
	Contralateral hemiplegia	Cerebral peduncle
	Paresis of vertical eye movements, sluggish pupillary response to light	Supranuclear fibers to cranial nerve III
	Contralateral ataxia or postural tremor	
Internal carotid artery	Variable signs according to degree and site of occlusion—middle cerebral, anterior cerebral, posterior cerebral territory	Uncertain
Basilar artery	Ataxia	Middle and superior cerebellar peduncle
Superior cerebellar artery	Dizziness, nausea, vomiting, horizontal nystagmus	Vestibular nucleus
	Horner's syndrome on opposite side, decreased pain and thermal sensation	Descending sympathetic fibers
		Spinal thalamic tract
	Decreased touch, vibration, position sense of lower extremity greater than upper extremity	Medial lemniscus
Anterior inferior cerebellar artery	Nystagmus, vertigo, nausea, vomiting	Vestibular nerve
	Facial paralysis on same side	Cranial nerve VII
	Tinnitus	Auditory nerve, lower cochlear nucleus
	Ataxia	Middle cerebral peduncle
	Impaired facial sensation on same side	Fifth cranial nerve nucleus
	Decreased pain and thermal sensation on opposite side	Spinal thalamic tract
Complete basilar syndrome	Bilateral long tract signs with cerebellar and cranial nerve abnormalities	—
	Coma	—
	Quadriplegia	—
	Pseudobulbar palsy	—
	Cranial nerve abnormalities	
Vertebral artery	Decreased pain and temperature on opposite side	Spinal thalamic tract
	Sensory loss from a tactile and proprioceptive	Medial lemniscus
	Hemiparesis of arm and leg	Pyramidal tract
	Facial pain and numbness on same side	Decending tract and fifth cranial nucleus
	Horner's syndrome, ptosis, decreased sweating	Decending sympathetic tract
	Ataxia	Spinal cerebellar tract
	Paralysis of tongue	Cranial nerve XII
	Weakness of vocal cord, decreased gag	Cranial nerves IX and X
	Hiccups	Uncertain

Adapted from Adams RD and Victor M: *Principles of neurology,* New York, 1981, McGraw-Hill Inc.

Table 24-2. Clinical symptoms and laboratory findings for neurovascular disease

Disease type	Clinical picture	Laboratory findings

Thrombosis	*Extremely variable*
	Proceeded by a prodromal episode
	Uneven progression
	  Onset develops within minutes, hours, or
	    over days ("thrombus in evolution")
	60% occur during sleep—awaken unaware of
	  problem, rise, and fall to floor
	Usually no headache, but may occur in mild
	  form
	Hypertension, diabetes, or vascular disease elsewhere
	  in body
		Cerebrospinal fluid pressure is
		  normal
		Cerebrospinal fluid is clear
		EEG: limited differential diagnostic
		  value
		Skull radiographs are not helpful
		Arteriorgraphy is the definitive
		  procedure, it demostrates site
		  of collateral flow
		CT scan is helpful in chronic
		  state when cavitation has occurred

TIAs	Linked to atherosclerotic thrombosis Proceeded or accompanied by stroke Occur by themselves Last 2-30 minutes Experience a few attacks or hundreds Normal neurological examination between attacks If transient symptoms are present on awakening, may indicate future stroke	Usually none

Embolism
Cardiac
Non cardiac
  Atherosclerosis
  Pulmonary thrombosis
  Fat, tumor, air
	Extremely variable
	Occurs extremely rapidly—seconds or minutes
	There are no warnings
	Branches of middle cerebral artery are involved
	  most frequently, large embolus will block
	  internal carotid artery or stem of middle cerebral
	  artery
	If in basilar system, deep coma and total paralysis
	  may result
	Often a manifestation of heart disease, including
	  atrial fibrillation and myocardial infarction
	Headache
	As embolus passes through artery, client may
	  have neurological deficits that resolve as embolus
	  breaks and passes into small artery supplying
	  small or silent brain area
		Generally same as thrombosis
		  except for following:
		  If embolism causes a large
		    hemorrhagic infarct, cerebro-
		    spinal fluid will be bloody
		  30% of embolic strokes produce
		    small hemorrhagic infarct
		    without bloody cerebrospinal
		    fluid

Hemorrhage
Hypertensive hemorrhage
	Severe headache
	Vomiting at onset
	Blood pressure >170/90; usually "essential"
	  hypertension but can be from other types
	Abrupt onset, usually during day, not in sleep
	Gradually evolves over hours or days according
	  to speed of bleeding
	No recurrence of bleeding
	Frequency in blacks with hypertensive hemorrhage
	  is greater than frequency in whites
	Hemorrhaged blood absorbs slowly—rapid improvement
	  of symptoms is not usual
	If massive hemorrhage occurs, client may survive
	  a few hours or days secondary to brainstem
	  compression
		CT scan can detect hemorrhages
		  larger than 1.5 cm in cerebral
		  and cerebellar hemispheres;
		  they are diagnostically superior
		  to arteriography; they are especially
		  helpful in diagnosing small
		  hemorrhages that do not spill
		  blood into cerebrospinal fluid;
		  with massive hemorrhage and
		  increased pressure, cerebrospinal
		  fluid is grossly bloody; lumbar
		  puncture is necessary when
		  CT scan is not available
		Radiographs occasionally show
		  midline shift (this is not true
		  with infaction)
		EEG shows no typical pattern,
		  but high voltage and slow
		  waves are most common with
		  hemorrhage
		Urinary changes may reflect
		  renal disease

Ruptured saccular
aneurysm
	Asymptomatic before rupture
	With rupture, blood spills under high pressure
	  into subarachnoid space
	  Excruciating headache with loss of con-
	    sciousness
	  Headache without loss of consciousness
	  Sudden loss of consciousness
	Decerebrate rigidity with coma
	If severe—persistent deep coma with respi-
	  ratory arrest, circulatory collapse leading to
	  death; death can occur within 5 minutes
	If mild—consciousness regained within hours
	  then confusion, amnesia, headache, stiff neck,
	  drowsiness
	Hemiplegia, paresis, homonomous hemiano-
	  psia, or aphasia usually absent
		CT scan detects localized blood
		  in hydrocephalus if present
		Cerebrospinal fluid is extremely
		  bloody
		Radiographs are usually negative
		Carotid and vertebral arteriography
		  are performed only if certain
		  of diagnosis

Adapted from Adams RD and Victor M: *Principles of neurology,* New York, 1981, McGraw-Hill Inc.

cerebral palsy (see Chapter 9). The development of abnormal movement patterns in the trunk begins with lack of control and weakness and an inability to maintain weight evenly on the pelvis. In the acute phase, when the upper extremity lacks control and "hangs" by the side of the body, the trunk on the affected side may appear to be laterally flexed.

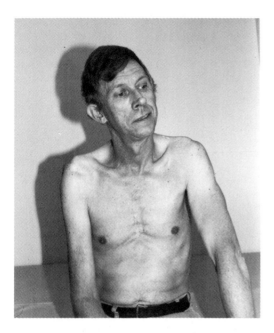

Fig. 24-1. Side bending of the head toward the affected side with the face directed away from the affected side.

Loss of control of the upper trunk over the lower trunk results in abnormal upper trunk forward flexion or rib cage rotation backwards on the affected side. The thoracic vertebrae follow and rotate in a compatible direction, giving the body an appearance of being "retracted" as described by Bobath.[10] The initial development of abnormal movement in the trunk, the downward pull of gravity and its effect on joint alignment, and the lack of skilled extremity control may be responsible for the emergence of the "typical synergistic" patterns seen in the extremities.

Upper extremity. With a severe insult to the central nervous system (CNS), the upper extremity has no active movement and the scapula assumes a downwardly rotated position (the superolateral angle moves inferiorly and the inferior angle becomes adducted). With scapular downward rotation, the glenoid fossa orients downward, and the passive locking mechanism of the shoulder joint is lost. The loss of this mechanism, the loss of postural tone, and the stretch on the shoulder capsule result in an inferior humeral subluxation of the hemiplegic shoulder. The humerus hangs by the side in internal rotation and the elbow is extended (Fig. 24-2).

A second pattern develops as the trunk gains more extension control than flexion control. An increase in cervical and lumbar extension becomes evident. The head and neck assume a position of ipsilateral flexion and contralateral rotation. The rib cage loses its abdominal "anchor" and rotates backward. The patterns of muscle return in the scapula and humerus are strongly influenced by this rib cage deviation. The downwardly rotated scapula

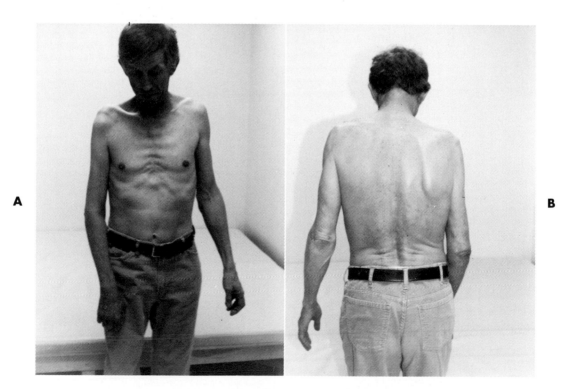

Fig. 24-2. A, Right arm dangles from the client's side. **B,** Scapula is rotated downward.

begins to move superiorly on the thorax, and the humerus hyperextends with internal rotation. This combination of rib cage rotation, humeral hyperextension, and internal rotation allows the humeral head to sublux anteriorly (Fig. 24-3).

Because humans function in the upright position, the battle against gravity is often responsible for compensations. If a person with hemiplegia is in an unsupported sitting position and exhibits the previously described upper extremity pattern and has poor trunk control, the body will try to keep from falling backward by pulling the head forward (turtlelike) and rounding the shoulders. This forward compensation accentuates the internal rotation of the humerus and with the continued development of tightness or muscle activity in the pectorals to give peripheral stabilization, the humerus may be pulled forward across the thorax in horizontal adduction (Fig. 24-4).

The third movement pattern is characterized by abnormal coactivation of the limb muscles. This gives an appearance of "mass" flexion in the hemiplegic upper extremity. The head and neck control in clients with this upper-extremity pattern contains elements of both flexion and extension. The control patterns are not sufficiently integrated to allow selective combinations of movement. The scapula is usually elevated and abducted on the thorax. The head of the humerus is held tightly beneath the acromial process. Although the deltoid and biceps attempt to initiate humeral motion, no dissociation occurs between the humerus and scapula. The upper extremity pattern available as a result of the position of the scapula and humerus is shoulder elevation with humeral abduction, internal rotation, and elbow flexion (Fig. 24-5).

Lower extremity. In the acute stage of recovery or after a severe stroke, when the client's motor control is one of low postural tone and little motor activity, the movement pattern is strongly influenced by gravity. As the client attempts to assume a standing position, the pelvis will either tilt anteriorly or posteriorly, and will list downward on the affected side. As a result of this position and the loss of motor control, the hip and knee will flex. This hip and knee flexion combined with an inability to bear weight on the affected side places the ankle in plantarflexion. Because the calcaneus becomes non-weight-bearing, any weight that is placed on the leg will be borne by the forefoot.

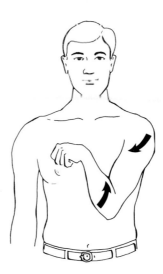

Fig. 24-4. Humeral adduction, internal rotation, elbow flexion, forearm pronation, and wrist and finger flexion.

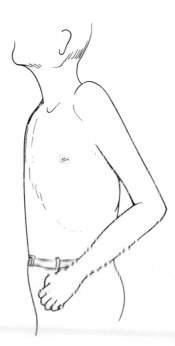

Fig. 24-3. Humerus hyperextends with internal rotation and subluxes anteriorly.

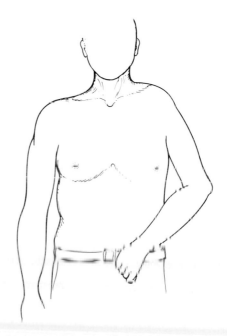

Fig. 24-5. Humerus abducts with internal rotation and subluxes superiorly.

As functional training for activities such as transfers, standing, and walking is begun, clients are often encouraged to put the heel down on the ground. If this is done without correction of the proximal trunk and hip problems, the knee will move into recurvatum and the ankle will continue to move in the direction of plantarflexion.

During recovery or with a less severe stroke, a second pattern becomes evident. Motor return causes an imbalance of control between trunk flexor and extensor muscle groups. Due to brainstem and spinal motor generator control spinal extensor patterns seem more available to the client than spinal flexor patterns. Clients use these extensor patterns unilaterally as they attempt functional activities. In standing, active use of pelvic hikers causes the pelvis to be tilted anteriorly and elevated (listed upward). The knee will extend unless the client has been taught to push the knee into flexion. If the knee moves into recurvatum, the ankle will plantarflex and the talus will move anteriorly relative to the calcaneus. If soft tissue tightness develops, ankle dorsiflexion range is lost.

These clients use this lower trunk extension and pelvic hiking to initiate the swing phase of gait. Pelvic hiking prevents any lower trunk rotational component from occurring. The hip and pelvis become a unit (with no dissociation present), the knee is extended stiffly, and the ankle is "pushed" into plantarflexion as the client attempts to swing the leg forward. As the client tries to clear the foot from the floor, the foot will begin to supinate. Whether the motor pattern is a compensatory response due to lack of lower extremity stabilization or a synergistic response due to lack of regulated control is not known.

At heel strike, the client's forefoot strikes the ground first. When body weight is placed on the foot, the midfoot collapses and weight is transferred back toward the heel. As weight shift during stance is attempted, the knee remains in recurvatum, hip extension is blocked, and the pelvis is not able to initiate a forward diagonal movement pattern. Therefore these clients compensate with either the upper trunk or the unaffected side to initiate weight shift over the stance limb. The pelvis stays elevated, tilted anteriorly, and rotated backwards. The hip is in relative flexion and varying degrees of internal rotation. There is a strong, rigid push of the leg into the ground.

The third movement pattern is characterized by abnormal coactivation of muscles. This gives the appearance of "mass flexion" during movement of the lower extremity. The trunk control in clients with this lower extremity pattern contains elements of both flexor and extensor patterns, but the control of these patterns is not integrated enough to allow selective movement patterns (i.e., lateral flexion, upper or lower trunk rotation, or counter rotation). Such clients recruit flexor patterns during swing phase of gait and extensor patterns during stance. Recruitment of distal motion is used to reinforce the proximal motions, especially during non-weight-bearing movements.

Clients who move with this third control pattern initiate the swing phase with a posterior pelvic tilt. The hip moves into relative flexion, but the most noticeable hip movement is abduction.[62]

Another pattern is often seen in clients whose tone remains low and whose active movement control is minimal. This client will tend to sit more than walk. In the sitting position, the pelvis may roll to a position of posterior tilt. Because the activity level of these clients is low, the pelvis often becomes fixed in this position. When standing, these clients tend to hold the pelvis in this familiar posterior position and will flex the upper trunk forward over the pelvis to counterbalance themselves. The posterior tilt of the pelvis tends to place the hip in a position of relative external rotation.

Although the main tonal movement problems of stroke are spasticity, flaccidity, or combinations thereof, other motor disturbances, such as ataxia, do occur. In ataxia, the main movement problem is one of low, fluctuating tone, which results in instability of the trunk, shoulder, and girdles. The compensation for this central instability is excessive movement of the extremities. Voluntary extremity movements are usually present but uncoordinated. The person with ataxia has low trunk and girdle tone. Occasionally, high tone is present in the extremities as a result of compensatory movements (see Chapter 23).

Sensory disturbances. A cerebrovascular accident with resultant hemiplegia and sensory loss is a devastating event. It is best appreciated by the client. Whereas some clients with hemiplegia experience a total loss of tactile and/or proprioceptive sensation, a majority experience partial impairment, which usually affects the higher discriminatory sensations. A client may feel touch but be unable to localize it, may interpret pressure as light touch, or may be unable to distinguish variations in temperature. Sensory deficit may be so complete as to lead to a loss of recognition of the affected side. The suddenness of the sensory loss leaves the two sides of the body with different sensory messages, thus providing the brain with different forms of sensory feedback. This loss of control and disturbed sensory feedback also results in disturbances of movement in the "good" side of the body.[11]

Even if the client has suffered no loss of sensation but has experienced an abnormality of muscle tone, the abnormal sensations from the spastic muscles and the resultant abnormal feedback provided from the joints result in abnormal sensory feedback from the periphery to the CNS.

Sequential stages of recovery from acute to long-term care

Evolution of recovery process. The evolution of the recovery process from onset to the return to community life can be divided into three stages—acute, active (rehabilitation), and adaptation to personal environment.

The acute state involves the stroke-in-evolution, the completed stroke, or the TIA and the decision whether or not to hospitalize.

The stroke-in-evolution develops gradually with distinct demarcation of the events over 6 to 24 hours. The thrombosis, the most common cause for stroke, results first in ischemia and finally in infarction. Its gradual onset has led researchers to believe that a "cure" may be found for this type of stroke. If ischemic tissue can be treated and saved before infarction occurs, the neurological damage may be reversible. Small hemorrhages also may become a stroke-in-evolution by effusing blood along nerve pathways and by attracting fluid.[44] A completed stroke has a sudden onset and produces distinct nonprogressive symptoms and damage within minutes or hours. In contrast, the TIA has a brief duration of neurological deficit and spontaneous resolution with no residual signs. TIAs vary in number and duration.

The need for hospitalization is decided by the physician. The trend to hospitalize is more common today than years ago.[75] However, a mild stroke or TIA may produce minimal physical-mental symptoms, and the person may not even seek medical help.

Once the stroke is completed the clinical symptoms begin to decrease in severity. Stroke caused by an embolic episode may have symptoms that reverse completely in a few days; more frequently however, improvement takes place very slowly with a marked deficit. The fatality rate is high within the first day but decreases substantially in the following months of recovery.[75]

The Framingham study population has revealed that long-term stroke survivors have a good chance of returning to independent living. The greatest deficit in those persons with hemiplegia who have recovered basic motor skills and who have returned home is in the psychosocial and environmental areas.[27]

Recovery of motor function. Recovery of motor function after a stroke was thought historically to be complete after 3 to 6 months of onset. Research has shown that functional recovery from a stroke can continue for months or years.[5,74]

The initial functional gains following the stroke are attributed to reduction of cerebral edema, absorption of damaged tissue, and improved local vascular flow. However, these factors do not play a role in long-term functional recovery.[5] The brain damage that results from a stroke is thought to be circumvented rather than "repaired" during the process of functional recovery. The CNS reacts to injury with a variety of potentially reparative morphological processes. Presently, the two mechanisms underlying functional recovery after stroke are collateral sprouting and the unmasking of neuropathways.[1,9] Research will continue to provide important insights into the fundamental capabilities of the brain to respond to damage. Therapeutic intervention and retraining of functional skills also improve the functional ability of the person after a stroke.

Predictable traits. The CNS has some predictable traits in response to injury. Because the developing nervous system is more plastic than the adult nervous system, a stroke in an 8-year-old child is usually characterized by good recovery of function. However, a stroke at 80 years of age may be more devastating as a result of poorer functional recovery. Second, the less complete the lesion, the more likely significant recovery will occur. Third, damage to primary motor or sensory pathways is more likely to result in greater functional deficit than is damage to other areas.[47] Clinically, we have found some predictable events after a stroke. Twitchell, in his classic study, first documented the initial loss of voluntary function.[12] Although flaccidity initially exists, there is seldom if ever total flaccidity.[12] He reported both an increase in deep tendon reflexes after 48 hours and the emergence of synergistic patterns of movement. The synergistic movement patterns of the upper extremity and lower extremity have been described in detail by many, including Bobath,[10] Brunnstrom,[13] and Knott and Voss.[35] Although the descriptions at first glance may seem at odds with each other, each is describing the same phenomenon. Semantics, differences in British and American terminology, and the degree of completeness of description cause the confusion. Verbal description of a visual phenomenon often leads to differences in written and spoken communication, yet the visual array or behavioral patterns may be exactly the same.[8]

The severity of the stroke, compensations, and deformity as well as the type of treatment may cause variations in or combinations of these described patterns of movement.

Synergistic patterns do not allow normal functions to occur. Synergistic patterns are not the same as the movement combinations necessary for function. Although it is said that the leg recovers more quickly or better than the arm, a leg that is bound by an extensor synergy and that is as "rigid as a pillar" during gait has not recovered quicker and/or better than an arm that is flexed and held across the chest and that can only grasp in a gross pattern with no ability to release.[48]

Although the relationship of voluntary movement to spasticity has not been clearly defined, clinical evidence demonstrates that as voluntary function increases, the dependence on synergistic movement decreases and spasticity decreases.[64] Twitchell concluded that at the point of complete motor recovery, the only remaining deficit may be an increased tendency to fatigue.[13]

With the knowledge that the CNS is capable of reacting to injury with a variety of morphological processes, we should no longer view the effect of a stroke as a negative event. The brain immediately institutes neuromechanisms that reconstitute normal function. Therapy should emphasize normality through long-term events and direct treatment goals and should attempt to achieve the highest level of function by concentrating on the quality, not the quantity, of recovery.

Medical management and pharmacological considerations

Acute medical care

Thrombosis and TIAs. Although infarcted tissue cannot be restored presently, medical management of the acute stroke from thrombosis or TIA is geared toward restoring the cerebral circulation as quickly as possible to prevent ischemic tissue from becoming infarcted tissue. Cerebral circulation is maintained by preventing upright posture for the first few days, avoiding dependency in the systemic circulation, maintaining blood pressure, and correcting anemia.

Anticoagulant drugs may prevent TIAs and may stop a stroke-in-evolution. Before anticoagulant drugs are used, an accurate differential diagnosis is necessary because of the danger of excessive bleeding if hemorrhage is present. Heparin is often used in the early stage of the stroke, and warfarin (Coumadin) is commonly used in the months following the stroke. Cerebral edema, if present, is managed pharmacologically during the first few days. Antiplatelet drugs such as aspirin, dipyridamole (Persantine), and sulphin pyrazone (Anturane) are being used, and their effects are being studied as a means to prevent clotting by decreasing platelet "stickiness."[1]

Surgical treatment, thromboendarterectomy, or grafting are used when TIAs are the result of arterial plaques. Areas accessible and suitable for surgery include the carotid sinus and the common carotid, innominant, and subclavian arteries. Although surgery and anticoagulant therapy is used in TIA, Adams and Victor[1] extensively reviewed the wide divergence of opinions. For clients who have had a stroke yet recovered quickly and well, medical care focuses on prevention. Prevention usually includes maintaining blood pressure and blood flow, monitoring hypotensive agents (if given), and avoiding oversedation, especially for sleep, to prevent cerebral ischemia.

Embolic infarction. Management of embolic infarction is similar to that of thrombotic infarction. The primary emphasis is on prevention. Long-term anticoagulant therapy is effective in preventing embolic infarction in clients with cardiac problems such as atrial fibrillation, myocardial infarction (MI), and valve prostheses. The diagnostic use of CT scans is important in anticoagulant therapy to rule out hemorrhage after the infarct.

Hypertensive hemorrhage. Medical procedures for hypertensive hemorrhage parallel those for thrombosis and embolus. Surgical removal of the clot and lowering of the systemic blood pressure to decrease hemorrhage have generally not been helpful. Again, the preventive use of antihypertensive drugs in clients with essential hypertension is the soundest medical management available.[1]

Ruptured aneurysm. Comatose clients are not good candidates for surgery. However, if the client survives the first few days and if the state of consciousness improves, surgical intervention whether extracranial or intracranial is the treatment of choice. Medical treatment consists of lowering arterial blood pressures. Bed rest for 4 to 6 weeks with all forms of exertion avoided is prescribed. Antiseizure medication may be used. Often a systemic antifibrinolysin is given to impede lysis of the clot at the site of rupture.

Vasospasm, resulting in severe motor dysfunction, is present with the use of drugs such as reserpine (Serpasil) and kanamycin (Kantrex).

Regardless of the cause of the stroke, comatose stroke clients are managed by (1) treatment of shock; (2) maintenance of clear airway and oxygen flow; (3) measurement of arterial blood gases, blood analysis, CT scan, and spinal tap; (4) control of seizures; and (5) gastric tube feeding (if coma is prolonged). Hypertensive hemorrhage is one of the most common vascular causes of coma.[72]

Medical management of associated problems with hemiplegia

Hypertonicity. **Hypertonicity** and its treatment present a major medical problem because there are several types of hypertonicity and because the relationship between hypertonicity and movement has not been universally accepted. Various pharmacological, surgical, and physical means have been used to decrease hypertonicity and therefore ameliorate the problems it causes. The pharmacological and surgical means are examined here, and the physical treatment is discussed later.

Three types of drugs are currently being used to counter the effects of hypertonicity. Centrally acting drugs (barbiturates and tranquilizers) have been used to depress the lateral reticular formation and thus its facilitory action on the gamma motor neurons. This form of drug is used widely to treat spasticity, even though the greatest disadvantage of centrally acting drugs is the fact they depress the entire CNS. Drowsiness and lethargy often result.

Peripherally acting drugs also have been used to block a specific link in the gamma group. Procaine blocks selectively inhibit the small gamma motor fibers, resulting in a relaxation of intrafusal fibers. The effect of procaine blocks is transient. Intramuscular neurolysis with the injection of 5% to 7% phenol has been used to destroy the small intramuscular mixed nerve branches.[18] Phenol blocks relieve hypertonicity and improve function, especially when followed by an intensive course of therapy.[57] They can provide relief from 2 to 12 months, and their effects have been documented to last as long as 3 years.[18,57] Disadvantages of phenol use include its toxicity to tissue and the complications of pain that occasionally result.

Dantrolene sodium has been used recently to interrupt the excitation-contraction mechanism of skeletal muscles. Trials have shown that it has reduced spasticity in 60% to 80% of clients while improving function in 40% of these clients. The side effects—drowsiness, weakness, and fatigue—can be decreased through gradation of dosage. Serious side effects, including hepatotoxicity, precipitation of seizures, and lymphocytic lymphoma, have been reported when the drug has been used in high dosages over a long time.[18]

The surgical treatment of spasticity through tenotomy or neurectomy has been considered when all other treatments fail, and it has been carried out for the purposes of correcting deformity, especially of a hand or foot, and improving function. A peripheral nerve block is often used as a diagnostic tool to evaluate the effect of surgical treatment. If anatomical or functional gains are made through a temporary nerve block, considerations are given for surgical release. In the client with hemiplegia, the most common surgical sites include the hip adductors, ankle plantar flexors, and toe, wrist, and finger flexors.

Botulinum toxin A (Botox) has been used to decrease the effects of hypertonicity on the quality of movement in hemiplegia.[17,68] Local injection of the toxin into spastic muscles produces selective weakness by interfering with the uptake of acetylcholine by the motor endplate. The effect of the toxin is temporary, depends on the amount injected, and to this date is associated with minimal side effects.

Respiratory involvement. Fatigue is a major problem for the person with hemiplegia. This fatigability, which interferes with everyday life processes and active rehabilitation, is attributed to respiratory insufficiency resulting from paralysis of one side of the thorax. Haas and others[29] studied respiratory function and hemiplegia and found decreased lung volume and mechanical performance of the thorax to be significant factors, in addition to abnormal pulmonary diffusing capacity. Clients with hemiplegia consume 50% more oxygen while walking slowly (regardless of the presence or absence of orthotic devises) than subjects without hemiplegia.[29] The decreased respiratory output and the increased oxygen demand that result from abnormal movement patterns are responsible for early fatigue in persons with hemiplegia. Treatment objectives and techniques must reflect the understanding of this respiratory problem. The use of standard respiratory functions as an objective measure of the efficacy of treatment techniques must not be overlooked.

> **EXAMPLE:** Clients with left hemiplegia initially ambulate 5 to 20 feet with no ability to accept or bear weight on the left side.
> *Treatment objective:* To facilitate weight acceptance onto left hip during standing and walking.
> *Results:* Initial oxygen consumption 50% greater than normal; following treatment, oxygen consumption improved to 30% greater than normal.
> *Assessment:* Gait deviations may not have changed dramatically, but the ability to shift weight onto the left hip did improve; the rate of oxygen consumption approached normal.
> *Conclusion:* The functional ability of the client improved.

Common breathing pattern problems of the person with hemiplegia include clavicular breathing, a "breathy" quality of exhalation, inability to switch from oral to nasal breathing, and asymmetrical trunk control and tone.

Trauma. If the hemiplegic client is not trained in weight shifting and weight bearing to both sides, poor balance and resultant falls will occur.[51] Protective mechanisms may not be present, and the person often falls to the affected side. Frequent fractures include the humerus and femur. Treatment of femoral fractures is complicated by spasticity in the hip musculature. In addition to the loss of balance and protective mechanisms, the development of osteoporosis from disuse is a precipitating factor for fractures as a result of falls.[49]

Thrombophlebitis. Thrombophlebitis may occur in the early stages of rehabilitation. Vascular changes may have been present before the stroke, and they can be aggravated by the inactivity and dependent postures of the extremities.

Reflex sympathetic dystrophy. Medical treatment of reflex sympathetic dystrophy includes the use of chemical sympathetic blocks and oral or intramuscular steroids. The use of blocks and steroids often stops the burning pain. The length of time of the relief varies from client to client. Adverse reactions occur about 20% of the time.[14]

Pain. The pharmacological management of pain resulting from hemiplegia includes the use of corticosteroids. (For additional information regarding pain and its management see Chapter 31.)

EVALUATION PROCEDURES
General evaluation

Following or during the evolution of a stroke, a thorough medical examination is conducted; all systems are surveyed, with emphasis placed on the level of consciousness, mental, affective, and emotional states, cranial nerves, communication, perceptual ability, sensation, and motor function.

Scales of varying types are used to measure the client's level of consciousness, to assess the initial severity of brain damage, and to prognosticate recovery curves. The Glasgow Coma Scale, devised by Teasdale and Jennett[72] in collaboration with Plum, has been used for nontraumatic comas caused by stroke and cardiac disease. This scale records motor responses to pain, verbal responses to auditory and visual clues, and eye opening; it assigns numerical values according to graded scales.[75] Plum and Caronna[58] and Levy and others[41] have also established criteria for correlating clinical signs of coma with prognosis.

The standard descriptions of level of consciousness—normal, semistupor, stupor, deep stupor, semicoma, coma, deep coma—are categorized by objective medical data but often leave a gap in the understanding of how the client functions in life.[72] This gap was closed by the creation of a scale, "Levels of Cognitive Functioning," devised at Rancho Los Amigos Hospital. This behavioral rating scale is not a test of cognitive skill but an observational rating of the client's ability to process information.[43]

The history portion of the neurological evaluation leads to an assessment of the mental, emotional, and affective state. The client's ability to describe the illness gives information on memory, orientation to time and place, the ability to express ideas, and judgment. If the examiner suspects a particular problem, a more thorough review is undertaken of the higher cortical function: serial subtraction, repetition of digits, and recall of objects or names. Emotional or behavioral traits are also documented. Clients with right hemiplegia may be cautious and disorganized in solving a given task, and clients with left hemiplegia tend to be fast and impulsive and seemingly unaware of the deficits present. These different response patterns stem from hemispheric involvement and prior hemispheric specialization. Loss of emotional control often exists after a stroke. Crying is a common problem. Although excessive, inappropriate, or uncontrollable crying is usually a result of brain damage and a sign of emotional lability, crying can also be an expression of sadness as a result of depression. This difference is distinguishable by the ease with which the crying can be stopped (see Chapter 8). Other signs of emotional lability in persons with hemiplegia from stroke include inappropriate laughter or anger.

A general evaluation of communication disorders is noted while taking the history. Cerebral disorder resulting from infarct or hemorrhage can produce a loss of production or comprehension of the spoken word, the written word, or both. Specific evaluation of aphasias and dysarthrias can be found in Chapter 26. The therapist should be familiar with all types of communication disorders and with alternate modes of communication to establish a good client interrelationship. The interrelationship between the therapist and client is critical for the retraining of the sensory, motor, and perceptual problems of hemiplegia.

Thorough cranial nerve evaluation is necessary in hemiplegia because a deficit of a particular cranial nerve helps to determine the exact size and location of the infarct or hemorrhage. In hemiplegia, it is imperative to check for visual field deficits, pupil signs, ocular movements, facial sensation and weakness, labyrinthine and auditory function, and laryngeal and pharyngeal function.

Standard areas of reflex testing include the triceps, biceps, supinator, quadriceps, and gastrocnemius muscles. According to Adams,[1] there are four plantar reflex responses: (1) avoidance—quick, (2) spinal flexion—slow, (3) Babinski—toe grasp, and (4) positive support.

Perceptual deficits in clients with hemiplegia are complex and are intimately linked to the sensorimotor deficit. Normal development has shown us that the acquisition of motor function is related to perceptual function.[4]

> **EXAMPLE:** In the sitting position, a 6- to 8-month-old child learns to hold midline with his or her trunk and then explores reaching up, reaching down, reaching from side to side, and reaching behind. As motor function allows exploration of the space around midline, the child's perception of midline up, down, side, front, and back is established.
>
> Sensory integration theory has begun to establish norms and objective data for testing and documenting perceptual deficits in children. Presently, norms and testing procedures for adults have not been standardized, but perceptual deficits have been identified in clients with hemiplegia. Common perceptual deficits found in left and right brain damage can be found in the accompanying box.

Perceptual retraining without standardized norms for the deficit is at best difficult. The soundest course presently available appears to be one that relates perceptual and motor learning rather than retraining perception in isolation (see Chapters 11 and 27).

Perceptual deficits in CNS dysfunction

Left hemiparesis: right hemisphere—general spatial-global deficits

Visual-perceptual deficits
  Hand-eye coordination
  Figure-ground discrimination
  Spatial relationships
  Position in space
  Form constancy
Behavioral and intellectual deficits
  Poor judgment, unrealistic behavior
  Denial of disability
  Inability to abstract
  Rigidity of thought
  Disturbances in body image and body scheme
  Impairment of ability to self-correct
  Difficulty retaining information
  Distortion of time concepts
  Tendency to see the whole and not individual steps
  Affect lability
  Feelings of persecution
  Irritability, confusion
  Distraction by verbalization
  Short attention span
  Appearance of lethargy
  Fluctuation in performance
  Disturbances in relative size and distance of objects

Right hemiparesis: left hemisphere—general language and temporal ordering deficits

Apraxia
  Motor
  Ideational
Behavioral and intellectual deficits
  Difficulty initiating tasks
  Sequencing deficits
  Processing delays
  Directionality deficits
  Low frustration levels
  Verbal and manual perseveration
  Rapid performance of movement or activity
  Compulsive behavior
  Extreme distractability

Traditional sensory testing is used to assess sensory deficits in the adult with hemiplegia, that is, light touch, deep pressure, kinesthesia, proprioception, pain, temperature, graph esthesia, two-point discrimination, appreciation of texture and size, and vibration. A comparison of the differences in the two sides of the body and qualitative as well as quantitative measurements are important features of sensory testing in clients with hemiplegia. Sensory testing is difficult because it relies on the client's interpretation of the sensation, the client's general awareness and suggestibility, as well as the client's ability to communicate a response to each test item.

The presence and quality of sensory loss must be considered during the process of reeducating motor control. Sherrington established the principle of interdependence of sensation and movement; current researchers have refined the concept and hypothesize that sensation modifies ongoing movement by providing feedforward, feedback, and corollary discharge; yet sensation is not an absolute prerequisite for movement.[12,71] Motor learning can occur in the absence of sensation through the learning of a "set," which is an equilibrium point between agonist and antagonist.[8] Although clinical investigations have correlated severe sensory loss with poor prognosis for motor function, the reason for this correlation may not be a cause-and-effect relationship but rather the state of the art of therapy. On the other hand, directing therapy only at movement will not give functional results if sensory preparation is not included. The ability to tolerate and appreciate light touch and pressure is related to the ability to tolerate weight bearing, to conform to objects, and to explore the environment.

Motor system evaluation

An evaluation of motor behavior can be broken down into three distinct but interrelated parts. The first part is an assessment of movement possibilities, postural mechanisms, and functional activities. The second part is an assessment of joint function, including pain. The third is an assessment of the sensory systems. This systematic evaluation of the client's motor capabilities must be conducted before beginning to plan a treatment program. Because human beings are motor driven creatures who achieve functional activity through movement, a motor system evaluation must be carried out with function in mind.

Assessment of movement possibilities

Active movement. When assessing active movement patterns in the trunk and the upper and lower extremities, the therapist should be aware not only of whether the activity can be initiated or accomplished, but of how the movement is carried out. The quality of the movement pattern indicates which muscles are functioning and which are not. Active movement patterns should be noted by joints and by position (supine, side-lying, sitting, and standing) because the effect of gravity and reflexes will influence the control of movement during changes of position.

> **EXAMPLE:** Active movement patterns—sitting, shoulder flexion to 60 degrees, downward rotation of the scapula, and internal rotation of the humerus.
> For the function of forward reach the missing components would be upward rotation and protraction of the scapula and external rotation of the humerus.
> If the hemiplegic client is asked to perform a functional activity that requires use of components he or she does not have control of, a compensation will occur.
> **EXAMPLE:** The client in the previous example cannot perform the function of forward reach. He or she will compensate for a lack of forward reach by recruiting shoulder elevators or by side bending away from the affected side, which gives the appearance of greater forward flexion and reach. If allowed to occur repeatedly, compen-

sations for function will become habits, and habits will eventually lead to contractures. These contractures have the potential to become a fixed deformity. The presence of a fixed joint deformity rules out the possibility of facilitating new functional movement patterns.

The assessment of active movement in hemiplegia is commonly documented by therapists through the use of the synergistic stages as outlined by Brunnstrom[13] or by Bobath's long evaluation form, which relates postural abilities (righting, equilibrium, protection) to selective movement activities.[10] Each of these assessment methods lacks a numerical score to standardize the postural and motor performance of hemiplegic clients. Numerical rating scales for evaluating neuromotor performances are being devised.[23]

Postural mechanisms. The loss of postural control (**postural instability**) includes the loss of trunk control, an alteration in the tonal state of body musculature, and a loss of the ability to integrate trunk and limb movements into functional tasks.

Trunk control. Trunk control allows us to change our body position in space, to control movements against the constant pull of gravity, and to change and control our body position for balance and function while we are upright. Trunk control allows us to shift our weight to free our extremities for function. For some functional movements, such as sitting, trunk control keeps the upper and lower trunk stable as we shift our weight and balance. For other tasks, such as reaching across midline, the upper trunk must be rotating, with the reaching arm, on a relatively stable lower trunk.

The demands of trunk control increase with the complexity of the task. At least four levels of trunk control can be described:

Level I: Experiencing the upright posture. This is the most basic level of postural control and has an important sensory/perceptual component.

Level II: Reestablishment of trunk movements. The trunk moves in three planes and can initiate movement in these planes from either the upper trunk or the lower trunk.

    Flexion/extension—upper trunk initiated
            —lower trunk initiated
    Lateral flexion —upper trunk initiated
            —lower trunk initiated
    Rotation   —upper trunk initiated—flexion
            —extension
            —lower trunk initiated—flexion
            —extension
    Counterrotation

Level III: Adapting to extremity movement. This level of control allows the trunk to remain stable yet move in response to the task of reaching around and away from midline.

Level IV: Power production. This is the highest level of trunk control. The movement and control of the trunk is used to increase the power production of the extremities for propulsive activities such as running, jumping, throwing, hitting, and rowing.

In our clients with hemiplegia, the loss of trunk control results in poor balance and a decreased ability to perform functional activities. The lesion may produce movement deficits related to weakness, improper sequencing of muscles, and altered timing of muscle contraction. Asymmetries, poor joint alignment, and soft tissue changes may appear as secondary problems that must be addressed in treatment along with the primary movement deficits.

Tone. The evaluation of postural mechanisms must always include an assessment of tone. Over the years, the great physiologists have split into two camps over the definition of tone. During the first half of the century, tone was thought of as postural reflexes. In the 1950s the concept of tone was thought of as a state of light excitation or a state of preparedness.[25] Granit[26] recently encouraged us to think of the relatedness of both these views. He felt that the same spinal organization is mobilized by the basal ganglia to produce *both* manifestations of tone, a state of preparedness and the postural reflexes. Today it is known that the cerebellum plays a crucial component over the regulation of tone (see Chapter 23).

It is heartening to hear such discussions occurring among physiologists, because therapists are also questioned about their notations of and changes in tone, and they often have

no objectively derived standard clinical system for quickly measuring tone. The debate over tone continues, but clients with CNS dysfunction clinically display changes of muscle tone that the therapist must identify.

The first noticeable change in tone is the change from the premorbid state. Clients in the acute phase of hemiplegia all exhibit, for varying periods of time, a lower than normal tonal state. After the first 24 hours postinjury, the client with hemiplegia begins to become more alert and more active. Because the client has moved before, he or she is motivated to move and will use whatever movement patterns are available. In the severe stroke, there is only one side to use for movement. Moving with half the body is hard, stressful work, and with that slow, laborious effort comes an increase in tone. The hemiplegic client's first automatic movement response is often one of primitive trunk extension on the affected side (a C curve, concavity to the affected side) and a weight shift to the unaffected side (Fig. 24-6).

A universally satisfactory definition of "tone" is hard to come by. For therapists retraining motor function in clients with CNS dysfunction, it is important to distinguish between postural tone and muscle tone. Postural tone is tone that is "high" enough to keep the body from collapsing into gravity, but "low" enough to allow the body to move against gravity. It is influenced by the input from the corticospinal tracts, the vestibular system, the alpha and gamma systems, and peripheral-tactile and proprioceptive receptors.[20] Normal postural tone allows a constant interplay between the various muscle groups in the body and imparts a constant readiness to move and to react to changes in the environment (internal and external). It provides us with an ability to adjust automatically and continuously to movements. These adjustments provide the proximal fixation necessary to hold a given posture against gravity while allowing voluntary and selective movements to be superimposed without conscious or excessive effort. Fig. 24-7 illustrates this concept in diagrammatical form.

Muscle tone is defined as the passive resistance derived from the series and parallel elastic elements of a muscle. Although controversy now exists (see Chapter 3), hypertonicity (or increased muscle tone) is classically defined as

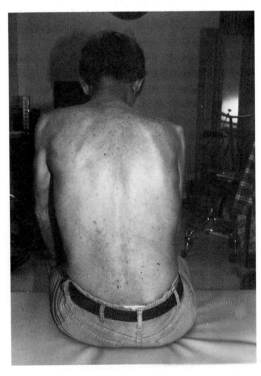

Fig. 24-6. This client with a right hemiplegia shows the tendency to shift weight to the unaffected side and the beginnings of a C curve of the spine with the concavity to the affected side.

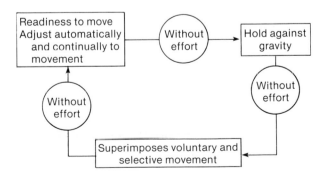

Fig. 24-7. Model for normal postural tone.

increased resistance to passive stretch. Severe hypertonicity makes coordinated movements impossible.[59] Moderate hypertonicity can be defined clinically when movements are possible but characterized by great effort, slow velocity, and abnormal coordination. Slight hypertonicity allows gross movement patterns to occur with smooth coordination, but combined, selective movement patterns will be incoordinated or not possible.[10]

Differences in tonal states lower than normal are also present in hemiplegia. The "floppy," or "almost zero," state is characterized by a feeling of total "dead weight" upon passive lifting. A limb with low tone feels heavy, but some "following" of passive movement patterns can be detected. When assessing and treating movement disorders, therapists should be aware of changes in both postural tone and muscle tone.

Righting and equilibrium reactions. Righting reactions enable a person to change position, such as rolling, rising from a lying position, and moving from a sitting to a standing position. The righting reactions are mediated by sensory receptors and begin to develop at birth. The five groups of righting reactions are:

1. Labyrinthine righting on the head
2. Body righting acting on the head
3. Neck righting
4. Body righting acting on the body
5. Optical righting

Equilibrium reactions develop as we become upright creatures, that is, as we are placed in a sitting or standing position. Equilibrium reactions help us to maintain or regain our balance by keeping the center of gravity within the base of support. Both the trunk and limbs are involved with equilibrium. Equilibrium reactions are often referred to as the body's first line of defense against falling. They occur when the body has a chance of winning the battle against gravity. If equilibrium reactions cannot preserve balance, the second line of defense emerges: protective reactions. One of the best known protective responses in the arm is the "parachute reaction." Protective responses in the leg include hopping, staggering, or stepping.

The maintenance of balance or posture involves many postural reactions besides righting and equilibrium. In fact it is most difficult to quantify where a righting reaction stops and where an equilibrium reaction begins. Antigravity control is an integral part of all skilled movement. The antigravity mechanism, first manifested as a supporting reaction, allows us to support the weight of our body against gravity. Righting reactions and equilibrium reactions supplement this to allow us to move and stay upright. The postural fixation of varying parts of the body (the head on the trunk, the trunk on the pelvis, the shoulder girdle on the trunk) is maintained so that a movement can be made elsewhere while balance is maintained. This phenomenon has also been called "weight shift," "body sway," and "mobility superimposed on stability."

These baseline postural reactions must be evaluated following a stroke. For righting reactions to occur, rotation must be available and the ability to shift weight must be present. Rotation, a balance between flexors and extensors, occurs naturally at the extremes of pure lateral motion. The ability to shift weight in straight planes and in diagonal planes assumes the ability to accept and bear weight. Therefore to assess postural reactions, therapists must focus on available range, weight shift, and movement control.

For the person with a stroke, the presence of righting and equilibrium reaction varies according to the degree of abnormal tone and the amount of active movement present. As with head injury and cerebral palsy, a severe stroke can cause an absence of a righting reaction, but with a mild stroke, righting reactions are present but decreased in quality and timing and/or delayed. Although only one side of the body seems impaired, the unaffected side of the body often loses the ability to normally right itself—in part because the inability of the affected side to accept and bear weight.

Hemiplegic clients with decreased or absent righting reactions move slowly and often stay in one position for uncomfortably long periods of time. When they do move, their movement is not automatic and smooth but willed, cautious, and jerky. Without righting reactions, the person with a hemiplegia thinks at a conscious level about how he or she will change position and has learned the one or two patterns of movement that are safe. If any unexpected change in the environment or learned patterns occurs, he or she will no longer be safe and may stumble or fall.

Righting reactions can be assessed in the person with hemiplegia. The following outline specifies positions and functional patterns:

1. Supine position
   a. Rolling
2. Side-lying position (forearm and extended arm support)
   a. Moving into the sitting position from side-lying position*
   b. Moving into the side-lying position from a sitting position*
3. Sitting position
   a. Transferring to the left and right
   b. Sitting position to the standing position
      (1) Bilateral—moving from a chair to a standing position
      (2) Unilateral—moving from a kneeling position to a half kneel to a standing position

---

* Assessing righting reactions from both of these functional patterns is necessary because motor control of the upper body may be different from that of the lower body and thus affect the presence and/or quality of the reaction.

4. Standing position
   a. Right step to a stance
   b. Left step to a stance

Care should be taken to observe reactions of the head, neck, and trunk. When righting reactions are absent or diminished, the following questions should be addressed:

1. Is range of motion available?
2. Can the person accept some weight on each side?
3. Can the person bear full weight on each side?
4. Can the person shift weight to each side?
5. How does the person shift weight?

When assessing equilibrium or balance reactions in the client with hemiplegia, the therapist must remember the distinction between equilibrium reactions and protective reactions. Equilibrium reactions should be assessed while slowly moving either the limb or trunk away from the base of support. The size of the base of support, the size of the supporting surface, and the range of joint movement of the joint supporting the body weight as well as the evaluator's handling skills will affect the quality and the timing of the reaction (Fig. 24-8). Refer to Chapter 28 for additional information on balance.

Protective reactions can be tested in the prone position if the supporting surface is tilted and in the sitting, kneeling, half kneeling, and standing positions. Protective reactions are elicited by moving the person forward, backward, downward, and/or sideways quickly. Protective reaction consists of two parts—extension of the limb and acceptance of weight on the supporting part.

Functional activities. Skilled functional activity is performed against a background of these postural reactions. The person with hemiplegia has a disturbance of the postural mechanism that affects the ability to perform functional skills in a normal fashion. If the hemiplegic side is left untreated or untrained in normal movement, the person with a hemiplegia can become adept at solving most functional tasks using only the sound side of the body. However, exclusive use of one side of the body for function results in asymmetry, poor balance, and an eventual deterioration of function of the unaffected side. This deterioration results from excessive stress and weight bearing and the marked exaggeration of movement patterns required to balance and simultaneously function with only one side of the body. Overcompensation is one reason for the abnormal movements seen on the unaffected side of hemiplegic clients.

Functional movement. To retrain motor function appropriately, it is necessary to evaluate motor function not only quantitatively but qualitatively. To assess how a functional activity is performed, it is important to measure the active movement components, the changes in tone, the available range, the ability to shift weight, and the need for adaptive devices.

Active movement components are identified descriptively at every joint involved. Limitation of degrees of movement and the movement's relations to gravity are documented. The movement components that are necessary for function to occur can then be assessed.

> **EXAMPLE:** If in a sitting position, a person can move the humerus to 60 degrees of shoulder flexion only with abduction and internal rotation, the missing components of the *shoulder* for the function of finger feeding would be: shoulder external rotation, protraction, forward flexion, and neutral abduction/adduction.

In CNS lesions, tonal changes occur with stress, effort, fear, or change of position. Documentation of the degree and type of tonal change at specific points in a functional activity will aid treatment planning.

> **EXAMPLE:** Mrs. J. rises from a chair to a standing position; pushing down an armrest with the sound hand causes the involved leg to shoot out in an extensor pattern, which causes the pelvis and trunk to push back into the chair. Problem: The excessive effort and stress of trying to rise from the chair pushing with one hand increases the

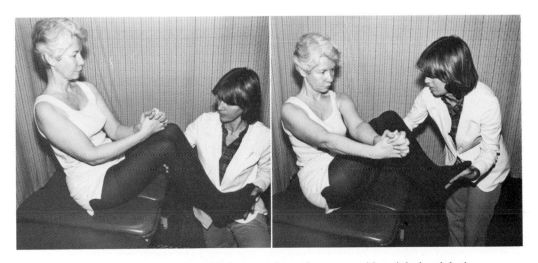

Fig. 24-8. Assessment of equilibrium reactions of a person with a right hemiplegia.

tone in the trunk and pelvic girdle, thus decreasing the chance of performing the function of rising from the chair independently.

The ability to shift and bear weight onto each side determines whether a functional activity can be performed and how it is performed.[39] To assess the ability to bear weight, the therapist can place a person with hemiplegia in the desired position, and the cocontraction pattern necessary to actively maintain the desired position can then be assessed.

EXAMPLE: To assess the ability of a client's hip to bear weight in the sitting position, the client's pelvis can be controlled and the trunk can be aligned over the hip. As the therapist's hands are removed, the question asked is, "Are the hip muscles working enough to maintain unilateral weight bearing?" Ability to shift weight can be noted both passively, with the therapist moving the client's body through the weight shift, and actively, with the client moving through the desired pattern.

If assistive devices are used, the following questions should be asked:

1. Is the device always used? If not, when is it used?
2. How is the device used?
3. Could the device be used in another fashion that would foster symmetry and weight bearing on the affected side?

When evaluating functional activities, three phases of the movement pattern can be assessed. The first phase is the initiation of the act, which includes the initial weight shift and the establishment of antigravity control. The transition phase, the second phase, represents the point in the functional activity at which there is a switch in the muscle groups that provide antigravity control. The third phase is the completion of the activity, involving a final weight shift and the ability to maintain postural control.

Passive range of motion. Passive range of motion (ROM) is important in the assessment of hemiplegia because the knowledge of the degree of movement available at a joint will help the therapist decide whether a normal movement pattern is possible. True, limited, passive range points to either a contracture or deformity. Treatment plans and goals for contracture and deformity are very different from treatment plans to correct compensatory movements. With normal ROM, normal movement patterns can be experienced independently or with assistance. Preferred posturing exhibited by the person with hemiplegia can be noted in the category of passive range. Some people with hemiplegia hold their head laterally flexed to the sound side, and some hold their head laterally flexed to the involved side. ROM may be normal initially, but as a result of the preferred "hold" of a position, it may at a later date cause loss of joint motion and eventually result in a contracture.

The presence of pain is detrimental to any movement patterns. A person with a hemiplegia should not be allowed to experience joint pain. Pain, if present, must be accurately assessed by answering the following questions:

1. Where is the pain? Pinpoint the location.
2. When does the pain occur?
3. What type of pain? Pins and needles, sharp, dull, stabbing?
4. How does pain relate to the joint or to the adjacent joints? Are there joint limitations?
5. How does active movement relate to pain?
6. What is the tone in the body part experiencing pain?

For an in-depth discussion of the topic of pain management, see Chapter 31.

Motor evaluation forms

The previous information, once gathered, can be placed on an evaluation form in many ways. Every medical institution seems to have its own evaluation form and its own system of recording data. At one hospital the documentation of pain may be descriptive, and at another it may be numerical. Active movement at the shoulder joint may be described in one institution in terms of percentages of synergistic stages, at another institution by a narrative of degrees and planes of movement, and at still another by functional outcomes of shoulder movement. It is important to keep in mind the substance of the evaluative material, not the form in which it is described. A detailed motor evaluation form is necessary for the establishment of realistic goals and for subsequent treatment planning, but the specific form depends on both the needs of the specific clinical setting and on the clinician's choice.

ESTABLISHING REALISTIC GOALS
Process

The process of establishing realistic goals for functional recovery for the person with hemiplegia is difficult because of the incomplete knowledge of underlying neurophysiological repair mechanisms in the CNS. The brain is incapable of myotactic regeneration, and it is probably incapable of axonal regrowth as occurs in peripheral nerves. Currently accepted "theories" that explain the reasons for long- and short-term recovery in CNS deficits include renewed circulation, decreased edema, collateral sprouting, and unmasking. Despite existing and changing reasons for neuroplasticity, we know from clinical experience that functional recovery can occur for months or years after a stroke. Although some persons recover spontaneously from hemiplegia, in those persons with a residual deficit, rehabilitation offers the most effective means to reestablish a quality life.[3]

Although established means to restore functional movement deficits exist, cognitive and emotional barriers, such as the inability to learn or retain information, disoriented integrative skills, and disoriented emotional behavior, may interfere with the recovery process. With this in mind, we can begin to examine the needs of the person with hemiplegia. The key to establishing realistic goals lies in the accurate

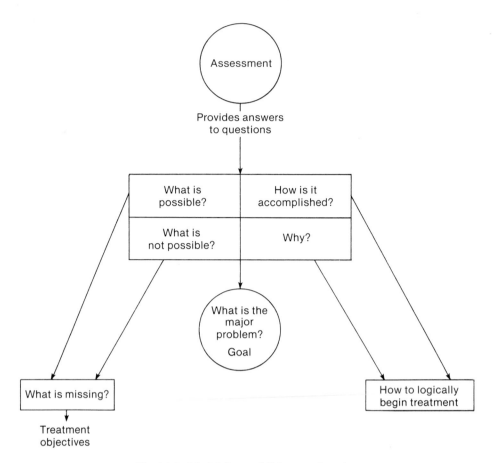

Fig. 24-9. Model for establishment of goals.

collection and interpretation of data from the assessment of the client. Fig. 24-9 presents a model that illustrates a framework for establishing realistic goals.

Recognizing needs

The information obtained from the total evaluation provides the basis for answers to the questions: What movements and functions are possible? What movements and functions are not possible? By understanding the movement components a person with hemiplegia uses to move, the therapist can answer the question: What movement components are missing? The answer to this question becomes the objective for treatment. *How* the *possible* is accomplished and *why* the *impossible* exists will provide logical suggestions for treatment procedures. *How* and *why* will give answers that ensure quality in treatment. A person with hemiplegia needs to know not only how to roll, stand, or walk but the safest and most efficient way to roll, stand, and walk. *Safest* ensures the closest to normal biomechanical and *efficient* means—the closest to symmetry and bilaterality.

The answer to the question: "What is the major problem?" provides the therapist with a *short-term goal*. The *major problem* of a person with a hemiplegia is related to what is possible and what is not possible. A realistic

short-term goal should be the result of a change the therapist can produce in one or two treatment sessions that helps to eliminate or ameliorate the major problem. The *long-term goal* will be a functional skill that is directly linked through movement components to the short-term goal.

EXAMPLE: In the client with left hemiplegia, *What is possible?* The client sits unsupported and rises to a stand with assistance. *How?* With weight on the right side, he or she pushes up to a stand with the right hand, the left leg shoots out into extension, the trunk pushes back in the chair, and the head is in a forward position. *What is not possible?* Symmetrical sitting, symmetrical rise to a stand, and normal tonal situation in the left leg during rise to a stand is not possible. *Why?* Client cannot bear weight on left leg in sitting or standing position. *Why?* Because of lack of left hip control, lack of pelvic girdle control, lack of appropriate trunk reactions, and because spasticity rises dramatically with effort. *What is missing?* The ability to shift and bear weight on the left side.

Treatment objective: Facilitate weight shift and weight bearing to both sides, especially to the left.

Logically begin treatment

1. Weight on left side.
   a. Side-lying position—function rolling.
   b. Sitting—assisted weight shift to both sides.
2. Increase motor control of the left hip.
   a. See 1 above.
   b. Lateral and diagonal weight shifts in sitting position with assistance.

Table 24-3. Goals for the three recovery phases

Acute	Completed	Long-term
Maintain mobility	Maintain mobility Teach client	→
Give feeling of normal movement patterns	Begin to reproduce normal movement patterns	Move as normally as possible
Begin establishing symmetry in posture and movement	Allow symmetry to occur	Provide continued use of symmetry
Provide normal sensory input	→	→
Bedside care	Living skills	Maximal level of independence
Monitor changes in tonal states	Teach client to be aware of changes in tone and how to influence it	→

→, Indicates continuation of same goal.

    c. Initiating the rise to a stand with assistance with weight equally distributed on both lower extremities.

Major problem: The ability to bear weight and shift weight onto the left hip in the sitting position and in *coming* to a stand.

Short-term goal: Shift weight onto left and right hips with appropriate trunk elongation and shortening.

Long-term goal: Shift weight to both sides while standing, and bear weight on the left side in the left step stance and in the right step stance.

Goals for recovery phases

Two distinct types of goals may be established for a client with hemiplegia: functional goals and treatment goals. Functional goals are based on the needs and desires of the client and on the functional impairments that have been identified by the therapist during the initial assessment. Functional goals require movement sequences of both the trunk and limbs; therefore, to achieve functional improvement, the therapist must treat the trunk in relationship to the limbs or the limbs in relationship to the trunk. Functional goals should represent significant changes in the patient's level of independence. Compensatory strategies are often needed to function due to loss of movement control, but if they are used, they should incorporate the use of the involved extremities and should activate as much normal trunk movement as possible to maximize the eventual use of muscle return.

Treatment goals are based on reeducation of movement and control in the hemiplegic trunk and extremities. Treatment goals are focused on the primary movement problem resulting from the stroke and the ensuing secondary problems of alignment, muscle shortening or shifting, edema, and pain. Treatment goals should be established in relationship to the functional goal, so that improvement in strength and control will result in improved functional performance. The goals for three recovery phases in hemiplegia are suggested and identified in Table 24-3.

TYPICAL CLINICAL SIGNS AND PROBLEMS WITH POSSIBLE TREATMENT ALTERNATIVES
Hypertonicity

There is considerable debate in the academic and clinical therapy community over the clinical relevance of hypertonicity and the need to address it in treatment. In the 1950s, it was suggested that increased tone, spasticity, interfered with normal motor performance and that it needed to be and could be changed as the primary focus of treatment so that the client could acquire selected movement patterns.[10] In the 1980s, motor learning theorists stressed the importance of relearning through task-specific training and deemphasized the need to include the problem of spasticity when formulating treatment goals.[15]

Although not a primary movement problem in hemiplegia, hypertonicity is a secondary problem that interferes with movement control and must be considered during treatment planning. Hypertonicity has been classified or categorized in at least seven different ways in the research community.[38] Clinically, at least three different situations result in a client's increase in tone: (1) increased tone as a result of proximal instability, either insufficient trunk control for the task, or instability of proximal limb musculature; (2) increased tone due to poor joint alignment and the resultant shortening, shifting of muscles; and (3) increased tone that is voluntarily produced during attempts at active movement, especially in the extremities.

Regardless of the type or cause of hypertonicity, its presence or a sudden increase in its intensity is easily recognized by the therapist and client. If hypertonicity is left untreated, the task of muscle reeducation becomes more difficult and additional secondary problems result such as joint dysfunction, pain, and asymmetrical weight-bearing patterns.

Although patterns of hypertonicity are very consistent, different body parts often display varying degrees of high tone. The hemiplegic hand and fingers may demonstrate more hypertonicity than the scapula, and the shoulder girdle may demonstrate more hypertonicity than the pelvic girdle. In treating this increase in tone, it is often easier to achieve success treating the less high-toned part first. It will be capable of more voluntary movement, and that movement, along with inhibition of the hypertonicity, will lead to a decrease in tone in the muscle groups with the highest tone.

The physical procedures available for the treatment of hypertonicity include complete elongation of the shortened muscle groups, weight bearing or moving the body on the elongated limb, cooling, vibratory stimulation, and biofeed back. The elongation of the shortened muscle groups at the point of maximally tolerated muscle length has proven effective in inhibiting hypertonicity.[54] In the client with hemiplegia, elongation of the shortened muscle groups is followed by weight bearing or moving the body as a whole over the elongated limb (Fig. 24-10). The pattern of elongation for an upper extremity that displays hypertonicity in the scapular downward rotators and adductors, shoulder adductors and internal rotators, elbow flexors, forearm pronators, and wrist and finger flexors is one of scapular protraction and upward rotation, shoulder external rotation and abduction, elbow extension, forearm supination, and wrist and finger extension (Fig. 24-11). Once elongation has been achieved, weight can be placed on the heel of the hand (Fig. 24-12, *A*) or the hand can be placed in the weight-bearing position, such as against a wall, while the body moves on the arm (Fig. 24-12, *B*). Many of the proprioceptive neuromuscular facilitation (PNF) patterns, which in-

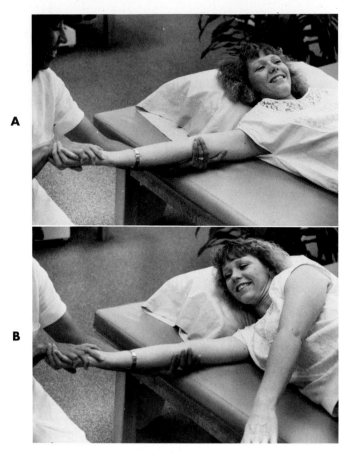

Fig. 24-10. A, Arm is externally rotated and abducted. **B,** Body moves over the elongated right arm.

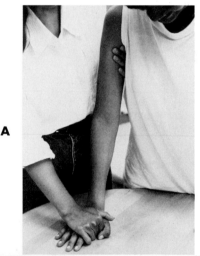

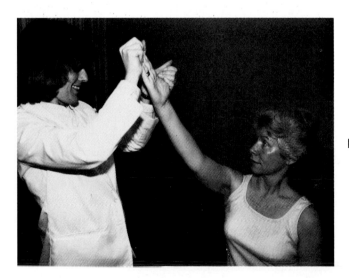

Fig. 24-11. Pattern of elongation for an arm that displays spasticity in the scapular downward rotators, shoulder adductors, internal rotators, elbow flexors, and wrist and finger flexors.

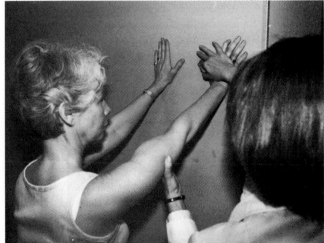

Fig. 24-12. A, Weight bearing on an extended right arm. **B,** Weight bearing of the right arm against the wall.

clude movements of the body on the limbs, also can be incorporated.[35]

Vibration and other techniques that facilitate the antagonist can be used to inhibit the hypertonic agonist. The perceptible reduction of hypertonicity occurs during the vibration, and at that point reeducation of the muscle groups can begin.[7]

Biofeedback can be used to reduce electromyographic (EMG) levels in the hypertonic muscles of clients with hemiplegia. The electrodes are placed over affected muscle groups, and the client's goal is to achieve electrical silence or a 0 reading on the biofeedback equipment during varying environmental and movement situations[76] (see Chapters 29 and 30).

Cold has been used historically to temporarily decrease hypertonicity. The study on the effects of cold on the stretch reflex and H-response on hemiplegic clients revealed that local cooling might decrease, increase, or exert no effect on hemiplegic hypertonicity.[73] Thus for ice to be a useful tool in treatment of hypertonicity, careful assessment of the client must first be conducted.

As in biofeedback, many clients can learn to slightly decrease their hypertonicity through a process of conscious relaxation similar to that taught by Jacobson.[30] This learned ability to change hypertonicity is often enough to allow the client to place an extremity in a position of weight bearing while performing a functional task. For example, placing the affected arm on the edge of a sink while brushing the teeth

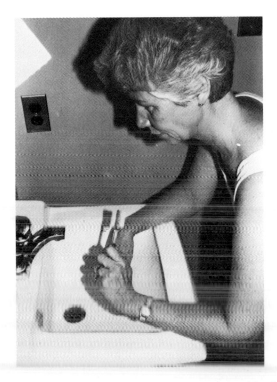

Fig. 24-13. Weight bearing on the affected right side during functional skills.

enables a better weight shift through the pelvis and both lower extremities (Fig. 24-13).

The temporary decrease of hypertonicity that occurs with any of these methods does not by itself directly lead to an increase in function. They must be immediately followed by therapeutic exercise to create a learning environment that improves motor performance.[10,64,76]

Loss of mobility—decreasing range of motion

Loss of ROM can lead to decreased function in clients with hemiplegia. Documentation of affected joints should be followed by an assessment of the active movement present in the involved joint. A loss of active movement at one joint may biomechanically cause a loss of passive movement at another joint.

For example, if assessment reveals a decreasing passive movement in dorsiflexion of the ankle and a loss of pelvic mobility in a posterior direction, resulting in a fixed posture of the pelvis in an anterior tilt, an analysis of the problem may reveal that the position of anterior pelvic tilt causes a shift of weight forward from the heel toward the toe, thus placing the foot in more plantar flexion. If this pelvic posture persists, a decrease in ROM of dorsiflexion of the ankle will result. To maintain correct ankle ROM, pelvic mobility and control will need to be established.

While classic "orthopedic" stretching procedures have been advocated for use in clients with hemiplegia, consideration must be made for the reasons behind the loss of joint range.[48] In hemiplegia slow, maintained stretching or elongation through weight bearing (i.e., functional stretching) in conjunction with the retraining of motor control is more effective than "orthopedic" stretching in reestablishing joint range and in preventing the future loss of joint range. (See Chapter 6 for discussion of mobilization.)

> **EXAMPLE:** If a pelvis is anteriorly tilted, the hip flexors may be tight. From an analysis of the development of abnormal tone, we know that the paravertebral musculature on the affected side is often the first to demonstrate high tone. An analysis then reveals that if the paravertebral muscles are tight and if a client with hemiplegia is stood without appropriate support before motor control of the hip extensors and abdominals is sufficient to maintain a neutral pelvic posture, the pelvis will be pulled by the paravertebral muscles and by gravity into an anterior tilt. Stretching the hip flexors will not correct this problem as quickly or as permanently as will supporting the lower extremities and pelvic girdle in a standing position and moving the upper body over the lower body to facilitate abdominal and hip extensor musculature.

Pain

In the client with hemiplegia, pain can be caused by an imbalance of muscles, improper movement patterns, joint dysfunction, improper weight-bearing patterns, and muscle shortening; or it may be of CNS origin. An assessment of the type of pain, the exact anatomical location of the pain, the presence of soft tissue dysfunction, a description of the body position during the active movement that causes pain, or the exact passive movement that causes pain is necessary before treatment planning can begin.

Joint pain. During functional movement, weight-bearing patterns are usually accompanied by normal joint alignment. If, during weight bearing, hypertonicity is allowed to occur, the muscle pull will stress the joint, the soft tissues, or the tendon and will eventually lead to inflammation. For example, if weight bearing on an extended upper extremity occurs with severe shoulder internal rotation and elbow extension, biceps tendonitis and/or anterior shoulder joint pain can occur. When joints are improperly aligned, passive or active movement of the joint will result in joint or referred pain. This pain is usually sharp.

Pain from muscle imbalance or improper movement patterns is related to biomechanics and joint dysfunction. If, when raising the arm in forward flexion, a sharp pain is reported on the superior portion of the shoulder joint at approximately 60 degrees of forward flexion, the therapist immediately suspects an inability of the scapula to upwardly rotate and protract. If the glenohumeral rhythm is not present above 60 degrees of forward flexion, an impingement of the shoulder capsule between the humerus and scapula occurs and sharp pain results. If pain is present, the therapist should lower the humerus immediately upon complaint of pain, assess the mobility of the scapula, and if this mobility is normal, ask for forward flexion again while passively rotating and protracting the scapula upward and externally rotating the humerus. The movement will then proceed above 60 degrees of forward flexion without pain (Fig. 24-14). Pain itself decreases muscle function. Thus the therapist must differentiate pain caused by peripheral instability or tightness from pain due to motor systems influence on muscle contraction caused by the vascular insult.

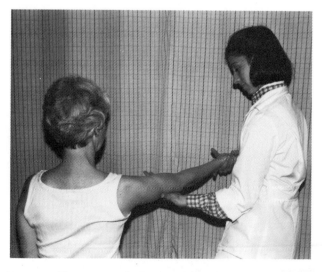

Fig. 24-14. To ensure pain-free movement of the arm, forward flexion must be accompanied by scapula protraction and upward rotation and external rotation of the humerus.

Muscle pain. When a hypertonic or shortened muscle is slowly stretched, a strong "pulling" type pain is often reported in the region of the muscle belly being stretched. If the amount of stretch is decreased a few degrees, the reported pain subsides.

Shoulder dysfunction

The primary shoulder problems of the person with hemiplegia are subluxation, pain, and a lack of functional movement patterns. To plan treatment programs, an understanding of normal anatomy, biomechanics, and kinesiology must be reviewed in conjunction with the problems that result from CNS damage.[14]

Shoulder subluxation occurs when any of the biomechanical factors contributing to glenohumeral joint stability are interrupted. In persons with hemiplegia, subluxation is related to a change in the angle of the glenoid fossa. In the frontal plane the scapula is normally held at an angle of 40 degrees. When the slope of the glenoid fossa becomes less oblique (and more vertical), the humerus will "slide" down the slope of the fossa and "subluxation" occurs.[6]

This change in obliquity of the glenoid fossa occurs in both the flaccid and hypertonic stage of hemiplegia. In the flaccid, or low-tone, stage, the scapula, which no longer has stability of its muscular attachments, loses its normal orientation on the thorax and is rotated downward by gravity. Downward rotation occurs as a result of (1) low tone in the rotator cuff and serratus anterior muscles, (2) the depression and downward rotation of the scapula when sitting or standing is allowed without scapular support, and (3) the spinal curvature that occurs with unilateral weight bearing to the sound side. Downward rotation orients the glenoid fossa vertically and the humerus is subluxed inferiorly (Fig. 24-15). The client in Fig. 24-16, *A,* has low-tone upper extremity and a downwardly rotated scapula resulting in large subluxation of 2-year duration. In Fig. 24-16, *B,* the scapula is passively rotated upward, and the subluxation is markedly reduced. As subluxation occurs, the shoulder capsule is vulnerable to stretch, especially when the humerus is dependent and resting by the side of the body. In this position, the capsule is taut anteriorly, so any downward distraction of the humerus will place an immediate stretch on the upper part of the capsule. As the humerus is abducted the capsule has more slack anteriorly (Fig. 24-17); thus a greater degree of subluxation in this position is necessary before capsule stretching occurs. The superior portion of the capsule is reinforced by the coracohumeral ligament, which is crucial for shoulder stability. Jenson[32] has discussed the implications of rupture of this ligament as a result of forced abnormal passive motion as a cause of shoulder pain in subluxation.

During the hypertonic stage, the strong downward pull of the latissimus dorsi and the active use of shoulder elevators initially cause the glenoid fossa to be vertically oriented and the scapula to begin to elevate on the rib cage. As the humerus postures or moves into hyperextension and internal rotation, the humeral head will sublux anteriorly.

A third type of subluxation, a superior subluxation, occurs if the pattern of active return includes deltoid biceps firing. In these clients the scapula is downwardly rotated and elevated on the rib cage while the humeral head is internally rotated and pulled up under the acromial process.[33,63]

Prevention of subluxation requires (1) proper assessment (ribcage/scapula/humeral position), (2) appropriate treatment in accordance with assessment, and (3) prevention of shoulder capsule stretch, including support and positioning against the pull of gravity.

Pain occurs in the hemiplegic shoulder as a result of muscle imbalance, with loss of joint range from severe

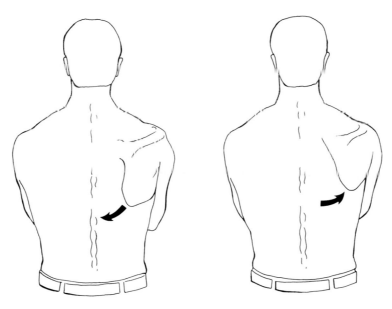

Fig. 24-15. As the scapula rotates downward, the slope of the glenoid fossa becomes less oblique and the humerus "slides" downward.

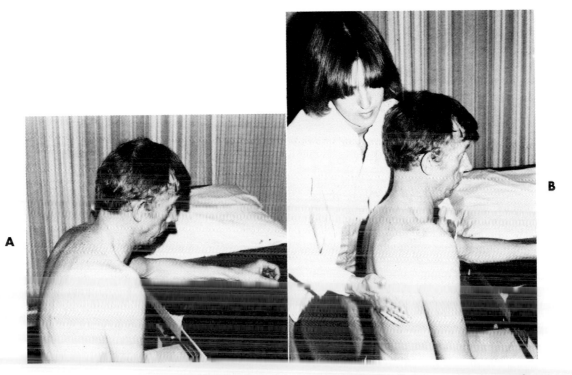

Fig. 24-16. A, Downwardly rotated scapula with a subluxated humerus. **B,** If the scapula is rotated upward to a normally aligned position, the humerus is no longer subluxated.

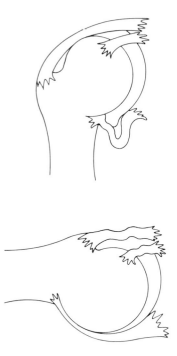

Fig. 24-17. As the humerus abducts, the anterior portion of the shoulder capsule has more slack.

long-standing subluxation and from all the possible causes of nonhemiplegic shoulder pain. The combination of loss of active and passive motion, loss of the ability to bear weight, and long-standing subluxation without support eventually leads to what is termed *sympathetic pain.*

Shoulder-hand syndrome

The shoulder-hand syndrome begins with tenderness and swelling of the hand and diffuse aching pain from altered sensitivity in the shoulder and entire arm.[63] This pain interferes with the reeducation of movement patterns and causes a general desire on the part of the client to "protect" the arm by not moving it. Limited shoulder and wrist and finger ROM soon occurs.

The second stage of shoulder-hand syndrome includes further loss of shoulder and hand ROM, severe edema, and loss of skin elasticity. This is followed by the third stage, which includes demineralization of bone, severe soft tissue deformity, and joint contracture.[63]

Not every edematous hemiplegic hand leads to a shoulder-hand syndrome. Hand edema results from an upper extremity that remains dependent and that does not move for long periods of time. It is essential to teach the person with hemiplegia how to properly care for the hand and to give the responsibility for the care of the hand and arm to the client.

Hand dysfunction. The grasp reflex in the hand normally disappears before voluntary grasp develops. A grasp reflex occurs when a stimulus is placed in the palmar surface of the hand and the fingers close quickly and tightly around it. The client with a grasp reflex requires desensitization through firm pressure and weight bearing.

A hand that is tightly closed can be loosened by proper alignment and by applying pressure on the "heel" of the hand. When opening the thumb, the therapist should place pressure at its base rather than pull from the distal tip of the thumb, which may result in subluxation of the interphalangeal (IP) or metacarpophalangeal (MP) joints. Although the prone position is usually advocated in children to achieve weight bearing through shoulders, elbows, and/or hands, it often is not a comfortable position for older adults with hemiplegia. The same beneficial weight-bearing pattern can be achieved in the sitting position by leaning forward onto the elbows and forearms, in the standing position by leaning on extended arms, or in the side-lying position by rotating onto forearms (Fig. 24-18).

To maintain a flexible, open hand and normal joint motion, the importance of proper alignment of the shoulder and arm and the experience of weight bearing through the hand cannot be stressed enough.

Hip, knee, ankle, and foot problems

Problems of the hip, knee, ankle, and foot in the client with hemiplegia are interrelated. These problems often become evident when the client is placed in a standing position or when he or she attempts to walk; yet these same problems appear minimal or mild when the client is sitting or kneeling. If this is the case, the exaggeration of the problems with higher-level activities is the result of a lack of postural control of the lower trunk and pelvis, which leads to an increase of hypertonicity in the lower extremity. Lack of control and the presence of excessive tone in one muscle group leads to abnormal postures in neighboring joints. For example, (1) hip flexion may be the result of an anteriorly tilted pelvis resulting from lack of abdominal control and/or hypertonic paravertebral muscles; (2) knee flexion may be the compensation to avoid falling forward, if exaggerated anterior pelvic tilt and hip flexion are present; (3) knee hyperextension may result from an excessive anterior tilt of the pelvis with the resulting biomechanical line of gravity falling in front of the knee joint; (4) knee flexion or knee hyperextension may be the compensation for excessive tone in the gastrocnemius-soleus muscle group; and (5) ankle plantar flexion can be the result of excessive pelvic lordosis and hip flexion.

Therefore problems of instability should be assessed in light of neighboring compensatory mechanisms before treatment is planned. All too often the excessive knee hyperextension in a person with hemiplegia is blamed on poor knee control. It is usually the result of poor pelvic, hip, and trunk control; spasticity or tightness in the plantar flexors of the ankle; and/or poor ankle and foot control.

Although great emphasis is placed on the ability to dorsiflex the ankle in a client with hemiplegia, the need for the calcaneous to properly bear weight is of greater importance. Proper calcaneal alignment and heel strike allow the ankle to move appropriately. In hemiplegia, in non-weight-bearing situations, the calcaneus frequently is in

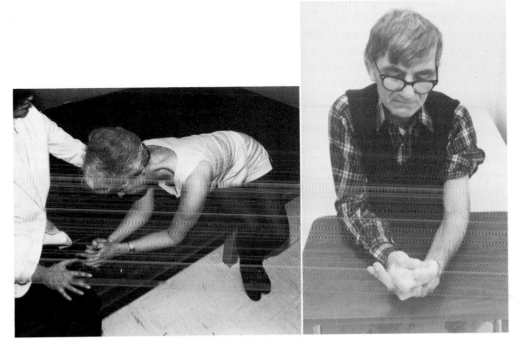

Fig. 24-18. Examples of the forearm weight bearing.

equino varus, the midfoot supinates, and the forefoot adducts. When the foot makes ground contact, the client has difficulty bearing weight on the heel. The calcaneous remains in equinus and varus while the midfoot pronates in relation to the rearfoot to seek the ground and the forefoot abducts.[62] Both abnormal foot positions must be corrected before ankle joint range can be assessed. Conventional double upright metal braces, prefabricated or custom-molded polypropylene braces, and inhibitory plaster casts that do not hold forefoot and rearfoot correction will not ameliorate the problems presented by an equinovarus foot. See Chapter 32 for an in-depth discussion of orthotics and their therapeutic implications.

Toe clawing. Toe clawing occurs for two reasons: loss of biomechanical alignment and as part of an equilibrium reaction.

If the calcaneus moves into equinus (because of shortened or spastic gastrocnemius/soleus muscles), the midfoot will shift and the metatarsal heads will become depressed. As the metatarsal heads depress, the phalanges hyperextend proximally and flex distally.[33]

During functional movement, especially during walking, clients with hemiplegia are attempting to move the body's center of gravity over a new base of support. If trunk and pelvic control is not appropriate for the task, the body will recruit an equilibrium reaction and as part of this reaction, the toes will claw.

Problems of blistering and pain in the toes occur in the intermediate and long-term stage of hemiplegia as the result of the toes rubbing on the tops of the shoes and the constant struggle of pushing clawed toes into shoes. In treatment,

clawing can be temporarily relieved by realigning the metatarsals and slowly lengthening the shortened long-toe flexor muscles. This often allows a shift of weight from the toes to the heel of the foot, thus allowing a more normal weight-bearing pattern. The problems of pelvic and hip control can then be more easily approached. Inhibition and carry-over can be maintained through shoe inserts, toe extensions in polypropylene orthoses, or removable metatarsal pads.

Scoliosis

The appearance of an uncorrectable scoliosis in the sitting position is one of the largest problems of clients with long-standing hemiplegia. Once the person with hemiplegia is placed in a sitting position, the tendency for spinal curves begins as a result of unequal weight distribution, muscle tightness, and rib cage rotation. The presence of the scoliosis will affect the positioning of the scapula and pelvis, which in turn affects the movement possibilities of the upper and lower extremities. Therefore alignment and movement control of the spine and rib cage must be achieved before extremity treatment can be effective.

Gait

The evaluation of gait patterns includes the assessment of the temporal characteristics of each gait cycle, the description of gait deviations, and ideally the assignment of a numerical score representing the efficiency of ambulation.

The temporal characteristics of gait—step time, cycle time, step length, and stride length—can be measured with a piece of chalk and a stopwatch or with more sophisticated equipment such as a gait analyzer.[51,56] These temporal parameters provide an objective measurement of performance and a baseline from which the efficacy of treatment procedures and client progress can be assessed.

Gait deviations in persons with hemiplegia have been described according to their biomechanical and kinesiological abnormalities and in terms of the loss of centrally programmed motor control mechanisms.[36,56] Perry[56] has described common problems of the hemiplegic person's gait as loss of controlled movement into plantar flexion at heel strike, loss of ankle movement from heel strike to midstance (resulting in loss of trunk balance and forward momentum for push off), and loss of the normal combination of movement patterns at the end of stance (hip extension, knee flexion, and ankle extension) and at the end of swing (hip flexion with knee extension and ankle flexion).

Knutsson and Richards[36] classified the motor control problems of the hemiplegic gait into three types. Type I is characterized by inappropriate activation of the calf muscles early in the gait cycle with corresponding low muscular activity in anterior compartment muscles. Type II consists of an absence or severe decrease in EMG activity in two or more muscle groups of the involved lower extremity. Type III activation patterns consist of abnormal coactivation of several limb muscles with normal or increased muscular activity levels in the muscle groups of the involved side.

In the type I activation pattern, the calf musculature is activated before the center of gravity passes over the base of support. This thrusts the tibia backward instead of propelling the body forward in a push-off as normally occurs. The client with hemiplegia compensates for the backward thrust of the tibia by anteriorly tilting the pelvis and/or flexing forward at the hip. Type II activation patterns, markedly decreased muscular activity, result in compensatory mechanisms to gain stability. Type III activation patterns result in a disruption of the sequential flow of motor activity.

The isolation of at least three different motor control problems in the gait of clients with hemiplegia underscores the importance of proper assessment. The major problem is not the same in all clients; therefore retraining programs should be selective to the problem.

The functional ambulation profile (FAP) is a system that attempts to relate the temporal aspects of gait to neuromuscular and cardiovascular functioning and that converts this relationship to a single numerical score.[51,52]

TREATMENT PROCEDURES

The treatment of the deficits in motor control of the person with hemiplegia centers on improving function and preventing greater disability through secondary complications. Much debate exists over the type of treatment that should be used. Two broad and divergent schools of thought exist: Some people believe that hemiplegic clients should be trained to use only their residual motion, whereas others believe that new learning can be achieved that will provide a more normal foundation on which function can occur. Within the latter school of thought, debate continues over which neurophysiological approach is optimal and whether approaches should be combined. At the present time, none of these questions can or have been objectively answered through well-documented studies. This section does not attempt to answer these controversial questions, but it gives a structure on which each therapist can choose the treatment technique best for him or her. As Mossman[48] so accurately stated, "It is what you do, not what you call it, which matters."

Objectives

Objectives for selective treatment procedures that are based on neurophysiological principles and that are designed to help the client relearn basic postural control and functional movement patterns include the following:

1. Reestablishing postural control and reeducating movement control for basic functional movement tasks and refined extremity skills in safe, efficient patterns.
2. Training functional skills with as much trunk symmetry and extremity bilaterality as possible to maximize use of muscle return.
3. Preventing secondary problems of muscle shortening, joint malalignment, pain, and contracture.

Treatment procedure is divided into two sections. First, procedures and considerations necessary for reestablishing postural control are described. Second, the projections are given for improving selective functional skills.

Reestablishing postural control

Head, neck, and trunk control. In normal movement, postural control of the head, neck, and trunk frees all extremities for function. A 3-month-old baby, in the prone position, develops the ability to control his or her head and upper trunk and to shift weight from one arm to the other. The skill of shifting and bearing weight over one arm frees the remaining arm for the function of reach, grasp, and release. So too, the person with hemiplegia must develop the ability to control his or her head and trunk so that he or she can shift and bear weight on each side to free an extremity for function.

Along with sensory information (tactile, proprioceptive, kinesthetic, visual, and vestibular), movement requires a point of stability or base of support, a point of mobility, and a weight shift. Weight shift, which can be anterior, posterior, lateral, or diagonal, is followed by one or more of the following: righting reactions, equilibrium reactions, protective reactions, or falling. Establishing head and neck control allows for dissociation of the shoulder and pelvic girdles from the trunk and dissociation of the extremities from the girdles (Fig. 24-19).

Motor skills are learned or relearned through experiencing the movement; the movement must be performed

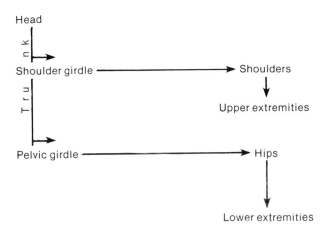

Fig. 24-19. Flowchart establishment of central motor control frees distal components for movement.

actively.[12] We do not always move the exact same way when performing a functional motor skill, but we always achieve the same purpose. Therefore for the establishment of motor control, the body must be prepared to automatically adjust posture to allow a movement to achieve its purpose.

Treatment should include mobility and active control of straight plane as well as rotational movements. Although rotation is a combination of anterior or posterior and lateral movement, the therapist need not always wait until anterior, posterior, or lateral control is established before working toward or in a rotational pattern. If the spinal vertebrae are not aligned properly, however, true rotation will not occur.

Head and neck control. Vision, hearing, and labyrinthine influences are essential for normal head control. To establish head and neck control these systems should be incorporated in treatment. It is often necessary to use auditory clues to orient the client to his or her position in space. An auditory stimulus can be presented in midline and, if necessary, the client can be assisted to "find" midline, then allowed to move out of midline to see if he or she can then "find" midline again.

EXAMPLE: "I will help you find the middle. Can you stay here? Now you are falling to the left. I will move you back to the middle, to the right. Can you move back to the middle?" Each time the client is moved out of midline a weight shift will be occurring. This shift can often be reinforced with proprioceptive clues such as deep pressure. Progression from verbal commands to automatic correction of position is desirable in order to shift from a declarative learning task to a procedural motor plan

To establish good head and neck control, axial extension (i.e., a chin tuck), not a forward head, should be facilitated along with upper thoracic extension and normal alignment of the shoulder girdle. Weight bearing through symmetrically positioned arms will help organize the body and orient the head to midline

Although head and neck control is often treated before trunk control is well established, the trunk must be supported

in good alignment before treatment of the head and neck can begin. While children are placed in the prone position for this purpose, the adult with hemiplegia may need alternate positions, for example:

1. The client can be seated on a firm surface (on a mat table or in a wheelchair with a solid seat) with the trunk and upper extremities supported by leaning forward onto a table top or forward onto a wedge or bolster resting on the table (Fig. 24-20, *A*).
2. The therapist can support the client's trunk from the front with the hands controlling the upper trunk and scapula (Fig. 24-20, *B*).
3. The therapist can support the trunk from behind the client (Fig. 24-20, *C*).
4. The client can be placed in the side-lying position with forearm support to one side.

The use of the sitting position requires that the pelvis, hips, and knees be properly aligned and that the feet be able to rest on the floor. If trunk control is not yet established, it is imperative that support be given to the upper extremities, scapula, and upper trunk before facilitation of head and neck control begins.

Trunk control. Trunk movements are encouraged through weight shifts anteriorly, posteriorly, laterally, and diagonally. A gradual lateral weight shift onto the right hip results in an elongation of the right trunk musculature and a shortening of the left trunk musculature (Fig. 24-21).

In hemiplegic clients, this righting response will be impaired on each side, so weight shift and appropriate trunk movements to each side must be included in the treatment process. Before lateral trunk movements can occur, however, the pelvis must be able to be aligned in a neutral position (anterior superior iliac spine and iliac crest in the same plane). If the pelvis is tilted posteriorly or anteriorly, a weight shift will not occur through the hips and the trunk will not be able to respond appropriately. Lateral and diagonal trunk control will occur more easily if anterior and posterior pelvic and lumbar spine movements are available first. If the spine can be aligned passively, rotational and diagonal movements can be facilitated. If the spine cannot be aligned passively, true rotation never occurs. In persons with hemiplegia, spasticity in the lower extremity and loss of pelvic mobility often contribute to a "fixed" lumbar spine. If this occurs, most movement of the trunk will be upper trunk movement with the axis of movement centered around T10 or a point on the spine that is hypermobile.

Girdle control. Dissociation of the shoulder and pelvic girdles from the trunk means the ability to separate shoulder and pelvic girdle movements from the trunk. Lack of dissociation results from soft tissue tightness, spasticity, or lack of motor control. After the reasons for lack of dissociation have been assessed, treatment can be chosen appropriately. To dissociate a girdle from the trunk, the therapist can (1) hold or stabilize the trunk through weight

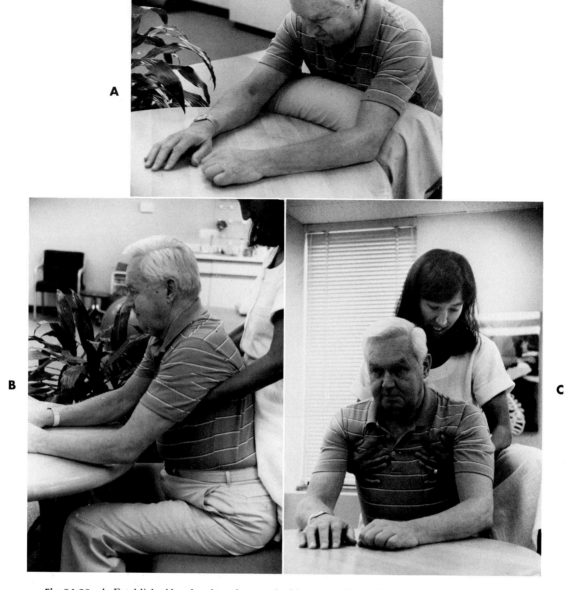

Fig. 24-20. **A,** Established head and trunk control with support from table and bolster. **B,** Establishing head and trunk control with therapist controlling from upper trunk and scapula. **C,** Establishing head and trunk control with therapist supporting from behind.

bearing and then facilitate movement from the girdle or (2) hold or stabilize the girdle and then facilitate movement from the trunk.

If the scapula will not move on the rib cage, the humerus will not move properly, and any passive movement of the humerus will result in pain or discomfort. If the pelvis will not move on the spine, the femur will not move properly in the acetabulum and sitting, standing, and walking will be abnormal.

Extremity control. As in normal development dissociation of the extremities from the girdles occurs through weight bearing as the girdles dissociate from the trunk. Treatment of the hemiplegic arm and leg is made easier by

examining this development. As a baby learns to extend the head and neck in the prone position, the scapula and upper extremities move from the position of adduction, downward rotation, hyperextension, and internal rotation to abduction, upward rotation, forward flexion, and external rotation as weight bearing is increased. The adult with hemiplegia whose scapula is downwardly rotated and adducted and whose humerus is hyperextended and internally rotated can use varying positions of weight bearing and weight shift to facilitate scapular movements on the trunk. Normal scapular movements will allow the humerus to dissociate from the scapula through the facilitation of humeral external rotation and forward flexion.

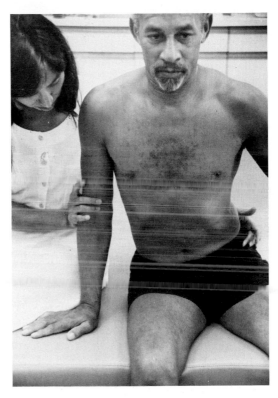

Fig. 24-21. Pelvic initiated weight shift to right to lengthen right trunk musculature.

During weight-bearing treatment, the upper extremity moves toward or into a position of external rotation as the scapula protracts and abducts on the thorax. If during weight bearing with the arms flexed or extended, the shoulder internally rotates or the head of the humerus rolls forward, dissociation will not occur.

Once dissociation begins, normal weight shifting and weight bearing movements can be reeducated and functional training of the extremities can begin.

The extremities participate in both open-chain and close-chain activities and should be specifically trained for each. A closed-chain activity is one where the distal end is fixed to a supporting surface and the body moves across the distal fixed part. This is also referred to as "mobility superimposed on stability" or "mobility in a weight bearing position."[70] The stance phase of gait is an example—the foot is fixed and the body moves over the foot.

An open-chain extremity movement is one in which the extremity moves in space. "Stability superimposed on mobility" or "mobility in a non-weight-bearing position" are synonomous terms. Examples of such movements would be reaching, feeding, bathing, throwing a ball, or the swing phase of gait.[67] When training open-chain extremity movement in clients with hemiplegia, the therapist begins with the arm at or above 90 degrees because in this position the depressors and downward rotators of the scapula and humerus are elongated, allowing optimal position for facilitating the scapula upward-rotators and forward-flexors of the humerus.

During close-chain activities the weight-bearing hand is open and flat. During the reach and grasp of an open-ended activity, the hand displays more of a palmar arch with varying degrees of wrist extension and finger movement.

Functional activities

The goal of all treatment is to restore or optimize function. Keeping in mind the concepts of head and trunk control and extremity dissociation mentioned earlier, treatment procedures to train selected basic functional skills are reviewed.

Bedside care. Although textbooks have provided lists of how to position clients with hemiplegia,[14] these lists are not always applicable. Hemiplegic clients are not all alike, and problems change in the days after the stroke. Some clients need the affected side of the trunk lengthened in bed; others just need the trunk placed in the neutral position; and still others require the upper extremity and shoulder girdle to be positioned in an upward-rotated, forward-flexed, protracted position with the arms overhead supported by a pillow.

Symmetry and midline need to be encouraged and reinforced in the person with hemiplegia. Much of the early intervention can be carried out by the client and family. Family members should be encouraged to sit, visit, talk, feed, and touch the person with the hemiplegia from the client's affected side, unless visual impairment is present. Because family members are often afraid to touch or move the client's affected side, they should be educated quickly to be made a part of the treatment process. The forward and laterally flexed head so commonly seen in the client with hemiplegia can be treated at the bedside initially through proper pillow placement and the facilitation of axial extension (chin tucking). Bilaterality and sensory awareness can be encouraged by bringing both hands to midline and to various body parts, especially the head, face, and mouth. Pressure on the heel of the affected hand will begin to prepare the hand for future weight bearing and eventual function (Fig. 24-22).

The lower extremities can be positioned in many ways with the goals of mirroring functional patterns. Proprioceptive input through the heel of the foot is encouraged during bedside care when hip and knee are held in flexion to prepare the foot for weight bearing in sitting and standing. This flexed position also avoids eliciting total extension or extensor hypertonicity. To prepare for ambulation, the lower extremities can be positioned out of total synergistic patterns. For example, position the affected leg in hip extension with knee flexion and ankle dorsiflexion while in the side-lying position (Fig. 24-23).

To avoid later shoulder problems, the therapist can plan bedside treatment that includes scapular positioning and scapular facilitation to ensure protraction and upward rotation of the scapula as the humerus is raised above 60 degrees of forward flexion or abduction. The shoulder pain

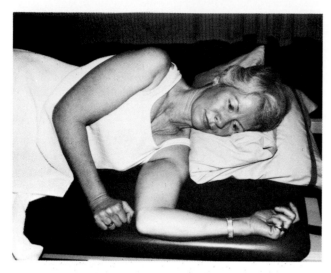

Fig. 24-22. Pressure on the "heel" of the hand prepares the hand for weight bearing and eventual functional tasks.

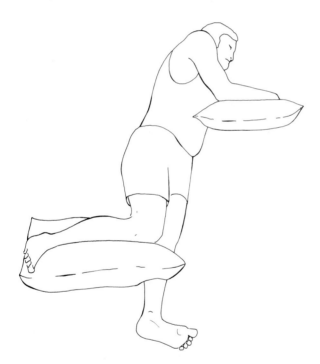

Fig. 24-23. This side-lying position for the right leg mirrors the leg position needed for late stance phase of gait.

that occurs when the client is lying on the affected side can be relieved immediately by moving the body so that the scapula lies in a normal position on the thorax.

Feeding and swallowing. Symmetry and weight bearing can be encouraged during meals. Before normal head and mouth control and normal feeding can be established, it is necessary to have a degree of trunk and girdle control. Although detailed facilitation and inhibition of oral and neck musculature for feeding and articulated language are a specialty of speech pathologists, the therapist must be able

to prepare the trunk and girdles so that feeding and speech is possible. The following outline lists typical head and neck problems and related trunk problems in persons with hemiplegia.

1. Oral problems
   a. Forward head, poor lip closure, loss of saliva and food
   b. Facial asymmetry during function greater than at rest
   c. Inability to swallow
   d. Inability to chew
   e. Inability to lateralize foods
   f. Inability to take liquids from cup or spoon
   g. Poor muscle tone
2. Central problems
   a. Asymmetry of trunk
   b. Poor balance
   c. Upper body retraction leading to facial asymmetry
   d. Unable to feed self
3. Compensations
   a. Use of gravity—with head and neck extension the food flows down the throat
   b. Chewing on one side only
   c. Using the hand to place food in the mouth
   d. Using the hand to pull food from the cheek
   e. Using thicker food, which is much easier to handle than soft food (soft food is used often)
   f. Labiodental closure versus lip closure

In the majority of cases, swallowing problems are transient in persons with hemiplegia. Following the initial insult and during the flaccid period, many clients exhibit a decreased gag reflex (see Chapter 26).[6] Precautions to consider during early recovery include proper trunk, pelvis, and head position before feeding. Liquids, especially water, are often encouraged at this time because they do less damage than nonwater items if they are aspirated to the lung. However, liquids are the hardest for persons with hemiplegia to control because of their thinness and slipperiness. Water, because of its tastelessness, is especially difficult for hemiplegic clients with a decreased gag reflex to control.

The presence of a nasogastric tube will depress and/or diminish the gag reflex. Because the indications for use of a nasogastric tube include an inability to swallow, oral treatment to stimulate the mouth cavity is often indicated when a nasogastric tube is present. To help the person with a decreased but present gag reflex to eat, the therapist should provide a solid surface on which to control the pelvis, trunk, and head. If the person with hemiplegia is eating in bed, the therapist should make sure that the trunk is held over a level pelvis, establish some trunk balance, provide symmetry of the shoulder girdles, and assist with head control, if needed, while providing a diet that will coincide with the hemiplegic person's ability to feed and swallow. Drooling occurs for the following reasons:

1. Poor lip closure as a result of a forward head from lack of trunk control and/or spasticity in cervical paravertebral area
2. Problem number 1 above plus a sensory loss
3. Normal head and mouth control but a primary swallowing problem

Specific feeding programs are noted in Chapters 6 and 26. There are three differences between feeding adults and feeding children. First, when feeding adults it is imperative to remember that someone else's hands in or near the mouth is an invasion of privacy and a very uncomfortable experience. Second, automaticity is a greater factor with adults; it is abnormal for us to chew and swallow on command. Third, adults use many more conscious compensations than children. In acute care settings, where liquid diets are often routinely given to persons with hemiplegia, education of hospital staff to the merits of using thicker foods should be considered. Thicker, chopped food is easier to swallow than soft food. Soft food is easier to swallow than liquids. Liquids with distinct taste or texture are easier to swallow than water.

Drooling from the side of the mouth that is paralyzed often presents a problem. The client with hemiplegia may not be able to maintain lip closure, and in addition, may not feel the saliva running out of the mouth's corner. He or she does not identify a need to swallow. Telling the client to swallow does not treat the problem—it only treats the symptom. If lip closure cannot be maintained as a result of imbalance of muscle tone leading to a forward head, swallowing cannot occur easily. Treating the correct problem, not only the symptom, will result in an automatic improvement of the drooling.

If the client is sitting on a soft mattress with the bed raised to 60 degrees, the pelvis cannot be controlled. This may result in a forward head, poor jaw closure, and thus difficulty in swallowing. Therefore for feeding to be successful and therapeutic, the client needs a firm sitting surface and a neutral pelvic position. If possible, the affected upper extremity should be up on a table in a position to accept weight; it should at least be within the visual field.

Dressing activities require the ability to control the head and trunk against gravity and to shift weight. If these prerequisites are not present, dressing will be stressful, frustrating, and most likely impossible. Assisted dressing should be carried out with as much trunk support as possible. Perceptual problems often prevent success at dressing skills. Thorough understanding of perceptual integration is paramount to understanding development of skill in any complex activity of daily living.

Leisure activities at the bedside throughout the day should be reviewed to establish carry-over of treatment principles. Alternate positions for watching television, reading, and resting should be given. If the person with hemiplegia thinks of ways of positioning himself or herself and of moving throughout the day, deformity and pain can be avoided and the repetition necessary for motor learning can be established.

Rolling or bad mobility. When rolling from the supine to the side-lying position, the person with hemiplegia tends to avoid initiating the roll from the involved side. Rolling should be practiced to both sides to promote symmetry and weight bearing on the affected side. Bilateral reaching can be easily incorporated during rolling. This will encourage scapula protraction and also will place the affected arm within the visual field (Fig. 24-22). While lying on the unaffected side, the affected hand can be placed on the bed to encourage weight bearing.

Pillow height affects head position in the side-lying position. If the person with hemiplegia prefers to hold the cervical spine in a position of side bending to the affected side when lying, a high pillow can be placed under the head on the affected side to elongate the shortened muscle groups. Similarly, when positioned on the unaffected side, a low pillow will elongate the shortened muscles.

Facilitating and maintaining trunk rotation while rolling will have a dramatic effect on extremity tone. Rotation within the body axis helps release the extremities' dominant synergistic patterns and free the limbs for more purposeful activities.

After the client has rolled from the supine to the side-lying position, the function of forearm support on the affected side requires that graduated, appropriate support be given to the weight-bearing scapula, shoulder, and trunk until antigravity control is established (Fig. 24-24). When the affected side is uppermost, the affected upper extremity should be encouraged to move forward or be placed forward so that weight can be placed on the extremity, allowing it to function as an assist.

Sitting. The establishment of pelvic control, especially in the anteroposterior plane, is essential for good sitting. The pelvis must be actively controlled in a neutral position for lateral weight shift and appropriate trunk movements to occur. The position and control of the pelvis will influence the position of the lower extremity of the hemiplegic client: If the pelvis is held in a posterior tilt, the lower extremity will tend to abduct, and if the pelvis is held in an anterior tilt, the hemiplegic leg will tend to adduct. While in the sitting position, the hemiplegic client with severe lower-extremity extensor hypertonicity may demonstrate an anterior tilt of the pelvis and a lower extremity that is pushing into adduction, internal rotation, knee extension, and plantar flexion. This pushing of the lower extremity is often accompanied by pushing of the entire trunk, usually into the back of the chair or other supporting surface. In treatment, the dampening of hypertonicity, allowing the pelvis to come to a neutral position, and weight bearing and weight shifting to each side will help reestablish control of the sitting posture. When establishing trunk control in the sitting

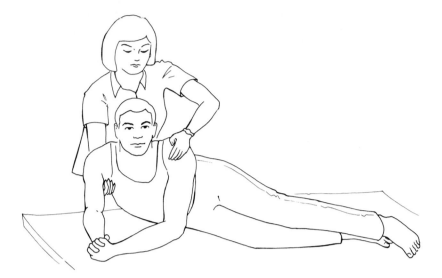

Fig. 24-24. Support is given to the upper trunk to grade the amount of weight taken by the affected right shoulder in the side-lying position.

position, the therapist can place the affected foot on the floor in line with, but not in front of, the nonaffected foot so that in weight shift appropriate weight can be accepted and borne through the feet and normal motor plans practiced as the client normally shifts weight.

The affected upper extremity should not be allowed to hang unsupported or retract severely during sitting activities. A bilateral weight-bearing position for both upper extremities appropriate to the level of the client can be selected and varied during sitting activities. A few ideas include hands placed on knees, hands fisted or opened down on the chair at the sides of the body, elbows and forearms placed on a lap board or table in front of the client, and tapping procedures over the glenohumeral joint. Care must be taken to keep the scapula in normal alignment during sitting activities.

Transfers. The hemiplegic person should be taught to transfer to all objects (chair, bed, toilet) from each side. This will promote symmetry through weight shift, weight bearing, and rotation to each side and will allow the person to function in any environment regardless of furniture placement.

The pelvis initiates the forward weight shift of a transfer and is accompanied by spinal extension. This same antigravity motor control pattern is present during sit-to-stand activities. If the shoulders are allowed to initiate the forward weight shift of the transfer, the spine will flex, which is not compatible with the upright posture (Fig. 24-25, *A* and *B*).

In treatment, the following points should be considered:

1. Pelvis and trunk movements should be facilitated during the transfer.
2. The upper extremity should not be allowed to hang unsupported.
3. Full standing should not be attempted until pelvic and

trunk control is established and until the client can take the "little" steps required to turn the entire body through the transfer.

A partial stand followed by pelvic and lower trunk initiation onto the new supporting surface is necessary in the early stages of recovery (Fig. 24-26).

Transfers to the affected side have the advantage of:

1. Retraining motor control through weight shift and weight bearing to the affected side.
2. Inhibiting the extensor synergy in the lower extremity through the deep pressure obtained by maintaining weight on the affected lower extremity. This can also be accomplished by maintaining some knee flexion to inhibit extension.
3. Directing vision and attention to the hemiplegic side.
4. Protracting and rotating the affected shoulder girdle forward as the upper trunk rotates away from the hemiplegic side during the transfer.

Transfers to the unaffected side have the advantage of being familiar to hospital staff because they are the "traditional" textbook way of transferring the person with hemiplegia. Nevertheless, transfers to the affected side are as easy and as safe to teach as transfers to the unaffected side. The dampening of the extensor thrust in the affected lower extremity and the facilitation of normal movement patterns contribute to the reestablishment of righting and equilibrium reactions. The result is better motor control and balance.

Coming to a stand. The ability of the trunk to extend and the pelvis and trunk to flex over the hips (anterior pelvic tilt) is crucial to the function of rising to a stand. Hemiplegic clients often push their trunk backward when trying to stand

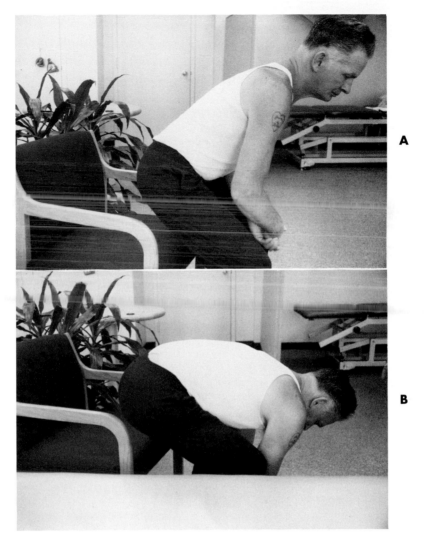

Fig. 24-25. **A,** Transfer with pelvic initiation and spinal extension. **B,** Transfer with shoulder initiation and spinal flexion.

as a result of a posterior pelvic tilt and the extensor spasticity demonstrated in the lower extremity. If the hemiplegic client pushes back instead of leaning forward and flexing from the hips, tightness of the hips and hamstrings should be assessed.

Along with controlling the trunk in a forward position, weight must be shifted from the pelvis to the feet. This weight bearing through the heel of the affected foot helps inhibit the extensor thrust in the lower extremities and allows retraining of motor control of the knee, hip, and ankle musculature.

The upper extremity should be symmetrically supported during the rise to a stand to take the weight off the trunk and to encourage even weight shift through the lower extremities. Bilateral pushing off from the surface, reaching forward with or without clasped hands, and pushing up with both hands from a table placed in front are possible strategies.

As a full standing position is approached, the abdominal muscles and the hip extensors need to be facilitated to allow

the pelvis to return to a neutral position and to allow weight to be borne appropriately through the lower extremity.

Kneeling to half-kneeling. The process of moving from a kneeling to a half-kneeling position requires the facilitation of or the active control of diagonal trunk patterns. The half-kneeling position is a transitional component of the full stand and should be encouraged to both sides.

When half-kneeling with the unaffected leg forward, the person with hemiplegia will shift his or her weight and bear the majority of weight on the affected side. Hip extension, the most important component of gait for the person with hemiplegia, can be facilitated easily in this position. Weight shift and weight bearing on the affected hip are important for the development of lateral hip control. Half-kneeling with the affected leg forward is a favorable position to facilitate ankle movements and to increase proprioceptive input through the heel. Although kneeling and half-kneeling are not generally functional patterns in adults in regard to

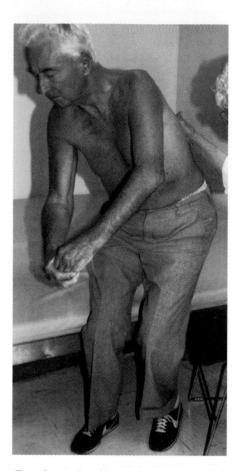

Fig. 24-26. Transfers to the affected side encourage weight bearing onto the leg. This partial stand is followed by pelvic and lower trunk rotation.

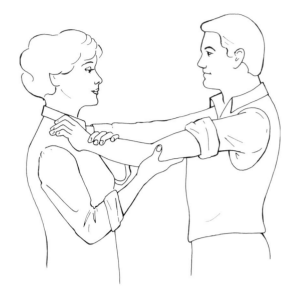

Fig. 24-27. While the client is standing, upper body control is provided to allow training of lower extremity movement control.

normal activities of daily living, they are very important in motor plans used when coming to stand after falling.

Standing. Treatment considerations given for the pelvis in preceding sections hold true for pelvic control in standing. With the feet placed in a parallel and even position, weight shift (anterior, posterior, lateral, and diagonal) and weight bearing can begin. This weight shift should be done with the feet parallel and in right step stance and left step stance. The person with hemiplegia will tend to avoid weight bearing onto the affected side, especially in standing. The use of external supports is necessary when standing is practiced before good control is established. If trunk and extremity control is poor, as with a severe stroke, the hemiplegic client will use spasticity in the extremities and girdles to "hold" himself or herself in the standing position. To compensate for the lack of central stability in the trunk, the leg will become a rigid pillar. Therefore total inhibition of extensor hypertonicity in the lower extremity in standing without facilitation of active movement patterns may result in a "collapse" of the lower extremity. The affected foot must be correctly aligned and ankle movement (tibia moving over the fixed foot) must be possible for functional standing to be achieved.

It is often necessary to prepare the foot for standing by aligning the foot, facilitating weight transfer through the heel, inhibiting clawing of the toes, and facilitating ankle and forefoot movement. This preparation can be done in the sitting position, the half-kneeling position, or during transfers.

In the standing position, the alignment of the scapula and arm should be maintained, and the upper extremity should be allowed to weight bear when possible (Fig. 24-27) to add stability in the upper trunk while practicing lower trunk and lower extremity movements. Thus guarding the client on the affected side while maintaining the upper extremity in a weight-bearing pattern encourages pelvic mobility and appropriate trunk movements while providing dampening to the hypertonic upper-extremity patterns.

Gait. If one of the obvious features of walking is its automaticity, gait training should reflect this factor. Before independent walking is achieved, the hemiplegic client should have practiced and regained partial control of the trunk and lower extremities in parallel standing, in step stance, and in unilateral weight bearing on each leg.

Common problems in walking can be separated into problems of trunk control, problems of lower extremity control, and problems of the upper extremity. The problems in stance phase differ from the problems in swing phase, but are interrelated. Categories of problems include the influence of postural deviations, inadequate postural preparation resulting in abnormal alignment and control, and atypical firing patterns and weakness in the lower extremity.

Once a particular gait disturbance is identified, specific treatment procedures can be instituted. For example, in a type I motor control problem with premature activation of the calf muscles, treatment might facilitate forward hip rotation during swing to allow the center of gravity to advance ahead of the foot before the activation of calf muscles pulls the lower leg backward. With a type II disturbance, training to improve control and power of the leg in standing and walking may be indicated. In a type III problem, treatment would be directed at facilitation of trunk control.

When retraining gait in the client with hemiplegia, the therapist should focus on three critical areas: weight acceptance (heel strike to foot flat), double-single limb support (mid-stance to heel off), and limb-length adjustment (swing).

In the weight acceptance phase, the task is weight shifting on a forward diagonal initiated from the pelvis. The heel should strike the ground first, the upper and lower trunk remain aligned, and the hip move from flexion toward extension.

During double-single limb support, the task is shifting weight from the lateral aspect of the heel to the medial aspect of the forefoot. The foot should not supinate excessively, weight must be accepted on the ball of the foot, and appropriate movement components of the hip and knee should be facilitated.

Swing phase of gait requires that the foot "lead" the movement and reach ahead of the body. Prerequisites for swing include (1) the ability to dissociate (separate) the hip from the pelvis and the pelvis from the rib cage, (2) that the pelvis and lower extremity be in their most posterior position to the trunk for the pendulum action of the leg to perform most efficiently, and (3) that the body continue to move forward in space.

Hand reach, grasp, and release. Treatment of the hand requires normal alignment and reeducation of the wrist, forearm, elbow, and shoulder. Motor reeducation of the hand should be accompanied by tactile, proprioceptive, and visual stimulation. Examples include rubbing or sliding, touching (or pushing the hand into) different surfaces, and encouraging the hand to conform to objects. Grasp is encouraged when carpal, wrist, and forearm alignment can be maintained. Upper-extremity movements should focus on initiation from the hand, especially when the hand is grasping an object. In hemiplegia, clients commonly grasp an object and then initiate the movement from the shoulder, which places the hand in a nonfunctional position.

When trunk control is not established and when prolonged sitting is accompanied by an increase in spasticity that results from associated reactions, hand treatment can be performed in the supine or side-lying position. In these positions, the trunk is fully supported with the arm protracted, forward flexed, or abducted, and the scapula is in normal alignment on the thorax.

Treatment of hand function also can begin in sitting, with the trunk being supported forward against a high table, with good pelvic and trunk positioning and weight bearing through the elbows and forearms.

If active functional movements of the hand are not possible, treatment should aim at decreasing the associated reactions that occur in the involved upper extremity as a result of one-handed activities. The affected arm and hand can be placed in a weight-bearing position in the visual field, and one-handed activities can be graded to help decrease these undesired associated reactions, which often interfere with symmetry and weight bearing. If they persist over long periods of time, the posturing that results may lead to deformity, contracture, and pain.

Equipment

Equipment for persons with CNS dysfunction can be thought of as supports or as an "extra" hand used to allow the client to be more properly aligned or controlled so that he or she can move and function in a more normal or desired way. Too much support or equipment will prevent the person's participation in an activity and will hinder the development of new motor control. Equipment should never be a substitute for treatment and should not be given without first being used during treatment. Ongoing assessment of the appropriateness of the equipment's relation to gains made in therapy must be made so that equipment always contributes to independence and so that it is not a substitute for development of new motor control. Equipment for adults with hemiplegia should be appropriate to the individual and should consist of items commonly found in the individual's environment.

Bedside equipment. When severe hypertonicity is present, air or water mattresses are used for clients with hemiplegia to provide a movable surface for the facilitation of head and trunk motion.

In acute and rehabilitation settings, pillows, blankets, or towels are used to position the client in bed. With the client in the supine position, the head pillow can be angled so that it slips under the shoulder and scapula to prevent scapular adduction and downward rotation. Towel rolls are used under the greater trochanter to maintain normal alignment of the affected pelvis and lower extremity. If the hip of the hemiplegic client is kept in a neutral position, pressure will not be placed on the lateral malleolus and pressure sores will be avoided.

Foot boards have been used traditionally in the flaccid stage of hemiplegia. A disadvantage of foot boards is that if the foot is firmly placed against the board and hypertonicity develops, the extension or "pushing" of the lower extremity may increase, facilitating the positive supporting reaction or extension synergy. A pillow placed in front of the foot board gives a soft surface so "pushing" will not be reinforced. The foot board can also be removed as soon as any hypertonicity develops. As extensor hypertonicity develops in the lower extremity, loss of ankle range of movement is avoided by changing position frequently, using the sitting position with the feet placed firmly on the floor, and, if possible, lying in the prone position with the knees flexed and the lower legs raised on pillows so that gravity will contribute to the position of ankle dorsiflexion.

Sitting and standing supports. Sitting, coming to a stand, and standing, if attempted before postural control is established, can be extremely frightening for the person with hemiplegia. In treatment care is given to provide appropriate support through external means to allow the function to be achieved without a severe increase in hypertonicity. A large increase in tone may render the desired function impossible.

In the sitting position, support may be given through a chair. The sling seats and backs of hospital wheelchairs do not provide a stable surface for the pelvis or trunk. In clients with hemiplegia, sling seats place the affected lower extremity in adduction and internal rotation, and the sling back allows either the pelvis to roll back into a posterior tile or the trunk to lean back over an anteriorly tilted pelvis. Solid seats and backs allow the pelvis, trunk, and extremities to be more normally aligned.

Foam wedges with a thicker edge uppermost can be used in solid chairs to encourage the trunk to remain upright over a neutral pelvis. The therapist can give support to the client's upper body and shoulders by standing in front of the client in the sitting position and placing his or her arms under the axilla and onto the thorax. As the client gains control in the sitting position, support can be gradually withdrawn until only the client's arms are held. Forward sitting can be achieved by having the client with hemiplegia lean against a table. High tables can be used for maximal support, and lower tables can be used as control of sitting improves.

While the client is sitting, lap boards, pillows, and arm rests are used to support the upper extremity. Lap boards and pillows should be used to promote symmetry. The use of a clear plastic lapboard maintains visual body image continuity, which can be an important component of treatment. When the hands are resting at midline, they are in the visual field. The client with hemiplegia should be encouraged to touch and move the affected arm. Arm rests do not offer the advantage of promoting symmetry and, if used, should be placed forward on the wheelchair arm so that the client's upper extremity is not placed in a position of humeral hyperextension, scapular adduction, and/or downward rotation.

Smith and Okamoto[67] offer a review of shoulder slings for hemiplegic clients. Slings should be assessed carefully to see whether, following treatment, they "hold" the corrected scapulohumeral position. Slings should not be expected to inhibit spastic muscles or to facilitate the movement necessary to achieve normal alignment of the scapula and humerus.

The ideal shoulder sling maintains the normal angular alignment of the glenoid fossa, decreases the tendency of the humerus to internally rotate, yet allows the upper extremity freedom of movement. In the acute stage, if lap boards and pillows are used when the client is seated, slings need to be used only during standing and walking activities when the arm may be dependent.

When the client is coming to a stand, his or her trunk can be supported from under the axilla bilaterally or unilaterally from the affected side. A table, walker, or chairback can be used to control the upper trunk through bilateral arm support as the client practices coming to a stand. Canes or hemiwalkers placed in front of the client provide moderate support through bilateral upper extremity weight bearing during the rise to a stand.

Standing supports for the motor reeducation of dynamic standing should be vertical (i.e., parallel to the body's line of gravity). Supports with forward or backward tilts are indicated only to decrease hip, knee, or ankle contractures. Supported standing is easily achieved through the use of a wall (Fig. 24-28, A and B). When early standing is attempted, the client's chair can be placed close to the wall so that only a small transfer is necessary before the body is supported.

Activities that can be used in treatment when using this type of support include sliding up and down the wall, moving only the upper body away from the wall, moving only the lower body away from the wall, and moving the entire body away from the wall. Standing forward against a high counter, dresser, or dining room buffet with bilateral upper-extremity weight bearing also can be used as a support.

Equipment used to encourage movement and prevent deformities

Canes. Canes are given to clients with hemiplegia to provide "extra" balance, not as a means to support body weight. Therefore canes should be provided after the ability to shift and bear weight to each side has been established. Four-pointed or "quad" canes are used because they can remain upright and do not wobble when leaned on heavily. However, they foster asymmetry, lack of weight bearing on the affected side, and loss of postural control. Single canes can be modified through the use of elastic bands or wrist loops to eliminate the problem of the cane falling or interfering with use of the unaffected hand.

Braces and shoe modifications. Although the use of knee, ankle, foot orthoses (KAFOs) in hemiplegia is no longer common practice, ankle, foot orthoses (AFOs) are frequently used to ensure clearance of the foot in the swing phase of gait and to provide medial-lateral ankle and forefoot stability. Metal, double, upright, short leg braces have the disadvantage of being heavy and of not holding calcaneal-forefoot alignment. Custom-molded AFOs that maintain heel and forefoot alignment are indicated for clients who display a strong pull into inversion, supination, and plantar flexion (Fig. 24-29, A and B). If a client lacks dorsiflexion, a light prefabricated AFO may be very appropriate (see Chapter 32).

All AFOs should allow the tibia to move forward over the fixed foot. If normal movement cannot occur passively while the foot is in the orthosis, normal patterns of motor control for ambulation will not be established. Clients should be encouraged to spend time standing without the brace so that dependence on the brace is not established. When possible, short periods of walking without the brace can be practiced.

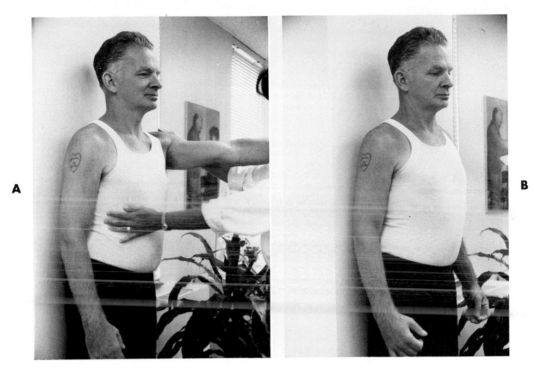

Fig. 24-28. Supported standing against a wall.

Ace elastic supports can be worn on the ankle to provide some support but less support than provided with the orthoses (Fig. 24-29, *C*). The use of an orthosis can be withheld until good standing is achieved. As motor control of the trunk, hip, knee, and ankle improves, less foot support is appropriate.

Foot control orthoses, such as a supramalleolar foot orthosis or a University of California at Berkeley Laboratory (UCBL) insert, which maintain alignment of the rearfoot, midfoot, and forefoot, are recommended over shoe modifications such as sole or heel wedges.

In the acute stage after a stroke, knee supports are not necessary if trunk, hip, and ankle movements are controlled. In the chronic stage, however, if the knee joint has become weakened or destroyed through inappropriate weight bearing, elastic knee supports or firm knee cages can be used to maintain the knee joint in normal alignment.

Movable surfaces. Movable surfaces such as inflatable balls of varying sizes, large rolls, and castered adjustable stools are used to help increase mobility while postural control is maintained (Fig. 24-30, *A*). To facilitate automatic trunk balance reactions, the client with mild or minimal hemiplegia can sit on a large ball at a table while performing upper-extremity functional activities (Fig. 24-30, *B*).

Large inflatable balls can provide support to the trunk in an all-fours position and to the upper trunk and upper extremities in the kneeling and half-kneeling positions. Use of the large balls helps to facilitate straight plane and diagonal weight shift while incorporating bilateral upper-extremity weight bearing.

Hand splints. The practice of splinting the hemiplegic hand is controversial and has undergone change since the introduction of neurophysiological approaches.[53] Controversy exists over whether rigid one-surface dorsal or volar splints facilitate or inhibit hypertonicity. Hand and wrist splints that are designed to maintain bone alignment and normal length of both flexor and extensor tendons and yet block abnormal muscle pull will decrease hypertonicity and allow appropriate motor reeducation. One surface dorsal or volar splinting in a functional position does not allow function (reach, grasp, release) to occur because the splint is in the way. Thumb abductor bars or opponents splints often provide some inhibition of flexor hypertonicity in the hemiplegic hand, but allow functional grasp and release to occur. MacKinnon's splint allows use of functional hand patterns while providing inhibition of flexor hypertonicity through deep pressure at the metacarpal heads.[42] These devices, however, do not provide carpal support or alignment.

Two approaches for casting the hemiplegic ankle and foot and wrist and fingers exist—orthopedic casting and inhibitory casting. Orthopedic or static casting takes the joint close to its limit and immobilizes it. Inhibitory or dynamic casting not only places the joint at the end of its limited range, but also provides a weight-bearing surface for movement. Inhibitory casting requires treatment during the period of immobilization, including weight bearing and muscle retraining. Fiberglass plaster is lighter and more appropriate for upper-extremity casting because the weight of regular plaster places a great stress on the hemiplegic shoulder joint. Farber[19] thoroughly discusses the advantages and disadvan-

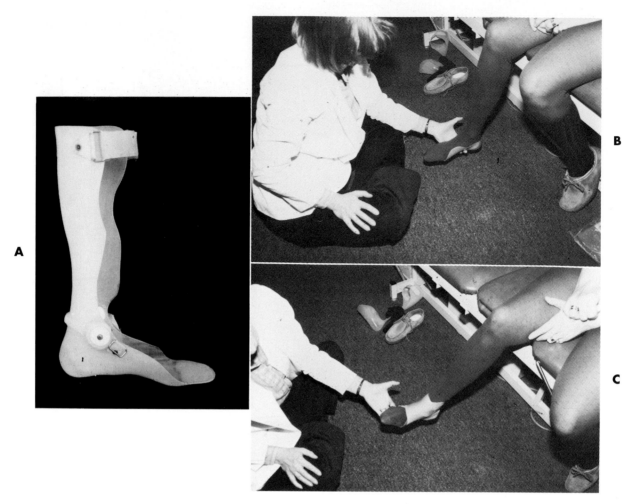

Fig. 24-29. Ankle, foot orthosis (AFO) designed to control equinovarus.

tages of adaptive equipment, as well as a variety of possible alternatives when selecting specific assistive devices and splints.

PSYCHOSOCIAL ASPECTS AND ADJUSTMENTS

The suddenness of a stroke and the dramatic change in motor, sensory, visual, and perceptual performance and feedback may leave the person with hemiplegia confused, disoriented, angry, and fearful. With a stroke, time is not allowed for gradual adjustment to the resulting disability. The usual psychosocial adjustments to disability are compounded in persons with hemiplegia resulting from stroke by the problem of increasing age (see Chapter 7).

The difficulties resulting from deficits in speech, movement, vision, sensation, and perception cause varying degrees of stress and frustration during the performance of functional activity.

Psychosocial adjustments may be more detrimental than functional disability to long-term stroke survivors.[28] Decreased interest in social activity inside and outside the home and decreased interest in hobbies attributable to psychosocial

disability hamper the hemiplegic person's return to a normal social life.[37] Feelings of rejection and embarrassment may interfere with the hemiplegic person's interaction with peers or nonpeers outside the home environment. Persons with long-standing hemiplegia often become clinically depressed with symptoms of loss of sleep and appetite, self-blame, and a hopeless outlook. Suicide can result.

Family members and spouses may have difficulty assessing the capabilities of the hemiplegic person and may be overprotective. Overprotection among spouses may be a sign of affection and support or a sign of guilt.[34,50] Long-standing marriages do not tend to dissolve when one member experiences a stroke. However, previous marriage problems and personality traits may become exaggerated as a result of the presence of increased and changing demands and stresses that occur when the person returns home.

A comparison of occupational status of long-term stroke survivors in the United States and Sweden reveals that 40% of the Swedes returned to a form of employment (including part-time work), but none of the United States group returned to work.[21] The scarcity of part-time work

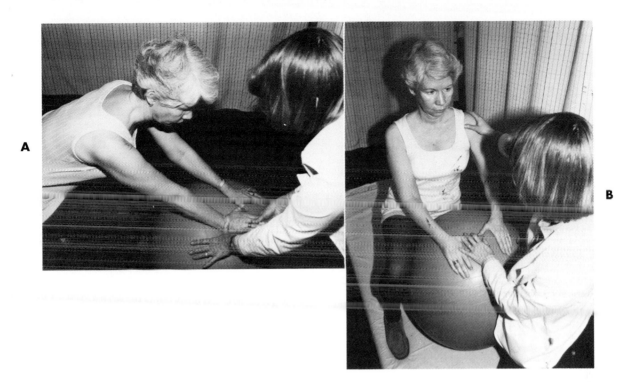

Fig. 24-30. Movable surfaces, such as balls, can be used to encourage dynamic upper extremity weight bearing for the affected right arm.

and a shorter treatment period dictated by third-party payers in the United States may account for this discrepancy.

Age is a general predictor for return to employment, and younger people are more attractive to employers. Barriers to return to work for the person with hemiplegia include speech, perceptual, and cognitive deficits along with a need for psychosocial support. Architectual barriers also can create severe problems to hemiplegic clients with regard to both work and recreational activities. Stroke clubs, usually organized through hospitals, the Easter Seal Association, or the American Heart Association provide educational, social, and recreational support for the hemiplegic person and his or her spouse.

The impact of psychosocial disability and the need for its long term treatment is great. Programs need to be established and continued for years to allow clients and their families to deal with the many problems that result from the stroke.

Sexuality

The majority of persons with hemiplegia experience a decline in sexuality through a decrease in frequency of sexual intercourse without a change in the level of prestroke sexual desire.[22] On return home, the person with hemiplegia faces the uncertainty of sexual skills and the risk of failure. Sexual dysfunction that results from a stroke depends on the amount of cerebral damage and includes a decreased ability

to achieve erection and ejaculation in men and decreased lubrication in women.[60] The sensory, motor, visual, and emotional disturbances of hemiplegia may cause awkwardness, but these disturbances can be overcome through the education of the spouse in alternate positioning and ways to provide appropriate sensory experiences. The normal factors of aging also interfere with the sexual performance of persons with hemiplegia. The closeness between partners achieved through satisfactory sexual relationship can add to the quality of a hemiplegic person's life (see Chapter 7).

SUMMARY

Treatment of the person with hemiplegia poses special clinical problems. Although one-sided motor and functional skills may appear to accomplish a "function," such skills will never contribute to the redevelopment of normal postural and movement control. The process of establishing goals and treatment plans for the person with hemiplegia requires a careful assessment of the existing movement patterns.

Active movement patterns, postural control, and functional activities have been reviewed to help the therapist establish a foundation on which an understanding of the hemiplegic person's problems can be established. Guidelines have been given to help the therapist translate assessment findings to short- and long-term goals and into appropriate treatment plans.

REFERENCES

1. Adams RD and Victor M: *Principles of neurology,* New York, 1981, McGraw-Hill.
2. Adler MK and others: Stroke rehabilitation: is age a determinant? *J Am Geriatr Soc* 28:499, 1980.
3. Anderson TP and others: Stroke rehabilitation: evaluation of its quality by assessing patient outcomes, *Arch Phys Med Rehabil* 59:170, 1978.
4. Ayres AJ: *Sensory integration and learning disorders,* Los Angeles, 1979, Western Psychological Services.
5. Bach-y-Rita P: *Recovery of functions: theoretical considerations for brain injury rehabilitation,* Baltimore, 1980, University Park Press.
6. Basmajian JV: *Muscles alive: their functions revealed by electromyography,* Baltimore, 1978, Williams & Wilkins.
7. Bishop B: Spasticity: its physiology and management, *Phys Ther* 57:396, 1977.
8. Bizzi E and Polit A: Characteristics of motor programs underlying movement in monkeys, *J Neurophysiol* 42:183, 1979.
9. Bjorklund A and others: Regeneration of central neurons as studied in cerebral iris implants. In Scheinberg P, editor: *Cerebrovascular disease,* Tenth Princeton Conference, New York, 1976, Raven Press.
10. Bobath B: *Adult hemiplegia: evaluation and treatment,* ed 3, London, 1990, William Heinneman Medical Books.
11. Brodal A: Self-observations and neuroanatomical considerations after a stroke, *Brain* 96:675, 1973.
12. Brooks VB: Motor programs revisited. In Talbott RE and Humphrey DR, editors: *Posture and movement,* New York, 1979, Raven Press.
13. Brunnstrom S: *Movement therapy in hemiplegia,* New York, 1970, Harper & Row.
14. Cailliet R: *The shoulder in hemiplegia,* Philadelphia, 1980, FA Davis.
15. Carr J and others: *Movement science: foundations for physical therapy in rehabilitation,* Rockville, Md, 1987, Aspen Publishers.
16. Chine N: Electrophysiological investigation of shoulder subluxation in hemiplegics, *Scand J Rehabil Med* 13:17, 1981.
17. Das TK and Park D: Effect of treatment with bolutlinum toxin on spasticity, *Postgrad Med J* 65:208, 1989.
18. Easton JKM and others: Intramuscular neurolysis for spasticity in children, *Arch Phys Med Rehabil* 50:155, 1979.
19. Farber S: Adaptive equipment. In Farber S, editor: *Neurorehabilitation: a multisensory approach,* Philadelphia, 1981, WB Saunders.
20. Fiorentino M and Schultz J: *NDTA Adult hemiplegia course manual,* Hartford, Conn, 1982.
21. Fugl-Meyer AR: Post-stroke hemiplegia—occupational status, *Scand J Rehabil Med* (suppl) 7:167, 1980.
22. Fugl-Meyer AR and Jaaskor L: Post-stroke hemiplegia and sexual intercourse, *Scand J Rehabil Med* 7(suppl):158, 1980.
23. Fugl-Meyer AR and others: The post-stroke hemiplegic patient: a method for evaluation of physical performance, *Scand J Rehabil Med* 7:13, 1975.
24. Granger CV and others: Stroke rehabilitation: analysis of repeated Barthel Index measures, *Arch Phys Med Rehabil* 60:14, 1979.
25. Granit R: Comments. In Granit R, editor: *Progress in brain research,* Netherlands, 1979, North Holland Biomedical Press.
26. Granit R: Interpretation of supraspinal effects on the gamma system. In Granit R, editor: *Progress in brain research,* Netherlands, 1979, North Holland Biomedical Press.
27. Gresham GE and others: Epidemiologic profile of long-term stroke disability: the Framingham study, *Arch Phys Med Rehabil* 60:487, 1979.
28. Gresham GE and others: ADL status in stroke: relative merits of three standard indexes, *Arch Phys Med Rehabil* 61:355, 1980.
29. Haas AL and others: Respiratory function in hemiplegic patients, *Arch Phys Med Rehabil* 48:174, 1967.
30. Jacobson E: *You must relax,* New York, 1962, McGraw-Hill.
31. Jennett B: Predictors of recovery in evaluation of patients income. In Thompson RA and Green JE, editors: *Advances in neurology,* ed 22, New York, 1979, Raven Press.
32. Jenson M: The hemiplegic shoulder, *Scand J Rehabil Med* 7(suppl):113, 1980.
33. Kapandji IA: *The physiology of the joints,* ed 2, London, 1970, Churchill Livingstone.
34. Kinsella GJ and Duffy FD: Attitudes towards disability expressed by spouses of stroke patients, *Scand J Rehabil Med* 12:73, 1980.
35. Knott M and Voss DE: *Proprioceptive neuromuscular facilitation,* New York, 1976, Harper & Row.
36. Knutsson E and Richards C: Different types of disturbed motor control in gait of hemiparetic patients, *Brain* 102:405, 1979.
37. Labi ML and others: Psychosocial disability in physically restored long-term stroke survivors, *Arch Phys Med Rehabil* 61:561, 1980.
38. Landau WM: Spasticity: the fable of a neurological demon and the emperor's new therapy, *Arch Neurol* 31:217, 1974.
39. Lane RE: Facilitation of weight transference in the stroke patient, *Physiotherapy* 64:260, 1978.
40. Lehmann JF and others: Stroke rehabilitation: outcome and prediction, *Arch Phys Med Rehabil* 56:383, 1975.
41. Levy DE and others: Prognosis in nontraumatic coma, *Ann Intern Med* 94:293, 1981.
42. MacKinnon F and others: The MacKinnon splint: a functional hand splint, *Can J Occup Ther* 42:157, 1975.
43. Malkmus D: Levels of cognitive functioning, Ranchos Los Amigos Hospital, Inc.
44. Marshall J: *The management of cerebrovascular disease,* ed 3, Oxford, 1976, Blackwell Scientific Publications.
45. Miller L and Miyamoto A: Computed tomography: its potential as a predistor of functional recovery following stroke, *Arch Phys Med Rehabil* 60:108, 1979.
46. Moore J: Remarks at Mary Fiorentino Symposium, 1987, Windsor Locks, Connecticut.
47. Moore RY: Response to injury in the mammalian central nervous system. In Scheinberg P, editor: *Cerebrovascular disease,* Tenth Princeton Conference, New York, 1976, Raven Press.
48. Mossman P: *A problem oriented approach to stroke rehabilitation,* Springfield, Ill, 1976, Charles C Thomas.
49. Mulley G and Espley AJ: Hip fracture after hemiplegia, *Postgrad Med J* 55:264, 1979.
50. Mykyta LJ and others: Caring for relatives of stroke patients, *Age Aging* 5:87, 1976.
51. Nelson AJ: Functional ambulation profile, *Phys Ther* 54:1059, 1974.
52. Nelson AJ: Personal communication, Nov 1981.
53. Neuhaus B and others: A survey of rationales for and against hand splinting in hemiplegia, *Am J Occup Ther* 35:83, 1981.
54. Odeen I: Reduction of muscular hypertonus by long-term muscle stretch, *Scand J Rehabil Med* 13:93, 1981.
55. Ostfeld A: A review of stroke epidemiology, *Epidemiol Rev* 2:136, 1980.
56. Perry J: Clinical gait analyzer, *Bull Prosthet Res* 188, Fall 1974.
57. Petrillo CR and others: Phenol block of the tibial nerve in the hemiplegic patient, *Orthopedics* 3:871, 1980.
58. Plum F and Caronna JJ: Can one predict outcome of medical coma? In Outcome of severe damage to the central nervous system, *Ciba Foundation Symposium* 34, Amsterdam, 1975, The Foundation.
59. Primbram KH: *Languages of the brain,* Englewood Cliffs, vol 5, 1971, Prentice-Hall.
60. Renshaw DC: Stroke and sex. In Comfort A, editor: *Sexual consequences of disability,* Philadelphia, 1978, George F Stickley.
61. Roland PE: Quantitative assessment of cortical motor dysfunction by measurement of the regional cerebral blood flow, *Scand J Rehabil Med* 7(suppl).27, 1980.
62. Ryerson S: The foot in hemiplegia. In Hunt G, editor: *The foot and ankle in physical therapy,* New York, 1987, Churchill Livingstone.
63. Ryerson S and Levit K: The shoulder in hemiplegia. In Donatelli R, editor: *The shoulder in physical therapy,* ed 2, New York, 1991, Churchill Livingstone.

64. Sahrmann S and Norton BJ: The relationship of voluntary movement to spasticity in the upper motor neuron syndrome, *Ann Neurol* 2:460, 1977.

65. Sahs AL and Hartman EC, editors: *Fundamentals of stroke care,* Washington, DC, 1976, DHEW Publication.

66. Schoenberg BS: Epidemiology of cerebrovascular disease, *South Med J* 72:31, 1979.

67. Smith RO and Okamoto GA: Checklist for the prescription of slings for the hemiplegic patient, *Am J Occup Ther* 35:91, 1981.

68. Snow B and others: Treatment of spasticity with botulinum toxin: a double-blind study, *Ann Neurol* 28:512, 1990.

69. Stern PH and others: Factors influencing stroke rehabilitation, *Stroke,* 1971.

70. Stockmeyer SA: An interpretation of the approach of Rood to the treatment of neuromuscular dysfunction, *Am J Phys Med* 46:900, 1967.

71. Taub E: Motor behavior following deafferenation in the motorically mature and developing monkey. In Rerman RM and others, editors: *Advances in behavioral biology,* New York, 1976, Plenum.

72. Teasdale G and Jennett B: Assessment of coma and impaired consciousness: a practical scale, *Lancet* 2:81, 1974.

73. Urbscheit N and others: Effects of cooling on the ankle jerk and H-response in hemiplegic patients, *Phys Ther* 51:983, 1971.

74. Wall JC and Ashburn A: Assessment of gait disability in hemiplegics, *Scand J Rehabil Med* 11:95, 1979.

75. Weinfeld D, editor: The national survey of stroke, *Stroke* 12(suppl 1):2, 1981.

76. Wolf SL and others: EMG biofeedback in stroke: a 1-year follow-up on the effect of patient characteristics, *Arch Phys Med Rehabil* 61:351, 1980.

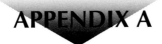

APPENDIX A

Audiovisual resources

Inner World of Aphasia—35 minute film
American Journal of Nursing Film Library
267 W. 25th Street
New York, NY 10001

Candidate for Stroke—35 minute film
American Heart Association

I Had a Stroke—35 minute film
Filmakers Library, Inc.
290 West End Avenue
New York, NY 10023

Living with Stroke
Rehabilitation Research and Training Center
The George Washington University
2300 EYE St., N.W., Suite 714
Washington, D.C. 20037

Evaluation of the Hemiplegic Patient (Sensory/Motor)
Audio-Visual Department
School of Allied Health
University of Maryland
32 Greene Street
Baltimore, MD 21201

Children's book

First One Foot, Then The Other—Tomie de Paola
This book explores the feelings and fears of children to a relative who has had a stroke.

CHAPTER 25

Brain Function, Aging, and Dementia

Osa Jackson-Wyatt

LEARNING OBJECTIVES

After reading this chapter the student/therapist will:

1. Define the basic terminology and discuss the prevalence of cognitive disturbances seen in older persons.
2. Describe normative changes in brain function with normal aging and the relevance for diagnoses of delirium and dementias.
3. Discuss how symptoms are altered with normal aging (i.e., specifically related to Arndt-Schultz Principle, law of initial values, habitual biorhythms for an individual).
4. Describe normal sensory changes with aging and how this alters the overall ability to adapt to stress.
5. Describe how, and for what type of patient, to use the Mini-Mental State Examination as a part of the physical therapy assessment.
6. Describe common sensory changes with dementia and implications for adapting physical therapy evaluation and treatment.
7. Discuss common changes in learning styles with aging and implications for adapting physical therapy intervention so as to enhance the patient's ability to perform to his or her highest functional level.
8. Describe how the environmental design/ergonomics can enhance patient performance in ADL/IADL.

9. Describe strategy to evaluate patient's emotional capacity to participate in a learning task and clinical relevance for physical therapy.
10. Describe criteria for delirium and reversible dementia and sample strategies for modifying physical therapy evaluation and treatment procedures.
11. Discuss symptomology and disease progression in irreversible dementia.
12. Discuss therapist's role on the treatment team in educating key caregiver(s) and/or support personnel and sample training strategies.
13. Discuss treatment skills that are helpful in working with irreversible dementia.
14. Describe research activities/new findings that affect physical evaluation/treatment of the patient with dementia/delirium.

FRAMEWORK FOR CLINICAL PROBLEM SOLVING

The therapist has a key role as a member of the geriatric rehabilitation team and as a resource for other caregivers for the older patient with cognitive deficits. The therapist can teach, solve problems, and adapt movement and activities related to special self care and recreation needs that are the result of impairments caused by cognitive deficits. The clinician can help the patient with cognitive deficits who may need to learn or relearn basic functional skills. In addition, therapy can be adapted to compensate for the cognitive impairments of each patient. The therapist working with patients with cognitive impairments needs to have had adequate advanced training in assessment of communication skills, neurological functioning, and gerontology, so that he or she can work with maximal efficacy and also enjoy clinical interactions with each patient. This chapter reviews in detail the rationale for the modification of **physical therapy assessment and treatment** for patients with cognitive deficits, *or* as well as the changes in the aging brain and the impact of these changes on cognition and behavior. It also discusses aspects of delirium and **dementia** and specific modifications in the physical therapy assessment and treatment.

In 37 BC, the Roman poet Virgil stated: "Age carries all things, even the mind, away."[24] Nearly 400 years ago, Shakespeare described the last stage of human life as: "second childishness and mere oblivion,/Sans teeth, sans eyes, sans taste, sans everything."[87] This pessimistic view of the fate of the elderly continues to persist amongst health care workers today[91] despite the fact that significant cognitive deficits affect only between 6.1% and 12.3% of the elderly in the United States.[35]

The clinician should not assume that an older person has impaired cognitive functioning. Perhaps the most crucial concept for clinical problem solving is that the clinician must not accept at face value what she or he sees. When a patient is observed to have altered brain **function,** it is necessary to describe the extent and type of the distortion of intellectual capacity and to determine the cause(s) to allow appropriate and effective treatment and care.

Definition of terms

There are three major categories of intellectual impairment: mental retardation, delirium, and dementia. A definition of terms is necessary to ensure that all personnel use the same framework for clinical problem solving.

Mental retardation. A person with mental retardation (also called developmental disability) has had some degree of intellectual impairment all her or his life. A person with mental retardation also can develop a delirium and/or a dementia. A delirium or dementia differs from mental retardation in that there has been a change from the baseline level of functioning for that person.

Delirium. A person with delirium usually shows a change both in intellectual function and in level of consciousness.[64] The patient may be perplexed, disoriented, fearful, and/or forgetful. The patient is often less alert than normal and may be sleepy or obtunded; however, many patients with delirium are hyperalert and may be extremely agitated and suspicious. Delirium frequently occurs in the presence of a concurrent dementia. Early identification of the symptoms and formal medical assessment and treatment are critical to ensure the return of a normal level of alertness and of intellectual functions and to prevent the development of secondary functional impairments and possible dementia.[65]

Dementia. Dementia is an impairment in some or all aspects of intellectual functioning in a person who is fully alert. Some diseases that can cause dementia are treatable, and if treated early and aggressively, the patient's deterioration of intellectual function may be either reversed or prevented from worsening. Dementia usually involves cognitive impairment affecting memory and orientation and at least one of the following:

- Abstract thinking
- Judgment and problem solving skills
- Other complex cognitive functions such as language use, ability to perform complex physical tasks (i.e., bathing), ability to recognize objects or people, or to construct objects
- Personality[4,53,71]

Alzheimer's disease. The term Alzheimer's disease is not synonymous with dementia but rather one of the many causes of dementia. The term should be used only as a diagnosis when a complete clinical evaluation has been performed, a diagnosis of dementia has been made, and all other possible causes of the dementia have been ruled out. It is not possible to definitely ascertain whether a patient has this disease until an autopsy or brain biopsy has been performed. Although multiple putative cause(s) of the disease have been proposed, the etiology and pathogenesis of the disease are unknown. Although currently there is no curative treatment for Alzheimer's disease, at least one drug, tacrine, may slow the process of cognitive deterioration in some patients, and patients and their families can be helped to cope better with the vicissitudes of the disease* (see Chapter 5).

Epidemiology

It is estimated that today more than 1 million Americans with a dementia reside in nursing homes. An additional 1.5 to 2.5 million individuals with severe dementia are estimated to live at home, although they require continual care. An estimated 5 million persons live at home who suffer from mild or moderate dementia and who require partial care and supervision.[74,108] It is expected that disorders causing cognitive deficits will continue to be a growing public health problem for at least the next 50 years. The actual number of people with severe dementia is expected to increase by 60% by the year 2000. The projected statistics, assuming there are no cures or effective means of preventing the common causes of dementia, are that by the year 2040, there will be five times as many cases of dementia (7.4 million Americans) as today. This increase is partially the result of the increased life expectancy of elderly Americans.[45] (The most rapid population growth in this country is in the oldest age groups, which leads to an increase in the prevalence of severe dementia. Dementia figures rise from approximately 3% [ages 65 to 74] to 18.7% [ages 75 to 84] to 47% [over age 85]).[29] The large increase in the number of persons over age 85 will increase the incidence of dementia.

More than 70 known conditions can cause dementia.[52] Secondary behavioral problems in the patient with dementia can be interpreted as a response of the individual to somatic, psychological, and/or existential stress.[92,99] As memory impairments, impairments of abstract thinking or judgment, or global cognitive impairments in an elderly individual may be a symptom of acute physical illness,[1] the patient's physical, emotional, social, and cognitive status and the patient's physical and affective environment need to be evaluated systematically.

*Gradual or sudden changes in intellectual capacity or memory function are not a normal part of the **aging** process.* Any change, whether it develops slowly over time or happens suddenly, should be diagnosed and, where possible, the underlying cause(s) of the delirium or dementia should be treated. Even if the cause of the dementia is untreatable, it is always possible to teach the patient and significant others strategies to make the patient's activities of daily living (ADL), instrumental activities of daily living (IADL), and the effects of the cognitive deficits easier to manage.

Physical and occupational therapists are important in the comprehensive evaluation, treatment, and ongoing care of the patient with delirium and/or dementia. It is critical that all treatment planning occur as a part of a team effort, in which the patient, the family or significant others, the physician, nurses, social worker, physical therapist, and occupational therapist collaborate so that a consistent treatment plan and orientation is followed.

PHYSIOLOGY OF AGING: RELEVANCE FOR SYMPTOMATOLOGY AND DIAGNOSIS OF DELIRIUM AND DEMENTIAS
The normal brain

The brain of a normal person at age 80 shows several significant anatomical, physiological, and neurochemical changes when compared with the brain of a younger person. It has been noted that there is a decrease in brain weight with advancing age. For example, the mean brain weight for women age 21 to 40 is 1260 g; for women over the age 80, it is 1061 g.[78] Brody and Vijayashankar[17] have noted that although the brain loses thousands of cells daily, the areas of the brain involved in language, memory, and cognition are relatively spared of significant loss of neurons.

In experimental settings, these changes are manifested by a decrease in the ability to register, retain, and recall certain recent experiences, a slower rate of learning new material, slower motor performance on tasks that require speed, and difficulties with fine motor coordination and balance.[23,105,106] However, a normal, motivated, elderly person who is not experiencing emotional stress will not only show few negative changes in intellectual capacity, but may actually demonstrate increases in intellectual functioning over time.[47,63,84,87]

Because many of the variables that need to be considered as part of the clinical evaluation of the **rehabilitation** potential of the person with dementia are affected by both aging and disease, it is important for therapists working with the aged patient to be aware of these variables. The therapist can explore ways to compensate for these changes, and the patient will have a greater possibility of achieving his or her potential for self-care and a meaningful existence.

A slowing of the natural pace of movement is commonly noted in individuals over age 80. This slowdown is manifested in the brain as a slowing of resting electroencephalogram (EEG) rhythms. At age 60, the mean frequency of the occipital rhythm is 10.3 Hz; at age 80, the mean frequency is 8.7 Hz. The average change in EEG frequency is about one cycle per second per decade during these years.[111] The speed of nerve conduction in the elderly can be 10% to 15% slower than in younger persons.[11] Because of these physiological changes, if the process and structure of evaluation and care of the healthy older person emphasize speed of execution or timed activities, the aged will appear less capable than they really are. Therefore the therapist requires more time when working with persons over the age of 70 than is generally required for the average younger adult.

---

* References 3, 24, 66, 72, 89, 92, and 99.

The function of a normal brain requires a delicate synchronization of a large number of variables. To make normal intellectual function possible, the brain must have the following:

- No genetic defects
- A constant supply of nutrients, neurotransmitters, and other neurochemicals
- An unfailing supply of oxygen (implying appropriate blood count, collateral circulation, normal respiratory exchange, and adequate cardiac output)
- Normal blood biochemistry, especially fluid and electrolytes
- Normal hepatic and renal function
- Freedom from noxious stimuli such as trauma, infection, or toxins (including medications)
- Optimal levels of sensory stimulation
- Optimal levels of intellectual stimulation

The brain is the most physiologically active organ in the body. It represents only 2% of the total body weight, and yet it consumes up to 20% of the oxygen and 65% of the glucose available in the circulation in the entire body.[24] The minimum cardiovascular output required to deliver this is 0.75 Ls/minute, which is equal to 20% of the total circulation. Because of the high level of nutrient utilization by the brain, it is one of the organs of the body most likely to be affected by any acute change in its tenuous homeostasis. The homeostasis of the elderly brain physiology is more vulnerable to disruption because of the normal age-related changes already discussed, as well as increased permeability of the blood-brain barrier and increased sensitivity of neurons to the effects of outside agents such as drugs.

Arndt-Schultz Principle

The Arndt-Schultz Principle summarizes the changes between the younger and the aged brain's ability to respond to stimuli:[62]

1. The elderly require a higher level and/or a longer period of stimulation before the threshold for initial physiological response is reached.
2. The physiological response in the aged is rarely as big, as visible, or as consistent as is noted in the younger age groups.
3. The only similarity between the response of the young and the elderly to stimuli is that once the threshold is reached, the more stimuli that are provided, the greater the response.
4. On average, the range of safe therapeutic stimulation is narrower for the elderly than for the young.

The implication of the Arndt-Schultz Principle for clinical problem solving is that the level of a stimulus (e.g., heat, cold, sound, light, or emotional input) needs to be adjusted to compensate for the altered physiology of the aging patient. It is possible that a level of stimulus that is therapeutic for the young may not be for the older patient because it does not reach the threshold for generating a physiological response or it goes beyond the safe therapeutic range for the older adult and becomes harmful. Therefore when an elderly patient does not respond to treatment or presents with an unusual physical response, the clinician must ascertain whether the strength of the stimulus is too strong or too weak, and if modification of the stimulus is necessary because of factors associated with the aging process or the patient's cognitive deficits.

Law of initial values

The law of initial values is both a physiological and a psychological principle that states that, with a given intensity of stimulation, the degree of change produced tends to be greater when the initial value of that variable is low. In other words, the higher the initial level of functioning, the smaller is the change that can be produced.[112-114] The law of initial values, when defined and applied to younger persons, presumes that homeostasis is a stable and consistent process. When the law is used to describe physiological and psychological responses in older persons, it cannot be presumed that homeostasis for any variable is predictable or consistent from one person to the next or within a 24-hour day for the same individual. In the young, it is possible to define the average times of peak activity for most physiological processes as well as for intellectual capacity. In the clinical assessment of the aged, it is necessary to define the peak times of the day for awareness and intellectual capacity for each individual. For example some patients are best able to participate in learning a new skill in the early morning and some only in the late afternoon.

Biorhythms

The body has a biological clock that controls all physiological functions in a precise temporal course, whether it be daily (e.g., secretion of some hormones), monthly (e.g., menstruation), or during a certain period of the life cycle (e.g., ability to become pregnant). Before evaluating a geriatric patient who presents with dementia or disturbance of intellectual functioning, it is helpful to examine the patient's premorbid biorhythm. The patient assessment must allow for and assess the current and past variability of individual biorhythms. It is essential to acknowledge and clearly document these biorhythms, and then maintain and reinforce their stability as much as possible. For example if a woman has worked for 40 years as a night nurse, being primarily active from 11 AM to 7PM she will most likely be alert and best able to participate in a rehabilitation program during those hours. In most cases, it is possible to let the patient choose the best time for treatment. For those patients whose dementia is too severe to make this determination, the staff, by monitoring the patient's behavior, can choose a time for treatment when the client is most alert. For the elderly, and particularly for those who have a dementia, the time of assessment and treatment must be documented and taken into account to maximize the client's rehabilitation potential.[50]

Sensory changes with aging

Aging also can be defined in terms of adaptation. Aging is the progressive and usually irreversible diminution, with the passage of time, of the ability of an organism or one of its parts to perform efficiently or to adapt to changes in its environment. The consequence of the process is manifested as decreased capacity for function and for withstanding stresses.[33] As the rehabilitation evaluation identifies functional problems, it is necessary to examine the possibility that sensory losses or disturbances (e.g., vision, hearing, touch, taste, smell, proprioception, temperature, and kinesthesia) are contributing to the functional impairments.[62] A partial or total loss of one or more of the normative sensory inputs can result in a disturbance of an individual's mental status.

The more sudden the loss of a sensory function, the more difficult the adaptation to the sensory disability. This is especially true for elderly persons. Normally adaptation to a sensory loss in one function is accomplished through an increased sensitivity of the other senses. For example, a young blind patient can adapt by using hearing and kinesthesia and usually learns to function well in spite of the loss of visual input. The older the patient is when blinded, however, the more difficulty she or he will have in making this adaptive crossover to other senses. At some time in any person's life, adaptive crossover from one sense to another becomes exceedingly difficult, if not impossible, and psychopathological or behavioral changes may occur if a sensory impairment develops.[55] This situation becomes more likely if the disruption of neurosensory input occurs in several senses and occurs abruptly.

The polio epidemics of the early 1950s demonstrated the relationship between sensory input and abnormal behavior. Patients with poliomyelitis who were placed in tank-type respirators developed intermittent disruptions in mental state, including hallucinations, delusions, and dreamlike experiences while awake.[33] These patients were deprived of the senses of kinesthesia and proprioception and had severely restricted vision and hearing because of the nature of the construction of and the noise that emanated from the respirator. Called the sensory deprivation psychosis by Solomon,[100] this clinical situation may include cognitive changes in addition to psychotic symptoms.

Bender and others note that the sensory changes associated with normal aging can lead to the same degree of loss or distortion of significant sensory input as described above.[32,59] A bilateral loss of vision may lead to agitation and disorientation. Elderly individuals with hearing impairments often have grave difficulty relating to the world. It is common for elderly persons who become deaf to experience some episodes of paranoid behavior.[55] The problems for

hearing-impaired elderly persons are often exacerbated by health care professionals who do not know how to place a hearing aid in a patient's ear, recognize a dead battery, adjust the volume on the hearing aid, clean the aid of excess cerumen, or recognize a malfunctioning hearing aid. Finally, sensory impairments may become exacerbated by surgical or medical interventions with a patient.

Certain medications, as well as some diseases, also can distort kinesthesia and/or retard the activity and movement of the patient. Movement is significant in the maintenance of an efficient nervous system. Anything that denies a person the ability to perform physical movement (e.g., drugs, restraints, or architectural design not adapted to the aged) hastens and increases the difficulty of adapting to functional limitations. Movement is necessary for accurate sensation.[30,32] Psychophysicists have demonstrated that if movement of the eyes does not occur properly, vision becomes ineffective. The same is true to a lesser degree for hearing. If movement does not occur in the course of the hearing process, hearing can become distorted and misrepresented at the central level.

Cognitive changes in normal aging

As noted previously, it is a myth that cognitive decline is a necessary part of aging. This belief has been debunked by research on crystallized and fluid intelligence.[41] Crystallized intelligence involves the ability to perceive relations, to engage in formal reasoning, and to understand one's intellectual and cultural heritage. Crystallized intelligence can be shaped by the environment and the attitude of the individual.[22] It is therefore possible, with self-directed learning and education, that crystallized intelligence can increase as long as a person is alive. The measurement of crystallized intelligence is usually in the form of culture-specific items such as number facility, verbal comprehension, and general information.

Fluid intelligence is not closely associated with acculturation. It is generally considered to be independent of instruction or environment and depends more on the genetic endowment of the individual.[75] The items used to test fluid intelligence include memory span, inductive reasoning, and figural relations, all of which are presumed to be unresponsive to training. Because fluid intelligence involves those intellectual functions that are most affected by changes in neurophysiological status, they have been generally assumed to decline with age. This myth is not true, as noted in several studies, one of which noted that during middle age, scores on tests for fluid intelligence are similar to scores in mid-adolescence.[56]

Botwinick[13] described the classic pattern of changes in intelligence with aging. In the adult portion of the life span, verbal abilities decline very little, if at all, whereas psychomotor abilities decline earlier and to a greater extent. Although the period between ages 55 and 70 is a transition time and some decreases in performance are noted on many cognitive tests, a substantial decline on laboratory tests of cognitive function is generally limited to those over 75 years of age.[45] In these latter years, however, the decline in fluid intelligence is offset by the growth in crystallized intelligence for most people, unless a dementia is present. Thus although changes may be demonstrated in the laboratory, they are not significant in the "real world," and the elderly are as capable as the young to participate in rehabilitation training. For elderly people to benefit maximally, however, they must control the pace of training, as the tasks that are the most difficult for the aged are those that are fast-paced, unusual, and complex.[56] *All physical therapy treatment with older patients needs to be structured to encourage the patient to self-pace.* Interventions should be predictable and progress by adding one new concept at a time.

Another type of cognitive change differs from the types of changes that occur in normal aging and those that occur in patients with dementia. This type of cognitive change, the "terminal drop," involves a decline in IQ scores by individuals within a year before death. This change in intellectual function is thought to result from some predeath changes in brain physiology. It is likely that research studies that show drastic decreases in intellectual function with advanced age have a large percentage of subjects who were near death as a part of the sample.[12] If the data from these subjects are deleted, the findings are similar to those studies on normal elderly persons.

Stress and intellectual capacity

Selye[86] defined stress as the nonspecific response of the body to any demand made on it. All human beings require a certain amount of stress to live and function effectively. When a stressor (stimulus) is applied, the body predictably goes through the three stages of response called the "general adaptation syndrome." The first response is a general alarm reaction, a "fight or flight" response that mobilizes all senses in an effort to make a judgment about the response that is needed. The next stage involves judgment and the selective adaption to the stressor. A decision is made as to which body action is needed, and all other body activities return to homeostasis. If the stimulus continues and goes beyond the therapeutic level, then the body system or part will gradually experience physiological exhaustion. A person in physiological exhaustion is likely to manifest abnormal responses to any new stimulus. Paradoxical reactions can result in unusual physiological and/or psychological responses to stimuli (e.g., erythematous response when an ice pack is applied or a patient becoming more agitated after receiving a sedative).

With aging, the body undergoes physiological changes, noted later, that make the older individual less physiologically efficient in her or his response to stressors. The general alarm reaction is poorly mobilized and takes longer to become activated (Arndt-Schultz Principle). The stage of resistance should yield a series of responses that allows the

body to economize its response to stress. In persons of all ages who are receiving too many different stimuli, and in the elderly experiencing normal levels of stimuli, the body becomes less efficient at turning off the general alarm response and replacing it with more appropriate and limited responses. Because the body and mind are easily overwhelmed by these stressors, the individual may demonstrate mild global or specific cognitive impairments, especially mild short-term memory loss.

The assessment of an elderly person, with or without dementia, must include a determination of the type, number, and severity of the individual's current stressors. It is important to realize that positive life events (e.g., marriage or the birth of a grandchild) are also stressful life events. Using scores that rate various stressful life events, it is possible to predict which patients are at greatest risk of physiological and emotional exhaustion.[46] Elderly patients, with their numerous psychosocial problems and chronic and acute illnesses, are likely candidates for physiological and emotional exhaustion and the development of psychopathology.* Thus the environment and process of rehabilitation care need to be modified to counteract the effect of stress on the intellectual capacity of the older patient. Any action that modifies stressors so that a deterioration in intellectual function is stopped or reversed is an efficient and cost-effective part of the total rehabilitation effort.

STRATEGIES FOR ASSESSING, PREVENTING, AND MINIMIZING DISTORTIONS IN INFORMATION PROCESSING

Each person acts on the available data at a specific moment. This stimulus-response cycle has four major steps, and at each step, there is a possibility for distortion and/or error. When a person is presented with a stimulus, all data (physiological, psychological, sociological, and environmental) are collected, and then integrated with data based on past experience. Based on the results, a response is determined, which is then followed by the behavioral concomitant of this response.

At the very outset of the process of patient assessment, it is necessary to examine the amount of verbal and written stimuli processed by the patient in relation to the amount used as a part of the testing process. Using an overview of the patient's cognitive capacity, it is possible for the rehabilitation staff to modify the process of evaluation to maximize the patient's performance. A basic assessment of the patient's fluid and crystallized intelligence at a given moment (to allow a comparison of cognitive capacity at other times in the 24-hour cycle) provides the clinician with a specific description of what aspects of intellectual function appear to be impaired and pinpoints those aspects of intellectual functioning that are still intact. Based on this

* References 92, 94, 96-99, 102, and 115-118.

approach, it is possible to proceed with the rehabilitation evaluation in a language and at a pace that is comfortable for the patient.

The Mini-Mental State Examination

The Mini-Mental State Examination (MMSE) was developed as a result of a study noting that 80% of cognitive disorders among elderly people were not detected by the general practitioner.[37,91,115] Most professionals on the rehabilitation team (physicians, nurses,[20,44] physical therapists,[49] and social workers[18]) are likely to have had only minimal specialty training in gerontology and the unique symptoms and needs of the very old.

The MMSE provides a screening test for identifying unrecognized cognitive disorders in the elderly.[34,35,110] The MMSE (Fig. 25-1) assesses only cognition and does not examine other aspects of the traditional mental status examination such as mood, delusions, or hallucinations. The test can identify if the patient is oriented; remembers (short-term); and can read, write, calculate, and see the relationship of one object or figure to another. The examination is used to screen for cognitive dysfunctions, much as a measurement of blood pressure or blood sugar is used to screen for significant medical disorders. The MMSE also may be used in a serial fashion to quantitate changes in a patient's cognitive status over time. This examination can

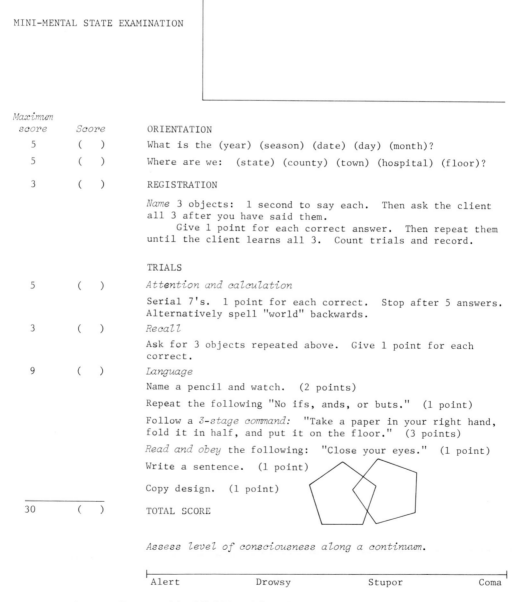

Fig. 25-1. Form used for Mini-Mental State Examination to assess cognition.

be used as a springboard for planning how to carry out the traditional rehabilitation evaluation on a patient who has some intellectual dysfunction.[15,67]

The MMSE has been standardized for elderly persons living in the community. The scores on this test correlate significantly with the Weschsler Adult Intelligence Scale and the Wechsler Memory Test. The MMSE is reported to have a test-retest reliability for both normal and psychiatric samples of 0.89 or greater.[34] It has been found that when a cut-off score of 24 is used for the detection of dementia, the MMSE had a sensitivity of 87.6% and a specificity of 81.6%.[44] Several studies have found that interviews with informants are highly consistent with elderly persons' scores on the MMSE.[48]

The examination takes only a few minutes to administer, is scored immediately, and can be administered by any member of the rehabilitation team. The entire examination grades cognitive performance on a scale from 0 to 30. A score of 24 or less usually indicates some degree of cognitive dysfunction, but some patients with dementia may score above 24, and some with depression or delirium may score significantly below 24. A low score on this examination can mean that the patient is probably suffering from a dementia, delirium, mental retardation, amnestic syndrome, or aphasia.[31] A low score on the MMSE indicates the areas of specific cognitive impairment and gives the rehabilitation team data about how to best communicate with the patient.

A shortened version of the MMSE has been developed (using only 12 of the 20 original variables). Although the original study suggested that the shortened version of the MMSE is equally as effective as the full MMSE in identifying elderly patients with cognitive deficits,[13] several more recent studies have questioned these findings.

Sensory changes with dementia

Patients with dementia may have specific problems that inhibit the integration of sensory input. Aphasias and disruption of association pathways may inhibit the patient's ability to integrate accurately perceived sensory information in a meaningful way. Bassi and others[10] and Fozard[36] have demonstrated that patients with Alzheimer's disease, multi-infarct dementia, and alcoholic dementia may demonstrate disturbances in visual acuity, depth perception, color differentiation, and differentiation of figure from ground when compared with normal aged-matched controls and normal younger individuals.

When a patient has a distortion in cognitive capacity, all neurosensory stimuli must be minimal. An assessment of specific sensory systems is also necessary. The challenge in rehabilitation is to design a process and environment of care so that there is compensation and modification that maximizes the ability of the elderly patient with sensory deficits to adapt to most life situations.

The example of visual deficits is a case in point. One out of every two blind persons in the United States is over 65.[117]

Techniques of environmental adaptation and special measures to organize care to help elderly blind individuals have allowed many of them to live independently in the community.[42] However, many elderly individuals with visual impairments are not blind. Some of the structural changes that result in mild to moderate deficits of vision include yellowing, uneven growth, striation, and thickening of the lens; increasing weakness of the muscles controlling the eye; alteration of the perception of color (especially fine distinctions in tone and brightness); and slower adaptation to light.[36] Modifications of the environment includes good, nonglare lighting, dark and clear large-size print, low-vision aids (e.g., magnifying glass), verbal orientation and escort by persons accompanying patients in a new environment, consistent furniture placement, explanation when changes occur, clear hallways, a systematic storage system for clothes and toilet articles, and the use of contrasting colors to identify doors, windows, baseboards, and corners.[20,21,36,39,40]

Older adult learning styles and communication

Learning occurs throughout life.[56] In rehabilitation the client learns new and/or relearns old adaptive skills. As with intelligence, the learning process does not change abruptly when an individual reaches old age, but differences in performance have been reported. One challenge for rehabilitation therapy is to find ways to improve the efficiency of learning by the older person.

Botwinick[13] has noted that learning and performance are not the same. Poor performance on a learning task may mean that insufficient learning has occurred or that the performance does not accurately reflect the extent of learning achieved.[75] The key variables that affect a person's ability to participate in a learning situation are intelligence, learning skills acquired over the years, and flexibility of learning style. Noncognitive factors also can have a strong bearing on an individual's performance. The noncognitive factors include visual and auditory acuity, health status, motivation to learn, level of anxiety, the speed at which stimuli and learning are paced, and the meaningfulness of the items or tasks to be learned. Therefore a rehabilitation assessment must include a review of the common alterations in learning styles seen among the elderly. This is particularly essential before discontinuing a patient from a rehabilitation program, as a lack of progress may not reflect the patient's lack of capacity for rehabilitation, but rather, may reflect a dissonance between the patient's learning style and skills and the presentation of materials in the treatment program (i.e., verbal input has not been adapted to match the patient's level or pace of comprehension).

Interference

Interference can make the learning process less efficient in two major ways.[27] First, interference can result from a conflict between one's present knowledge with the new knowledge to be learned. Second, if two learning tasks are undertaken at the same time, they can interfere with each other. The elderly have special difficulties if they must concentrate on intake, attention, and retrieval processes at the same time.[27] Therefore the process and **therapeutic environment** of rehabilitation for the elderly patient must not be distracted by such things as background noise, other stimuli in the environment, or personal anxiety. When learning a new task, the elderly patient may require a quiet room with no other stimuli than those offered by the therapist. The need to rid the environment of distractions is particularly important when working with an elderly patient with dementia, as this patient will have greater difficulty filtering out irrelevant sensory inputs, even when compared with elderly patients without dementia.

Pacing

The pacing of therapeutic intervention is a significant variable in helping an elderly person learn. Elderly persons (with or without dementia) perform best if they are given as much time as they need, when learning is self-paced.[13] The major drawback of a fast pace (as perceived by the patient) is that the elderly person generally chooses not to participate rather than risk making a mistake. Nonresponse in the treatment environment is often interpreted as apathy, poor motivation, or "confusion."[6] Nonresponse is reduced when extra time to complete a rehabilitation task is offered. Following the individual assessment, group work (where concepts can be presented, reviewed, and examined at leisure) also can be used to reduce the psychological pressure of faster-paced learning. The details of therapy must be planned carefully, including how questions are asked (this includes asking clear and precise questions in nonmedical language), and, most important, including planning for enough treatment time so the patient can respond at a leisurely pace.

Organization

If data are organized in the brain as part of the learning process, the retrieval of these data becomes easier. Older persons are less likely than members of other age groups to spontaneously organize data to facilitate learning and later retrieval (memory) of that learning.[7] Elderly people who are highly verbal show fewer weaknesses in the ability to organize stimuli. Elderly persons with poor verbal skills show significant improvement when strategies for organization of data are provided from others (e.g., the therapist). Arenberg and Robertson-Tchabo[7] noted that older learners have difficulty following content because they cannot anticipate what will be taught and do not see the whole that is being presented.

Thus it is helpful to organize therapy by beginning with an overview of the entire lesson to be learned in outline form. This presents the patient with a conceptual map of the upcoming experience. The use of purposeful organizing also can help to bridge the gap between what the older person

---

Techniques for maximizing the efficiency of older adult learners

1. Use mediators—the association of word, story, mnemonics, or visual inputs to help the person remember.
2. Choose learning activities that are meaningful for the client.[19]
3. Use concrete examples to make learning easier.[13]
4. Provide a supportive learning environment to prevent stress that can interfere with efficient learning.[28]
5. Use supportive or neutral feedback and avoid feedback that is presented in a challenging tone.[83]
6. Reward all responses, but reward correct responses more than incorrect responses. This can encourage elderly persons to decrease the number of errors by omission, which are often interpreted as apathy or lack of cooperation.[50]
7. Use combinations of auditory and visual input to facilitate the learning process.[6] This is only effective if the data presented are similar because variation between the two kinds of messages can result in interference and a decrease in the efficiency of learning.
8. Active learning is known to be more effective. A patient who moves the involved body part while getting verbal and visual input is likely to be more efficient in mastering the new skill.[75]
9. Design the learning situation so that successful completion of the task is likely.[6] Older people are more likely to focus on errors, which increases anxiety and lowers the self-concept. Worst of all, with all the energy focused on the error, there is a strong chance of repeating the error.

---

knows and the new information or task to be learned. The use of neurolinguistic programming (NLP) is especially effective with elderly patients or with patients with cognitive deficits because it builds consciously—through language, kinesthesia, and visual input—a picture of a new concept from a known and familiar frame of reference.[8]

Inefficient learning, and at times an inability to learn, occurs in the older adult if material is presented in one way and the older person is expected to apply it some other way. Instructions need to be provided in the format in which they are to be used. If possible, one piece of new data should be presented at a time. A conscious transition needs to be made by the therapist from the patient's current frame of reference to the understanding of the new data, and the pace needs to be set by the patient.

There are several other strategies for maximizing the efficiency of older adult learners based on awareness of normal age-related changes. Some of the more frequently used techniques are summarized in the box above.

The research findings and techniques discussed previously describe many of the aspects of the Feldenkrais approach to learning.[30,31] The Feldenkrais Method has been applied to the needs of elderly persons with good results. The principle that learning needs to be pleasurable is especially applicable to patients (with and without dementia) because they are not as likely to be as motivated as young persons. Despite changes in learning style, the older person (with or without dementia) can be helped to learn more efficiently through well-planned instruction. The use of techniques to increase learning efficiency for the elderly has been demonstrated to decrease the stress that at times may result in emotional or cognitive overload and abnormal cognitive reactions.[30,31]

Environmental considerations

Hypothermia. The temperature of the living environment must be carefully controlled because aged clients may not perceive that they are chilled, as they may not experience shivering. Accidental hypothermia can develop in an older person even at temperatures of 60°F (15.5°C) to 65°F (18.3°C). Accidental hypothermia is a drop in the core body temperature to below 95°F (35°C). Patients at risk for hypothermia are presented in the box at the right.

The symptoms of hypothermia may include a bloated face, pale and waxy or pinkish skin color, trembling on one side of the body without shivering, irregular and slowed heartbeat, slurred speech, shallow and very slow breathing, low blood pressure, drowsiness, and symptoms of delirium. The two principles of treatment of hypothermia are that the person will stay chilled unless rewarmed slowly and the patient should be evaluated by a physician, regardless of the apparent severity of the hypothermia.[16,75]

If a person is determined to be at risk for hypothermia, specific preventive measures can be taken to prevent subsequent distortions of cognitive status. First, the room temperature should be set at least to 70°F (21°C). Second, the person should wear adequate clothing; this may include long underwear and undershirt. In addition, adequate nutrition also may be a factor in preventing hypothermia.

Patients and their caregivers often may attempt to save money by lowering room temperatures and thus inadvertently cause accidental hypothermia. It is also common to find institutions with central air conditioning. To prevent accidental hypothermia, special accommodations for the elderly, such as special wings or individual temperature controls in the rooms, are required.[117]

Transplantation shock. It is known that some elderly persons seem to function well in a familiar environment, but they become severely disoriented and unable to perform their ADL if taken out of their own homes. As a general rule, these individuals suffer from very mild symptoms of dementia, which are not readily apparent when they remain in a structured, familiar, stable environment and maintain a consistent daily routine. When faced with the need to adapt to a new environment and being bombarded with multiple unfamiliar sensory stimuli, however, the diseased brain is unable to make sense out of this large volume of new stimuli. If a patient was oriented before admission to an institution

---

> ### Patients at high risk for hypothermia
>
> - Persons over the age of 65
> - Persons showing no signs of shivering or pale skin in response to cold
> - Persons taking medications containing a phenothiazine (to treat psychosis or nausea)
> - Persons with disorders of the hormone system, especially hypothyroidism
> - Persons with head injuries, strokes, Alzheimer's disease or other dementias, Parkinson's disease, or other neurological conditions
> - Persons with severe arthritis
> - Persons with arteriosclerotic peripheral vascular disease, chronic ulceration, or amputation

and then becomes disoriented, it is not unusual for the patient's cognitive functioning to return to its baseline level of functioning upon return to the familiar environment. Therefore all moves by a patient from one hospital room to another or from one institution to another, or all changes in a treatment regimen need to be carefully planned. If a change is anticipated, the patient should be involved in the decision making. If the change is a permanent move, the patient should have a chance for one or two trial visits before the actual move. The patient should be informed of all changes well in advance of any change, and this information needs to be given repeatedly to the patient with dementia. The precautions mentioned can help the patient relocate without creating transplantation shock and related cognitive changes.

Emotional capacity to participate in a learning task

Many elderly persons who come for physical therapy are in a state of emotional overload, as evidenced by disorientation, depression, anger, or a withdrawn and apparently uncooperative attitude. A person who is at or near the point of emotional overload needs to be evaluated as to his or her ability to participate in learning tasks that require active input. If the patient is in an emotional overload, forms of therapeutic intervention that allow the patient temporarily to be a passive recipient of therapeutic intervention can be used. Various types of therapeutic interventions, including massage, connective tissue massage, heat, breathing exercises, relaxation exercises, and Feldenkrais Functional Integration can promote a relaxation response, lower the anxiety level, reinforce self-pacing of activity, and thereby prepare the patient to participate in more physically active types of therapeutic exercise. If asked directly, most patients will state whether they feel able to actively participate.

If for any reason, the patient is not able or willing to state her or his feelings, it is still possible to evaluate the patient's ability to participate. If it is possible to get a patient's cooperation, the following movements can be attempted and then evaluated. (These should be used only if active diseases involving the eyes are not present and there is no pain in doing the movements.)

1. Close eyes.
2. Close eyes and keep them closed for 30 seconds; then for 1 minute.
3. Close eyes; move eyes to the right and left slowly (slow movements with control is the goal).
4. Close eyes; move eyes in diagonals, right and up, then left and down; then left and up, right and down.

If a patient is unable to perform these movements, feels it requires much effort, or feels it is uncomfortable, a high level of tension is present. When the patient is very tense, it is necessary to begin treatment using passive therapeutic procedures. If a person can comfortably execute the movements, the individual (i.e., central nervous system and the body) is able to receive and integrate new data and act with ease. When physical therapy requires active participation by the patient, it is important to verify psychomotor readiness to participate by using a simple set of actions to be performed.

Distortions in intellectual and emotional capacity to receive input, integrate input, and then act on the input affect a person's ability to participate in a learning task. This section has described the most common sources of distortion in information processing that are external to the patient and therefore under the direct control of the rehabilitation team. It is possible for the rehabilitation team to make the choice to acknowledge the common age-related changes and common sources of stress response in the elderly and then to design a process and environment of care that maximizes the elderly patient's potential.

DELIRIUM/REVERSIBLE DEMENTIA: EVALUATION AND TREATMENT

The following discussion focuses on the patient's *internal* environment (physiological, psychological, spiritual and pathological) and presumes that all unnecessary external environmental stressors have been removed. Delirium and dementia have been defined earlier in this chapter. A delirium usually becomes manifested suddenly, or over a period of hours or days. Occasionally, a delirium may be chronic, but this is relatively infrequent. A dementia, whether reversible or irreversible, usually has a much longer time of onset, although an acute onset can occur.

The establishment of the diagnosis of the underlying cause of the dementia or delirium is the key to effective care. Although the diagnostic process is primarily medical, the therapist can obtain information, as part of a team evaluation, that will help establish the underlying diagnosis. Historical information needs to be obtained about the amount of time that has elapsed since the onset of symptoms; the course of progression or lack of progression of symptoms; associated functional impairments; associated medical signs and symptoms; use of prescription, over-the-counter, and illegal drugs, alcohol, caffeine, and nicotine; exposure to occupa-

tional or avocational toxins; and a developmental history. Even in a patient with cognitive disturbances, this information can frequently be obtained and be corroborated by obtaining history from significant others.

The possible causes of delirium and reversible dementias are many. In the elderly person, however, certain causes are more common than others (see the box on p. 733). Alcohol and drugs (prescribed, over-the-counter, illegal, and home remedies) are prime offenders as causative agents of delirium. The delirium may be the result of intoxication, side-effects, or withdrawal syndromes.[90,104] Indeed, one set of clinical symptoms that differentiate elderly addicts from younger addicts is the presence of cognitive deficits.[93] Benzodiazepines are among the most commonly prescribed offenders, as even a single dose of a medication in this class may cause demonstrable cognitive changes.[84] Other common drugs that cause delirium or reversible dementia are alcohol, oral narcotics, psychotropic medications, steroids, antineoplastic drugs, digoxin, anesthetic agents, anti-Parkinsonian drugs, and anti-histamines. However, all classes of drugs have the potential of causing significant cognitive problems in the elderly.[60] These symptoms often resolve with discontinuation of the offending agent or treatment of the withdrawal syndrome. According to Chaprone, for some patients, a medication holiday of longer than 24 hours may be needed before a positive change in cognition can be noted.[50]

At times, the symptoms may be correlated clearly with the pharmacokinetic profiles of the medications taken by the client. The dose and/or frequency of administration of medications can be contributing factors to a delirious state.[88] Each member of the rehabilitation team needs to document the patient's ability to participate in learning tasks and the time of the assessment, because timing of medication administration can affect functional performance. The rehabilitation team needs the input of a clinical pharmacologist who can help the team focus on concepts such as biological half-life, clearance, bioavailability of drugs, and time course of drug concentration in plasma as a function of dose and frequency.

Several medical diseases are quite likely to cause symptoms of delirium or reversible dementia, which will also reverse with treatment of the underlying disease. Urinary tract infections, more common in women, are the cause of delirium in 23% of patients.[68] Fecal impaction is another common cause of acute cognitive changes in elderly persons. Other common causes include distended bladder caused by prostatic enlargement or drug-induced urinary retention, dehydration, malnutrition, cardiovascular disorders,[16] metabolic disturbances (particularly undiagnosed diabetes mellitus[24]), endocrine diseases, renal diseases, hematological diseases, pneumonia or bronchitis,[16] and vitamin B_{12} deficiency.

Transient (and usually mild) cognitive deficits may be the result of a cerebrovascular accident. The cognitive deficits

---

Common causes of delirium/reversible dementia

Alcohol/drug abuse/dependence

Intoxication
Toxicity
Side effects
Withdrawal

Cardiovascular/pulmonary

Congestive heart failure
Cardiac arrhythmia
Hypertensive crisis
Hypoxia
Chronic obstructive pulmonary disease

Metabollic/endocrine

Electrolyte disturbance
   (especially hyponatremia)
Hypercalcemia
Dehydration
Overhydration
Renal failure
Hypoglycemia
Diabetic ketoacidosis
Hypothyroidism
Hyperthyroidism
Malnutrition
Vitamin B_{12}/folate deficiency
Hepatic failure
Wernicke-Korsakoff syndrome
Cushing's syndrome

Infection

Urinary tract infection
Pneumonia/acute bronchitis
Tuberculosis
Other acute infections

Neurological

Stroke
Head trauma
Mass lesion (e.g., tumor, hematoma)
Seizure

Pharmacological

Benzodiazepines
Barbiturates and other
   sedative/hypnotics
Antidepressants
Neuroleptics
Antihistamines
Anticholinergics
Cardiac glycosides
Steroids
Antineoplastic drugs
Narcotics
Antiarrhythmics
Antihypertensives

Miscellaneous

Sensory deprivation
Sensory overstimulation
Acute or chronic pain
Constipation/fecal impaction
Urinary retention

---

after a cerebrovascular accident are often reversible, although they may last for several months after the stroke. The rehabilitation team needs to evaluate and regularly reevaluate the patient's cognitive capacity and build a program of care around those current abilities. A program of therapeutic intervention, which allows the older person to work in a self-paced program for 1 to 3 months, can yield good therapeutic results and also prevent unnecessary secondary deconditioning until part or all of the patient's cognitive capacity returns.[82]

Depression is commonly misdiagnosed as dementia in the elderly.[16,102] For many years, it was thought that depression was a form of "pseudodementia" or false dementia.[61] Depression can result in mild and subtle cognitive changes affecting immediate recall, attention, and the ability to perform basic ADL. Some older reports noted that as many as 31% of those thought to have dementia have depression instead.[89] However, recent research has clarified the close relationship between structural changes in the elderly brain and the onset of depression in the elderly,[43,57] thus bringing

the concept of pseudodementia, or depression as a reversible dementia, into disrepute. Depression is a treatable disorder, and many patients with cognitive impairments show some improvement in their cognitive functioning if the depression is treated; however, the underlying cognitive problem does not resolve with treatment of the depression.[106]

Because the presence of depression can affect the process of rehabilitation through cognitive deficits or its effects on motivation, it is important for this disorder to be diagnosed early and accurately. The Geriatric Depression Scale,[119] a 30 item yes-no questionnaire that can be asked of the patient, allows the treatment team to screen for this disorder. Although there is no sharp cut-off score that signifies depression, most individuals with a score of 13 or higher suffer from this disorder. The higher the score, the more likely that the patient not only suffers from depression, but that the severity of the depression is greater.

In particular, post-stroke major depression can produce a reversible decline in cognitive performance.[41] Post stroke depression is more likely to occur in patients with left hemisphere lesions, and is more likely to occur as the site of the lesion moves toward the frontal pole.[81] This relationship between site of lesion and depression also has been noted on neuropsychological testing.[12]

The treatment of major depression generally involves pharmacotherapy, psychotherapy, and environmental manipulation, which can require support from the entire rehabilitation team.[107] In the treatment of a patient with depression, therapeutic techniques that promote a relaxation response and a decrease in anxiety level (massage, heat, or Feldenkrais Functional Integration) can help bring the patient to the point where it is possible to begin involvement in aerobic training, which is known to have a beneficial effect. All aerobic training for the elderly person should begin with a stress test, modified as necessary to determine the patient's exercise target heart rate. The modifications most commonly required are that the upper extremities are used to achieve the training effect because lower extremity function may be limited or that major ADL involving the upper extremities are used as the training program to achieve the training effect.

The causes of delirium and reversible dementia are usually treatable, and if diagnosis and care are provided in a timely fashion, it is likely that the patient can regain full command of his or her cognitive processes. When this does not happen, it is likely that the patient had a mild irreversible dementia that had remained hidden until the onset of an acute problem that uncovered the poor cognitive functioning. The length of time in an institution (hospital or nursing home) needs to be kept as short as possible to avoid learned dependency and learned helplessness,[95,101] which makes a return to both full cognitive functioning and independent living difficult.[102]

Therapy for elderly persons who are experiencing delirium or reversible dementia consists of treating the underlying causes of the cognitive changes. A close working relationship among all members of the rehabilitation team, including a geriatric psychiatric consultant is necessary. Even before the cause of the disorder is elucidated, the patient should receive the same emotional and physical support as any patient with an irreversible dementia. The therapist must adapt all activities to the extent and types of cognitive losses that are present. The patient needs to feel secure, live in an environment that has as few changes as possible, and have a consistent and stable schedule for activities.

IRREVERSIBLE DEMENTIA

The course of an irreversible dementia is unique for each patient. The variation in clinical course will occur based on the cause of the underlying disease and superimposed biological and psychosocial factors, including but not limited to medications, concurrent illnesses (including delirium), the nature of the social support system, and the patient's premorbid personality structure. The causes of irreversible dementia are summarized in the box below.

Regardless of the cause of the dementia, the clinical course of these disorders has several commonalities.[109] Most of these diseases are progressive. As the patient's insight is often impaired and symptoms may be subtle early in the course of the illness, the onset of the disease is usually noted by the person with the disorder, family members, friends, and/or colleagues at work, rather than by a physician. The signs of impairment of mental ability are commonly memory loss, poor judgment, or incompetence at work. The patient can often succeed at hiding his or her symptoms for a while. The social consequences of the cognitive impairment usually brings the patient to the attention of health care professionals. In addition the patient with dementia can manifest a variety of psychiatric symptoms, including mood disturbance, agitation, violent behaviors, socially inappropriate behaviors, delusions, hallucinations, catastrophic reactions, and perseveration.[66,67] The pattern of onset and the types of psychiatric symptoms are often directly related to the underlying pathological condition.

When a physician is finally consulted, the diagnostic process can begin. When a complete diagnostic evaluation,

---

Common causes of irreversible dementia

Degenerative

Alzheimer's disease
Parkinson's disease
Huntington's disease
Pick's disease
Fahr's disease
Multiple sclerosis

Other

Normal pressure hydrocephalus
Mixed dementia
Alcoholic dementia
Toxins
Head trauma
Mass lesions

Infectious

Neurosyphilis (general paresis)
Tuberculosis
AIDS
Creutzfeldt-Jakob disease

Vascular

Multi-infarct dementia
Stroke
Binswanger dementia
Anoxia
Arteriovenous malformation

including a complete history, physical examination, neurological examination, neuropsychological testing, and laboratory testing (see the box below), are performed, an accurate diagnosis can be made in about 90% of patients,[52] although experienced geriatric psychiatrists can make an accurate diagnosis in over 95% of patients.

Once the diagnostic process is completed, treatment can be started. Medications can assist in reversing underlying causes in only a small percentage of cases; patients in whom this tactic is successful usually have had a potentially reversible dementia that has gone untreated and now have permanent sequelae of the disorder. Medications may only be able to slow down the process of an irreversible disorder (e.g., tacrine for Alzheimer's disease) or prevent further deterioration (e.g., aspirin for multiinfarct dementia). Psychotropic drugs may reverse depression or the behavioral symptoms associated with dementia.[72,89,103] Medical management also involves the prevention and treatment of any comorbid medical conditions.

Thus the foci of medical management of irreversible dementias are maximizing the patient's remaining functions and roles, rehabilitation of some lost functions, and family education and support.[67] Training caregivers to adapt to the patient (i.e., how to get the patient out of bed, bathing), simplifying the individual's living space, and referring relatives to family support services are some of the major techniques used to accomplish these goals.[116]

The treatment of irreversible dementias is a long-term process. Recent studies have found that the average duration of illness from first onset of symptoms to death was 8.1 years for Alzheimer's disease, 6.7 years for multiinfarct dementia,[9] and 5.6 years for Pick's disease.[51] In addition, good medical and nursing care can extend the life expectancy of patients with dementia for up to 20 years or more.

In 1907, Alzheimer[3] described the case and the neuropathology of a 54-year-old woman who developed morbid jealousy, which was followed by loss of memory, inability to read and understand, and death 4.5 years after onset of the illness. Since then, it has been noted that 50% of patients with dementia suffer from Alzheimer's disease.[2] In making the diagnosis of Alzheimer's disease, all other causes of cognitive dysfunction must be ruled out. The disease can occur any time (the junior author has seen a patient in whom the diagnosis was made at age 28), but the onset of the disease is almost always after age 65. The prevalence of the disease gradually increases to a rate of 20% in individuals over the age of 85.[54]

Alzheimer's disease can be clinically described with the use of staging instruments. The use of these instruments enables the family and health care team to plan ahead for the individual's needs. Staging helps the family prepare themselves for the process of interacting with the patient longitudinally. It makes it possible for the treatment team to plan for the appropriate levels of services as an individual's abilities decline. Finally, it allows the health care team to quantitate change in functional and cognitive abilities over time, which will help assess the efficacy of the patient's treatment plan. The use of staging instruments requires an accurate description of the patient's behavior (without the use of jargon), as well as an assessment of the patient's mental state.

Traditionally, the symptoms of Alzheimer's disease have been thought to progress in three stages. Stage 1 lasts from 2 to 4 years and involves loss of functional skills or orientation, memory loss, and lack of spontaneity. The patient is often aware of the losses and is, in many cases, able to cover up the cognitive losses by talking around the issues. During this stage the patient and family may need to deal with the issue of giving up a job, hobbies, or other types of meaningful activity because of the inability to carry them out safely and independently. The patient begins to lose the ability to handle money and a personal budget, will not be able to drive a car safely, and will lose the ability to tell time. The family or meaningful others may have to come to terms with the question of whether the patient can live alone. Depression is common during this stage of the disorder.[103]

In stage 2, there is progressive memory loss and the presence of a variety of neurological symptoms. Aphasias, apraxias, wandering, repetitive movements and stereotypes, increased or decreased appetite, constant movement, and a peculiar wide-based gait can occur. Psychotic symptoms (especially paranoid delusions and hallucinations), agitation, violent behaviors, and uncontrollable screaming are common symptoms during this stage of the disorder.

In stage 3, the patient develops vegetative symptoms. The patient may become mute, stop eating, and become incontinent of bowel and bladder. Muscle twitches or jerks, spasms of the diaphragm, and an inability to walk generally occur. The patient may develop seizures, and emotional

---

Laboratory evaluation for delirium/dementia

Complete blood count
Thyroid function tests
Vitamin $_{12}$/folate levels
Urinalysis
Blood levels of drugs patient is taking
Urine drug screen
Electrocardiogram
MRI scan of head (CT scan if MRI contraindicated)
Automated chemistries (including electrolytes, glucose, renal functions, hepatic functions, protein/albumin, cholesterol/triglycerides)
Blood alcohol level
HIV titer
Chest radiograph

responsiveness, if present, is at a very primitive level. Eventually, the patient dies from the disease.

The MMSE also may be used as a staging tool. Scores of 26 or more are generally associated with minimal, if any dementia, scores of 21 to 25 with mild, 15 to 20 with moderate, 10 to 14 with severe, and scores of 9 or less with profound dementia. The severity of most other symptoms correlates well with the MMSE score.

Reisberg and co-workers[79-80] have developed a scale that defines seven stages, many with substages, of Alzheimer's disease. This scale is probably the most accurate staging system for Alzheimer's disease. In addition, the staging used by this scale closely correlates with the progression of different sets of symptoms through the course of the disease.

STRATEGIES FOR TREATMENT AND CARE

Because changes in cognitive function and behavior happen to a person who is a part of a circle of friends and family support, the rehabilitation team needs to include the caregivers and the patient as much as possible in treatment planning. A very large majority of elderly people with decreased cognitive abilities live with family or friends and not in institutions. The goal of rehabilitation is to ensure that the patient remains safe, independent, and able to perform ADLs and IADLs for as long as is reasonable. The planning to reach these goals is best done within the context of the patient's social support system.

The rehabilitation process begins while the diagnostic workup is still in progress. At this stage of treatment, the rehabilitation plan includes basic training for the patient in performing and adapting the ADLs. It also includes **caregiver training and support** for significant others, so that they can make needed environmental modifications to ensure safety for the patient with dementia.

Once the diagnosis is established, treatment planning for long-term care at home or in an institution must be carefully made. No matter where the patient will be living, involvement of the caregivers and significant others is crucial. It is necessary to ascertain the emotional and physical resources of the patient and family and/or significant others who will be the caretakers. A review of the caretakers' willingness to perform basic tasks or visitation, willingness to be taught needed skills, and the realistic need for respite must be determined.[58] Family training and orientation manuals that deal with all the details of caring for a person with dementia are available.[67,70] The same detailed orientation is needed for institutional staff who are to care for elderly patients with dementia. It is possible, by the structure and process of care, to help patients to be maximally active in their self-care and to prevent unnecessary anxiety and catastrophic reactions.

As a part of the rehabilitation program, physical therapy treatment for this group of patients needs to emphasize reassurance, hands-on interventions, and communication to allow treatment to proceed at a pace perceived as reasonable by the patient.[50] In the early and middle stages of all

dementias, physical therapy intervention usually can prolong the ability to move with ease for ADL/IADL and maintain the ability to participate in some social activities. This is extremely important for caregivers, as deficits in patients' abilities to perform ADLs and IADLs[118] often relate to their inability to physically perform these acts under supervision. The ability to walk is lost late in most dementias,[26,38] but gait and coordination disturbances are common and can benefit from physical therapy. Therapy intervention to assist the patient and train the caregivers involves facilitation of ease of movement and motor planning and developing or refining environmental and cognitive cues to assist in carrying out complex tasks. Ultimately, caregivers will need training in how to move, lift, and otherwise assist the patient.

Cognitive impairment is a key limiting factor in both the performance of ADLs and IADLs, as well as a limiting factor for participating in rehabilitation. An accurate assessment and training by the therapist helps the caregiver provide only the help that is absolutely needed, with patients continuing to perform for themselves as many ADLs as possible. For example to brush the teeth, a patient needs to be able to remember the command, to recognize the toothbrush, and to perform a complex but repetitive motor action. The patient may only need the help of someone placing the toothbrush in his or her hand and slowly guiding it to the mouth to be able to safely brush the teeth.

The accurate assessment of IADLs and ADLs is more reliable than medical diagnosis for predicting the amount of assistance and interaction a person will need in a nursing home. The first goal of rehabilitation for patients with dementia is to create a supportive emotional and physical environment. In other words, the environment must work actively to compensate for the patient's specific cognitive/functional losses as they gradually occur. The ultimate goal is to help patients feel that they are capable, so that they will continue to try to do those things for themselves that they can do safely, whether they remain in their home or live in an institution. It is equally important to orient and train significant others so that they feel comfortable allowing the patient to participate safely in activities and basic self-care tasks modified to their cognitive level.

The Alzheimer's Association is a resource for professionals and caregivers of individuals with dementia. The goals of the association are to support research related to the diagnosis, therapies, causes, and cures for Alzheimer's disease and related disorders; to aid in organizing family support groups; to educate and assist affected families; to sponsor educational programs for professional and lay persons on the topic of Alzheimer's disease; to advise government agencies of the needs of the affected families to promote federal, state, and private support of research; and to offer help in any manner to patients and their caregivers to promote the well-being of all involved. Through the efforts of the association, it is hoped that humane care can be provided to the patient with dementia and related disorders throughout the course of the illness. Other models of support groups have been tried in communities where spouses have worked to develop ongoing respite care.[14]

As a member of the rehabilitation team, the physical therapist needs to conduct an inventory of services as a part of their annual review of the quality of care that is provided for patients with dementia. A survey of persons caring for patients with dementia listed the following services in their perceived order of importance:[76,109]

1. A paid companion who can come to the home a few hours each week to give caregivers a rest (respite)
2. Assistance in locating people or organizations that provide patient care
3. Assistance in applying for government programs, such as Medicaid, disability insurance, and income support programs
4. A paid companion who can come to the home for overnight care so caregivers can go away for one or more days (respite)
5. Personal home care for the individual with dementia to help with activities such as bathing, dressing, or feeding in the home
6. Support groups composed of others who are caring for individuals with dementia and other cognitive deficits
7. Special nursing home care programs only for individuals with dementia
8. Short-term respite care in nursing homes or hospitals to take care of individuals with dementia and other cognitive deficits while the caregiver is away
9. Adult day care providing supervision and activities away from the home
10. Visiting nurse services for care at home

In-home care, information about the availability of services and government programs, and various forms of respite care were also ranked high in the survey. Overall, caregivers (family and friends) of the patient are often able and willing to provide care for the patient throughout the illness if appropriate professional consultation can help them solve problem situations and if adequate respite time is provided to the caregiver(s).

Not mentioned in this study was the need for psychological support for caregivers. The stress on caregivers is extreme, and symptoms of anxiety and depression are common. Because of the relative lack of counseling services for caregivers, however, the use of (and probable abuse of and dependence on) psychotropic medications by caregivers is quite high.[14] As these medications may impair the cognitive functioning of caregivers, the risk of harm to the patient with dementia is also high.

DEMENTIA/DELIRIUM—NEW FRONTIERS

Most current research in delirium and dementia is focused on Alzheimer's disease. Research is underway to explore possible causes of dementias, including work that examines the roles of neurotransmitters, structural brain changes, nutrition, viruses, drugs, immunological deficits, and the role of heredity in the etiology of Alzheimer's disease. Studies to increase the diagnostic accuracy of different dementias, including a distinction between cortical and subcortical dementias, or the use of DSM-III-R criteria,[5,77] DSM-IV criteria,[4] or neuropsychological criteria, are also underway. Newer models of dementia, including those caused by stage II or III HIV infection,[73] are also being studied.

The most exciting area of research is pharmacological treatment.[105] The advent of tacrine, a drug that slows down the progression of Alzheimer's disease in some patients, has produced an explosion of research on drugs to try to stabilize or reverse the symptoms of this disease. Although no cures are available, some drugs, such as physostigmine, ondansetron, and nerve growth factor, have shown some promise in the treatment of this disorder. These studies have spawned a search for new drugs not only to treat Alzheimer's disease, but to treat the symptoms of other dementias.

SUMMARY

In working with the patient with dementia or delirium, the therapist can do much to make the quality of life better for the patient and the caregivers.[67] A detailed listing of the "how tos" has been described in other texts, and it is anticipated that the details needed to develop an environment and process of care for elderly persons with cognitive deficits can be found in those sources.[66,67,70]

Specific examples of modifications of physical therapy assessment and treatment may include working in collaboration with other members of rehabilitation team and developing a consultative relationship with key caregivers (professional and nonprofessional, and all shifts of institutional staff) to encourage **problem solving** and patient participation in self-care. Another important modification includes the evaluation of each patient's communication abilities before the therapy assessment to adapt assessment in such a way as to promote patient participation.

Modifications of treatment include the use of neurological rehabilitation techniques (e.g., Feldenkrais, neurodevelopmental therapy [NDT], or Brunnstrom techniques) to decrease the presence of abnormal muscle tone and to increase the ease of movement, to increase ease of breathing (to enhance endurance and minimize the related sense of anxiety) if the rib cage is carried with massive muscle tightness, and to increase patient coordination. The therapist needs to modify the process of neurological facilitation to enhance the patient's sense of safety and motivation for self-care within the security of a supervised environment. Tasks may need to be simplified so that the patient can perform them and/or the caregiver is trained to perform only those tasks that the patient cannot perform.

Each month the therapist, treatment team, patient, and caregiver should identify safe physical activities that the

CASE 1 ▼   The Complexity of Aging

The patient was a 78-year-old woman who had the following deficits on the Mini-Mental State Examination: was not aware of where she lived, date or year, had poor short-term memory and could not spell the word "world" backwards, could not copy the two overlapping hexagons. The patient was generally happy and enjoyed having someone sit with her. The patient fractured her femur and because of the location of the fracture site, a surgical procedure was performed to allow total weight bearing. The surgeon and the psychiatrist decided that partial weight bearing would not be a concept that the patient could understand. The physical therapist and assistant worked together with the family and caregivers in the nursing home to develop a plan of care. At the initial care conference, the big question was whether the patient should receive physical therapy. The family was fearful that the patient would fall again if she were taught how to walk. The focus of the conference was to educate the family and other staff as to the importance of physical therapy so the patient could learn how to participate and eventually perform transfers from wheelchair to toilet as well as to bed. The decision was made to begin physical therapy, with the initial goal being to achieve all functional ADL transfers with standby physical assistance.

The patient was not interested in walking and was fearful of falling. The key change in physical therapy intervention was in the style of communication that was used to teach basic bed mobility and the components of transfer skills. Using trial and error, it was found that the patient responded best to a smile, verbal encouragement, hand signals and gentle manual pressure to indicate the desired task to be performed. If the task was broken down and components were identified, the patient became frustrated and refused to participate. If the patient was invited by manual cues and verbal reassurance to stand up and sit on the bed, the patient would hesitate for up to 1 minute and then she would attempt to perform the task. It became obvious that the patient needed at least 30 to 60 seconds of waiting time between verbal requests given by staff and when she was ready to act on the request. It was also discovered that if additional input were given, the patient appeared to get frustrated and would refuse to cooperate. A sign was placed over her bed with the instructions for communication: smile, reassure, use your hands to guide her to perform the desired action, and wait 60 seconds: Let her feel there is plenty of time.

A sliding board was introduced in therapy, and the patient enjoyed the idea. The board allowed transfers for all ADL to involve no lifting for the staff. The patient would lean her head on the shoulder of the staff member while sitting and then she would assist in sliding across on the board. All transfers for ADL using the sliding board were possible within five visits of physical therapy. A bed was located that was 17 inches high to facilitate bed-to-wheelchair transfers. The bed could be raised to assist the nursing aide in cleaning activities. The decision was made to leave the bed at 17 inches unless the nursing staff needed to perform special in bed procedures with the patient. The wheelchair foot rests were modified so that they formed a solid flat surface to allow the patient to rest in a natural position. The patient was only 5'2" tall and the standard wheelchair only allowed her to comfortably put both feet on one foot pedal and sit with her weight mostly on one pelvis. A smaller wheelchair and the adapted foot rest gave the patient an equal pressure on both sitting bones, and the patient began to sit at rest in a natural upright posture. The other goal of physical therapy was to teach the patient wheelchair mobility using her hands to push the chair. Once the patient was given gloves for her hands (she did not like germs), she was willing to try to push the wheelchair. The patient was instructed in the physical therapy department during two visits. The patient was next seen by the therapist on the unit to allow the nursing aide to be a part of the physical therapy instruction. The rationale was that the nursing aide would need to help reinforce the skills and encourage practice of the wheelchair mobility skills as a part of daily activities. During the last visits the physical therapist watched daytime, afternoon, and evening staff practice with the patient and problem solve new situations that arose. It is critical to train all caregivers on three shifts to ensure consistency of verbal and manual cuing for the patient.

Before discharge to restorative nursing, the patient's current level of functional abilities was documented using an ADL chart that specified time of day when tasks were easiest, task(s), equipment needs, special positioning, clothing and other assistive devices, verbal cuing, or other communication requirements for each critical task that had been mastered in physical therapy. The cataloguing of functional skills reminded the nursing aide of the ingredients involved in order for the patient to successfully perform ADLs. The other advantage of the detailed discharge summary to the nursing staff is that new staff could use the document and as needed, contact physical therapy for clarifications if the patient suddenly were not able to perform the tasks (a signal of possible medical/psychosocial problems).

Key points
1. Common goals identified and agreed on between all team members and patient's significant others.
2. Education provided as needed to allow for consistency of verbal and manual cuing for the patient.
3. Physical therapy treatment began in a quiet, undisturbed area where the patient could concentrate. As mastery of a skill was achieved, the skill was practiced with supervision and teaching of other staff in the patient's real living situation with adaptations as needed.
4. Equipment/furniture was adjusted to help the patient perform tasks with minimal assistance.
5. Discharge from therapy involved providing nursing staff with a detailed description of functional abilities and the conditions required to help maximize patient participation, sense of safety, and control (as had already been reviewed with all aides working with patient).
6. The physical therapist should be viewed as a resource person for nursing staff for simplifying functional tasks in patient care; consultation for problem solving should be encouraged.

CASE 2   A Client in Early Stage of Alzheimer's Disease

The patient was a 64-year-old man who until 1 month ago was working. He was forced to retire because he would forget the natural sequences of the work tasks. For example his partner would see him direct someone to wait for him in the waiting room and then he would forget the person was in the waiting room. On the Mini-Mental State Examination, he had difficulty with date and year, would try to redirect the question in an apparent attempt to cover up for loss of short-term memory. He could or would not spell the word "world" backwards, and he poorly copied the overlapping hexagons (looked more like squares). He was a runner but now he apparently would not remember how to get home, and he would pretend to be hurt and get someone to drive him home. The man reported feeling restless.

The patient, his wife and two sons were seen by the team at a psychiatric clinic. The wife was very upset and the family was asking for help. The role of therapy at this early stage of Alzheimer's disease involved:

1. a. Functional assessment of basic ADL/IADL activities and home assessment.
   b. Orientation of spouse/significant caregivers as to the functional changes that may occur in the near future and how to compensate for current functional losses (i.e., patient had difficulty dressing in morning and would get frustrated).
2. Orientation to the role of physical therapy in hands-on treatment related to techniques to help the patient relax. After initial evaluation, it was decided to teach caregivers massage techniques identified by the therapist as soothing and relaxing for the patient. NOTE: The emphasis in the hands-on intervention is to create slow, predictable, and nurturing contact that is perceived by the patient as soothing and relaxing.
3. Orientation of caregivers to the use of manual contact and hand signals to communicate and reinforce the intention. Kinesthetic contact and the ability to follow kinesthetic cues can help the patient with ADL tasks at home. At this time the kinesthetic cuing may not be critical for the patient, but the caregivers need to get in the habit of cuing the patient as a compensatory tool for future cognitive losses.
4. Orientation of caregivers to the benefits of a ritualized schedule of daily events for the patient and assistance in developing the daily schedule. The predictability of the ritual will help the patient feel safe and in control. The ritualizing is especially helpful initially to address the frustrations with dressing in the morning.
5. Written information about local support groups, day treatment centers, and the availability of the rehabilitation team/including therapy for problem solving.
6. Participate in evaluation of patient/family need for placement in a day treatment center or use of home health aide. Supervision was needed for cooking (would leave burners on), working in the woodshop (would leave power tools running), and in self care repair to ensure his safety. It was decided to use

supervision in the home, with family members sharing the load. The idea of leaving the home to go to a new place was not positively received by the patient. NOTE: patient may often function better in the environment where he or she has lived for a long time due to the familiarity with the details of the surroundings.
7. Therapist participated in development of the home care plan and provided four home visits to accomplish tasks described in numbers 1-6.

The next contact that the family made with therapy was to address the patient's inability to settle himself down and be able to go to sleep at night. A home visit was made to evaluate the bedtime ritual, the relaxation strategies being used, and communication with the physician about current medications taken. It became obvious that the patient disliked bathing and undressing for bed. After discussion with caregivers, the patient was allowed to go to bed in his clothes without bathing and undressing (bathing and undressing would be carried out in the morning when he was less tired). Relaxation massage was modified to involve the face, neck, hands, and feet; and the caregivers were instructed and practiced during two visits under the supervision of the therapist. A satisfactory bedtime ritual was developed and home health care for the patient was workable for the patient and the caregivers.

The next request for therapy consultation came 14 months later when the wife and the daughter-in-law (who had been taking turns being the primary caregiver) both felt the need to hire and train an attendant/companion for the patient for 8 hours a day. At this time the patient preferred to be in the home, walk in the yard, or take long walks in the local park. The therapist, in cooperation with other team members, trained the patient/aide in how to sequence for ease in ADL tasks; use of kinesthetic cuing; how to problem solve ADL, bathing, dressing using slow pace and ritualized format; and sequencing the tasks and relaxation techniques to help the patient settle down and go to sleep. Foot massage was the only technique that the patient now allowed and appeared to enjoy. After three physical therapy visits over a 2-week period, the attendant was able to carry out home health care effectively for the patient.

The last request for help occurred when the family was concerned because the patient was "trying to run away." The therapist made a home visit and found that the patient sat most of the day. Mini-Mental State Examination showed that he could not give his own first or last name and had no short-term memory. Based on the evaluation, it was proposed that the family/attendant go with the patient for a walk when the patient showed an interest in leaving the house. This strategy worked for a few months but then the patient began to sit down on the sidewalk when he was tired. Another visit was made after a wheelchair was ordered to train the caregivers in use of the wheelchair and to orient the patient to the desired procedures and to reassure the patient. After this visit the patient showed gradually less interest in leaving the home over the next few months until he eventually stayed in the house constantly. At this time the patient also became incontinent of

Continued.

CASE 2   A Client in Early Stage of Alzheimer's Disease–cont'd

bowel and bladder. The patient refused to use the toilet and the decision was made to seek nursing home placement.

Key points:

1. Physical therapy is a part of the caregiving team for the patient and family of the patient with Alzheimer's disease.
2. Evaluation of functional skills, communication related to functional skills, and home modifications to enhance patient participation in self-care can be continued as long as the caregivers request the support and problem solving.
3. Problem solving with caregivers and educating caregivers are the primary roles once the therapist has identified the intervention of choice to solve the key functional problems.
4. All therapy intervention needs to be coordinated with actions of other members of the caregiving team.

---

patient can be encouraged to do for recreation, relaxation, and overall fitness and to enhance the performance of simple ADL and IADL tasks (e.g., wash out own socks, set the table) to enhance patient self-esteem. In addition the physical therapist, along with other members of the rehabilitation team and caregivers, need to monitor the patient for new signs and symptoms of a concurrent delirium or reversible dementia so that treatment can be initiated early and further deterioration prevented.

The Hospital Patients Bill of Rights and the Nursing Home Patients Bill of Rights define the minimum quality of care required for any patient. The concepts presented in the two bills apply to the care of patients with cognitive deficits, no matter what the setting. The provision of considerate and respectful care for the person afflicted with dementia or other cognitive deficits is possible and necessary. Well-planned and gentle care prevents unnecessary distortions in cognitive function brought on by feelings of fear or being rushed, and thereby maximizes all remaining cognitive function. To use his or her remaining emotional and cognitive resources, the patient with cognitive deficits needs to live in an environment and experience a process of care that is modified to meet the special needs created by delirium and/or dementia.

Physical therapy is a key resource for the creation of a therapeutic environment and for the effective and timely assessment and treatment for the patient with cognitive deficits. The goal of therapy is to create a process of care where the patient feels safe and the caregivers are given the training and support in problem solving so as to guide the patient to participate in self-care and recreation as long as it is safe and functionally possible.

REFERENCES

1. Agate J: *The practice of geriatrics,* ed 2, London, 1970, William Heinemann Medical Books.
2. Allison RS: *The senile brain,* London, 1962, Edward Arnold.
3. Alzheimer A: Über eine eigenartige Erkrankung der Hirnrinde, *Allgemeine Zeitschrift für Psychiatrie und Psychish-Gerichtliche Medizin,* 64:146-148, 1907.
4. American Psychiatric Association: Delirium, dementia, amnestic and other cognitive disorders. In *DSM-IV draft criteria,* Washington, 1993, American Psychiatric Association.
5. American Psychiatric Association: Organic mental syndromes and disorders. In *Diagnostic and statistical manual,* ed 3, revised, Washington, 1987, American Psychiatric Association.
6. Arenberg D: Concept problem solving in young and old adults, *J Gerontol* 23:279-282, 1968.
7. Arenberg D and Robertson-Tchabo EA: Learning and aging. In Birren JE and Schaie KW, editors: *Handbook of the psychology of aging,* New York, 1977, Van Nostrand Reinhold Co.
8. Bandler R and Grinder J: *Frogs into princes,* Cupertino, 1979, Real People Press.
9. Barclay LL and others: Survival in Alzheimer's disease and vascular dementias, *Neurology* 35:834-840, 1985.
10. Bassi CJ, Solomon K, and Young D: Vision in patients with Alzheimer's disease, *Optom Vision Sci* 70:809-813, 1993.
11. Birren JE: *Handbook of aging and the individual,* Chicago, 1973, University of Chicago Press.
12. Bolla-Wilson K and others: Lateralization of dementia of depression in stroke patients, *Am J Psychol* 146:5:627-634, 1989.
13. Botwinick J: *Aging and behavior—a comprehensive integration of research findings,* New York, 1978, Springer.
14. Brache CI: The aging client and their family network. In Jackson O, editor: *Physical therapy of the geriatric patient,* New York, 1983, Churchill Livingstone.
15. Braekhus A, Laake K, and Engedal K: The mini-mental state examination: identifying the most efficient variables for detecting cognitive impairment in the elderly, *J Am Geriatr Soc* 40:1139-1145, 1992.
16. Brocklehurst JC: *Textbook of geriatric medicine and gerontology,* ed 2, New York, 1985, Churchill Livingstone.
17. Brody H and Vijayashankar N: Anatomical changes in the nervous system. In Finch CE and Hayflick L, editors: *Handbook of the biology of aging,* New York, 1977, Van Nostrand Reinhold.
18. Busse EW and Pfeiffer E, editors: *Mental illness in later life,* Washington, 1973, American Psychiatric Association.
19. Calhoun RO and Gounard BR: Meaningfulness, presentation rate, list length and age in elderly adults paired association learning, *Educ Gerontol* 4:49-56, 1979.
20. Campbell ME: Study of the attitudes of nursing personnel toward the geriatric patient, *Nurs Res* 20:141-151, 1971.
21. Carroll K, editor: *Human development in aging—compensation for sensory loss,* Minneapolis, 1978, Ebenezer Center for Aging and Human Development.
22. Cattell RB: Theory of fluid and crystallized intelligence—a clinical experiment, *J Educ Psychol* 54:1 22, 1963.
23. Cerella J: Aging and information-processing rate. In Birren JE and Schaie KW, editors: *Handbook of the psychology of aging,* ed 3, San Diego, 1990, Academic Press.
24. Charatan FB: *Management of confusion in the elderly,* New York, 1979, Roerig.

25. Clipp EC and George LK: Psychotropic drug use among caregivers of patients with dementia, *J Am Geriatr Soc* 38:227-235, 1990.

26. Coons D and others: *Final report of project on Alzheimer's disease: subjective experience of families,* Ann Arbor, 1983, Institute of Gerontology.

27. Craik IM: Age differences in human memory. In Birren JE and Schaie KW, editors: *Handbook of the psychology of aging,* New York, 1977, Van Nostrand Reinhold.

28. Elias MF and Elias PK: Motivation and activity. In Birren JE and Schaie KW, editors: *Handbook of the psychology of aging,* New York, 1977, Van Nostrand Reinhold.

29. Evans DA and others: Prevalence of Alzheimer's disease in a community population of older persons: higher than previously reported, *JAMA* 262:2551-2556, 1989.

30. Feldenkrais M: *Awareness through movement,* New York, 1972, Harper & Row.

31. Feldenkrais M: *The elder citizen,* Berkeley, 1989, Feldenkrais Resources. (Pamphlet and audio cassette tapes.)

32. Fields WS, editor: *Neurological and sensory disorders in the elderly,* New York, 1975, Stratton Intercontinental Medical Book Corp.

33. Foley JM: Sensation and behavior. In Fields WS, editor: *Neurological and sensory disorders in the elderly,* New York, 1975, Stratton Intercontinental Medical Book Corp.

34. Folstein MF, McHugh PR, and Folstein SF: Mini-Mental State—a practical method for grading the cognitive state of patients for the clinician, *J Psychiatr Res* 12:189-198, 1975.

35. Folstein MF and others: The meaning of cognitive impairment in the elderly, *J Am Geriatr Soc* 33:228-235, 1985.

36. Fozard JL: Vision and hearing in aging. In Birren JE and Schaie KW, editors: *Handbook of the psychology of aging,* ed 3, San Diego, 1990, Academic Press.

37. Galesko D and others: The MMSE in the early diagnosis of disease, *Arch Neurol* 47:49-52, 1990.

38. George LK: *The dynamics of caregiver burden,* Washington, 1984, Association of Retired Persons—Andrus Foundation.

39. Gobetz GE: *Learning mobility in blind children and the geriatric blind,* Cleveland, 1967, Cleveland Society for the Blind.

40. Gobetz GE and others: *Home teaching of the geriatric blind,* Cleveland, 1969, Cleveland Society for the Blind.

41. Grant I and Adams K, editors: *Neuropsychological assessment of neuropsyc disorders,* New York, 1986, Oxford University Press.

42. Gross AM: Preventing institutionalization of elderly blind, *Vis Impairment Blindness* 2:49-53, 1979.

43. Grossberg GT, Manepalli J, and Solomon K: Diagnosis of depression in demented patients. In Morely JE and others, editors: *Memory functioning and aging-related disorders,* New York, 1992, Springer.

44. Gunter LM: Student attitudes toward geriatric nursing, *Nurs Outlook* 19:466-469, 1971.

45. Hertzog C and Schaie KW: Stability and change in adult intelligence: simultaneous analysis of longitudinal means and covariance structures, *Psychol Aging* 3:122-130, 1988.

46. Holmes TH and Rahe RH: The social readjustment rating scale, *J Psychosom Res* 11.213-218, 1967.

47. Hultsch DF and Dixon RA: Learning and memory in aging. In Birren JE and Schaie KW, editors: *Handbook of the psychology of aging,* ed 3, San Diego, 1990, Academic Press.

48. Jackson JF and Ramsdell JW: Use of the MMSE to screen for dementia in elderly outpatients, *J Am Geriatr Soc* 36:662, 1988.

49. Jackson O: Physical therapy and the geriatrics patient—a descriptive study of cross-cultural trends in Denmark and the United States, doctoral dissertation, Ann Arbor, 1979, University of Michigan.

50. Jackson O: *Physical therapy and the geriatric patient,* New York, 1987, Churchill Livingstone.

51. Jung R and Solomon K: Psychiatric manifestations of Pick's disease, *Int Psychogeriatr* 5:187-202, 1993.

52. Katzman R: Alzheimer's disease, *New Engl J Med* 314:964-973, 1986.

53. Katzman R: Clinical presentation of the course of Alzheimer's disease: the atypical patient. In Rose CF, editor: *Modern approaches to the dementias,* Part II, Basel, 1985, Kraeger.

54. Kay DWK and others: Old age mental disorders in Newcastle-Upon-Tyne: a study of prevalence, *Br J Psychol* 110:146-158, 1964.

55. Kay DWK and others: The differentiation of paranoid from affective psychoses by patient's premorbid characteristics, *Br J Psychiatry* 129:207-215, 1976.

56. Knox AB: *Adult development and learning,* San Francisco, 1977, Jossey-Bass.

57. Krishnan KRR: Neuroanatomic substrates of depression in the elderly, *J Geriatr Psychiatry Neurol* 6:39-58, 1993.

58. Lang R and Jackson O: Model demonstration of a comprehensive care system for older people, Project Grant Number 90-A-1618, Administration of Aging, 1980, Washington, DC.

59. Leighton DA: Special senses—aging of the eye. In Brocklehurst JC, editor: *Textbook of geriatric medicine and gerontology,* New York, 1985, Churchill Livingstone.

60. Levinson AJ, editor: *Neuropsychiatric side effects of drugs in the elderly,* New York, 1979, Raven Press.

61. Libow LS: Pseudo-senility: acute and reversible organic brain syndromes, *J Am Geriatr Soc* 21:112-120, 1973.

62. Licht S: *Therapeutic heat and cold,* New Haven, 1960, Elizabeth Licht.

63. Light LA: Interactions between memory and language in old age. In Birren JE and Schaie KW, editors: *Handbook of the psychology of aging,* ed 3, San Diego, 1990, Academic Press.

64. Lipowski ZJ: Delirium (acute confusional states), *JAMA* 258:1789-1792, 1987.

65. Lipowski ZJ: Delirium in the elderly, *New Engl J Med,* 320:578-582, 1989.

66. Mace NL, editor: *Dementia care: patient, family, and community,* Baltimore, 1990, Johns Hopkins University Press.

67. Mace NL and Rabins PV: *The 36 hour day—a family guide to caring for persons with Alzheimer's disease, related dementing diseases and memory loss in later life,* Baltimore, 1981, Johns Hopkins University Press.

68. Manepalli J and Grossberg GT: Recognition and treatment of depression. In Szwabo PA and Grossberg GT, editors: *Problem behaviors in long-term care. Recognition, diagnosis, and treatment,* New York, 1993, Springer.

69. May BJ: An integrated problem solving curriculum for physical therapists, Washington, 1976, American Physical Therapy Association.

70. McDowell FH, editor: *Managing the person with intellectual loss (dementia or Alzheimer's disease) at home,* White Plains, 1980, Burke Rehabilitation Center.

71. McKahann G and others: Clinical diagnosis of Alzheimer's disease, *Neurology* 34.939-944, 1984.

72. Meyers BS and Cahenzli CT: Psychotropics in the extended care facility. In Szwabo PA and Grossberg GT, editors: *Problem behaviors in long-term care. Recognition, diagnosis, and treatment,* New York, 1993, Springer.

73. Morgan MK, Clark ME, and Hartman WL: AIDS-related dementia: a case report of rapid cognitive decline, *Psychology,* 44:1024-1028, 1988.

74. Nissen T and others: Dementia evaluated by means of the Mini-Mental State Examination, clinical neurological patient material, *Hasskr Nor Laegeforen* 109:1138-1182, 1989.

75. Peterson D and Orgren RA: Older adult learning. In Jackson O, editor: *Physical therapy of the geriatric patient,* New York, 1983, Churchill Livingstone.

76. Rabins PV and others: Emotional adaptation over time in care givers for chronically ill elderly people, *Age Aging* 19:185-190, 1990.

77. Rebok GW and Folstein MF: Dementia, *Neuropsychiatry* 5:265-276, 1993.

78. Reichel W, editor: *Clinical aspects of aging,* Baltimore, 1978, Williams and Wilkins.

79. Reisberg B: Clinical presentation, diagnosis, and symptomatology of age-associated cognitive decline and Alzheimer's disease. In Reisberg B, editor: *Alzheimer's disease: the standard reference,* New York, 1983, Free Press.

80. Reisberg B and others: The Global Deterioration Scale (GDS): an instrument for the assessment of primary degenerative dementia (PDD), *Am J Psychiatry* 139:1136-1139, 1982.

81. Robinson RG and others: Mood disorders in stroke patients, *Brain,* 107:81-93, 1984.

82. Rodstein M: Characteristics of nonfatal myocardial infarction in the aged, *Arch Intern Med* 98:84-90, 1956.

83. Ross E: Effect of challenging and supportive instructions in verbal learning in older person, *J Educ Psychol* 58:261-266, 1968.

84. Salzman C, Fisher J, and Nobel K: Cognitive improvement following benzodiazepine discontinuation in elderly nursing home residents, *Int J Geriatr Psychiatry* 7:89-93, 1992.

85. Schaie KW: Intellectual development in adulthood. In Birren JE and Schaie KW, editors: *Handbook of the psychology of aging,* ed 3, San Diego, 1990, Academic Press.

86. Selye H: *Stress without distress,* New York, 1974, JB Lippincott.

87. Shakespeare W: As you like it, III,i. In Craig WJ, editor, *The complete works of William Shakespeare,* London, 1922, Humphrey Milford Oxford University Press.

88. Simonton DK: Creativity and wisdom in aging. In Birren JE and Schaie KW, editors: *Handbook of the psychology of aging,* ed 3, San Diego, 1990, Academic Press.

89. Sky AJ and Grossberg GT: Aggressive behaviors and chemical restraints. In Szwabo PA and Grossberg GT, editors: *Problem behaviors in long-term care. Recognition, diagnosis, and treatment,* New York, 1993, Springer.

90. Solomon K and others: Alcoholism and prescription drug abuse in the elderly: St. Louis University Grand Rounds, *J Am Geriatr Soc* 41:57-69, 1993.

91. Solomon K and Vickers R: Attitudes of health workers toward old people, *J Am Geriatr Soc* 27:186-191, 1979.

92. Solomon K: Behavioral and psychotherapeutic interventions in the nursing home. In Szwabo PA and Grossberg GT, editors: *Problem behaviors in long-term care. Recognition, diagnosis, and treatment,* New York, 1993, Springer.

93. Solomon K and Stark S: Comparison of older and younger alcoholics and prescription drug abusers: history and clinical presentation, *Clin Gerontol* 12(3):41-56, 1993.

94. Solomon K: The depressed patient: social antecedents of psychopathologic changes in the elderly, *J Am Geriatr Soc* 29:297-301, 1981.

95. Solomon K: Learned helplessness in the elderly: theoretic and clinical implications, *Occup Ther Ment Health* 10(3):31-51, 1990.

96. Solomon K: Mental health and the elderly. In Monk A, editor: *Handbook of gerontological services,* ed 2, New York, 1990, Columbia University Press.

97. Solomon K: The older man. In Solomon K and Levy NB, editors: *Men in transition: theory and therapy,* New York, 1982, Plenum Publishing.

98. Solomon K: Psychosocial dysfunction in the aged: assessment and intervention. In Jackson OL, editor: *Physical therapy of the geriatric patient,* ed 2, New York, 1989, Churchill Livingstone.

99. Solomon K and Szwabo P: Psychotherapy for patients with dementia. In Morley JE and others, editors: *Memory functioning and aging related disorders,* New York, 1992, Springer Publishing.

100. Solomon P: *Sensory deprivation,* Cambridge, 1961, Harvard University Press.

101. Solomon K: Social antecedents of learned helplessness in the health care setting, *Gerontologist,* 22:282-287, 1982.

102. Solomon K: The elderly patient. In Spittel JA Jr, editor: *Clinical medicine,* vol XII, Hagerstown, Md, 1981, Harper and Row.

103. Solomon K: The subjective experience of the Alzheimer's patient, *Geriatr Consultant* 1:22-24, 1982.

104. Solomon K and Shackson JB: Substance use disorders in nursing home patients. In Reichman WE and Katz PR, editors: *Psychiatric care in the nursing home,* New York, in press, Oxford University Press.

105. Spirduso WW and MacRae PG: Motor performance and aging. In Birren JE and Schaie KW, editors: *Handbook of the psychology of aging,* ed 3, San Diego, 1990, Academic Press.

106. Stern RG and Davis KL: Treatment approaches in Alzheimer's disease: past, present, and future. In Weiner MF, editor: *The dementias: diagnosis and management,* Washington, 1991, American Psychiatric Press.

107. Sunderland T and others: A new scale for the assessment of depressed mood in demented patients, *Am J Psychiatry* 145:955-959, 1988.

108. US Bureau of the Census: *Statistical abstract of the United States,* ed 110, Washington, 1990, US Bureau of the Census.

109. Office of Technology Assessment: *Losing a million minds: confronting the tragedy of Alzheimer's disease and other dementias,* Washington, 1987, US Government Printing Office.

110. Vander Camman TJM and others: Value of the Mini-Mental State Examination and informants' data for the detection of dementia in geriatric outpatients, *Psychol Rep* 71:1003-1009, 1992.

111. Wang HS: Special diagnostic procedures—the evaluation of brain impairment. In Busse EW and Pfeiffer E, editors: *Mental illness in later life,* Washington, 1973, American Psychiatric Association.

112. Wilder J: Basimetric approach (law of initial value) to biological rhythms, *Ann NY Acad Sci* 98:1211-1220, 1968.

113. Wilder J: Basimetric approach to psychiatry. In Arieti S, editor: *American handbook of psychiatry,* New York, 1966, Basic Books.

114. Wilder J: *Stimulus and response: the law of initial value,* Bristol, 1967, John Wright and Sons.

115. Wolf W, editor: Rhythmic functions in the living system, *Ann NY Acad Sci* 98:753-1326, 1962.

116. Winograd CH and Jarvik LF: Physician management of the demented patient, *J Am Geriatr Soc* 34:295-308, 1986.

117. Worden H: Aging and blindness, *New Outlook for the Blind* 70:433-437, 1976.

118. Yankelovich, Shelley, and White, Inc: *Caregivers of patients with dementia,* Washington, 1986, Office of Technology Assessment.

119. Yesavage JA and others: The Geriatric Depression Rating Scale: comparison with other self-report and psychiatric rating scales. In Crook T, Ferris S, Bartus R, editors: *Assessment in geriatric psychopharmacology,* New Canaan, 1983, Mark Powley Associates.

APPENDIX A   *THE BARTHEL INDEX*

The Barthel Index (BI) is another profile scale (see box); it includes 10 self-care, sphincter control, and mobility factors (Table 25-1).[18] The specific details used in scoring this index are presented in the boxed material. The advantage of the Barthel Index is its simplicity and usefulness in evaluating patients before, during, and after treatment. It is functionally oriented and may be best used accompanied by a clinical evaluation.[12]

Rating guidelines for Barthel Index*

1. Feeding
   10 = Independent. The patient can feed himself a meal when someone puts the food within his reach. He must put on an assistive device if this is needed, cut up the food alone. He must accomplish this in a reasonable time.
   5 = Some help is necessary (with cutting up food, etc., as listed above).

2. Moving from wheelchair to bed and return
   15 = Independent in all phases of this activity. Patient can safely approach the bed in his wheelchair, lock brakes, lift footrests, move safely to bed, lie down, come to a sitting position on the wheelchair, if necessary, to transfer back into it safely, and return to the wheelchair.
   10 = Either some minimal help is needed in some step of this activity or the patient needs to be reminded or supervised for safety of one or more parts of this activity.
   5 = Patient can come to a sitting position without the help of a second person but needs to be lifted out of bed, or if he transfers with a great deal of help.

3. Doing personal toilet
   5 = Patient can wash hands and face, comb hair, clean teeth, and shave. He may use any kind of razor but must put in blade or plug in razor without help as well as get it from drawer or cabinet. Female patients must put on own makeup.

4. Getting on and off toilet
   10 = Patient is able to get on and off toilet, fasten and unfasten clothes, prevent soiling of clothes, and use toilet paper without help. If it is necessary to use a bedpan instead of a toilet, he must be able to place it on a chair, empty it, and clean it.
   5 = Patient needs help because of imbalance or in handling clothes or in using toilet paper.

5. Bathing self
   5 = Patient may use a bathtub, a shower, or take a complete sponge bath. He must be able to do all the

steps involved in whichever method is employed without another person being present.

6. Walking on a level surface
   15 = Patient can walk at least 50 yards without help or supervision. He may wear braces or prostheses and use crutches, canes, or a walkerette but not a rolling walker. He must be able to lock and unlock braces, if used, assume the standing position and sit down, get the necessary mechanical aids into position for use, and dispose of them when he sits. (Putting on and taking off braces is scored under dressing.)
   10 = Patient needs help or supervision in any of the above but can walk at least 50 yards with a little help.

6a. Propelling a wheelchair
   5 = If a patient cannot ambulate but can propel a wheelchair independently. He must be able to go around corners, turn around, maneuver the chair to a table, bed, toilet, etc. He must be able to push a chair at least 50 yards. Do not score this item if the patient gets score for walking.

7. Ascending and descending stairs
   10 = Patient is able to go up and down a flight of stairs safely without help or supervision. He may and should use handrails, canes, or crutches when needed. He must be able to carry canes or crutches as he ascends or descends stairs.
   5 = Patient needs help with or supervision of any one of the above items.

8. Dressing and undressing
   10 = Patient is able to put on and remove and fasten all clothing, as well as tie shoe laces (unless it is necessary to use adaptions for this). The activity includes putting on and removing and fastening corset or braces when these are prescribed.
   5 = Patient needs help in putting on and removing or fastening any clothing. He must do at least half the work himself. He must accomplish this in a reasonable time. Women need not be scored on use

Mahoney FI and Barthel DW: Md State Med J 14:61, 1965
*A score of 0 is given in the activity when the patient cannot meet the criteria as defined.

Continued.

Rating guidelines for Barthel Index–cont'd*

of a brassiere or girdle unless these are prescribed garments.

9. Continence of bowels
   10 = Patient is able to control his bowels and have no accidents. He can use a suppository or take an enema when necessary.
   5 = Patient needs help in using a suppository or taking an enema or has occasional accidents.

10. Controlling bladder
    10 = Patient is able to control his bladder day and night. Patients who wear an external device and leg bag must put them on independently, clean and empty bag, and stay dry day and night.
    5 = Patient has occasional accidents or cannot wait for the bedpan or get to the toilet in time or needs help with an external device.

Table 25-1. Barthel Index*

	With help	Independent
1. Feeding (if food needs to be cut = help)	5	10
2. Moving from wheelchair to bed and return (including sitting up in bed)	5-10	15
3. Personal toilet (wash face, comb hair, shave, clean teeth)	0	5
4. Getting on and off toilet (handling clothes, wipe, flush)	5	10
5. Bathing self	0	5
6. Walking on level surface	10	15
(or if unable to walk, propel wheelchair)	0†	5
7. Ascend and descend stairs	5	10
8. Dressing (include tying shoes, fastening fasteners)	5	10
9. Controlling bowels	5	10
10. Controlling bladder	5	10

From Mahoney FI and Barthel DW: *Md State Med J* 14:61, 1965.

*A patient scoring 100 BI is continent, feeds himself, dresses himself, gets up and out of bed and chairs, bathes himself, walks at least a block, and can ascend and descend stairs. This does not mean that he is able to live alone. He may not be able to cook, keep house, and meet the public, but he is able to get along without attendant care.

†Score only if unable to walk.

PART THREE

Special Topics and Techniques for Therapists

CHAPTER 26

Disorders in Oral, Speech, and Language Functions

Nina Newlin Simmons-Mackie

KEY TERMS

language	oral-motor function
speech	dysphagia
communication	aphasia
apraxia of speech	language disorder
dysarthria	

LEARNING OBJECTIVES

After reading this chapter the student/therapist will:

1. Acquire basic facts regarding normal communication including physical structures and developmental sequences.
2. Learn characteristics of commonly encountered communication problems in the neurologically impaired population.
3. Learn the role of the physical or occupational therapist in neurological communication disorders including four management goals.
4. Recognize the interaction between communicative and physical development and rehabilitation.
5. Learn appropriate methods of working with communicatively impaired individuals.
6. Appreciate the complexity of communication disorders and the need for a team approach.

The use of **language** to reconstruct the past, represent the present, and consider the future has been a most remarkable human accomplishment. The need to communicate is so compelling that sophisticated and complex systems of **speech**, gesture, writing, and graphics have been developed to relay ideas. Through language we learn about things that we have never experienced and impart our own experiences. Language plays a role in solving problems, expressing feelings, and relating to other human beings.

Language is an organized set of symbols used for **communication.** Speech is the oral manifestation of language, as writing is the graphic form and sign language is the gestural form. Without a language system speech does not develop. The development of language in turn depends on the ability to organize and symbolize concepts. This cognitive or conceptual development is based on integration and association of sensory experiences learned through interaction with the environment. Obviously speech and language are intimately related and depend on sensorimotor development.

The development of language is a complex process. Consider the difficulty of learning a language. Assuming an intact conceptual and cognitive system, one must perceive, retain, and produce a variety of speech sounds requiring precise and coordinated activity of the lips, tongue, palate, larynx, and respiratory system. One must sequence the sounds to form words, remember and order the words in an accepted and meaningful way, use syntax appropriate to the intended meaning, inflect and stress words correctly to portray correct meanings and attitudes, and then monitor the production through sensory channels. The rules of communicating that govern acceptability as a speaker and listener must also be learned. Appropriate speaking distance, cues to turn-taking such as eye and hand movements, and sensitivity to the listener's prior knowledge of the subject are examples of pragmatic rules of communication that are learned through interaction. We develop an appreciation for context and intonation that can indicate meaning beyond the literal spoken words. For example, the same words can be spoken seriously, humorously, or sarcastically.

Communication is accomplished through facial expression, body movement, and gestures. These nonverbal components are of great importance in the communication process. Information about attitudes and feelings is portrayed in posture, gaze, and voice inflection. If oral and written language is disrupted, facial expression and body language may be the only means of communication. On the other hand, individuals with severe neuromuscular problems may be unable to project body language information.

The therapist undoubtedly will encounter individuals representing all types and degrees of communication disorders. Any combination of the above described aspects of communication can be disrupted through developmental or acquired disorders. It is imperative that the therapist understand not only how to communicate best with these clients but also how therapy can assist or detract from the development or restoration of communication. This chapter presents concepts fundamental to understanding speech and language disorders typically seen in the physical therapy clinic. Although communication obviously includes speaking, listening, reading, writing, and even signing, discussions are limited primarily to oral communication or speech. This chapter reviews the sensory and motor systems necessary for normal speech and language development; discusses the characteristics, assessment, and treatment of neurogenic speech and language disorders; and summarizes the role of the therapist.

OVERVIEW OF NORMAL ORAL COMMUNICATION
Physical structures

The physical structures used for speech serve the primary survival functions of breathing, food intake, chewing, and swallowing. Speech is a sophisticated volitional function that shares the oral mechanism with these vegetative functions. The physical structures composing the speech mechanism include the lips, tongue, cheeks, jaw, pharynx, larynx, palate, and respiratory system (Fig. 26-1). The muscles of the speech mechanism are controlled at various levels within the nervous system, including lower motor neuron, extrapyramidal, upper motor neuron, and cerebellum.[19,59,80] At the highest level, cortical control of speech appears to be lateralized to the dominant, usually left, hemisphere of the brain.[9,29]

The *respiratory system*, consisting of inspiratory and expiratory muscles, is responsible for transfer of air to and from the lungs. Vegetative breathing involves regular cycles of inhalation and exhalation involuntarily controlled at the brainstem level.[20] This automatic activity must be modified for speaking. Breathing for speech requires considerable control and coordination. During speech the inhalation cycle is shortened and the exhalation phase is prolonged as the exhaled air is shaped into sound. The loudness of speech and the length of utterances can be controlled by altering the amount or force of exhaled air.[19]

The *larynx* is a cartilaginous structure at the superior aspect of the trachea that acts as a valve by action of the vocal folds. The vocal folds remain in an open position to allow passage of air through the larynx during breathing.[19,34] When swallowing is initiated, the vocal folds close automatically to prevent food from entering the respiratory tract.

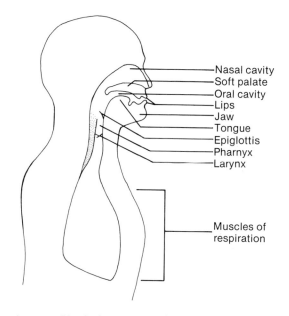

Fig. 26-1. Physical structures of the speech mechanism.

For speaking the laryngeal valve must be opened, closed, tensed, and relaxed in a finely coordinated fashion to produce the necessary tone for speech.[22] Voice or phonation is produced as the breath stream sets the closed vocal folds into vibration. The pitch of the voice is altered by the tension and length of the folds. Because many speech sounds (such as /s/, /f/, and /p/) do not require voice, rapid opening of the vocal folds must be coordinated with articulation of these sounds, followed by rapid closing for production of voiced sounds (such as /z/, /v/, and /b/).

The *pharynx* is a tube extending from the nasal and oral cavities to the esophagus and larynx.[34] The muscles of the pharynx assist in the transport of food into the esophagus during swallowing. The shape, size, and tension of pharyngeal walls influence the voice quality produced in speaking.

The *palate* consists of the bony hard palate and muscular soft palate, which separate the oral and nasal cavities. During vegetative breathing, the soft palate remains open, allowing air to pass from the pharynx into the nasal passage.[22] As a protective measure during feeding, the soft palate elevates, closing off the nasal passages. All English speech sounds are produced with the soft palate elevated, with the exception of /m/, /n/, and /ng/.

Opening, closing, and lateral movements of the *jaw* allow mastication of food. During speech mandibular opening, closing, and stabilization are rapidly and finely adjusted in the production of speech sounds.[19]

The *cheeks* enclose the oral cavity. The muscles of the cheeks aid the tongue in mixing food with saliva and pushing food onto the teeth during chewing. The cheeks also assist in shaping the oral cavity during speaking.

The *tongue* is made up of intrinsic muscles for altering tongue shape and extrinsic muscles that lift, lower, protrude, and retract the tongue.[19,22] It is capable of an extremely wide variety of complex and fine movements. The tongue moves food in the mouth, mixing it with saliva, placing it for chewing, and finally transporting it to the back of the mouth for swallowing. It also removes food lodged between the teeth and gums. In speech the tongue is responsible for producing speech sounds by rapidly assuming different shapes and contact points in the mouth.

The *lips* form the opening of the mouth cavity. They take food in and retain it within the mouth. The lips open and purse for sucking and close during swallowing. For speech the lips assist in formation of sounds by changing shape and size of the opening.[19,34] The lips, along with the cheeks and eyes, also contribute to communication through facial expressions.

Sensory input for speech production. Speech is not produced or developed solely by movement of the physical structures. Sensory input is responsible for eliciting and maintaining the vegetative responses of sucking, chewing, and swallowing. Sensation produces and maintains a continuous feedforward and feedback system during production of speech.[34] The sensory systems of primary importance to oral communication include oral sensation, audition, and vision.

Development of oral sensation

The tongue and lips are extremely sensitive to touch, temperature, and pressure to prevent ingestion of inappropriate substances.[34] In addition, texture, size, and position information is required to detect what is in the mouth and where. This provides the lips with feedback to maintain closure and prevent drooling.[55] Sensory input tells the tongue tip where to place material for chewing, when material is too dry and needs moistening, and when food has reached the appropriate consistency for swallowing. Developmentally, these assistive tongue tip motions of feeding promote sensory experience that forms a basis for the selective refined movement of speech. The tip of the tongue is more generously endowed with touch receptors than the back of the tongue or palate.[34,52] The tongue is more sensitive than the lips. The back of the tongue and posterior walls of the oral cavity respond to pressure that induces swallowing.[55] Pressure at the back of the mouth also elicits the gag reflex. In addition, the tongue is keenly sensitive to taste, especially along the edges[52]; some tastes mobilize the tongue into activity for feeding; others cause a protective response.[52]

Oral sensation is extremely important for speech. Sensory feedback relative to positions and contacts assumed for sound production and pressure of air across structures provides a continuous monitoring and correction loop.[34] It seems that oral sensory function is related to the quality of oral motor proficiency.[65] Neuromotor deficits that change early feeding habits can diminish oral sensory experience and cause impairments in sensorimotor integration. For instance, chewing and swallowing problems of the cerebral-palsied baby may result in continuation of soft or liquid diets, which fail to provide normal sensory variety. Experimental disruption of oral sensation seems to produce deterioration of articulatory proficiency in normal subjects,[34] and poor oral sensory function in cerebral-palsied individuals seems to be associated with defective chewing, drinking, and articulatory ability.[64] Oral sensory deficits have been associated with **apraxia of speech**[51,60] and **dysarthria.**[15]

Audition. Audition is possibly the most important sensory component of oral communication. The ravages of disturbed auditory input on speech development are most apparent in the markedly deficient or sometimes nonexistent speech of individuals with profound congenital hearing loss. Auditory input is of extreme importance in learning speech and language and in maintaining adequate speech production. During speech we continuously monitor what we say and how we say it via audition. The smooth flow of speech depends on the auditory system's satisfaction that all is going well. An excellent way of gaining respect for auditory monitoring of speech is to speak into a delayed auditory feedback system. These systems, available in many speech clinics, provide several milliseconds of delay between word utterance and hearing that utterance via headphones. The response of most normal speakers is immediate and dramatic difficulty in the fluent production of speech.

In addition to its role in monitoring speech production, audition plays an obvious role in the comprehension of speech. A listener must receive and perceive the sounds in appropriate order, retain the sound sequences for mental processing, and associate meaning to the retained sequences. In addition, undesired sounds (background noise) must be filtered out while desired sounds are localized and processed. Difficulty in auditory sensation, perception of speech sounds, or processing speech for meaning will affect verbal communication.[34]

Vision. Although not primary to monitoring speech production, visual input is important in oral communication. Visual input from the environment provides information on language context, gesture, facial expression, turn-taking cues, and feedback about listener reaction. Seeing a speaker's face also greatly assists in the actual understanding of speech. Information on lip placement and tongue position (lip reading) assists our perception of what is heard. This is apparent at noisy parties when we pay particular attention to watching the speaker's face. Moreover, compensatory production of speech sounds that look wrong but sound exactly like the target sound are often considered error productions. Obviously we see speech as well as hear it.

Development of oral communication. The development of speech and language is a complex process that has been extensively studied and described.[4,8,12,13,24,44] It is imperative that the physical or occupational therapist grasp the process of language and speech development in relation to overall motor development. The acquisition of speech and language is intertwined with the acquisition of motor skills. The physical or occupational therapist can play an important role in promoting language and speech development and in reducing the potentially destructive effects of neuromuscular deficits on communication. Too often rehabilitation results in a division of responsibility such that the physical or occupational therapist works on motor development and the speech-language pathologist works on language development. In reality, the two develop as an integrated process; treatment should be focused accordingly.

Early oral development. At birth the infant demonstrates the vegetative responses of sucking, swallowing, and breathing that will later be modified for oral communication. The infant's first vocalizations consist of crying in response to discomfort and hunger. Motor responses, including **oral-motor function,** are diffuse and undifferentiated. Yet already the infant is responding to a remarkable range of sensory stimuli that are the building blocks of cognitive and communicative development. For instance, sucking produces tactile stimulation of the mouth, which elicits further sucking. Repetitions of this cycle soon generate integrations in which activity in one modality leads to sensory feedback in another modality.[54]

The motor organization of the speech structures in infancy is similar to the extension-flexion pattern of the extremities.[78] Gently stroking a baby's cheek causes the head to turn toward the stimulus. The jaws open, the lips purse, the tongue protrudes, and sucking begins. An unpleasant stimulus causes the head to turn away, the jaws to close, and the lips and tongue to retract.[22] As the baby matures, the patterned, diffuse oral motions differentiate into an array of movements needed to accommodate solid food.[46] Structural and motor changes in the growing mechanism promote new movements with functional autonomy of structures possible. Although these early developments serve feeding, their importance as the raw material for motor control of speech is obvious.[55] For instance, the lip rounding of sucking can also serve to produce an "oo" sound, while tongue retraction is involved in producing "ah."[22]

Introduction of solid food for chewing and biting provides a similar framework of motor patterns, including lip closure, jaw stabilization, and tongue tip elevation. Speech requires fine control of the lips and tongue tip while reference structures, such as jaw and tongue body, are stabilized. Precursors of these movements are being developed in infancy. With the eruption of the first teeth, the infantile swallow (jaws open and tongue thrust forward) usually begins to give way to an adult swallow (teeth together with tongue retraction). The constant sensory feedback from the changing texture, temperature, and consistency of foods and the oral exploration of objects and body parts and vocalization promote the integration of sensory and motor systems that will ultimately subserve language.

Auditory-vocal development. Although individual timetables of development vary, the infant's use of hearing and vocalization develops in an orderly sequence (Table 26-1). Initially the infant shows a startle response to sudden loud sounds.[78] It has been shown that within the first 2 weeks the child's body movements are synchronized with the pleasant sound of organized adult speech.[14] Babies as young as 1 month old tune in to speech and discriminate between speech and nonspeech sounds.[7] By 2 months the infant ceases body activity to "listen" to interesting sounds. During the second month facial expressions develop. The child begins to associate familiar sights and sounds and to produce sounds of pleasure.[7] Sound localization, tracking, and discrimination become possible as the child develops better head control. The development of head and trunk control also lays the foundation for effective feeding, exploration of the surroundings, and vocalization.[11]

Often the first vocalizations other than crying are sounds produced with the back of the tongue ("goo, goo"), perhaps because myelination of the primary motor cortex proceeds from the back of the mouth to the front.[24] These cooing sounds diversify into a wider variety of sound sequences

Table 26-1. Approximate developmental milestones for speech and language[44,46,55,78]

Age of child	Behavior
0-3 months	Startles to loud noise
	Becomes still with sound of moderate loudness
	Cries and fusses
	Facial expression develops
	Sucking-swallow reflex present
	Tongue-thrust swallow present
3-6 months	Sounds vary and begins to babble; vocal play
	Recognizes familiar persons and objects
	Watches faces; turns to sounds
	Begins intonation patterns
	Early reflexes begin to diminish
6-8 months	Lip and tongue sounds predominate
	Uses voice to influence environment
	Babbling becomes more volitional
8-12 months	Imitates sounds and words
	First word
12 months	Receptive vocabulary increases
	Follows directions
12-24 months	May imitate and echo adult speech
	Uses two- to three-word phrases
3 years	Simple sentences and questions

called babbling. Initially, choice of sounds is probably biologically dictated by growth of the vocal tract and increases in basic motor control. Infants seem to discover their own sounds and movements and their variations as they move, twist, turn, and breathe. The imitation of these body movements and vocalizations can eventually lead to movements and sounds that serve language. The biologically determined sounds come more and more under self-control.[24]

At this time adults are playing an important role. They imitate the infant's sounds, reinforce productions, and provide models of appropriate intonation patterns. In addition to auditory-vocal stimulation, the infant receives tactile, visual, kinesthetic, and vestibular sensations that contribute to an integrated communication system. The child's movements in space and relationship to objects in space form the basis for mental representations of objects.[7] Children learn that objects that disappear from their zone of vision continue to exist. This mental memory for objects or understanding of object permanence seems important to the development of symbols for objects.[7] The learning of language is closely tied to the learning of the identity of objects, discrimination of object differences, and classification of object similarities. Sensorimotor experience is necessary in the development of these concepts.[1] Objects children see, hear, and manipulate are frequently the ones for

which they first learn language symbols.[54] Touch, pressure, and movement during feeding, dressing, and washing form the basis of early perceptual learning and develop the nonverbal framework for interaction.[7] Also, caretakers typically talk to their babies during these activities, instilling the need and pleasure of verbal communication. Exchange of gaze and turn-taking are outgrowths of such interpersonal activities. Children develop a sense of self and body schema and learn to control their environments for their own satisfaction.[3,4]

The child's first means of environmental control (crying) gives way to more sophisticated approaches. Bates and others[5] suggest that functional use of language is a form of tool usage. Initial schemes of tool use (using a stick to obtain another object) precede use of gesture as a tool (pointing to obtain an object), which in turn precedes use of verbalization as a tool (uttering the name of an object to obtain it). Gestures serve an important role in early language learning. Gestures such as showing, giving, eye contact, reaching, and pointing are examples of the capacity for controlling others and a manifestation of emerging communication. During the first year the child begins to use babbling-like sounds with meaningful intonation; these sounds develop as part of the sensorimotor action schemes equivalent to gestures.[3,4]

Around 12 months of age the first real word is often produced.[8] The first words teach us a great deal about the way the child perceives the world. A common attribute of children's first words is that they reflect action (roll, bark, fall). Often words for moving, changing, or manipulating objects are learned earlier than names for static objects.[8] Obviously salient sensory stimulation (sight, sound, touch, or movement) dictates early language learning. Impairment in the ability to manipulate objects and receive sensory information about objects has the potential for disrupting language acquisition.[1]

During the first year the child's receptive language and attention span for speech grow steadily. Receptive language exceeds speech production; the child understands more about words than use of words indicates.[8] The child who calls all dogs, horses, cats, pigs, and even birds "doggie" is often swift to point to the horse when asked "Where is the horse?" The child often understands sentences and grammatical constructions before acquiring their productive use.

Developing word production requires increasingly fine motor control. Some children attempt to imitate adult productions. Fortunately, adults seem to intuitively simplify models from which children draw early words. These can be refined as motor control improves.[24] Developing language also requires organization of perceptual experiences. Shape, sound, size, movement, texture, taste, and smell contribute to distinguish concepts.[7] For instance, perception of the particular attributes of dog-ness distinguishes all dogs from cups or cats or objects with different distinct characteristics.

During the second year the child begins to utter words in

sequence to represent a chain of events.[7] Later, words are tied into phrases to represent a thought. Early sentences represent action or object relations ("push car" or "mama chair") without descriptors (such as *red* car) or use of adult syntax ("I am *pushing* the *car*" or "*Mama* is sitting on the *chair*").

Receptive vocabulary grows rapidly as does the acquisition of rules of grammar and conversational skills. As the child grows language development is measured by the complexity of syntax, by the clarity of speech production, and by the ability to use language in a variety of ways in different conversational settings.

AN OVERVIEW OF DISORDERS IN ORAL, SPEECH, AND LANGUAGE FUNCTION

Impaired communication can be caused by influences present before, during, or after this developmental process. These influences can be external to the individual, such as poor speech models or environmental deprivation, or internal, such as brain dysfunction; or they may represent an interaction between external and internal factors. A breakdown in any of the processes contributing to oral communication, such as oral motor function, sensory integration, cognition, or language processing, can interfere with speech (Table 26-2). Impaired communication can be classified in a variety of ways depending on the aspect of communication that is deficient (e.g., language, motor speech production, motor speech planning, fluency, or pragmatic skills) or on the cause of the deficit (e.g., neurological deficit, emotional problem, experiential deprivation, sensory deficit, or structural abnormality). Often there are multiple deficits and causes. Such is the case when the primary neuromotor deficit in cerebral palsy causes diminished experiential and sensory input resulting in secondary effects on language.

Acquired versus developmental problems

Although there are many similarities between the acquired and the developmental versions of communication disorders, they cannot be considered synonymous. The failure to develop speech or language must be approached clinically in a very different manner from interference to a fully learned system. Mental and emotional side effects of abnormal development and sudden loss are quite different. The clinician needs to be aware of the developmental level at which communication is arrested and the amount of cognitive and language resources that have been acquired. For instance, the infant demonstrating flaccid weakness of the oral mechanism with diminished ability to suck or swallow has not developed the sensorimotor patterns necessary for speech. Although cortical structures may be unimpaired, the normal learning process may be disrupted by a limited ability to orally explore objects, express pleasure through babbling, or interact normally during feeding. The adult with a similar flaccid weakness of the speech musculature has the benefit of an intact language system, developed cortical association paths, and prior fund of sensory data on which to rely. Because developmental and acquired disorders present different problems, they will be considered separately.

Acquired neurogenic communication disorders

Understanding the communication disorder is of utmost importance in the proper handling of the patient. Disorders of speech, hearing, language, and cognition each require a different approach. Misdiagnosis of the nature of the disorder not only disrupts appropriate interaction and stimulation but also promotes emotional maladjustment and motivational decline. The following section will briefly define and categorize the most typical acquired neurogenic communication disorders.

Table 26-2. Primary areas of impairment in neurogenic communication disorders[24,50]

| Diagnostic label | Primary deficit areas | | | | | |
	Receptive and expressive language	Nonverbal intelligence	Hearing	Motor speech production	Interpersonal interaction	Orientation
Developmental aphasia	X	?	—	—	—	—
Acquired aphasia	X	?	—	—	—	—
Apraxia of speech	—	—	—	X	—	—
Dysarthria	—	—	—	X	—	—
Dementia	X	X	—	—	?	?
Mental retardation	X	X	—	—	—	—
Confusion	?	?	—	—	X	?
Schizophrenia	X	?	—	—	X	—
Autism	X	?	—	—	X	—
Rightsided brain damage	—	—	—	—	X	—
Hearing impairment	X	—	X	—	—	—

X, Primary associated deficit; —, not a primary cause; ?, unknown.

Motor speech disorders

Dysarthria. The dysarthrias are "a group of speech disorders resulting from disturbances in muscular control—weakness, slowness, or incoordination—of the speech mechanism due to damage to the central or peripheral nervous system or both."[76] Dysarthria occurs in children and adults. Although it may coexist with other communication disorders, dysarthria per se has no effect on language, intelligence, or orientation. The causes of dysarthria are varied.[22,76] The speech characteristics of the dysarthric client are a direct reflection of neuromuscular function and neurophysiological status.[22] Just as the therapist tests range, speed, and strength of lower-extremity musculature and then observes function through gait, so the speech pathologist tests the range, speed, and strength of the oral musculature and then listens to speech to infer function. Speech symptoms produced by neuromuscular conditions vary considerably from one type of dysarthria to another. Therefore proper identification is imperative to appropriate management. The following dysarthria classification system, developed by Darley and others,[22] relates perceived motor and speech symptoms to underlying neurological processes.

Flaccid dysarthria. Produced by a lower motor neuron lesion, flaccid dysarthria can affect one or more aspects of the oral motor system, depending on the site and extent of the lesion. Table 26-3 presents the functional relationship of the bulbar nuclei and cranial nerves to speech production and implies location. The neuromuscular conditions associated with this dysarthria are flaccid paralysis or weakness, hypotonicity, and impairment of both voluntary and involuntary movement.[22] Swallowing may be disturbed, and the gag reflex may be impaired or absent.

Spastic dysarthria. Spastic dysarthria is caused by upper motor neuron damage. Because of the bilateral innervation of the speech mechanism above the level of the bulbar system, it has been suggested that bilateral impairment of the corticobulbar tract is required to produce spastic dysar-thria.[22] This form of dysarthria (sometimes known as pseudobulbar palsy) affects voluntary movements of the speech mechanism, causing spasticity, weakness, and slowness of movement. A hyperactive gag reflex, sucking reflex, and jaw jerk are often present. Drooling and swallowing difficulty is common because of the slowness and inefficiency of motor mechanisms. A disinhibition of the motor mechanism of crying and laughing is often associated with spastic dysarthria, resulting in what is sometimes called emotional lability, but in fact this is a disinhibited motor reflex. The speech of the client with spastic dysarthria sounds as if it is being produced against considerable resistance. The slow, labored articulation and strangled voice quality reflect limited range and spasticity of musculature.

Ataxic dysarthria. Ataxic dysarthria, resulting from cerebellar system dysfunction, is characterized by inaccurate and uncoordinated movement of the speech mechanism.[22] The loss of smooth control results in what has been described as scanning speech: Each syllable seems to be given equal stress. The loss of speech rhythm and the equalized pattern is reminiscent of the slow, wide-based gait of the ataxic individual, a step-by-step approach devoid of natural timing. Because of loss of speed and efficiency of movement, there is also an irregular breakdown in articulation of sounds.[22] Moreover, the client has difficulty coordinating rapid articulatory movements with respiration and phonation. The speech of the ataxic client may sound like that of an intoxicated person.

Hypokinetic dysarthria. Hypokinetic dysarthria is seen in disorders of the motor system, such as Parkinson's disease. Increased muscle tone, rigidity, and paucity of movement are apparent in the lack of facial expression and limited movement of lips and tongue during speech.[22] The rapid rate of speech, monotone, quiet voice, and imprecise consonant production are probably a reflection of limited range and paucity of movement. Hesitations, inappropriate silences, and then progressive blurring of articulation seem

Table 26-3. The relationship of cranial nerves to motor speech production

Nerve	Function for speech	Lower motor neuron lesion effects on speech
Phrenic and spinal intercostal nerves	Control exhaled breath stream	Short phrases Reduced loudness
Trigeminal (V)	Open and close jaw Maintain mouth closure Stabilize jaw for lip and tongue movement	Poor articulation
Facial (VII)	Regulate lip movement for producing sounds	Imprecise articulation of lip sounds
Vagal (X)	Regulate palatal movement for directing air through the mouth or nose Regulate opening and closing of the vocal folds for phonation	Hypernasality Breathy or whispered voice Monotone Short phrases
Hypoglossal (XII)	Regulate tongue movement for producing sounds	Imprecise articulation

to be the vocal correlate of festination of gait. Palilalia, the repeating of words or syllables, is often present.

Hyperkinetic dysarthria. Hyperkinetic dysarthria is characterized by excess and involuntary movement.[22] Chorea and myoclonus are examples of disorders producing quick, involuntary movements and variable muscle tone, which interfere with the smooth, rapid execution of speech movements. The slow hyperkinesia of athetosis, dyskinesia, or dystonia causes distorted movements and postures, slowed movement, and variable hypertonicity of the speech musculature. The effect on speech depends on the extent and severity of the movement disorder.

Mixed dysarthria. Mixed dysarthria includes characteristics of two or more of the above dysarthrias and is commonly seen in traumatic head injuries, multiple cerebrovascular accidents, amyotrophic lateral sclerosis, and multiple sclerosis. Often one type of dysarthria predominates.

Neurogenic swallowing disorders (dysphagia). The client with weakness, slowness, or incoordination of the oral-pharyngeal motor system commonly has a swallowing disorder, termed **dysphagia.** Dysphagia can refer to a range of disorders from inefficient handling of food or liquid because of oral motor deficits to severe compromise of nutritional and pulmonary status caused by penetration of food or liquid into the airway (aspiration). The pattern of deficits in swallowing will reflect the neurophysiological cause of the disorder and frequently correlates with observed speech motor symptoms. Signs of oral-stage swallowing problems might include difficulty chewing, maintaining a lip seal, and clearing food or liquid from the spaces in the oral cavity. Signs of aspiration include coughing and choking during meals, excess mucus production, a "wet" voice quality, fever, weight loss, and rejection or spitting out of food. Clients might be unaware of swallowing problems; those with decreased pharyngeal sensation might even aspirate silently[47] with no coughing or outward symptom of laryngeal penetration.

Apraxia of speech. A disruption of speech motor planning caused by brain damage is called apraxia of speech or verbal apraxia.[22] Positioning and sequencing for the voluntary production of sounds are impaired, although there is no significant weakness, slowness, or uncoordination of the speech muscles during automatic activities such as chewing, swallowing, and coughing. Damage to the left hemisphere in Broca's area (premotor area) has been associated with this motor programming deficit.[21] Impaired oral sensation is often a correlate of apraxia of speech as well. Because of the proximity of Broca's area to the motor strip, hemiparesis, especially involving the right upper extremity, is often seen.

By definition, the client with pure apraxia of speech shows no decrement in orientation, intelligence, or auditory comprehension; however, apraxia of speech often coexists with aphasia.[22] Inconsistent, variable articulation errors are often preceded by groping movements and struggle behav-

ior. The disability can range in severity from difficulty only on multisyllable tongue twisters to inability to program the mechanism for production of a single syllable or sound. Often the client with apraxia of speech will fluently and accurately produce automatic speech (e.g., cursing or overlearned phrases).

Language disorders: aphasia. Acquired **aphasia** is an impairment caused by brain damage in the ability to process and/or produce language. Aphasia affects auditory comprehension, reading comprehension, verbal expression, writing, and symbolic gesturing. The disorder is not caused by general intellectual deficits, sensory loss, or motor dysfunction.[76] By definition, aphasia affects both receptive and expressive language, although the degree of involvement in each system can vary.[9] The lesion producing aphasia most often is found in the dominant (usually left) hemisphere of the brain, and the type of behavior varies according to the location and extent of damage.[70] One classification system[30] divides the acquired aphasias into fluent and nonfluent categories depending on the amount and flow of verbal output. The nonfluent client typically struggles to think of words and often uses content words only ("man uh-uh water uh . . . uh boat"). The fluent aphasic person verbalizes but may substitute words or produce empty speech ("This one here is a snorker for water and I use it over there"). The client with aphasia may or may not be aware of errors, depending on auditory monitoring. The aphasic client is typically not confused or hard-of-hearing. Language is disrupted, not general intelligence. Usually nonlinguistic communication, such as facial expression, turn-taking, and affective tone, is preserved because this aspect of communication seems to be a right hemisphere function. Automatic speech (profanity, greetings, common expressions) may be preserved as well. The aphasic client is alert and oriented, but orientation is often impossible to test in the standard question-answer format.[70] To ensure appropriate management, aphasia must not be confused with dementia, retardation, confusion, or psychotic illness.

Related communication disorders

Dementia. Because cognition and concept development form the infrastructure for language, any factor that hinders cognition will affect speech. Such is the case when speech and language abilities diminish with progressive dementia[5] and organic brain syndrome. The communication deficit is one symptom of a more generalized intellectual deficit.[76] Although the client with dementia often exhibits aphasic-like language, these symptoms coexist with a variety of behavioral changes not attributable to a language disorder. Aphasia is not an appropriate diagnosis in these cases. Nonverbal performance, orientation, memory, affect, and judgment are impaired. The brain dysfunction causing a generalized deficit is widespread, disseminated, or diffuse, often because of disease (such as Alzheimer's), multiple infarcts, or generalized vascular insufficiency.

Confusion. The language of the confused person is often

impaired; however, the disorder is not language specific. The communication reflects "reduced recognition, understanding of and responsiveness to the environment, faulty memory, unclear thinking, and disorientation in time and space. Structured language events are usually normal . . . open-ended language situations elicit irrelevance and confabulation."[76, p.2] Confusion seems to be associated with relatively diffuse brain dysfunction and is frequently a sequela of traumatic brain injury (TBI) or metabolic imbalance.

Traumatic brain injury. A TBI can result in any number of communication deficits depending on the locus and extent of lesion; however, when diffuse injury occurs, the communication disorder is secondary to underlying cognitive disorganization rather than a specific speech or **language disorder,** such as aphasia or apraxia of speech.[33] In such cases attention, memory, organization, and other cognitive deficits affect both verbal and nonverbal processing. The array of symptoms might include reduced initiation of communication, reduced ability to follow directions, rambling and confabulatory speech, poor organization of thinking reflected in speech and writing, reduced verbal problem solving, poor use of social conversation rules, and inappropriate nonverbal communication.[71]

Frequently, staging systems are used to describe recovery in TBI and to assist in targeting treatment appropriately. For example the Ranchos Los Amigos Levels of Cognitive Function[33] provide a behavioral description of recovery stages that can be correlated with typical communication patterns. Others have identified behavioral symptoms associated with early, middle, and late phase recovery patterns.[71] Table 26-4 identifies potential communication behaviors associated with each recovery phase.

Schizophrenia. Language disruption is often associated with schizophrenia. Failure to use language interpersonally seems to be the overriding characteristic of schizophrenia.

However, irrelevant neologistic output is somewhat reminiscent of fluent aphasia. Because fluent aphasia is often caused by a posterior parietal or temporal lobe brain lesion and may not be associated with hemiplegia, sudden incidence of fluent aphasia may be mistakenly considered a psychiatric problem. The clinician must be careful to avoid misdiagnosis.

Right hemisphere damage. The client with damage to the nondominant (usually right) cerebral hemisphere often shows adequate oral language; however, interactive and affective aspects of communication are disrupted.[27,56,59] The client may exhibit a decreased awareness of the rules of communication, such as turn-taking, eye contact, listener sensitivity, and attention to and use of affective cues such as inflection and facial expression. Language is often literal so that humor, sarcasm, metaphors, or implied meanings may be missed.[28] Gardner has described the right-brain-damaged client as "a language machine, a talking computer that decodes literally what is said and gives the most immediate response . . . insensitive to the ideas behind the question, the intentions or implications of the questioner."[27,p.296]

Developmental neurogenic communication disorders

It is difficult to isolate a single cause-and-effect relationship in developmental problems because the interaction of learning, environment, and central nervous system (CNS) dysfunction creates a constantly changing and complicated picture. The learning and behavior deficits found in children with CNS dysfunction encompass a wide range of diagnostic labels, such as developmental language disorder, learning disability, hyperactivity, and developmental delay. The child seen in the speech clinic as exhibiting language disorder may be perceptually impaired to the occupational therapist or tactilely defensive to the physical therapist. The arbitrary fragmentation of development into isolated functions fails to recognize the integrated process of learning. Although the

Table 26-4. Recovery stages in TBI and examples of potential cognitive and communicative behaviors

Stage	Cognition	Communication
Early	Reduced arousal and alertness	Mute or minimal verbal and nonverbal communication Following directions may be nonexistent or delayed Emerging communication may be mouthed words, random vocalizations, or gestures; Might not make sense
Middle	Poor attention Disoriented, confused, possibly agitated Poor memory Poor organization and sequencing	Needs short, simple inputs Emerging speech may be inappropriate, irrelevant, confabulated, or abusive Dysarthria might be apparent Impaired social interaction
Late	Oriented but impaired learning and memory Reduced self-monitoring, insight and self-awareness Impaired abstract and multistep thinking	Poorly organized discourse and texts Pragmatic language impairment (e.g., rude comments, immature interactions) Reduced academic language skill Problems picking out main points

following section refers to typical diagnostic labels associated with neurogenic communication problems, the therapist should not lose sight of the multiple interacting variables that hinder or facilitate development of the child as a whole. Often the primary problem, such as motor, sensory, cognitive, memory, or attentional deficit, inhibits the language learning process, which is then complicated by emotional overlay, overprotection, and/or maladjustment.

Deficits in motor development. Failure to acquire normal oral motor patterns at any level of development influences speech development. Defective early vegetative function of swallowing, sucking, and chewing may preclude normal speech. Once vegetative motor functions develop, failure to develop voluntary motor control of the speech mechanism hinders speech development. Absence of sensory feedback and sensorimotor integration impedes acquisition of articulation. When speech does not develop normally, negative influences on language, emotion, and affect result.

The most widely recognized childhood neuromotor disorder affecting speech occurs in cerebral palsy. Much has been written about this oral motor dysfunction.[44,46,55,72,78] The dysarthrias described in the previous section generally apply to the developmental motor speech disorders of cerebral palsy. However, the sensory, perceptual, or intellectual problems found hinder direct comparison to the acquired dysarthrias. The dysarthrias of cerebral palsy are often mixed, with one condition (e.g., spastic or athetoid) predominating. Compensatory movements, secondary deficits produced by prolonged incorrect postures, sensory deprivation, and lack of experience are potential contributors to the clinical symptoms.

Defective motor planning results in developmental *apraxia of speech.*[51,72] Children with apraxia of speech show auditory abilities and general cognitive development far superior to verbal expression. The primary disability has been described as a sensorimotor deficit because it is frequently associated with disrupted oral sensation. The child has difficulty producing and ordering the rapid sequential articulatory movements that compose words. The result is often unintelligible speech characterized by omission or substitution of consonant sounds.

Deficits in language development

Developmental language disorder. Developmental language disorder is an impairment in the capacity to process language because of brain dysfunction. There is no apparent oral motor deficit or generalized mental retardation, yet language development is disturbed. The disturbed development of verbal language is often associated with auditory perception and processing deficits. Nonverbal cognitive development usually far exceeds the development of language, distinguishing this child from the mentally retarded child. The child attempts to communicate and interact through nonverbal channels and is alert to situational cues.

The term *childhood aphasia* was popular in the 1970s and is sometimes used to refer to a developmental language disorder associated with brain damage. *Delayed language* is a more general term used to encompass failure to acquire language normally for a variety of reasons such as minimal brain dysfunction, hearing loss, emotional disturbance, and experiential deprivation. *Learning disability* is associated with language learning disorders because it can affect one or more of the basic psychological processes involved in language.

Because terminology used for developmental disorders affecting speech and language is confusing, it is important to avoid focusing on specific labels and view the constellation of symptoms that hinder the learning process.[25] This includes awareness of the interrelated effects of visual, auditory, vestibular, and tactile-kinesthetic systems, motor development, and cognition. Auditory processing, hyperactivity, and tactile defensiveness cannot be pigeonholed into separate categories for treatment.

Attention deficit disorder. Attention deficit disorder (ADD), also called hyperactivity syndrome, hyperkinetic disorder, or minimal brain dysfunction, is characterized by short attention span, poor concentration, impulsivity, and a high level of motor activity. A high prevalence of speech and language disorders and academic learning problems have been identified among children diagnosed with ADD.[10]

Mental retardation. Mental retardation reduces the capacity for verbal as well as nonverbal intelligence. Because cognition and concept development form the foundation for language, defective cognitive development precludes normal language acquisition. The degree of mental retardation affects the potential for language learning.

Autism. Autism has been associated with disturbed language development as well as disrupted use of pragmatic or interactive skills. The autistic child often demonstrates literal, echolalic, or bizarre language patterns in conjunction with a constellation of behavioral and interpersonal problems. Many fail to develop language and are mistakenly suspected of being hearing impaired early in development.

EVALUATION OF COMMUNICATION
Role of the therapist

The therapist working with neuropathologies will undoubtedly encounter clients with communication disorders. The therapist's role in the evaluation and remediation of these disorders will vary depending on the setting, nature of the disorder, availability and role of speech pathologists, and individual experience and expertise. Generally, however, the goals of the therapist working with the communication-disordered client are fourfold.

The first goal is recognition and identification of the communication problem. Often the therapist is the first professional to note speech and language problems and begin the referral process. Awareness of normal communication and development and the effects of disease or injury assist in the identification process. All too often families, physicians, or health care professionals take a wait-and-see attitude when early intervention could reverse the course of a disorder. Recognition of a problem not only directs attention to needed services but also allows the therapist to incorporate appropriate communication-related activities into the program. The clinician should avoid labeling the communication disorder. The therapist must recognize the problem, but actual diagnosis of the communication problem should be in the hands of the speech pathologist.

The second goal is to determine how to communicate with the client. Assessment procedures, information gathering, and direction giving require communication between the client and therapist. Clinicians must learn how to alter the situation or their own speech to maximize communication and how to best understand client needs. This goal can best be accomplished if there is a complete understanding of the communication disorder. Information provided by the speech pathologist, family, and caregivers, as well as by direct observation, can be of great help in learning to communicate with the individual.

The third goal involves determination of the effects of stimulation, movement, and positioning on the communication of the client. This information is helpful in planning a program and can be relayed to the family and other therapists. For instance, the therapist who observes the calming effect of a particular form of sensory stimulation on a hyperactive child might relay this information to the teacher or speech pathologist. Based on this information, a treatment schedule may evolve.

The fourth goal involves determining how therapists can assist in stimulating speech and language. This requires programming prespeech or communication activities into the therapy regimen and eliminating tasks that might interfere with development of communication. Although the job of the therapist is not to remediate the communication disorder per se, the clinician can provide a sound physiological framework for speech production. For instance, the use of an associated movement to increase activity in a hemiplegic client may also increase laryngeal tone. If the client exhibits spastic dysarthria, this increased laryngeal tone can be destructive to speech. On the other hand, such activity with a flaccid dysarthric client might facilitate voicing. Encouraging the aphasic client to communicate by providing a supportive atmosphere and appropriately structuring a natural conversation facilitates language, while asking an aphasic client to name objects in the room is rarely an appropriate activity for the physical or occupational therapy clinic. An awareness of tasks that aid communication is imperative in a holistic approach to treatment.

Motor activities make excellent contexts for language stimulation. Children need to experience objects and events referred to by the speech they hear to learn the relationships between sound and meaning.[7] The therapist can provide part of this experience in the clinic. Adults and children

with neuromuscular impairments need a background of physiological support upon which to build speech. The therapist can provide this support. Communication is a social function. The therapist can reinforce positive attitudes and promote interaction. A facilitatory and supportive environment promotes functional reorganization of a disturbed communication system. The therapy clinic can provide an environment conducive to reorganization and integration.

The organization of nervous system function does not take place piecemeal. The overlap of function extends the role of the therapist beyond that of a motivator, supporter, and stimulator of communication. The neural processes underlying movement cannot be separated from speech and language. As McDonald Critchly so eloquently stated, "The headstream of language overflows into every possible channel."[16,p.299] The reverse is also true. We speak with our mouths and our bodies.

Unfortunately, speech has been considered a special and separate function by many. However, research and clinical experience suggest that speech is intimately related to the motor system as a whole.[41] Not only is oral-motor function an outgrowth of early vegetative function, but also it seems intricately tied to other motor functions.

It seems to be no coincidence that the cerebral hemisphere that controls speech also usually controls a person's dominant hand. It has been proposed that left-hemispherical specialization for speech is a consequence not so much of an asymmetrical evolution of symbolic functions as it is a consequence of the evolution of certain motor skills that happen to lend themselves readily to communication.[40] In other words, the left hemisphere evolved language not because it gradually became more symbolic or analytical per se but because it became well adapted for some categories of motor activity.[41] There is an obvious relationship between speech and hand use. Babies punctuate crying with hand movements and begin early manual stressing gestures in time with speech.[14] The pairing of verbal and motor output is not random. There seems to be an interconnection between verbal and nonverbal systems. It is difficult for normal speakers to speak with hand movements that are *not* in synchrony with the rhythm of their speech. Kimura[39] found that gestures occurring during the speech of right handers were associated almost exclusively with the right hand. Such gestures were not observed during humming. Kinsbourne[41] extended this idea to a presumably biologically preprogrammed linkage between language functions and skilled movements of the right side. This is related to an early association between infant vocalizations and body-orienting response. With maturation, speech is detached from overt body orientations. However, the philosophy that language evolves in a motor context and that there is a neurophysiological link between speech and the right extremities cannot be ignored. While evaluating and treating the motor system, the effects on speech and language should be closely monitored. Moreover, specific knowledge of the functioning of the speech mechanism will assist in heightening awareness of the interrelationships of sensorimotor systems.

Communication screening

Evaluation and diagnosis of communication disorders are complicated and time-consuming procedures for which the speech-language pathologist is specially trained. A staggering array of standardized and nonstandardized test materials are available to assess auditory perception, comprehension, reading, memory, verbal expression, verbal problem solving, motor speech, and writing in both children and adults. Results of a complete evaluation form the basis for decisions regarding diagnosis, prognosis, and treatment. This information can be of great value to the therapist. Therefore communication with the speech pathologist is necessary. Often, however, the therapist must gain preliminary information before a speech evaluation is completed. Therefore familiarity with informal assessment and observation procedures is needed. Assessment of the functional level of communication can be carried out by (1) observing the client communicate; (2) interviewing family or caregivers; (3) reviewing biographical, medical, and historical information; and (4) requiring that the client perform certain screening tasks. The following section presents a variety of areas that influence communicative adequacy. The age, behavior of the client, and cause of the disorder help dictate the type and extent of assessment. Information acquired should be used to assist in the delivery of therapy services, not for the diagnosis and treatment of the communication disorder.

Assessment of oral-motor function. Structural and functional integrity of the speech mechanism is obviously required for adequate speech. Requiring speech of a deficient oral-motor mechanism is like requiring walking before adequate strength, movement, or coordination of the trunk and extremities is obtained. The devastating effects of neuromuscular impairment on speech quality and intelligibility are obvious when we hear the severely dysarthric cerebral-palsied individual attempt to squeeze speech from an uncooperative oral mechanism. The speech mechanism should not be overlooked in the therapy clinic. Knowledge of the condition of the motor system as a whole is imperative to suitable treatment.

The following section briefly addresses movements necessary for speech production. Although knowledge of the range of movement, strength, and accuracy of muscle groups is of extreme importance, actual muscle testing and grading of movement is not covered because this information is available elsewhere.[18,38]

The child or adult should be assessed both at rest and while engaged in activity. Symmetry of the face and lips, muscle tone, alignment of the teeth and jaws, involuntary or overflow movement, and facial expression should be observed. The oral cavity can be inspected to note the size, shape, and mobility of the tongue and soft palate. Obvious deviations, such as cleft palate, gross malocclusions, tremors, and deformities, are likely to affect speech.

Oral reflexes should be tested and determination made of appropriateness to the individual's age (Table 26-5). Because the motor functions required for sucking, chewing, swallowing, coughing, and breathing are necessary prespeech movements, knowledge of these activities is needed. Questioning the client or family and directly observing breathing, eating, and drinking provide valuable information regarding (1) adequacy of the motor pattern itself, (2) positions assumed during activity, and (3) interference of movement of extremities and reflexes on oral-motor functions.

Often simple vegetative or voluntary movements are performed adequately; yet movement cannot be combined into smooth, rapid, fine transitions required for speech. Voluntary movements can be tested with and without visual cues using imitation as well as spontaneous production. Observation of facial expression is helpful in determining functional use of patterns also.

Respiration. Vegetative breathing can be observed with the individual in the supine position by looking across the chest. Infants often demonstrate belly breathing, but by 2 years of age most children begin lifting the upper chest during inhalation. Continued belly breathing may indicate that muscles of upper chest and neck are not able to fix the rib cage against pressure created by diaphragm movement.[78] The breathing pattern should be smooth and rhythmical.

Notation of head and sitting balance contributes to information on respiration because both assist with air intake. For instance, sitting in a flexed position may inhibit upper chest movement and initiation of phonation. Proper support and positioning can dramatically alter breathing and speech.

Breath support for speech requires voluntary control and sufficient air capacity to sustain exhalation through a sentence. Voluntary control can be tested in the older child or adult by taking a deep breath and sustaining the outflow of air as long as possible. Any involuntary motion or lack of

Table 26-5. Normal and pathological oral reflexes[46,55]

Reflex	Normal (approximate ages)	Abnormal
Rooting	Up to 4 months	In adult
Suck-swallow	Up to 5 months	In adult
Bite reflex	Up to 5 months	In adult
Mature swallow	Normal after 1 year	
Gag	Always normal	
Cough	Always normal	
Cephalic		Abnormal
Chew reflex		Abnormal
Jaw jerk		Abnormal

smoothness should be noted. The same exercise should be repeated as the client moves one arm, then the other, to see if involuntary activity is triggered.

Laryngeal system. Involuntary function can be inferred from the pitch, quality, and loudness of crying or vocalizations. Coughs should be rapid and sufficiently loud to indicate vocal fold activity; a weak or dragged out cough is a sign of laryngeal problems.

Voluntary vocal fold activity can be tested by having the individual sustain a tone (the proverbial "ah") for as long as possible. Phonation for 10 seconds or less is probably inadequate for normal connected speech. The loudness and pitch of the voice should be noted. A whispered or breathy sound suggests inadequate closing of the vocal folds. The ability to rapidly start and stop phonation can be tested by having the individual produce "ah ah ah . . ." like a machine gun as fast as possible.[78] The ability to alter the length of the vocal folds can be tested by having the client intone "ah" beginning at a low pitch and building to high pitch.

Palate. Involuntary motion of the palate is easily observed by eliciting the gag reflex. Hyperactivity or hypoactivity and symmetry can be noted. Activity for speech is observed by watching the movement of the palate on production of "ah." The head should not be tilted back because gravity would then assist with palatal movement.

Tongue. With the lips held apart, the involuntary motion of the tongue can be observed during eating. Food can be placed at corners of the mouth, on the upper lip, and in between the cheeks and teeth to observe the mobility of the tongue. Drooling or ejection of food from the mouth or presence of a primitive tongue-thrust swallow should be noted.

Voluntary movement can consist of elevation and lateralization of the tongue tip and protrusion and retraction. With the jaw stabilized open, the client should touch the tongue tip behind the upper teeth. Rapid side-to-side and up-and-down movement is requested with notation made of speed, range, and accuracy or any shift into an extensor retraction pattern. The clinician should note if resistance to movement elicits improved function or overflow activity.

Lips. Adequate sucking requires lip closure as well as action of the cheeks. Drooling or difficulty removing food from a spoon may indicate poor lip closure. Lip closure should be maintained for swallowing in an adult swallow. Lip movements tested for speech include retraction, pressing lips together, and lip rounding. Rapid motion is observed by pursing and smiling or by opening and closing as fast as possible.

Assessment of oral sensation. Because no aspect of voluntary motor activity is independent of its sensory component, the integrity of tactile and kinesthetic feedback should be assessed. This can include light touch and pressure to the face, lips, and palate and tongue tip, sides, and body. The clinician should note presence of hypersensitivity or

hyposensitivity or elicitation of abnormal reflexes during testing. When drooling persists in spite of ability to achieve lip closure and tongue movement, decreased sensation is suspect. Oral tactile hypersensitivity may result in gagging, choking, or even an extensor thrust of the tongue when something is introduced into the mouth.[78] Often tactile defensiveness is especially noted on stimulation around the mouth.[1]

Oral stereognosis has been tested by use of small plastic shapes attached to a cord.[64] The shapes are placed in the mouth and the client picks an identical shape from an array. Such procedures must be used with extreme caution by trained professionals because of the potential risk of airway obstruction. Taste and temperature sensitivity are often assessed to assist in swallowing programs and neuromuscular facilitation.[52]

Assessment of speech. In addition to evaluating oral-motor and sensory integrity, an impression of the functional use of these structures for speech is important. When the language system is intact yet the neuromotor system fails to sufficiently support speech (as in dysarthria), the output can be described in terms of intelligibility (how easy it is to understand) and perceived characteristics (such as monotone, breathiness, and excessive loudness). The intelligibility gives an overall impression of the individual's ability to use speech to communicate. The perceived characteristics explain what has gone wrong to disrupt speech. The usefulness of this approach to assessment can be understood with the following treatment example. The therapist observes a cerebral-palsied client with shallow, uncoordinated breathing patterns, excessive overflow movement, and deviant positioning. The speech pathologist observes unintelligible speech characterized by short phrasing, reduced loudness, imprecise consonants, and variable breakdown. The therapist might work on positioning, facilitate breathing, increase isolated muscle control, and diminish overflows. The speech pathologist might build on this improved speech support by focusing on altering phrasing, rate of speech, and articulation of specific sounds to improve intelligibility.

An impression of the function of oral structures for speech can be gained by having the client imitate isolated syllables, words, and sentences and engage in conversation. It is not uncommon to observe minimal difficulty in producing isolated oral movements, such as elevating the tongue while the system is unable to produce the motion rapidly and in coordination with the rest of the speech mechanism. The speech pathologist usually tests motor speech in ascending levels of motor speech difficulty; for instance, the ability to produce vowels (ah), combine vowels and consonants (pa), rapidly sequence syllables (papapa . . .), rapidly alternate syllables (pataka . . .), produce simple words (pie, cat), produce multisyllabic words of varying length (cat, catnip, catastrophe), produce sentences, and converse. During these tasks notation is made of the range, speed, and accuracy of movement, the intelligibility of the product, and the perceived characteristics of the output.

Assessment of mental status. The overall approach to understanding a communication disorder requires carefully ruling out possible contributing variables. The problems must be pinpointed to ensure appropriate goal setting and treatment. For instance, the child with a language learning disorder resulting from inability to attend and from hyperactivity might be overstimulated by exaggerated multimodal sensory stimulation, while the child with aphasia may require exaggerated multimodality sensory input. Biographical, medical, and historical information, as well as observation of specific behaviors, will help delineate the deficits.

Levels of consciousness. Level of alertness can be determined by observing the individual's response to stimuli and his or her interaction with the examiner. Drifting off to sleep, inattention, and decreased awareness of surroundings are typical of the lethargic client.[70] Specific assessment of speech and language skills are not valid in reduced levels of consciousness because communication disturbance varies with level of alertness and awareness.

Attention. The ability to attend to a specific stimulus without distraction should be observed and described. Inattention caused by hyperactivity and distractibility (midbrain lesion) should be distinguished from that caused by indifference, perseveration, or abulia (frontal lobe lesion).[70] Inattention confined to specific modalities should be noted also.

Visual and auditory sensitivity. Knowledge of the integrity of vision and audition are prerequisites of communication testing. If the client cannot clearly visualize objects used to elicit speech, then errors may result from vision, not language. Similarly, the client who does not follow a spoken command may be hearing impaired rather than language impaired.

Mood/nonverbal communication. Observation of nonverbal behavior assists greatly in determining the type of communication problem. Use of facial expression, voice tone, gestures, and body position should be noted. Does the individual watch carefully as though searching for information? Does the client appear motivated to communicate? Aphasic adults and children attempt to relate to others nonverbally through gesture and affective tone. Individuals with generalized intellectual deficits often display shallow or flat affect, bland depression, indifference, or general dullness. A discrepancy between the level of nonverbal and verbal development is an extremely important clinical observation.

Orientation. Orientation is classically assessed in adults by asking name, date, and location information. Too often aphasic clients are mistakenly labeled confused because of this kind of testing. Such an assessment of a language disordered person is not valid. Orientation must be observed functionally, and great caution should be used in interpreting observations.

Memory. Several types of memory disturbance are associated with neuropathological conditions. Immediate recall is often tested using digit repetition tasks.[70] Remote memory of general knowledge is assessed by asking biographical questions. Prior knowledge of correct information is imperative. The author has been fooled more than once by confused clients who provide beautiful, believable information that is totally confabulated. Tasks that require the client to recall information provided earlier in the session, remember a string of words, or tell what was served for lunch all provide data on memory. However, the client with speech or language problems may be unable to perform such tasks accurately in spite of adequate memory. It might be helpful in such cases to compare responses to nonverbal memory tasks. Informal tests may be performed, such as placing the client's cane or jacket behind a door while the client is looking and noting later if the individual remembers where it is. A more formal method is to hide objects while the client watches, then in several minutes show a duplicate object and see if the client recalls the location of the hidden object. Observation of information that enhances memory should be made using visual, auditory, and tactile input, repetition, or exaggeration of the stimulus. For instance, some clients (and therapists) will be more likely to remember information if they have seen it in writing, had it repeated several times during the session, or have been shown pictorial examples. Auditory-verbal information must not be required during such tasks because this tests the speech or language problem rather than memory.

Nonverbal intelligence. Observation of the way the adult or child relates to the environment, solves problems, or performs nonverbal tasks such as visual matching helps distinguish between specific speech and language problems and more generalized cognitive deficits. Observation of play is very useful in children. Symbolic play is an important prerequisite for language.

Assessment of language

Auditory comprehension. As noted previously, before assessing auditory comprehension the examiner must determine if peripheral hearing is intact. Does the client turn toward an auditory stimulus or startle to loud noises? Is there differential reaction to varying tone of voice? Does the individual respond differently to speech versus environmental sounds (such as sirens or phone ringing)? When an audiological evaluation rules out hearing impairment yet the client fails to follow commands consistently, the clinician should attempt to determine the degree of comprehension problems.

Comprehension should be assessed without requiring verbal responses from the client and with full knowledge of the correct answer. Questions such as "Did you like breakfast?" may elicit socially appropriate "yes" or "no" responses, but the examiner has no way of knowing if they reflect accurate understanding. Typical comprehension testing usually requires pointing to objects named or carrying out simple directions. Responses are often better for whole body or axial commands ("get up"; "sit down") than for distal commands ("point"; "pick up"). If a motor response is facilitated, does the individual respond better to the verbal command? The clinician should be aware of situational or inadvertent gestural cues that may be assisting the client and note if responses are more accurate when visual, tactile, or situational cues are used.

Verbal expression. Areas generally covered in speech and language evaluations by the speech pathologist include verbal repetition of words or phrases of increasing length, describing a picture, naming and describing the function of common objects, reading aloud, answering questions, and completing sentences. The most obvious informal approach to gaining an impression of an individual's language is to engage in conversation. The approach will vary considerably depending on age. The young child rarely responds well to question-answer interaction, engaging the child in play, using parallel talk, or providing a context in which the child needs to speak (e.g., to ask for a toy) are preferable to approaches asking "What is this?" Adults can be asked open-ended questions, such as "What brought you into the hospital?" A general idea of function can be gained from the amount, accuracy, and appropriateness of spontaneous speech and the ability to interact. In addition, the clinician can check serial speech, repetition, and confrontation naming.

A brief screening of gesturing and writing may be helpful if verbal expression is nonfunctional. Language impaired clients rarely write better than they speak. However, if this channel along with gesturing can add information to verbal output, awareness of the skill is helpful.

Motor function and alternate communication systems. The influence on communication of neuromotor dysfunction can range beyond specific speech and language problems. The ability of the individual with nonfunctional speech to adapt to an alternate form of communication, such as a communication board or signing, can dictate the possibility of functional communication. The range, strength, and fine control of, for example, extremities and sitting balance determine the appropriateness of various alternate communication systems. The physical or occupational therapists will need to work closely with the speech pathologist and the family to ensure that an alternative communication system is appropriate physically, mentally, and socially to the individual.

Environmental variables. The physical characteristics of the environment can markedly affect verbal communication.[49] The therapist must be acutely aware of the influences of setting on the interaction with the client. Common sense dictates that anything that hinders normal communication will interfere with disordered communication. Attempting to speak in a noisy, bustling environment can be distracting to anyone. It can be chaotic and overwhelming to the individual with communication problems. The positions of the client

and therapist can inhibit or facilitate interaction. Face-to-face, eye-level communication maximizes the client's and the therapist's use of all cues. Nonverbal information, such as gestures, facial expression, and calming voice quality, can assist. Lighting should be adequate to promote visualization of the speaker and the environment. Attitude and motivation can be enhanced by the appearance of the environment and the therapist. For instance, a child who has been poked, probed, and stuck by physicians for the past year may react negatively to anyone in a laboratory coat. An adult who has suffered a stroke may resent being treated with baby toys.

TREATMENT CONSIDERATIONS

The treatment goals of the therapist will be to improve the physiological support for speech production, maximize the client's use of existing communication, and reinforce and stimulate the development of a functional communication system. These goals should be incorporated within the context of therapy. The therapist must not attempt to do speech or language therapy. Rather, a close working relationship with the speech pathologist and occupational therapist will help in defining roles and ensuring unified, holistic treatment. The following section briefly highlights areas of treatment. The purpose is to familiarize the reader with the variety of treatment needs of the speech impaired client, rather than prepare the clinician to implement such treatment. Clinical experience and education will be necessary to fully appreciate the variety and complexity of treatment variables that influence speech and language learning.

Oral-motor dysfunction

Techniques such as inhibiting, resisting, and facilitating movement, positioning, and muscle strengthening are appropriate for the speech mechanism (see Chapter 6).[60,61] However, appropriateness of techniques will depend on the specific type of motor dysfunction or dysarthria. Treatment of the speech mechanism will obviously affect feeding and swallowing. In fact, treatment often centers around feeding activities. Awareness of oral-motor dysfunction should not be limited to these activities. However, during all treatment the effects on the speech mechanism should be noted. Overflow of activity to the oral mechanism should be observed when using techniques to facilitate movement elsewhere. The approach to training oral-motor function should take into account the total pattern of the target movement and the concomitant sensory experiences. Learning proceeds best when a trained, isolated movement is incorporated into meaningful activity with appropriate feedback to allow for discrimination and generalization.[2] At all times the goal is to help the individual initiate, sustain, and terminate oral movement while approximating normal function as closely as possible.[57]

Posturing. Exploring postural influences on speech can provide information on needed modifications. To perceive the pattern of a new speech movement, competing feedback from tension and involuntary movement elsewhere in the body must be reduced. Postures will vary depending on the disorder, the target movement, and the needs of the individual. Postures that inhibit reflexes may help the neurologically impaired individual practice movement patterns for speech that might otherwise trigger massive primitive movement patterns. Correct posturing is also important in preventing abnormal development. For example, a persisting asymmetrical tonic neck reflex could cause deviation of the mandible and restrain articulation. Stabilization techniques may be necessary in extreme cases when overflow movement precludes speech learning.

Vegetative to voluntary activity. Targeting the more primitive movements of sucking, chewing, swallowing, and vegetative breathing allows the establishment of correct prespeech patterns, with the goal of gradually achieving voluntary control. Feedback through all sensory modalities will heighten awareness of the movement and assist in modifying these for speech.

Respiration and phonation. Prolongation and control of respiration can be stimulated to improve phonation and speech phrasing. Assuming an antigravity position, such as sitting, often helps stimulate lung expansion. Rotation within the body axis tends to decrease spasticity and increase respiratory output. For speech purposes, the client who cannot sit alone should be positioned with adequate support to maximize breathing, assist phonation, and allow eye contact. As trunk and head control increases, vocalization often occurs spontaneously during movements, yawning, or sighing. This phonation can be encouraged and shaped to build toward volitional sound production. Respiratory muscle strengthening can be accomplished during activities to improve trunk stability, head control, and sitting balance. During such activities, breathing can be facilitated, progressing from passive to resisted motion. Voluntary control can be encouraged by activities such as blowing a match without extinguishing it, blowing a ping pong ball across a table, or taking a deep breath, holding it, and prolonging a sound.

Sucking and swallowing. When vegetative responses are absent or diminished, facilitatory techniques can often be used to improve function. Effective control of swallowing implies use of the lips, cheeks, tongue, palate, larynx, and respiratory systems. Therefore it is an excellent focus for therapy (see Chapter 6). Food is one of the primary facilitators of oral movement because it can stimulate sensations of touch, taste, and temperature, as well as providing visual and olfactory input.

Swallowing is usually approached in a sitting position with the head flexed slightly forward to avoid aspiration. Because aspiration, nutritional imbalance, and negative feelings can be produced by improper techniques, foods, or positions, it is recommended that the clinician become well versed in swallowing therapy[31,32,45,47,55] and seek assistance from allied professionals specifically trained to conduct

videofluoroscopic swallow studies and assess swallow dynamics before initiating this treatment. In conjunction with swallowing therapy or when a full feeding program is not necessary, an array of facilitory and inhibitory techniques can be used to stimulate the speech mechanism.[44,47,60,75] Various tastes can be introduced to elicit responses. Typically, salt mobilizes the tongue, bitter tastes cause protrusion, and sweets elicit retraction.[52] Movement elicited by various tastes, textures, temperatures, and pressures can be shaped toward functional patterns.

Lips. Lip closure is necessary to prevent drooling and produce speech sounds.[55] Lip closure can be stimulated by activities such as holding the fingers above and under the lips, stretching the lips, attempting closure against resistance, and pulling a small metal spoon out between closed lips to create resistance.[52] Shaking the lip sometimes reduces spasticity.[55] Lip closure and rounding can be stimulated by sucking a gloved finger or through straws of progressively smaller diameter.[60]

Tongue. Tongue movement can be stimulated by passive then resisted motion, and stretching.[61] Elevation may be assisted by brushing the ridge behind the teeth and walking down the midline with a tongue blade, then releasing the pressure and elevating the tongue with the blade. The client can be encouraged to lick food from the roof of the mouth, corners of the mouth, or lips after facilitatory activities. A tongue blade can be used for tactile cues, tapping, or sustained pressure as appropriate.

Jaw. Control of jaw stabilization is needed for speech. Using a bite block during tongue and lip exercises will prevent associated jaw movement until isolated tongue and lip movement is achieved. Once this is achieved attention can be directed to the voluntary control of the jaw. Motion can be assisted during chewing movements, and the range and rate can be slowly increased.

In cases of pathological bite reflex, pressure at the temporomandibular joint or under the chin might reduce the reflex.[55] Extensor thrust of the jaw often accompanies athetosis, and positioning can often diminish this problem. Passively opening and closing the jaw while slowly initiating phonation may help disassociate the jaw thrust from voicing.[78]

Treatment considerations in dysarthria

The following section attempts to orient the reader in a general direction for treatment rather than delineate the treatment of each dysarthria type. The therapist is well aware of techniques for physical restoration. Obviously these principles apply to the speech mechanism. In some cases the speech pathologist will prefer doing the physical restoration specific to the speech mechanism. However, the therapist might incorporate appropriate treatment tasks into the general therapy regime. The ideal situation involves an overlap of roles because the speech pathologist rarely has the setting or the expertise to explore body position and the therapist may need guidance in choice of speech movements relative to difficulty, developmental level, and importance to speech. Obvious precautions should be taken relative to medical diagnoses and to ensure that strengthening and positioning maintain muscle balance and symmetry. Therapy activities must be designed with the purposeful goal of improving the physiological support for verbal communication. The speech pathologist will simultaneously attempt to maximize the client's use of the impaired neuromotor system for speech production. Feedback should be sufficient to allow for generalization. In other words, appropriate sensory input must be given to allow the client to develop an awareness of the movements being facilitated or trained.

The physical management of *flaccid dysarthria* requires increasing muscle tone, strength, and range through facilitation techniques or through techniques such as biofeedback.[17] Oral movements can be practiced in positions that allow gravity to assist in the motion (such as producing tongue tip movements with head bent forward or prone), then slowly guiding the tongue tip to work against gravity, then against active resistance. Increased activity of hypotonic speech musculature is observed when clients exert effort elsewhere, as in lifting themselves off a chair, bridging, or sustaining a pushing action with arms against resistance. Vocalizing during such activities sometimes allows the client to learn the feeling of modified tone and may heighten reflexive closure of the vocal folds. Incorporation of such speech activities into general strengthening programs and transfer training can be helpful and efficient.

Muscle strengthening, increasing speed and range of motion, and inhibiting excess tone are the primary targets of treatment in *spastic dysarthria*. Relaxation, slow stroking, and pressure have been recommended as inhibitory techniques[52] as well as exploring effects of postures on muscle tone and speech. Jaw shaking for relaxation and working from the vegetative function of chewing to build volitional motor function has been recommended.[26] Exercises to increase control, such as sustained, relaxed exhalation and voicing, are used. While exercise programs geared to improve speed and range of motion (e.g., repetitive tongue tip elevations) are underway, the speech pathologist often teaches the client to slow down the rate of speech. These procedures are not contradictory. A similar circumstance might be seen when the hemiplegic client is attempting to increase speed and strength of lower-extremity movement yet is required to walk slowly and deliberately to accommodate the remaining neuromotor deficit. Biofeedback is a possible technique for reducing hypertonicity and undesired overflow activity.[58]

The client with *ataxic dysarthria* usually shows improved speech as general stability increases. The primary goal with ataxic speakers is improving the coordination of the speech mechanism. Imposing conscious cortical control over the movements for speech seems to improve the quality and intelligibility of the speech output.

The management of the individual with *hypokinetic dysarthria* requires increasing the range of motion and decreasing the excess tone caused by rigidity. Movement seems to increase when the client is asked to exert extra effort. For instance, clients with Parkinson's disease can be asked to take very deep breaths and exaggerate their speech. Using multiple input and output systems often helps, such as touching a colored square each time a word is spoken.[35,50] Movement improves speech and speech improves movement. Therefore gait or exercise activities might logically incorporate speech. Answering a question by saying one word with each step or counting repetitions out loud are examples of this.

The treatment of the client with *hyperkinetic dysarthria* will focus largely on inhibiting involuntary movements that interfere with speech. Postures and positioning will be of utmost importance in eliminating abnormal activity and tone during speech exercises, and stabilization may be necessary when movements of the extremities continually trigger mandible or tongue extension. Relaxation and sensory stimulation or biofeedback[23] may be useful in inhibiting excess movement in some cases.

Developmental communication disorders

Although the speech pathologist will evaluate and plan actual language remediation, when needed, other health professionals and family members should assist in language learning. Knowledge of development of communication and learning theory will prepare clinicians for this assistive role.

Several general principles are helpful in approaching language learning. Easy language structures for adults may not be easy language structures for children. Language used with children should be simplified according to developmental levels. The young child is more likely to imitate "Push ball" than "Who is funny?" Therefore simple structures and words geared to the child's functional level can be incorporated into therapy in the form of parallel talk. The therapist describes what is going on ("roll the ball . . . bounce the ball") and reinforces any attempts at communication or imitation by the child. Correcting should be avoided. Rather, positive reinforcement is used to model closer and closer productions. Copying the child immediately after a behavior is produced often encourages increased production. Repetition improves learning. The same words and phrases can be repeated over and over in context by the therapist ("roll ball . . . push ball . . . ball fell down") during routine activities. Expanding children's utterances can introduce slightly more difficult sentence structures ("Joey rolled the ball"). Providing appropriate speech models and rewarding attempts to repeat or respond are preferable to requiring the child to say "ball." Imitation of speech in the absence of meaningful context is not useful.[7]

The situation and interaction should be structured to

764 SPECIAL TOPICS AND TECHNIQUES FOR THERAPISTS

motivate communication. Encouraging independence by allowing choices increases a sense of self and desire to control the environment. All forms of communication should be encouraged, such as gestures, facial expression, and eye contact. Songs and rhythm can be combined with movement to tap right hemisphere processing. The therapist should maximize input by combining auditory, gestural, facial, and inflection information.

Subtle responses in severely communication impaired clients can be shaped to form a basis for social interaction. For example a child with severe cognitive, sensory and motor problems might "communicate" by attending to a moving wind-up toy and glancing at the therapist when the toy stops—a subtle request to rewind the toy. Reinforcement by rewinding the toy and repeating the scenario begins to mold the child's emerging "requesting" behavior into a communicative interaction.

Learning proceeds best when the sensory input is adequate to build associations. Combining speech with active motion can reinforce concepts. Real objects can be used to provide tactile, visual, and auditory input, such as banging, throwing, or rolling.[8] Assuming various positions in relation to objects assists in integrating experiences while the therapist verbalizes. Young children can be guided into conceptualizing object permanence and building early symbolic memory with simple hide-and-seek activities. Older children can build concepts of directionality by crawling *into* the box and sitting *on* the box.[7] Motion allows active involvement and often helps focus attention. Therefore activities geared appropriately to the child's developmental level are natural for physical therapy. Treatment should be dynamic, with texture, sight, and sound integrated into motion. Sensory and perceptual integration will promote language learning. Using sand, water, colorful toys, or music can motivate and heighten input.[1]

A note of caution is in order: The clinician must determine which sensory stimulation is consistent with learning and which interferes with learning. Children with auditory or tactile defensiveness may need specific work on reducing this defensiveness. Insufficiently inhibited sensory input in one modality can interrupt learning in another modality.[1] On the other hand, sensory stimuli can facilitate learning in another modality. Such is the case when we remember someone's name (auditory) by remembering a distinctive facial feature (visual). The amount of sensory stimulation can help or hinder language processing also. A listener usually attends more carefully to a question accompanied by a soft touch on the arm; the listener would probably miss the question entirely if simultaneously punched in the arm! Exploring the type and amount of sensory stimulation that facilitates motor and language learning can have far-reaching effects. Ayres[1] has observed that vestibular stimulation contributes to sensory integration, often elicits vocalization, and serves as a precursor to more cognitive approaches to learning.

Constant awareness of the many variables that influence learning must be maintained. Nonverbal information projected by the therapist can influence the child's responses. For instance, a loud voice or a fearful, tense clinician inadvertently might increase hyperactivity in a child. Activities building fine hand control may contribute to motor planning overall. However, speaking during such activities can be an interference unless the speaking activity is expressly geared to mediate motor planning.[42,43,48]

Treatment considerations in dementia

Frequently, the bizarre or tangential verbalizations and apparent learning problems of the patient with dementia make structured treatment a considerable challenge. In such cases, several general principles for communicating with the individual might prove valuable. First, the goal is rarely to actually "teach" better or more appropriate communication, but rather to provide an atmosphere that lightens the demands on the ravaged "cognitive system" so that the individual can use what cognitive "strengths" remain. For example, providing a predictable structure (treatment at the same time each day with the same activities and instructions) will minimize the demands on memory, allowing the individual to focus mental energy on acquiring the target skill. Also consistency, repetition, and redundancy in verbal and nonverbal communication can facilitate memory and new learning. The tendency to engage in normal "chit chat" with the confused patient during an activity can actually promote increased confusion and agitation; if this appears to be the case, using simple descriptions of what is being done while working with the individual might help inhibit misunderstanding and orient the client to the activity. Spoken instructions or information might be supplemented with simple written instructions to facilitate understanding and attention. Body language (e.g., smiling) and speech tone that is gentle and supportive can reduce confusion. In addition, in some cases anticipating clients' needs rather than requiring them to communicate a need can help lighten the demands.

Conversing with the confused or demented client is a true art. Many clinicians feel the need to correct and "teach" the individual by pointing out memory errors or repeatedly "testing" orientation. In fact, this approach serves more to discourage communication than to facilitate it. Orientation should be provided in a natural, supportive, conversational manner; orientation information should be given to, rather than requested of, the client (e.g., "My goodness . . . it is already December. 1993 is almost over" versus "What month is it?"). Redirecting is preferable to challenging or calling attention to inappropriate, inaccurate, or tangential verbalization. Topics that the client enjoys and remembers should be encouraged even if they represent remote memories. It is often quite satisfying and reinforcing to the client to talk about the same happy memory every day. Although possibly tedious to the clinician, reinforcement of these lucid memories can form a nonthreatening framework for introducing new information.

Treatment considerations in traumatic brain injury

As with the client with dementia, the communication of the patient with a traumatic brain injury is a direct reflection of underlying cognitive disruption. Techniques to lighten the processing load and facilitate cognitive organization are required. The clinician can use communication as a barometer to the client's cognitive state and adjust treatment accordingly. For example verbal outbursts, agitation, and inappropriate utterances represent confusion and agitation in middle stage TBI. A usually quiet, passive client who begins yelling obscenities when transported into the gym might be reacting to sensory overload. Such agitation might be reduced by limiting distractions (treating at bedside, reducing verbal input) and providing structure and familiarity. Soft voice, a familiar caretaker, short simple sentences, and repetition can be soothing to a confused patient. Asking open-ended or memory-loaded questions to a confused or memory-impaired patient is likely to elicit confabulation or bizarre responses.

Therapists working with confused TBI clients will need to avoid provoking and heightening cognitive disorganization by overloading the system with sensory input. Conversely, early stage TBI requires high levels of stimulation to promote arousal and alertness. At all times goals and techniques of physical restoration must be adjusted to accommodate simultaneous cognitive reorganization. Refer to Chapter 14 for additional suggestions regarding treatment of clients with TBI.

Treatment considerations in adult aphasia

The primary goal of the speech pathologist with the aphasic adult is to work toward functional communication. Language training is based on graded levels of difficulty and a variety of specific techniques, such as melodic intonation therapy[68] or visual action therapy.[36] Normal speech and language is rarely achieved in cases of residual aphasia. The goal of the physical therapist is to maximize the client's use of remaining communication ability, provide a motivating and supportive setting to avoid development of maladaptive attitudes, and stimulate the reorganization of physiological processes for language. Because management varies considerably with the type and severity of the aphasia, the physical and occupational therapists will want to work closely with the speech pathologist.

To maximize comprehension in the aphasic adult, certain general principles should be followed. The client's level of auditory comprehension will dictate the alterations needed in communication. One common error seems to be assuming no comprehension and excluding the client from the conversation. Another problem occurs when it is assumed that the client understands everything. Usually this type of client receives visual and inflectional information or responds in a socially appropriate manner with only partial understanding. The therapist must be sure that the client is not receiving faulty or damaging information. Distraction and background noise will interfere with auditory comprehension. This includes conflicting tactile or visual input as well as noise. Asking a client an important question while ranging a painful arm is not conducive to comprehension. Aphasic individuals have difficulty switching tasks. Therefore the therapist must be sure that sufficient time and information (visual, gestural, and auditory) are provided to mark a change in task or topic. Speaking from the front at eye level facilitates comprehension. When important information is given, conversation should be one on one. Involving several people, as is done on medical rounds, requires rapid switching, changing speaking distances, and distraction. Gestures, situational cues, visual prompts, voice inflection, and facial expression can enhance or destroy comprehension. The client who hears a loud, clipped "Sit on the mat" may comprehend anger rather than the direction; the client's negative response may appear confused or hostile to the imperceptive clinician. Alerting cues can be used, such as a soft touch, verbalizing the client's name, or using a starter word ("Now . . . push my hand").

Communication should be maintained in a calm, matter-of-fact manner. Sentences should be short and simple; phrasing should allow for processing pauses. The tendency seems to be for people to ask a question, then panic and rephrase, repeat, or answer themselves immediately. Above all, the client should have extra time to listen and to talk. Directions can be formulated to use high-imagery action words, assuming there is right hemisphere processing, and axial commands such as "Pretend you're *swimming*" versus "Move your arms."[77] The organizaion of proximal versus distal muscle groups seems to have a language correlate. That is, axial commands seem to be easier than distal commands. Altering speech to maximize communication and responsiveness should become a habit. For instance, the following direction could be confusing: "I want you to put your arms over my shoulders and I'm going to lift you up. Then I want you to pivot your feet and we'll lower you onto the mat." This could be rephrased to: "Watch me (gesture) . . . we will *stand up* . . . *turn* . . . and *sit down*" (demonstrate as each verb is said).

Communication is a social, interactive activity. People talk because they have something to say. Unfortunately, many people seem to forget the rules of polite conversation when confronted with a communication-disordered client. Asking an acquaintance "What is my name?" or holding up a banana and asking "What is this?" would be considered bizarre behavior indeed at a dinner party. It is no less inappropriate with an aphasic client. The skill of conversing without making excessive demands enhances the enjoyment of working with aphasic people. Relating an interesting story with questions or comments interspersed or talking about activities without directly requesting a response allows the client to participate when able. Questions can be phrased to allow "yes," "no," or pointing responses. Asking a question that requires a complicated answer and then waiting for a response is insensitive. Instead of asking the client with severe expressive problems "What did you do in Occupational Therapy?" several questions and comments can be used to converse: "Did you go to Occupational Therapy?"; "How *was* OT today?"; "Hard work, I'll bet."; "Did you do some arm work (gesture)?"; "Exercises can be tiring!" Although the details of the questions may not be fully understood, the interaction is reinforcing and social.

Encouraging expressive language should not be restricted to verbal communication. If speech is not available, ask the client to show a response. Upper-extremity gestures sometimes facilitate verbalization. This does not imply that aphasic clients have normal use of pantomime or signs. All channels (writing, speaking, and gesturing) are affected to some degree in aphasia. However, speech pathologists often pair hand movements with verbalization to build verbal expression in nonfluent aphasic clients. Voluntary movement of an extremity promotes neurophysiological reactions in the contralateral cortex.[41] Perhaps activation of the anterior speech areas in the brain is enhanced when neighboring motor and premotor hand areas are activated.

Attempts at speech should not be corrected per se. If the therapist does not understand, an honest statement to that effect or request for repeat is usually best. Sometimes narrowing the field with yes/no questions will help: "Is it about a person? . . . family? . . . your son?" Sometimes tactfully changing the subject avoids frustration when failure continues. When the therapist understands but the utterance was faulty, modeling the correct production unobtrusively is suggested. For example, the client points to the cane and says "My coat"; the therapist might say "OK, here's your cane." Helpful communication strategies are discussed further by Lubinski.[49]

Alternative communication systems

A variety of alternatives to verbal communication are available when speech is not possible.[6,66,73,74] The type and complexity of the system will be dictated by physical, linguistic, and cognitive requirements. The financial situation and attitude of the client will influence the choice also. Systems in popular use include sign languages and communication boards.

Obviously sign languages require fairly fine control of the upper extremities, although simple systems have been adapted for one-handed use with apraxia of speech.[67] Adequate memory and language is needed to learn the signs. Most sign systems are used by the hearing impaired community. However, the increased use of signs to facilitate language development in autistic, mentally retarded, and aphasic clients[53,67,79] suggests that physical and occupational therapists may be called upon to provide information on praxis and fine hand control as prerequisite to sign usage.

Communication boards—surfaces upon which letters, objects, or actions are represented—range from simple photocopied alphabet or picture boards to expensive computerized electronic devices.[66,73] The nonverbal client picks out the pictures or words that represent the thought to be communicated. Communication boards can be small, portable lap boards or large systems. A full evaluation by a team of professionals is the best approach because an inappropriate choice is not only a waste of time and money but also an emotionally debilitating experience for the client. The psychologist can determine nonverbal memory, intelligence, emotional maturity, and attitude of the client. The speech pathologist can determine the interactive needs and language capacities. The physical and occupational therapists can determine sitting balance and tolerance, fine and gross motor control, appropriate method of responding (pointing, arm press, head pointer), best positions for responding, placement of the board for maximizing motor function, and fatigability.

Psychosocial implications of communication disorders

As has been mentioned previously, communication is social. However, the reverse is probably more accurate—society is formed through communication. The individual who does not communicate normally is not easily assimilated into society. People tend to feel uncomfortable and avoid communication-impaired individuals. Reactions often reflect prejudices, such as "People who do not speak well are retarded or crazy." Reactions of this kind promote feelings of self-doubt and inadequacy. The need to talk about feelings often goes unfulfilled. In a typical day in a normal person's life, basic needs are communicated quickly and easily. Most speech serves as social, emotional, or intellectual stimulation. The person with a significant communication problem has difficulty communicating even the most basic needs. The result can be embarrassment, discomfort, and humiliation. The enjoyment of expressing one's ideas and opinions and revealing intelligence and emotion is unavailable. If family and friends fail to provide affection and understanding, withdrawal from contact with others often occurs. The result is depression, loneliness, and anxiety.

In many cases the emotional difficulties caused by verbal language problems further reduce the adequacy of communication. Anxiety and stress diminish communicative performance. Reduced communication also affects an individual's ability to participate in school, employment, and social activities. The families of communication-impaired clients often report that friends and social activities diminish markedly with the onset of the disorder. The communication disorder becomes a family problem and a financial problem. Professionals working with the communication-disordered client should take into account these frustrations and fears. Therapists can provide a warm, supporting atmosphere, where attempts at communication are welcomed and feelings are accepted. Families can be counseled on the need to develop outside interests, to promote independence, and to foster feelings of self-worth. Communication is maximized when psychosocial difficulties have been minimized.

SUMMARY

Neurological disorders frequently involve deficits in some aspect of communication. Because communication is an integral aspect of behavior and learning, holistic treatment of the neurologically impaired client should include attention to hearing, speech, and language. Understanding communication and its disorders can add an exciting dimension to practice. It is hoped that this chapter will serve as the scaffolding upon which the clinician can begin to build knowledge through further reading, observation, and interaction with experienced professionals in a team approach to rehabilitation.

REFERENCES

1. Ayres AJ: *Sensory integration and learning disorders,* Los Angeles, 1973, Western Psychological Services.
2. Basmajian J: *Therapeutic exercise,* Baltimore, 1978, Williams & Wilkins.
3. Bates E and others: The acquisition of performatives prior to speech, *Merrill-Palmer Q* 21:205, 1975.
4. Bates E and others: From gesture to the first word: on cognitive and social prerequisites. In Lewis M and Rosenblum L, editors: *Interaction, conversation and the development of language,* New York, 1977, John Wiley & Sons.
5. Bayles K: Language and dementia. In Holland A, editor: *Language disorders in adults,* San Diego, 1984, College Hill Press.
6. Beukelman DR and Yorkston K: A communication system for the severely dysarthric speaker with an intact language system, *J Speech Hear Disord* 42:265, 1977.
7. Bloom L and Lahey M: *Language development and language disorders,* New York, 1978, John Wiley & Sons.
8. Bowerman M: Words and sentences: uniformity, individual variation and shifts over time in patterns of acquisition. In Minifie FD and Lloyd LL, editors: *Communicative and cognitive abilities—early behavioral assessment,* Baltimore, 1978, University Park Press.
9. Brookshire RH: *An introduction to aphasia,* Minneapolis, 1978, BRK Publishers.
10. Cantwell D and Baker L: *Psychiatric and developmental disorders in children with communication disorder,* London, 1991, American Psychiatric Press.
11. Carr J and Shepherd R: *Physiotherapy in disorders of the brain,* London, 1980, William Heinemann Medical Books.
12. Clark E: Some aspects of the conceptual basis for first language acquisition. In Schietelbusch R and Lloyd L, editors: *Language perspectives—acquisition, retardation and intervention,* Baltimore, 1974, University Park Press.
13. Cohen IB and Salapatek P: *Infant perception: from sensation to cognition.* Vol 2. *Perception of space, speech and sound,* New York, 1975, Academic Press.
14. Condon W and Sander L: Neonate movement in synchronized with adult speech: interactional participation and language acquisition, *Science* 183:99, 1974.
15. Creech RJ and others: Oral sensation and perception in dysarthric adults, *Percep Mot Skills* 37:167, 1973.
16. Critchley M: *Aphasiology and other aspects of language,* London, 1970, Edward Arnold.
17. Daniel B: EMG feedback and recovery of facial and speech gestures following neuroanastomosis, *J Speech Hear Disord* 43:9, 1978.
18. Daniels L and Warthingham C: *Muscle testing,* Philadelphia, 1980, WB Saunders.
19. Daniloff R and others: *The physiology of speech and hearing: an introduction,* Englewood Cliffs, NJ, 1980, Prentice-Hall.
20. Darby J: The interaction between speech and disease. In Darby J, editor: *Speech evaluation in medicine,* New York, 1981, Grune & Stratton.
21. Darley FL: A retrospective view: aphasia, *J Speech Hear Disord* 42:161, 1977.
22. Darley FL and others: *Motor speech disorders,* Philadelphia, 1975, WB Saunders.
23. Farrar WB: Using electromyographic biofeedback in treating orofacial dyskinesia, *J Prosthet Dent* 4:384, 1976.
24. Ferguson C: Learning to pronounce: the earliest stages of phonological development in the child. In Minifie FD and Lloyd LL, editors: *Communicative and cognitive abilities—early behavioral assessment,* Baltimore, 1978, University Park Press.
25. Flower R: Neurodevelopmental disorders in children. In Darby J, editor: *Speech evaluation in medicine,* New York, 1981, Grune & Stratton.
26. Froeschels E: Chewing method as therapy, *Arch Otolaryngol* 61:427, 1952.
27. Gardner H: *The shattered mind,* New York, 1974, Random House.
28. Gardner H and others: Comprehension and appreciation of humorous material following brain damage, *Brain* 98:399, 1975.
29. Gilman S and Newman S: *Menter and Gatz's essentials of clinical neuroanatomy and neurophysiology,* ed 7, Philadelphia, 1987, FA Davis.
30. Goodglass H and Kaplan E: *The assessment of aphasia and related disorders,* Philadelphia, 1972, Lea & Febiger.
31. Griffin KM: Swallowing training for dysphagic patients, *Arch Phys Med Rehabil* 55:467, 1974.
32. Groher M: *Dysphagia: diagnosis and management,* Boston, 1984, Butterworth Publishers.
33. Hagen C: Language disorders in head trauma. In Holland A, editor: *Language disorders in adults,* San Diego, 1984, College Hill Press.
34. Hardcastle W: *Physiology of speech production,* London, 1976, Academic Press.
35. Helm N: Management of palilalia with a pacing board, *J Speech Hear Disord* 44:350, 1979.
36. Helm N and Benson F: Visual action therapy for global aphasia, Unpublished paper presented to the Academy of Aphasia, Chicago, 1978.
37. Jones-Owens JL: Prespeech assessment and treatment strategies. In Langley M and Lombardino L, editors: *Neurodevelopmental strategies for managing communication disorders in children with severe motor dysfunction,* Austin, TX, 1991, Pro-ed.
38. Kendall H and others: *Muscles: testing and function,* Baltimore, 1971, Williams & Wilkins.
39. Kimura D: Manual activity during speaking. I. Right handers. II. Left handers, *Neuropsychologia* 1:45, 1973.
40. Kimura D and Archibold Y: Motor functions of the left hemisphere, *Brain* 97:337, 1974.
41. Kinsbourne M, editor: *Asymmetrical function of the brain,* Cambridge, England, 1978, Cambridge University Press.
42. Kinsbourne M and Cook J: Generalized and lateralized effects of concurrent verbalization on a unimanual skill, *Q J Exp Psychol* 23:341, 1971.
43. Kinsbourne M and Murray J: The effect of cerebral dominance on time sharing between speaking and tapping by preschool children, *Child Dev* 46:240, 1975.
44. Langley M and Lombardino L, editors: *Neurodevelopmental strategies for managing communication disorders in children with severe motor dysfunction,* Austin, TX, 1991, Pro-ed.
45. Larsen GL: Rehabilitation for dysphagia paralytica, *J Speech Hear Disord* 37:187, 1972.

46. Levitt S: *Treatment of cerebral palsy and motor delay,* London, 1977, Blackwell Scientific Publications.
47. Logemann J: *Evaluation and treatment of swallowing disorders,* San Diego, 1983, College Hill Press.
48. Lomas J and Kimura D: Intrahemispheric interaction between speaking and sequential manual activity, *Neuropsychologia* 14:23, 1976.
49. Lubinski R: Environmental language intervention. In Chapey R, editor: *Language intervention strategies in adult aphasia,* Baltimore, 1981, Williams & Wilkins.
50. Luria AR: *Traumatic aphasia,* The Hague, 1970, Mouton Publishers.
51. Macaluso-Haynes S: Developmental apraxia of speech. In Johns D, editor: *Clinical management of neurogenic communicative disorders,* Boston, 1978, Little, Brown.
52. May A and Hudgens D: Selected proprioceptive neuromuscular facilitation techniques in dysarthria treatment, Unpublished paper presented to the American Speech and Hearing Association Annual Conference, Chicago, 1977.
53. Miller A and Miller EE: Cognitive developmental training with elevated boards and sign language, *J Autism Child Schizophr* 3:65, 1973.
54. Minifie FD and Lloyd LL: *Communicative and cognitive abilities: early behavioral assessment,* Baltimore, 1978, University Park Press.
55. Mueller H: Facilitating feeding and prespeech. In Pearson P and Williams C, editors: *Physical therapy services in the developmental disabilities,* Springfield, Ill, 1972, Charles C Thomas.
56. Myers P and Mackisack L: Right hemisphere syndrome. In Lapointe L, editor: *Aphasia and related neurogenic language disorders,* New York, 1990, Thieme.
57. Mysak ED: *Pathology of the speech system,* Springfield, Ill, 1989, Charles C Thomas.
58. Netsell R and Cleeland CS: Modification of lip hypertonia in dysarthria using EMG feedback, *J Speech Hear Disord* 38:131, 1973.
59. Pimental P and Kinsbury N: *Neuropsychological aspects of right brain injury,* Austin, TX, 1989, Pro-ed.
60. Rembisz L and Gribin S: Neuromuscular facilitation therapeutic techniques in treating the dysarthric patient, Exhibit presented at the American Speech and Hearing Association Annual Convention, Washington, DC, 1975.
61. Rembisz L and Gribin S: Neuromuscular facilitation and techniques in treating dysarthria for the cerebral palsied, Exhibit presented at the American Speech and Hearing Association Annual Convention, Chicago, 1977.
62. Rosenbek J and others: Oral sensation and perception in apraxia of speech and aphasia, *J Speech Hear Disord* 16:22, 1973.
63. Rosenberg S: Disorders of first language development: trends in research and theory. In Gollin E, editor: *Malformations in development: biological and psychological sources and consequences,* New York, 1984, Academic Press.
64. Rutherford D and McCall G: Testing oral sensation and perception in persons with dysarthria. In Bosma J, editor: *Symposium on oral sensation and perception,* Springfield, Ill, 1967, Charles C Thomas.
65. Scott CM and Ringel RL: The effects of motor and sensory disruption on speech: a description of articulation, *J Speech Hear Res.* 14:819, 1971.
66. Silverman J: *Communication for the speechless,* Englewood Cliffs, NJ, 1980, Prentice-Hall.
67. Skelly M: *Amer-Ind gestural code based on universal American Indian hand talk,* New York, 1979, Elsevier North Holland.
68. Sparks RW: Melodic intonation therapy. In Chapey R, editor: *Language intervention strategies in adult aphasia,* Baltimore, 1981, Williams & Wilkins.
69. Springer S and Deutsch G: *Left brain, right brain,* San Francisco, 1981, WH Freeman.
70. Strub RL and Black FW: *The mental status examination in neurology,* Philadelphia, 1977, FA Davis.
71. Szekeres S, Ylvisaker M, and Holland A: Cognitive rehabilitation therapy: a framework for intervention. In Ylvisaker M, editor: *Head injury rehabilitation: children and adolescents,* San Diego, 1985, College Hill Press.
72. Thompson C: Articulation disorders in children with neurogenic pathology. In Lass N and others, editors: *Handbook of speech-language pathology and audiology,* Philadelphia, 1988, BC Decker.
73. Vanderheiden GC: *Non-vocal communication resource book,* Baltimore, 1978, University Park Press.
74. Vanderheiden GC and Grilley K: *Non-vocal communication techniques and aids for the severely physically handicapped,* Baltimore, 1976, University Park Press.
75. Vaughn G and Clark RM: *Speech facilitation: extraoral and intraoral stimulation technique for improvement of articulation skills,* Springfield, Ill, 1979, Charles C Thomas.
76. Wertz RT: Neuropathologies of speech and language. In Johns D, editor: *Clinical management of neurogenic communicative disorders,* Boston, 1978, Little, Brown.
77. West J: Heightening the action imagery of materials used in aphasia treatment. In Brookshire RH, editor: *Clinical aphasiology conference proceedings,* Minneapolis, 1978, BRK Publishers.
78. Westlake H and Rutherford D: *Speech therapy for the cerebral palsied,* Chicago, 1961, National Society for Crippled Children.
79. Wilbur RB: *American sign language and sign system,* Baltimore, 1979, University Park Press.
80. Zemlin WR: *Speech and hearing science, anatomy and physiology,* Englewood Cliffs, NJ, 1968, Prentice-Hall.

ADDITIONAL READINGS

Beasley D and Davis GA: *Aging, communication processes and disorders,* New York, 1980, Grune & Stratton.
Bradford L and Hardy W: *Hearing and hearing impairment,* New York, 1979, Grune & Stratton.
Leitch S: *A child learns to speak,* Springfield, Ill, 1977, Charles C Thomas.
Simmons-Martin A and Calvert D: *Parent-infant intervention: communication disorders,* New York, 1979, Grune & Stratton.
Werner H and Kaplan B: *Symbol formation,* New York, 1963, John Wiley & Sons.

APPENDIX A　　*AUDIOVISUAL RESOURCES*

Neuromuscular Facilitation Techniques in Treating Dysarthria (slides) and A Feeding Program for the Dysarthric Patient (slides):

Director, Education Department
Children's Specialized Hospital
New Providence Road
Westfield-Mountainside, NJ 07091

CHAPTER 27

Disorders of Vision and Visual Perceptual Dysfunction

*Laurie Efferson**

* With special thanks to Mary Jane Bouska for her contributions to previous editions, especially the discussion of visual perceptual disorders in this chapter.

KEY TERMS

anatomy of the eye	eye diseases
functional visual skills	visual screening
refractive error	treatment
strabismus	visual perceptual dysfunction

LEARNING OBJECTIVES

After reading this chapter the student/therapist will:

1. Understand visual anatomy and physiology as they pertain to visual function.
2. Understand the functional visual skills and how visual dysfunction may affect functional performance.
3. Understand the symptoms of visual dysfunction.
4. Develop ability to take visual case history using behaviors and clinical observations.
5. Understand the difference between a phoria and a strabismus.
6. Understand the difference between a visual field loss and a unilateral neglect.
7. Be familiar with various pediatric and age-related disease conditions that may affect vision.
8. Learn nonoptical and be familiar with optical adaptations for patients with low vision.
9. Understand basic tools for vision screening.
10. Understand when to refer and document.

Vision is an integral part of development of perception. Some aspects of vision such as pupillary function are innate, but many other aspects are stimulated to develop by experience and interaction with the environment. Visual acuity itself has been demonstrated to rely on the presence of a clear image focused on the retina. If this does not occur, a "lazy eye" or amblyopia will result. Depth perception develops as a result of precise eye coordination and will not occur unless eye alignment is corrected within the first 7 years of life. Research has demonstrated that, in fact, most visual skills such as acuity, binocular coordination, accommodation, oculomotilities, and depth perception are largely intact by 6 months to 1 year.[51] Visual skill development parallels postural reflex integration and provides a foundation for perception.

Early in infancy visual input is associated with olfactory, tactile, vestibular, and proprioceptive sensations. The infant is driven to touch, taste, smell, and manipulate what he or she sees. Primitive postural reflexes such as the asymmetrical tonic neck reflex help to provide visual regard and attention.

At some point the young child is able to look at an object and determine both the texture and the shape without having to touch or taste it. As adults, vision has moved to the top of the sensory hierarchy in providing full multisensory asso-

ciations from sight alone. Even the visualized image of eating an apple can recreate the smell, sound of crunching, taste, and feel of the experience.

Early visual impairment and later acquired impairment can affect the quality of the image presented to the brain and thus affect the learning process. In addition damage to association centers involved with spatial perception, figure-ground, and directionality can interfere with learning and performance. It is important therefore to isolate the primary visual processes of seeing from the secondary or associational processes of perceiving in the evaluation of perceptual disorders. The identification of a vision problem becomes part of the differential diagnosis of a perceptual deficit. It is just as important to eliminate vision as a contributing factor to a perceptual problem as it is to find a possible vision problem.

ANATOMY OF THE EYE

An operational analogy of the eye as a camera may be useful in understanding the physical function of the structures. Once the image hits the retina and image enhancement begins, however, metaphors change to match our ever-changing comprehension of brain function.

Eye chamber and lens

Structures and function are discussed from anterior to posterior (Fig. 27-1). The first structure that light hits after it is reflected from an image is the cornea. Corneal tissue is completely transparent. Light is refracted, or bent, to the greatest degree by the cornea, as the light rays must pass through a change in media, or a change in density, as from air to water.[39] One can observe the refraction of light by observing how a stick, when placed into water, appears bent where it enters the water (Fig. 27-2).

Damage to the cornea from abrasions, burns, congenital, or disease-related processes can alter the spherical shape of the cornea and disturb the quality of the image that falls on the retina. In keratoconus, the cornea slowly becomes steeper and more cone-shaped, distorting the image and causing reduced vision.[38]

Iris

Behind the cornea is the iris, or colored portion, which consists of fibers that control the opening of the pupil, the dark circular opening in the center of the eye. The constriction and dilation of the pupil control the amount of light entering the eye in a similar fashion to the way the F stops on a camera change the size of the aperture to control the amount of light and depth of field.[22] Under bright light conditions the opening constricts, and under dim light conditions it dilates, allowing as much light in to stimulate the photoreceptor cells of the retina. This constriction and dilation are under autonomic nervous system (ANS) control with both sympathetic and parasympathetic components.[46] Under conditions of sympathetic stimulation (fight or flight)

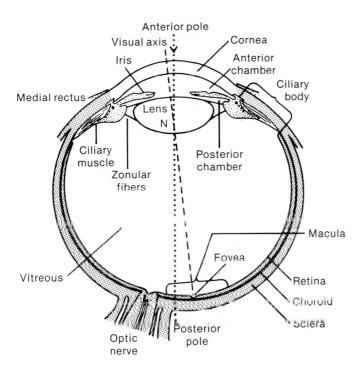

Fig. 27-1. Horizontal section of the eye. (Modified from Wolff E: *Anatomy of the eye and orbit,* ed 7, London, 1976, HK Lewis & Co, Ltd.)

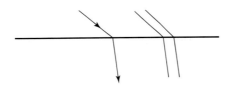

Fig. 27-2. Refraction: bending of light at air-water interface.

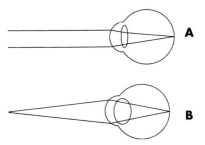

Fig. 27-3. Accommodation. **A,** Looking far away. **B,** Looking up close.

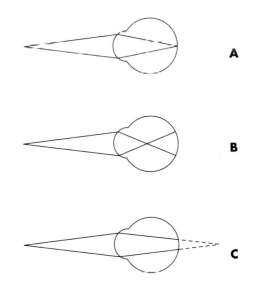

Fig. 27-4. Blur circle. **A,** Image focused on retina. **B,** Blur circle, formed if eyeball is too short, e.g., hyperopic eye. **C,** Blur circle, formed if eyeball is too long, e.g., myopic eye.

the pupils dilate, perhaps giving rise to the expression "eyes wide with fear." Under parasympathetic stimulation the pupils constrict. The effect of drugs that stimulate the ANS can be observed.[6] For example someone who has taken heroin will have pinpoint pupils.

Exercise 1
Observe pupilary dilation and constriction on a willing subject (or on yourself in a mirror) by flashing a penlight at his or her pupil. Observe the decreased size of the pupil. Remove the light and watch the pupil dilate.

Lens

Behind the iris is the lens. The lens is involved in focusing, or accommodation. It is a biconvex, circularly shaped, semirigid, crystalline structure, which fine-tunes the image on the retina. In a camera, the lens is represented by the external optical lens system. The ability to change focus on the camera is achieved by turning the lens to change the distance of the lens from the film, which effectively increases or decreases the power of the lens, allowing near or distance

objects to be seen more clearly. The same effect, a change in the power of the lens, is achieved in the eye by the action of tiny cilliary muscles, which act on suspensory ligaments, thereby changing the thickness and curvature of the lens. A thicker lens with a greater curvature produces higher power and the ability to see clearly at near. A thinner lens and flatter curvature produces less optical power, which is what is needed to allow distant objects to be clear (Fig. 27-3). The process of lens thickening and thinning is accommodation.[22,46]

Ideally, the lens will bring an image into perfect focus so that it lands right on the fovea, the area of central vision. If the focused image falls in front of the retina, however, then a blurred circle will fall on the fovea (Fig. 27-4). In this case the lens is too thick, having too high an optical power. This can be one cause of myopia (nearsightedness). One simple remedy is to place a negative (concave) lens externally in front of the eye in glasses to reduce the power of the internal lens and allow the image to fall directly on the fovea. A similar type of problem can occur in hyperopia (farsightedness), where the image

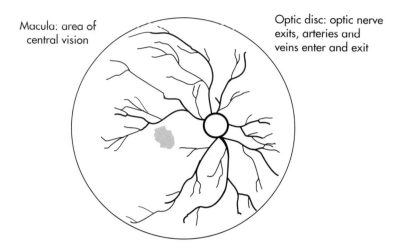

Macula: area of
central vision

Optic disc: optic nerve
exits, arteries and
veins enter and exit

Fig. 27-5. Retinal topography.

falls in back of the retina. In presbyopia (old eyes) the flexibility of the lens fibers decreases, and the lens becomes more rigid.[51] Accommodation gets weaker until the image can no longer be focused on the retina. When this occurs, a plus (positive) lens may be worn externally to aid in reading.[22]

The lens also can be affected by cataracts, where the general clarity of vision is impaired due to a loss of transparency of the chrystalline lens. Incoming light tends to scatter inside the eye causing glare problems.

Vitreous chamber

The space behind the lens is filled with a gel-like substance and is called the vitreous chamber.[46]

Retina

The retina at the back of the eye is the photosensitive layer, like the film in a camera, receiving the pattern of light reflected from objects. The topography of the retina (Fig. 27-5) includes the optic disc, which is where the optic nerve exits and arteries and veins emerge. This is also the blindspot because there are no photoreceptor cells on the disc. The macula is temporal to the optic disc and contains the fovea, or central vision. The surrounding retina is considered peripheral vision and defines a 180-degree half sphere.[46]

Exercise 2

Your blindspot may be observed by doing the following: draw two dots 3 inches (7.5 cm) apart on a piece of paper. The dots can be ¼ inch (.5 cm). Cover your left eye and look at the dot on the left. Starting at about 16 inches (40 cm), slowly bring the paper closer. Make sure you can see the two dots—one you are looking at directly and the other peripherally. At approximately 10 inches (25 cm) the dot on the right will disappear. This is your blind spot! Why can this exercise only be done monocularly, (with one eye)?

Visual pathway

The visual pathway begins with the photoreceptor cells, which begin a three-neuron chain exiting through the optic nerve. This chain consists of the rods and cones, which synapse with bipolar cells that synapse with ganglion cells (Fig. 27-6).[28,46]

There are two types of photoreceptor cells: rods and cones. The cone or rod shape is the dendrite of the cell. Its variation in shape and slight variation in pigment give each one different sensitivities. The rod cell has greater sensitivity to dim light, but less sensitivity to color, whereas the cone cell has greater sensitivity to color and high intensity light and less to reduced light conditions. The highest concentration of cone cells is in the fovea and macula, with decreasing concentration of cone cells and increasing concentration of rod cells moving concentrically away from the macula.

The phenomenon responsible for the high degree of neural representation of the foveal region and that accounts for the tremendous conscious awareness one has of the central view is called convergence.[46] At the periphery of the retina the degree of convergence is great; many photoreceptor cells synapse on one ganglion cell, which accounts for poor acuity, but high light sensitivity. The closer to the macula, the less the degree of convergence, until finally, at the fovea there is no convergence. This means that one photoreceptor cell synapses with one bipolar cell and one ganglion cell.

The awareness of what is seen is directly related to the amount of convergence, which reflects the extent of neural representation. The 1:1 correspondence between photoreceptor and ganglion cell at the fovea means that there is a very high degree of neural representation of the foveal image in the brain. It is even greater than the neural representation of the lips, tongue, or hands.[48] This accounts for one's primary awareness of what is in the foveal field and

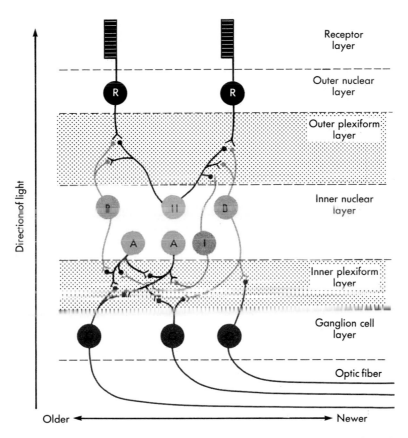

Fig. 27-6. The connections among retinal neurons and the significance of prominent layers. The neurons shown are photoreceptors *(R)*, horizontal cells *(H)*, bipolar cells *(B)*, interplexiform cells *(I)*, amacrine cells *(A)*, and ganglion cells *(G)*. It has been suggested that ganglion cells dominated by amacrine cell inputs represent phylogenetically older circuitry and that ganglion cells dominated by bipolar cell inputs represent newer circuitry. The arrow indicates the direction of light as it passes through the retina to reach the photoreceptors. (From Berne RM and Levy MN, editors: Visual systems, p. 107. In *Physiology*, St. Louis, 1988, Mosby.)

secondary awareness of the peripheral field. Conscious awareness of the environment is whatever is in the foveal field at the moment. But continuous information about the environment is flowing over the peripheral retina, usually subconsciously. Attention quickly shifts from foveal to nonfoveal stimulation when changes in light intensity or rapid movement are registered. This type of stimuli rouses attention immediately because it could have specific survival value. For example, one is driving down the street and picks up rapid motion off to the right. The foveas swing around immediately to identify a small red ball bouncing into the street. This information goes to the association areas where small ball is associated, with small child soon to follow. Frontal cortical centers are aroused and a decision is made to initiate motor areas to take the foot off the accelerator and onto the brake.

Exercise 3
Peripheral central awareness.

We have a unique ability to change our awareness by consciously shifting attention from our foveal awareness to our peripheral awareness. For example, as you read these words become aware of the background surrounding the paper, notice colors, forms, shapes; continue to expand your awareness to include your clothes, the floor, walls and ceiling if possible. You are consciously stimulating your primitive, phylogenetically older visual system. The ability to do this has considerable therapeutic value, as a typical pattern of visual stress is associated with an overfoveal concentration. The ability to expand the peripheral awareness at will is a skill that can help you to relax while you drive, can improve reading skills, and can be used in visual training techniques.

The moment light hits the retina, the photographic film model must be abandoned for the image processing or computerized image enhancement model. The primary visual pathway at the retinal level is a three-neuron chain. From back to front the first neuron is the photoreceptor cell, rods or cones. They synapse with a bipolar cell, which in turn synapses with a ganglion cell. The axon of the ganglion cell exits via the optic nerve. Image enhancement occurs at the two junctions between the three nerve cell pathway. Lateral cells at the neural junctions have an inhibitory action on the primary three-neuron pathway, and through the inhibition of an impulse the image is modulated. For example, at the first junction between photoreceptor cell and bipolar cell, there are horizontal cells. These cells enhance the contrast between light and dark by inhibiting the firing of bipolar cells at the very edge of an image. This makes the edge of the image appear darker than the central area, which increases the contrast, and thereby increases attention-getting value. After all it is by perceiving edges that we are able to maneuver around objects. In a similar manner amacrine cells act at the second neural junction between bipolar and ganglion cell to enhance movement detection.[29]

This image enhancement process continues throughout the visual pathway. The process has been likened to the way in which a computer enhances a distorted picture of outer space received from a satellite. The image goes through a series of processing stations in the inner workings of the computer. The computer-generated, enhanced image shown on the screen is like the end product in the brain: the perceived image.

The visual pathway continues through the brain (Fig. 27-7). The ganglion cell axons exit the eyeball via the optic nerve, carrying the complete retinal picture in coded electro-chemical patterns. From there the patterns project to different sites within the central nervous system (Fig. 27-8). Projections to the pretectum are important in pupillary reflexes; projections to the pretectal nuclei, the accessory optic nuclei, and the superior colliculus are all involved in eye movement functions.[46] The largest bundle, called the optic tract, projects to the lateral geniculate body (LGB) in the hypothalamus, where additional image enhancement and processing occurs. The next group of axons continue on to the primary visual cortex, and from there to visual association areas.

At what point does the retinal image become a perception, and with what part of the brain does one see? Current theory regarding visual perception is the result of Nobel Prize winning research by Hubel and Wiesel in the 1960s called the "receptive field theory."[36] This theory states that different neurons are feature detectors, defining objects in terms of movement, direction, orientation, color, depth, and acuity. Recent research by Hubel and Livingstone[35a] was

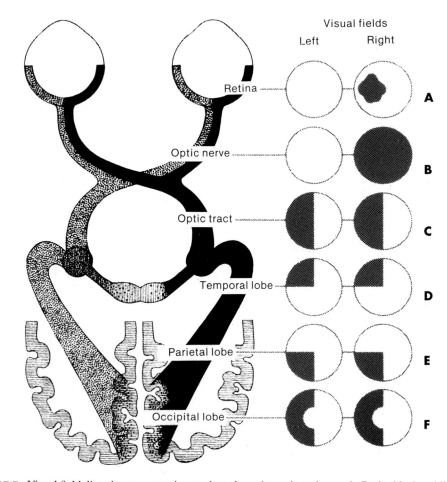

Fig. 27-7. Visual field disturbances at various points along the optic pathway. **A,** Retinal lesion: blind spot in the affected eye. **B,** Optic nerve lesion: partial or complete blindness in that eye. **C,** Optic tract or lateral geniculate lesion: blindness in the opposite half of both visual fields. **D,** Temporal lobe lesion: blindness in the upper quadrants of both visual fields on the side opposite the lesion. **E,** Parietal lobe lesion: contralateral blindness in the corresponding lower quadrants of both eyes. **F,** Occipital lobe lesion: contralateral blindness in the corresponding half of each visual field, but with macular sparing. (Courtesy Smith, Kline & French Laboratories, Philadelphia, Penn.)

able to locate a segregation of function at the level of the LGB. They identified two types of cells, one type being larger and faster magno cells, which are apparently phylogenetically older and color blind, but which have a high contrast sensitivity, and are able to detect differences in contrast of 1% to 2%. They also have low spatial resolution (low acuity). They seem to operate globally and are responsible for perception of movement, depth perception from motion, perspective, parallax, stereopsis, shading, contour, and interocular rivalry. Through linking properties (objects having common movement or depth) emerges figure-ground perception. Much of this perception occurs in the middle temporal lobe.

The other type of cells called parvo cells, are smaller, slower, color sensitive, and have smaller receptive fields. They are less global and are primarily responsible for high resolution form perception. Higher level visual association occurs in the temporal-occipital region, where learning to identify objects by their appearance occurs. It appears that these two types of cells are functionally and structurally related to the two visual systems represented in retinal topography—the foveal (central) and peripheral visual systems.

Eye movement system

The eye movement system consists of six pairs of eye muscles: the medial recti, lateral recti, superior and inferior recti, and superior and inferior oblique (Fig. 27-8). Together they are controlled by cranial nerves III (oculomotor), IV (trochlear), and VI (abducens). The eye movement system has both reflex and voluntary components. Reflexive movements are coordinated through vestibular interconnections at a midbrain level. The vestibular ocular reflex (VOR)

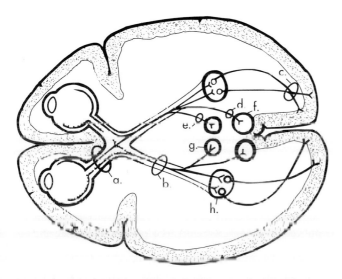

Fig. 27-8. Visual tract system. *a,* Optic nerve. *b,* Optic tract. *c,* Geniculate-occipital radiators. *d,* Retino-colliculo radiation. *e,* Retino-pretecto tracts. *f,* Superior colliculus (Midbrain). *g,* Pretectal area (Tegmentum). *h,* Lateral geniculate.

functions primarily to keep the image stabilized on the retina. Through connections between pairs of eye muscles and the semicircular canals, movement is analyzed as being either external movement of an object or movement of the head or body. From this information the VOR is able to direct the appropriate head or eye movement.[46]

Two types of eye movements are the result. Smooth, coordinated eye movements are called *pursuits,* and rapid localizations are called *saccades.* Voluntarily control of both these motions indicates cortical control. Pursuits are used for continuously following moving targets and are stimulated by a foveal image. Saccades are stimulated by images from the peripheral system, where a detection of motion or change in light intensity results in a rapid saccadic eye movement to bring the object into the foveal field. Difficulties in either the eye movement system or underfunctioning of the vestibular system can affect the coordinated, efficient functioning of eye movement skills.

A third type of eye movement is specifically related to eye aiming ability. This is the coordinated movement of both eyes inward towards the nose, as in crossing the eyes, or outward towards midline, as when looking away in the distance. The inward movement is called convergence, and the outward is divergence. The most important result of efficient vergence abilities is depth perception, or stereopsis. Very small errors in aiming can dramatically affect stereopsis. Problems such as double vision, wandering eyes, and *strabismus* are discussed in greater depth in a later section.

Exercise 4

Pursuits: Follow a moving target such as a pencil point as you move it across your field of gaze. Continue to move it in different directions, vertically, horizontally, diagonally, and circularly to stimulate all pairs of eye muscles. For a more challenging demonstration find a fly and follow its flight path around the room. If you lose sight of it, notice that the detection of the movement of the fly will signal your eye movement directly toward it.

Saccades: Hold two pencils about head width apart. Shift your eyes from pencil to pencil. Notice that your awareness is of the two pencils, not of the background between them. Generally perception occurs the moment the eyes are still, rather than while moving during saccades. For a more challenging exercise, move the pencil you are not looking at, then shift quickly to it, move the other pencil while looking at the one you just moved. In other words, you will pick up the location of the other pencil peripherally and direct your eyes to the foveal region. The size and degree of blur of the peripheral image will tell the brain where the image is and how far to move the eyes. This ability again is due to the function of neural convergence, which is related to neural representation.

Convergence: Hold a pencil at arm's length along your midline. Slowly bring the pencil closer in toward you along your midline. Feel your eyes moving in (crossing). Try to bring the pencil to your nose, keeping the pencil single. (It's okay if you can't). Move the pencil away now and your eyes are diverging.

FUNCTIONAL VISUAL SKILLS
Refractive error

Before discussing binocular coordination and the individual visual skills, it is important to describe **refractive**

errors and how they can affect binocular coordination. Three common types of refractive errors are myopia or nearsightedness, hyperopia or farsightedness, and astigmatism.[29,46]

The myopic eye is too long, so that the focused image falls in front of the retina. It is easily corrected with a negative or minus lens, which optically moves the image back onto the retina.

The hyperopic eye is too short, and the focused image falls behind the retina. A positive or plus lens optically moves the image onto the retina.

An eye will have astigmatism if it is not perfectly spherical. An aspherical eye will cause the image to be distorted, where part of the focused image will be in front of the retina and part in back. A person with astigmatism may see vertical lines clearly and horizontal lines as blurry, depending on the specific aspherical shape. A cylindrical type of lens is used to correct astigmatism. This lens corrects the distortion of the image so that it is placed right on the retina.

Following are examples of different refractive errors:

−5.50 D.S. (diopter sphere): Myopia
+4.00 D.S.: Hyperopia
+1.50 −1.50 ×180: Astigmatism. Note: "x" stands for the axis of the cylinder correction.

When significant refractive errors are uncorrected, they can reduce vision. Uncorrected refractive error also can interfere with binocular coordination. The symptoms are described in greater detail in the next section.

Binocular coordination is the end result of the efficient functioning of the visual skills (see the box). The individual visual skills include accommodation, eye alignment or vergence, eye movements, stereopsis (depth perception), and peripheral/central coordination. During normal activities, all the skills are inseparable.

Accommodation

Accommodation is the ability to bring near objects into clear focus automatically and without strain. Relaxation of accommodation allows distant objects to come into focus. The primary action is that of the ciliary muscles acting on the lens, and the primary system of control is the ANS with sympathetic and parasympathetic components.[46]

Accommodation is reflexly related to pupillary constriction and dilation.[22] As one focuses on a near object, the

---

Binocular coordination
Corrected refractive error
Accommodation
Eye alignment
Stereopsis
Central and peripheral coordination
Efficient eye movement skills

---

lenses thicken, allowing the near object to come into focus. At the same time the pupils constrict to increase depth of field (just as in a camera). As one looks into the distance, the lens gets flatter, relaxing accommodation, and the pupil dilates, decreasing the depth of field.

Accommodative ability is age related. A young child can focus on small objects just a few inches in front of the eyes. At about the age of 9 years, the accommodative ability slowly begins to decrease. By the mid-40s the reserve focusing power diminishes to the point that near objects begin to blur. At this stage reading material is pushed farther away until the arms are not long enough, and then reading glasses are needed. This is called presbyopia (old eyes).

Problems in accommodation may contribute to myopia, hyperopia, and presbyopia. Symptoms include blurriness, either at near or far depending on the age and the problem.

Accommodation is important mainly for up-close activities; reading, hygiene, dressing—specifically fasteners, use of tools, typing, table top activities, and games.

Exercise 5

Accommodation cannot be directly observed, but it can be implied indirectly, through observation of pupillary constriction while doing an accommodative task.

Cover one eye. Hold a finger in front at about 10 inches (25 cm). Focus on the finger, making sure that the fingerprint is clear. Shift focus to a distant object. Continue shifting far to near and near to far while a partner observes the pupil. He or she should be able to observe pupillary constriction/dilation as the focus is shifted.

Vergence

Vergence ability includes convergence and divergence. It is the ability to smoothly and automatically bring the eyes together along the midline in order to observe objects singly at near (convergence), or conversely to move the eyes outward for single vision of distant objects (divergence). Specific brain centers control convergence and divergence.

Vergence is reflexly associated with accommodation: convergence with accommodation, and divergence with relaxation of accommodation. The function of this reflex is to allow objects to be both single and clear, either at near or far.

Vergence has both automatic and voluntary components. Most of the time it is not necessary to think about moving the eyes inward as one looks at a close object, yet if asked to cross the eyes, most people can do this at will.

Problems can occur in vergence ability when the eye movement system is out of coordination with accommodation or from damage to cranial nerves III, IV, or VI. Problems can be slight, where there is merely a tendency for the eyes to converge in or out too far, or they can be gross. Tendencies to underconverge or overconverge are called phorias, and are not visible to the observer. An individual may be asymptomatic, but problems may be elicited under conditions of increased stress or fatigue such as excessive reading, computer terminal activity, or from drug side effects (licit or illicit).

Some phorias may worsen to the extent that binocularity

breaks down, at which point the individual has a strabismus. There are two main types of strabismus, esotropia and exotropia. An esotropia is an inward-turning of the eye, and an exotropia is a visible outward-turning. A third, less common, type of strabismus is hypertropia, where one eye aims upward. Strabismus and dysfunctional phorias are discussed in greater detail in the next section.

Vergence ability is needed for singular binocular vision; thus it is basic to all activities. At near, the patient may have difficulty finding objects, eye-hand coordination may be decreased affecting self-care and hygiene tasks, and reading may be difficult. Distance tasks that may be affected include driving, sports, movies, communication, and frequently ambulation. Individuals with impaired vergence ability may also have difficulty focusing and may have decreased or no depth perception. Interpreting space can be quite difficult and confusing. If decreased vergence is a result of traumatic head injury or stroke, it may contribute to the patient's confusion, and he or she may not be able to identify or communicate the problem.

Exercise 6

Hold a pencil in front of you at eye level at about 12 inches (30 cm). Look at the pencil. Look away into the distance. Looking at the pencil is convergence and looking into the distance is divergence. As you converge and diverge slowly back and forth notice any changes you may feel: changes in how relaxed you feel, how focused or spaced out you feel, feelings of dreaminess, or nothing at all. Observe a partner's eyes as they shift back and forth as well.

Pursuits and saccades

Eye movement skills consist of pursuits and saccades. Pursuits are the smooth, coordinated movement of all eye muscles together, allowing accurate tracking of objects through space. Perception is continuous during pursuit movements. Saccades are rapid shifts of the eyes from object to object, allowing quick localization of movements observed in the periphery. The systems involved in eye movement skills are the oculomotor system with the VOR, in conjunction with coordination of the central and peripheral visual systems. The peripheral visual system is finely tuned for detecting changes in light levels and small movements.

Problems in pursuits and saccades can be the result of a dysfunctioning of any individual muscles or of the VOR. Because the VOR helps to stabilize the image on the retina and to differentiate image movement from eye movement, simple tracking can be more difficult.

In addition visual field loss, either central or peripheral, can dramatically affect localization ability. People with blind half or quarter fields can be observed to do searching eye movements rather than direct jumps to the object.

Activities affected include searching for objects, visually directed movement for fine-motor tasks and gross movement and ambulation tasks, eye-hand coordination, self-care, driving, and reading.

Memory also may be affected by an eye movement dysfunction. Research by Adler-Grinberg and Stark[1] examined patterns of eye movements as subjects looked at a picture. Distinct eye movement patterns, called scan paths, became apparent. When asked to recall the picture, the same eye movement pattern was elicited as the subject recalled the picture. Perhaps a type of oculomotor motor planning is involved in recall. Applying this idea to the clinical setting, if a patient has inaccurate eye movement, inability with undershooting and overshooting, or uses 30 saccades to scan a picture rather than 10, then perhaps the stored memory is less efficiently stored, and consequently more difficult to reconstruct from memory. Additionally, if a patient has a type of brain damage with generalized dyspraxia, the eye movement system could quite likely be affected and might be involved in the patient's perceptual dysfunction.

SYMPTOMS OF VISUAL DYSFUNCTION
Case history

The identification of a visual problem begins with case history. It is important to get some idea of the client's prior visual status or any history of eye injury, surgery, or diseases. Information can be elicited by direct questioning of the client or family members or by clinical observation. Sample questions include the following:

- Are you having difficulty with seeing, or with your eyes?
- Do you wear bifocals?
- Do your glasses work as well now as before the (stroke, accident, etc.)?
- Have you noticed any blurriness? Near or far?
- Do you ever see double? See two? See overlapping or shadow images?
- Do you ever find that when you reach for an object that you knock it over, or your hand misses?
- Do letters jump around on the page after reading for a while?
- Are you experiencing any eye strain or headaches? Where and when?
- Do you ever lose your place when reading?
- Are portions of a page or any objects missing?
- Do people or things suddenly appear from one side, that you didn't see approaching?
- Do you have difficulty concentrating on tasks?

Clinical observations of the client while performing various activities are a valuable source of problem identification. Therapists in general are in an ideal position to observe clients in a variety of functional tasks that require near vision, far vision, spatial estimations, depth judgments, and oculomotor tasks. This situation varies considerably from the doctor's observations in the more contrived environment of the examination room. Additionally, the therapist's initial observations can be used in documenting difficulties within the therapy realm that may be amenable to visual remediation in terms which can be applied to reimbursement of therapy.

Clinical observations include the following:

- Head tilt during near tasks
- Avoidance of near tasks
- One eye appears to go in, out, up or down
- Vision shifts from eye to eye
- Seems to look past observer
- Closes or covers one eye
- Squints
- Eyes appear red, puffy, irritated, or have a discharge: Notify nurses or doctor of these observations
- Rubs eyes a lot
- Has difficulty maintaining eye contact
- Spaces out, drifts off, daydreams
- During activity neglects one side of body or space
- During movement bumps into walls, objects (either walking or in a wheelchair)
- Appears to misjudge distance
- Under- or over-reaches for objects
- Has difficulty finding things

Near point blur

The first area of symptomatology is near accommodative problems. The primary symptom is near point blur. This symptom alone is not indicative of a problem in any one area, but could indicate farsightedness (hyperopia), astigmatism, or reduced accommodative ability (insufficiency). The client may move objects or the head farther or closer, may complain of eye strain or headaches, may squint, or may even avoid near activities as much as possible. One might observe excessive blinking, and the patient may complain of glasses not working well.

Distance blur

The next problem could also indicate a number of different etiologies. Distance blur could indicate nearsightedness (myopia), pathology (such as beginning cataracts), or accommodative spasm. Most people have some experience with accommodative spasm. After spending long periods of time either studying or reading a novel and then glancing up at the wall across the room, it may be blurry, and then clear up very slowly. For some individuals, this spasm eventually becomes one component in their nearsightedness if the reading habits continue for a long time.

The client experiencing distance blur may make forward head movements and frequently squint in an attempt to see. They may not respond or orient quickly to auditory or visual stimuli beyond a certain radius. One may also note excessive blinking and a withdrawn attitude because the patient cannot see well enough to interact with the environment.

Visual hygiene can be recommended to assist in the development of good visual habits. Good lighting and posture, taking frequent breaks, and monitoring the state of clarity of an environmental cue such as a clock across the room are all useful.

Phoria and strabismus

The next area of eye alignment problems can be divided into two types of problems: phorias and strabismus. Phorias can be defined as a natural positioning of the eyes where there is a tendency to aim in front of or behind the point of focus. It may or may not be associated with symptoms. Fusion is intact to some degree and depth perception may also be intact.

Everyone has a phoria just as everyone has a posture. It may be within normal range, or, just as someone may have scoliosis, a high phoria may cause problems. The following phorias may cause problems:

Esophoria: eyes are postured in front of the point of focus.

Exophoria: the eyes are postured in back of the point of focus.

Phoria is measured in units of prism diopters, which indicates the size of the prism needed to measure the eye position in or out from the straight ahead position.[22]

Phorias tend to produce subtle symptoms. They include having difficulty concentrating, frontal or temporal headaches, sleepiness after reading, and eyes stinging after reading.

A **strabismus** or tropia is a visible turn of one eye, which may be constant, intermittent, or alternating between one eye and the other. The person may have double vision, or if the strabismus is long-term, the person may suppress or "turn off" the vision in the wandering eye. Suppression is a neurological function that is an adaptation to the intolerable situation of double images. It is only exhibited in long-term strabismus, because apparently the brain cannot learn to suppress past the time of peak plasticity (up to age 7 years). The developing brain must choose which eye has the visual direction, which is confirmed by motor and tactile inputs as being the "real" image. The other fovea's image is then neurologically suppressed. The peripheral vision in the suppressing eye is still normal, and the eye is not by any means blind.

The essential concept in understanding the difference between phoria and strabismus is that in strabismus *fusion and depth perception are not present.* Definitions of different types of strabismus are presented in the box on p. 779. It is not a conclusive list; many other types and permutations are beyond the scope of this discussion. The intent here is to expose the therapist to different terms that may be used by the doctor in diagnosing the type of strabismus.

In strabismus one eye appears to go in, out, up or down, and there is frequently an obvious inability to judge distances, especially if the strabismus is of recent onset (acquired). The client may under- or over-reach for objects, cover or close one eye, complain of double vision, or exhibit

Types of strabismus

Esotropia: one eye turns in.

Exotropia: one eye turns out.

Hypertropia: one eye turns up relative to the other eye.

Intermittent: the person is strabismic at times and phoric (fusing) at times. Fatigue or stress may bring out the strabismic state.

Alternating: The person switches from using the right eye to using the left eye. The person also switches the suppressing eye. If using the right eye, the person suppresses the left, while using the left eye the person suppresses the right, otherwise the person would see double.

Constant strabismus: one eye is always in or out, always the same eye.

Comitant strabismus: the amount of eye turn is the same regardless of whether the person is looking up, down, right, left, or straight ahead. People who have had it for a long time are usually comitant. New or acquired strabismics, i.e., from stroke or head injury, are usually noncomitant, where the amount of eyeturn changes depending on which direction the eyes are looking.

a head tilt or turn during specific activities. He or she may appear to favor one eye, have difficulty reading, appear spaced out, or avoid near activities. Additionally, especially if the patient sees double but is unable or unwilling to talk about it, he or she may be confused or disoriented.

Oculomotor dysfunction

A client with an oculomotor dysfunction will have difficulty with activities that require smooth pursuits, tracking, and convergence and divergence. During reading tasks these patients may lose their place, skip lines, or reread lines or have poor ball skills, poor eye-hand coordination, decreased balance, and clumsiness.

Visual field loss

Visual field loss could implicate damage at the optic chiasm, post-chiasmic, in the visual radiations of the thalamus, or in the visual cortex. The resultant visual field loss is characteristic (even diagnostic) in each case. It could be bitemporal (outer half of each field), half-field (hemianopsia) with or without macular involvement, or quarter field loss (see Fig. 27-7). Some symptoms of field loss are an inability to read or starting to read in the middle of the page, ignoring food on one half of plate, and difficulty orienting to stimuli in specific area of space.

Unilateral neglect

Some clients also may have a concomitant unilateral neglect. Differentiating a neglect from a hemianopsia is difficult. One test to differentiate between the two involves the extinction phenomenon. Presenting first stimuli on one side followed by simultaneous presentation of stimuli on both sides and comparing the results can differentiate a hemianopsia from a neglect if the client has a neglect, but not a hemianopsia. Please see section on inattention in visual perception.

Generally, if the patient has a field loss, it will be possible to conduct a field test and obtain fairly reliable results. The client will be able to respond more easily, and tell you where the test item appears and disappears. Additionally, when doing compensation training, the client with a field loss can grasp the techniques, whereas a client with a neglect cannot without quite a bit of additional training. The client with a neglect frequently has proprioceptive and tactile loss on the neglected side, and that area of space including that half of the body does not provide feedback. Therefore if the client also has a field loss, test results are unreliable and invariably inaccurate.

EYE DISEASES

Areas addressed in this section are common ocular and systemic disease of the pediatric and geriatric populations, an introduction to low vision, and recommendations for adaptations of the treatment plan. If reduced vision (low vision) is a result of eye disease the client may be assisted by magnification aides. Also, the therapy treatment program may need to be altered to accommodate any special visual needs of the client (lighting, working distance, inclusion of magnifiers, use of filters, contrast enhancing devices).

Pediatric conditions

Retinopathy of prematurity. The incidence of retinopathy of prematurity is increasing because of the improved survival of premature infants due to improved ventilation. Immature retinal vessels are sensitive to high oxygen tension. The effect on the vessels is vasoconstriction, eventually leading to obliteration of the vessels. This creates a state of ischemia, which stimulates the growth of new blood vessels. These small, fragile vessels bleed easily and lead to fibrosis and traction on the retina. As a result of the traction, the macula gets stretched, interferring with the function of central vision.

The temporal vessels are most affected because they develop last. The degree of damage may be mild or quite severe, depending on the amount of prematurity.[51]

Retinoblastoma. Retinoblastoma is the most common malignant tumor in children.[51] The current incidence is 1 in 20,000 live births, a rate that has been increasing over the last 30 years, apparently due to inheritance of a mutated gene.

The young child may have a strabismus due to impaired vision in the eye from the tumor. As the tumor grows the pupil may appear milky white. If not detected early, it will lead to loss of the eye, and if the tumor invades the brain death will occur. Clearly, early detection is critical.

Mental retardation. There is a higher association of

visual problems with mentally retarded populations.[51] These individuals have a higher incidence of refractive error (myopia, hyperopia, astigmatism), strabismus, nystagmus, and optic atrophy than children with normal intelligence.

Cerebral palsy. Therapists who work with children with cerebral palsy have noticed a high incidence of vision problems. Many studies confirm these observations. A study by Scheinman examining the incidence of visual problems in children with cerebral palsy and normal intelligence found the following incidences: strabismus in 69%, high phorias in 4%, accommodative dysfunction in 30%, and refractive errors in 63%.[51,52]

Hydrocephalus. Various studies have found that the most common visual problem in children with hydrocephalus is strabismus, with an incidence of 30% to 55%. The strabismus may develop either from the hydrocehalus itself or from the shunting procedure.

Fetal alcohol syndrome. Children affected by fetal alcohol syndrome have several characteristic features and visual problems. Visually, they have a higher incidence of strabismus, myopia, astigmatism, and ptosis. These children frequently have some degree of mental retardation as well, and are of small stature.

Age-related conditions

Cataracts. The most common malady affecting vision of elderly persons is cataracts. General clarity of vision is impaired due to a loss of transparency of the chrystalline lens of the eye.

In the senile cataract the lens slowly loses its ability to prevent oxidation from occurring, and liquification of the outer layers begins. The normally soluble proteins adhere together causing light scatter.[38] Vision slowly declines as light scatter increases until the lens must be removed.

Age-related macular degeneration. Age-related macular degeneration is the leading cause of blindness in the Western world and is the most important retinal disease of the aged (28% of the 75 to 85 age group).[52]

There is loss of central vision from fluid that leaks up from the deeper layers of the retina, pushing the retina up and detaching it from the nourishing layer. New vessel growth and hemorrhage and atrophy further destroy central vision.

This condition has significant implications for independent functioning. Mobility tends to be less impaired, because the peripheral visual system is still intact. All activities involving fine detail such as reading, sewing, and cooking are affected. Safety also can be affected.

Arteriosclerosis. In arteriosclerosis, vision may or may not be affected. There is a hardening of the retinal arteries, which may eventually lead to ischemia, with the areas of retina deprived of sufficient oxygen eventually dying.

Hypertension. Hypertension is usually accompanied by arteriosclerosis. There may be retinal bleeding and edema, which can affect central vision if macula involved.

Diabetes. Diabetes can affect the lens. In the diabetic "sugar cataract" sorbital collects within the lens causing an osmotic gradient of fluid into the lens, which leads to disruption of the lens matrix and loss of transparency. As the fluid increases and decreases within the lens, the patient's vision also can fluctuate, depending directly on the sugar level. This makes prescribing glasses during this time quite difficult.

The retinal effects include microvascular damage and the development of microaneurysms. Central vision may be reduced due to retinal ischemia. The ischemia leads to new vessel growth (neovascularization). These new vessels are very weak, frequently leaking and causing hemorrhage. The hemorrhage attracts fibrotic development, which puts traction on the retina, pulling it off and leading to retinal detachment and blindness. Laser treatment may destroy the neovascularization, preventing retinal detachment.

Glaucoma. Glaucoma occurs 7.2% in the 75 to 85 age group.[52] It is caused by an increase in the intraocular pressure. This pressure interferes with the inflow and outflow of blood and nutrients at the optic disc. If severe enough, glaucoma can cause field loss and eventually complete blindness.

In one type of glaucoma called open-angle glaucoma, the outflow of aqueous humor is reduced, leading to increased intraocular pressure. There are no overt symptoms. In another type, closed-angle glaucoma, the outflow is blocked by the iris. Symptoms are a painful, red eye, which may be confused with conjunctivitis. Because steroids are used to treat many conditions in the elderly for long periods of time, it is useful to be aware that side effects can include glaucoma and cataracts.

Eye muscle dysfunctions. Eye muscle dysfunctions causing double vision may result from several disease conditions including thyroid disease (Graves' and others), multiple sclerosis, myasthenia gravis, and tumors. The underlying condition must be diagnosed and treated.

Visual field loss. Visual field loss may be either central (macular degeneration glaucoma or retinal disease) or peripheral field loss due to retinal damage or stroke at any point in the visual pathway. This is potentially the most functionally disabling form of visual impairment (see Fig. 27-7).

Implications for functional performance

Lighting. Lighting conditions are important and vary depending on the nature of the condition. The person with presbyopia requires more light because the aging pupil gets smaller. The smaller pupil has the advantage of increasing the depth of focus, allowing the presbyope to see clearly over a wider range, but has the disadvantage of eliminating more light from the eye. Thus providing a good source of direct lighting, especially on fine print, is very helpful. Direct lighting from a halogen source is helpful for some low-vision patients as well.

Glare. People who have problems with glare, such as

those developing cataracts or other disease conditions, can be helped by several approaches. Incandescent lighting is preferred over fluorescent lighting. The use of a visor or wide-brimmed hat also can be helpful. For some individuals who have trouble reading because of the glare coming off the white page a black matte piece of cardboard with a horizontal slit in it (called a typoscope) can be used to reduce the surrounding glare and enhance reading. Special antiglare lenses developed by Corning are available by prescription through the eye doctor. An antireflective coating may also help.

Low vision aids. Many types of low-vision optical and nonoptical aids are available, usually by prescription by a low-vision specialist. Clients who have experienced damage to their central vision as in age-related macular degeneration or diabetic maculopathy, and who still have some reduced central vision, may be able to use various types of magnification aids. One type is a stand magnifier, which leaves the hands free for other activities. It also is useful for patients who have a tremor. Hand magnifiers are another type of aid. Some are equipped with their own internal illumination.

A telescope system can be attached to the patient's glasses frames, allowing distance viewing. High magnification also can be incorporated into special reading glasses. Some patients may need a closed circuit TV, which allows large and variable magnification, without the distortion caused by optical magnifiers.

Nonoptical aids include large print materials, available at many libraries, typoscopes mentioned earlier, and reading stands. Talking books are available for those for whom reading is an important hobby. New developments include text-to-speech synthesizers, large print computers, and image intensifiers.

For clients with field losses, specially designed prism or mirror systems may be used. These frequently require a bit of training to get used to and are not useful for everyone. Compensation training also can be helpful. Margin markers, reading slits, or holding the book sideways so that the print is vertical are other helpful techniques.

VISUAL SCREENING

Primary visual dysfunction must be differentiated from a visual perceptual disorder so that appropriate treatment can be addressed for each problem. Gianutsos and others[26] found that over half of the individuals in their study admitted for general head injury rehabilitation who were eligible for cognitive services had visual sensory impairments sufficient to warrant further evaluation. Visual screening can identify the need for referral for a complete eye examination. The results of the examination become part of the differential diagnosis regarding a perceptual dysfunction. See the box for key elements in vision screening.

The following discussion describes vision screening tools and adaptations for various populations.

Key elements in vision screening

1. Distance and near visual acuities
2. Oculomotilities (pursuits, saccades, near point of convergence)
3. Some measure of eye alignment to detect a strabismus or high phoria
4. Some measure of depth perception (stereopsis)
5. Some measure of the visual fields

Acuities: Acuities should always be tested first because decreased acuities will bias other tests except for oculomotilities and the peripheral field test.

Positioning: The body and head should be in good alignment or straightened with positioning devices, with the head in midline.

Glasses: If the client normally wears glasses, either for distance or near, the patient should be wearing glasses for tests for which spectacle correction is required. When in doubt, try it both ways, record the best response, and note if glasses were worn.

Observations during testing

The client's response during the test can provide important qualitative information about the patient's visual system, including postural changes (head forward or back, body forward or back, head tilts or rotation [turning to either side]), squinting, closing one eye, excessive blinking, rubbing, signs of strain or fatigue, and holding breath. Clients should be encouraged to relax, breathe normally, and not squint.

Distance acuities

Equipment Needed: Distance acuity chart, occluder, 20 ft measure, and patient's corrective lenses if worn for distance.*
Set Up: Tape distance chart on well-lighted wall at patient's eye level. Measure off 20 ft.
Procedure: Cover one eye and ask patient to read smallest letters that he or she can see. Exposing one letter or line at a time can help if tracking or attention is a problem. **Encourage the patient to guess and instruct patient not to squint.** Note how many letters were missed on the smallest line that the patient is able to see. Repeat by covering the other eye. Then proceed with both eyes.
Record: Record smallest line patient was able to read. If the client missed any letters on that line record minus number of letters missed. For example, if the client read four letters

* Bernell Corp., P.O. Box 4637, South Bend, IN, 46634-4637. Complete Vision Screening Kit: Laurie Efferson, O.D., O.T.R., 5918 Greenridge Rd., Castro Valley, CA 94552.

Interpretation/referral

20/20 is considered normal.
20/40 is required by most Department of Motor Vehicles (DMV) for full-time day and night driver's license, although requirements vary in different states.
20/80 is required by DMV for daytime driver's license.
20/40 or worse indicates referral to eye doctor.
20/200 corrected (with spectacle prescription) is considered legally blind.
A difference of 2 lines or more between the 2 eyes indicates referral to an eye doctor, e.g. right eye is 20/20, left eye is 20/30.

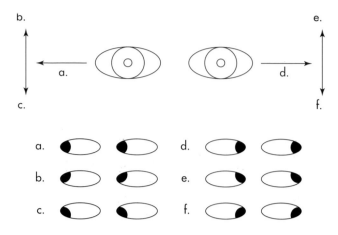

Then move from e→f, b→f, f→b, c→e to observe diagonal and midline pursuit patterns.

Fig. 27-9. Pursuit patterns.

correctly on the 20/30 line, but missed the other two, then record 20/30-2. Record the score for the client's right eye, left eye, and for both eyes together.

If the *patient* is unable to see the top line at 20 ft, ask the patient to move forward until he or she is able to identify the top letters. Then record: test distance/letter size (top line). For example, if the patient had to move up to 4 ft to see the top line, record 4/100. To calculate 20 foot equivalence, set up an equation where X equals size of letter (e.g., $4/100 = 20/X$); cross multiply: $4X = 2000$; divide 2000 by $4 = 500$. Client's vision is 20/500 (see the box).

Note: For clients whose attention is very poor, testing distance may need to be as close as 2 ft.

Note: Other testing stimuli can be used for children such as the Broken Wheel Test* or the Lighthouse cards.* Very low functioning client's or infant's acuity can be evaluated by using preferential looking methods. Targets are usually high contrast grating patterns of decreasing size. One such type is the Teller cards.†

Implications: A patient who fails this test may require glasses, or a change in current prescription.

Near acuities

Equipment: Near point test card, occluder, and client's corrective lenses if normally if normally worn for near.
Procedure: Same procedure as for distance acuity. The standard test distance is usually 16 inches (40 cm).
Record: Record smallest line read.
Interpretation/Referral: 20/20 is considered normal, 20/40 is required for reading newspaper size print, 20/100 for large print. Referral to an eye doctor should be made if vision is 20/40 or worse, or if a difference of 2 lines exists between the 2 eyes. Neurological damage can affect the accommodative system. Sometimes it corrects itself spontaneously, but not always.

---

* Bernell Corp., P.O. Box 4637, South Bend, IN 46634-4637.
† Vistech Consultants, 4162 Little York Rd., Dayton, OH 45414-2566.

Visual retraining of the focusing system may be appropriate, depending on the patient's age. This can be determined by an eye doctor familiar with vision therapy.

Pursuits

Equipment: Any target that holds the patient's attention can be used, such as a pencil or small toy.
Set Up: Patient seated facing screener.
Procedure: Using one pencil held approximately 16 to 20 inches in front of the client, ask the client to look directly at one part such as the eraser. Instruct the client to keep the head still, holding it if necessary. Move pencil around, in the pattern shown in Fig. 27-9, which is designed to incorporate all directions of gaze. Observe for smooth following; notice and record jerks and jumps, where they occur, or if the eyes stop at a certain point. If one or both eyes stop tracking, encourage the client to look at the pencil. If the patient is unable, repeat movement pattern with each eye separately, recording where movement stops.

Note: Clients who have had cerebral vascular accident (CVA) or head injury should be tested first monocularly (each eye separately).

Record: Poor = Difficulty following target with any accuracy, very jerky or jumpy, nystagmoid movements, incomplete range of motion (ROM)

Fair = Generally able to follow target, but goes off target occasionally (one to two times), with slight jerkiness

Good = Eye movements are smooth with no jerkiness

If one eye stops tracking at a certain point, or the client reports double vision (diplopia) in certain directions, record which eye or in which direction the problem is noticed (e.g., right eye does not pass midline when moving from left to right; or diplopia reported on upward right gaze). This specific information can be helpful to the examining doctor.

Saccades

Equipment: Tracking pencils can be used, although a few saccadic tests are available. One is the King Devick Saccadic Test, the other is the Developmental Eye Movement Test.* These both require form perception (number reading) and may be difficult, depending on the client's cognitive level.
Set Up. Patient seated facing screener.
Procedure: Hold a pencil in each hand about 17 to 20 inches from the client. Tell the client you are going to ask him or her to look at one ball while you move the other pencil, but the client is not to look at it until you tell him or her to look at the other ball. Tell the client to move the eyes only, keeping the head still. While the client looks at the first ball, move the other pencil, saying "shift" or "look at this ball." Move the other pencil, say "shift," then move, say "shift," then move, etc. until a pattern of movement can be discerned.

Repeat this call-move call-move about 10 times, moving into different fields of gaze. Continue until you see how the client is responding. Observe for overshooting or undershooting the target, ability to isolate the eyes from the head (hold head still), for controlled eye movement, and ability to wait until the verbal command to look. Observe for the client's ability to shift to all fields of gaze.

Note: A lower level would be to ask the client to move the eyes from one target to the other as quickly as possible.
Record: Poor = Inability to control eyes with verbal command, consistent undershooting or overshooting, inability to isolate eyes from head.

   Fair = Client able to maintain eyes on target with verbal command 50% of the time, with slight undershooting or overshooting, and able to isolate eyes from head with verbal reminders.

   Good = Client able to follow verbal commands 90% of the time, with no undershooting or overshooting, and complete eye from head isolation.

Near point of convergence (NPC)

Procedure: Present pencil along client's midline, about 20 inches away. Ask client if the pencil is single. If not, move it further away. Tell the client that you will be moving the pencil toward him or her, and that it will be getting blurry,

* Bernell Corp., P.O. Box 4637, South Bend, IN, 46634-4637. Complete Vision Screening Kit: Laurie Efferson, O.D., O.T.R., 5918 Greenridge Rd., Castro Valley, CA 94552.

but to keep watching it as far in as he or she can. When the pencil is single, move the pencil in toward the nose, at a moderately slow rate (but not too slow). Watch the client's eyes. As long as the eyes are tracking the pencil, continue to move it in toward the nose. At the point where one eye moves out, both eyes move out, or the eyes simply stop tracking, measure the distance of the pencil to the nose. If the client is wearing bifocals make sure the patient is looking through the reading segment.
Record: The break point is the distance at which the eyes were observed to stop tracking the pencil in. If the client was able to track all the way into the nose, record tracking to the nose.
Interpretation/Referral: A score of poor or fair on saccades or pursuits suggests the need for training. NPC with a break point of 5 inches or more is suggestive of convergence problems, and recommendations for referral should be made.
Implications: Difficulties with smooth pursuit, accurate saccades, or convergence can all present tracking difficulties for the patient. These difficulties can cause loss of place in reading, rereading of words or lines, skipping lines, and lower comprehension and concentration. Inaccurate eye movements also may affect visual memory.

An eye movement problem may be the result of direct damage to the eye muscles themselves (Fig. 27-10), or the nerves controlling them, as in the case of a head injury. Damage to the vestibular center also may involve visual components. Neurons from cranial nerves III, IV, and VI synapse in the vestibular nuclei. Reflex control of eye movements occurs through the vestibuloocular reflex and the optokinetic system.

Cover test

Purpose: There are two cover tests.

The cover/uncover test is used to determine whether a strabismus is present. The alternate cover test determines what type of phoria is present. The magnitude of the phoria generally determines the extent of the client's symptoms.
Equipment: Occluder, one tracking pencil or small, distinct target.
Set Up: Client seated facing screener, who is also seated.
Procedure: Hold pencil approximately 16 inches in front of client. Ask client to look directly at the target and to keep it in focus.

Near cover tests:

Cover/Uncover: **Observe movement of the uncovered eye.** Cover the client's right eye and observe the left eye for movement in, out, upward, or downward. Repeat a few times, allowing the eyes to be uncovered for about 2 seconds between trials. Repeat with left eye covered, observing for movement in the right eye.

Alternate Cover Test: **Observe eye movement as the eye is uncovered.** Hold occluder over right eye for a few seconds while client looks at near target. Move the occluder from the

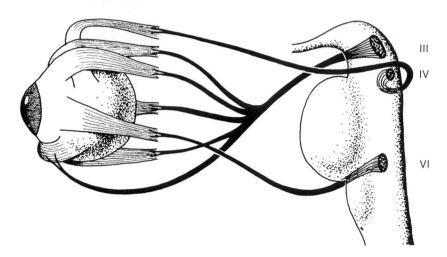

Fig. 27-10. Cranial nerves III, IV, and VI: Oculomotor, troclear, and abducent nerves and their innervation of the extraocular eye muscles. (Courtesy Smith, Kline, & French Laboratories, Philadelphia, Penn.)

right eye to the left eye while observing the right eye for movement in, out, up, or down. Wait a few seconds, move the occluder back to the right eye, observing the left eye for movement. Repeat back and forth several times until examiner is sure of what is seen.

Far cover tests:

Repeat preceding procedure with patient looking at distant target.

Interpretation/Referral: Any visible eye movement seen during the cover/uncover test with good maintenance of fixation on the target indicates a strabismus. If there is no previous history of strabismus, referral is indicated. A large eye movement seen with the alternate cover test, along with the presence of symptoms such as eye strain, headaches, or apparent difficulty in making spatial judgments, also indicates referral. In the clinic the therapist may notice that the client has difficulty finding objects in a drawer, that the client appears cross-eyed or seems to be looking past the target. He or she may have difficulty with spatial judgments in reaching for objects or in mobility, especially with stairs or curbs.

A visible eye movement may be part of a post-CVA client's premorbid pattern. This should be determined by asking the client or the family before making a referral. Or it may be the result of neurological damage to cranial nerves III, IV, or VI from CVA, head injury, or cerebral palsy. Eye muscles are striated muscles, under voluntary control. Like other striated muscles that can be affected by neurological damage, they may recover spontaneously, they may not recover at all, or they may benefit from visual retraining. Many learning-disabled children with vestibular dysfunction have poor binocular skills. An eye doctor specially trained in visual remediation can determine a patient's potential for vision therapy. Some published research has demonstrated the success of vision therapy for post-CVA patients.[16]

Stereopsis (depth perception)

Equipment: Any test that uses either Polaroid or red/green filters can test for stereopsis ability. Examples are the Titmus Stereo Fly, Rheindeer, or Butterfly.*

Procedure: Ask client to point to or say which test object appears closer. If the client is able to grasp for the object in space, some stereo ability is present.

Record: The client's response should be immediate. Long delays could indicate borderline ability.

Interpretation/Referral: If client fails this test, a referral is recommended. The patient must have best corrected acuities for this test; otherwise the results are invalid.

Implications: A deficit in depth perception can interfere with all activities involving spatial judgments, in particular fine motor and eye-hand type activities where judgments of relative depth are required (e.g., threading a needle, placing toothpaste on a toothbrush, hammering). Although ambulation itself may not be affected, ambulation involving curbs or stairs would be affected.

Vision therapy training can be helpful for clients with problems in binocular coordination. Proper diagnosis and therapy prescription are essential.

Visual field screening

Equipment: Occluder or eyepatch, black dowels with white pins on the ends, or just a wiggling finger can be used as a peripheral target.

Set Up: Client seated facing examiner.

Procedure: Client holds occluder over left eye. Examiner explains that he or she is going to wiggle a finger out to the

---

* Bernell Corp., P.O. Box 4637, South Bend, IN, 46634-4637. Complete Vision Screening Kit: Laurie Efferson, O.D., O.T.R., 5918 Greenridge Rd., Castro Valley, CA 94552.

side and that patient is to say "now" when he or she first detects the movement of the wiggling finger. The client should look at the screener's nose the entire time and ignore any arm movement. Begin with the hand slightly behind the client about 16 inches away from the patient's head. Slowly bring the hand forward while wiggling a finger. Continue randomly testing different sections of the visual field in 45-degree intervals around the visual field. Proceed to the left eye, asking patient to occlude the right eye. Alternatively, if using the dowel, slowly bring it in from the side until the patient reports seeing the small pin at the end of the dowel.

Note. These confrontation fields are considered a gross test as compared to a visual field perimeter test. Many clients cannot do the perimeter test because it requires a higher cognitive level. Confrontation fields will reveal a hemianopsia and a quadrantanopsia (quarter field cut).

Note: For lower functioning clients one can observe their eye movements in the direction of the target once they have seen it to get a general idea of peripheral function.

Record: Note the portion of field missing for each eye.

Interpretation/Referral: Refer for any hemianopsia or quadrantanopsia.

Implications: A visual deficit has significant implication for the safe performance of many functional activities, including driving and mobility. Visually guided movement through space becomes impaired, as well as efficient eye movements, and if central field loss is present, reading and any near activity are affected.

Refer to the discussion on assessment of unilateral inattention for differentiation between a "neglect" and a hemianopsia.

REFERRAL CONSIDERATIONS

The final outcome of the visual screening is referral to a doctor. It is important not to make diagnostic statements, but rather to indicate whether the client passed or failed the vision screening. By law, only optometrists or ophthalmologists can diagnose visual conditions.

It is not always clear-cut when to refer or to whom. Many doctors do not test all areas of visual function. Generally, behavioral or developmental optometrists have a functionally oriented philosophy quite similar to occupational therapy models of functional performance.*

Recommended referral guidelines are shown in the box.

Visual intervention

Early intervention is recommended where possible to identify ways in which a vision problem may be interferring with other therapies.[2,16,27] Some treatments may be applied early on as well. For example if the client has an eye muscle

---

* College of Optometrists for Vision Development has a list of behavioral doctors: P.O. Box 285, Chula Vista, CA 91912 or Optometric Extension Program, 2912 South Daimler Street, Santa Ana, CA 92705-5811

> ## Referral guidelines
>
> 1. Failure of either the distance or near acuity tests (with glasses on). This could indicate either an uncorrected refractive error, disease process, or neurological problem.
> 2. Failure of the oculomotility section only would not indicate referral because treatment of oculomotor dysfunction is currently within the scope of practice for rehabilitation.
>   EXCEPTION: Failure of the pursuit test due to a reduced ocular range of motion in any direction of gaze, which would indicate cranial nerve involvement.
> 3. Failure on the cover/uncover test indicates a strabismus, and should be referred unless there is a prior history of an eye turn.
> 4. A large eye movement seen on the alternate cover test, along with apparent difficulties in stereopsis, such as spatial judgments, or symptoms, such as headaches, eyestrain, or difficulty with comprehension, would indicate referral.
> 5. Failure of the stereopsis test alone would indicate a referral if there is no previous history of an eye turn, and there is movement on either cover test.
> 6. Quarter field loss and half field loss (hemianopsia) should be referred.

paresis, ROM exercises to the involved muscle can prevent the development of a contracture of the unopposed muscle.

In cases where the client experiences double vision, a patching regimen can be instituted. One regimen is to alternate daily, allowing some time to experience diplopia, so that the eyes may attempt to make a fusion response. The stimulus to fusion is double vision. If one eye is always patched, spontaneous recovery may be slowed. Another patching regimen is binasal taping, and another is occlusion using partially opaque materials to allow peripheral vision in the occluded eye. The patching regimen should be prescribed by an eye doctor.

In some cases of double vision a temporary plastic prism (Fresnell prism) can be applied to the client's glasses to reduce or eliminate the diplopia. This could significantly enhance the client's functioning in other therapies, particularly where spatial judgments are being made, e.g., fine motor tasks or ambulation.

Documentation

Vision problems should be documented in functional performance terms, i.e., how does the vision problem affect activities of daily living. Improvement can then be monitored according to function. This will also help in reimbursement. For example, a client with an eye muscle dysfunction will have difficulty with spatial judgments such as placing toothpaste on a toothbrush, spearing objects, reaching for a cup handle, doing pegboard tasks, and using vision for balance.

THERAPEUTIC CONSIDERATIONS

Once a referral has been made, the client has been seen, and the examination report has been received, what else can be done? How the dysfunction affects therapy can be considered and some visual training can be initiated.

Accommodative dysfunction

If the client has an accommodative dysfunction, the **treatment** may be prescribed glasses for reading or table top tasks or possibly near/far focusing exercises,[4] depending on the age of the client. "Flipper bars" are special lenses that exercise the focusing system.[4]

If the client needs glasses for near, but cannot get them for some reason, try moving the task farther away, and increasing the lighting on the task.

Eye alignment dysfunction

If the client has a problem in the eye alignment system, several factors should be considered. If the client is able to fuse some of the time, but loses fusion, seeing double when stressed or tired, then the most difficult tasks should be attempted when the client is least fatigued. Otherwise, if the client has constant double vision, or the client is seeing double at the time you are working with him or her, patching may be prescribed by the doctor. This will reduce the client's confusion and increase attention to the task. For clients with an acquired double vision, however, it is important to provide time without a patch so that they will attempt to regain fusion. Wearing the patch constantly will discourage any attempts by the brain to overcome the double vision.

Certain postures may facilitate fusion for some clients. The doctor will be able to determine which head position may be best. Frequently, many clients will automatically move around to the best position. At other times, however, head position will be used to avoid using one eye. Head and body position therefore are important aspects to consider.

Many convergence problems are amenable to vision therapy, but some are not.[14] Whether a particular problem can be helped by vision therapy can be determined by an eye doctor who can prescribe specific exercises.

Oculomotor dysfunction

If the client has a vestibular dysfunction, tracking activities should be combined as much as possible with vestibular stimulation.

While doing any sort of tracking activity, encourage the client to maintain peripheral awareness. This technique will help the client keep his or her place. The oculomotor system is guided by the peripheral location of an object.

Hemianopsia

For clients with hemianopsia, compensation training is frequently required to allow the client to resume activities such as reading. Compensation techniques include margin markers, or reading with a card with a slit in it to isolate one line (typoscope) or a couple of lines at a time. Holding reading material vertically also can help.

SUMMARY

Table 27-1 summarizes primary visual deficits. Once a therapist or specialist has eliminated the possibility of primary visual deficits, the clinician must assess whether the identified problem is due to central associative processing that is causing visual perceptual dysfunction.

VISUAL PERCEPTUAL DYSFUNCTION

This discussion of visual perceptual disorders is divided into a number of categories: unilateral spatial inattention; cortical blindness, defective color perception, and visual agnosia; visuospatial disorders; visuoconstructive disorders; and visual analysis and synthesis disorders. Cortical blindness is a disorder of primary visual input; however, because variations of it may influence perceptual interpretation, it is discussed here. All other disorders listed involve direct problems with the interpretation of visual stimuli. Although each of these terms represents symptoms recognized by many authors, the reader is reminded that there are no clear boundaries between one deficit and another or one system and another. Apraxia and body image disorders are not discussed under separate categories because they are not considered "visual" perceptual disorders per se even though their presence may influence and complicate an already dysfunctional visual perceptual system.

Problems of unilateral spatial inattention

Identification of various clinical subproblems

General category. In its purest form, unilateral spatial inattention is defined as a condition in which an individual with normal sensory and motor systems fails to orient toward, respond to, or report stimuli on the side contralateral to the cerebral lesion. Although this condition is not often seen in its pure form, inattention has been documented in persons who demonstrate no accompanying visual field defect (homonymous hemianopsia) or limb sensory or motor loss.[18] In most cases, however, unilateral spatial inattention is not seen alone but is associated with (although not caused by), accompanying sensory and motor defects such as homonymous hemianopsia, decreased tactile, proprioceptive, and stereognostic perception along with paresis or paralysis of the upper limb.

It is easy to become confused by the numerous terms used in the literature, for example, unilateral spatial agnosia, unilateral visual neglect, "fixed" hemianopsia, hemiinattention, or hemiimperception. All terms describe the same deficit. *Unilateral spatial inattention* is used in this chapter because (1) in severe cases the syndrome most likely involves tactile and auditory as well as visual unawareness (i.e., a total spatial unawareness) and (2) the syndrome

Table 27-1. Primary visual deficits associated with central lesions, functional symptoms, management, and treatment

Visual deficit	Functional deficit	Management	Treatment
Decreased visual acuity (distance or near)	Decreased acuity for distance or near tasks (reading)	Provide best lens correction for distance and near	May not be correctable
Inconsistent accommodation	Inconsistent blurred near vision	Ensure appropriate lenses are worn for appropriate activities Determine if bifocal is usable; if not, provide separate lenses for distance and near Enlarge target, control density, use contrast, task lighting	Accommodation training may be appropriate
Cortical blindness	Marked decrease in visual acuity Severe blurring uncorrectable by lenses	Evaluated by vision specialist to determine areas and quality of residual vision Present targets of appropriate size/contrast in best area of visual field	Use headlamp to improve visual localization, i.e, functional use of residual vision
Visual field deficits include: Homonymous hemianopsias Quadrantanopsias Scotomas Visual field constrictions	Blindness or decreased sensitivy in affected area of visual field	Be aware of normal field position in all meridians of gaze Ask patient to outline working area before beginning task Partial press-on FRESNEL prism to facilitate compensation	Scanning training to facilitate compensation Training in use of prism
Pupillary reactions	Slow or absent pupillary responses	Sunglasses to control excess brightness	—
Loss of vertical gaze (external opthamoplegia)	Inability to move eyes up or down	Raise target or working area to foveal level Teach patient head movement to compensate	Prism glasses to allow objects below to be seen as directly in front
Conjugate gaze deviation	Inability/difficulty moving eyes from fixed gaze position		—
Lack of convergence	Diplopia or blurred vision for near tasks Decreased depth perception for near tasks		Convergence exercises prescribed by vision specialist
Oculomotor nerve lesion (strabismus)	Intermittent or consistent diplopia in some or all meridians of gaze Loss of depth perception	FRESNEL prism to fuse image in select cases Occlude deviant eye	Oculomotor and binocular exercises with prism use prescribed by vision specialist
Pathological (motor) nystagmus	Movement/blur of image during reading/near activities/decreased activities	Enlarge print/target to decrease blur Contact lens provides feedback, reduces movement, and increases activity	Rigid gas permeable contact lens prescribed by vision specialist
Poor fixations, saccades or pursuits	Erratic scanning Unsteady fixation	Decrease density of material Isolate targets during evaluation and treatment	Oculomotor exercises prescribed by vision specialist Sensory integration activities Scanning training Use of kinesthetic and tactile systems to lead visual system (eye movements)

© Copyright by Mary Jane Douska, OTR/L, 1988
Modified by Laurie Ellerson, OD, OTR.

results in an *involuntary* lack of attention to stimuli contralateral to the lesion whereas the term *neglect* implies a voluntary choice not to respond.

Unilateral spatial inattention occurs most frequently in individuals with diagnoses of CVA, traumatic brain injury, and tumor. Most authors agree that unilateral spatial inattention occurs more often with right hemisphere than with left hemisphere lesions.[13,18,30] This frequency supports theories that the right hemisphere is dominant for visuospatial organization. It is clear, however, that inattention may be present in individuals with left hemisphere lesions. The clinician should remember that even though the chances are statistically less, the client with right hemiplegia may exhibit inattention to right stimuli.

Unilateral spatial inattention has been associated with lesions in both cortical and subcortical structures. It is most commonly seen in inferior parietal lobe lesions[18] but has also been observed in lesions in the dorsolateral frontal lobe, the cingulate gyrus,[32] and in thalamic[61] and putamenal hemorrhage.[34] Finally, lesions in the brainstem reticular formation have induced inattention in cats[50] and monkeys.[61]

Although a number of theories have been postulated regarding the mechanism underlying unilateral spatial inattention, no mechanism has been validly documented in human subjects. The one fact that is clear from all theoretical postulates is that inattention is a hemispheric deficit. LeDoux and Smylie[42] demonstrated this point effectively in an interesting case study of a right-sided lesion. During full visual exposure (bilateral hemispheric) of visual perceptual slides, the individual made visuospatial errors in left space. However, when the same slides were directed only to the right visual field (left hemisphere), performance improved substantially. It is as if the deficient hemisphere fails to receive or orient toward incoming information while the intact receiving hemisphere remains oblivious and goes about its own business. Treatment for inattention is problematic mainly because the mechanisms underlying unilateral spatial inattention are not clearly understood.

Theories on mechanisms underlying unilateral spatial inattention have attempted to explain it as an integrative associative defect as opposed to simply a problem of decreased sensory input. Theories include a unilateral attentional hypothesis suggesting that inattention results from a disruption in the orienting response; that is, the corticolimbic hemisphere is underaroused during bilateral input and therefore stimuli presented to that hemisphere are neglected.[32,33] Another theory is the oculomotor imbalance hypothesis, which suggests that individuals with inattention have a visuospatial disorder worsened by oculomotor imbalance. The hypothesis suggests that the lesion disconnects the frontal eye fields in the damaged hemisphere from their sensory afferent nerves, resulting in an oculomotor imbalance deviating the gaze toward the lesion. This imbalance can be compensated for only momentarily by a voluntary effort to gaze toward the opposite hemispace (i.e., neglected space).[15]

Unilateral spatial inattention with homonymous hemianopsia. Inattention occurs more commonly with visual field defects and is generally worse when the macula is not spared. Individuals with pure hemianopsias are aware of their visual loss and spontaneously learn to compensate by moving their eyes (foveae) toward their lost visual field to expand their visual space and thereby gather information right and left of midline. On visual examination other individuals may demonstrate no visual field defect on unilateral stimulation; however, during bilateral stimulation, they extinguish the target contralateral to their lesion. Other persons may perceive both targets simultaneously, yet when engaged in activity, they may not respond to visual stimuli in one half of visual space contralateral to their lesion. These individuals are unaware of their inattention. Careful observation of their activity reveals a paucity of eye movements into the neglected space. The fovea does not appear to be directed to gather information in this space.

Unilateral visual, auditory, and tactile inattention. Inattention has been described as a multimodal sensory associative disorder involving not only visual but also tactile and auditory unawareness. Clinicians are well aware of the client with left inattention who continues to direct the head and eyes toward the right throughout an entire conversation even though the therapist is standing on the client's left side. When one conceptualizes unilateral spatial inattention as a dynamic decrease or loss of sensory information within one half of the sensory-perceptual sphere (irrespective of hypothetical mechanism), the peculiar behaviors exhibited by these clients are more easily understood.

Unilateral spatial inattention and body image. Body image is often disturbed in individuals with inattention. The defect in these persons is unusual because it affects only that half of the body that is contralateral to the lesion, for example, the left side of the body in right-sided lesions. There appears to be a lack of spatial orientation and attention for one half of intrapersonal space. Those with severe inattention fail to recognize that their affected extremities are their own and function as though they are absent. They may fail to dress one half of their body or attempt to navigate through a door oblivious to the fact that the affected arm may be caught on the doorknob or door frame. In severe cases, individuals may deny their hemiparesis, or they may deny that the extremity belongs to them. This phenomenon is called *anosognosia.*

Behavioral manifestations of unilateral spatial inattention. Persons with inattention orient all their activities toward their "attended" space. The head, eyes, and trunk are rotated toward the side of the lesion during much of the time, including during gait. Careful observation of eye movements (scanning saccades) during activities indicates that all or almost all scanning occurs on only one side of the midline within the attended space; the individual never spontaneously brings the eyes or head past midline into contralateral "unattended" space. Oculomotor examination always shows full extraocular movements and no apraxia for eye movements.

Inattention, as all other perceptual disorders, may be viewed on a scale from mild to severe. Mild cases of inattention may go unrecognized unless behavior is carefully observed. Scanning is symmetrical except during tasks requiring increasingly complex perceptual and cognitive demands. Leicester and co-workers[13] believe that inattention occurs mainly when the individual has a general perceptual problem with the material, that is, some other problem with processing the task. This performance difficulty or stress brings on the additional inattention behavior, for example, neglect for matching auditory letter samples is more common in those with aphasia than in those with right hemisphere involvement without aphasia.

Independence in activities of daily living is often impossible because of inattention to both the intrapersonal and extrapersonal environment. The individual may eat only half of the food on the plate, dress only half the body, shave or apply makeup to only half the face, brush teeth in only half the mouth, read only half the page, fill out only one half a form, miss kitchen utensils, carpentry tools, or items in the store if they are located in the unattended space, collide with obstacles or miss doorways on the unattended side, and when walking or driving a wheelchair, veer toward the attended space rather than navigating in a straight line.

Assessment. Because most tests used to measure cognitive, language, perceptual, and motor skills require symmetrical visual, auditory, and tactile awareness, it is most important to rule out inattention early in the evaluation process of any client with a central lesion. The two most common methods used to distinguish inattention from primary sensory deficits are double simultaneous stimulation testing and assessment of optokinetic nystagmus (OKN) reflexes. Double simultaneous stimuli should be applied in three modalities: auditory, tactile, and visual. Initially, stimuli should be presented to the abnormal side. If primary sensation is impaired (e.g., a visual field loss), one cannot proceed because double simultaneous stimulation testing is invalid in that modality. If responsiveness is normal, however, bilateral simultaneous stimuli should be applied. Unilateral stimuli should be interspersed with bilateral stimuli to ensure valid responses. Lack of awareness (extinction) of stimuli contralateral to the lesion during bilateral stimulation should be noted. Clients with extinction in only one sensory system often do not demonstrate inattention behaviors; however, those with extinction in more than one modality (e.g., tactile and visual) often demonstrate these behaviors. If critical diagnosis of inattention is necessary, the client may be referred for OKN testing.

One of the best evaluation tools is a keen sense of

observation. The position of the client's head, eyes, and trunk should be observed at rest and during activity. Persistent deviation toward the lesion may indicate unilateral inattention. The individual should be asked to track a visual target from space ipsilateral to the lesion into contralateral space and maintain fixation there for 5 seconds. The therapist may ask the client to quickly fixate visual targets on command both right and left of midline. Problems with searching for targets in contralateral space should be noted. Some erratic oculomotor searching is normal when making saccades into a hemianoptic field because saccades are centrally preprogrammed by peripheral input. Very slow searching or failure to search should be considered indicative of inattention.

Asymmetries in performance should be noted during spatial tasks. Specific spatial tasks have been designed to detect inattention, including:

1. *Cancellation tasks.* The client may be given a sheet of paper with horizontal lines of numbers or letters and asked to cross out all the *eights* or *As.*
2. *Crossing out tasks.* In this test, standardized by Albert,[2] the client is asked to cross out diagonal lines drawn at random on an unlined sheet of paper.
3. *Line bisection tasks.* The client is asked to bisect a 4-inch–8-inch line on a piece of paper placed at his or her midline.
4. *Drawing and copying tasks.* The client may be asked to draw or copy a house, clock, or flower or to fill in the numbers of a clock drawn by the examiner. For copying tasks, it is important that the copy be placed in the client's attended space.

Clients with inattention demonstrate one or more of the following behaviors: failure to cancel figures or cross out lines in the unattended space; bisecting the line unequally, placing their mark toward the side of the midline ipsilateral

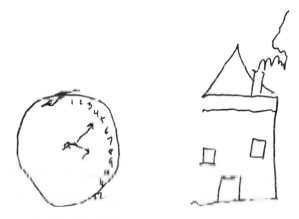

Fig. 27-11. Drawings of a clock and house by a client with a right hemisphere parietal lobe tumor. Note the left unilateral spatial inattention in the drawings.

to their lesion; placing their drawing toward the edge of the paper ipsilateral to their lesion rather than in the middle of the page; drawing only the right or left half of the house, flower, or clock; crowding all the numbers of the clock into the right or left half of the clock; or completing numbers on only one half of the clock (Fig. 27-11). When interpreting performance, the examiner is looking specifically for asymmetries in performance. Clients with inattention often have other visual perceptual deficits that result in faulty performance on these tasks; however, these deficits are always symmetrical, that is, evident in any space to which the individual attends.

Asymmetries in performance should be carefully observed during functional activities such as eating, filling out a form, reading, dressing, and maneuvering through the environment. The therapist may note unawareness of doorways and hallways in the unattended space; turns may be made only toward one direction. As a result, these clients lose their way in the hospital or even in the therapy clinic. This behavior should be distinguished from a topographical perceptual deficit in which the individual cannot integrate or remember spatial concepts well enough to find his or her way without getting lost. The Behavioral Inattention Test has recently been published as a standardized measure of functional inattention.[62]

Finally, various studies have shown that inattention may occur during testing that requires visual processing and therefore may invalidate test results.[12,13,24] Unresponsiveness to figures on one side of the page during visual, perceptual, cognitive, or language assessments may be subtle but must be documented to rule out the influence of inattention on raw score; that is, if the patient did not see the entire test display in an item, that test item is invalid. Responses to figures on the right half and left half of the test page should be counted. If the frequency of answers is noticeably less on one half of the page than would normally be expected, one may suspect that inattention may have occurred during testing. This may be used as additional evidence of inattention; but more important, this factor should be accounted for when computing test score. Only those test items in which the correct answer was located in the attended space should be scored, that is, only those items in which the correct answer was right of midline in a client with left inattention.

Treatment. As previously stated, the mechanisms underlying unilateral spatial inattention have not been clearly elucidated. This has made treatment rationales difficult. A number of studies, however, have investigated the remediation of unilateral spatial inattention. They have attempted to (1) define effective remediation techniques and (2) measure changes in trained tasks as well as generalization to untrained tasks; that is, does inattention training in one task carry over to other unrelated tasks such as activities of daily living. Treatment techniques used in all of these studies

resulted in less inattention in trained tasks.[21,41,57] An overview of these studies suggests that training may decrease inattention, although extent of change and generalization to other tasks may vary widely. Discrepancies in these results may be related to neurological variables in the various client samples, severity of inattention, sample size, or tasks measured. General principles of remediation follow.

1. Effort should be made to increase the client's cognitive awareness of the inattention. The individual should be made keenly aware of what a peripheral visual field loss is and how it is affecting his or her view of the world. The person with normal visual fields but with visual extinction should be treated the same as the individual with an actual visual field loss because the visual experience is similar. Pictures of the visual field deficit may be drawn for illustration. Actual performance examples in the environment should be pointed out to the client to demonstrate the biased field of view.

2. Visual scanning should be emphasized. Initially, the client should be made aware of how eye and eye-head movements may be used to compensate for the deficit. The individual should be trained to make progressively larger and quicker pursuits and saccades and longer fixations into the unattended space. Training may be accomplished with interesting targets held by the therapist, for examples, targets, secured to the tips of pencils, such as changeable letters, colored lights, or bright small objects. Pursuit or tracking movements of the target leading the eye from attended into unattended space should be stressed first, followed by saccades into the unattended space. Initially, the client may be allowed to move the head during scanning exercises; however, eye movements without head movements should be the major goal. Individuals with inattention often move their head into the unattended space while their eye remains fixed on a target in their attended space (i.e., the visual field remains the same). The client should be taught to independently carry out a daily right-left scanning program with targets appropriately positioned by the therapist. Eventually, these targets can be moved farther into the unattended space.

3. Increased awareness and scanning abilities should be incorporated in increasingly complex visual perceptual and visual motor tasks. Because inattention often increases as task complexity increases, the therapist must select and structure tasks carefully. Examples of simple yet specific scanning tasks might include surveying a room repetitively, rolling toward and touching objects right and left of midline, assembling objects from pieces strewn on a table or the floor, completing an obstacle course, or selecting letters from a page of large print.

4. Scanning should be stressed during functional activities, for example, dressing, shaving, and moving through the environment. The client may be taught to constantly monitor the influence of inattention on functional performance, for example: "When something doesn't make sense, look into the unattended space and it usually will."

5. Diller[20] has designed a number of specific training techniques to decrease inattention during reading and paper and pencil tasks. With a little creativity, these techniques may be applied to other activities. For example, when the client is reading, a visual marker is placed on the extreme edge of the page in unattended space. The individual is instructed not to begin reading until he or she sees the visual marker. The marker is used to "anchor" the client's vision. As inattention decreases, the anchor is faded. Each line may also be numbered and the numbers used to anchor scanning horizontally and vertically. To control impulsiveness, which often accompanies inattention, clients are taught to slow down or pace their performance by incorporating techniques such as reciting the words aloud. Underlining and looping letters/words can also be used as a method to slow down impulsive scanning (see Fig. 27-12). Finally, density of stimuli is reduced; decreased density appears to decrease inattention in these tasks.

To stimulate tactile awareness in clients with tactile extinction, Anderson and Choy[3] suggest simulating the affected arm as the individual watches. A rough cloth, vibrator, or the therapist's or client's hand may be used. Eventually, this activity may be done before activities that require spontaneous symmetrical scanning, such as dressing and walking through an obstacle course.

During the early phases of treatment, when inattention is still moderate to severe, the client should be approached from the attended space during treatment for inattention or other deficits such as apraxia, balance, or speech. This ensures that the individual comprehends and views all demonstrations and treatment instructions. Subsequently, as orientation and scanning improve, activities should be moved progressively into the unattended space and the therapist should be positioned in the unattended space during treatment. In the final stages of treatment the client should be able to symmetrically scan regardless of the therapist's position (i.e., the therapist should vary position).

To enhance the integration of scanning behavior during functional tasks such as gait and dressing, the client should be reminded of scanning principles and carried through a series of scanning exercises before initiation of the activity. If inattention reappears during the activity, the therapist should stop and assist the client in becoming *reoriented* before resuming the activity. Inattention results in confusion, and confusion increases inattention. As will be pointed out repeatedly in the following pages, the therapist must control the perceptual environment continuously so that the client is able to sequence bits of information together meaningfully in order to learn or relearn.

Problems of cortical blindness, color imperception, and visual agnosia

Identification of clinical problems

Cortical blindness. Cortical blindness is considered a primary sensory disorder as opposed to a secondary associative disorder. It is discussed here, however, because of the many variations of this lesion that may result in problems with interpretation of visual stimuli. Cortical blindness, also known as central blindness, is a loss of total or almost total vision resulting from bilateral cerebral destruction of the visual projection cortex (Area 17). Similar destruction limited to one hemisphere results in a hemianopsia.[18] The lesion may be ischemic, neoplastic, degenerative, or traumatic in nature. The client may perceive the

						0	①	2	4	5	6	7	8	9	10					
1.	①	2	3	5	4	9	7	8	0	6	3	2	10	①	2	3	5	4	9	7	1
2.	3	4	9	6	7	10	8	①	2	5	0	6	4	9	6	7	10	8	2	8	2
3.	8	0	6	2	①	3	5	4	7	9	10	①	8	0	6	2	①	3	5	7	3
4.	5	7	3	9	6	①	2	8	4	10	0	3	5	5	7	3	6	①	?	5	4
5.	6	5	①	4	2	3	8	10	9	7	9	0	6	5	①	4	2	3	8	9	5
6.	4	8	10	0	7	6	9	1	3	2	5	6	3	4	8	10	0	7	6	9	6
7.	9	6	5	3	8	4	2	0	10	1	7	2	4	9	6	5	3	8	2	4	7

Fig. 27-12. Underlining during visual discrimination tasks helps control eye movements (scanning).

defect as a "blurring" of vision, a marked decrease in visual acuity, or may be unaware of the complete nature of the disability and even deny it, blaming the problem on glasses that are too weak or a room that is too dark.

Color imperception. Color perception may be impaired in the client with brain damage. This symptom is usually associated with right hemisphere or bilateral lesions.[54] This deficit is different from color agnosia in which there is a problem with naming colors correctly. Clients with defective color perception may see colors as "muddy" or "impure" in hue, or the color of a small target may fade into the background, decreasing the ability to differentiate it from the background.[45,55] Total loss of color (achromatopsia) is rare but can occur.

Visual agnosia. A lesion circumscribed to the visual associative areas (Areas 18 and 19) results in a number of unique visual disorders that are categorized as some form of visual agnosia. Lesions are usually bilateral with combined parietooccipital, occipitotemporal, and callosal lesions. Visual agnosia is defined as a failure to recognize visual stimuli (e.g., objects, faces, letters) even though visual sensory processing, language, and general intellectual functions are preserved at sufficiently high levels.[53] It also has been described as perception without meaning; perception apparently occurs, but the percept seems "disconnected" from previously associated meaning. In this pure form, visual agnosia is a relatively rare syndrome, and there is controversy as to whether it is simply an extension of primary visual sensory deficits (variations of cortical blindness) or whether it should be considered as a separate neuropsychological entity.

Three types of agnosia have been recognized: visual, tactile, and auditory. Agnosia is most often modality specific; that is, the individual who cannot recognize the object visually will usually give an immediate and accurate response when touching or hearing the object in use. In visual agnosia, then, poor recognition is limited to the visual sphere.

Visual agnosia is divided into a number of types: visual object agnosia, simultanagnosia, facial agnosia, and color agnosia. These deficits may be seen in isolation or in various combinations, depending on size and location of lesion.

Visual object agnosia. During evaluation for the presence of visual object agnosia, the individual is presented with a number of common objects (e.g., key, comb, brush) and asked to name them. The evaluator may assume that the object is recognized if the client (1) names, describes, or demonstrates the use of the object or (2) selects it from among a group of objects as it is named by the examiner. If the person recognizes (describes or demonstrates) but is unable to name the object, failure is most likely a result of an anomia rather than an agnosic defect. Individuals with real visual agnosia have no concept of what the object is.[53]

Simultanagnosia. Along the same vein are visual disorders that constrict or "narrow" the visual field during active perceptual analysis (i.e., when perceptions are tested separately, the visual field is within normal limits). Simultanagnosia is a disorder in which the person actually perceives only one element of an object or picture at a time and is unable to absorb the whole. As the individual concentrates on the visual environment, there is an extreme reduction of visual span. The problem is functionally similar to tubular vision. The narrowing of the functional perceptual field decreases the ability to simultaneously deal with two or more stimuli. It appears as if the person has bilateral visual inattention with macular sparing, although perimetric testing reveals full visual fields. A typical example is the individual whose visual attention is focused on the tip of a cigarette held between his or her lips and fails to perceive a match flame offered several inches away.[31]

Facial agnosia. Another special type of agnosia that has been documented is failure to recognize familiar faces. The disorder is also known as *prosopagnosia.* The individual is able to recognize a face as a face but is unable to connect the face and differences in faces with people he or she knows. This person is unable to recognize family members, friends, and hospital staff by face. One must be careful not to confuse this with generalized dementia. There may be categorical recognition problems of items involving special visual experience, for example, recognition of cars, types of trees, and emblems. Facial agnosia is usually seen in combination with a number of other deficits including spatial disorientation, defective color perception, loss of topographical memory, constructional apraxia, and a left upper quadrant visual field loss. These other symptoms are most likely not causative but rather a result of the similar neurological location of these functions.[8]

Color agnosia. Finally, the individual may have difficulty recognizing names of colors—that is, an inability to name colors that are shown or to point to the color named by the examiner. This defect is considered agnosic (as opposed to a defect in color perception) because the client is able to recognize all colors in the Ishihara Color Plates[37] and is also able to sort colors by hue. The determining factor here appears to be a problem with visual-verbal association. Color agnosia is most common in left hemisphere lesions and is often accompanied by the syndrome of alexia without agraphia.[53]

Assessment. Cortical blindness and variations of it should be thoroughly assessed by the vision specialist. Assessment for agnosia must be preceded by a thorough visual acuity, visual field, and unilateral visual inattention assessment, because these primary visual sensory and scanning deficits are often mistaken for agnosic performance. Next, basic color perception should be measured using the Ishihara Color Plates and color-sorting or color-matching tasks. Individuals with defective color perception will have difficulty with some visual perceptual tasks since contextual cues related to color and shading are unavailable to them. Agnosia is a valid diagnosis only if (1) the aforementioned primary visual skills are intact and (2) language skills are intact (that is, there should be no word-finding difficulty in spontaneous speech).

Although there are no standardized tests for agnosia, commonly used assessment methods have been included. The presence of simultanagnosia is determined by keen observation of performance that indicates perception limited to single elements within objects, for example, describing only the wheel of a bicycle or, within the environment, describing only one part of a room or an activity.

Object agnosia is tested by placing common real objects (e.g., comb, key, penny, spoon) in front of the client and asking him or her to name or point to the item chosen by the examiner. In pointing and naming tasks, the therapist must be sure that the client is fixating on the appropriate target. This response is considered normal if the object is named correctly, described, or its functional use demonstrated. Abnormal responses will be confabulatory or perseverative, the individual often giving the name of a previous or similar object. Responses may also be completely bizarre and unrelated. The examiner may also present objects at an unusual angle. Abnormal responses will show lack of recognition and/or rotation of the head or body to try to view the object in the "straight on" position. The diagnosis of visual object agnosia is further confirmed if the individual can identify the object by touch or by hearing it in use. Both should be done with vision occluded.

Color agnosia is evaluated by having the client name a color and point to colors named by the examiner. Facial agnosia is evaluated by presenting the individual with photographs of famous world figures, actors, politicians, and family members.[55]

Treatment. There are no reliable studies regarding treatment of cortical blindness, color imperception, or visual agnosia. Treatment principles presented here are based on Bouska's and other clinicians' experience. If cortical blindness or simultanagnosia is suspected, the therapist must first attempt to increase the client's knowledge of foveal versus peripheral vision, that is, where the individual is fixating. A small headlamp attached to the client's forehead may be used under conditions of subdued lighting. This should not be used in a completely darkened room because the client needs to use normal spatial cues from the environment. The movement of the projected light in the environment and kinesthetic input from the neck receptors augment knowledge of where the eye is fixed. To carry out this task, the client must learn to position the eyes in midline of the head. The individual is asked to move the light (his head and eyes) to locate and discriminate fairly large, bright stimuli placed on a plain background (e.g., yellow block on a brown table). As acuity and localization skills improve, stimuli and background should be made smaller and more complex (e.g., paper clip on a printed background or letters printed at different locations on a large page). The client should be encouraged to accurately point to and/or manipu

late targets once located with the light or to keep the light on a target as he or she slowly moves the target with one hand. In this mode, the kinesthetic input from the limb can augment visual localization abilities.[41] In patients with color imperception, treatment should initially involve materials/tasks with sharp color contrasts with minimal detail and progress to less contrast (more hues) with more detail.

If the assessment has revealed a narrowing of the perceptual field, treatment should be aimed at progressively increasing the perception of large, bright, peripheral targets. For example, the client may be asked to fixate a centrally placed target while another bright target is brought in slowly from or uncovered in the periphery.[5,63] The individual is encouraged to maintain fixation on the central target while remaining alert for the presence of another target somewhere in the periphery. As the client improves, targets should be smaller, multiple, and exposed for briefer periods. Peripheral targets should always have bright surfaces that reflect light since the peripheral receptors in the retina are mainly rods (light as opposed to color receptors).

The treatment of clients with object agnosia should progress according to the abilities that return first in spontaneous recovery from agnosia. Common real objects should be used before line drawings in treatment. Presentations should be given "straight-on" rather than at an angle or rotated. The client should be asked to point to objects named by the examiner before being asked to name them. Manipulation of the object with simultaneous visual input should be attempted. This may help recognition, or it may simply confuse the client; each case is unique. In general, tactile input with or without simultaneous visual input should be encouraged as a compensation method even though it may not be helpful during treatment sessions.

Color and facial agnosia may be approached by simply drilling the individual with regard to two or three names of colors or names of faces of people important to him or her. The client may be helped to pick out or memorize cues for associating names with faces.[55]

Problems of visuospatial disorder

Identification of clinical problems. Individuals with brain lesions, particularly in the right posterior parietal and occipital areas, may have difficulties with tasks that require a normal concept of space.[18] Disorders of this nature have been termed visuospatial disorders, spatial disorientation, visuospatial agnosia, spatial relations syndrome, and numerous other terms. Visuospatial abilities are complexly interwoven within the performance of many perceptual and cognitive activities, such as dressing, building a design, reading, calculating, walking through an aisle, and playing tennis. An attempt is made here, however, to discuss spatial disorders in their purest form—that is, basic disorders—before dealing with visuoconstructive disorders and disorders of analysis and synthesis. Constructional tasks require spatial planning, a type of planning that involves the building up and breaking down of objects in two and three dimensions. Constructional apraxia is viewed as a particular type of spatial perceptual disorder and, therefore, will be discussed separately under visuoconstructive disorders and disorders of analysis and synthesis. Similarly, although perceptual skills such as figure-ground, form constancy, complex visual discrimination, and figure closure involve spatial concepts, tasks involving these skills often require the intellectual operations of synthesis and deduction. They too will be discussed in the section dealing with analysis and synthesis.

All visuospatial disabilities involve some problem with the apprehension of the spatial relationships between or within objects. Benton[7] has categorized them as the following disabilities:

1. *Inability to localize objects in space, to estimate their size, and to judge their distance from the observer.* The client may be unable to accurately touch an object in space or indicate the position of the object (e.g., above, below, in front of, or behind). Relative localization may be impaired so that the individual may be unable to tell which object is closest to him or her. There may be difficulty determining which of two objects is larger or which line is longer. Holmes[35] reported cases of gross disorder in spatial orientation revealed through walking, with individuals who, even after seeing objects correctly, ran into them. In another example, a man, intending to go toward his bed, would invariably set out in the wrong direction. Difficulty in estimating distances may also extend to judgments of distances of perceived sounds and lead to overly slow and cautious gait or fear of venturing into public areas.

2. *Impaired memory for the location of objects or places,* as in recalling the position of a target previously viewed or the arrangement of furniture in a room. Individuals with this difficulty often lose things because they have no spatial memory to rely on for recall.

3. *Inability to trace a path or follow a route from one place to another.* Persons without this ability, known as topographical orientation, have difficulty understanding and remembering relationships of places to one another so that they may have difficulty finding their way in space, locating the therapy clinic in a hospital, locating the housewares department in a store previously familiar to them. Normally functioning individuals often experience mild signs of topographical disorientation. Everyone is familiar with the disoriented feeling of not knowing how to get out of a large department store or losing a sense of direction in a familiar city. Many of the topographical errors made by clients result from unilateral spatial inattention. For example, someone with left inattention may make only right turns. Topographical disorientation,

however, may be seen in a person with no signs of unilateral inattention. This individual will demonstrate route-finding difficulties at certain points and apparently randomly choose a direction.

4. *Problems with reading and counting.* These high-level tasks require directional control of eye movements and organized scanning abilities. Eye movements (saccades) during reading bring a new region of the text on the fovea, the part of the retina where visual acuity is the greatest and clear detail can be obtained from the stimulus. During reading, the line of print that falls on the retina may be divided into three regions: the foveal region, the parafoveal region, and the peripheral region. The foveal region subtends about 1 degree to 2 degrees of visual angle around the reader's fixation point, the parafoveal region subtends about 10 degrees of visual angle around the reader's fixation point, and the peripheral region includes everything on the page beyond the parafoveal region. Parafoveal and peripheral vision contribute spatial information that is used to guide the reader's eye.[49] Visuospatial disorders appear to interfere to varying degrees with the spatial schema of a page of type or numbers and the dynamic organizational scanning that must take place to gather information appropriately. Clients with unilateral spatial inattention will miss words or numbers located on one half of the page. Other spatial problems unrelated to unilateral inattention include skipping individual words within a line or part of a line, skipping lines, repeating lines, "blocking" or the inability to change direction of fixation, particularly at the end of a line, and generally losing the place on the total page. Performance usually deteriorates progressively as the individual continues to read. Eventually, such persons cannot make sense of what they read or, if counting, they complain of being lost or confused. This type of reading or counting disorder has nothing to do with recognition or interpretation of letters or numbers or their spatial configuration; rather it represents a problem with dynamic sequential visuospatial exploration during cognitive processing.

Other visuospatial problems may include loss of depth perception, problems with body schema, and defective judgment of line orientation. There may also be difficulties with discrimination of right and left. Although unilateral spatial inattention is considered a visuospatial disorder by many, it has been discussed separately in this chapter to increase clarity. Problems with judging line orientation (slant) and/or unilateral spatial inattention often interfere with a client's spatial ability to tell time when using a standard watch or clock. Perception of the vertical may also be considered a visuospatial skill. Verticality perception is the interpretation of internal and external cues to maintain body balance. This maintenance is a complex neuromuscular process involving visual, proprioceptive, and vestibular systems. Clients with right lesions, particularly in the parietooccipital region, have more difficulty perceiving verticality than those with left lesions. This may affect posture and ambulation.[19]

Assessment. The client should be asked to accurately touch a number of targets in all parts of the visual field while fixating on a central point. Mislocalization should be noted as well as that part of the visual field in which it occurred. Mislocalization within the central field is infrequent; however, defective localization of stimuli on one or both extraocular fields is more frequently seen.[18] The client should be asked to determine which of a number of small cube blocks (placed perpendicularly in front of him or her) is closest, which is farthest, and which is in the middle. Differences in binocular (stereoscopic) and monocular viewing should be measured in this and other tasks. Impairment in both of these types of depth perception and subsequent inaccuracy in judging distances have been described in individuals with brain injury.[7]

With regard to memory for the location of objects or places, clients should be asked to describe the position of objects in their room from memory. They may also be asked to duplicate from memory the position of two or more targets (on a table or piece of paper) that have been presented for a 5-second period. As the number of targets increases, individuals with short-term memory for spatial localization will begin to make errors in spatial placement. Visual memory per se should be ruled out as a conflicting variable.

Topographical sense is assessed by asking clients to describe a floor plan of the arrangement of rooms in their house or to describe familiar geographical constellations, such as routes, arrangement of streets, or public buildings. After therapy these persons may also be asked to find their way back to their room after being shown the route several times. Failure suggests a topographical orientation problem. Finally, such a client may be asked to locate states or cities on a large map of the United States. In all of these procedures, the examiner must be sure to separate unilateral spatial inattention errors from topographical errors.

The influence of spatial dysfunction on reading and counting written material may be measured simply by asking the client to read a page of regular newsprint. The examiner should observe performance carefully and document type and frequency of errors. If errors occur, eye movements should be observed to gather additional information. Pages of scanning material (letters or numbers) often give additional information on spatial planning during reading. These are pages of print in which the size and density of the print are controlled. Scanning behavior may be demonstrated by asking the client to circle specific letters. Switching direction in the middle of a line, skipping letters or lines, perseveration, or any other abnormal performance behavior should be noted. Benton's Judgment of Line Orientation Test[9] may be used to document problems with directional orientation of

lines. If there is no indication of apraxia, the client may simply be given a ruler and asked to match it to the directional orientation of the examiner's ruler.

Treatment. Treatment for visuospatial deficits should follow basic developmental considerations progressing from simple to more complex tasks. As with children, if the evaluation suggests disorders in body scheme, tactile or vestibular input, or right-left discrimination, these should be dealt with first.

Clients who do not know where they are in space need to internalize a spatial understanding before they can make judgments regarding the space around them. In gross motor spatial training, clients can be asked to roll and reach toward various targets. In supine, prone, sitting, and standing, with vision occluded, clients should try to localize tactile stimuli (various body locations touched by the therapist) and auditory stimuli (snapping fingers or ringing bell) presented above, below, behind, in front of, and right and left of their bodies. The individual should state where the stimulus is and then point, roll, crawl, or walk toward it; this verbal, kinesthetic, and vestibular input augments spatial learning. In the occupational therapy kitchen the client, once oriented to the room, may be asked to retrieve one type of object (e.g., cup) from "the top cupboard above your head," from "the bottom cupboard below your waist," from "the table behind you," or from "the drawer on your right or left." These clients may also place objects in various positions within a room. They should then stand in the middle of the room, close their eyes, and from memory visualize, verbalize, and point to where the objects are in relation to themselves. Having localized them, the clients should then walk through the space and retrieve the objects in sequence. Functional carry-over should always be emphasized, such as having individuals remember through visualization where they put their glasses in the living room before they begin searching. Visualization is defined as the internal "seeing" of something that is not present at that moment: a vision without a visual input or internal visual imagery.[23] Visualization (spatial and other) is part of all perceptual tasks and may be used effectively as a treatment strategy. As previously discussed, a small feedback light placed in the middle of the client's forehead can help teach spatial localization through eye-hand movements.

More complex spatial skills may be taught by asking clients to "partition" space and then localize within it. An excellent activity is one in which clients use a yardstick to divide a blackboard into four or more equal parts and then number each section.

Objects may be presented to clients, who must select the largest, the farthest away, or the one placed at an angle; they may be asked to place various objects in certain relationships to each other. As shape, size, and angle begin to "make sense" to these individuals, form boards, simple puzzles, and parquetry blocks may be added to training.

Topographical abilities should improve as clients begin to

better conceptualize space; however, they may be trained directly. The therapist may help such clients organize a basic floor plan of their hospital room and the furniture within it while looking at the room. They may then be asked to do this from memory. Activities can progress to drawing plans or larger areas with a number of rooms. These clients should first "navigate" tactually through the area with their finger. Eventually, they should walk or wheel through the route themselves, visualizing and repeating the route until spatial concepts are learned. Imaginary routes also may be taken through maps of cities, states, or countries.

Organized visuospatial exploration (eye movements) during reading or other scanning and cancellation tasks may be taught. Number and letter scanning sheets may be used for such training. Initially, size of numbers and spaces between numbers should be large; this places less stress on visual acuity while training scanning. Before beginning, clients should orient themselves to the page spatially by numbering the right and left edge of each line. These numbers are used as additional spatial localization cues if needed during the scanning task.[20] Clients should then be asked to circle a specific number (or numbers) whenever it occurs. To control erratic or impulsive eye movements, they should be instructed to use a pencil to underline each line and then loop the selected letter as it comes into view (Fig. 27-12). They may also be asked to read each letter. Underlining allows the kinesthetic and tactile receptors of the arm to control eye movements; verbalization allows the language and auditory systems to influence eye movements. Visuospatial exploration exercises should progress to large-print magazines, books, or newspapers. The *New York Times* and *Reader's Digest* are both available in large print.

In all training activities it is most important that, before the activity begins, clients fully comprehend the total space in which they will work. It is equally important that they reorient themselves at any point where errors occur. Those who lose their place during reading will eventually lose it again if the therapist simply points to where they should be. Chances are better that they will not lose their place again if they reorient themselves to the page spatially when an error occurs.

Problems of visuoconstructive disorders

Identification of clinical problems. Clients with lesions in either the right or left hemisphere may have problems when trying to "construct." Lesions in the parietal, temporal, occipital, and frontal lobes have been documented in individuals with visuoconstructive disorders.[18,44] The normal ability to construct, also known as visuoconstructive ability and constructional praxis, involves any type of performance in which parts are put together to form a single entity. Examples include assembling blocks to form a design, assembling a puzzle, making a dress, setting a table, or simply drawing four lines to form a square (graphic skills). The skill implies a high level of dynamic, organized,

visuoperceptual processing in which (1) the spatial relations are perceived and sequenced well enough among and within the component parts to (2) direct higher-level processing to sequence the perceptual motor actions so that eventually (3) parts are synthesized into a desired whole. Visuoconstructive ability may be compromised if any part of this process is disturbed.

Typical tasks used to measure this ability include building in a vertical direction, building in a horizontal direction, three-dimensional block construction from a model or a picture of a model, or copying line drawings such as house, flower, and geometric designs.[8]

Clients with visuoconstructive deficits, especially those with right lesions, often also have visuospatial deficits. These individuals may rotate the position of a part erroneously, place it in the wrong position, space it too far from another part, be oblivious to perspective or a third dimension, or simply be unable to complete more than two or three steps before becoming entirely confused. This is usually evidence of breakdown because of faulty or inadequate spatial information.

Other clients, usually those with left lesions, have an "executional" or apraxic problem; they seem to have difficulty initiating and conducting the planned sequence of movements necessary to construct the whole. The problem seems to be in planning, arranging, building, or drawing rather than in spatial concepts. This deficit in its purest form is known as constructional apraxia. Constructional apraxia lies clinically outside the category of most other varieties of apraxia and is considered a special kind of "perceptual" apraxia. It occurs frequently in aphasic individuals; therefore the underlying mechanisms of aphasia and constructional apraxia may be related.[56]

Assessment. Constructional abilities are generally measured through tasks that require (1) copying line drawings such as a house, clock face, flower, or geometric designs (drawing may also be done without copy); (2) copying two-dimensional matchstick designs; (3) building block designs from copy or model; or (4) assembling puzzles. (Table 27-2 lists common tests.) The more complex the picture or design to be copied, the more complex the constructional tasks. The following are examples of drawing and block construction deficits.

1. Clients may crowd the drawing or design on one side of the page or in one corner of the page or available space on the working surface, usually a result of the influence of unilateral spatial inattention.
2. Lines in drawings may be wavy or broken, too long or short.
3. One line may not meet another accurately or lines may transect each other; in block designs, parts may not be neatly placed but rather may have small gaps.
4. There may be "overdrawing" of angles or parts of the figure because of graphic perseveration (scribble),

Table 27-2. Common tests used to assess visuoconstructive skills

Test	Standardization
Drawing pictures or shapes with or without copy	Not standardized
Reproducing matchstick designs	Not standardized
Assembling puzzles	Not standardized
The Bender Visual Motor Gestalt Test	Standardized for children only
Kohs' Blocks Test	Standardized for adults
WAIS Block Design Test	Standardized for adults
Benton's Three-Dimensional Constructional Praxis Test	Standardized for adults

spatial indecision, or problems with executive planning.

5. Clients may superimpose their copy on the model or superimpose one of their drawings on top of another. In block design construction, they may become confused between the model and their reproduction and use part of the model to complete their design. This has been termed the "closing-in" phenomenon, a failure to distinguish between model and reproduction.[18]

6. Parts of the drawing or design may be reversed. Horizontal reversals are more common than vertical reversals.

A note might be appropriate here regarding dressing apraxia. This problem occurs most frequently with right hemisphere damage. It is considered a "perceptual" apraxia rather than a motor apraxia because the inability to dress is believed to result from body scheme, spatial, and visuoconstructive deficits rather than difficulty in motor execution. Persons with dressing apraxia cannot correctly orient their clothes to their body. They often put clothes on backward or inside out. Failure to dress one side of the body is also often noted and is directly related to unilateral spatial inattention.

Treatment. It must be remembered that both visuoconstructive and visual analysis synthesis skills are often used almost simultaneously during task performance. Thus treatment should not separate the two skills but rather be a precise interrelationship of activities that require finer and finer levels of each facility. For example arranging an office filing system is both an analytical/synthetical and a visuoconstructive task. The individual must first analyze overall needs and translate them into an imagined visuospatial plan (preliminary synthesis of the whole) that will help organization. Then the organizer begins to use his or her hands to categorize (segment visual space). This building is a visuoconstructive task. Intermittently during building, new ideas of the whole surface, and visuoconstructive tasks change in response to a "better idea" (final synthesis of the whole). Task perfor-

mance, except for tasks that are rote, usually follows similar perceptual processes. Treatment therefore must be integral. Visuoconstructive skills, however, may be emphasized more than visual analysis and synthesis skills or vice versa.

As previously mentioned, visuoconstructive disorders are thought to result from different underlying problems in different individuals (e.g., visuospatial disorders in persons with right hemisphere lesions and executive, planning, or synthetic disorders in those with left hemisphere lesions). There are few reliable studies on treatment strategies for visuoconstructive disorders. One possible treatment strategy is known as *saturational cuing.*[10] *This method involves presenting controlled verbal instruction on task analysis and sequence and presenting cues on spatial boundaries, (cuing is also response related).*

If there are problems with planning and sequencing of steps necessary to accomplish a visuoconstructive task, the therapist should begin with simple tasks that require only three to four steps, such as positioning one place setting at a table. The client should discuss the plan and sequence of steps before initiating the activity, while looking at the parts to be used, such as silverware, plate, and glass. These steps may even be written down for additional input. The client should be helped to reorient the plan at any point during task breakdown. Eventually, tasks should increase in complexity (e.g., setting a table for five), and the client should be encouraged to function more independently. Another technique often used by clinicians is known as *backward chaining.* This involves presenting a partially completed task and asking the client to complete the final steps—for example, placing the knife and glass on a partially completed place setting. The perceptual cues of the task already begun appear to stimulate constructional abilities. As the client progresses, he or she should complete more steps.

Treatment for problems with spatial planning during visuoconstructive tasks should begin with simple spatial exercises discussed previously. If problems still exist, the individual may be asked to draw around shapes (blocks) one by one. These shapes should first have been placed in a simple two-dimensional design. The client is then asked to rebuild the design with the shapes alone. Therapy should progress from horizontal to vertical to oblique designs, from two-dimensional to three-dimensional designs, and from tasks with common objects to tasks involving abstract designs. For example, spatial problems with drawing, such as placing windows in a house or numbers on a clock face, are usually a result of underlying spatial disorder. The client should use a ruler or protractor to segment the space and plan placement before drawing. Dot-to-dot tasks may be designed that actually lead and sequence the drawing into a spatial whole. Simple puzzles also may be used to increase visuospatial abilities during visuoconstructive tasks. Finally, if task breakdown results from impulsive visual or motor behavior, these symptoms should be dealt with before further visuoconstructive treatment continues.

Examples of visuoconstructive tasks that may be designed for therapeutic use are:

Setting a table for one to five people
Wrapping a gift
Assembling a piece of woodwork, a toy, a tool, a motor
Changing a tire on a car
Organizing a shelf in a library or a kitchen
Organizing a filing system or cabinet
Putting pieces of a sewing pattern together
Addressing an envelope
Rearranging furniture according to a preset plan
Assembling a craft according to a preset plan
Drawing from memory or copy
Copying two-dimensional block designs
Copying three-dimensional designs with oblique components

The key to effective visuoconstructive learning, however, is not the task itself but rather how carefully the therapist organizes it and monitors performance. Clients with visuoconstructive disorders are often visually or motorically impulsive; they often move or draw parts before analysis has taken place. Once a part is placed inappropriately, it begins to confuse the whole visuoperceptual process. This confusion increases anxiety and contributes to further breakdown in analysis and synthesis. Treatment should be directed at the underlying causes of task breakdown if these can be determined.

Problems of visual analysis and synthesis disorders

Identification of clinical problems. This separate discussion of visual analysis and synthesis is arbitrary. There is never any clear demarcation between the processes of visuospatial orientation, visuoconstruction, and visual analysis and synthesis. Analysis of likes and differences, relationships of parts to one another, and reasoning and deduction occur simultaneously with more basic spatial and constructive percepts. The final visual concept of a task (e.g., what a place setting on a table should look like) is necessary before the task is begun. Similarly, synthesis of one part of a task may be necessary before synthesis of the entire task can occur. For example the person who is setting a table for four people must be able to conceptualize one place setting before conceptualizing the table with four place settings. Those points during perceptual processing when there is a colligation or blending of discrete impressions into a single perception are known as synthesis. This final stage of coordination and interpretation of sensory data is thought to be deficient in many individuals with perceptual problems. Deficits may be present with either left or right hemisphere damage but are more common and more severe with right lesions.[47,60]

Visual perceptual skills considered to be analytical and synthetic in nature include making fine visual discriminations, particularly in complex configurations; separating figure from background in complex configurations (figure-ground); achieving recognition on the basis of incomplete information (figure closure); and synthesizing disparate elements into a meaningful entity as, for example, conceptualizing parts of a task into a whole.[8]

Assessment. Many tests have been designed to measure the capacity for analysis and synthesis. Test items include complex figures in which small parts of a figure differ from another figure. The client is asked to select the one that is different. Studies have shown that basic discrimination of single attributes of a stimulus such as length, contour, or brightness are intact in many clients.[11,58,59] The problem appears when these individuals are asked to discriminate between more complex configurations with subtle differences. Tests also measure figure-ground ability; the client must select the embedded figure from the background. Functional examples of this problem are the client who cannot find his or her glasses if they are lying on a figured background, cannot find his white shirt on a white bedspread, and cannot find his wheelchair locks. Figure closure is measured by asking the client to complete an incomplete figure, such as part of the outline of a common shape. Finally, synthesis of parts into a whole, also known as visual organization, is measured by asking the client to conceptualize and organize the whole picture by, for example, looking at separate segments of the picture (such as cup or key) that have been divided and placed in unusual positions. This type of synthesis is necessary for high-level constructional tasks. Table 27-3 outlines examples of tests used to evaluate visual analysis and synthesis.

Treatment. Treatment for deficits in visual analysis and synthesis should follow developmental considerations described in the children's section. Visual discrimination tasks should begin with simple figures and obvious differences in complex figures. Color, size, texture, lighting, and verbal direction may help the client "cue in" on subtle differences among objects or figures. The therapist should determine the threshold at which the client is capable of discriminating differences and vary the dimension, contrast, and functional activity at this level. For example, if the individual cannot select a can of vegetables from a kitchen shelf stocked with

Table 27-3. Common tests used to assess visual analysis and synthesis

Test	Use
Hooper Visual Organization Test	Standardized for adults
Motor-Free Visual Perception Test	Standardized for adults
Raven's Progressive Matrices	Standardized for adults
The Embedded Figure Test	Standardized for adults
Southern California Figure-Ground Test	Standardized for children only

cans of similar size, the therapist may simply change the task to fit that person's level of visual discrimination by removing some of the cans (decreasing the density of the display), replacing some of the cans with boxes of food (increasing the spatial contrast), moving the can to be selected forward or to one edge of the display (decreasing figure-ground difficulty), removing the label from the can (increasing the light and color contrast), or giving cues regarding what to search for (verbal direction). This example is described not as a method of compensation but rather as an approach to be used therapeutically in slowly building the client's visual discrimination abilities. Eventually, high-level visual discrimination skills should be incorporated within tasks requiring three or more steps, such as selecting a can of vegetables, opening the can (which involves selecting the can opener from the utensil drawer), and emptying the vegetables into a specific bowl (which involves selecting the bowl from among other bowls). Visual discrimination and figure-ground skills may appear normal until the client is required to do multiple-step activities, is given time constraints, or becomes anxious or confused. Tabletop games that require high levels of visual discrimination along with cognitive strategies may be therapeutic and motivating. Examples include Monopoly and card games such as solitaire. Matching and sorting tasks also may be helpful in enhancing visual discrimination. Examples include matching picture cards or sorting laundry, tools, silverware, or files.

Drawings of figures with subtle differences also may be used for therapy. The client should be encouraged to point to, verbalize, or outline the subtle differences in two or more pictures; this enhances visual attention to detail. If the individual cannot select the discrepant detail(s) among three or more figures, the problem most likely results from an inability to select one feature and compare it with elements in the other figures. This is a fairly high-level skill that requires selective attention and analysis with internal visualization while the individual is still viewing the complete figures. This type of client should practice feature detection and then begin systematic comparisons of likes and differences between two figures, eventually progressing to three or more figures. The therapist may number or outline similar areas of each figure to help the client (1) direct attention to similar areas of all figures and (2) sequence comparisons appropriately. The client should verbalize, draw, or write details concerning similarities and differences in individual aspects of the figures. This enhances visual analysis and also informs the therapist as to how the individual is selecting and comparing features. Eventually, speed should be stressed, the highest level being presentation of tachistoscopic designs.

Visual organization may be emphasized by presenting the client with activities that have multiple parts that must be sequenced together into a whole. Activities involving this type of synthesis are discussed in the preceding section on treatment of visuoconstructive disorders. Figure closure may be emphasized by presenting parts of figures or objects (e.g., half a plate covered by a towel) and asking the client for identification. Figure-closure task difficulty may be increased by placing many objects on a table, some of which partially occlude others. Identification of objects in such a task requires figure closure simultaneous with figure-ground abilities.

Visual analysis and synthesis deficits reflect a disruption in cognitive function with specific regard to visual perceptual features. The affected client may function normally when analytical tasks require another system, for example, language. In others with generalized brain damage (e.g., traumatic head injury and senile dementia), general cognitive analysis and synthesis may be at fault rather than visual analysis. Because most cognitive performance requires visual processing, however, increased ability to analyze and synthesize visual perceptual material often generalizes to an increase in cognitive function.

PERCEPTUAL RETRAINING WITH COMPUTERS

During the last 10 years, numerous computer programs have been developed for rehabilitation of brain damage symptoms including cognition (e.g., attention, sequencing, or memory) and perception. Because the computer is so highly visual, it becomes an obvious tool for treatment of visual perceptual dysfunction. Treatment with computers has been coined "computer-assisted therapy." No large treatment studies have yet defined the outcome significance of computer-assisted therapy versus conventional treatment programs. However, reports indicate that computer-assisted therapy is very motivating for patients with poor attention and motivation. Advantages of computer-assisted therapy include control/flexibility of perceptual variables during treatment (e.g., number, size, speed), immediate feedback of performance, and automatic control for learning (i.e., items are repeated if incorrect to facilitate learning). Visual perceptual training with computers should be viewed as one part of a patient's treatment program if used. One should always remember that the computer, monitor, and keyboard are just that: They do not require the many perceptual, vestibular, and motor responses typical of daily performance (e.g., scanning requirements may be bilateral, but they are not global and associated with head movement). A patient's total program may include computer-assisted therapy as an additional tool; however, it should never be substituted for more significant training within the multidimensional environment. Some computer programs for visual perceptual training are listed in the box on p. 800.

SUMMARY

Careful organized evaluation should delineate deficits well enough to result in a visual perceptual function profile for each client, including both primary and associative visual skills. Clients rarely come with isolated visual perceptual deficits; more often they exhibit a combination of visual

Computer programs for visual perceptual training

Visual Perceptual Diagnostic Testing and Training Programs
H. Greenberg and C. Chamoff
Educational Electronic Techniques, Ltd.
1886 Wantagh Avenue
Wantagh, NY 11793

Captain's Log Cognitive Training System
J. Sandford and R. Browne
Computability Corporation
101 Route 46 East
Pine Brook, NJ 07058

Psychological Software Services Programs
Odie Bracey
Psychological Software Services
P.O. Box 29205
Indianapolis, IN 46229

Life Science Associates Programs
R. Gianutsos
Life Science Associates
1 Fenemore Road
Bayport, NY 11705 (Diagnosis and Training)

Cognitive Rehabilitation Series
Hartley Courseware
2023 Aspen Glade
Kingwood, TX 77339

perceptual deficits usually interrelated with motor, language, and cognitive dysfunctions. For example, a visual perceptual function profile may reveal a strabismus, left unilateral visual inattention, visuospatial deficits, visuoconstructive deficits, and problems with visual analysis and synthesis—all affecting daily function. Treatment should be organized to progressively build skills emphasizing one component more than another. The goal of treatment is eventual generalization of improvements in individual skills to spontaneous high-level function.

The presentation of information in this chapter is an attempt to use isolated and mechanistic terms to define a system that is extremely subtle, integrated, and complex. The reader is reminded that much of the normal and abnormal perceptual system has not been well defined. Preliminary studies cited throughout this chapter, however, suggest that disorders may be responsive to management and treatment. Research is needed to standardize evaluation procedures well enough to further define deficits and to investigate the effectiveness of various treatment approaches with varied client populations.

REFERENCES

1. Adler-Grinberg D and Stark L: Eye movements, scanpaths & dyslexia, *Am J Optom Phys Optics* 55:557-570, 1978.
2. Aksionoff E and Falk N: Optometric therapy for the left brain injured patient, *J Am Optom Assoc* 63:564-588, 1992.
3. Anderson E and Choy E: Parietal lobe syndromes in hemiplegia: a program for treatment, *Am J Occup Ther* 24:13, 1970.
4. Andrezejewska W and Baranowska G: Accommodative disorders after head injury and cerebral contusion, *Klin Oczna (Poland)*.
5. Balliet R and others: Rehabilitation of visual function in occipital lobe infarctions, Paper presented at the American Congress of Rehabilitation Medicine and the 43rd Annual Assembly of the American Academy of Physical Medicine and Rehabilitation, San Diego, Nov 1981.
6. Bartlett J and Jaanus S: *Clinical ocular pharmacology,* ed 2, London, 1989, Butterworths.
7. Benton A: Disorders of visual perception, disorders of higher nervous activity. In Vinken PJ and Bruyn GW editors: *Handbook of clinical neurology,* vol 3, Amsterdam, 1975, North-Holland Publishing.
8. Benton A: Visuospatial and visuoconstructive disorders. In Heilman K and Valenstein E, editors: *Clinical neuropsychology,* New York, 1979, Oxford University Press.
9. Benton A and others: Judgment of Line Orientation Test, Forms H and V, Department of Neurology, University Hospitals, Iowa City, 1975, University of Iowa Press.
10. Ben-Yishay Y and others: Ability to profit from cues as a function of initial competence in normal and brain-injured adults: a replication of previous findings, *J Abnorm Psychol* 76:378, 1970.
11. Bisiach E and others: Hemispheric functional asymmetry in visual discrimination between invariate stimuli: an analysis of sensitivity and response criterion, *Neuropsychologia* 14:335, 1976.
12. Bouska MJ and Biddle E: The influence of unilateral visual neglect on diagnostic testing, Paper presented at the American Speech, Language and Hearing Association Annual Conference, Atlanta, Nov 1979.
13. Bouska MJ and Kwatny E: Manual for application of the Motor-Free Visual Perception Test to the adult population, Temple University Rehabilitation Research and Training Center No 8, Philadelphia, 1980.
14. Carroll R and Seaber J: Acute loss of fusional convergence facility following head trauma, *Am Orthop J* 24:57-59, 1974.
15. Chedru F and others: Visual searching in normal and brain-damaged subjects: contribution to the study of unilateral visual inattention, *Cortex* 9:94, 1973.
16. Cohen A: Optometric management of binocular dysfunction secondary to head trauma: case reports, *J Am Optom Assoc* 63:569-575, 1992.
17. Cohen A and Rein L: The effect of head trauma on the visual system: the doctor of optometry as a member of the rehabilitation team, *J Am Optom Assoc* 63:530-536, 1992.
18. Critchley M: *The parietal lobes,* New York, 1966, Hafner Publishing Co.
19. DeCencio DV and others: Verticality perception and ambulation in hemiplegia, *Arch Phys Med Rehabil* 51:105, 1970.
20. Diller L: The development of a perceptual remediation program in hemiplegia. In Ince L, editor: *Behavioral psychology in rehabilitation medicine,* Baltimore, 1980, Williams & Wilkins.
21. Diller L and others: Studies in cognition and rehabilitation in hemiplegia, Rehabilitation Monograph No 50, New York, 1974, New York University Press.
22. Fannin T and Grosvenor T: *Clinical optics,* Boston, 1987, Butterworths.
23. Forrest EB: Visualization and visual imagery: an overview, *J Am Optom Assoc* 51:1005, 1980.
24. Gianotti G and Tiacci C: The relationship between disorders of visual perception and unilateral spatial neglect, *Neuropsychologia* 9:451, 1971.
25. Gianutsos R and Ramsey G: Enabling rehabilitation optometrists to help survivors of acquired brain-injury, *J Vision Rehabil* 2:37, 1988.
26. Gianutsos R, Ramsey G, and Perlin R: Rehabilitative optometric

services for survivors of acquired brain injury, *Arch Phys Med Rehabil* 69:573-578, 1988.

27. Gianutsos R and Ramsey G: Enabling survivors of brain injury to receive optometric services, *J Vis Rehabil,* 37-58:1988.

28. Glaser J: *Neuro-ophthalmology,* Philadelphia, 1990, JB Lippincott.

29. Gregory RL: *Eye and Brain,* ed 2, New York, 1972, World University Library, McGraw-Hill Book Co.

30. Hacean H: Aphasic, apraxic and agnosic syndromes in right and left hemisphere lesions, disorders of speech perception and symbolic behavior. In Vinken PJ and Bruyn GW, editors: *Handbook of clinical neurology,* vol 4, Amsterdam, 1969, North-Holland Publishing Co.

31. Hacean T and de Ajuriaguera J: Balint's syndrom (psychic paralysis of visual fixation) and its minor forms, *Brain* 77:373, 1954.

32. Heilman K: Neglect and related disorders. In Heilman K and Valenstein E, editors: *Clinical neuropsychology,* New York, 1979, Oxford University Press.

33. Heilman K and Valenstein E: Mechanisms underlying hemispatial neglect, *Ann Neurol* 5:166, 1979.

34. Hein DB and others: Hypertensive putamental hemorrhage, *Ann Neurol* 1:152, 1977.

35. Holmes G: Disturbances of visual orientation, *Br J Ophthalmol* 2:449, 1918.

35a. Hubel DH and Livingstone MS: Color and contrast sensitivity in the lateral geniculate body and primary visual cortex of the macaque monkey, *J Neurosci* 10:2223-2237, July, 1990.

36. Hubel DH and Wiesel TN: Receptive fields and functional architecture of monkey striate cortex, *J Physiol* 195:215-243, 1968.

37. Ishihara color plates, Tokyo, 1977, Kanehara & Co, Ltd. Available from Berneil Corp, P.O. Box 4637, South Bend, Indiana, 46634-4637.

38. Kanski JJ: *Clinical ophthalmology: a systematic approach,* ed 2, London, 1989, Butterworth-Heinemann.

39. Keating M: *Geometric, physical and visual optics,* Boston, 1988, Butterworths.

40. Krohel GB, Kristen RW, Simon JW, and Barrows NA: Post traumatic convergence insufficiency, *Am J Ophthalmol* 18(3):101-102, 104, March, 1986.

41. Kwatny E and Bouska MJ: Visual system disorders and functional correlates: final report, Temple University Rehabilitation Research and Training Center No 8, Philadelphia, 1980.

42. LeDoux JE and Smylie C: Left hemisphere visual processes in a case of right hemisphere symptomatology: implications for theories of cerebral lateralization, *Arch Neurol* 37:157, 1980.

43. Leicester J and others: Some determinants of visual neglect, *J Neurol Neurosurg Psychiatry* 32:580, 1969.

44. Luria AR: *Higher cortical functions in man,* ed 2, New York, 1980, Basic Books, Inc.

45. Meadows JC: Disturbed perception of colors associated with localized cerebral lesions, *Brain* 97:615, 1974.

46. Moses R and Hart W: *Adler's physiology of the eye, clinical application,* St Louis, 1987, Mosby.

47. Newcombe F and Russell WR: Dissociated visual perceptual and spatial deficits in focal lesions of the right hemisphere, *J Neurol Neurosurg Psychiatry* 32:73, 1969.

48. Nilsson L: *Behold man,* Boston, 1973, Little, Brown.

49. Rayner K: Eye movements in reading and information processing, *Psychol Bull* 85:618, 1978.

50. Reeves AG and Hagman WS: Behavioral and EEG asymmetry following unilateral lesions of the forebrain and midbrain of cats, *Electroencephalog Clin Neurophysiol* 30:83, 1971.

51. Rosenbloom A and Morgan M, editors: *Vision and aging, general and clinical perspectives,* New York, 1986, Professional Press Books, Fairchild Publications.

52. Rosenbloom A and Morgan M: *Principles and practice of pediatric optometry,* San Francisco, 1990, JB Lippincott.

53. Rubens A: Agnosia. In Heilman K and Valenstein E, editors: *Clinical neuropsychology,* New York, 1979, Oxford University Press.

54. Scotti G and Spinnler H: Colour imperception in unilateral hemisphere-damaged patients, *J Nurol Neurosurg Psychiatry* 33:22, 1970.

55. Seiv E and Freishat B: *Perceptual dysfunction in the adult stroke patient: a manual for evaluation and treatment,* Thorofare, NJ, 1976, Charles B Slack.

56. Semenza C and others: Analytic and global strategies in copying designs by unilaterally brain-damaged patients, *Cortex* 14:404, 1978.

57. Stanton K and others: Teaching compensation for left neglect through a language-oriented program, Paper presented at the American Speech, Language and Hearing Association Annual Conference, Atlanta, Nov 1979.

58. Taylor AM and Warrington E: Visual discrimination in patients with localized brain lesions, *Cortex* 9:82, 1973.

59. Teuber HL and Weinstein S: Ability to discover features after cerebral lesions, *Arch Neurol Psychiatry* 76:369, 1956.

60. Warrington E and James M: An experimental investigation of facial recognition in patients with unilateral lesions, *Cortex* 3:317, 1967.

61. Watson RT and Heilman RM: Thalamic neglect, *Neurology* 29:690,1979.

62. Wilson B, Cockburn J, and Halligan P: Behavioral Inattention Test, Hants, England, 1988, Thames Valley Test Co.

63. Zihl J: Blindsight: improvement of visually-guided eye movements by systematic practice in patients with cerebral blindness, *Neuropsychologia* 43:71, 1980.

ADDITIONAL READINGS

Arnadottir G: *Neurobehavioral assessment in adult CNS dysfunction,* St Louis, 1989, Mosby.

Humphreys G and Riddoch MJ: *To see but not to see: a case study of visual agnosia,* Hillsdale, 1987, Laurence Erlbaum.

Zolton B, editor: Visual system dysfunction, *Head Trauma Rehabil* 4(2) (entire issue), June, 1989.

CHAPTER 28

Balance Disorders

Leslie Allison

KEY TERMS

impairment
disability
balance
center of gravity (COG)
base of support
limit of stability
sensory environment
systems model or systems approach

sensory conflict
automatic postural responses
strategies
anticipatory postural responses
volitional postural movements
motor learning stages

LEARNING OBJECTIVES

After reading this chapter the student/therapist will:

1. Understand the relationship between impairments and disabilities.
2. List common postural control impairments found in neurological clients.
3. Describe both central and peripheral sensory and motor components of the postural control system.
4. List commonly used balance tests.
5. Understand how test results are used to identify impairments and disabilities.
6. Know the stages of motor learning.
7. Understand the interaction of individual, task, and environmental factors that affect balance.
8. Describe how to progress balance exercise programs to increase the use of, or compensation with, remaining sensory inputs.
9. Describe how to progress balance exercise programs to increase the control of center of gravity in upright postures.

No matter what the neurological diagnosis, a disease or injury that affects the nervous system is likely to compromise one or more of the postural control mechanisms. Clients with stroke, head trauma, spinal cord injury, peripheral neuropathy, multiple sclerosis, Parkinson's disease, cerebellar dysfunction, cerebral palsy, Guillain-Barré, etc. all experience disequilibrium problems. The common thread between all of these different *diagnoses* is the presence of balance *impairments*. Clients with different diagnoses may have the same balance impairments; clients with the same diagnosis may have different balance impairments, depending on which portions of the postural control system are involved. To optimally understand and manage balance problems, an evaluation of each balance component and the interactive nature of the components is important. The traditional medical "diagnostic" model does not provide this information and may not be the most beneficial model for balance rehabilitation interventions. The diagnosis *is* relevant: It is critical, for example, to know whether deficits are permanent or temporary, or whether recovery or progressive decline is expected. This prognostic information will assist in goal setting and treatment planning.

An alternative model, which may better explain balance disorders, is the concept of "impairment" and "disability" described by the World Health Organization (see Chapter 1 Fig. 1-5). **Impairments** are problems that result from the diagnosis, such as the loss of strength, sensation, or flexibility that may follow a stroke. **Disabilities** are the functional limitations that result from the impairments, i.e., "unable to walk" or "needs moderate assistance to transfer." Therapists perform functional tests (transfers, walking, lifting, etc.) to determine whether treatment is indicated, and if so, *what tasks* need to be learned. They also strive to identify neuromusculoskeletal problems through the assessment of strength, sensation, range of motion, etc. to discern *what impairments* are causing the reduced function. To improve the functional level of their clients, therapists treat both impairments and disabilities. For example, weakness of the quadriceps may interfere with the ability to rise from a chair; sufficient strength in the quadriceps will contribute to the independent achievement of standing. Treatment might include both strengthening exercises and practice of sit-to-stand tasks from different surfaces.

Balance impairments negatively affect function, leading to disability. These impairments often restrict activity levels, produce abnormal compensatory motor behaviors, and may require support from devices or assistance from others. When imbalance is severe, falls can result, leading to secondary injuries. To avoid these consequences and advance the functional status of their clients, therapists should understand the demands that functional tasks place on the postural control systems, and the impairments that may diminish the ability of those systems to respond adequately.

BALANCE
Definitions of balance

Balance is a complex process involving the reception and organization of sensory inputs, and the planning and execution of movement, to achieve a goal requiring upright posture. It is the ability to control the **center of gravity (COG)** over the **base of support** in a given sensory environment.[20,21] The COG is an imaginary point in space, calculated biomechanically from measured forces and moments, where the sum total of all the forces equals zero. In a normal person standing quietly, it is located just forward of the spine at about the S2 level. With movement of the body and its segments, the location of the COG in space will change constantly. The base of support is the body surface that experiences pressure as the result of body weight and gravity; in standing, it is the feet, in sitting, the thighs and buttocks. The size of the base of support will affect the difficulty level of the balancing task. A broad base of support makes the task easier; a narrow base makes it more challenging. The COG can travel farther while still remaining over the base if the base is large. The "shape" of the base of support will alter the distance that the COG can move in certain directions.

With any given base of support, there is a limit to the distance a body can move without either falling (as the COG exceeds the base of support) or establishing a new base of support by reaching or stepping (to relocate the base of support under the COG). This perimeter is frequently referred to as the **"limit of stability"** or "stability limit."[13,20] It is the farthest distance in any direction a person can lean (away from midline) without altering the original base of support by stepping, reaching, or falling.

Environmental context

This biomechanical task (keeping the COG over the base of support) is always accomplished within an environmental context, which is detected by the sensory systems. The **sensory environment** is the set of conditions that exist, or are perceived to exist, in the external world that may affect balance. Peripheral sensory receptors gather information about the environment, body position in relation to the environment, and body segment positions in relation to the self. Central sensory structures process this information to determine the opportunities and limitations present in the environment. Gravity is one environmental condition that must be reckoned with to remain stable. For all except the astronauts, it is a constant condition. Surface and visual conditions, however, may vary significantly and may be stable or unstable. Unstable surface conditions might include the subway, a sandy beach, a gravel driveway, or an icy parking lot. Common unstable visual conditions are experienced on mass transit, in crowds, or on a boat. Rapid head movements may render even a stable visual environment unusable for postural cues, and darkness may preclude the use of vision. The more stable the environment, the lower the demand on the individual for balance control. Unstable environments place greater demands on the postural control systems.

Balance is also affected by an individual's intentions to achieve certain goals and the purposeful tasks that are undertaken. Volitional balance disturbances are self-initiated almost constantly, such as shifting from foot to foot, reaching for the telephone or catching an object that is falling from a high shelf. Even reactions to involuntary balance disturbances, such as a slip or trip, will be modified based on the immediate task. A man carrying a bag of groceries who slips may drop the bag to reach with both hands and catch himself. If he is instead carrying his infant child, he may reach with only one hand, or even suffer the fall if by doing so he can protect the baby from harm.

All of these variables—the location of the COG, the base of support, the limit of stability, the surface conditions, the visual environment, the intentions and task choices—are inconstant, producing changing demands on the systems that control balance. The integrity and interaction of postural control mechanisms allow a wide range of movements and functions to be achieved without loss of balance.

HUMAN CONTROL OF BALANCE

Early studies of postural control mechanisms using selectively lesioned cats and primates focused on reflexive and reactive equilibrium responses that are relatively "hard-wired."[27] These valuable studies brought to light certain stereotypical motor responses to specific sensory stimuli, such as the "crossed extension" reflex or tonic neck reflexes. Earlier balance treatment methods based on this neurophysiological science sought to "inhibit" abnormal reflexes and "facilitate" normal responses.[3,16] These tech-

niques are not without merit, but recent research advances make it clear that this view of the nervous system and resultant scope of treatment are too narrow.[19,33] Balance abilities are heavily influenced by higher level neural circuitry, and by other systems (cognitive, musculoskeletal, etc.) as well.[13] Current theory attempts to include all of these facets in a **"systems model or systems approach"** to dynamic equilibrium.[1,25] Contemporary testing and treatment methods based on this systems model have consequently begun to evolve.[14,25] Prior techniques have been modified and expanded to allow for a more comprehensive approach.

The systems approach

The systems model for dynamic equilibrium recognizes that balance is the result of *interactions* between the individual, the task the individual is performing, and the environment in which the task must be performed. These interactions are represented in Fig. 28-1. Within the individual, both sensory inputs and processing systems (left side of figure) and motor planning and execution systems (right side of figure) are critical. Both peripheral components (lower level of figure) and central components (upper level of figure) of the systems are involved in the cycle. The cycle is driven both by purposeful choices of the individual and demands placed on the individual by the environment. Successful function of the sensory systems allows recognition of body position in relation to self and the world. The desired outcome from the motor systems is the generation of movement sufficient to maintain balance and perform the chosen task.

Peripheral sensory reception. The three primary peripheral sensory inputs contributing to postural control are the bilateral receptors of the somatosensory, visual, and vestibular systems.[1,21] Somatosensory receptors located in

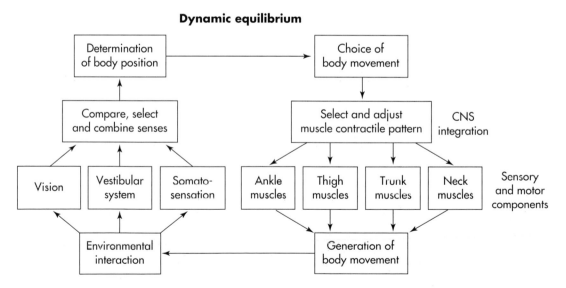

Fig. 28-1. The systems model of postural control illustrates the constant cycle that occurs simultaneously at many levels. (Reprinted with permission from NeuroCom International, Inc.)

the joints, ligaments, muscles, and skin provide information about muscle length, stretch, tension, and contraction; pain, temperature, pressure; and joint position. The feet, ankles, knees, hips, back, neck, and eye muscles all furnish useful information for balance maintenance. Visual receptors in the eyes perform dual tasks. Central (or focal) vision allows environmental orientation, contributing to the perception of verticality and object motion, as well as identification of the hazards and opportunities presented by the environment.[1] For example, a canoeist may see rocks in a stream as a hazard to be avoided, whereas a hiker who wants to cross the stream may see the same rocks as a welcome opportunity. Peripheral (or ambient) vision detects the motion of the self in relation to the environment, including head movements and postural sway,[1] whereas central visual inputs tend to receive more conscious recognition. Both are normally used for postural control.[1] Orientation to the environment allows "feedforward," or anticipatory, actions; detection of head movement and body sway provide feedback for responsive actions. Vestibular receptors in the inner ears provide information regarding the position of the head in relation to gravity and the linear and angular accelerations of the head during movement. Pitch (neck flexion/extension), yaw (right/left head rotation), and roll (right/left neck sidebending) describe angular accelerations experienced with head movements, and riding in a car or an elevator produces horizontal or vertical accelerations, respectively.[12]

Disease of, or damage to, the peripheral sensory receptors impairs or removes the detection capabilities of the system, rendering sensory information unavailable for use in postural control. Many patients with neurological diagnosis have peripheral sensory impairments. Peripheral somatosensory loss occurs after spinal cord injury, peripheral neuropathy, tabes dorsalis, amputation, etc. Peripheral vision loss may result from diabetic retinopathy, cataracts, glaucoma, etc. Peripheral vestibular loss is experienced with temporal bone fracture, acoustic neuroma, Meniere's disease, etc.[12]

Central sensory perception. All of the environmentally available sensory information gathered by the peripheral receptors is processed in varying degrees by the brain. This processing is usually referred to as sensory integration or sensory organization.[1,21] Central sensory structures function first to *compare* available inputs between *two sides* and between *three sensory systems*. For example, with head movement, firing from one vestibular organ will increase, whereas in the other, firing will decrease proportionately. The inputs from the two sides "match." Using the same example, if the eyes are open while the head moves, the rate of the visual flow will be equal, and the direction of the visual flow will be opposite to rate and direction information from the vestibular inputs. The inputs from the two systems are congruent. If both sides and all three systems provide compatible inputs, the process of organization is simplified.

Sensory conflict can arise when information between sides or between systems is not synchronous. Sensory

organization processing then becomes more complex, as the brain must then *recognize* any discrepancies and *select* the correct inputs on which to base motor responses. For example a driver stopped still at a red light suddenly hits the brake when an adjacent vehicle begins to roll: Movement of the other car detected by the peripheral visual system is momentarily misperceived as self-motion. In this situation, the vestibular and somatosensory systems do not detect motion, but the forward visual flow is interpreted as backward motion. Because the brain failed to suppress the (mismatched) visual inputs, the braking response was generated. Other examples of external sensory conflict situations include escalators, elevators, trains, and airplanes. Intrinsic central sensory processing impairments also can produce sensory conflict. An adult hemiplegic patient with pusher syndrome illustrates an inability to integrate visual, vestibular, and somatosensory inputs for midline orientation. Within a single system, discrepancies between the sides are also problematic. Vertigo, for example, may result from unilateral vestibular hypofunction, with the "mismatch" causing a spinning sensation when no real motion is occurring.[12]

Finally, the central processing mechanisms *combine* any available and accurate inputs to answer the question "Where am I?" This includes both an internal relationship of the body segments to each other (e.g., head in relation to trunk, trunk in relation to feet), and an external relationship of the body to the outside world (e.g., feet in relation to surface, arm in relation to handrail). Central nervous system (CNS) disease or trauma may impair these processing mechanisms, so that even available, accurate sensory inputs are not recognized or incorporated into determinations of position and movement.[8,15] Impairments of central sensory processing may occur after stroke, head trauma, tumors, or aneurysms, with disease processes such as multiple sclerosis, and with aging.

Central motor planning. Whereas sensory processing allows the interaction of the individual and the environment, motor planning underlies the interaction of the individual and the task. Aside from reflexive activity such as breathing and blinking, most motor actions occur because some goal is to be achieved. That is not to say that reflexes occur separately from volitional movements; for example, the vestibuloocular reflex is active concurrently with tracking activity,[12] but that most actions occur because of some purposeful intent. These task intentions precede motor actions.[16] Wrist and hand movements will vary depending on what is to be grasped (a cup versus a doorknob), foot placement and trunk position will vary depending on what is to be lifted (a heavy suitcase versus a laundry basket). The initiation of volitional motor actions depends on intention, attention, and motivation.[1,26]

Once an objective ("Where do I want to be? What do I want to do?") has been chosen, the next step in motor planning is to determine how to best accomplish the goal given the many options that are potentially available. For example, when the task demands fine skills or accuracy, the dominant hand is preferred; when the task involves lifting a large or heavy object, both hands are preferred. In addition to which limbs, joints, and muscles will be used, motor planning also adjusts the timing, sequence, and force modulation. This can be demonstrated in various reaching tasks. Reaching to remove a hot item from the oven will occur slowly, whereas reaching to put an arm through a sleeve will occur more quickly. Optimal motor plans are developed with knowledge of self (abilities and limitations), knowledge of task (characteristics of successful performance), and knowledge of the environment (risks and opportunities).[26]

The motor plan must be transmitted to the peripheral motor system to be enacted. A copy of the intended movement plan is sent to the cerebellum during the transmission. When the movement begins, incoming sensory inputs ("feedback") about the actual movements and performance outcome are compared to the intended movements and performance outcome. Movement errors (the difference between the intended and the actual movement) and performance errors (desired goal not achieved) are detected and plans for correction are then formed and transmitted. This process of error detection and error correction is the foundation of motor learning.

Clients with CNS disorders often have central motor planning impairments. After a stroke clients may have spasticity; clients with head trauma may have difficulty initiating or ceasing movements; clients with Parkinson's disease exhibit bradykinesia, and those with cerebellar ataxia display modulation problems.[5]

Peripheral motor execution. Movement is accomplished through the bilateral joints and muscles. Normal range of motion, strength, and endurance of the feet, ankles, knees, hips, back, neck, and eyes must be present for the execution of the full range of normal balance movements. Decreased ankle dorsiflexion, for example, will restrict the forward limits of stability. Weakness of the hip extensors and abductors will impede successful use of a hip strategy. Initially adequate toe clearance may diminish with fatigue. Some clients with peripheral motor nerve involvement, such as spinal cord injury or Guillain-Barré syndrome, have primary weakness, whereas other clients with central motor involvement often develop weakness as a result of force modulation deficits or disuse.[25] Many neurological clients also develop stiffness and contractures as a result of persistent weakness or spasticity. Restrictions in range of motion also may limit balance abilities.

The ability to achieve static postural alignment, although necessary for normal balance, is not sufficient to allow volitional functions. Adequate strength (to control body weight and any additional loads) through normal postural sway ranges is needed to permit dynamic balance activities such as reaching, leaning, and lifting. Postural control

demands are increased during gait as the forces of momentum and the relationships of recruitment, timing, and velocity also must be regulated.[23] Traditionally considered *orthopedic* problems, deficits in strength, range of motion, and endurance have a great impact on balance abilities. Attention must be given to these musculoskeletal losses in assessment and treatment of clients with neurological diagnosis.

Influence of other systems. Balance abilities also are influenced by other systems. Attention, cognition, and memory, often impaired in hemiplegic and head-injured clients, are critical for optimal balance function. Attentional deficits reduce awareness of environmental hazards and opportunities, interfering with anticipatory postural control. Cognitive problems such as distractibility, poor judgment, and slowed processing increase the risk of falls. Memory loss may preclude recall of safety measures. Emotional lability, agitation, or denial of impairments also can increase the risks for loss of balance. In addition to having a direct impact on balance abilities themselves, these cognitive and behavioral problems impede motor learning processes, which are crucial for the *relearning* of balance skills.

Constant cyclic nature. The systems model of postural control presented previously illustrates the constant cycle that occurs simultaneously at many levels. Attention and intention allow feedforward processing for active sensory search of the environment and motor planning, both needed for anticipatory postural control. Movements are initiated and executed, with resultant sensory experiences and error detection, or feedback. Successful movements are repeated and refined; unsuccessful ones are modified. The nature of this cycle presents the clinician with opportunities for intervention. Through feedback and practice, balance abilities can improve.

Motor components of balance

Reflexes. Many levels of neuromuscular control must be functioning to produce normal postural movements. At the most basic level, reflexes and righting reactions support postural orientation. The vestibuloocular reflex (VOR) and the vestibulospinal reflex (VSR) contribute to orientation of the eyes, head, and body to self and environment.[1] The VOR allows the coordination of eye and head movements. When the eyes are fixed on an object while the head is moving, the VOR supports gaze stabilization. Visuoocular responses often work concurrently with the VOR. They permit "smooth pursuit" when the head is fixed while the eyes move and visual tracking when both the eyes and the head move simultaneously.[1] The VSR permits stability of the body when the head moves and is important for the coordination of the trunk over the extremities in upright postures. Righting reactions support the orientation of the head to the trunk and the head position relative to the ground and include labyrinthine head righting, optical head righting, and body-on-head righting.[1]

Automatic postural responses. At the next level, **automatic postural responses** operate to keep the COG over the base of support. They are a set of functionally organized, long-loop responses that act to keep the body in a state of equilibrium.[20,21] Functionally organized means that the responses, though stereotypical, are matched to the stimulus in direction and amplitude. If the stimulus is a push to the right, the response is a shift to the left, toward midline. The larger the stimulus, the greater the response. Automatic postural responses always occur in response to a stimulus. Because they occur rapidly, in less than 250 msec, they are not under volitional control.

There are four commonly identified automatic postural responses, or **strategies.** Ankle strategy describes postural sway control from the ankles and feet. The head and hips travel in the same direction at the same time, with the body moving as a unit over the feet (Fig. 28-2, A). Muscle contractile patterns are from distal to proximal (i.e., gastrocnemius, hamstrings, paraspinals). This strategy is used whenever sway is small, slow, and near midline. It occurs when the surface is broad and stable enough to allow pressure against it to produce forces that can counteract sway to stabilize the body.

Hip strategy describes postural sway control from the pelvis and trunk. The head and hips travel in opposite directions, with body segment movements counteracting one another (Fig. 28-2, B). Muscle contractile patterns are from proximal to distal (i.e., abdominals, quadriceps, tibialis anterior). This strategy is observed when sway is large, fast and, nearing the limit of stability, or if the surface is too narrow or unstable to permit effective counterpressure.

Suspensory strategy describes a lowering of the COG toward the base of support via bilateral lower extremity flexion, or a slight squatting motion (Fig. 28-2 C). By shortening the distance between the COG and the base of support, the task of controlling the COG is made easier. This strategy is often used when a combination of stability and mobility is required, as in windsurfing.

Stepping and reaching strategies describe steps with the feet or reaches with the arms in an attempt to re-establish a new base of support with the active limb(s) when the COG has exceeded the original base of support (Fig. 28-2 D).

Anticipatory postural responses. Anticipatory postural responses are similar to automatic postural responses, but they occur before the actual disturbance.[6] If a balance disturbance is predicted, the body will respond in advance by developing a "postural set" to counteract the coming forces. For example, if an individual lifts an empty suitcase thinking it is full and heavy, the anticipatory forces generated before the lift (to counter the anticipated weight) will cause excessive movement and brief instability.

Volitional postural movements. Volitional postural movements are under conscious control. Weight shifts to reach the telephone or put the dishes in the dishwasher, for example, are self-initiated disturbances of the COG to accomplish a goal. Volitional postural movements can range from simple weight shifts to complex balance skills of skaters and gymnasts. They can occur after a stimulus or be self-initiated. Volitional postural movements can occur quickly or slowly, depending on the goal at hand. The more complex or unfamiliar the task, the slower the response time. A broad variety of movements that might successfully achieve a goal is possible. Volitional postural movements are strongly modified by prior experience and instruction. Automatic and anticipatory postural responses allow the continuous unconscious control of balance, whereas volitional postural movements permit conscious activity.

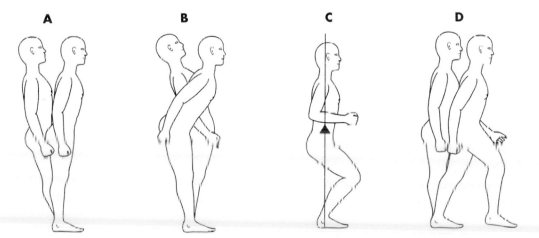

Fig 28-2. Automatic postural strategies: **A,** ankle strategy, **B,** hip strategy, **C,** suspensory strategy, **D,** stepping strategy. (From Hasson S: *Clinical exercise physiology,* St Louis, 1994, Mosby.)

CLINICAL ASSESSMENT OF BALANCE
Objectives of testing

When present, disabilities need to be identified and measured: Functional scales are usually used to determine the presence and severity of disabilities. From these functional tests, decisions can be made about whether to treat, and if so, what tasks need to be practiced. If treatment is indicated, clinicians must make judgments about what to treat. Further testing to identify and measure impairments is then necessary to know what systems are involved. A comprehensive evaluation of balance includes both functional and impairment tests.

There is no single, simple test for balance because balance is a complex sensorimotor process.[9] Many balance tests exist, but not all tests are appropriate for all clients. Different tests may be needed to answer specific questions. For example, several good tests have been developed to determine the risk for falls in elderly people. These would be totally insufficient to discern whether an injured dancer can resume practice, or an injured roofer is ready to return to work. Clinicians should understand the advantages and limitations of different balance tests to be able to select appropriate evaluative tools.

In general, a balance test will not be useful unless it challenges the postural control system being tested. Tests for stability ("static balance") are appropriate for clients who are having difficulty just finding midline and/or holding still in sitting or standing. They are of much less value for higher level clients. Conversely, single-leg stance tests or sensory tests using a foam surface may be far too difficult for lower-level clients to perform.

A word of caution about interpreting test results is indicated. Most clinical tests rely on observations of motor behavior to arrive at some conclusion about impairments. There are many possible causes for abnormal motor behavior, and clinicians should be careful before concluding that an observed behavior is due to problems in a certain, single system. For example the Romberg test is commonly assumed to test the use of vestibular inputs. Yet during the test, both somatosensory and vestibular inputs are (normally) used for balance control. If balance control is impaired, is it certain that the vestibular system is the culprit? Could somatosensory system deficits also result in a poor test result? Or alternatively, because the Romberg test is performed with feet together, what effect would hip weakness have on the ability to stand with a narrowed base of support? When using a test whose results may be altered by problems in more than one system, any relevant system should be evaluated. If multiple system deficits exist, and they often do in neurological clients, then use caution in making "commonly assumed" conclusions based on clinical test results.

Because there are so many balance tests from which to choose, several questions must be asked to determine whether a test is appropriate for use.[9] For what purpose and population was the test designed? Is it appropriate to use that test for a different purpose or with a different population? Is it valid? Is it repeatable by different examiners or by the same examiner multiple times? Are results reliable? In what populations are they reliable? How sensitive is this test, i.e., how large must changes be before this test can detect them? Are there normative data for comparison? Most of these questions have not been answered yet as they relate to the clinical balance tests commonly used by therapists.

Types of balance tests

Balance tests can be grouped or classified by type. There is no single test that can adequately measure all the components of balance. Different types of tests measure different facets of postural control (Table 28-1). Quiet

Table 28-1. Types of balance tests

Type	Tests
Quiet standing	Romberg
	Sharpened Romberg/Tandem Romberg
	One-legged-stance-test (OLST)
	Postural Sway
	Nudge/Push
	Postural Stress Test
	Motor Control Test
Active standing	Functional Reach
	Limits of Stability
	Rhythmic Weight Shifts
Sensory manipulation	Sensory Organization Test (SOT)
	Clinical Test for Sensory Interaction on Balance (CTSIB)
	Vertiginous Positions
	Hallpike-Dix Maneuver
	Vestibular-Ocular Reflex (VOR)
	Ocular-Motor Tests
	Fukuda Stepping Test
Functional scales	Berg Balance Scale
	Mobility Skills Assessment
	Get Up and Go/Timed Get Up and Go
	Tinetti Performance Oriented Assessment of Balance
	Tinetti Performance Oriented Assessment of Gait
	Gait Assessment Rating Scale (GARS)
Combination test batteries	Fregley-Graybiel Ataxia Test Battery
	Fugl-Meyer Sensorimotor Assessment of Balance Performance
	Speechley's Physical Therapy Checklist

standing (static) refers to tests where the patients is standing, and the movement goal is to hold still. Disturbances to balance, called perturbations, may or may not be applied. Active standing (dynamic) tests also position the patient standing, but the movement goal involves voluntary weight shifting. Sensory manipulation tests use various body and head positions, eye movements, or stepping to stimulate or restrict visual, vestibular, and somatosensory inputs. Functional balance, mobility, and gait scales involve the performance of whole-body movement tasks, such as sit-to-stand, walking, and stepping over objects. Finally, a few test batteries offer a combination of the preceding tests. A commonly accepted test for sitting balance in adults is not yet available, although clients with neurological problems may often need sitting balance retraining in early stages. Usually, clinicians modify standing tests or pediatric sitting tests to assess sitting balance in adult neurological clients.

Quiet standing. The classic Romberg test was originally developed to "examine the effect of posterior column disease upon upright stance."[22] The client stands with feet parallel and together and then closes the eyes for 20 to 30 seconds. The examiner subjectively judges the amount of sway. Quantification of sway can be accomplished with a videotape or forceplate. Excessive sway, loss of balance, or stepping during this test is abnormal. The sharpened Romberg,[22] also known as the tandem Romberg, requires the client to stand with feet in a heel-to-toe position and arms folded across the chest, eyes closed for 60 seconds. Often four trials of this test are timed with a stopwatch, for a maximum score of 240 seconds.

One-legged-stance-tests[22] are commonly used. Both legs must be alternately tested, and differences between sides are noted. The client stands on both feet and crosses the arms over the chest, then picks up one leg and holds it with the hip in neutral and the knee flexed to 90 degrees. This test is scored with a stopwatch. Five 30-second trials are performed for each leg (alternating legs) with a maximum possible score of 150 seconds per leg. Normal young subjects are able to stand for 30 seconds, but this may not be a reasonable expectation for older clients.[22]

Objective postural sway measures can be obtained through the use of computerized forceplates.[10,18] The client is asked to adopt a standardized foot placement if possible (varies with manufacturer) and to stand quietly with arms at sides or hands on hips for 20 or 30 seconds. Sway with both eyes open and eyes closed is commonly measured. Graphic and numeric quantification is provided (Fig. 28-3 on p. 810). Normative data may be provided.

Automatic postural responses are assessed through the client's response to perturbations. The client is asked to stand quietly, and the examiner disturbs the balance, either manually or via equipment. Most commonly used are nudge/push tests.[28] The examiner gives the client slight to moderate pushes backward at the sternum or pelvis, and then forward between the shoulder blades or at the pelvis. The

clinician subjectively notes any losses of balance and the use of recovery strategies (e.g., ankle, hip). Scoring involves rating the responses as normal, good, fair, poor, or unable. These nudge/push tests should be performed both predictably (i.e., "Don't let me push you") to judge anticipatory postural control and unpredictably (no cues) to judge automatic postural responses.

The Postural Stress test[35] was developed to examine elderly people and determine risk for falls. It is essentially a quantifiable, repeatable nudge/push test. The client stands wearing a waist belt attached posteriorly to a line that travels through a pulley and is attached on the other end to one of three weights. The weights are 1.5%, 3.0%, or 4.25% of the client's body weight. Each of these weights is dropped from a standard height, pulling the line that displaces the client backward. The expected response is a compensatory forward adjustment. Clients are videotaped, and the videotape is reviewed to assign scores to the balance responses (Fig. 28-4 on p. 811), from 0 (no response/fall) to 9 (appropriate response). If videotape is not available, a second examiner may be asked to observe the responses during the test.

The motor control test[20] perturbs the client through surface displacement (Fig. 28-5 on p. 811). The client stands on the forceplate, which is movable, with feet parallel and arms at sides. The support surface very rapidly rotates toes up or toes down, or translates (slides) forward or backward. Both of these surface displacements result in a rapid shift in the relationship between the COG and the base of support. The expected responses are directionally specific (to the direction of the stimulus) forces generated against the surface to bring the COG back to the center. Response latencies and postural sway are measured. Normative data are available.

Active standing. Volitional control of the COG is evaluated by asking the client to make voluntary movements that require weight shifting. The functional reach test[4] was developed for use with elderly people to determine risk for falls. The client stands near a wall with feet parallel. Attached to the wall at shoulder height is a yardstick. The client is asked to make a fist and raise the arm nearest the wall to 90 degrees of shoulder flexion. The examiner notes the position of the fist on the yardstick. The client is then asked to lean forward as far as possible, and the examiner notes the end position of the fist on the yardstick (Fig. 28-6 on p. 812). Beginning position is subtracted from end position to obtain a change unit in inches. Three trials are performed. Normative data are available.

The limits of stability test[10] uses a computerized forceplate to measure postural sway away from midline in eight directions. Clients assume a standardized foot position and control a cursor on the computer monitor by shifting their weight. They are asked to move the cursor from midline to eight targets on the screen (Fig. 28-7 on p. 813). Measures include movement time, path sway (length of the trajectory of the COG), and accuracy of target achievement (COG position). Normative data are available.

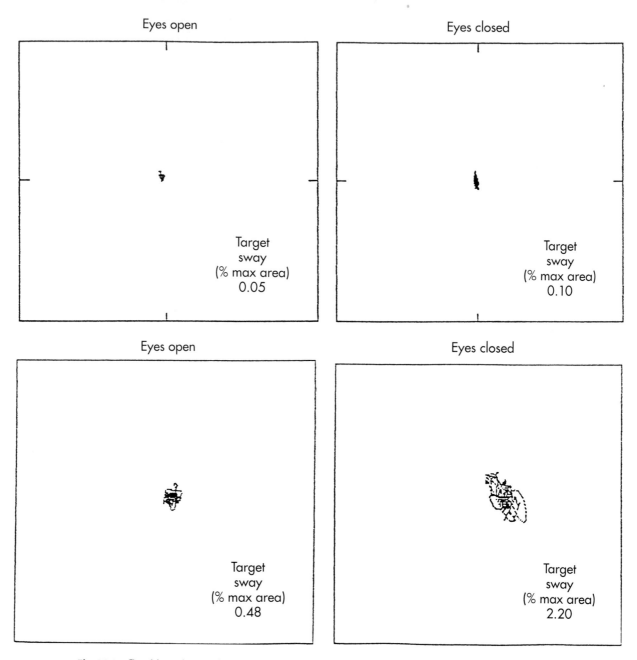

Fig. 28-3. Graphic and numeric postural sway measures using a computerized forceplate system. Top left: Normal subject, eyes open. Top right: Normal subject, eyes closed. Bottom left: Parkinson's client, eyes open. Bottom right: Parkinson's client, eyes closed. (Reprinted with permission from NeuroCom International, Inc.)

Rhythmic weight shift tests[10,18] also use a computerized forceplate and add a timing component to volitional sway measures. Clients assume a standardized foot position, controlling a cursor on the computer monitor by shifting their weight. They are asked to rhythmically shift a limited distance to the right and left, or forward and backward, in time to an audio cue. Movement at three different speeds is tested (Fig. 28-8 on p. 814). Velocity and consistency of sway are measured.

Sensory manipulation. Sensory inputs play a critical role in postural control, but tests to measure their use to produce a balance performance outcome have only recently been developed. The sensory organization test[20,21] uses a computerized movable forceplate and movable visual surround to systematically alter the surface and visual environments. The client stands with feet parallel and arms at sides on the forceplate and is asked to stand quietly. Three 20-second trials under each of six sensory conditions are

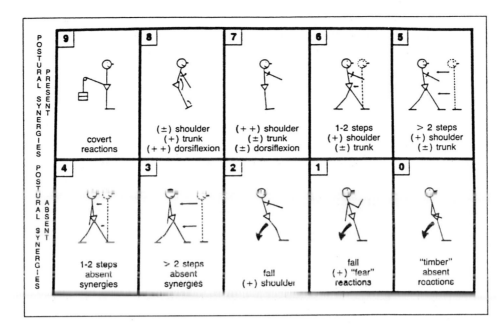

Fig. 28-4. Ratings of balance strategies used by elderly subjects during the postural stress test after a backward postural perterbation. (+) and (++) symbols indicate very frequently visible and invariably visible synergistic responses, respectively. (±) refers to less frequently seen components. Frames 2 to 0 show essentially absent coordinated activity followed by a fall. (Reprinted from Whipple R and Wolfson LI. In Duncan P: *Balance: proceedings of the APTA Forum,* Alexandria, Va, 1990, American Physical Therapy Association.)

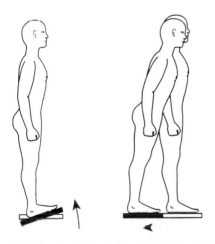

Fig. 28-5. Surface perterbations during the motor control test using computerized dynamic posturography. Forceplate measures include latency and amount of response, and adaptation of the response to repeated perterbations. (From Hasson S: *Clinical exercise physiology,* St Louis, 1994, Mosby, p 210.)

performed (Fig. 28-9 on p. 815). In conditions one, two, and three the support surface (forceplate) is fixed. During conditions four, five, and six the support surface is sway referenced to the sway of the client. In other words, the movement of the surface is matched to the movement of the client in a 1:1 ratio. This responsive surface movement maintains a near-constant ankle joint angle despite body

sway, rendering the somatosensory information from the feet and ankles inaccurate for use in balance maintenance. Visual inputs are undisturbed in conditions one and four. Vision is absent (eyes are closed) in conditions two and five. The movable visual surround is sway referenced in conditions three and six. This responsive visual surround movement maintains a near-constant distance between the eyes and the visual environment despite body sway, rendering visual inputs from the eyes inaccurate for balance maintenance in those two conditions.

Under condition one, all three senses (vision, vestibular, and somatosensory) are available and accurate. Body sway is measured via the forceplate; this initial measurement forms the baseline against which subsequent measures are compared (Fig. 28-10 on p. 816.) Under condition two, the eyes are closed, so only somatosensory and vestibular cues remain. In a normal subject, the somatosensory inputs will dominate in this condition. By comparing sway during condition two to sway during condition one, it is possible to detect how well the client is using somatosensory inputs for balance control. Clients with somatosensory loss due to spinal cord injury, diabetes, and amputation have difficulty in condition two. Functional situations with inadequate lighting or unusable visual cues (e.g., busy carpeting) are similar to condition two.

Under condition four, the support surface is sway referenced (somatosensory cues are available but are inaccurate), so only visual and vestibular cues remain. In a normal sub

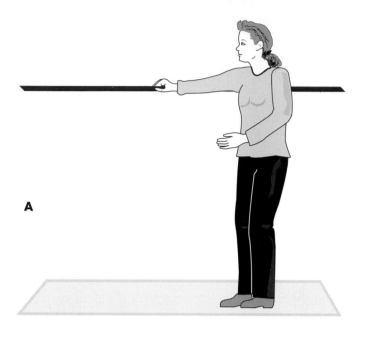

A

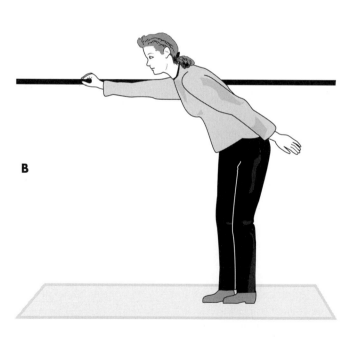

B

Fig. 28-6. During the functional reach test, the client is asked to reach forward as far as possible from a comfortable standing posture. The excursion of the arm from start to finish is measured via a yard stick affixed to the wall at shoulder height. **A,** Functional reach—starting position. **B,** Functional reach—ending position.

ject, the visual inputs will dominate in this condition. Comparing sway during condition four to sway during condition one indicates how well the client is using visual inputs for balance control. Clients with visual loss due to diabetes, cataracts, or field loss have difficulty in condition four. Functional situations that correlate with condition four include compliant surfaces (beach, soft ground, gravel driveway) and unstable surfaces (boat deck, slipping throw-rug).

Under condition five, the eyes are closed (visual cues are absent) and the support surface is sway referenced (somatosensory cues are inaccurate), leaving the vestibular inputs as the only remaining sense that is both available and accurate. Comparison of sway during condition five to sway during condition one indicates how well the client is using vestibular inputs for balance control. Clients with vestibular loss due to head injury, multiple sclerosis, and acoustic neuroma may have difficulty with condition five. Many elderly clients also may be unstable in this condition. Functional situations where these clients may be at risk for falls would have both inadequate lighting and compliant or unsteady surfaces, i.e., walking on a gravel driveway or thick carpet in the dark.

Under both conditions three and six, the visual surround is sway referenced (visual cues are available but inaccurate). By comparing sway during these two conditions to sway in the absence of vision (conditions two and five, with eyes closed), it is possible to determine how well the client can recognize and subsequently suppress inaccurate visual inputs when they conflict with somatosensory and vestibular cues. Some clients with CNS lesions (e.g., head injury, stroke, tumor) may have difficulty with this condition. Clients who cannot recognize and ignore inaccurate visual cues cannot distinguish whether they are moving or the environment is moving. If they perceive that they are moving (away from midline) when in actual fact they are not, they may often actively generate postural responses to "right" themselves. These responses, invoked to bring the COG to midline, then result in movement away from the midline. The inaccurate perception leads to a self-initiated loss of balance. Functional situations that correlate with this test condition include public transportation, grocery and library aisles, and moving walkways.

The sensory organization test is valid and reliable in the absence of motoric problems, which increase sway for reasons unrelated to sensory reception and perception. Normative data are available.

The Clinical Test for Sensory Interaction on Balance (CTSIB)[29] is a clinical version of the sensory organization test that does not use computerized forceplate technology. The concept of the six conditions remains intact (Fig. 28-11 on p. 817). Instead of sway measures, the examiner uses a stopwatch and visual observation. A thick foam pad substitutes for the moving forceplate during conditions four, five, and six. A modified Japanese lantern substitutes for the moving visual surround in conditions three and six. The

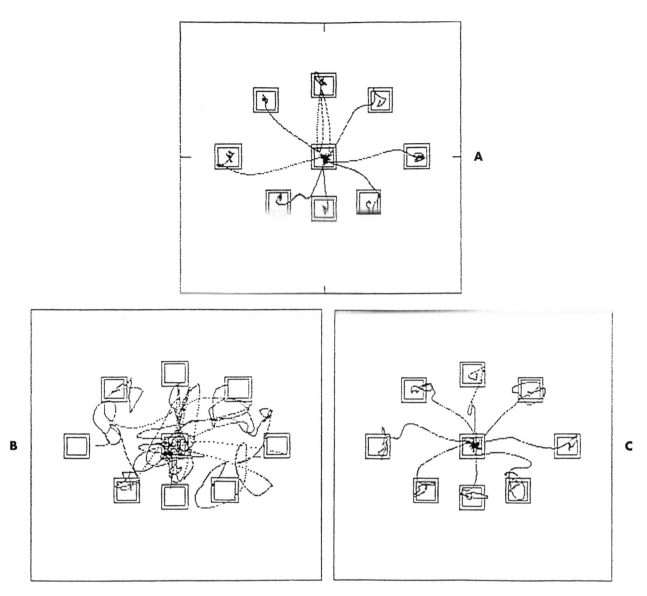

Fig. 28-7. Graphic postural sway measures from the limit of stability test using a computerized forceplate system (numeric measures not shown). Clients are asked to move away from and return to midline. **A,** Normal subject. **B,** Hemiplegic client on initial evaluation. **C,** Hemiplegic client on discharge evaluation. (Reprinted with permission from NeuroCom International, Inc.)

client is asked to stand with feet parallel and arms at sides or hands on hips. Five 30-second trials of each condition are performed.[8] The watch is stopped if the client steps, reaches, or falls during the 30 seconds. A maximum score for five trials of each condition is 150 seconds. Normal subjects are able to stand without loss of balance for 30 seconds per trial per condition. In normal subjects and clients with peripheral vestibular lesions, measures using foam correlate to moving forceplate measures.[34] Studies have not shown that measures using the Japanese lantern correlate with the moving visual surround measures. The CTSIB may not be a reliable measure in clients with hemiplegia.[7]

Tests that attempt to stimulate the vestibular semicircular canals are usually called vertiginous positions tests because they move or place clients in various positions and monitor for vertigo, dizziness, nausea, and nystagmus.[12] No single list of positions is used consistently across sites, but in general most of these tests have 10 to 20 provoking movements that are performed in order from least to most disturbing (Fig. 28-12 on p. 818.) A standardized method of scoring is not used across sites, but the examiner usually monitors the number of positions that induce symptoms (i.e., 10/16), the number of repetitions of the maneuver that can be performed before symptoms begin to increase, the intensity of the symptoms as rated by the client (i.e., 0 = no symptoms up to 10 = severe symptoms with near vomiting),

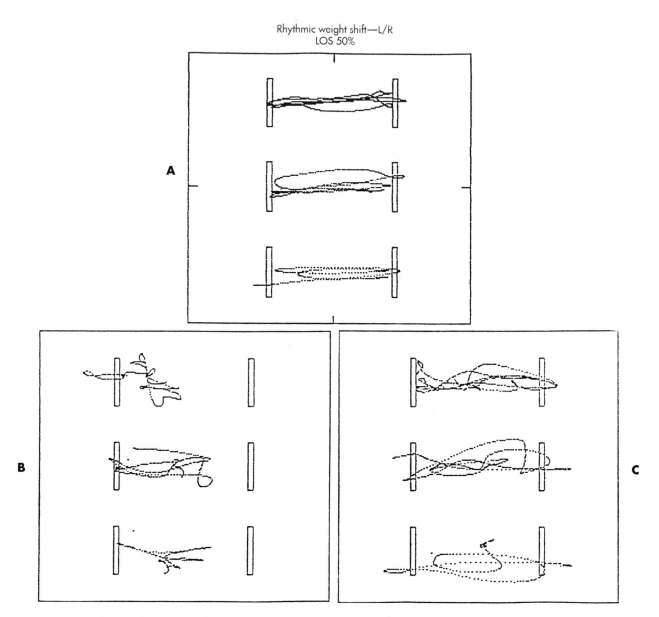

Fig. 28-8. Graphic postural sway measures from a medial-lateral weight shift test at three speeds using a computerized forceplate system (numeric measures not shown). Clients are asked to shift between the right and left lines (across midline) six times at each speed. **A,** Normal subject. **B,** Hemiplegic client, initial evaluation. **C,** Hemiplegic client, discharge evaluation. (Reprinted with permission from NeuroCom International, Inc.)

and the duration of the change in symptom level (e.g., client began at intensity level two and symptoms increased with the positioning maneuver to a level seven; it took 26 seconds for the symptoms to return to a level two). Improvement is noted by fewer provoking positions, a greater number of repetitions before symptom exacerbation, lower intensity of symptoms, and shorter duration of symptoms.[30]

The Hallpike-Dix maneuver is a vertiginous position test to stimulate the posterior semicircular canal[12] (Fig. 28-13 on p. 819). The client is positioned in long-sitting on a mat or plinth such that, when supine, the head and neck extend over the upper edge of the surface. The examiner holds the head of the sitting client between both hands, then rapidly moves the client backward and down with the head turned to the side and the neck extended 30 to 45 degrees below the horizontal. The head is held in this position for 20 to 30 seconds. The examiner monitors for symptoms of vertigo and observes the eyes for nystagmus.

The vestibular-ocular reflex (VOR) test examines the interaction of the visual and vestibular systems for eye and head orientation. The ability to hold the eyes fixed on a target while the head is moving (gaze stabilization), and the ability

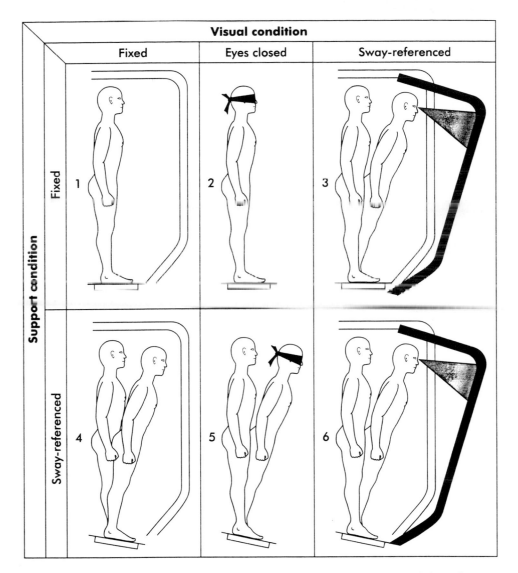

Fig. 28-9. The six sensory organization test conditions. The SOT determines the relative reliance on visual, vestibular, and somatosensory inputs for postural control using computerized dynamic posturography. (From Hasson S: *Clinical exercise physiology,* St Louis, 1994, Mosby, p 216.)

to synchronize eye and head movements in the same or opposite directions rely on the VOR. The client is asked to perform these tasks in horizontal, vertical, and diagonal planes (Fig. 28-14 on p. 820). The examiner observes eye movements for velocity and smoothness. The client reports any perceived inabilities as well. The client may be asked to read words on the targets to establish more objectively any problems with eye/head movements or velocities.

Ocular motor tests are performed to determine the ability of the eyes to fixate.[12] Saccades, or the ability for the eyes to move suddenly to locate a point in space, are tested by asking the client (head fixed) to look at one target. The examiner then suddenly presents a second target on the opposite side of the visual field. The client must look at this second target as quickly as possible without moving the head. In normal subjects, a single rapid jump of the eyes

occurs. Abnormal responses include an undershooting or overshooting of the visual target, which must be adjusted with subsequent smaller jumps. The examiner observes for these multiple attempts to exactly locate the visual target. Smooth pursuit, or the ability for the eyes to move at various speeds to follow a moving visual target, is tested by asking the client (head fixed) to follow a moving object held by the examiner. The examiner moves the object at different speeds and in different directions throughout the visual field and observes for any inability to follow the object. Normal subjects have no difficulty following the moving target.

The Fukuda stepping test was developed to assess labyrinth function.[22] A grid is drawn on the floor (Fig. 28-15 on p. 821) with two concentric circles (one and two meters in diameter, respectively) divided into 30-degree sections. The client is placed standing in the center of the circles, is

SENSORY ANALYSIS			
RATIO NAME	**TEST CONDITIONS**	**RATIO PAIR**	**SIGNIFICANCE**
SOM Somatosensory	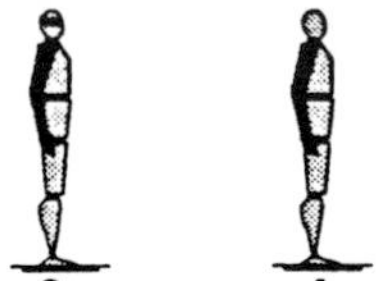 2 1	Condition 1 / Condition 2	Question: Does sway increase when visual cues are removed? Low scores: Patient makes poor use of somatosensory references.
VIS Visual	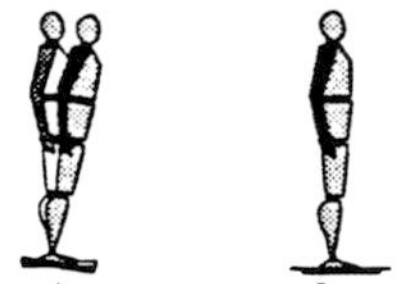 4 1	Condition 4 / Condition 1	Question: Does sway increase when somatosensory cues are inaccurate? Low scores: Patient makes poor use of visual references.
VEST Vestibular	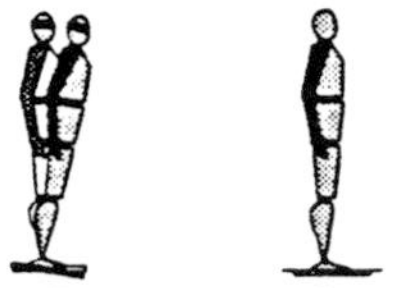 5 1	Condition 5 / Condition 1	Question: Does sway increase when visual cues are removed and somatosensory cues are inaccurate? Low scores: Patient makes poor use of vestibular cues, or vestibular cues unavailable.
PREF Visual Preference	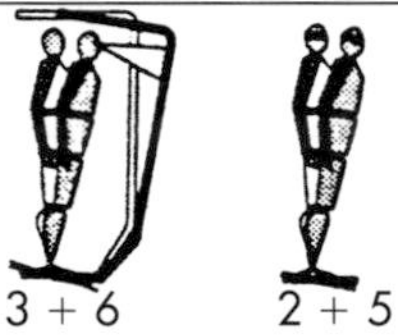 3 + 6 2 + 5	Condition 3 + 6 / Condition 2 + 5	Question: Do inaccurate visual cues result in increased sway compared to no visual cues? Low scores: Patient relies on visual cues even when they are inaccurate.

Fig. 28-10. Postural sway measures from each of the six SOT conditions are compared and the ratios are used to identify impairments in the use of sensory inputs for postural control. (Reprinted from Jacobson GP, Newman CW, and Kartush JM: *Handbook of Balance Function Testing,* 1993, with permission of Mosby.)

blindfolded, and raises the arms outstretched to shoulder height. The examiner instructs the client to take 100 marching steps (knees high) in place, then observes for postural sway and deviations of position of the head, arms, and body. Once the client has stopped, the examiner quantitatively measures the angle of rotation, angle of displacement, and the distance of displacement. Per Fukuda, normal subjects are able to take 100 steps without traveling more than one meter and without rotating more than 45 degrees, whereas clients with peripheral vestibular dysfunction deviate outside this range toward the side of the deficit. Reliability studies of this test have not yet been published. Obviously, the client being tested must be motorically very high level to perform this test, and the examiner must be sure that any observed deviations are not due to motoric (versus vestibular) causes.

Functional scales. A comprehensive balance evaluation must include both impairment measures and disability measures. Functional scales help to address the latter. By asking the client to perform functional tasks that demand balance skills, the clinician can determine the presence of disabilities and identify the tasks that the client needs to

practice. Four mobility scales and two gait scales focus on postural control; all six were developed for the elderly population to determine risk for falls. Many clinicians also are using them to assess neurological clients, although their usefulness with neurological populations has not been formally evaluated.

The Berg balance scale is a list of 14 tasks that the client is asked to perform.[2] The examiner rates the client on each task using a scoring scale of 0-1-2-3-4, where zero is unable to perform and four is able to perform without difficulty. The mobility skills assessment is a similar list of 10 items.[4] Clients are rated by the examiner using a scoring scale of 0-1-2, where zero is unable to perform, one is performed with abnormality or difficulty, and two is performed without difficulty. The *Get-Up-and-Go test* is made up of seven items scored on a scale of 1-2-3-4-5, where one is normal, and five is severely abnormal.[17] The Tinetti Performance Oriented Assessment of Balance is a list of nine items scored on scales of either 0-1 or 0-1-2, with the higher numbers reflecting better (more normal) performance.[32] The best possible score is a 16. The score value is specific to the item. Most balance

VISUAL CONDITIONS

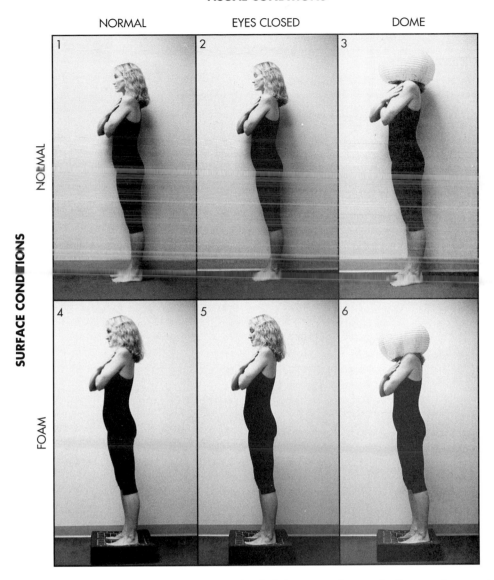

Fig. 28-11. The clinical test for sensory interaction in balance uses foam and a Japanese lantern to replicate the six sensory conditions. A stopwatch is used to time trials.

and mobility scales have been developed to assess risk-for-falls in the elderly. Many share similar items. See Table 28-2 on p. 822 for a summary of scale items.

The Tinetti Performance Oriented Assessment of Gait is a list of seven normal aspects of gait that are observed by the examiner as the client walks at a self-selected pace and then at a rapid but safe pace.[32] Scoring scales are again either 0-1 or 0-1-2, and higher numbers indicate better performance. Score values are specific to the item being observed (Table 28-3 on p. 823). The best possible score is a 12. When combined, the Tinetti balance and gait scales offer a best possible score of 28. The Gait Assessment Rating Scale (GARS) is a list of sixteen abnormal aspects of gait observed by the examiner as the client walks at a self-selected pace (35) (See

Table 28-3 on p. 823). These abnormalities are commonly seen in elderly people who fall. The items are scored on a scale of 0-1-2-3, with lower numbers reflecting better (less abnormal) performance. The best possible score is a zero. This gait scale provides some relative numerical indication of the quality of gait. These two gait scales were developed to assess risk-for-falls in the elderly. They focus on elements of postural control during gait.

Combination test batteries. Because no single test can give a complete picture of a client's balance abilities, three commonly used test batteries combine several types of tests. The Fregley-Graybiel Ataxia Test Battery is a list of eight test items that the client must perform[22] (Fig. 28-16 on p. 823). Standing trials in tandem stance both off and on a

UNIVERSITY OF MICHIGAN VESTIBULAR TESTING CENTER HABITUATION TRAINING

NAME: _____ MRN: _____ AGE: _____ SEX: _____

DATE: _____	INTENSITY	DURATION	SCORE
BASELINE SYMPTOMS			
1. Sitting → Supine			
2. Supine → Left Side			
3. → → Right Side			
4. Supine → Sitting			
5. Left Hallpike			
6. → → Sitting			
7. Right Hallpike			
8. → → Sitting			
9. Sitting → Nose To Left Knee			
10. Sitting → Erect Left			
11. Sitting → Nose To Right Knee			
12. Sitting → Erect Right			
13. Sitting → Head Rotation			
14. Sitting → Head Flex. And Ext.			
15. Standing → Turn To Right			
16. Standing → Turn To Left			

INTENSITY: SCALE FROM 0 TO 5 (0=NO SX, 5=SEVERE SX)
DURATION: SCALE FROM 0 TO 3 (5-10 SEC=1 POINT, 11-30 SEC=2 POINTS, ≥30 SEC=3 POINTS)

MOTION SENSITIVITY QUOTIENT: $\dfrac{POSITIONS \times SCORE}{2048} \times 100 =$ _____ 28-12.

TOTAL

Fig. 28-12. An example of a standardized list of vertiginous positions tests. Intensity of dizziness is rated by the client and duration of dizziness is measured with a stopwatch. (Reprinted with permission from the University of Michigan Vestibular Testing Center.)

rail with eyes open and closed are timed. Timed single leg stance trials also are performed for each leg. Walking 10 steps with eyes closed is included. Five trials of each task are given. Trials are stopped if the client uncrosses the arms, opens eyes (during eyes closed trials), steps (during standing trials), or falls. Trials are judged on a pass/fail basis. This test battery is valid for use with clients who have peripheral vestibular dysfunction. Normative data are available from a normative database comprised primarily of young men. As noted earlier, clients must be motorically very high level to perform these tasks. Interpretations regarding clients use of sensory inputs when motor involvement is also present cannot be made with certainty.

The Fugl-Meyer Sensorimotor Assessment of Balance Performance is a subset of the Fugl-Meyer Physical Performance Battery, which was designed for use with hemiplegic clients[8] (Fig. 28-17 on p. 824). Three sitting and four standing balance activities are listed. The items are scored on a 0-1-2 scale, with score values specific to each item. Higher scores indicate better performance; the maximum (best) score is 14; however, a client could achieve this score [14] and still not have normal balance.

The physical therapy checklist is a combination of risk-factor items relating to the status of neuromuscular systems, foot problems, balance skills, and walking abilities[31] (Fig. 28-18 on p. 824). It was designed to assess risk for falls in elderly clients. Items are scored either normal (0) or abnormal (1) for neuromuscular and foot items, and negative (0) or positive (1) for balance and gait problems. This test has not been validated. Normal subjects would receive the best possible score of zero.

Considerations in the selection of balance tests

Many of the functional scales reviewed previously were designed to determine whether balance is abnormal in elderly clients who have no diagnosis, in other words, as

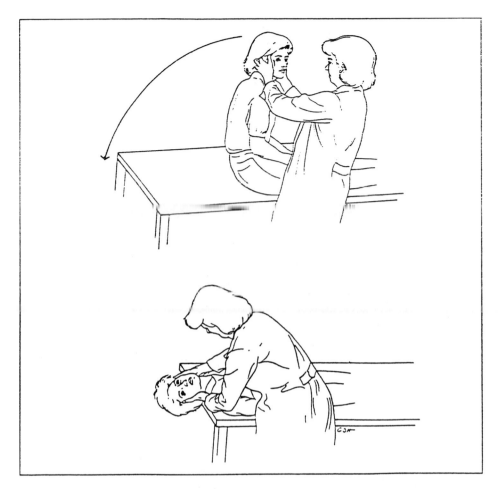

Fig. 28-13. The Hallpike-Dix maneuver. Moving the patient rapidly from a sitting to a supine position with the head turned so that the affected ear is 30 to 45 degrees below the horizontal will stimulate the posterior canal and may produce vertigo and nystagmus. (Reprinted from Herdman S: Treatment of benign paroxysmal positional vertigo, *Phys Ther* 70:381-388, 1990, with permission of the American Physical Therapy Association.)

screening tools. Clinicians working with clearly diagnosed neurological clients often do not need such tools to establish that balance skills are abnormal because the deficits are patently obvious. These tools can be useful, however, to identify disabilities, to establish a baseline, and to monitor progress.

Many clinical facilities have therapy evaluation forms that include a section on balance. Usually, items and scoring are defined by the facility, and client performance on each task is rated either normal, good, fair, poor, unable, or as requiring no-supervision-minimal-moderate-maximal assistance (Fig. 20-19 on p. 025). These are essentially functional rating scales, although they are not standardized across sites as are published scales. It is important to use some sort of functional balance rating scale in the evaluation of neurological clients. To be sensitive enough to measure change in clients who clearly are not (and may never be) clinically normal, scales should have at least five to seven possible relative scores.

In addition, it is necessary to perform additional tests to assess the systems which may affect postural control to help identify and measure impairments (e.g., range of motion, strength, sensation and sensory organization, motor planning and control). These types of measures should be sensitive, objective, and quantifiable. Unfortunately, there are some systems for which objective, quantifiable clinical measures have not been developed (e.g., peripheral somatosensation and motor planning). In these cases, clinicians must continue to use subjective rating scales.

Other factors to include when deciding what tests to use are the time it takes to perform the test, the number of staff who must be present, and the space and equipment needed. Clinicians must now weigh the potential benefits of technological tools (e.g., computerized electromyography, forceplates, isokinetics, motion analysis) against their cost and practicality, i.e., their cost-effectiveness. The test must be suitable for the client's level of functioning (physical and cognitive). Many head-injured clients, for example, cannot

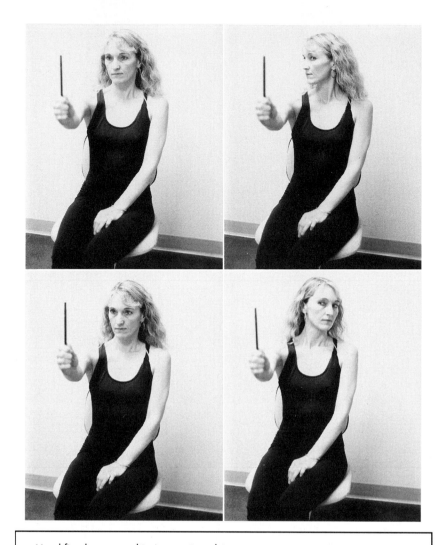

Head fixed, eyes tracking a moving object.

Eyes fixed on an object, head moving. (see corresponding sequence of photos)

Eyes and head and object moving while focusing on the moving object.

Vertical movements of the eyes with the head stable and moving.

Eyes diagonal with the head stable and moving.

Eye movements incorporated with trunk movements.

Fig. 28-14. Eye and head motions are assessed to determine whether symptoms associated with the vestibular-ocular reflex mechanism are present. (Reprinted from Whitney S: Dizziness and balance disorders, *Clin Manage* 11:42-48, 1991, with permission of the American Physical Therapy Association.)

initially participate in traditional forms of testing due to cognitive limitations.

PROBLEM IDENTIFICATION, GOAL SETTING, AND TREATMENT PLANNING
Clinical decision making

Treatment of clients with neurological diagnosis is based on the particular set of impairments and disabilities pos-sessed by each individual. Remediation of balance deficits similarly must be specific to the involved systems and functional losses in each client. Clinicians should generate an overall problem list for each client; if imbalance is a listed problem, then a sublist of balance problems also can be developed (Fig. 28-20 on p. 825).

To direct and establish priorities for treatment, clinicians must review the problem list and ask themselves the

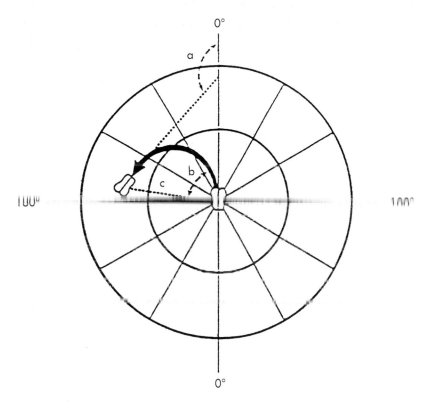

Fig. 28-15. The Fukuda stepping test for peripheral vestibular clients uses a floor grid to detect the extent of drift that occurs during an eyes-closed stepping task. (Reprinted from Newton R: *Brain Injury* 3:335, 1989.)

following questions: Which impairments are temporary and can be remedied? How much improvement can be expected? How soon will it occur? Which impairments are permanent and must be compensated for? What other systems can be counted on to substitute? What external compensations may be needed (Fig. 28-21 on p. 826)? For example, consider two clients, both with vestibular diagnosis. One client has unilateral peripheral vestibular hypofunction. This situation may be temporary, or the contralateral vestibular organ may be able to compensate. In either case the use of vestibular inputs for balance control could improve, so exercises to stimulate the vestibular system are indicated. The other client has total bilateral vestibular loss secondary to neurotoxic medication. This condition is permanent, and no use of vestibular inputs is possible, so exercises must focus on improving the use of remaining inputs (somatosensory and visual).

With some neurological clients, it is often not possible to know whether a problem is permanent or temporary, as in recovery from a stroke or head injury. In others with progressive diseases such as Parkinson's disease or multiple sclerosis, the rate of decline is unknown and abilities may fluctuate. In these cases the clinician should consider the following issues: Would a consult provide me with the information I need to know? If so, referral is appropriate. Are there any contraindications to treatment? What are the risks and benefits of providing versus withholding treatment? Is

some amount of functional improvement possible? If there are no contraindications, the benefits outweigh the risks, and there is an expectation of functional improvement, then a trial of treatment may be given if it cannot be known for certain whether the problem(s) will respond to the treatment. In these cases especially, a baseline must be established against which to measure any change. Change for the worse or no change after a reasonable trial period indicates that treatment should be altered or discontinued.

Using the systems model to identify postural control impairments

To develop a balance problem list the systems approach is useful because it can be applied to different diagnosis equally well and allows deficits in multiple systems to be recognized. Table 28-4 on p. 826 illustrates several examples of ways this framework is used to identify balance deficits in clients with different neurological diagnosis.

For each client, problems affecting postural control should be described in objective, measurable terms whenever possible. For example, writing "impaired vision" is too vague; "two-line drop on eye chart" is more specific. "Poor use of visual inputs for balance control" is an interpretation; the objective result could be stated "Loss of balance after less than 15 seconds on 5/5 trials of standing on foam, eyes open." Documenting problems in this manner makes goal writing (and consequently, treatment planning) much easier

Table 28-2. Balance and mobility scale items

Activity	Berg test	Mobility skills	Get up and go	Tinetti balance
1. Sit unsupported	√	√		√
2. Sit to stand	√	√	√	√
3. Stand to sit	√		√	√
4. Transfers	√			
5. Stand unsupported	√	√	√	√
6. Stand with eyes closed	√			√
7. Stand with feet together	√			
8. Tandem stand	√			
9. Stand on one leg	√			
10. Trunk rotation while standing	√			
11. Retrieve object from floor	√	√		
12. Turn 360 degrees	√			√
13. Stool stepping	√			
14. Reach forward while standing	√	√		
15. Sitting reach		√		
16. Walk		√	√	
17. Abrupt stop		√		
18. Walk then turn		√	√	
19. Step over obstacle		√		
20. Stairs		√		
21. Sternal nudge				√

Writing goals based on impairments and disabilities

Goals also should be stated in objective and measurable terms so that their achievement can be judged. "Improved balance" is open to anyone's interpretation, whereas "Able to stand on right leg for 30 seconds on 3/3 trials" and "Walks tandem entire length of balance beam without misstep 7/10 times" are measurable goals. These types of goals may be helpful to the clinician, who understands the link between impairments and function but may seem nonfunctional (and therefore unnecessary) to others who read them (e.g., case managers, third-party payers). It is beneficial from their standpoint to incorporate into the impairment goal the functional task that will be affected positively by its achievement. For example: "Able to stand on right leg for ....*so that* stairs can be ascended/descended step-over-step without railings," or "Walks tandem on balance beam ....*to demonstrate* ability to avoid falls using hip strategy." By describing the impairment/function relationship in the treatment objectives, clinicians force themselves to focus on functional outcomes and illustrate for others *why* these goals are meaningful. The need for and validity of the treatment is then more likely to be perceived clearly.

If a problem cannot be improved and requires compensation, the goal(s) should reflect this as well. For example, a client with diabetes has progressive peripheral neuropathy with somatosensory loss and ineffective ankle strategy. If the client's visual and vestibular sensory systems and proximal strength are relatively intact, however, then the goals might mention improved use of visual cues and successful substitution of hip strategy. Educational and environmental modification goals for safety also are appropriate in these situations.

Developing a treatment plan

Once the goals are listed and priorities established, the treatment plan is developed. *The most effective and efficient treatments will focus first on those problems with the greatest impact on function and address more than one problem at a*

Table 28-3. Gait Scale Items

Gait activities	Tinetti gait scale	Gait assessment rating scale
1. Initiation (hesitancy)	√	√
2. Step length	√	√
3. Step height	√	
4. Step symmetry	√	√
5. Step continuity	√	√
6. Path deviation	√	√
7. Trunk	√	√
8. Walking-heel distance	√	
9. Staggering		√
10. Heel Strike		√
11. Hip ROM*		√
12. Knee ROM*		√
13. Elbow extension*		√
14. Shoulder extension*		√
15. Shoulder abduction*		√
16. Arm-heelstrike synchrony		√
17. Forward head*		√
18. Shoulders held elevated*		√
19. Forward flexed trunk*		√

*During gait.

time. Training balance on an unstable surface not only contributes to the use of visual and vestibular inputs, but also (1) to the use of hip strategy, (2) increased lower extremity strength, and (3) increased motor control (skill) on that type of surface. Training gait on a treadmill with eyes closed or head movements increases (1) the use of somatosensory and vestibular inputs, (2) endurance, and (3) lower extremity strength. Creative clinicians develop comprehensive treatment plans with this type of multiproblem approach to maximize the time available with clients.

The clinician must thoughtfully choose *environments* and *tasks* that together stimulate and challenge the appropriate postural control systems. To stimulate one sensory system, the other systems must be placed at a disadvantage to force reliance on the targeted system. The environment is then structured to disadvantage the other systems, i.e., training with eyes closed or in the dark puts vision at a disadvantage and forces the use of somatosensory and vestibular inputs. If one side or limb is significantly more affected, such as in hemiplegia, then the other side must be disadvantaged to force reliance on the targeted side. Tasks are then selected to disadvantage the less affected side. For example, placing the less affected leg up on a step or small ball makes it more difficult to use for balance and forces the transference of weight to the more affected leg. To achieve optimal function, however, all systems and all sides must be capable of working together, so training to improve balance impairments must be incorporated and interspersed with training functional tasks. For carry-over of improvements into "real-life" situations, training tasks should be varied enough to promote motor problem solving on the part of the client. For example, sitting balance and transfers should be taught to stable and unstable surfaces, of different heights and firmnesses, with and without armrests and back supports, or to both right and left sides. This technique may improve the

FREGLEY TEST

Condition	Trials				
	1	2	3	4	5
1. Sharpened Romberg, EC (60 sec; feet in tandem)					
2. Walk on Rail, EO (5 steps; best 3/5 trials)					
3. Stand on Rail, EO (3 trials; 60 sec/trial)				x	x
4. Stand on Rail, EC (3 trials; 60 sec/trial)				x	x
5. Stand on Right Leg, on Floor, EC (5 trials; 30 sec/trial)					
6. Stand on Left Leg, on Floor, EC (5 trials; 30 sec/trial)					
7. Walk on Floor, EC (3 trials; 10 steps each)				x	x
8. Stand sideways on rail (characterize sway)†					

†Added by the author to observe the movement strategy used by the individual
EO, eyes open; EC, eyes closed.

Fig. 28-16. A combination of tasks (Romberg, OLST walking) and environments (EO, EC, rail) are included in the Fregley-Graybiel ataxia test battery. (Reprinted from Newton R: *Brain Injury* 3:335, 1989.)

FUGL-MEYER

Test	Scoring	Maximum Possible Score	Attained Score
1. Sit without support _____	0—Cannot maintain sitting without support 1—Can sit unsupported less than 5 minutes 2—Can sit longer than 5 minutes		
2. Parachute reaction, non-affected side _____	0—Does no abduct shoulder or extend elbow 1—Impaired reaction 2—Normal reaction		
3. Parachute reaction, affected side _____	Scoring is the same as for test 2		
4. Stand with support _____	0—Cannot stand 1—Stands with maximum support 2—Stands with minimum support for 1 minute		
5. Stand without support _____	0—Cannot stand without support 1—Stands less than 1 minute or sways 2—Stands with good balance more than 1 minute		
6. Stand on unaffected side _____	0—Cannot be maintained longer than 1–2 seconds 1—Stands balanced 4–9 seconds 2—Stands balanced more than 10 seconds		
7. Stand on affected side _____	0—Scoring is the same as for test 6		
	Maximum Balance Score		

Fig. 28-17. The Fugl-Meyer Sensorimotor Assessment of Balance Performance includes both very low level and very high level tasks. (Reprinted from DiFabio RP and Badke MB: *Phys Ther* 70:20, 1990.)

PHYSICAL THERAPY CHECKLIST*

Item/Criteria		Scoring
Neuromuscular		Normal = 0 Abnormal = 1
Shoulder strength/ROM		☐
Hand grip strength		☐
Hip flexion		☐
Knee flexion		☐
Knee extension		☐
Ankle dorsiflexion		☐
Ankle plantar flexion		☐
Foot problems		Absent = 0 Present = 1
Grossly long nails		☐
Severe callouses		☐
Any bunions		☐
Any toe deformities		☐
Balance items		Negative = 0 Positive = 1
Nudge	Subject standing at full height, examiner pushes gently on sternum three times. Positive score is staggering or struggling for balance.	☐
Single leg balance	Subject asked to balance on each leg for 5 seconds. Positive score is touching ground with other foot.	☐
360° turn	Subject asked to turn one complete revolution on the spot. Positive score is any unsteadiness.	☐
Chair sit	Subject asked to sit down in a firm armless chair. Negative score is safe smooth motion, else positive.	☐
Gait items		Negative = 0 Positive = 1
Path deviation	Subjects asked to walk straight line over a 3 m course (or use of walking aid).	☐
Trunk sway	Subjects observed over 3 m straight course. Positive score is trunk sway, flexion of knees or back, abduction of arms, (or use of walking aid).	☐
Pick up speed	Subjects asked to walk at as fast a pace as they feel is safe. Positive score is inability to pick up speed.	
	Total (Max. = 18)	☐

* These items, derived from a variety of sources 1-4, 6-8, 11-13 are included because they have been both associated with falling and are potentially modifiable through physical therapy. This checklist may prove useful in identifying those who are at increased risk of falling because of deficits that may be remediable through physiotherapy.

Because this is not a validated scale, the score has no standard meaning. It is not recommended for use as a comprehensive risk assessment instrument.

Fig. 28-18. Designed as a risk-for-falls screening tool for use with the elderly, Speechley and Tinetti's physical therapy checklist covers both impairments (strength, ROM) and functional tasks (stand-to-sit, walking). (Reprinted from Speechley M and Tinetti M: *Physiother Can* 42:75, 1990.)

BALANCE

Sitting—Static/Dynamic
- Normal
- Good dynamic—Able to reach to floor to pick up shoe; able to cross one leg over other (to both sides) as needed to put on shoes.
- Fair dynamic —Able to turn side to side with ability to pick up clothing on both sides.
- Poor dynamic —Unable to complete above. Loses balance with this activity.
- Good static —Able to maintain balance for at least 3 minutes *without* hand hold; feet on or off floor; able to turn head but not trunk side to side.
- Fair static —Able to maintain balance approximately 5 minutes *with* hand hold; foot on floor. Able to turn head—not trunk side to side.
- Poor static —Unable to sit without assistance; touching patient or movement by patient causes him to fall over.

State tendency to lose balance forwards, backwards, (R) or (L).

Standing Balance—Static/Dynamic
- Normal
- Good dynamic—Able to maintain balance while picking ball off floor.
- Fair dynamic —Able to maintain balance while turning head/trunk; lifting arms.
- Poor dynamic —Unable to complete above without loss of balance. Requires handhold.
- Good static —Able to maintain a statue position without handhold.
- Fair static —Requires handhold unilateral or bilateral to maintain upright.
- Poor static —Requires handhold and assistance from another to maintain upright.

Fig. 28-19. Example of intrafacility balance rating scale. (Reprinted with permission from Mills-Peninsula Hospitals.)

EXAMPLE OF BALANCE PROBLEM LIST

General Problem List	Balance Problem List
1. Decreased strength (L) side	
2. Decreased ROM (L) shoulder	
3. Decreased endurance	
4. Impaired sensation (L) side	
5. Decreased balance	a. Decreased weight bearing on left (L) LE b. Unable to maintain midline orientation c. Extraneous sway with eyes closed d. Unable to stand on (L) LE e. Decreased limits of stability to 40/100% f. Unable to shift to (L) side g. Unable to establish stable base of support h. Unable to stand on unstable surface i. Unable to perform hip strategy
6. Increased tone (L) side	
7. Synergistic movement (L) side	
8. Min. assist transfers	
9. Mod. assist ambulation	

Fig. 28-20. An example of a balance-specific problem list (as a subset of a general problem list), which should be developed to guide balance rehabilitation treatments.

client's abilities to perform safe sitting and transfers in new situations not previously practiced in therapy.

Tables 28-5 through 28-7 on pp. 827-829 illustrate the process of test choice, problem identification based on test results, goal setting based on impairments and disabilities, and treatment planning based on goals in three different types of clients. Note that for each client, only selected tests were performed. Goals were directly related to the problems that were identified by the tests, and treatment plans followed directly from the goals.

Table 28-4. Examples of impairments and diagnosis

Impairments from systems model:	Client with diabetic stroke	Client with Parkinson's disease	Client with incomplete paraplegia
Peripheral sensory			
Vision	Retinopathy	Cataracts	
Vestibular		Hair cell loss	
Somatosensory	Peripheral neuropathy	Slowed transmission time	Complete loss
Central sensory			
Vision	Hemianopsia	Vision dominant	Needs superior use to compensate
Vestibular	Failure to use inputs		Needs superior use to compensate
Somatosensory	Failure to use inputs	Failure to use inputs	
Strategy selection	Step dominant	Ankle dominant	Hip dominant
Perception of position in space	Midline shift (L) neglect	Restricted cone of stability	
Central motor			
Timing	Increased reaction time	Bradykinesia	
Sequencing	Disordered	Co-contraction	
Force modulation	Spasticity	Rigidity	
Error correction	Use (R) side only		
Peripheral motor			
ROM	Knee hyperextension	Bilateral ankle PF contractures	Hip flexion contractures
Strength	Decreased (L) side	Decreased bilateral LE	Severe weakness bilateral lower extremity (LE) and trunk
Endurance	Severely impaired	Moderately impaired	Mildly impaired

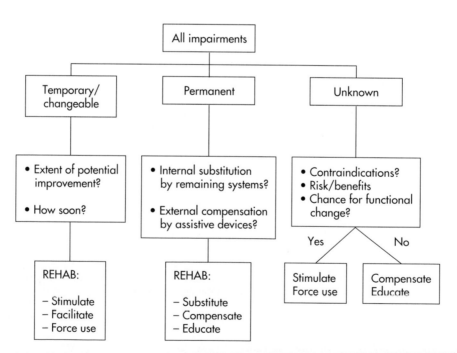

Fig. 28-21. A clinical decision-making tree to illustrate the treatment-planning process in balance rehabilitation.

Table 28-5. An example of test selection, problem identification, goal setting, and treatment planning in a client with a peripheral vestibular deficit

Patient Profile:
- 50-year-old woman
- DX: Uncompensated (R) unilateral peripheral vestibular deficit, X 6-7 years
- ENT → Psychol → Neuro Otol → Outpatient PT

Test	Problems identified	Goals set	Treatment plan
Visual acuity	- 2 line drop on chart	- Able to read chart with only 1 line drop	Gaze stabilization exercises
Ocular motor • Saccades • Pursuit • Nystagmus	- + nystagmus with Frenzel lenses		
Gaze stabilization • Vis./vest. interaction • VOR cancellation • Hallpike	- unable to perform test - ↓ fixation with horizontal + vertical head movements after 5-10 sec	- Able to rotate head horizontally 2 min. without problems - Able to perform visual/vestib interaction test	Gaze stabilization exercises
Sensory Organization Test (SOT)	Decreased use of somatosensory inputs 70/100 - Decreased use of visual inputs 55/100 - Absent use of vestibular inputs 0/100 - Unable to resolve visual conflict 0/100	- Somatosensory use 100/100 Vision use 90/100 - Vestibular use 70/100 - Visual conflict resolution 90/100	Sensory environment stimulation
Limits of stability	- Restricted anteriorly and posteriorly to 35% LOS - Slow movement time	- Limits of stability expanded to 85% ant. and post. at 5 sec pacing	COG control training
ROM/strength	None		
Gait - Eyes open - Eyes closed - Head turning - Pivots - Abrupt stops	- Deviates to (R) with eyes closed - Weaves side-to-side and dizzy with horizontal head turns - Loss of balance and dizzy with (R) pivot - Very unsteady with abrupt stop—feels "off"	- Walks in a straight line with eyes closed - Walks with only slight deviation with eyes closed and head turning - Spins to (R), (L) with eyes closed - Comes to abrupt stops steadily	Gait training

Reprinted with permission from NeuroCom International, Inc.

BALANCE RETRAINING TECHNIQUES
Motor learning concepts

Although it is not within the scope of this chapter to cover the principles of motor learning, it is not possible to approach balance retraining methods without some consideration of several motor learning concepts that must be incorporated into treatment. The clinician must remember that successful treatments address the *interaction* of the individual, the task, and the environment (Fig. 28-22 on p. 830).

Individual Therapists should know their client's impairments, sensory and motor, peripheral and central. Whenever possible, therapists should know which impairments can be rehabilitated and which will require compensation. Due to the nature of neurological insult, this includes an awareness of cognitive and perceptual impairments that may affect the ability to relearn old skills or develop new

ones. Optimal learning of skilled movement requires that the client have (1) knowledge of self (abilities and limitations), (2) knowledge of the environment (opportunities and risks), (3) knowledge of the task (critical components), (4) the ability to use those knowledge sets to solve motor problems, and (5) the ability to modify and adapt movements as the task and environment changes. To the extent that a client is missing these characteristics, the clinician should attempt to support their development, or even to supply them until they are present. Different types of clients will vary in which characteristics are likely to be missing. For example, a cognitively impaired head-injured client may lack awareness of self and environment, even though his or her physical abilities make it quite possible for him or her to modify and adapt movements. Conversely, a quadriplegic client may be very aware of his or her limitations, the environment, and the

Table 28-6. An example of how treatment planning flows from test results in an elderly client with frequent falls

Patient Profile:
- 72-year-old woman
- DX: Disequilibrium of aging, frequent falls
- Cardiologist → Neurologist → PT Outpatient

Test	Problems identified	Goals set	Treatment plan
Peripheral sensory • Somatosensory • Vision	↓ Acuity-cataracts ↓ Depth perception Mildly decreased vibration sense bilateral LE	- Compensate for permanent sensory loss	Educate about safe surfaces and lighting Home safety evaluation
Sensory Organization Test (SOT)	- Absent 0/100 use of vestibular inputs - Decreased use of somatosensory inputs 60/100 - Dependent on vision	- Increase use of vestibular inputs to 30/100 - Increase use of somatosensory inputs to 75/100	Somatosensory and vestibular stimulation*
Static postural sway	- Excessive sway—2 standard deviations outside normal range for age	- Standing sway WNL for age	COG control training
Nudge/push test	- No use of ankle or hip strategy - Steps immediately	- Survives 5/10 pushes with hip strategy	Hip strategy exercises*
Limit-of-Stability (LOS)	- No ankle strategy—all hip - Sway to 45% LOS anterior, 35% LOS posterior, - Slow movement time	- Uses ankle strategy to reach 40% LOS ant/post - Reaches 8/8 targets at 75% LOS using hip or ankle within 4 sec.	Ankle strategy exercises* COG control training
R.O.M.	↓ neck ext 0-10° ↓ lumbar ext 0-15° ↓ hip ext 0-5°	↑ spinal extension neck 0-20° lumbar 0-20° ↑ hip ext 0-10°	ROM exercises*
Strength	Flex 4/5 (B) Hip Abd 3⁺/5, Ext 3/5 (B) Knee Ext 4⁺/5, Flex 4/5 (R) Ankle DF 3⁻/5 (L) Ankle DF 2/5, (B) Ankle PF 3⁺/5	↑ (B) hip abd/ext to 4/5 ↑ (B) ankle DF to 4⁻/5	Progressive resistive exercises, including bicycle*
Gait (GARS)	- Score 25/51 - Deviations-forward flexed trunk -double stance bilaterally prolonged -short step length	- GARS Scales 35/51 - (I) amb with walker in home/ community	Gait training* 1-starts, stops, turns 2-treadmill 3-uneven surfaces, curbs, stairs, carpet, outdoors
Endurance	- Fatigue after ambulating 60'	- Ambulates >200' without stopping	Gait training as above
Tinetti Balance Scale	- 6/16 score	Tinetti Balance score 10/16	Gait training as above
Tinetti Gait Scale	- 5/12 score - Falls and catches self	Tinetti Gait score 8/12	Gait training as above

*Also included in Home Exercise program
Reprinted with permission from NeuroCom International, Inc.

task demands, but may initially have limited experience to know how to solve a motor problem and limited physical ability to modify movements.

The clinician must also ask what **motor learning stage** the client is in for different tasks. Skill acquisition is the first stage. The objective is for the client just to "get the idea of the movement[11]," to begin to acquire the skill. In this stage, errors are frequent, and performance is inefficient and inconsistent. Within the nervous system, only temporary

changes are occurring. Skill refinement is the second stage. The goal is for the client to improve the performance, reducing the number and size of the errors, and increasing the consistency and efficiency of the movements. Skill retention is the final stage. The ability to perform the movements and achieve the functional goal has been accomplished, and the new objective is to retain the skill (across time) and transfer the skill to different settings. Retention and transfer are the hallmarks of true learning,

Table 28-7. An example of how treatment planning flows from test results in a client with right hemiparesis

Patient Profile:
- 69-year-old woman
- DX: Left CVA with right hemiparesis
- Acute Rehabilitation → Home Health → Outpatient Rehab

Test	Problems identified	Goals set	Treatment plan
Peripheral somatosensory	None		
Sensory Organization Test	- Average overall stability 47/100 - Absent use of vestibular inputs 0/100	- Average stability 60/100 - ↑ use of vestibular inputs 15/100	Vestibular stimulation with forced use and head movements
Postural sway			COG control training
—Functional reach	- Forward lean restricted to 5 inches	- Able to reach forward 8 in	
—Static	- Weigh shift asymmetry to left in static standing and medial/lateral sway, 25% LOS to left of midline	↑ control of COG: • Stands midline • ↑ forward LOS to 50% • ↑ right LOS to 50% • ↓ extraneous sway scores by 50%	
—Limit of stability	- Forward weight shift restricted to 25% LOS		
—Rhythmic weight shift	- Extraneous sway off desired path		
OLST	- Unable on right leg - 30 seconds on left leg	- Stands on left leg 10 sec	COG control training
Nudge/push (motor strategy selection)	- Switch from ankle to hip strategy noted but unable to withstand perturbation	- Able to stand upright after mild perturbations 5/10X - Able to "catch" self by stepping/reaching 5/10X	Hip and stepping strategy training
ROM	None		
Strength: right leg	4/5 Knee ext 3/5 Knee flex 2/5 Ankle dorsiflx 3/5 Ankle plantarflx	↑ R.LE strength • 5/5 Knee • 4/5 Ankle	Progressive resistive exercises
Endurance	Standing tolerance less than 10 minutes	- Able to stand unaided for 15 minutes	Standing tolerance tasks
Gait	- ↓ step length—R.LE - ↓ step height—R.LE - ↓ heel strike—R.LE - ↓ toe off—R.LE	- Symmetrical step height and length 5/10X - ↑ Heel strike R.LE 5/10X	Gait training on treadmill

Tinetti Gait Scale	4/12 score
	Unable to turn, reach or bend without loss of balance
	Falls: uneven surfaces
	    low lighting
	    head turning
	No community ambulation
	Requires cane
	Requires supervision for household ambulation
		8/12 score
		No falls
		Gait independent without cane in household; with cane in community
			Gait training on uneven surfaces, with head movements, with low lighting
			Safety education

where some relatively permanent changes have occurred within the nervous system. A client may have attained the skill retention phase for sitting balance tasks, be in the skill refinement stage for standing balance tasks, and in the skill acquisition stage for locomotor balance tasks.

Therapists use practice and feedback to teach motor skills. Repetition is necessary to develop skill; feedback is necessary to detect and correct errors. During skill acquisition, frequent repetition of a movement or task and frequent feedback are beneficial to help the client begin to be able to

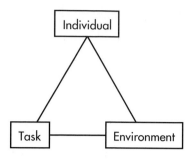

Fig. 28-22. Interactions of the individual, the environment, and the task are critical to postural control skills. Although they may be isolated in the mind of the clinician for assessment purposes, they are never isolated in the function of the client.

perform the desired movements and tasks. As the client progresses to the skill refinement stage (the clinician observes reduced errors and less variable performance), however, then practice should be varied and feedback briefly delayed. For example the task of standing and reaching to one side to take an object from the therapist might initially be repeated to the same side and at the same height several times. Then the therapist should begin to gradually vary the task demands: reach farther, or faster; take different objects of various weights, shapes, and sizes; and take the object from higher and lower heights and reach to right and left sides alternately. This variation introduces a problem-solving demand for the client: modifications in timing, force, sequencing, etc. are now necessary.

Feedback, which is especially helpful for those with sensory reception or perception problems, initially may contain information to assist the client in detecting errors about the goal achievement (knowledge of results, i.e., "you did not lean far enough to reach this last time") or about a movement error (knowledge of performance, i.e., "you did not straighten your knee enough last time"). Early feedback also may contain cues about what to do better next time, such as "straighten your knee before you shift weight onto that leg." If feedback is always provided by an external source, such as the therapist, a mirror, or a computer monitor, then the client is not given the opportunity to develop internal error detection/error correction mechanisms and will not be as likely to retain or transfer the skill. By delaying the feedback and asking the client to estimate or describe their own errors, and afterward providing the feedback, clients are allowed to compare their own developing internal frame of reference with the (correct) external frame of reference. By asking clients to suggest what might be done to correct the errors, the error correction process shifts from the external source to the clients, supporting motor problem-solving processes. As clients progress to the skill retention level, variations should increase (including task and environmental demands) and feedback delays should be longer. The clinician must develop a sense of how to therapeutically use practice variation and feedback delay to progress clients through the stages of motor learning. Too much variation and

too little feedback early on impedes skill acquisition; insufficient variation and excessive feedback later on hamper skill retention and transfer.

Task. Functional rating scales performed as a part of the evaluation yield information about what tasks, or functional activities, are limited by the postural control impairments. Bed mobility, sitting, sit-to-stand, transfers, standing, walking, working, and sports participation may be affected. Repeating the problematic tasks over and over is one approach; however, it is far more productive for the clinician to analyze the tasks to determine what postural control demands are placed on the client when undertaking that task. Does the task demand predominantly stability? Mobility? Both? For example standing to take a photograph demands the ability to hold still, standing to move laundry from the washer to the dryer requires weight-shifting, and standing to don a pair of pantyhose calls for both steadiness and movement. All three are standing tasks, but each places different postural control demands on the client. By using task analysis, the therapist may consciously select or design tasks to place specific demands on the client such that the postural control systems that need improvement will be challenged to respond.

Analysis of mobility tasks includes attention to timing, force, and duration of movements. Consider the different timing demands for weight-shifting and reaching to (1) catch an item falling from a shelf, (2) take a hot casserole out of the oven, or (3) open a door. Compare the different amounts of force necessary to pick up a heavy suitcase, pick up a baby from a crib, or replace a ceiling lightbulb. The duration of a balance demand may be brief, as in recovering from a trip, or extended, as in walking across an icy parking lot. Clinicians should choose tasks that vary these parameters to prepare clients for activities with various mobility demands.

Therapists also need to consider whether the elements of the task are predictable or unpredictable. In other words will the postural control demand be a voluntary movement (sweeping the porch), an automatic postural response (missing the last step on a flight of stairs), or an anticipatory postural preparation (preceding a lift, for example)? Clients need to learn to respond in all three conditions, which are often combined. For instance, lifting is a voluntary movement. Predicting the load to be lifted leads to anticipatory postural preparation. Counteracting the destabilizing force of a greater-than-predicted load requires an automatic postural response. If, during therapy, the clinician says "don't let me push you" before nudging the client, the demand is for anticipatory postural preparation. If the disturbance is provided without warning, the demand calls for automatic postural reactions. If the clinician requests a lean to the right, that is a voluntary postural adjustment.

Environment. Just as tasks can be purposefully selected to promote postural control responses, environmental conditions also must be included in the design of the therapy plan to stimulate the necessary systems. Gravity cannot be manipulated by the clinician, but the client needs to learn to counteract it at different speeds and from different positions, among other things. Familiarity with how gravity can aid movement, as in walking, is also important. The surface conditions can be varied by the therapist. They may be stable, even, and predictable (hospital hallway, sidewalk), unstable (boat, subway, gravel driveway), uneven (grass, curbs, stairs), or compliant (beach, padded carpeting). Visual conditions also may be manipulated. Visual cues may be available and accurate (daylight, florescent lighting), unavailable (darkness or poor lighting, or lack of environmental cues such as a busy carpet pattern on a stairway), unstable (moving crowd, public transportation), used for purposes other than balance (fixation on a ball in tennis), or dependent on head movements. Clinicians should help prepare their clients to function in the real world by training them to maintain balance under different combinations of surface and visual conditions. This includes situations where cues from the environment agree, i.e., visual, somatosensory, and vestibular inputs are all sending the same message, so to speak, as well as in sensory conflict environments, where cues from one system may disagree (not match) cues from the other sensory systems. Functional situations where sensory conflicts may exist include elevators, escalators, people movers, airplanes, and subways.

Treatment progressions

To treat each problem that may contribute to a balance disorder individually would not be practical. The therapist must address several problems at a time, not just for efficiency, but because these systems should be able to function together to perform functional activities in real-world environments. Treatment then, is multiimpairment oriented, with tasks and environments selected to stimulate involved or compensatory systems.

Sensory systems. In general the less sensory information available, the more difficult the task of balancing. A treatment progression then, might start with full sensory inputs (vision, somatosensory, and vestibular = 3/3) available in the environment, and perhaps augmented feedback if intrinsic sensory channels are deficient. Challenge is added by manipulating either visual or somatosensory inputs, so that equilibrium must be maintained using only 2/3 senses (vision and vestibular, or somatosensory and vestibular). If both vision and somatosensory inputs are manipulated, then only the vestibular inputs are a reliable source of sensory information, and balance is accomplished with only 1/3 senses. High-level clients may even tolerate the addition of eye and head movements, challenging the vestibular system further.

To stimulate the use of somatosensory inputs, environments are designed to disadvantage vision while providing reliable somatosensory inputs (stable surfaces). Having the client close the eyes, or practice in low lighting or darkness, removes visual inputs. Vision can be destabilized by

requiring head and eye movements during the balance task (catching/passing a ball, reading) or by practice in a moving visual environment (crowded hallway, optokinetic stimulation with moving lights, moving striped curtains, sliding wall stripes, or moving visual surrounds).

To stimulate the use of visual inputs, environments are designed to disadvantage somatosensation while providing reliable visual cues (stable visual field with landmarks). Somatosensation cannot be removed like vision, but it can be destabilized by sitting/standing on unstable surfaces (rocker board, BAPS board, randomly moving platforms), or confused by sitting/standing on compliant surfaces that "give way" to pressure, such as foam, space boots, responsively moving platforms.

To stimulate the use of vestibular inputs, environments are designed to disadvantage both vision and somatosensation while providing reliable vestibular cues (detectable head position). Practicing on unstable or compliant surfaces, with vision either absent (eyes closed), destabilized (eye movements), or confused (i.e., optokinetic stimulation) provides challenging combinations. Difficulty can be increased by adding neck extension and rotation to place the vestibular organ at a disadvantaged angle. Vestibular habituation exercises involve repeated head movements in the directions that provoke dizziness, with increasing speed and number of repetitions to continue to provoke the system.

Remember that each sensory system has two peripheral receptors. In cases where the sensory loss is unilateral and permanent, the other side should be stimulated to compensate for the loss. If the sensory loss is unilateral and temporary, however, the other side should be placed (temporarily), when possible, at a disadvantage to force reliance on the underused side. As the affected side improves, integration of the two sides and the three systems is the desired outcome.

Many neurological clients have temporary difficulty with head control early on in their recovery, and others have chronic head control problems. Their ability to properly orient the vestibular organs, eyes, and neck proprioceptors is impaired, which negatively affects the ability to perceive internal and environmental cues that could assist in balance maintenance. Clients with spasticity or contractures of the ankles and feet who cannot place their feet in full contact with the floor are not only at a biomechanical disadvantage, but also have difficulty receiving somatosensory inputs that could support postural control processes. The more accurate and reliable sensory information available, the greater the chances that the sensory-perceptual processes that contribute to balance can fulfill their role. Treatment progressions should include attention to increasing the client's ability to receive and process sensory information pertinent to balance control, through ocular motor, head, and peripheral limb positioning and movement.

Control of the center of gravity. Effective control of the COG depends on biomechanical and musculoskeletal systems. Trunk and head control abilities are primary. For clients with paralysis or degenerative disease, which limit the ability of arms and legs to assist with postural stability, head and trunk control may be the dominant means of balance. Both the head/neck and trunk need to be able to (1) achieve and hold a midline position, (2) rotate around this midline axis, and (3) move away from and return to the midline without loss of balance. The term *midline* here refers not to a line between right and left sides, but to a point where right/left and forward/backward components are centered in all planes—medial/lateral, anterior/posterior, rotary, and sidebending (shortening/elongation on either side).

Sitting balance. In sitting, the pelvis and posterior thighs form the primary base of support, with additional stability provided by the feet in contact with the floor. The axis of anteroposterior movement rotates around the greater trochanter, and forward/backward leans are achieved via pelvis and trunk movement. Anterior pelvic tilt with upper trunk extension allows forward reaching and begins the sit-to-stand transition. Lateral weight shifts with trunk elongation precede right/left reaching and scooting. Lateral weight shifts with trunk rotation permit cross-midline reaching and begin the sit-to-supine progression. The use of arms to prop in sitting is an extension of the base of support.

In standing, the feet form the base of support. The axis of anteroposterior movement rotates around the medial malleolus. Weight shifts move the COG through space for reaching and lifting tasks as well as in preparation for stepping. Ankle strategy is most effective for movement of the COG through the limits of stability. As the COG nears the sway boundary, hip strategy works to restrict its travel. If this fails, stepping or reaching strategies are used to reestablish a new base of support. During gait, the COG follows a sinusoidal path as forward progression of the body mass combines with alternating lateral weight shifts to the stance foot (Fig. 28-23).[23] Each step creates a new base of support. Assistive devices such as canes, walkers, and crutches extend the base of support and thus reduce the demands on the intrinsic balance control system. In sitting, standing, and walking, control of the COG involves the ability to establish a stable base of support and to transfer weight over it. Treatment progressions for COG control, then involve, training to establish, maintain, and reduce the base of support and to produce automatic, anticipatory, and voluntary postural responses to restrict or produce weight shifts.

Early treatment progression for COG control includes neurodevelopmental sequence activities (e.g., prone on elbows, all-fours, kneeling, right/left sidesitting, half kneeling), not for the purpose of "reflex development" in the traditional sense, but because the tasks are to balance with progressively less surface contact, i.e., shrinking the base of support. It also is useful for simultaneously addressing impairments such as lower extremity extensor tone, trunk weakness and asymmetries, and head/neck extensor weak-

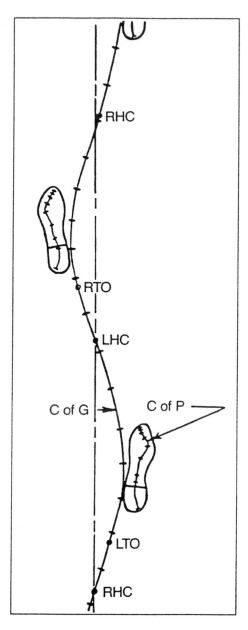

Fig. 28-23. The trajectory of the center of gravity (COG) and the center of pressure (COP) during a gait cycle. (RHC, right heel contact; RTO, right toe off; LHC, left heel contact, LTO, left toe off). (Reprinted from Patla AE and others: In Duncan P: *Balance: proceedings of the APTA forum,* Alexandria, VA, 1990, American Physical Therapy Association.)

ness. Functionally, bed mobility and floor-to-stand transfers are related to neurodevelopmental sequence exercises and should be practiced concurrently in low and high level clients, respectively.

Sitting balance can be progressed by removing upper extremity support (hands on firm surface—moveable surface, i.e., ball, bolster, rolling stool—one hand free—both hands free), making the seating surface less stable (mat - bed - rocker board - Swiss ball), for example, removing the use of one foot by crossing the leg or of both feet by raising the height of the seat so they do not touch the floor. Tasks might include multidirectional weight shifts with the hands in contact with a bolster or ball, which is pushed/pulled to and fro, reaching or passing objects, upper body tasks (grooming, dressing), and managing socks/shoes and wheelchair armrests/footrests, etc.

Sit-to-stand and transfer balance. Transitional movements such as sit-to-stand and transfers involve large COG excursions over a stable base of support. For sit-to-stand, the base of support must change from the seat to the feet. The feet begin to accept the weight first by downward pressure through the heels as the pelvis rolls anteriorly. The weight moves to the front of the feet as the trunk comes forward and the pelvis lifts from the surface, then backward toward midline as the trunk extends into standing. The COG stays near midline if both legs are participating equally, but will often deviate to a preferred side during the transition in clients with hemiplegia. Training should include disadvantaging the preferred leg (perhaps by moving it a bit forward) to allow the more affected leg and foot to experience the weight transference. During transfers a lateral weight shift is required in addition to the partial stand. The COG does not remain near midline, but instead moves forward to load the feet, then laterally toward the side of the transfer. Progression of balance skills in sit-to-stand and transfer tasks may involve gradually lowering the height of the surface, removing arm rests to preclude upper extremity assist, transfers to surfaces of different heights and firmnesses, etc. Remember that velocity is a normal part of sit-to-stand movements, as the momentum is used to assist the weight transfer from seat to feet, so the clinician must allow some speed during this task. If the client is unsteady upon arising (cannot dampen or slow the speed in a controlled manner), working gradually from stand-to-sit initially may be beneficial before progression to sit-to-stand.

Standing balance. Standing balance tasks also can begin with finding midline and becoming stable there. Controlled mobility (volitional) should be encouraged as soon as possible, at first on a stable surface with slow, small weight shifts. Challenge is added by increasing the distance traveled away from midline, moving toward restricted regions of the limits of stability, altering speed of sway, adding combined upper extremity activities (e.g., dribbling a basketball, reaching), adding resistance (manual, theraband), etc. Narrowing the base of support (Romberg, tandem, single leg) makes control of the COG more demanding. Placing the feet in a diagonal stride position is more desirable for pregait weight shifting than symmetrical double stance. Attention should be given to the stance (loading) leg regarding pelvic protraction, hip and knee extension, and ankle dorsiflexion, with the tibia traveling forward over the foot. Focus on the swing (unloading) leg should include pelvic drop with knee

flexion as the heel comes up and pressure through the ball of the foot and toes to maximally load the opposite leg. Standing balance exercises can be made more difficult by training on a less stable surface (carpet, foam, rocker board, BAPS board) and by adding combined head/eye movements tasks or closing the eyes. The goals for dynamic sitting and standing balance exercises are to increase the size and symmetry of the limits of stability and improve the ability to transfer weight to different body segments with control at different speeds and with varied amounts of force.

Strategy training. Training ankle, hip, and stepping strategies begins in a voluntary manner, but must progress to an automatic level of use to develop more normal balance and to prevent loss of balance. Before strategy training, the clinician should be sure that the client has the ability to develop the desired strategy(ies). The observed dominance of other strategies is appropriately compensatory, not dysfunctional, if a missing strategy cannot be effectively executed. Clients use these strategies to prevent loss of balance, so the clinician must take care not to reduce reliance on an effective strategy, but to add additional strategies to the repertoire.

Ankle strategy should be practiced on a firm, broad surface. Clients can be asked to sway slowly in anterior/posterior, right/left, and diagonal directions, first to and from midline, progressing to passing midline, and finally progressing to sway toward the periphery without return to midline. Head and pelvis should be traveling in the same direction at the same time. Clients can practice standing near a wall with a table in front of them, swaying forward to touch the table with their stomach (leading with the pelvis) and backward to touch the wall with the back of their head. Cues are given not to "bow" to the table and not to touch the wall with the buttocks. As soon as the client begins to be able to perform this protocol, functional meaning should be added with maneuvers such as forward or lateral reaching tasks, hands-over-head to take things off shelves, and leaning backward to rinse hair in the shower. To improve anticipatory and automatic ankle strategy use, add slight perturbations to the body or the surface when midline, progress to gentle perturbation when away from midline, and finally progress from predictable to unpredictable perturbations.

Hip strategy is practiced on a narrow surface, such as standing sideways on a balance beam or a half-slice foam roller, or an unstable surface such as foam or a rocker board. The head and pelvis travel in opposite directions to counterbalance each other, in a forward bow/backward bending motion for anterior/posterior sway. Rapid sway is requested in forward/backward, right/left, and diagonal directions. Using the wall and table setting mentioned previously, clients can be cued to bow to touch the nose toward the table while simultaneously touching the wall with the buttocks. Lateral hip strategy can be trained similarly, with the client standing sideways to the wall, touching the

CASE 1 ▼ Andy

Andy is a 27-year-old man who sustained a severe closed-head injury in a skiing accident. He was hospitalized for 2 months, and at a long-term care facility for 6 months, before cranial surgery for removal of bilateral subdural hygromas and revision of a ventriculo-peritoneal shunt. Postsurgically, he demonstrated marked improvement and was transferred to a rehabilitation unit. His initial physical therapy assessment revealed the following impairments, which had a negative effect on postural control: (1) oculomotor deficits (difficulty tracking to the right and upward); (2) disorientation; (3) very delayed and slow responses; (4) bilateral ankle plantar-flexion contractures (−10 degrees left, −15 degrees right); limited right shoulder flexion (0 to 100 degrees) and external rotation (0-20 degrees); (5) hypotonic trunk (right, moderate; left, mild), hypertonic (extensor) lower extremities (right, moderate; left, mild), hypertonic right upper extremity, mild; (6) fair head control; (7) poor trunk control with right scapular atrophy, shortened right side, strength 3−/5; (8) left upper and lower extremity movement isolated and coordinated but slow, strength 4/5 at shoulder, 4+/5 elbow/wrist/hand, 4/5 hip and knee, 3+/5 ankle, able to place and hold for weight bearing; (9) right upper extremity rests and moves in synergistic pattern but can move out of synergy with request or demonstration, strength 3−/5 at shoulder and 4−/5 distally, coordination is poor, can place and hold for weight bearing if cued but not spontaneously; (10) left lower extremity moves in flexor/extensor pattern, grossly 3+/5 in hip and knee flexion, 2+ hip extension, 3+/5 knee extension, no isolated ankle movement, cannot place or hold for weight-bearing. Functional tests found the following disabilities: (1) minimum assist supine to sit; (2) sitting balance, poor; (3) moderate assistance sit-to-stand; (4) standing balance, unable; (5) moderate assist transfers; (6) nonambulatory.

Impairment goals were the following: (1) increase range of motion to within normal limits (WNL) throughout; (2) increase trunk tone to normal and strength to 4+/5; (3) decrease right-sided tone to normal; (4) increase spontaneous use, isolated movement and strength (4+/5) in right extremities; (5) able to place and weight bear on right lower extremity. Short-term functional goals were the following: (1) independent in all bed mobility, (2) independent in wheelchair transfers, (3) good static and fair dynamic sitting balance,

(4) contactguard sit-to-stand, and (5) minimum assist static standing balance. Ambulation goals were temporarily deferred due to the ankle contractures and balance deficits.

Early treatments included (1) standing frame activities for head control, visual tracking, trunk control, reduced lower extremity extensor tone, and heelcord stretching with ultrasound; (2) neurodevelopmental sequence activities for head and trunk control, trunk strengthening, decreased lower extremity extensor tone, balance on all fours/heel-sitting/kneeling; (3) supine to-and-from sitting, especially over the right arm; (4) sitting balance with upper extremity functional tasks (e.g., putting glasses on/off, taking shirt off/on, wiping nose with tissue), with focus on right visual tracking, right trunk elongation, and incorporation of right lower extremity ground pressure for stability; (5) transfer training with incorporation of right upper extremity to push up, reach and grasp, and right lower extremity placing and weight bearing.

As soon as Andy's ankle dorsiflexion range of motion was near neutral on the right (was then 0 to 5 degrees on the left), neurodevelopmental activities were phased out and standing balance and pregait activities in the parallel bars were initiated with moderate assistance. He rapidly progressed to minimum assistance gait in the parallel bars, but with significant scissoring of the lower extremities. Gait outside the bars was begun with a quad cane on the left, but Andy was not able to organize the sequence for cane use and did not use it when loss of balance occurred, so it was discontinued. Gait without assistive device required moderate assistance from the therapist for balance. A line drawn on the floor provided a visual cue to remind him to keep his feet apart; when walking without this cue about 25% of his steps were close or crossed.

At discharge, 2 months after admission, Andy had good visual tracking; normal range of motion with the exception of right lower extremity dorsiflexion, which was limited to 0 to 5 degrees; normal tone in the left extremities; mildly increased tone in the right extremities with slight extensor patterning in the leg; good head and trunk control; and strength grossly 4+/5 throughout. Functionally, he was independent in bed mobility, wheelchair mobility, and sitting balance. He required supervision for safety in transfers and standing activities and minimum to moderate assistance for indoor ambulation without an assistive device, depending on his fatigue level.

---

table with one hip and the wall with the opposite shoulder. Sway close to the edge of the client's limit of stability should produce a shift from ankle to hip strategy, so to enhance the use of hip strategy, the client should practice sway control as far away from midline as possible without stepping. As soon as the client demonstrates the ability to perform this strategy, incorporate it into functional tasks such as low reaching (e.g., trunk of car, laundry dryer). To promote anticipatory and automatic use of hip strategy, begin with the client in midline and give moderate, rapid perturbations to the body or the surface such that ankle strategy will be insufficient to

counteract the force. Progress by increasing the size of the disturbance, and by having the client away from midline when the perturbation is given so that righting to midline is appropriate. Shift from predictable ("Don't let me make you step or fall") to unpredictable perturbations.

Stepping strategy can be practiced first from atop a step, curb, or balance beam. Both legs should be included in training, as real life situations such as a slip or trip often preclude the use of one limb and demand the use of the other. Progress to stepping on a level surface and then to stepping up onto a step or curb or over progressively larger obstacles

CASE 2   Doris

Doris is a 73-year-old woman with a long history of Parkinson's disease who had fallen four times within the 6 months before referral to physical therapy. As a result of her most recent fall, during which she hit her head, Doris developed ear pounding, light-headedness, and headaches. After referral to an otolaryngologist, she was diagnosed with unspecified peripheral vestibular dysfunction and referred to outpatient therapy. Her therapist found that Doris complained of increased light-headedness and dizziness, with anterior/posterior head movements, rolling in bed, sit-to-stand, and the Hallpike maneuver (worse to the right). Multiple impairments that could be contributing to her instability and falls, as well as symptoms related to the vestibular disorder, were also noted. Doris had mildly decreased range of motion in her left ankle, shoulders, and neck; mild left-sided weakness and lack of coordination; marked bilateral upper extremity tremor, and moderate forward flexed posture. She could not perform an ankle strategy at all and used hip strategy continually; she also used stepping strategy frequently with the least shift or sway. Static postural sway tests indicated that Doris had excessive sway when attempting to stand still, and that she kept her COG slightly posterior and to the right of midline. Sway increased tenfold with eyes closed. Doris could not perform repeated weight shifts in either anterior/posterior or medial/lateral directions. Her limits of stability were severely restricted to less than half of normal sway range anteriorly, and her movement time was very slow.

Functional testing revealed that Doris had several disabilities. She had to use a walker or have manual assistance to ambulate and could negotiate level surfaces only. Without her walker or handhold assistance, Doris could stand for less than 30 seconds and take a maximum of 10 steps. For community ambulation, Doris needed minimum assistance with her walker and could go only very short distances. She also required minimum assistance with bathing and home-making tasks.

Doris participated in therapy twice a week for 6 weeks and also performed a home exercise program daily. Her treatment plan included vestibular habituation exercises for the dizziness and balance retraining exercises for instability and falls. The habituation exercises she was given were designed to repeatedly provoke her symptoms, and included head turning in supine and sitting (progressed to standing), rolling in bed, rocking in a rocking chair, and sit-to-stand practice. As her dizziness subsided, her home program was modified to increase the number and rate of head movements. To improve her use of somatosensory and vestibular inputs, Doris also practiced standing on a firm surface with eyes closed (with family supervision). In the clinic, Doris did stretching, strengthening, and postural extension exercises to address her musculoskeletal limitations. Using postural sway biofeedback, she practiced achieving the midline position, controlled anterior and left-sided weight shifts at progressively faster speeds, and ankle strategy. Gait training included starts, stops, turns, and obstacle avoidance and progressed to community ambulation tasks such as curbs and ramps.

Despite her multiple problems, Doris was able to reduce the severity of her impairments and consequently improve her functional level. Her dizziness resolved completely. Although she still had excess sway during static standing, she was able to achieve and hold a midline position, and her sway with eyes closed reduced by more than half. Doris could weight shift in both anterior/posterior and medial/lateral directions at moderate speeds using ankle strategy, without stepping. Her limits of stability were expanded from 35% to 80% of normal, and she was able to shift much more quickly. Functionally, she could stand without the walker for 8 minutes and walk independently indoors on level surfaces without the walker for short distances. She was independent in community ambulation with the walker. At a 3-month follow-up visit, Doris reported that she had no further falls.

(appliance cord, shoe, phone book). All directions should be practiced. Large, rapid perturbations are given such that ankle and hip strategies will be inadequate and stepping/reaching is demanded. Progress from predicted to unpredictable disturbances.

Gait training. The initial focus for controlling the COG during gait is a stable base of support that can continually be reestablished quickly and reliably through stepping. Begin first in the forward direction, but also include backward and sideways directions (sidestepping, braiding, or hariolation). Challenge can be added by narrowing the base of support (tandem) or reducing the foot/surface contact (walk on toes or heels). Unlike standing balance, where the base is stable and the COG moves over it, during locomotion the base is moving and the COG moves to stay over the base. Achieving a symmetrical, smoothly oscillating COG movement is the objective, with the forces of

gravity and momentum being exploited. Speed assists in this process; excessively slow gait cannot take advantage of these forces. Treadmill training is gaining in popularity with neurological patients as the increased speed reduces some abnormal asymmetrics.[24] Training to integrate postural control with locomotor skills is best accomplished not through continuous, steady pace walking, but by starting, stopping, turning, bending, varying the speed, and avoiding or stepping over obstacles. Difficulty is added by increasing the abruptness, frequency, and unpredictability of these types of tasks and by adding tasks such as carrying or reading while walking. Altered surface conditions (carpets, ramps, curbs, stairs, grass, gravel) or reduced lighting conditions also heightens the challenge. Head and eye movements while walking should be added as the client improves. Walking quickly while reading signs on the wall or room numbers, for example, or looking toward and away from the therapist while walking makes it more difficult to use vision for stability. Walking in crowds or busy, cluttered environments is also challenging.

Other considerations

Treatment tools. Therapists use both high-tech and low-tech equipment in the remediation of balance deficits; each has advantages and disadvantages. High-tech options include forceplate systems with postural sway biofeedback, electromyographic (EMG) biofeedback, optokinetic visual stimulation (from visual surround or moving lights), video-taping, and treadmills. Computerized systems allow advanced monitoring of progress and biofeedback, which supports motor learning. Motorized systems provide the ability to manipulate the environment easily and efficiently and to safely graduate tasks and environmental challenges. Drawbacks to high-tech equipment include cost, space requirements, and operator training requirements. Low-tech options include mirrors, soft foam pads, hard foam rollers, rocker boards, BAPS boards, tilt boards, Swiss balls, minitrampolines, and wedges/incline boards. All of these items are accessible (low cost, easy to obtain), portable, and easy to use. They do not provide novel feedback, objective scoring, or graphic recording; and clinicians must be skilled and creative in their use for appropriate gradation of task difficulty and environmental conditions.

Safety education and environmental modifications. It is not always possible to remediate balance deficits, but it is the clinician's responsibility to ensure the safety of each client. When permanent deficits exist, the client and the family should be taught in what environments the client is at risk (i.e., a client with vestibular loss on a gravel driveway at night), what tasks are unsafe (e.g., ladder-climbing, changing ceiling light bulbs), how the client can compensate (use a cane at night or in crowds), and what changes in the home or workplace are needed (e.g., night lights, stair-stripes). Clinicians can ask the client (or family) to problem solve risky situations: What would they do? Home evaluations should be followed by a recommendation list of safety modifications. Falls are frightening and dangerous; clinicians should do their utmost to see that they do not occur. If falls are likely, clients and families should be taught what to do if a fall occurs, including floor-to-stand or floor-to-furniture transfers. Home monitoring services such as LifeLine may be indicated if the client lives alone and is prone to fall.

Home programs. Many balance exercises can (and should) be performed at home if safety and compliance can be ensured; however, unstable clients should always be supervised. Many standing tasks can be completed in a corner or near a countertop so that no other person is needed. The community setting is ideal for postural control training. Grocery or library aisles, public transportation, elevators, escalators, grass, sandboxes or beaches, ramps, trails, hills, and varied environmental conditions in general provide both challenge and functional relevance.

ACKNOWLEDGEMENT

Thanks to Kenda Fuller, PT, NCS; Janet Helminski, MS, PT, Linda Horn, PT, NCS, and Pat Huston, MS, PT, for their significant contributions to the development of this chapter. Gratitude is also extended to Darcy Umphred, PhD, PT, and David Ginsburg for their patience and support.

REFERENCES

1. Barnes ML and others: *Reflex and vestibular aspects of motor control, motor development, and motor learning,* Atlanta, 1990, Stokesville Publishing Co.
2. Berg K and others: Measuring balance in the elderly: preliminary development of an instrument, *Physiother Can* 41:304, 1989.
3. Bobath B: *Adult hemiplegia: evaluation and treatment,* ed 2, London, 1978, William Heinemann Medical Books.
4. Chandler J and Duncan P: Balance and falls in the elderly, issues in evaluation and treatment. In Guccione A, editor: *Geriatric physical therapy,* St Louis, 1993, Mosby.
5. Charness A: *Stroke/head injury: a guide to functional outcomes in physical therapy management,* Rockville, Md, 1986, Aspen Publications.
6. Cordo P and Nashner L: Properties of postural adjustments associated with rapid arm movements, *J Neurophysiol* 47:287, 1982.
7. Cromwell S and Held J: Test-retest reliability of three balance measures used with hemiplegic patients, *Neurol Rep* 17:24, 1994.
8. DiFabio RP and Badke MB: Relationship of sensory organization to balance function in patients with hemiplegia, *Phys Ther* 70:20, 1990.
9. Duncan P and others: Is there one simple measure for balance? *PT Magazine,* 1:74, 1993.
10. Flores AM: Objective measurement of standing balance, *Neurol Rep* 16:17, 1992.
11. Gentile AM: A working model of skill acquisition with application to teaching, *Quest,* 17:3, 1972.
12. Herdman S: *Vestibular rehabilitation,* Philadelphia, 1994, FA Davis.
13. Horak F, Shupert C, and Mirka A: Components of postural dyscontrol in the elderly: a review, *Neurobiol Aging* 10:727, 1989.
14. Horak F: Clinical measurement of postural control in adults, *Phys Ther* 67:1881, 1987.
15. Ingersoll C and Armstrong C: The effects of closed head injury on postural sway, *Med Sci Sports Exerc* 24:739, 1992.
16. Knott M and Voss D: *Proprioceptive neuromuscular facilitation: patterns and techniques,* ed 2, New York, 1968, Harper and Row.
17. Mathias S, Nayak U, and Isaacs B: Balance in the elderly patient: the "Get Up and Go" test, *Arch Phys Med Rehabil* 67:387, 1986.
18. Moore S and Woollacott M: The use of biofeedback devices to improve postural stability, *Phys Ther Pract* 2:1, 1993.
19. Morris SL and Sharpe MH: PNF revisited, *Physiother Theory Practice* 9:43, 1993.
20. Nashner L: Evaluation of postural stability, movement, and control. In Hasson S, editor: *Clinical exercise physiology,* Philadelphia, 1994, Mosby.
21. Nashner L: Sensory, neuromuscular, and biomechanical contributions to human balance. In Duncan P, editor: *Balance: proceedings of the APTA forum,* Alexandria, Va, 1990, American Physical Therapy Association.
22. Newton R: Review of tests of standing balance abilities, *Brain Inj* 3:335, 1989.
23. Patla AE and others: Identification of age-related changes in the balance control system. In Duncan P: *Balance: proceedings of the APTA forum,* Alexandria, Va, 1990, American Physical Therapy Association.
24. Rose DK and Guiliani CA: A comparison of overground walking and treadmill walking in patients with cerebral vascular lesion, *Neurol Rep* 17:23, 1993.
25. Schenkman M and Butler RB: A model for multisystem evaluation, interpretation, and treatment of individuals with neurologic dysfunction, *Phys Ther* 69:538, 1989.

26. Schmidt R: *Motor control and learning: a behavioral emphasis,* ed 2, Champagne, Ill, 1988, Human Kinetics.

27. Sherrington C: *The integrative action of the nervous system,* New Haven, 1961, Yale University Press.

28. Shumway-Cook A and Horak F: Vestibular Rehabilitation, unpublished course syllabus. 1991.

29. Shumway-Cook A and Horak F: Assessing the influence of sensory interaction on balance, *Phys Ther* 66:1548, 1986.

30. Shumway-Cook A and Horak F: Vestibular rehabilitation: an exercise approach to managing symptoms of vestibular dysfunction, *Semin Hearing* 10:194, 1986.

31. Speechley M and Tinetti M: Assessment of risk and prevention of falls among elderly persons, *Physiother Can* 42:75, 1990.

32. Tinetti M: Performance oriented assessment of mobility problems in elderly patients. *J Am Geriatr Soc* 41:479, 1986.

33. Van Sant AF: Should the normal motor developmental sequence be used as a theoretical model to progress adult patients? In Lister MJ, editor: *Contemporary management of motor control problems: proceedings of the II-STEP conference,* Alexandria, Va, 1991, Book-crafters.

34. Weber P, and Cass D: Clinical assessment of postural stability, *Am J Otol* 14:566, 1993.

35. Whipple R and Wolfson LI: Abnormalities of balance, gait, and sensorimotor function in the elderly population. In Duncan P: *Balance: proceedings of the APTA forum,* Alexandria, Va, 1990, American Physical Therapy Association.

CHAPTER 29

Electrodiagnosis in Neurological Dysfunction

Charlene M. Nelson

KEY TERMS

clinical electromyographical examination (EMG)
nerve conduction tests
evoked potential tests
reaction of degeneration (RD)

LEARNING OBJECTIVES

After reading this chapter the student/therapist will:
1. Identify electrodiagnostic tests used in neurological clients.
2. Describe general procedures for electrodiagnostic tests.
3. Recognize basic normal and abnormal findings of electrodiagnostic tests.
4. Discuss indications for electrodiagnostic tests in neurological clients.
5. Recognize the implications of findings of electrodiagnostic tests in planning and modifying treatment programs.
6. Appreciate the value of electrodiagnostic tests as part of overall client evaluation and management.

The goal of this chapter is to enhance the therapist's ability to recognize indications for the more commonly used electrodiagnostic tests and to integrate knowledge of these test indications and findings into the overall therapeutic management of clients with neuropathological dysfunction. To help the therapist attain this goal, the chapter presents a basic description of the electrophysiological tests and the neuroanatomical structures and functions involved in each test. Normal and abnormal test findings are discussed. The major emphasis is on explaining how knowledge of these

tests can assist the therapist in client evaluation, treatment program planning, and modification of treatment programs as follow-up test results are reviewed.

Rather than thinking of electrophysiological tests as a distinct and exclusive entity used by "others" for diagnostic evaluation, the therapist is encouraged to view these tests as both a basis for diagnosis and as useful adjuncts that can guide and enhance the logical planning and modification of treatment programs. In addition, having an informed perspective of the application of electrophysiological tests should benefit the therapist's interaction and communication with other members of the medical and health management community.

Most of the electrophysiological tests described here require application of an external electrical stimulus to a nerve or muscle, and observation and assessment of the muscle or nerve response. Exceptions are the **clinical electromyographical examination (EMG)** and the single-fiber electromyogram (SFEMG), which involve monitoring and recording the electrical activity produced by the muscle tissue, either while at rest or during muscle contraction.

Electrical tests commonly used at this time are motor and sensory nerve conduction tests, F-wave and H-reflex tests, repetitive stimulation, and somatosensory **evoked potential (SSEP) tests** and EMG. Another electrical test, which has been used in the past but is now rarely applied intentionally as a test, is the test for **reaction of degeneration (RD).**

Electrodiagnostic procedures are performed by physical therapists and other medical practitioners who have special education, training, and experience in the procedures. Several references at the end of the chapter should be useful to therapists with less experience with these procedures.

Before implementing electrodiagnostic examinations, a review of the client's history and a clarifying physical examination are invaluable. The clarifying examination should be directed toward evaluating those factors that will guide the examiner in planning the appropriate electrical tests and the sequence of test procedures. The client's neurological signs, muscle strength and tone, sensation, range of motion (ROM), and cognition are among the data important to the examiner in planning and administering electrical tests.

REACTION OF DEGENERATION TEST

Although the test for reaction of degeneration is infrequently used as a specific test, a brief description of its usefulness as a screening procedure is worthy of mention. Many therapists indirectly use a modified form of the RD test when they apply a neuromuscular electrical stimulator (NMES) to facilitate contraction of weak or paralyzed muscles. The standard, small, portable NMES units produce a relatively short duration electrical impulse (pulse), generally less than 0.5 msec in duration. These pulses are applied with a frequency and other predetermined parameters designed to produce controlled, physiological-like muscle contractions. For further description of NMES, see Chapter 30.

Recalling a fundamental feature of nerve and muscle electrophysiological response, an electrical stimulus applied to a motor nerve can result in muscle contraction only if the stimulus amplitude (strength or intensity) and duration meet minimal criteria. To evoke a muscle response, the duration of the stimulus pulse can be no shorter than the chronaxie value of the nerve supplying the muscle.[6,9,15] Rheobase (threshold) is the lowest amplitude of electrical stimulus required to produce a response in nerve or muscle when

using a pulse of long duration (over 100 msec). Chronaxie is the shortest pulse duration that can elicit a response when using a stimulus amplitude twice the rheobase value. Because the chronaxie of normal peripheral motor nerves is generally less than 0.5 msec, a stimulator with a pulse duration of 0.5 msec or less can produce an effective muscle contraction.

Chronaxie of muscle is considerably longer than that of nerve; therefore, a stimulator with a pulse duration longer than the muscle chronaxie is necessary to produce a contraction in a peripherally denervated muscle.[9] If a muscle contraction does not occur when using an NMES on a client with a weak or paralyzed muscle, the therapist must establish whether the technique of application should be modified, or if the muscle has a compromised peripheral innervation.

To determine whether the problem is procedural or in the equipment, the therapist should apply the stimulator to an uninvolved muscle, either on the same or another extremity. If a normal response is readily obtained from the uninvolved muscle, but no response is seen in the involved muscle, the therapist should suspect degeneration (a positive reaction of nerve degeneration) and decide whether further electrical testing is indicated. Muscles that are weak or paralyzed because of involvement of the central nervous system (CNS) should contract when the NMES is applied. This use of the NMES is similar to the first part of the traditional RD test.

Before development of nerve conduction testing and EMG, the part of the grossly qualitative RD test just described would be followed by a second part, i.e., application of a stimulus of infinitely long duration and assessment of the response of the muscle. The problem would then likely have been further evaluated using a strength duration test, which would provide somewhat more quantitative information on the electrical excitability of the muscle, namely, the chronaxie value, and a curve describing the interrelationship of the stimulus amplitude and duration.[6,15] Characteristics of this curve represent the status of the peripheral nerve supplying the muscle being tested. This may vary from normal innervation, partial degeneration or regeneration, to complete degeneration. The RD and strength duration tests have generally been replaced by the more objective nerve conduction and EMG tests; however, therapists should recognize the reason a response is not obtained and refer the client for electrodiagnosis.

NERVE CONDUCTION TESTS

A general overview of these tests is presented here to provide the reader with an understanding of their application and indications. For details of the techniques, many excellent texts are available.[12,14,16]

Motor and sensory nerve conduction tests (NCT) can provide data that are helpful in establishing the presence of pathological conditions in the peripheral nervous system (PNS). The tests may differentiate the anatomical level, such as a localized peripheral mononeuropathy, or a plexopathy.

In addition they may further localize the site of compromise, such as a median nerve compression at the wrist, a lesion of the lateral cord of the brachial plexus, or a cervical radiculopathy. The tests also are helpful in differentiating between lesions that primarily involve axonal degeneration and those that are primarily peripheral demyelination.[13,16] The severity or extent of the problem may be determined, e.g., a mild, localized compressive disorder of the myelin (neuropraxia), a more severe lesion in which the nerve and its surrounding connective tissue have been completely disrupted (neurotmesis), or a demyelinating and axonal degenerating polyneuropathy.[13,20] In the event that findings of the NCT and EMG are normal, the clinician may be able to rule out most conditions involving the PNS and look for CNS or other pathology. Knowledge of this rationale for NCT and EMG should help the therapist decide when the tests may be indicated and understand the reasoning behind reports of tests that have already been performed on their clients.

Motor nerve conduction

In motor nerve conduction tests (MNCT), the peripheral nerve is stimulated at various sites, and the evoked electrical response is recorded from a distal muscle supplied by the nerve. Surface electrodes are usually used for both stimulating and recording. Electrode configuration for MNCT is shown in Fig. 29-1. The response represents the electrical activity of muscle fibers under the recording electrode and is sometimes called the compound muscle action potential (CMAP). It is also called the "M" wave or response. Measurements are taken of latency (the time in milliseconds required for the impulse to travel from each stimulus site to recording site) and the amplitude of the response in millivolts (mV). The shape and duration of the response are assessed, and motor nerve conduction velocity (MNCV) is calculated for each segment of interest by dividing the distance between stimulus sites (in millimeters), by the difference in latency measured at each respective site. For example, to determine whether an ulnar nerve is compromised at the canal of Guyon, at the wrist, or in the ulnar groove at the elbow, the nerve is stimulated in the palm, at the wrist, and below and above the elbow. The latency of the response recorded from the abductor digiti minimi muscle is measured from each of these stimulus sites. Motor nerve conduction velocities are then calculated across the wrist and across the elbow, using the formula:

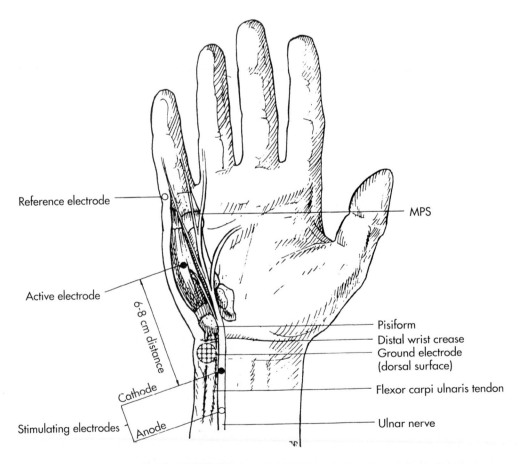

Fig. 29-1. Electrode location for ulnar motor nerve conduction. (Modified from: National Institute for Occupational Safety and Health (NIOSH), Performing motor and sensory neuronal conduction studies in humans, Washington, DC, 1990, U.S. Department of Health and Human Services, Public Health Service Center for Disease Control, p 17.)

$$NCV \ (M/S) = \frac{distance \ between \ 2 \ stimulus \ sites \ (mm)}{difference \ in \ latency \ between \ 2 \ sites \ (ms)}$$

These velocities, the latencies from the wrist and palm and the shape and amplitude of the responses, are studied and compared with established normal values and often with values taken from tests of the uninvolved extremity. Normal adult MNCT values of more commonly tested nerves are shown in Table 29-1. In infants and children, nerve conduction is slower than in adults and reaches adult values by age 4 years.[16] Nerve conduction time gradually slows after age 60 years[13,16] but generally remains within the outer limits of normal.

Sensory nerve conduction

Sensory nerve conduction can be measured from many superficial sensory nerves, such as the superficial radial and the sural nerves. It also can be measured from mixed motor and sensory nerves, by placing either the stimulating or the recording electrode over a sensory branch of a nerve. An orthodromic technique may be used, for example, stimulating the median nerve at the index or long finger, and recording the sensory (afferent) nerve action potentials (SNAP) as they travel centrally from the finger toward the spinal cord (Fig. 29-2). Response latencies and amplitudes are measured, and sensory nerve conduction velocities (SNCV) are calculated for each segment by dividing the distance between two adjacent stimulus and recording sites, or two stimulus sites, by the latency (conduction time) between these same sites. Normal sensory conduction values are shown in Table 29-2. Sensory nerve responses are

Table 29-1. Normal motor-conduction values of commonly tested nerves in adults

Nerve	Distal latency (ms)	Velocity m/sec (meters/second)
Median		
Wrist-muscle (8 cm)	<4.2	
Elbow-wrist		≧45
Ulnar		
Wrist-muscle (8 cm)	<4.0	
Elbow-wrist		≧45
Radial		
Forearm-muscle (8 cm)	<3.5	
Mid-humerus-forearm		≧45
Peroneal (deep) (7 cm)		
Ankle-muscle	<5.5	
Above fibular head-ankle		≧40
Tibial (10 cm)		
Ankle-muscle	<5.5	
Knee-ankle		≧40

From Nelson C. In Gersh MR, editor: *Electrotherapy in rehabilitation,* Philadelphia, 1992, FA Davis, p 116.

considerably smaller than motor responses, and their amplitudes are measured in microvolts (μV).

Another method of measuring sensory nerve conduction is the use of an antidromic technique, in which the stimulus is applied at proximal sites (e.g., the median nerve at the palm, wrist, and elbow) and recording from the index or long finger. This measures the SNAP as they travel distally to the finger, opposite to the direction of flow of the normal afferent nerve impulse, thus, the term *antidromic*. Latency and conduction velocity values for both techniques are similar.

F-wave

The F-wave latency is a measure of the time required for action potentials of alpha motor neurons elicited by stimulating a nerve in the periphery, to be transmitted centrally to the motor neuron cell body, and then return as a recurrent discharge along the same neuron, to activate the muscle from which the recording occurs.[13,15,16,21] No synapse is involved and therefore the F wave is not a reflex response, but rather only a measure of motor neuron conduction. Specific conditions of electropotential must exist at the somadendritic cell membrane to reactivate the efferent axon; therefore the occurrence of the F response is inconsistent and variable in latency and waveform.[21] Because the time required to produce a response in the muscle is considerably longer than that of the conventional M wave latency, the F response is sometimes referred to as a "late" response.

By subtracting the motor conduction latency (M wave latency) recorded at the axilla from the total F-wave latency using a specific formula proposed by Wu, central (or proximal) latency (i.e., from axilla to spinal cord) can be extrapolated.[25] Although F-wave latency is useful in evaluating conduction in conditions usually involving the proximal portions of the peripheral motor neurons (e.g., Guillain-Barré syndrome and thoracic outlet syndrome), its value is considered questionable by some authors because of its variability. Normal values of F-wave latency are 22 to 34 msec in the upper extremity (stimulating at the wrist), 40 to 58 msec in the lower extremity (stimulating at the ankle), and 12 msec central latency in the upper extremity, with a bilateral difference in latency of no greater than 1 msec. Formulas for calculating F wave velocity and F wave:M wave ratios have been proposed, however, because of variables in measuring distance over uneven body surfaces and other variables that may introduce error, latency measurements rather than velocities are more commonly reported.

H-reflex response

The H-reflex response latency is a measure of the time for action potentials elicited by stimulating a nerve in the periphery, to be propagated centrally over the Ia afferent neurons to the spinal cord, transmitted across the synapse to an alpha motorneuron, and then travel distally over this neuron to activate the muscle. The response therefore measures conduction in both the afferent and efferent

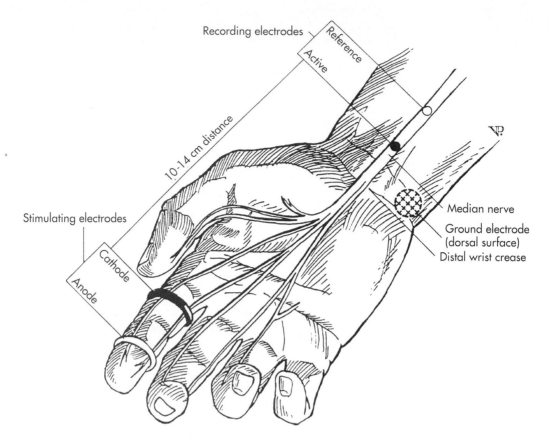

Fig. 29-2. Electrode location for median sensory nerve conduction. (Modified from: National Institute for Occupational Safety and Health [NIOSH], Performing motor and sensory neuronal conduction studies in humans, Washington, DC 1990, U.S. Department of Health and Human Services, Public Health Service Center for Disease Control, p 13.)

Table 29-2. Normal sensory nerve conduction values of commonly tested nerves in adults

Nerve		Distal latency (ms)	Velocity m/s
Median digit II-wrist	(14 cm)	<3.6	≧38
Ulnar digit V-wrist	(14 cm)	<3.6	≧38
Radial thumb-wrist	(14 cm)	<3.5	≧40
Superficial peroneal foot-leg	(14 cm)	<3.6	≧40
Sural lateral malleolus-leg	(14 cm)	<4.2	≧38

From Nelson C: In Gersh MR, editor, *Rehabilitation in electrotherapy,* Philadelphia, 1992, FA Davis, p 126.

neurons.[13,15,16] It also is referred to as a "late" response.

The H wave is readily identified, because it is constant in latency and waveform, and it occurs with a stimulus usually below the threshold level required to elicit the M response. This monosynaptic reflex response is found most easily by stimulating the tibial nerve at the popliteal area and recording from the soleus muscle. Therefore the H-wave latency is a valuable measure of conduction over the first sacral nerve root (S1) in suspected proximal plexopathy and radiculopathy. Sabbahi and Khalil[19] have reported a technique for recording the H wave from the flexor carpi radialis muscle when stimulating the median nerve. In normal

humans over the age of 1 year, the H wave is usually seen only in the tibial and median nerves. It can be elicited from several nerves in infants and in conditions of CNS dysfunction in adults.

Braddom and Johnson[2] described a technique for measuring H-wave latency in the tibial nerve and proposed a formula for predicting normal values, based on the high correlation they found with leg length and age. They report a mean latency of 29.8 msec (±2.74 msec) for the tibial nerve in normal adults, and a bilateral difference of no greater than 1.2 msec. The H-wave latency is most commonly used in evaluation of S_1 radiculopathy because it provides information about function of the dorsal spinal nerve root, which can be compromised by a herniated disc, and by foraminal impingement problems.

Repetitive stimulation tests

The repetitive stimulation (RS) test, used to evaluate the function of transmission at the neuromuscular junction, is a variation of motor nerve conduction testing. One protocol uses a series of supramaximal electrical stimuli applied to a peripheral nerve at a distal site, (e.g., median or ulnar nerve at the wrist) at a rate of three to five per second for five to seven responses, and the amplitude of the muscle response is measured. The test must be administered with particular attention given to firmly securing the stimulating and recording electrodes so that movement artifacts are completely avoided. Additional precise technical requirements are specified to prevent testing errors. Detailed descriptions of the RS test can be found in other texts.[13,17]

Under normal conditions, the amplitude does not change more than 10% from that of the initial response in a series of 10 stimuli, recorded before and after resistive exercise. An amplitude decrease in the fifth or sixth response of more than 10% is considered abnormal and is compatible with a physiological defect at the postsynaptic receptor site of the neuromuscular junction, such as in myasthenia gravis. If the test is negative when stimulating at the distal site, more proximal muscles, such as the deltoid or orbicularis occuli, are tested, stimulating the axillary and facial nerve, respectively.

In another RS protocol, stimuli are applied to a nerve, first at a slow rate, and then at a faster rate, usually 10 to 20 per second for up to 10 seconds. Normally, the amplitude can decrease up to 40% from the initial amplitude. In some defects at the presynaptic site, the response may be lower than normal with a slow stimulation rate, but show a significant amplitude increase at the higher rate. Amplitude increases greater than 100% over the initial response are consistent with presynaptic neuromuscular junction defects such as seen in small-cell bronchogenic carcinoma (Pancoast's tumor) and in botulism. In 1957 Eaton and Lambert[8] reported this phenomenon as a myasthenic syndrome.[8]

Gilchrist and Sanders[10] reported another protocol referred to as a double-step repetitive stimulation test, which measures amplitude before and after a temporarily induced ischemia of the extremity. They found the double-step RS test to be slightly more sensitive than the routine RS test, but only 60% as sensitive as the SFEMG technique. The SFEMG test is described later in this chapter. The RS test is a good alternative tool for neuromuscular transmission when the SFEMG is not available, but the examiner must meticulously adhere to technical details when conducting the test.

CLINICAL EVOKED POTENTIALS

Electrical potentials elicited by stimulation of nerves or sense organs in the periphery can be recorded from various sites as the impulses are transmitted centrally along the neuronal pathway and from the representative area on the brain.[3,4,11,13] Although demyelinating and axonal disorders involving peripheral nerves can be evaluated using conventional motor and sensory tests, evoked potential procedures are particularly useful in studying pathology in the CNS. They are helpful in differentiating between lesions in areas such as the plexus, spinal cord, brainstem, thalamus, and cerebral cortex. Evoked potential tests have the advantage of providing objective data about the integrity of both peripheral and central neuronal pathways, including transmission across axodendritic synapses.

The SSEP is particularly useful in assessing damage and continuity of spinal cord tracts in early spinal cord injury (SCI). For example, if an electrical stimulus is applied at the popliteal area over the tibial nerve, responses can be recorded with surface electrodes placed over the spine at the L3 and C7 spinal segments, and from the lumbar representation of the contralateral sensory cortical area. Conduction time and other parameters of the response waveforms can be measured from the recordings.

This simplified example of a SSEP illustrates how the function of both motor and sensory peripheral nerves and afferent pathways to the cerebrum can be studied. The median nerve is usually tested to evaluate the integrity of peripheral and central pathways and their synaptic connections as the impulses travel from the upper extremity to the contralateral cortical area. Evoked potential tests are particularly valuable in assessing function of afferent pathways in the CNS.

In visual evoked potential (VEP) procedures, visual stimuli, such as variable light flashes of changing patterns, are applied to one or both eyes under highly controlled conditions. The response is recorded from the scalp over the representative area of the cerebral cortex.[4,11,13] Pattern reversal evoked potentials (PREP), the more descriptive term for these procedures, is recommended by the American Electroencephalographic Society.[3] These tests and other visual evoked potential procedures are useful in assessing pathology of retinal photoreceptors, the optic nerve, the chiasma, and postchiasmal pathways. Abnormal conduction findings have been reported when using VEP studies in central demyelinating disorders such as multiple sclerosis and optic neuritis.

Auditory evoked potential tests are used to evaluate neurological function of the cochlear division of the auditory nerve (eighth cranial nerve), central auditory pathways and synapses in the brainstem, and the receptor areas on the cerebral cortex.[3,4,11,13] Brainstem auditory evoked potentials are frequently referred to as BAEP. A series of high-intensity clicks is applied to auditory receptors in the ears through headphones, and several components of the response waveforms are recorded using surface electrodes over the representative cortical areas. The BAEP is an effective test procedure for localizing and evaluating acoustic neuromas and other space-occupying lesions in the brainstem. It is also used for assessment of brain damage and determining the integrity of CNS pathways in patients who are comatose as a result of traumatic head injury. Robinson and Rudge[18] recommend caution when using BAEP tests for this purpose because other factors such as defective receptor organs can cause abnormalities in BAEP.

The evoked potential tests described in this chapter all require application of appropriate external stimuli, which are rapidly repeated many times, and the response is electronically averaged to sort out the desired signal from interference signals. The conduction times (latencies), waveform shape and amplitude, and sometimes conduction velocities are measured and compared with normal values. Absence of a response, increased latencies, decreased amplitudes, and slowing of conduction velocities are all abnormal findings. Normal values and details describing techniques for the evoked potential tests are described elsewhere.[3,4,11,13]

Therapists with special interest and training administer evoked potential tests for neurological applications—more frequently the SSEP. Because of the highly specialized techniques necessary to administer the VEP for ophthalmological applications and the BAEP for hearing dysfunction, these procedures are usually performed by specialists in these areas, or by other evoked potential specialists.

CLINICAL EMG

An understanding of the basis of findings reported in EMG studies should assist neurological therapists in planning and modifying therapeutic management programs of their clients. EMG is particularly useful in showing electrical changes that occur in skeletal muscle when there is pathology in lower motor neurons or in muscle itself. Certain patterns of motor unit recruitment activity also are associated with CNS disorders. Details of contraindications and special precautions are described by Currier and others.[7]

A small-diameter, sterile recording needle electrode is inserted in several representative muscles, and the electrical activity produced by the muscle is studied during relaxation or rest, slight contraction, and strong contraction. Characteristics of the muscle action potentials seen in these three conditions and the pattern of recruitment monitored during progressively stronger contractions are assessed by the examiner to determine whether they are normal, or whether electrical changes observed are consistent with those found in neuropathic, myelopathic, or myopathic conditions. EMG findings are not pathognomonic; therefore they must be carefully studied within the context of other laboratory and clinical findings. During acute stages of trauma or insult to the neurological systems, EMG is not usually indicated. As the client's condition stabilizes and as recovery begins, EMG may be valuable both for evaluation and for planning the therapeutic program. EMG can be useful, particularly with sequential follow-up testing, in determinations of progress

and prognosis. Many excellent resources are available for readers interested in details of the equipment and procedures for EMG.[1,5,7,12,13]

Explanation of the technique and clear communication of instructions to the client, along with patience on the part of the examiner, can allay the client's anxiety and minimize discomfort. Although client cooperation during EMG testing is important, some aspects of the muscle electrical activity can be studied in the client who is unable to move, or who has only involuntary or reflex activity. For example a client recovering from a head injury and with residual hemiplegia has abnormal extensor responses in the upper extremity and weak flexor responses in the lower extremity, except for flaccid ankle and foot responses. An EMG (and nerve conduction tests) of the leg and foot muscles may detect abnormal resting potentials, e.g., fibrillation and positive sharp waves, and no motor unit potentials in muscles normally innervated by the deep peroneal nerve, but normal potentials in the tibial nerve distribution. These findings would guide the physician and therapist in looking for a possible peripheral nerve lesion, concomitant with the CNS dysfunction. The treatment program in this situation would differ from a client without peripheral nerve pathology.

The term *motor unit potential* (MUP) is generally used to designate electrical activity detected in contracting muscle fibers surrounding the recording area of the needle electrode. Conventional EMG techniques actually record from fibers of more than one motor unit.[13] Potentials from single MUPs can only be recorded using the single-fiber EMG electrode and special techniques described later in this chapter. Motor unit potentials appear only during contraction of muscle fibers activated voluntarily or involuntarily, and in both isotonic and isometric contractions. In normal conditions, motor units are seen with voluntary movement; however, reflex activation of muscle also produces MUPs having certain normal characteristics. In CNS disorders with symptoms of spasticity, hypertonic or spastic muscles produce recordable MUPs only when they are actively shortening or contracting. Motor unit potentials are not seen in spastic muscles in a shortened but noncontractile condition. Other EMG findings in CNS disorders are discussed later in this chapter.

As shown in Table 29-3, MUPs are not seen in the normal, resting or relaxed muscle unless the needle is moved (insertion potentials); however, normal physiological endplate potentials are detected from selected sites, e.g., near the endplate zone. During minimum voluntary muscle contraction, specific parameters of MUP waveform amplitude, duration, and phase are studied. With progressively stronger contractions, increased firing frequency and recruitment pattern of MUPs are observed, until, with a very strong contraction, the baseline becomes nearly filled with overlapping potentials of maximum amplitude. This is referred to

Table 29-3. Characteristics of normal and abnormal EMG potentials

Neuro-muscular status	At rest		Minimum contraction			Strong contraction	
			Motor unit potentials (MUP)				
	Insertion activity	Spontaneous activity	Amplitude	Duration	Waveform	Recruitment	Interference pattern
Normal	Brief discharges	None Miniature endplate potentials Endplate potentials Endplate spikes	100-3000 uV (monopolar 5000 uV)	3-15 msec Average = 7 msec	Bi and triphasic 10% Poly-phasic	Normal	Full or complete
Abnormal	Absent response Increased or prolonged	Fibrillation Positive sharp waves Fasciculation	Absent Low or over 5000 uV	Less than 5 msec Longer than 15 msec	Polyphasic >10-15%	Decreased Single unit Early recruitment	Single unit Decreased number MUPs Partial or incomplete
	Decreased	Complex repetitive discharges Myotonic, myokymic potentials			Myotonic potentials		

Modified with permission from: Currier DP and others: Guidelines for clinical electromyography, *J Clin Electrophysiol,* 5:2,1993.

as a full or complete interference pattern, with normal recruitment.

The more commonly seen abnormal EMG findings are fibrillation potentials, positive sharp waves, fasciculation potentials, polyphasic potentials, high-frequency potentials, and MUPs, with various combinations of abnormal amplitude, duration and waveform, as shown in Table 26-3. The following brief description of these selected abnormal EMG potentials is only introductory; the reader should seek other sources for greater detail and explanation.[1,5,7,13]

Fibrillations are short duration, spontaneous biphasic or triphasic potentials produced by single muscle fibers. The first phase is in the positive direction (a downward tracing on the oscilloscope), and the total duration of the potential is not more than 5 msec. The amplitude is usually low, but may range from 20 to 1000uV. Because of their short duration, fibrillations are heard over the loud speaker as a high-pitched, crackling sound, similar to wrinkling cellophane or tissue paper.

Positive sharp waves are spontaneous, usually biphasic potentials. They have an initial positive phase, which gradually returns to the electrical baseline and then is followed by a lower amplitude negative phase. Fibrillations and positive sharp waves are thought to represent an unstable muscle fiber cell membrane. They appear in muscles in peripheral neuropathies such as peripheral nerve injuries and axonal neuropathies (e.g., diabetic neuropathy), motor neuron disorders, and in some myopathies, particularly acute inflammatory myopathies such as polymyositis and other conditions causing electrochemical instability of the muscle membrane. (See Chapter 13 on Musculoskeletal Problems.)

Fasciculations are spontaneously discharging MUPs from a few motor units or from bundles of muscle fibers. They may be of normal waveform or polyphasic, and may have increased or decreased duration and amplitude. Occasionally, they are seen in normal muscle, but usually do not appear as frequently or fire as arrhythmically as in the presence of pathology. Fasciculation potentials are seen in motor neuron disease and also in peripheral neuromuscular disorders.

High-frequency potentials or discharges have varying characteristics of firing frequency, amplitude, and duration. Myotonic-type potentials are characterized by fluctuations in amplitude and frequency, which increase and decrease, giving a waxing and waning appearance and a sound similar to a chain saw or a passing motorcycle. They can appear spontaneously or on mechanical stimulation such as percussion or needle movement and can occur with voluntary muscle activation. These myotonic potentials are associated with the myotonias, hyperkalemic periodic paralysis, and other diseases.[5,13] High-frequency potentials also can take on a form of continuous, complex repetitive discharges that spontaneously start and stop abruptly and do not vary in amplitude or frequency. They often have many phases and produce a sound similar to a rapidly firing automatic gun. Complex, repetitive discharges are seen in chronic denervating disorders, including motor neuron disease, polyneuropathy, radiculopathy, spinal muscular atrophy, Charcot-Marie-Tooth disease, and in myopathies (e.g., Duchenne muscular dystrophy and polymyositis).[5,13]

Normal MUPs are typically biphasic or triphasic. Occasionally, potentials of more than four phases, called polyphasic potentials, are seen and are considered within normal limits if they constitute no more than 10% to 15% of the MUPS detected in a muscle. A greater-than-normal number of polyphasics, which may have from 5 to 25 or more phases, are referred to as *increased polyphasia.* An increased number of polyphasics may indicate axonal sprouting and reinnervation, or axonal regeneration, which can occur in chronic neuropathies. Polyphasics potentials are nonspecific changes, because they can occur in neuropathy, including radiculopathy, motor neuron disease, and in myopathies.[1,5,13]

As electrical tests are being conducted, the findings are continuously studied and are used by the examiner as a guide in continuing with or modifying the plan for the examination. Data from EMG and nerve conduction studies are analyzed by the examiner to determine the extent and anatomical distribution of abnormal electrical responses. The examiner then interprets the findings to establish whether they fit the characteristics usually found in pathological groupings of abnormal patterns. As stated earlier, the results of electrodiagnostic tests must be correlated with the clinical findings.

SUMMARY OF CLINICAL EMG AND NERVE CONDUCTION STUDIES

Reviewing a summary of the more characteristic EMG and nerve conduction changes associated with selected groupings of neurological disorders may help the therapist use reports of these studies and recognize changes that may be seen in sequential tests during the course of the disorders. The reader is cautioned that the following is a simplified grouping of electrical changes and that actual electrodiagnostic studies show considerably more detail and frequent variations of these findings.[1,5,7,12,13]

Electrical testing in upper motor neuron disorders typically shows normal motor and sensory nerve conduction. In the EMG, spontaneous activity is seen infrequently, and individual motor units seen on muscle contraction usually have normal parameters. The recruitment pattern may show a slower than normal MUP discharge frequency, with an incomplete and irregular interference pattern. In the presence of tremor and other involuntary movements, bursts of MUPs occur, consistent with the muscle contraction pattern. The tests are important in differential diagnosis between a CNS and a PNS problem, but often are not used when clinical examinations demonstrate the problem to be definitely in the CNS.

In myelopathies, which include upper and lower motor neuron disorders (e.g., amyotrophic lateral sclerosis [ALS], poliomyelitis, cervical spondylitis, and syringomyelia), motor and sensory nerve conduction are usually normal, although there may be slight slowing.[13] The characteristic EMG changes, which usually appear in the more chronic stages of the disorders, are increased amplitude and duration of motor units because of the variable impulse conduction time in sprouting axon terminals. An increased number of polyphasic potentials with increased duration is usually found. Spontaneous activity is often seen, and on strong contraction, a reduced number of rapidly firing large MUPs are recruited, resulting in a single unit or partial interference pattern.

Peripheral neuropathies show different electrical changes, depending on the type and location of the pathology. In proximal pathologies (e.g., radiculopathies), motor and sensory nerve conduction generally remains normal, except for F waves and H-reflex responses in specific spinal cord segments. If motor nerve roots are compromised, spontaneous activity and increased polyphasics appear, and reduced recruitment of MUPs results in an incomplete interference pattern. In more chronic stages MUP amplitude and duration can be increased. As the lesion improves, spontaneous activity decreases and the recruitment pattern becomes more normal. If only sensory roots are injured, no EMG changes occur.

Lesions of peripheral nerves, which range from a focal mononeuropathy to plexopathy, frequently show abnormalities in motor and sensory nerve conduction, depending on which components of the nerve are involved. In the EMG, spontaneous activity, particularly fibrillation and positive sharp waves, is very common; if the lesion is complete, no MUPs are found. The presence of even a few MUPs suggests a more optimistic prognosis. Often the location of the lesion can be identified by the distribution of the electrical changes. With regenerating axons, low-amplitude polyphasic MUPs gradually appear. In the chronic stage, the amplitude and duration of MUPs are often increased. Spontaneous activity decreases with reinnervation, but may persist for several years.

In generalized, systemic peripheral polyneuropathies (see

Chapters 12 and 13) of the primarily demyelinating type, such as Guillain-Barré syndrome, motor and sensory nerve conduction and F waves become markedly slow. The EMG changes usually do not occur, except for a reduced recruitment pattern, consistent with weak muscle contraction. With primarily axonal polyneuropathies, such as uremic neuropathy, isoniazid and cisplatin toxicity, and lead poisoning, motor and sensory nerve conduction is mildly slowed or may remain normal. The duration and amplitude of the response, however, decrease. During advanced stages, many polyneuropathies develop both demyelinating and axonal pathology (e.g., diabetic neuropathy). On EMG, spontaneous activity is commonly seen. These electrical changes generally become more severe with worsening of the pathology, but also improve if the pathology is reversed.

With myopathic disorders, motor and sensory nerve conduction is generally normal unless neural tissue is also affected. In advanced stages, however, severely atrophied muscles can produce decreased amplitude and distorted nerve conduction responses. The characteristic findings on EMG are short-duration, low-amplitude potentials. Some spontaneous potentials, particularly fibrillations and positive sharp waves, may be found but are much more frequent in the inflammatory myopathies such as polymyositis. Spontaneous activity also is seen in some neuromuscular transmission disorders (e.g., botulism). Specific myotonic potentials appear in certain myopathic disorders (e.g., myotonia congenita). The recruitment pattern shows many low-amplitude MUPs, appearing in a full pattern, with little voluntary effort. This type of recruitment pattern is referred to as early recruitment.

CASE STUDIES

To clarify and apply the concepts, ideas and research presented in this chapter, a variety of case studies have been developed to aid the reader.

CASE 1 ▼ Rule Out Ulnar Nerve Injury: Electrophysiological Test Report

A 48-year-old man was in a motor vehicle accident 1 year ago and had nerve contusion of the right elbow with no fracture. For the past 3 months he has complained of increasing weakness of his right hand, numbness, and pain in the medial two digits.

Nerve conduction	Dist. latency (msec.)	Amp.	Velocity (M/sec.)
R ulnar motor	2.8	6mV	57 BE-W
			40 AE-BE
			59 AX-AE
R ulnar sensory	No response		
R median motor	3.0	15mV	50 E-wrist
R median sensory	3.2	18uV	43 index-wrist
L ulnar motor	2.6	11mV	55 BE-W
			51 AE-BE
L ulnar sensory	3.1	10uV	45 digit-wrist

Electromyography	Spontaneous activity	Motor units	Recruitment
R abd dig minimi	3+ fibrillation &	polyphasic	single
R flex carpi ulnaris	pos. sharp waves	incr. amp.	units
R abd pollicis brevis	none	normal	normal
R flex carpi rad brev	none	normal	normal

Impression: Slowing of right ulnar motor conduction across elbow and absent ulnar sensory conduction. Normal conduction in right median and left ulnar nerves. Nerve conduction and EMG findings are consistent with an incomplete lesion of right ulnar nerve at the level of the elbow.

BE-W is Below elbow to wrist; AE-BE is Above elbow to below elbow; AX-AE is Axilla to above elbow; E-wrist is Elbow to wrist.

Discussion: The electrophysiological evaluation confirms the presence of a partial ulnar nerve lesion at the right elbow. The physical examination conducted before electrical testing should show localized weakness and sensory changes in the ulnar nerve distribution. The plan for follow-up management includes a detailed manual muscle test and sensory examination in 4 to 6 weeks, and if the symptoms and physical examination show a progression of the nerve lesion, repeating the electrical test would be helpful in determining the extent of progression. The test results would be valuable to the referring physician in making decisions about intervention, including surgery.

In the interim, the client would be instructed to avoid excessive motions, which would aggravate the nerve compromise at the elbow, and to modify upper extremity (UE) activities, adopting protective positions and movements. If muscle weakness progresses, electrical muscle stimulation (EMS) may be incorporated into an exercise program (see Chapter 30).

CASE 2 ▼ Cervical Radiculopathy: Electrophysiological Test Report

A 48-year-old man was in a motor vehicle accident 1 year ago and had a nerve contusion of the right elbow with no fracture. For the past 3 months he has complained of weakness of his right hand, numbness, and pain and tingling in the medial three digits.

Nerve conduction	Dist. latency (msec.)	Amp.	Velocity (M/sec.)
R ulnar motor	2.8	6mV	59 AE-W
R ulnar sensory	2.8	10uV	50 dig V-wrist
R median motor	3.0	15mV	50 E-W
R median sensory	3.2	18uV	43 index-wrist
L ulnar motor	2.6	11mV	55 E-W
L ulnar sensory	3.1	10uV	45 dig V-wrist

Electromyography	Spontaneous activity	Motor units	Recruitment
R abd dig min	fibs, pos sharps 3+	incr polyphasics	reduced
R 1st dorsal interos	"	"	"
R flex carpi ulnaris	"	"	"
R abd pol brev	"	"	"
R ext carpi ulnaris	"	"	"
R flex pol longus	"	"	"
R flex carpi rad	none	normal	sl. reduced
R ext carpi rad	none	normal	normal
R biceps	none	normal	normal
R cervical parasp.	fibs, low cerv	incr polyphasics	normal
L flex carpi ulnaris	none	normal	normal
L abd dig min	none	normal	normal

Impression: Normal conduction in all nerves tested. EMG abnormalities seen in muscles innervated by C8,T1 spinal cord segment and lower cervical paraspinals. These findings are consistent with a C8,T1 cervical radiculopathy.

Discussion: The physical examination conducted before the electrophysiological evaluation should reveal clinical signs and symptoms consistent with the electrical changes, suggesting a C_8,T_1 radiculopathy. A detailed orthopedic musculoskeletal examination would be useful in further dfferentiating the cervical spine dysfunction and in determining a treatment plan. The referring physician can use the electrical test and musculoskeletal examination results to guide decisions about the need for additional tests, such as myelography, computerized tomography (CT) scans, magnetic resonance imaging (MRI) examinations, or other intervention.

Case study 1 and 2 intentionally use the same client history with only slightly different symptoms to illustrate how electrodiagnosis can provide objective data to support differentiation between a localized peripheral mononeuropathy and a more proximal cervical root disorder. Treatment of the two problems obviously would be different.

SINGLE-FIBER EMG

Electrical activity can be recorded from two or more muscle fibers innervated by the same motor unit using a specially designed single-fiber needle electrode. Single-fiber EMG (SFEMG) is, at this time, the most sensitive test for evaluating neuromuscular transmission defects, such as myasthenia gravis and myasthenic syndrome. It also is used to evaluate peripheral neuropathies, motor neuron diseases, and myopathies.[5,13,23]

During a carefully controlled minimal voluntary contraction, a 25 μm diameter needle is inserted into the muscle and several potentials from muscle fibers within the recording area are stored. Equipment with a trigger and delay line are necessary to time-lock the tracings of the potentials. The slightly different conduction time or interpulse interval (IPI) required for impulses to be transmitted from a single motor neuron to each of its terminal endplates, across the neuromuscular junction, and activate the muscle fiber is called "jitter." This time difference is collected from several tracings and is converted into a mean consecutive time difference (MCD), which normally ranges from 5 to 55 μsec. Values shorter or longer than this range are considered abnormal. The impulses from some axons to their muscle fibers may fail to be transmitted. This is referred to as *blocking.* Another capability of SFEMG is the measure of fiber density, i.e., the average number of muscle fibers within the needle recording area. Fiber density is increased in reinnervation and also with certain myopathies because of axonal collateralization or splitting.[5]

CASE 3 ▼ Peripheral Neuropathy: Electrophysiological Test Report

JR is a 36-year-old woman with an 8-year history of renal disease. She has been receiving dialysis for 14 months. Over the past 4 or 5 months she has developed increasing weakness and decreased feeling of both lower extremities. Bilateral lower extremity examination shows depressed deep tendon reflexes in knees and ankles, and markedly decreased sensation in a stocking pattern in legs beginning just below knees. Muscle strength is 3+ knee flexors and extensors, 1-2+ in muscles about the ankle, and 0 toe muscle function. Upper extremities are within normal limits and without symptoms.

Nerve conduction	Dist. lat. (msec.)	Amp.	Vel (M/sec.)	F waves (msec)
L peroneal motor	8.4	1.2 mV	27	absent
R peroneal motor	no resonse			
L tibial motor	7.2	2.0 mV	37	66
R tibial motor	7.8	1.8 mV	32	68
L sural	5.9	3.0 uV	24	
R sural	absent			
L ulnar motor	3.1	6.2 mV	55	26
R median motor	3.5	6.5 mV	52	27
L ulnar sensory	2.7	16 uV	52	
R median sensory	3	19 uV	47	

Electromyography	Spontaneous activity	Motor units	Recruitment
Left and right:			
tibialis ant	3 +fibrillation and pos. sharp waves	↑ polyphasics ↑ duration	markedly ↓
peroneus longus	"	"	"
gastrocnemius			
quadriceps	none	normal	normal
hamstrings	"	"	"

Impression: Slow motor and sensory nerve conduction in both lower extremities with normal conduction in upper extremities. EMG findings in distal leg muscles consistent with axonal changes. These findings are compatible with a diffuse sensorimotor polyneuropathy involving both lower extremities.

Discussion: The pattern of clinical findings is suggestive of a peripheral polyneuropathy (see Chapter 12). Findings are confirmed by the electrical test. Review of medical management by the referring practitioner would be a key factor in treatment decisions for this client. Some of the pathological changes seen in peripheral neuropathies may be reversible or at least reduced with good compliance and clinical management.

A soft ankle foot orthosis (AFO) for both lower extremities would enhance gait and also serve a protective function. A therapeutic exercise program, especially a home program, which may include NMES (see Chapter 30) would be designed to strengthen or at least maintain strength and ROM of both lower extremities. Client instruction should emphasize compliance with the medical plan and protective activities along with the exercise intervention.

MACRO EMG

A variation of SFEMG utilizes a macroelectrode to record the majority of muscle fibers of a single motor unit as they are triggered by an initial potential, which is then time-locked with all the other muscle fiber potentials recorded from a different part of the same or a nearby needle.[13,24] Two recording channels are used. Maximum amplitude of the potentials from several muscles has been reported by Stålberg.[24] The findings are analyzed, along with findings of jitter, fiber density, and conventional EMG, to evaluate the status and prognosis of various neurological and neuromuscular disorders, such as motor neuron disease, peripheral nerve lesions, and myopathies.

AUTOMATIC ANALYSIS

Instruments with computer-assisted analysis are now available for studying EMG signals in greater detail than in earlier years.[5,13,22] Parameters of the waveform, including amplitude, duration, frequency spectrum, number of turns, or phase polarity reversals and area—which is the integral or total voltage of a waveform—can be automatically analyzed. The data are then compared electronically with predetermined patterns of electrical changes, which correlate with categories of neuromuscular disorders such as myelopathies and neuropathies. Instruments with this capability are not in routine use in most clinics at this time, but rapidly changing technology will probably make this detailed automatic analysis more available in the near future.

A 52-year-old man with a 6-month history of progressive weakness and twitching of muscles of the extremities was referred for electrical testing. Examination showed fair to fair plus grade muscle strength in distal areas of both upper and lower extremities. Sensation was intact. Deep tendon reflexes were hyperactive throughout and Babinski response was + bilaterally. He was otherwise in good health.

Nerve Conduction and EMG test results: Motor nerve conduction in upper and lower extremities was within normal limits except for low-normal velocity in the peroneal nerves. Sensory nerve conduction was within normal limits. EMG showed many fibrillation potentials, positive sharp waves, and several arrhythmic fasciculations in the intrinsic muscles of the hands and in the leg muscles. Many motor units were of increased amplitude, up to 20 mV, and increased in duration. Recruitment pattern was reduced, with increased firing frequency of several units.

Impression: Nerve conduction and EMG findings are consistent with those seen in disorders of motor neurons.

Discussion: The results of the electrophysiological evaluation of this client would be correlated by the referring physician with the clinical examination and other laboratory tests to further differentiate a diagnosis. Management would then depend on the progression and prognosis of the disorder. For example, if the client is determined to have ALS, a plan for maintaining strength, ROM, and functional and social activities within limits of fatigue would be incorporated into a home program. Assistive devices would be used as needed. Referral to other health care professionals, including occupational therapy for activities of daily living (ADL), speech therapy for assistance with swallowing problems if they occur, and nursing care, would all be part of a coordinated team effort for client comfort and maintaining quality of life.

This 73-year-old woman sustained a right cerebrovascular accident (CVA) 3 weeks ago, with residual hemiparesis on the left. She is oriented, comprehension is slow but good, and she has moderate expressive aphasia. There is hypertonicity with a flexor synergy pattern in the upper extremity (UE). She is developing functional movement of shoulder flexors and abductors, elbow flexors, and extensors and slight movement of finger flexors. Activity cannot be elicited in wrist or finger extensors. There is active movement of all muscles of the lower extremity (LE) through partial range, with minimal hypertonicity. Passive ROM of left UE and LE is within normal limits (WNL) and sensation is intact to light touch. Right extremities have full ROM and at least functional strength throughout.

Specific problem is the complete absence of wrist and finger extension, which raises the question of a secondary radial nerve pathology. Nerve conduction and EMG studies are requested to help differentiate this problem.

Nerve conduction	Dist. lat. (msec.)	Amp.	Velocity (M/sec.)
L radial motor	3.3	3.2 mV	47
L radial sensory	3.3	8.0 uV	42
L ulnar motor	3.8	5.2 mV	48
L ulnar sensory	3.4	7.5 uV	41
R radial motor	3.4	3.5 mV	47
R radial sensory	3.2	8.0 uV	44

Electromyography	Spontaneous activity	Motor units	Recruitment
R ext digitorum ⎫ R ext carpi rad R ext pol brev R ext indicis ⎭	none	↓ amp, normal duration and phase	single units
R triceps	none	normal	mod reduced, irregular pattern

Impression: Nerve conduction approaching outer limits of normal but considered WNL for client's age. EMG shows no electrical evidence for peripheral denervation. A few single normal motor units were seen in wrist and finger extensors. These findings are consistent with an upper motor neuron disorder; however, clinical correlation is required.

Discussion: The nerve conduction values, which are approaching outer limits of normal, are not unusual for clients over 60 to 65 years of age. The normal nerve conduction is compatible with an upper motor neuron problem. On EMG, spontaneous activity is rarely seen with upper motor neuron lesions, and if motor units are found, they generally have normal characteristics. Therefore the EMG findings are also consistent with an upper motor neuron problem, rather than a PNS disorder.

The fact that radial nerve degeneration has been ruled out and the encouraging presence of some single motor unit potentials on EMG are important objective findings that should guide the therapist in management of this client.

Incorporating NMES or EMG biofeedback into the overall treatment plan can be useful in facilitating motor function and sensory awareness in the upper extremity. See Chapter 30 for details on supplementing therapeutic exercise programs with electrotherapy and EMG biofeedback.

REFERENCES

1. Aminoff MJ: *Electrodiagnosis in clinical neurology,* ed 3, New York, 1992, Churchill Livingstone.
2. Braddom RL and Johnson EW: Standardization of H reflex and diagnostic use in S_1 radiculopathy, *Arch Phys Med Rehabil* 55:161-166, 1974.
3. Chatrian GE: American Electroencephalographic Society:guidelines for clinical evoked potential studies, *J Clin Neurophysiol* 1:3-53, 1984.
4. Chiappa KH: *Evoked potentials in clinical medicine,* New York, 1990, Raven Press.
5. Chu-Andrews J and Johnson RJ: *Electrodiagnosis: an anatomical and clinical approach,* Philadelphia, 1986, JB Lippincott.
6. Cummings J: Electrical stimulation of healthy muscle and tissue repair. In Nelson RM and Currier DP, editors: *Clinical electrotherapy,* ed 2, Norwalk, Conn, 1991, Appleton & Lange.
7. Currier DP and others: Guidelines for clinical electromyography, *J Clin Electrophysiol* 5:2-19, 1993.
8. Eaton LM and Lambert EH: Electromyography and electrical stimulation of nerves in diseases of motor unit. Observations on myasthenic syndrome associated with malignant tumors, *JAMA* 163:1117-1124, 1957.
9. Electrotherapy Standards Committee of the Section on Clinical Electrophysiology: Electrotherapeutic terminology in physical therapy, Alexandria, Va, 1990, American Physical Therapy Association.
10. Gilchrist JM and Sanders DB: Double-step repetitive stimulation in myasthenia gravis, *Muscle Nerve* 10:233-237, 1987.
11. Halliday AM, editor: *Evoked potentials in clinical testing,* London, 1982, Churchill Livingstone.
12. Johnson EW: *Practical electromyography,* ed 2, Baltimore, 1988, Williams & Wilkins.
13. Kimura J: *Electrodiagnosis in diseases of nerve and muscle: principles and practice,* ed 2, Philadelphia, 1989, FA Davis.
14. National Institute for Occupational Safety and Health, Division of Safety Research: *Performing motor and sensory neuronal conduction studies in adult humans,* Washington, DC, 1990, US Department of Health and Human Services, Public Health Service Centers for Disease Control.
15. Nelson C: Electrical evaluation of nerve and muscle. In Gersh MR, editor: *Electrotherapy in rehabilitation,* Philadelphia, 1992, FA Davis.
16. Oh SJ: *Clinical electromyography: nerve conduction studies,* ed 2, Baltimore, 1993, Williams & Wilkins.
17. Ozdemir C and Young RR: The results to be expected from electrical testing in the diagnosis of myasthenia gravis, *Ann NY Acad Sci* 274:203-235, 1976.
18. Robinson K and Rudge P: Centrally generated auditory potentials. In Halliday AM, editor: *Evoked potentials in clinical testing,* London, 1982, Churchill Livingstone.
19. Sabbahi MA and Khalil M: Segmental H-reflex studies in upper and lower limbs of healthy subjects, *Arch Phys Med Rehabil* 71:216-222, 1990.
20. Seddon HJ: Three types of nerve injury, *Brain* 66:237-288, 1943.
21. Shiller HH and Stålberg E: F responses studied with single fibre EMG in normal subjects and spastic patients, *J Neurol Neurosurg Psychiatry* 41:45-53, 1978.
22. Stålberg E and others: Automatic analysis of the EMG interference pattern, *Electroencephalogr Clin Neurophysiol* 56:672-681, 1983.
23. Stålberg E and Trontelj J: *Single fibre electromyography,* Old Woking, Surry, UK, 1979, The Miraville Press Limited.
24. Stålberg E: AAEE minimonograph #20, macro EMG, *Muscle Nerve* 6:619-630, 1983.
25. Wu Y and others: Axillary central latency: simple electrodiagnostic technique for proximal neuropathy, *Arch Phys Med Rehabil* 64:117-120, 1983.

CHAPTER 30

Electrical Stimulation and Electromyographic Biofeedback

Applications for neurological dysfunction

Karen L. McCulloch and Charlene M. Nelson

KEY TERMS

neuromuscular electrical
  stimulation (NMES)
electrical muscular
  stimulation (EMS)
electromyographic
  biofeedback (EMGBF)

electric stimulation therapy
functional electrical
  stimulation (FES)
biofeedback

LEARNING OBJECTIVES

After reading this chapter the student/therapist will:
**(Relating specifically to clients with peripheral or
central nervous system disorders)**

1. Understand the basic mechanisms of neuromuscular
   electrical stimulation (NMES), electrical muscle
   stimulation (EMS), and electromyographic
   biofeedback (EMGBF).
2. Describe appropriate stimulus parameters for use of
   NMES, EMS, and EMGBF.
3. Discuss types of equipment available for NMES,
   EMS, and EMGBF.
4. Describe the potential benefits of NMES, EMS, and
   EMGBF.
5. List indications and contraindications for use of
   NMES, EMS, and EMGBF.
6. Provide examples of usage of these modalities for a
   variety of neurological problems:
   -peripheral nerve injury or peripheral neuropathy
   -altered muscular force production or
    control-hypertonicity
   -functional activity limitations
   -orthotic substitution (FES)
   -paralysis
7. Describe considerations for usage of these modalities
   with the following neurological client groups:
   cerebrovascular accident (CVA), spinal cord injury
   (SCI), traumatic brain injury (TBI), cerebral palsy
   (CP), spina bifida, and Guillain-Barré syndrome.
8. Describe decision-making process for evaluation of
   treatment efficacy; suggest modifications in NMES,
   EMS, and/or EMGBF program based on results.
9. Demonstrate awareness of feedback principles that
   relate to use of EMGBF.
10. Summarize research findings examining the efficacy
    of NMES, EMS, and EMGBF.

Among the tools available for facilitation of muscular control are **neuromuscular electrical stimulation (NMES), electrical muscle stimulation (EMS),** and **electromyographic biofeedback (EMGBF).** Although the mechanisms of action are different for these modalities, they may be used in conjunction with each other to meet goals of improving or modulating muscular activation, with the intent of improving client function. This chapter provides a basic introduction to the physiology, indications, contraindications, and applications of NMES, EMS, and EMGBF with clients exhibiting common neurological impairments. Specific protocols for treatment will not be detailed, as these are available elsewhere.[6,10,31,33,77] A review of the literature examining efficacy is also included to assist the therapist in making choices about the usage of these tools in the clinic.

EQUIPMENT AND STIMULUS PARAMETERS FOR NMES

Electrical stimulators designed for NMES may be either small, portable units or larger clinical models. The portable units are particularly convenient for use by the client who needs stimulation over a longer time, e.g., home treatment. Clinical models usually have the capability of setting more variables of wave form and modulations of the stimulus, and some can store customized programs in memory for individual patients. Many references are available for the reader interested in more detail on treatment.[41,76] For excellent discussions of neuromuscular electrical stimulation for clients with neurological impairment, the reader is referred to DeVahl[31] and Packman-Braun.[77]

Parameters of NMES

Waveform. The waveform of the stimulus of most NMES units is usually either a symmetrical or an asymmetrical biphasic pulse, with two phases in each pulse. The two phases continually alternate or reverse in direction between positive and negative polarity. With the asymmetrical biphasic pulse, the cathode (negative) and anode (positive) electrodes can be identified; therefore the therapist can selectively apply the negative electrode over the target muscle producing a more effective contraction. Because the polarity of the symmetrical biphasic waveform is continually reversing in direction and the two phases in each pulse are equal in amplitude, both electrodes alternately become active electrodes, and one is not more effective than the other.[1,36,73] Some stimulators use a monophasic waveform, which can be set as either a negative or a positive pulse at the active electrode. Using the negative polarity at the active electrode (over the target muscle) produces a muscle contraction with less current amplitude (intensity) than when using the positive polarity. While an ideal waveform for NMES has not been agreed upon, some studies have shown the symmetrical biphasic waveform to be more comfortable than either the asymmetrical biphasic or the monophasic waveform.[3,6,68]

Duration. Stimulators with a phase duration of 1 to 300 μsec (0.3 msec) can be used to activate muscles with intact innervation. A set duration of 300 μsec has been reported as preferred, compared with shorter durations.[20,44] Shorter duration waveforms require a greater current amplitude to produce a muscle contraction. Longer phase durations may be used, but are less comfortable.

Frequency. The stimulus frequency should be set at a rate sufficient to produce a smooth, sustained (tetanic) muscle contraction. While this varies with different muscles, a frequency of 30 to 50 Hz (pulses per second) is usually effective, although slower frequencies may be used if a satisfactory contraction is obtained.[36] Higher stimulus frequencies can cause fatigue, so the frequency should be set no faster than that which produces a smooth contraction.

Amplitude. Amplitude or intensity of the stimulus is gradually increased until the desired level of activation is obtained in the muscle(s) being stimulated. This level depends on the goal for the program. The client should be encouraged to participate actively by contracting the muscle(s) and synchronizing his or her effort with the timing of the external stimulus. With very weak muscles, a lower level of training is used, and it may be necessary to use gravity-eliminated positions to assist movement through as much of the available range as possible. With stronger muscles, higher current amplitudes are used, with a goal of activating the muscle to the strongest level of force indicated for the exercise program. In all situations, muscle fatigue should be avoided or minimized by using the lowest amplitude necessary to produce a satisfactory contraction.[14,15] The therapist must keep in mind that the NMES is being used to supplement, not substitute, for exercise.

Modulations. In addition to the parameters of the basic individual stimulus pulses (i.e., waveform, phase and pulse duration, pulse frequency, and amplitude), several modulations are necessary to enhance the effectiveness of the NMES program. The stimulus is applied in a repetitive "train" of pulses, which can be periodically interrupted or turned on and off in rhythmical "bursts" or cycles, ramped, and delivered with preset duty cycles.

On time and off time. Neuromuscular electrical stimulation for facilitation of muscle contraction should be used to supplement exercise, and goals for stimulation should be consistent with the goals of the exercise program. To simulate isotonic or isometric muscle contractions, as in voluntary movement for exercise, the stimulator must have the capability of setting bursts or cycles of on and off times; thus the period of muscle contraction is followed by a relaxation period[31,36] (Fig. 30-1). In most cases, a shorter on time than off time is desirable to avoid fatigue, for example, 5 second effective on time, and 25 second off time in a cycle, which would be an on/off ratio of 1:5.[78] If the goal is to reduce edema by providing a muscle pumping action, a ratio of 1:1 or 1:2 may be preferred.

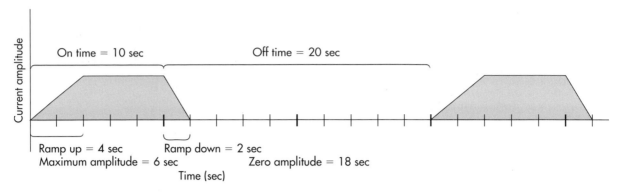

Fig. 30-1. Example of the relationship between ramp times and on/off times. Each division on horizontal axis equals 2 seconds. Note that the ramp-up time is considered part of the on time, while the ramp-down time is considered part of the off time. (From DeVahl J: Neuromuscular electrical stimulation (NMES) in rehabilitation. In Gersh MR: *Electrotherapy in Rehabilitation*, Philadelphia, 1992, FA Davis.)

Ramp time. Ramp time is another modulation to be set by the therapist. Ramp on is the time set for each train of pulses to increase from zero (no current flow) to maximum amplitude or intensity. Ramp off is the time set for the end of the train of pulses (at the end of the on time) to decrease from maximum amplitude to zero current flow (Fig. 30-1). Thus ramp time can be adjusted so that the stimulation more nearly resembles a pattern of gradually contracting and relaxing muscles. For clients with hypertonicity or spasticity and a goal of facilitation and strengthening of the antagonist muscle, a longer ramp-on time may avoid or minimize activation of the stretch reflex in the hyperactive agonist muscle. Shorter ramp times may be effective when the goal is to increase range of motion (ROM) or decrease edema.

Duty cycle. The term *duty cycle* is sometimes confused with the on/off time ratio. Duty cycle is the percentage of time a series or train of pulses is on, out of the total on and off time in a cycle.[6,36] As an example, if the train of pulses is on 10 seconds and off 30 seconds, the total cycle time is 40 seconds. The duty cycle would be 25%, i.e., 10 seconds of the total 40-second cycle. The actual on time and off time of the pulses in a cycle is a more informative description than using either the duty cycle or the on/off ratio.

NMES
Mechanisms

Muscle recruitment patterns triggered by **electric stimulation therapy** differ from those observed in normal muscle activation. In a voluntary muscle contraction, motor units fire asynchronously with a larger proportion of type I, fatigue-resistant muscle fibers of the smaller motor units being recruited first. The order of muscle fiber firing occurs as a result of the size of motor neurons and the anatomy of synaptic connections.[13] Conversely, an electrically stimulated muscle contraction elicits first response from larger motor units, with a greater number of fatigable, type II muscle fibers.[14] A study of healthy subjects demonstrates recruitment of these higher threshold motor units at

relatively low NMES training levels. This phenomenon is not possible with voluntary exercise, as much greater exercise intensity is required for activation of these larger motor units.[14] This provides support for observed increases in strength with low NMES training intensities, as muscle fibers usually only accessible by high intensity training participate in muscle activation and improve torque production.[97] Firing order in this scenario is a result of size of neuronal axon, proximity of the electrical stimulus, and the intensity of the stimulation.[42]

Synchronous recruitment of muscle fibers also may be obtained with electrical stimulation, a situation that does not occur with volitional activation. Careful attention to intensity of stimulation, stimulus frequency, and timing of rest periods is required to minimize fatigue.[14] Because the character of the muscle contraction is different with stimulation than with the physiological response of voluntary muscle activation, stimulation should be discontinued when the client can activate the muscle, so that active strengthening can occur.

Higher stimulus frequencies cause fatigue sooner than lower frequencies. In some instances, the frequency of stimulation may be dictated by the goal of NMES, for instance, sufficient stimulation intensity to move a limb through the desired range of motion. In general, stimulation intensity should be set at the lowest level possible to get the desired response to minimize fatigue.[14] *Numerous potential benefits are identified for NMES. Among them are improvement in ROM, edema reduction, treatment of disuse atrophy, and improvement of muscle recruitment for muscle reeducation.*[31]

Muscle reeducation

After an insult or injury affecting the central nervous system (CNS), problems with motor control are frequently manifest. One of the common goals of therapy is to facilitate movement in the areas where control is lacking. If active movement is not present, NMES allows movement to occur via stimulation, which may be followed by resumption of active movement, possibly triggered by the proprioceptive and sensory experience that accompanies the stimulation. When active movement is present, but weak or not well controlled, the therapist may choose to use NMES to supplement and "strengthen" the muscular contraction already present. In the presence of hypertonicity, the muscles serving as antagonists to the spastic muscle may be targeted for NMES, not only to strengthen the antagonist, but to inhibit the spastic muscle by reciprocal inhibition.[31,77]

Packman-Braun[78] investigated ratios of stimulation to rest time with NMES for wrist extension in a group of hemiplegic patients. Results supported the on-off time of 1:5 (stimulus time:rest time) as being the most beneficial in training programs of 20 to 30 minutes because of the deleterious effects of fatigue with lower ratios (1:1, 1:2, 1:3, 1:4). The question remains whether ratios with a greater proportion of rest time might prove more beneficial.

Functional electrical stimulation

The term **functional electrical stimulation (FES)** has been used casually to describe various applications of NMES; however, FES is defined by the Educational Standards Committee of the Section on Clinical Electrophysiology as the use of NMES (on innervated muscles) for orthotic substitution.[36] Baker and others[6] use the term to describe external control of innervated, paretic or paralytic muscles. . . to achieve functional and purposeful movements. While NMES generally is considered to have therapeutic applications, such as increasing ROM, facilitation of muscle activation, and muscle strengthening, the key to application of FES is to enhance or facilitate functional control. It is used with clients with spinal cord injury (SCI), traumatic brain injury, (TBI), cerebrovascular accident (CVA), and other CNS dysfunction, who have intact peripheral innervation.

A simple application of electrically stimulating the peroneal nerve to enhance ankle dorsiflexion during gait in patients with hemiplegia was reported by Liberson in 1961.[62] Numerous uses of FES have been described since then, ranging from single motor control activities, such as decreasing shoulder subluxation and reduction of scoliosis, to the highly technical computerized gait and bicycling capabilities, sometimes referred to as CFES.* The trigger to activate muscle contraction in synchrony with the functional activity can be initiated manually by the client, set within the stimulator to automatically trigger on and off cycles, or programmed into a complex computer system for bicycling or gait.

Stimulation is generally applied in short duration pulses with a frequency sufficient to provide smooth, tetanizing muscle contraction, e.g., 25 pps (pulse per second) and adjusted to cycle on and off with adequate ramp functions, as indicated by the speed and time needed to synchronize the stimulation with the functional activity. The length of

treatment or application sessions depends on the purpose and may vary from use only during the functional activity, to 30 minute daily sessions, repeated three to five times a week to several hours a day.[6]

An obvious goal and benefit of FES is to facilitate or substitute for specified functional activities. With the more complex, computerized systems, (e.g., the REGYS I or ERGYS I home model*) used with clients with complete spinal cord lesions, electrically activated functional movements are the mechanism to achieve physiological and psychological benefits, although in some situations, assisted function also is an important goal.† Hooker and others[50] evaluated physiological effects of using an ERGYS I leg-cycle ergometer on seven persons with paraplegia and seven with quadriplegia. Subjects were stimulated for 30 minutes with low power output levels to avoid fatigue. Compared with resting levels, significant increases were found in cardiac output, heart rate, stroke volume, respiratory exchange rate, pulmonary ventilation, and other physiological phenomena. They further concluded that no inappropriate or unsafe physiological responses occurred in their subjects. Computerized FES for cycle ergometry and ambulation also have been shown to increase muscle mass, electrically induce muscle strength and endurance,[81,87] increase circulation, decrease edema, and have a beneficial effect on self-image.[93]

The demonstrated benefits of FES clearly indicate it is a valuable tool for supplementing functional activities. The practicality and cost of applications of the more complex, computerized systems clearly need further study and technological development.

EMS
Mechanisms

For clients with peripheral nervous system (PNS) dysfunction (e.g., peripheral nerve injuries or peripheral neuropathy), EMS may be helpful in preserving the contractility and extensibility of the muscle tissue and in retarding muscle atrophy.[12,35,95] There is no doubt that literature highlights controversy on the benefits of EMS for peripheral neuropathies and continues to bewilder and lure therapists, physicians, and other researchers to deliberate and study its efficacy.[28,94] Many studies on animals,[58,84,100] and a few on humans[18,88,99] demonstrate that electrical stimulation enhances circulation and decreases venous stasis, thereby improving nutrition, reduces (not prevents) muscle atrophy, and assists in maintaining ROM and the contractile properties of muscle. The goal, then, is to keep muscle tissue healthier and viable until reinnervation is established. *Electrical stimulation does not hasten regeneration of injured nerve tissue.*

Opposing this goal are studies reporting that EMS may have the detrimental effect of retarding reinnervation at the

*Therapeutic Alliances Inc, 333N Broad St, Fairborn, OH, 45324.
†References 37, 50, 51, 79, 80, 82, 86, 93, and 98.

terminal endplate and neuromuscular junction.[63,83] In addition, the time and cost of treatment are major factors, because reinnervation at the rate of 1.5 to 2 mm/day dictates a recovery period of months or even 1 to 2 years. Others argue that studies are flawed and that stimulation is not detrimental to terminal nerve growth if stimulus parameters are wisely selected, and the amplitude is applied at a level that does not fatigue the regenerating nerve or stress the healing tissue. The following discussion should help the reader in making the decision of whether to use EMS for clients with denervated muscles.

Parameters

A number of electrical stimulators with pulses of sufficiently long duration to evoke contractions in denervated muscle are available. Pulse duration, usually monophasic, must be equal to or longer than chronaxie of the denervated muscle. Tests of chronaxie are rarely performed, but historically, tests have shown that pulse durations of 20 to 100 ms are required to produce responses in denervated muscle.[27,48] The shortest effective duration is preferred, because a lower amplitude is required to elicit a response, making the stimulation more comfortable and less fatiguing to the muscle. Therefore stimulators with adjustable durations are preferred, but few are available.

Pulse frequencies of 10 to 30 pps, applied in bouts of 5 to 20 stimulations to each involved muscle should be followed by a rest time longer than the stimulation time (on/off time ratio of no less than 1:5). The bouts of stimulation are then repeated two to three times in each session.[28,58,99] Treatment sessions are more effective if repeated two to three times a day and if initiated early in the course of the dysfunction.

Some reports advocate using a stimulus amplitude strong enough to cause a maximal contraction through the available ROM. Because of possible detrimental effects to the regenerating terminal axons and neuromuscular junction; however, strong submaximal muscle contractions may be a better choice. A stimulus amplitude high enough to produce at least a visible contraction is necessary.

If the prognosis for nerve regeneration is good, or at least fair, and the blood supply is viable, EMS may be useful in maintaining optimal conditions of blood flow, nutrition, and muscle tissue contractibility, so that if or when regeneration occurs, return of motor activation and function may be facilitated. If the EMS does not elicit an effective muscle contraction, stimulation should be discontinued after a 2- to 3-week trial period. If effective contractions can be elicited, the stimulation program should be continued 2 to 6 weeks past the time predicted for reinnervation to occur, as evidenced by visible active muscle contraction. Frequent visits to a physical therapy department for exercise and EMS over the long time awaiting reinnervation are not practical in terms of time or cost. Small, portable, and inexpensive EMS units that can deliver pulses of sufficiently long duration are available for home use. Supplementing a carefully planned therapeutic exercise home program with electrical stimulation should be seriously considered (Fig. 30-2).

EMGBF
Mechanisms

EMGBF has several well-documented applications including alteration of physiological responses such as heart rate, temperature, and muscle tension.[10] These applications may prove beneficial for clients with neurological dysfunction, if relaxation is required for pain reduction, for instance (see Chapter 31). The focus of this review is primarily the use of EMGBF for improvement of active movement, which may include hypertonicity reduction, in addition to muscle reeducation. Current technology provides for a variety of EMGBF units, from very basic single-channel portable models, to clinical units with multiple channels and multiple options for provision of feedback (audio or visual, or both).

EMGBF may be utilized to assist a client in attaining greater levels of muscle activation in a paretic muscle, lower levels of muscle activation in a spastic muscle, or to attain a balance between agonist and antagonist muscle pairs.[109] For the majority of practicing clinicians, EMG levels are monitored through the use of surface electrodes. Monitoring of activation of deep muscles therefore may not be feasible, but attention to size and specific electrode placement is critical to ensure feedback that will be most useful to the client. Smaller electrodes will allow more specific placement, although higher impedance also will be encountered, so skin must be carefully prepared to take this into account.[7] Because EMG recorded represents the sum of action potentials of a muscle between the electrodes, larger interelectrode distance will increase the volume of muscle recorded. Because of the risk of increased crosstalk as EMG from other nearby muscles may be recorded, smaller interelectrode distance is preferable. Basmajian and Blumenstein[7] provide an excellent review of electrode placements for the face, trunk, and upper and lower limbs.

EMGBF for hypertonicity reduction

DeBacher[30] has described a progression of treatment with EMGBF designed to reduce spasticity. It utilizes three stages of intervention: (1) relaxation of spastic muscles at rest even in the presence of distraction, mental effort, or use of muscles not targeted for EMGBF training; (2) inhibition of muscle activity during passive static and dynamic stretch of the spastic muscle, beginning with static stretch at the extremes of motion, then progressing to passive movement speed at a speed of 15 degrees per second, and gradually increasing movement speed at 15 degrees per second increments up to 90 degrees per second; and (3) isometric contractions of the antagonist to the spastic muscle, with relaxation of the spastic muscle, progressing to prompt muscle contraction and relaxation of the spastic muscle, and grading of muscle contractions with movement for various force output requirements. Application of a similar training approach with a group of four young adults with cerebral palsy demonstrated improvement in the resting levels of involuntary muscle activity, as well as reduction in resting and active tonic reflex activity.[75] Consistent functional improvements were not observed, however, as a result of these altered levels of EMG.

Investigation of agonist and antagonist upper extremity muscle activity in a population of stroke patients points to the importance of focusing attention on the weak agonist as opposed to relaxation of the antagonist.[43] EMG levels of targeted muscle groups were monitored in healthy control subjects during the performance of six upper extremity movements in order to describe the appropriate agonists and antagonists for each movement. Patients unable to perform movements demonstrated reduced levels of agonist activity as opposed to increased levels of antagonist muscle activa-

tion. Our presumptions about abnormal cocontraction preventing movement from occurring[16] may require further investigation.

The presence of hypertonicity and spasticity following neurological insult or injury may be problematic for some clients, as these problems may exist in conjunction with lack of active control. Assumptions about the functional importance of spasticity per se seem to be changing as studies demonstrate reduction of spasticity without improvement of motor control. Persistence of control problems may be related to lack of force production, deficits in speed of muscle activation, and lack of reciprocal interaction of muscle groups.[60] Nevertheless, EMGBF can be useful to help a client decrease abnormal muscle activation. Several questions remain: (1) Will the ability to relax a muscle at rest effect a change in muscle activation patterns with movement? and (2) Will alteration in EMG patterns result in functional improvement for the client?

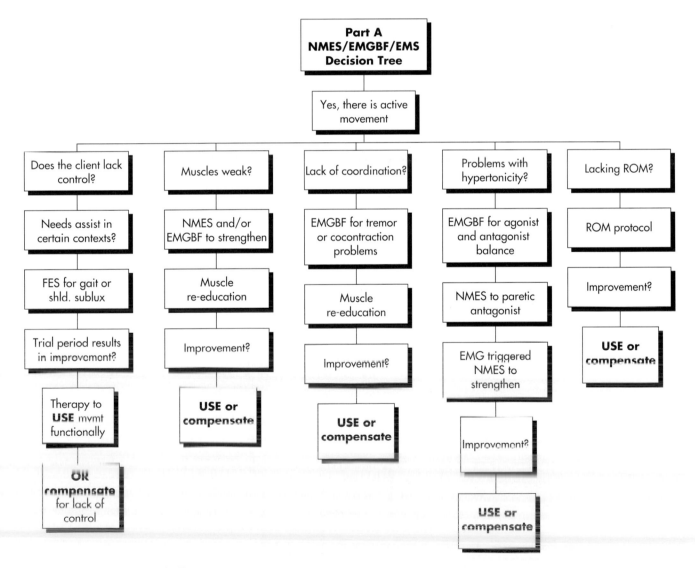

Fig. 30-2. A, Decision Tree for clients that exhibit active movement in the targeted treatment area.

Continued.

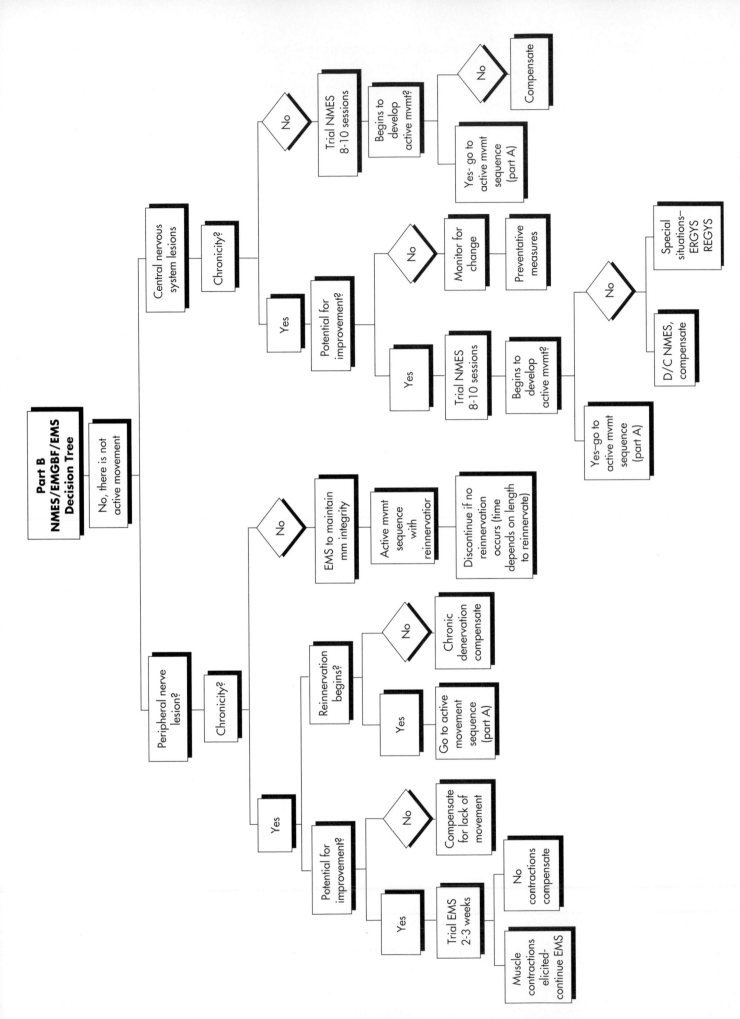

Fig. 30-2. **B,** Decision Tree for clients not yet demonstrating active movement as a result of peripheral nerve injury or central nervous system insult.

EMGBF for muscle reeducation

Therapists may opt to use **biofeedback** to provide information about the quality of the muscle contraction directly to the client. The client can then attempt to alter the contraction in accordance with guidelines provided by the therapist, whether the focus is to facilitate stronger contraction, decrease apparent hyperactivity, or modulate a balance of muscle activity during a functional task.

One such application of EMGBF is concurrent assessment of muscle activity (CAMA),[110] where the therapist utilizes biofeedback as an adjunct in evaluation of client response to therapeutic exercise. In this procedure, the therapist must decide which muscle group(s) are desired for activation and adjust client position or therapist intervention accordingly to achieve the desired muscular responses.[110] CAMA may allow judgment of efficacy of exercise intervention based on actual EMG responses rather than presumptions about what one expects to occur with a particular technique or activity.

Several authors suggest the use of biofeedback signals from homologous extremity muscles as a model for how the hemiplegic client needs to alter muscle activity in a particular function.[104,111] Described as a "motor copy" representation by Wolf and others,[111] this procedure was compared to a more traditional targeted training procedure in a group of 20 clients with stroke and 6 clients with head injury. Although improvements in functional activity level, ROM, and EMG activity were observed for both motor copy and targeted training groups, many of the improvements in the motor copy group appeared on follow-up evaluations (after a series of 10 treatments), whereas the improvements in the targeted training group were observed during the treatment process. Wissel and others[104] used a similar training procedure with monitoring of the uninvolved limb as a model for the hemiparetic upper or lower extremity in the functional tasks of grasping and drinking from a glass and ambulation. Most patients demonstrated improvements in maximum integrated surface EMG, upper extremity movement, multiple stage ratings of walking and drinking from a glass; but the subject group size (N = 11) was too small to draw conclusions statistically.

INTEGRATING NMES AND EMGBF FOR IMPROVED MUSCLE CONTROL

An alternative application that has merit is the use of EMG triggered NMES, where NMES is initiated once the client achieves a predetermined level of EMG activity in the targeted muscle. The threshold of EMG for onset of NMES can be manipulated by the therapist to engage increasing levels of client active control. The success of this application is emphasized for patients with hemiplegia in increasing levels of EMG (improvements in 90% of chronic patients with stroke selected for eight treatment sessions) and subsequent improvement in ROM in the involved arm and leg.[39] Threshold levels of EMG could gradually be increased

as the client gains the ability to activate muscles independently with eventual discontinuance of the NMES as strength and active control allows. A variation of this application is NMES triggered by positional feedback, such that NMES is initiated once the patient actively moves through a portion of the available ROM at a joint.[19] The therapist may set the threshold angle in accordance with the patient goals and abilities. This methodology was effective in improving wrist motion in patients following stroke, although not as effective in altering control of the knee in a similar patient group.[103]

Although discussions of EMGBF, EMS, FES, and NMES are often presented separately, the use of these modalities can be intertwined to achieve desired muscle control. Processes of clinical decision making are represented in Fig. 30-2, beginning with a determination of whether the movement control problem is a result of a CNS or peripheral nerve lesion (Refer to Chapters 12 and 29 for recommended testing to distinguish between the two). NMES or FES may be initiated in the absence of active control (although lower levels of muscle activation may be discovered and facilitated with EMGBF). Once active control begins to return, EMGBF may be utilized to refine the control. One may not assume that an increase in muscle EMG will automatically translate to an improvement in functional use of that muscle in daily activities. Consequently, NMES and EMGBF may be integrated into daily functional activities, so that appropriate muscle activity is elicited and used in a functional context.

CONTRAINDICATIONS AND PRECAUTIONS FOR NMES, EMS, AND EMGBF

NMES is contraindicated for clients that have epilepsy, demand type cardiac pacemakers, over the uterus in pregnancy, and in the area of cancer. Other factors require precaution, but are not strict contraindications such as sensory deficits, skin problems (sensitivity to stimulation/electrodes/gel, edema, open wounds), tolerance of stimulation intensity sufficient to elicit muscle contraction, capability of cooperative participation in the training process, and financial considerations.[27,31,41,76] Use of this modality outside of therapy sessions requires a degree of cooperation and motivation to take care of the stimulation unit, use it as instructed, and observe precautions. Long-term use of NMES (e.g., FES) may not be feasible for clients who do not have the financial resources (insurance or otherwise) to rent or purchase a unit, or do not have reasonable access to support for equipment maintenance.

EMGBF does not require as many precautions because the procedure only monitors muscle activity; but utilization of this form of feedback by the client requires a basic level of attention and cognitive skill to understand the meaning of the feedback, and to act on the feedback to effect a change in muscle performance. Client motivation and interest in use of this modality are also required, as the client must be able to develop sensitivity to the degree of muscle activation independently, so that the feedback is no longer required. EMGBF may be used in some instances that do not require the cognitive skills of the client to utilize this information, for example, as an evaluative tool for the therapist to gather information about muscle activation patterns in order to plan intervention strategies.[110]

FEEDBACK CONSIDERATIONS

Mulder and Hulstyn[70] provide a review of the features of feedback related to motor control and motor learning theories, with discussion of the characteristics of normal feedback. Feedback (in most instances provided verbally by the therapist) may be motivational, but relatively subjective and dependent on the skill of the therapist to attend to the client, observe accurately what occurs, and provide information to the client in a timely manner. Feedback in this form generally is provided with some delay after the activity. EMGBF has the benefit of being provided simultaneously with the client's movement, consisting of accurate and objective information about muscle activity (given careful electrode application and equipment in good working order), and not requiring the same level of therapist skill as verbal feedback provision. EMGBF therefore may be beneficial for clients with deficient sensory feedback systems. The frequency of feedback provision, however, may require close scrutiny by the therapist, as demonstrated by the following studies.

Experiments examining feedback frequency in the learning of motor tasks support the use of less than 100% relative frequency in order for the subject to learn the task. Feedback provided on every trial may improve performance but degrade learning in healthy subjects.[92] The application of this concept to the use of EMGBF was investigated by Bate and Matyas,[11] who used EMGBF with two groups of stroke patients attempting a pursuit tracking task. Comparisons were made of performance in a pretest, training test, and posttest phase. The biofeedback provided information about the contractions of the spastic antagonist (elbow flexors) for the movement task for the experimental group. The control group performed the task without the benefit of biofeedback. Posttesting revealed the use of continuous feedback had a negative transfer effect on learning of the movement task, suggesting that the experimental learners became dependent on the external feedback in performance of the task. It is imperative therefore that the clinician structure the use of external feedback carefully so that the client begins to develop a sense of muscle activation or relaxation which is present without the EMGBF apparatus. Biofeedback may be used with the screen turned away from the client (or audio signal turned off) so that the client can transfer the learning without feedback, and the clinician can evaluate client performance and judge actual client learning of the muscle activation patterns.

APPLICATIONS

The application of the common principles of EMGBF and NMES to different patient populations emphasizes the role of the therapist in tailoring intervention to meet specific client needs. Many investigators have evaluated the use of NMES and EMGBF in subjects with stroke. FES has been used extensively with clients with SCI. Other populations that demonstrate neuromuscular dysfunction have not been as thoroughly studied, as the heterogeneity of these groups may create difficulty in research design. Perhaps patients with cerebral palsy, brain injury, and Guillain-Barré syndrome gain or regain active control in therapy through conventional means; therefore therapists do not consider use of NMES or EMGBF. Nevertheless, there are documented applications of these modalities with a variety of patient populations. These results are reviewed.

Stroke

Wolf and colleagues[106] examined client characteristics that are critical to success with biofeedback retraining for upper and lower extremity control following stroke. In a group of 52 clients with stroke, no significant relationships between outcome and age, sex, number of EMGBF treatments, or side of hemiparesis were found. Lower extremity treatment was associated with a greater probability of success, and this success did not seem related to chronicity of stroke. In contrast, upper extremity treatment success did appear to be related to length of time since onset of stroke, and poorer outcomes were noted if clients had received physical therapy to the involved arm for more than 1 year before EMGBF training. Improvements in elbow and shoulder function were obtainable in this group of patients, but obtaining improvement in functional use of the hand was limited. Aphasia did emerge as a slight limitation to achieving improvement, but proprioception deficits were more significant in restricting functional gains. The role of client motivation in success with EMGBF training was emphasized. On follow-up over 12 months, the improvements made in the initial intervention were maintained in the 34 clients evaluated, with one exception, where deterioration in motor function was attributed to possible organic cause (transient ischemic attacks).[105]

A number of researchers have published papers discussing the muscle recruitment problems observed following CVA.[43,46,47,89] Knowledge of these problems is a prerequisite to determination of the appropriate application of EMGBF or NMES. It appears that delayed recruitment of agonist and antagonist is a relatively consistent finding. Some studies demonstrate delayed termination of muscle activity once initiated[89] and the presence of cocontraction of agonist and antagonist muscle groups.[46-47] Other investigators have discovered a lack of co-contraction[43] and problems with maintenance of agonist muscle contractions.[47] The possibility of these conflicting presentations underscores the benefit of usage of EMGBF so that the actual muscle activation patterns can be observed in a given client, and treatment can progress.

Upper extremity management. EMGBF has been studied extensively, but success of treatment is mixed, with difficulty in interpretation complicated by focus on measures that are not directly related to function in a number of studies. A reduction in co-contraction has been observed,[85] as well as improvement in several neuromuscular variables[54,107,108]; however, a lack of significant improvement in functional skill is noted. Given the challenge of improving upper extremity functional ability following stroke, Wolf Binder-Macleod suggest the consideration of several key factors in predicting which clients may benefit from EMGBF: "those patients who achieve the most substantial improvement in manipulative abilities initially possess voluntary finger extension; comparatively greater active ROM about the shoulder, elbow, and wrist; and comparatively less hyperactivity in muscles usually considered as major contributors to the typical flexor synergy."[108] Attention to the chronicity of motor dysfunction also appears critical in anticipating success with EMGBF, as clients 2 to 3 months after stroke demonstrated stronger functional gains following intervention with biofeedback as compared to clients 4 to 5 months after stroke.[8]

Common upper extremity applications of NMES for the stroke patient include reduction of shoulder subluxation (FES) and facilitation of elbow, wrist, and finger extension. Electrode placements for shoulder movements are detailed by Baker and Parker,[4] including shoulder extension, flexion and abduction, and scapular muscle stimulation.

FES was utilized with 63 stroke patients (mean of 46 days postonset for the control group, and 49 days postonset for the experimental group) to evaluate the effects of this treatment on shoulder subluxation as measured by radiography.[4] Treatment protocol included stimulation of the posterior deltoid and supraspinatus muscles to reduce shoulder subluxation, with gradual increases from three half-hour sessions to one 6- to 7-hour cycle per day with a 1:3 on/off ratio. The FES was used for 6 weeks. Radiographs at the end of the intervention period showed improvements in the study group from 14.8 to 8.6mm, with a 1 to 2mm loss of reduction when evaluated 3 months later. The control group began with a mean subluxation of 13.3mm, and the same amount of subluxation was noted after the 6-week intervention time. Three months after the study, the control group demonstrated no change in subluxation. No direct relationship between pain and amount of subluxation was noted. It may be argued that the chronicity of this patient population played a role in the success of the FES in altering shoulder subluxation, and that this intervention may prove more beneficial if used in the initial stages to prevent subluxation, rather than attempt to reduce it once it has occurred. Faghri and colleagues[48] implemented FES as a preventive measure in a group of acute patients. An experimental and control group each received conventional physical therapy, but the experimental group also received FES to reduce shoulder subluxation gradually increasing up to 6 hours per day and continuing for 6 weeks. Comparisons of arm function, arm muscle tone, posterior deltoid EMG activity, upper arm girth, shoulder ROM (to test for pain), and shoulder subluxation (by

radiography of both shoulders) were performed at the beginning of the intervention, at the completion of the 6-week program, and 6 weeks after the completion of the program. The experimental group exhibited significantly greater range without pain than the control group and significantly less subluxation (6mm initially, decreasing to 2.46mm after the treatment, and then increasing slightly to 3.46 mm 6 weeks later, as compared to values of 4 mm, 9.85mm and 9.35mm for the control group). Both groups demonstrated functional improvement with higher values (although not significantly different) for the experimental group.

FES for shoulder subluxation reduction appears beneficial for prevention of pain and subluxation, especially if utilized during the early stages of recovery. The functional benefits of this intervention are not clear; however, even in studies with relatively extensive intervention periods (6 weeks, with 6 to 7 hours of stimulation each day). Careful cost-benefit analysis is recommended when considering this modality for shoulder subluxation reduction.

FES also has been investigated as an upper extremity orthosis following hemiplegia utilizing movement of the uninvolved shoulder to trigger stimulation of elbow extension and hand opening.[66] After extensive training periods, patients were able to demonstrate functional use of the involved hand for basic reach and grasp. Systems with more than two channels of stimulation have proved difficult for patients to use.[115]

Three-month interventions with EMG triggered NMES, low intensity NMES, proprioceptive neuromuscular facilitation (PNF) exercises, or no treatment (control group) were compared in a group of chronic stroke patients.[59] Evaluations performed before treatment, at completion of treatment, and at 3- and 9-month intervals after treatment demonstrated improvements in those patients receiving therapy. Fugl-Meyer scores improved 18% for the PNF group, 25% for the patients receiving low-intensity NMES, and 42% for the group treated with EMG triggered NMES. The control group scores did not change.[59] These findings lend support to use of NMES as an adjunct to physical therapy.

Lower extremity management. Several studies evaluating EMGBF for retraining lower extremity control following stroke have focused on improvement of tibialis anterior control, and/or reduction of gastrocnemius muscle activity. Results support increases in strength and ROM in ankle dorsiflexion[9,21,90] with carry-over into ambulation[9] and maintenance of this improvement on follow-up evaluation.[9,21]

Wolf and Binder-Macleod[107] examined a number of variables at the hip, knee, and ankle in a controlled group study of the effects of EMGBF. Subjects were assigned to one of four groups: treatment of the lower extremity only with EMGBF, EMGBF treatment of the upper extremity only, general relaxation training, or no treatment. No significant changes were observed between experimental and control groups for EMG levels and ROM at the hip, but improvements were noted in knee and ankle active motion for the experimental group. Although subjects in the experimental group increased in gait speed, these changes were not significantly different from the comparison groups.

Utilization of EMGBF with the intent of improving ambulation may require use of the feedback during the task of ambulation instead of during static activity as demonstrated in this study. Positional biofeedback about ankle position and traditional EMGBF were compared in a group of hemiplegic patients.[65] A computerized system provided audiovisual feedback during ambulation for both groups. Pretreatment and posttreatment measures of ankle motion, gait, and perceived exertion were conducted for the two treatment groups and a control group. The group receiving positional biofeedback during ambulation increased their walking speeds relative to the other groups, with improvements maintained at follow-up intervals of up to 3 months. The consideration of integrating feedback into functional tasks bears further investigation.

Peroneal nerve stimulation has been documented as an assist for patients with hemiplegia to improve ambulation.[62,67,96,101] Chronic stimulation via implanted electrodes has proved effective in improving gait patterns, but not without significant drawbacks of difficulty eliciting balanced dorsiflexion, infection with nerve damage in a few cases, and problems with equipment maintenance.[101,102] In a few patients studied over a 10-year period, the need for stimulation eventually was eliminated, as patients regained the ability to dorsiflex independently.[102] Technology may provide smaller, more sophisticated versions of these devices so that such treatments are more realistic in the future.

Shorter term use of peroneal nerve stimulation as an adjunct to traditional physical therapy may be considered. In a controlled study examining the use of 20 minutes of peroneal nerve stimulation six times per week for 4 weeks the stimulated group demonstrated dorsiflexion recovery three times greater than the control group, as measured by an average of 10 maximal dorsiflexion contractions. These improvements were observed regardless of site of lesion, age, or time since lesion.[67] This type of stimulation is more easily applied than the chronic stimulation described earlier, and may prove more effective.

A series of studies from researchers in Ljubljana suggest the use of multichannel electrical stimulation as an intervention to expedite recovery of ambulation in hemiplegia following CVA or brain injury.[17,64,114] Through the use of stimulation (as an adjunct to traditional therapy) in daily sessions in a group of 10 patients over a 2- to 3-week period, a 61.6% increase in gait velocity, 46.3% increase in stride length, and significant decreases in mean stride time were observed during the use of FES. Carry-over of these effects to ambulation without the stimulation was observed to varying degrees.[17] A comparison of patients treated with this form of stimulation with patients treated by conventional rehabilitation demonstrated faster and greater recovery rates

for variables of step length and gait velocity in the stimulated group than the control group. At follow-up evaluation 8.4 months after the conclusion of therapy, however, the differences between groups had faded.[64]

Cozean and others[26] utilized NMES for ankle dorsiflexion triggered by heel switch contact during gait and biofeedback to improve active recruitment of ankle dorsiflexors and/or relaxation of ankle plantarflexors in a study with 36 hemiplegic patients. Patients were divided into four treatment groups: control, NMES, EMGBF, and combined EMGBF and NMES. Those patients assigned to the combined therapy group demonstrated significantly improved knee and ankle range parameters more rapidly than the NMES or EMGBF or control groups. This result was better maintained in the combined therapy group at follow-up 1 month later. Although all treatment groups improved in gait cycle times, the combined therapy group improved to a greater degree. The authors speculate that the reason for this success may be the benefit at the muscular level achieved by NMES and the focus on retraining central control through the use of EMGBF, which interact synergistically to allow the patient to use the hemiplegic limb more effectively.[26]

Upper and lower extremity management. A few studies have addressed upper and lower extremity retraining procedures simultaneously.[39,52,108,109] The use of actual EMGBF, simulated EMGBF, and no EMGBF were compared in a group of patients with stroke undergoing conventional physical therapy.[52] The simulated EMGBF was generated by the examiner contracting a muscle simultaneous to each patient attempt, so the feedback was positive, but not the actual patient EMG. After a 2-week treatment period, EMG responses from the deltoid and anterior tibial muscles and average ROM measures were compared. The two groups receiving feedback of some form in addition to physical therapy demonstrated significant improvements over the control group. Because the simulated feedback was provided by a therapist by observation of patient effort, it was not completely unrelated to the EMG activity of the limb. The specificity of the feedback did not appear to be critical, raising questions about the mechanism by which improvement occurs with this intervention.

Fields[39] used a technique of EMG-triggered electric muscle stimulation with a group of 69 outpatients with stroke, targeting wrist extension and ankle dorsiflexion initially, but progressing to other movements over the course of several months of four to five treatment sessions (45-minute sessions) per week. As previously described, the intervention allowed for setting gradually increased EMG threshold levels which subjects must meet before the onset of EMS to assist targeted muscle contraction. Peak unassisted voluntary EMG levels were used as quantitative indications of progress, despite difficulty normalizing these values. Measurable functional progress (improved active ROM and ambulation) was noted in greater than 90% of the patients treated in this study, with those patients unsuitable for this intervention being identified after the first several trials. This form of stimulation is commercially available (Electronic Medical Instruments, Bellevue, Washington), and may offer an alternative to traditional NMES or EMGBF.

Efficacy. Several reviews are available regarding the use of EMGBF with patients following stroke.[32,91,112,114] Well-designed studies with experimental and control groups support the efficacy of EMGBF in improving muscle activation and functional control of the upper and lower extremity, as demonstrated through a metaanalysis,[91] although only eight studies met the strict inclusion criteria for this analysis. Wolf[112] provides support for the use of biofeedback in retraining control of the upper and lower extremity following stroke, yet raises numerous questions for future investigation. Areas of possible study include correlation of feedback intervention with functional outcomes, carefully designed treatment protocols with control groups addressing acute and chronic stroke patients, clarification of site and extent of lesion as factors in the efficacy of EMGBF, and continued consideration of the factors of age, duration of previous intervention, and sensory and communicative skills in examination of treatment effects.[112,114]

Much of the literature evaluating the use of EMGBF and NMES involves patients with CVA. Although these studies have many significant results to share, interpretation of these findings with relation to what is recommended for clinical intervention is not so clear-cut. Improvements in generation of EMG activity and active movement appear well documented; the functional implications of these gains are

not as well established. Clearly in the current practice environment, much of the focus is on function, so that these techniques to improve muscle activation patterns must be put to functional use in the context of therapy. The therapist must consider the relevant factors that may predict success and critically evaluate outcome during trial usage of these modalities. Cost-benefit analyses must accompany intervention using technology, with the goal of regaining movement *without the use of the equipment* when practical, and as quickly as possible. These processes may be illustrated through the use of a case example (See Case 1.)

Spinal cord injury

NMES has a variety of applications for clients who have sustained SCI. Muscle strengthening may occur for muscles innervated by segments just above a complete spinal cord injury, or a variety of strengthening applications may be appropriate in the case of incomplete spinal cord injury. EMGBF may be used to identify muscle activity in very weak musculature, as a tool to judge improvement in muscle activation, and as a method of facilitating increased strength.[113] Applications of EMGBF for individuals with SCI also include facilitation of unassisted ventilation in high-level quadriplegia[69] and use of biofeedback for muscle reeducation with incomplete SCI in the acute stages when immobilization may be required.[74]

The use of NMES, EMGBF, and other physical therapy was examined in a group of clients with incomplete cervical spinal cord injuries over a total treatment period of 16 weeks. Clients were randomly assigned to one of four groups, receiving either physical exercise, NMES, or EMGBF administered in 8-week blocks. Group 1 re-

---

CASE 1 ▼ Left Middle Cerebral Artery CVA

A 68-year-old woman is referred to you 3 weeks s/p left middle cerebral artery CVA with residual right hemiparesis affecting the upper extremity to a greater degree than the lower extremity. Her left extremities appear well controlled with at least functional strength. She exhibits a two finger width right shoulder subluxation, with pain at the extremes of shoulder flexion (150°), abduction (135°) and external rotation (30°); and hypertonicity in a stereotypical flexor pattern affecting the shoulder horizontal adductors and internal rotators, elbow, wrist and finger flexors. She is beginning to develop upper extremity movement with the ability to shrug her shoulder, abduct and flex through partial range (with elbow flexed), full range elbow flexion, partial range elbow and wrist extension against gravity, and a very slight degree of finger extension with facilitation. Right lower extremity ROM is within normal limits, although control is limited at the ankle (dorsiflexion only with hip and knee flexion, no eversion actively) and knee control is decreased (reduced eccentric quadriceps control, difficulty isolating knee flexion with hip extension).

Ambulation is accomplished with use of a quad cane and an articulating ankle-foot orthosis (AFO) on the right for limited distances with stand-by assistance.

This client lives at home with her husband, who is very supportive of her rehabilitation. Both of them are retired, but have an active calendar of participation in volunteer and leisure activities. Insurance coverage is good.

Therapeutic intervention for this client would of course include extensive therapeutic exercise and functional activity training, but the following EMGBF and/or NMES options also may be considered (see the box on p. 864). The treatment of all of the problems listed may become confusing for the client because some of the stimulation may occur as part of a home program, and necessitates the use of a portable stimulator. Consequently, the client and therapist may need to discuss possible interventions and target one or two of these areas for concentrated effort, based on the goals of the client and your assessment of potential for improvement.

EMGBF/NMES options for Case 1

Client problems	Goals	Modality-Parameters	Measures to determine efficacy	Considerations
Shoulder subluxation.	Decrease subluxation to 1 finger width, with pain managable within patient's daily routine.	Portable FES for home use, begin with 10:30 second on/off ratio for 15 minute periods t.i.d., amplitude to generate mm contraction without shoulder elevation. Increase on time and treatment time as tolerated so that reduction is maintained majority of day.	Trial use x 1 month. Measure amount of palpable subluxation, painfree ROM; if improvement is not observed, discontinue FES, with instruction to maintain shoulder flexibility, consider lapboard or arm tray when sitting, support when standing.	1) Requires rental of portable FES unit, pt/family compliance is needed for success in home program. 2) Cost of rental of FES and supplies. 3) Frequent use for reduction of subluxation requires close monitoring of skin for possible reactions to stimulation, gel and/or electrodes. 4) Integrate scapular movement and stabilization exs into program.
Lack of active ankle dorsiflexion.	Increase active control of ankle dorsiflexion with knee extended, allowing heelstrike without AFO for short distance ambulation.	FES, b.i.d. for 15-minute duration; 10:20 second on/off ratio with slow ramping on/off; as active movement improves, consider EMGBF to further focus attention on balanced dorsiflexion (with eversion).	Monitor each session for increased active dorsiflexion in sitting, standing, and ambulation. Integrate use of heelswitch during ambulation without AFO. Trial use for 2-3 weeks, discharge if not seeing increase in voluntary control-compensate with AFO.	1) If pt rents unit for shoulder subluxation, may also use stimulator at home instead of requiring time during therapy session. 2) Similar cost, convenience issues as above. 3) Additional education necessary if stimulator settings are to be switched for dorsiflexion and shoulder subluxation interventions.
Lack of full active wrist and finger extension.	Control of active wrist and finger extension to allow release in gross grasp.	NMES and/or EMGBF b.i.d. for 10-minute sessions initially, with gradual increase in duration up to 20 minutes. Other parameters as described for ankle dorsiflexion.	Active movement in finger extensors with wrist in neutral position. Functional ability to release grasp of objects of varying shapes and sizes. Trial period of 2 to 3 weeks, discontinue if voluntary motion is not changing significantly.	May utilize portable stimulator as described for ankle or shoulder interventions, with similar considerations.
Muscle imbalance, lack of right upper extremity functional movement.	Decrease hypertonicity in flexor muscle groups, increase extensor control for gross arm movements (i.e., positioning).	EMGBF to decrease flexor muscle activity (resting and with passive movement), increase extensor activity. May utilize methodolgy described by DeBacher.[30]	Speed and control with reciprocal elbow motions, especially with extension. Use of this motion for functional activity (positioning the arm, reaching activity, etc.).	Focus on increased extensor control may prove more effective than simply decreasing flexor hyperactivity.

ceived EMGBF followed by physical exercise, group 2 received EMGBF followed by NMES, group 3 received NMES followed by physical exercise, and group 4 received 16 weeks of physical exercise only. Measures of muscle strength, self-care ratings, mobility scores, and voluntary EMG were conducted at baseline, treatment midpoint, and conclusion of the interventions. All groups demonstrated improvement across the treatment period on all measures except for voluntary EMG; however there were no significant differences among the four groups.[57] These results emphasize the need to carefully consider cost in planning treatment.

Upper extremity management. The use of electrically stimulated hand orthotic systems for patients with C-6 and higher level SCI have been refined to allow greater functional independence for a select group of patients.[56,79,80] Because hand function does not occur in a cyclical pattern, the onset and termination of stimulation must be controlled by the patient in some manner, with a myoelectric[80] or contact closing switch. Multiple channel stimulation is then applied with intramuscular electrodes for the flexors and extensors of the fingers and thumb, with computer configured interplay between the different muscles to achieve a functional grasp. A chest mounted position transducer (operated by shoulder elevation/depression and protraction/retraction) allows the user to initiate stimulation and "lock" the stimulation to maintain a grasp, as well as "unlock" for release. A toggle switch mounted on the chest allows a choice between electrically stimulated lateral or palmar grasp patterns.[56,79] Use of this type system may allow patients at the C-5 level to operate at the same or even higher level of independence as C-6 quadriplegia with tenodesis, gaining the ability to perform more activities of daily living without an attendant. Patients at the C-6 level may be able to manipulate a greater variety of objects without special adaptations.

Lower extremity management

Standing. In an excellent review of the utilization of FES for the purpose of standing patients with SCI, Gardner and Baker[40] describe the easiest approach of stimulating the quadriceps femoris in conjunction with upper extremity support to allow paraplegic clients to stand (see Chapter 16). More complex systems may incorporate stimulation of gluteus maximus, gluteus medius, hamstring, adductor magnus, gastrocnemius, and soleus muscles for longer duration and better quality standing performance. Despite these efforts, the duration of standing with electrically stimulated systems ranges from a few minutes to several hours. The client with SCI may be able to utilize this technology to perform functional activities that require standing. The use of these systems depend on the functions unavailable to a client without use of the technology, and the ease with which a system can be used and maintained.

Cycling. The use of systems to electrically stimulate reciprocal lower limb motions has increased for stationary cycling. The benefits of these interventions for the client with

SCI may relate to prevention of cardiovascular disease in the wheelchair-dependent client. Physiological changes noted with electrically stimulated cycling include improvement of peripheral muscular and cardiovascular fitness, as demonstrated by increased power output following training with leg cycle ergometry.[37,50,51,81] When testing of paraplegic and quadriplegic clients is conducted with arm crank ergometry following a training program with electrically stimulated leg cycle ergometry, clients do not demonstrate differences in pretest and posttest measures of hemodynamic and pulmonary responses. These findings may relate to the specificity of the leg exercise training or the presence of a peripheral rather than a central circulatory response to the training procedure.[51]

An additional possible benefit of use of lower extremity NMES with the SCI client is the improvement of circulation, as occurred in conjunction with cycling training in a case report.[98] Through the use of an initial program to strengthen the quadriceps femoris, stimulation can be applied with resistance added to the limb in gradual increments, until the client is able to tolerate the training protocol for electrically stimulated cycling (commercially available REGYS system). Further research is required to validate potential effects of decreased edema, increased blood flow, and concomitant improved wound healing as a result of electrically stimulated cycling.

Ambulation. As technology continues to progress, the use of electrically stimulated systems for ambulation[29,82] may become more practical and useful for the patient with SCI. Benefits of these systems may include increased muscle bulk, a reduced risk of pressure sores and osteoporosis, and psychological benefit. Drawbacks relate to the expense of the equipment and personnel and the lack of long-term efficacy studies. The speed with which a client with a complete SCI is able to walk with electrically stimulated systems remains relatively slow (2 to 54m/minute) as compared with a normal rates of 78 to 90m/min (1.3 to 1.5 m/sec).[71-72] Many of the published reports do not provide information about the maximal distance clients are able to walk with these systems, but reported distances range from 100 to 400 meters.

The use of electrically stimulated reciprocal thigh movements in conjunction with a reciprocating gait orthosis appears to be helpful in reducing the energy expenditure to ambulate (as compared with other orthotic interventions such as long leg braces or the reciprocating gait orthosis alone).[49] Despite these energy savings, the use of such a system at the current time is primarily for exercise as opposed to functional ambulation.

Some clients may perceive the technology of electrically stimulated standing, cycling, or walking as moving them toward a cure for their paralysis. With a complete injury, however, the stimulation occurs passively, without expectation that voluntary control will return. In cases of incomplete injury electrically stimulated ambulation may assist the client in using and bolstering active control, so that

CASE 2 ▼ C-6 Quadriplegia

An 18-year-old male client is referred to you for therapy 6 weeks after a diving accident, which resulted in fracture dislocation at C-6 with complete cord transection. The client is currently stabilized in a halo vest and has completed a course of inpatient rehabilitation, but continues as an outpatient for additional treatment. He exhibits dependent lower extremity edema, which is managed with thigh-high TED hose. Some difficulty with postural hypotension is present and is treated with an abdominal binder when he is in his wheelchair. Sensation is intact to light touch and pinprick through C-5 levels bilaterally, with impaired sensibility at C-6 and absent at C-7 dermatome and below. Passive ROM is full for both lower extremities, with the exception of neutral dorsiflexion (limited by ankle edema) and straight leg raises to 75 degrees bilaterally. Upper extremity range is full within the constraints of the halo vest.

He presents with the following manual muscle test grades:

Upper trapezius	4+/5 B	
Deltoid-middle	4+/5 B	
Biceps	5/5 R	4+/5L
Pectoralis major (clavicular)	4/5 B	
Pectoralis major (sternal)	0/5 B	
Wrist extensors	3+/5 R	3/5 L
Triceps	0/5 B	

No active motion below this level is obtained, although he occasionally demonstrates flexor spasms in his lower extremities in response to movement, including sustained ankle clonus, which interferes slightly with transfers. Functionally he is able to propel his manual wheelchair with rim projections for household distances on smooth surfaces. He requires maximal assistance with transfers. He is awaiting the arrival of his power wheelchair. He is using a R wrist orthosis for activities of daily living, but would benefit from increased ability to use tenodesis grasp without the orthosis (see box).

NMES options for C-6 quadriplegia

Client problems	Goals	Modality-Parameters	Measures to determine efficacy	Considerations
Decreased wrist extensor strength.	Increase wrist extensor strength and endurance to allow use of tenodesis grasp for manipulation of objects.	NMES to strengthen wrist extensors bilaterally, using b.i.d. sessions for 10-minute durations —two channels to work both wrists reciprocally; 10:20 second on/off ratio, amplitude to achieve strong contraction. May gradually increase duration to 20 minutes per session.	Ability to use tenodesis for functional grasp in ADL situations (timed manipulation tasks, or use of tool such as Jebsen Hand Function Assessment).	1) Access to portable stimulation for home use may accelerate process. 2) See considerations for CVA case (Case 1). 3) Integrate other strengthening exercises into home routine since active movement is already present.
Lower extremity edema.	Reduction of edema, with concomitant benefits of increased vital capacity, improved circulation and psychological benefit.	REGYS electrically stimulated cycling. Gradual increase of electrically stimulated cycling time as per manufacturer protocol.	Edema measurement, need for continued use of compression stockings.	1) Introduction of this idea must be carefully evaluated, as client may misinterpret potential for active movement return. 2) Cost of this intervention and access to the necessary equipment may preclude client involvement.

CASE 3 ▼ Traumatic Brain Injury

A 25-year-old man 8 weeks s/p TBI following a motor vehicle accident is transferred to your caseload in the rehabilitation unit of an acute hospital. He also sustained multiple trauma with a right distal femoral fracture, which was treated with internal fixation. He has been gradually regaining consciousness following coma duration of approximately 5 weeks, so that now he is at Rancho's Level V with bouts of agitation that occur after too much stimulation. He was serial casted at both ankles to prevent plantarflexion contractures while in a coma (range is neutral bilaterally), and now that these casts have been converted to resting splints, you have discovered a lack of ankle movement on the right. After diagnostic testing right common peroneal nerve injury is confirmed as a result of the femoral fracture and possible complication by bed positioning with the hip externally rotated while comatose.

Right upper and lower extremity movement is well controlled with the exception of the lack of ankle control. He exhibits increased flexor tone of the left upper extremity with only partial range extension and limited range to −30 degrees of elbow extension. He is beginning to develop some wrist and finger extension on the left, but currently flexion predominates. The left lower extremity demonstrates active control in muscle groups of the hip and knee, but movement is weak. Ankle motion is limited on the left with a tendency toward inversion and plantarflexion. In attempts to stand, his knee often buckles. He currently requires AFOs bilaterally for short-distance ambulation with the use of a large-based quad cane.

The use of electrical stimulation with a client who is confused presents some significant problems; however, several of these problem areas may be addressed with stimulation. A trial intervention with one of the problems is indicated, and if the client tolerates the stimulation well, it may be used in other contexts. As cognitive ability improves, more stimulation may be possible in addition to the use of EMGBF (see the box on p. 868).

---

movement without the stimulation is more feasible. In considering use of electrically stimulated cycling or ambulation, discussion of the goals of treatment and the costs of the procedure must be discussed openly with the client to allow an educated choice to be made about use of this expensive technology (See Case 2 on p. 866).

Other applications

Brain injury. NMES may be a useful tool with clients having sustained brain injury with potential benefits of managing contactures by increasing ROM, facilitation of active control, and reduction of spasticity by strengthening the antagonist to a spastic muscle.[5] In cases where an understanding of the purpose and principles of NMES is not feasible for the client, the comfort of the stimulation may be critical in ensuring its continued use. Comfort may be enhanced with increasing the ramp on time and selection of wave forms that allow stimulation at lower amplitudes yet obtain the desired muscle contraction.[116] Use of NMES with a client in Rancho Level IV and below is not appropriate, as the client may not be able to understand the purpose or meaning of the stimulus, and thereby perceive the stimulus as noxious.[116] The therapist may find greater success in use of NMES in functional activities if stimulation can be triggered by a heel switch or hand switch so that the stimulation coincides appropriately with the goal of therapy.

EMGBF applications for clients with brain injury can be similar to those used with stroke, given similar motor presentations.[61] Therapists must consider residual cognitive deficits following brain injury in determining the appropriateness of EMGBF (See Case 3).

Cerebral palsy. The use of NMES with children with cerebral palsy has been addressed to a limited degree, with several case study reports.[22,23,34] Carmick[22,23] described a variety of applications with children at 1.6, 6.7, and 10 years of age, integrating NMES into a treatment regimen that focuses on a "task-oriented model of motor learning." Improvements were noted in upper and lower extremity movement and functional use across a variety of tasks appropriate to the age and movement dysfunction each child demonstrated.

Advancements in technology allow for use of EMGBF in increasing contexts, such as the computer-assisted feedback (CAF) system, which can be used to provide feedback about muscle activity during ambulation.[25] Pilot data examining use of this system to provide feedback about the level of triceps surae activity during gait to children with cerebral palsy suggest potential improvements in gait symmetry, velocity and appropriate muscle activation patterns as a result of this intervention. Use of this modality as an adjunct to physical therapy may prove beneficial.

Spina bifida. Five children with spina bifida (aged 5 to 21 years) were treated with daily NMES over an 8-week period to strengthen the quadriceps femoris muscles. Increases in maximum quadriceps torque production were observed in two of the five subjects in the treated limb. Improvements in functional activity speeds were noted for all of the subjects. Lack of improvement in torque production by three subjects was speculated to be related to lack of adherence to the exercise regimen and the heterogeneity of the subject sample.[55] Further investigation of this modality with spina bifida is indicated.

Guillain-Barré syndrome. EMGBF in clients with

Use of stimulation for Case 3

Client problems	Goals	Modality-Parameters	Measures to determine efficacy	Considerations
Lack of right ankle movement secondary to common peroneal nerve injury with dorsiflexion ROM limited to neutral.	Increase ROM to 10 degrees of dorsiflexion. Maintain muscle integrity as reinnervation progresses. Begin active movement as soon as control is available.	EMS—low volt stimulation with long pulse duration, 2-3 pps, amplitude sufficient to obtain contraction, repeat 10-15 contractions per muscle b.i.d.; continue for number of weeks predicted for reinnervation to occur.	Attain muscle contraction with EMS. Monitor for reinnervation and return of active control.	1) Integrate positioning and weight-bearing activities into program. 2) As active movement begins to occur, switch to EMGBF to facilitate EMG activity or NMES to strengthen. 3) Time-consuming activity, more difficult to teach family or client to perform than NMES.
Elbow flexor hypertonicity and lack of full ROM in elbow extension (active and passive).	Active elbow flexion and extension through the full ROM. Able to move his arm functionally for activities such as reaching.	NMES to triceps muscle, 15 minute sessions with 10:20 second on/off ratio with slow ramping on/off, amplitude sufficient to attain strong triceps contraction.	Active and passive ROM elbow extension. Functional use of the arm for reaching, propping on the elbow with extension, etc.	May effectively be integrated into serial cast protocol to increase elbow extension range, with drop-out cast so that forearm is circumferentially casted, but upper arm is casted only on the flexor surface, leaving triceps area available for electrode placements and allowing elbow extension, but blocking flexion.
Lack of left lower extremity extensor control in standing.	Stability of knee extension for standing activities (weight shifting, sit to stand, balance in standing).	NMES to quadriceps during therapy activities in standing. Utilize therapist controlled onset to stimulate as appropriate.	Frequency of knee buckling with standing activities.	1) Ensure that biomechanical alignment is obtained in standing, so that buckling is a result of weakness as opposed to flexion moment at knee. 2) As attention and cognitive capacity improve may use EMGBF during standing to facilitate extensor control.
Lack of active wrist and finger extension on the left.	Refer to Case 1, wrist and finger extension parameters for specifics.			

Guillain-Barré syndrome demonstrated improvements in muscle strength in upper and lower extremities,[24,53] although inconsistent improvement in functional use of the upper extremities was noted.[53] Treatment regimens consisted of EMGBF for 10 trials per muscle, conducted in 45-minute treatment sessions twice a week, in one case for 78 weeks, and the other case for 46 weeks.[53]

SUMMARY

Clearly, there are numerous possibilities for the use of NMES and EMGBF with clients of all ages who have sustained neurological insult or injury. There is preliminary support for improvement of movement control in some applications, although the paucity of well-controlled group research in populations other than stroke and adult SCI underscores the need for further investigation to support efficacy of these modalities. As the therapy environment changes in response to time and funding constraints, therapists must carefully evaluate the benefits of a variety of available tools to assist their clients in regaining motor control and functional ability. An additional benefit of FES or EMGBF is the ability for the client to work autonomously (i.e., at home) after becoming familiar with the treatment regimen, with the therapist periodically updating a home program. This protocol allows therapy time to be used for direct intervention. NMES and EMGBF may efficiently assist in attaining improvement in control, and may also be used in the context of functional activities, but these tools alone will not effect functional changes. Trial use of EMGBF or NMES for 2 to 4 weeks (daily to three times a week) with careful outcome assessment may assist the therapist in judging treatment efficacy for each client.

REFERENCES

1. Alon G: Principles of electrical stimulation. In Nelson RM and Currier DP, editors: *Clinical electrotherapy,* ed 2, Norwalk, Conn, 1991, Appleton & Lange.
2. Axelgaard J and Brown JC: Lateral electrical surface stimulation for the treatment of progressive idiopathic scoliosis, *Spine* 8:242-260, 1983.
3. Baker LL, Bowman BR, and McNeal DR: Effects of waveform on comfort during neuromuscular electrical stimulation, *Clin Orthop* 233:75-85, 1988.
4. Baker LL and Parker K: Neuromuscular electrical stimulation of the muscles surrounding the shoulder, *Phys Ther* 66:1930-1937, 1986.
5. Baker LL, Parker K, and Sanderson D: Neuromuscular electrical stimulation for the head-injured patient, *Phys Ther* 63:1967-1974, 1983.
6. Baker LL and others: *Neuromuscular electrical stimulation: a practical guide,* ed 2, Downey, Calif, 1993, Los Amigos Research and Education Institute.
7. Basmajian JV and Blumenstein R: Electrode placement in electromyographic biofeedback, In Basmajian JV: *Biofeedback principles and practice for clinicians,* ed 3, Baltimore, 1989, Williams & Wilkins.
8. Basmajian JV and others: EMG feedback treatment of upper limb in hemiplegic stroke patients: a pilot study, *Arch Phys Med Rehabil* 63:613-616, 1982.
9. Basmajian JV and others: Biofeedback treatment of foot-drop after stroke compared with standard rehabilitation technique: effects on voluntary control and strength, *Arch Phys Med Rehabil* 56:231-236, 1975.
10. Basmajian JV: *Biofeedback principles and practice for clinicians,* ed 3, Baltimore, 1989, Williams & Wilkins.
11. Bate PJ and Matyas TA: Negative transfer of training following brief practice of elbow tracking movements with electromyographic feedback from spastic antagonists, *Arch Phys Med Rehabil* 73:1050-1058, 1992.
12. Bergmans J and Senden R: Electrical stimulation of denervated muscle. In Gorio A and others, editors: *Posttraumatic peripheral nerve regeneration: experimental basis and clinical implications,* New York, 1981, Raven Press.
13. Binder MD and Mendell LM: *The segmental motor system,* London, 1990, Oxford University Press.
14. Binder-Macleod SA and Snyder-Mackler L: Muscle fatigue: clinical implications for fatigue assessment and neuromuscular electrical stimulation, *Phys Ther* 73:902-910, 1993.
15. Binder-Macleod SA and McDermond LR: Changes in the force-frequency relationship in the human quadriceps muscle following electrically and voluntarily induced fatigue, *Phys Ther* 72:95-104, 1992.
16. Bobath B: *Adult hemiplegia: evaluation and treatment,* ed 3, Oxford, 1990, Heinemann Books.
17. Bogataj U and others: Restoration of gait during two to three weeks of therapy with multichannel electrical stimulation, *Phys Ther* 69:319-327, 1989.
18. Bowden REM and Gutmann E: Denervation and re-innervation of human voluntary muscle, *Brain* 67:273-309, 1944.
19. Bowman BR, Baker LL, and Waters RL: Positional feedback and electrical stimulation: an automated treatment for the hemiplegic wrist, *Arch Phys Med Rehabil* 60:497-502, 1979.
20. Bowman BR and Baker LL: Effects of waveform parameters on comfort during transcutaneous neuromuscular electrical stimulation, *Ann Biomed Eng* 13:59-74, 1985.
21. Burnside IG, Tobias HS, and Burnsill D: Electromyographic feedback in the remobilization of stroke patients: a controlled trial, *Arch Phys Med Rehabil* 63:217-222, 1982.
22. Carmick J: Clinical use of neuromuscular electrical stimulation for children with cerebral palsy, part 1: lower extremity, *Phys Ther* 73:505-513, 1993.
23. Carmick J: Clinical use of neuromuscular electrical stimulation for children with cerebral palsy, part 2: upper extremity, *Phys Ther* 73:514-527, 1993.
24. Cohen BA, Crouch RH, and Thompson SN: Electromyographic biofeedback as a physical therapeutic adjunct in Guillain-Barré syndrome, *Arch Phys Med Rehabil* 58:582-584, 1977.
25. Colborne GR, Wright V, and Naumann S: Feedback of triceps surae EMG in gait of children with cerebral palsy: a controlled study, *Arch Phys Med Rehabil* 75:40-45, 1994.
26. Cozean CD, Pease WS, and Hubbell SL: Biofeedback and functional electrical stimulation in stroke rehabilitation, *Arch Phys Med Rehabil* 69:401-405, 1988.
27. Cummings J: Electrical stimulation of healthy muscle and tissue repair. In Nelson RM and Currier DP, editors: *Clinical electrotherapy,* ed 2, Norwalk, Conn, 1991, Appleton & Lange.
28. Cummings JP: Electrical stimulation of denervated muscle. In Gersh MR: *Electrotherapy in rehabilitation,* Philadelphia, 1992, FA Davis.
29. Cybulski GR, Penn RD, and Jaeger RJ: Lower extremity functional neuromuscular stimulation in cases of spinal cord injury, *Neurosurgery* 15:132-146, 1984.
30. DeBacher G: Biofeedback in spasticity control. In Basmajian JV: *Biofeedback principles and practice for clinicians,* ed 3, Baltimore, 1989, Williams & Wilkins.

31. DeVahl J: Neuromuscular electrical stimulation (NMES) in rehabilitation. In Gersh MR: *Electrotherapy in rehabilitation,* Philadelphia, 1992, FA Davis.
32. DeWeerdt W and Harrison MA: The efficacy of electromyographic feedback for stroke patients: a critical review of the main literature, *Physiotherapy* 72:108-118, 1986.
33. Delitto A and Robinson AJ: Electrical stimulation of muscle: techniques and applications. In Snyder-Mackler L and Robinson AJ: *Clinical electrophysiology: electrotherapy and electrophysiologic testing,* Baltimore, 1989, Williams & Wilkins.
34. Dubowitz L and others: Improvement of muscle performance by chronic electric stimulation in children with cerebral palsy, *Lancet* 587-588, 1988.
35. Eichorn KF, Schubert W, and David E: Maintenance, training, and functional use of denervated muscle, *J Biomed Eng* 6:205-211, 1984.
36. *Electrotherapeutic terminology in physical therapy,* Section on Clinical Electrotherapy of the American Physical Therapy Association, Alexandria, Va, 1990, The American Physical Therapy Association.
37. Faghri PD, Glaser RM, and Figoni SF: Functional electrical stimulation leg cycle ergometer exercise: training effects on cardiorespiratory responses of spinal cord injured subjects at rest and during submaximal exercise, *Arch Phys Med Rehabil* 73:1085-1093, 1992.
38. Faghri PD and others: The effects of functional electrical stimulation on shoulder subluxation, arm function recovery, and shoulder pain in hemiplegic stroke patients, *Arch Phys Med Rehabil* 75:73-79, 1994.
39. Fields RW: Electromyographically triggered electric muscle stimulation for chronic hemiplegia, *Arch Phys Med Rehabil* 68:407-414, 1987.
40. Gardner ER and Baker LL: Functional electrical stimulation of paralytic muscle. In Currier DP and Nelson RM: *Dynamics of human biologic tissues,* Philadelphia, 1992, FA Davis.
41. Gersh MR: *Electrotherapy in rehabilitation,* Philadelphia, 1992, FA Davis.
42. Gorman PH and Mortimer JT: The effect of stimulus parameters on the recruitment characteristics of direct nerve stimulation. *IEEE Trans Biomed Eng* 30:407-414, 1983.
43. Gowland C and others: Agonist and antagonist activity during voluntary upper-limb movement in patients with stroke, *Phys Ther* 72:624-633, 1992.
44. Gracanin F and Trnkoczy A: Optimal stimulus parameters for minimum pain in the chronic stimulation of innervated muscle, *Arch Phys Med Rehabil* 56:243-249, 1975.
45. Grimby G and others: Changes in histochemical profile of muscle after long-term electrical stimulation in patients with idiopathic scoliosis, *Scand J Rehabil Med* 17:191-196, 1985.
46. Hammond MC and others: Co-contraction in the hemiparetic forearm: quantitative EMG evaluation, *Arch Phys Med Rehabil* 69:348-351, 1988.
47. Hammond MC, Kraft GH, and Fitts SS: Recruitment and termination of electromyographic activity in the hemiparetic forearm, *Arch Phys Med Rehabil* 69:106-110, 1988.
48. Harris R: Chronaxy. In Licht S, editor: *Electrodiagnosis and electromyography,* ed 3, New Haven, Conn, 1971, Elizabeth Licht Pub.
49. Hirokawa S and others: Energy consumption in paraplegic ambulation using the reciprocating gait orthosis and electric stimulation of the thigh muscles, *Arch Phys Med Rehabil* 71:687-694, 1990.
50. Hooker SP and others: Physiologic responses to prolonged electically stimulated leg-cycle exercise in the spinal cord injured, *Arch Phys Med Rehabil* 71:863 869, 1990.
51. Hooker SP and others: Physiologic effects of electrical stimulation leg cycle exercise training in spinal cord injured persons, *Arch Phys Med Rehabil* 73:470-478, 1992.
52. Hurd WW, Pegram V, and Nepomuceno C: Comparison of actual and simulated EMG biofeedback in the treatment of hemiplegic patients, *Am J Phys Med* 59:73-82, 1980.
53. Ince LP and Leon MS: Biofeedback treatment of upper extremity dysfunction in Guillain-Barré syndrome, *Arch Phys Med Rehabil* 67:30-33, 1986.
54. Inglis J and others: Electromyographic biofeedback and physical therapy of the hemiplegic upper limb, *Arch Phys Med Rehabil* 65:755-759, 1984.
55. Karmel-Ross K, Cooperman DR, and Van Doren CL: The effect of electrical stimulation on quadriceps femoris muscle torque in children with spina bifida, *Phys Ther* 72:723-730, 1992.
56. Keith MW and others: Functional neuromuscular stimulation neuroprostheses for the tetraplegic hand, *Clin Orthop* 223:25-33, 1988.
57. Klose KJ and others: Rehabilitation therapy for patients with long-term spinal cord injuries. *Arch Phys Med Rehabil* 71:659-662, 1990.
58. Kosmon AJ, Osborne SL, and Ivey AC: The influence of duration and frequency in electrical stimulation of muscles, *Arch Phys Med* 29:559-562, 1948.
59. Kraft GH, Fitts SS, and Hammond MC: Techniques to improve function of the arm and hand in chronic hemiplegia, *Arch Phys Med Rehabil* 73:220-227, 1992.
60. Landau WM and Hunt CC: Dorsal rhizotomy, a treatment of unproven efficacy. *J Child Neurol* 5:174-178, 1990.
61. Lazarus JC: Associated movement in hemiplegia: the effects of force exerted, limb usage and inhibitory training, *Arch Phys Med Rehabil* 73:1044-1049, 1992.
62. Liberson WT and others: Functional electrotherapy: stimulation of the peroneal nerve synchronized with the swing phase of the gait of hemiplegic patients, *Arch Phys Med Rehabil* 42:101-105, 1961.
63. Lomo R and Slater CR: Control of acetylcholine sensitivity and synapse formation by muscle activity, *J Physiol* 275:391-402, 1978.
64. Malezic M and others: Therapeutic effects of multisite electric stimulation of gait in motor-disabled patients, *Arch Phys Med Rehabil* 68:553-560, 1987.
65. Mandel AR and others: Electromyographic versus rhythmic positional biofeedback in computerized gait retraining with stroke patients, *Arch Phys Med Rehabil* 71:649-654, 1990.
66. Merletti R and others: Electrophysiological orthosis for the upper extremity in hemiplegia: feasibility study, *Arch Phys Med Rehabil* 56:507-513, 1975.
67. Merletti R and others: A control study of muscle force recovery in hemiparetic patients during treatment with functional electric stimulation, *Scand J Rehabil Med* 10:147-154, 1978.
68. McNeal DR and Baker LL: Effects of joint angle, electrodes and waveform on electrical stimulation of the quadriceps and hamstrings, *Ann Biomed Eng* 16:299, 1988.
69. Morrison SA: Biofeedback to facilitate unassisted ventilation in individuals with high-level quadriplegia: a case report, *Phys Ther* 68:1378-1380, 1988.
70. Mulder T and Hulstyn W: Sensory feedback therapy and theoretical knowledge of motor control and learning, *Am J Phys Med* 63:226-243, 1984.
71. Murray MP: Gait as a total pattern of movement, *Am J Phys Med* 46:290-329, 1967.
72. Murray MP, Koury RC, and Sepic SB: Walking patterns of normal women. *Arch Phys Med Rehabil* 51:637-650, 1970.
73. Myklebust BM and Kloth L: Electrodiagnostic and electrotherapeutic instrumentation: characteristics of recording and stimulation systems and the principles of safety. In Gersh MR: *Electrotherapy in rehabilitation,* Philadelphia, 1992, FA Davis.
74. Nacht MB, Wolf SL, and Coogler CE: Use of electromyographic feedback during the acute phase of spinal cord injury: a case report, *Phys Ther* 62:290-294, 1982.
75. Neilson PD and McCaughey J: Self-regulation of spasm and spasticity in cerebral palsy, *J Neurol Neurosurg Psychiatry* 45:320-330, 1982.

76. Nelson RM and Currier DP, editors: *Clinical electrotherapy*, ed 2, Norwalk, Conn, 1991, Appleton & Lange.

77. Packman-Braun R: Electrotherapeutic applications for the neurologically impaired patient. In Gersh MR, *Electrotherapy in rehabilitation*, Philadelphia, 1992, FA Davis.

78. Packman-Braun R: Relationship between functional electrical stimulation duty cycle and fatigue in wrist extensor muscles of patients with hemiparesis, *Phys Ther* 68:51-56, 1988.

79. Peckham PH, Keith MW, and Freehafer AA: Restoration of functional control by electrical stimulation in the upper extremity of the quadriplegic patient, *J Bone Joint Surg* 70:144-148, 1988.

80. Peckham PH, Marsolais B, and Mortimer JT: Restoration of key grip and release in the C6 tetraplegic patient through functional electrical stimulation, *J Hand Surg* 5:462-469, 1980.

81. Petrofsky JS and others: Bicycle ergometer for paralyzed muscles, *J Clin Eng* 9:13-19, 1984.

82. Petrofsky JS and others: Computer synchronized walking: an application of an orthosis and functional electrical stimulation, *J Neurol Orthop Med Surg* 6:219-230, 1985.

83. Pinelli P, Arrigo A, and Moglia A: In tibialis anterior reinnervation by collateral branching with or without electrotherapy, *Proceedings of the Fourth Congress of the International Society of Electrophysiology & Kinesiology* Boston, 1979 pp 106-107.

84. Pockett S and Gavin RM: Acceleration of peripheral nerve regeneration after crush injury in rat, *Neurosci Lett* 59:221-224, 1985.

85. Prevo AJH, Visser SL, and Vogelaar TW: Effect of EMG feedback on paretic muscles and abnormal co-contraction in the hemiplegic arm, compared with conventional therapy, *Scand J Rehabil Med* 14:121-131, 1982.

86. Ragnarsson KT: Physiologic effects of functional electrical stimulation-introduced exercises in spinal cord-injured individuals, *Clin Orthop* 233:53-63, 1988.

87. Ragnarsson KT and others: Clinical evaluation of computerized electrical stimulation after spinal cord injury: a multicenter pilot study, *Arch Phys Med Rehabil* 69:672-677, 1988.

88. Rosselle N and others: Electromyographic evaluation of therapeutic methods in complete peripheral paralysis, *Electromyogr Clin Neurophysiol* 17:179-186, 1977.

89. Sahrman SA and Norton BJ: Relationship of voluntary movement to spasticity in upper motor neuron syndrome, *Ann Neurol* 2:460-465, 1977.

90. Santee JL, Keister ME, and Kleinman KM: Incentives to enhance the effects of electromyographic feedback training in stroke patients, *Biofeedback Self Regul* 5:51-56, 1980.

91. Schleenbaker RE and Mainous AG: Electromyographic biofeedback for neuromuscular reeducation in the hemiplegic stroke patient: a meta-analysis, *Arch Phys Med Rehabil* 74:1301-1304, 1993.

92. Schmidt RA: Feedback and knowledge of results. In Schmidt RA: *Motor control and learning*, ed 2, Champaign, Ill, 1988, Human Kinetics Publishers.

93. Sipski MI, Delisa JA, and Schweer S: Functional electrical stimulation bicycle ergometry: patient perceptions, *Am J Phys Med Rehabil* 68:147-149, 1989.

94. Spielholz NI: Electrical stimulation of denervated muscle. In Nelson RM and Currier DP, editors: *Clinical electrotherapy*, ed 2, Norwalk, Conn, 1991, Appleton & Lange.

95. Sunderland S: *Nerves and nerve injuries*, ed 2, Edinburgh, 1978, Churchill Livingstone.

96. Takebe K and others: Peroneal nerve stimulator in rehabilitation of hemiplegic patients, *Arch Phys Med Rehabil* 56:231-240, 1975.

97. Trimble MH and Enoka RM: Mechanisms underlying the training effects associated with neuromuscular electrical stimulation, *Phys Ther* 71:273-282, 1991.

98. Twist DJ: Acrocyanosis in a spinal cord injured patient: effects of computer-controlled neuromuscular electrical stimulation: a case report, *Phys Ther* 70:45-49, 1990.

99. Valencic V and others: Improved motor response due to chronic electrical stimulation of denervated tibialis anterior muscle in humans, *Muscle Nerve* 9:612-617, 1986.

100. Wakim KG and Krusen FH: The influence of electrical stimulation on the work output and endurance of denervated muscle, *Arch Phys Med Rehabil* 36:370-376, 1955.

101. Waters RL, McNeal D, and Perry J: Experimental correction of footdrop by electric stimulation of the peroneal nerve, *J Bone Joint Surg* 57A:1047-1054, 1975.

102. Waters RL and others: Functional electric stimulation of the peroneal nerve for hemiplegia: long term clinical follow-up, *J Bone Joint Surg* 67A:792-793, 1985.

103. Winchester P and others: Effects of feedback stimulation training and cyclical electrical stimulation on knee extension in hemiparetic patients, *Phys Ther* 7:1096-1103, 1983.

104. Wissel J and others: Treating chronic hemiparesis with modified biofeedback, *Arch Phys Med Rehabil* 70:612-617, 1989.

105. Wolf SL, Baker MP, and Kelly JL: EMG biofeedback in stroke: a 1-year follow-up on the effect of patient characteristics, *Arch Phys Med Rehabil* 61:351-354, 1980.

106. Wolf SL, Baker MP, and Kelly JL: EMG biofeedback in stroke: effect of patient characteristics, *Arch Phys Med Rehabil* 60:96-102, 1979.

107. Wolf SL and Binder-Macleod SA: Electromyographic biofeedback applications to the hemiplegic patient: changes in lower extremity neuromuscular and functional status, *Phys Ther* 63:1404-1413, 1983.

108. Wolf SL and Binder-Macleod SA: Electromyographic biofeedback applications to the hemiplegic patient: changes in upper extremity neuromuscular and functional status, *Phys Ther* 63:1393-1403, 1983.

109. Wolf SL and Binder-Macleod SA: Neurophysiological factors in electromyographic feedback for neuromotor disturbances. In Basmajian JV: *Biofeedback principles and practice for clinicians*, ed 3, Baltimore, 1989, Williams & Wilkins.

110. Wolf SL, Edwards DI, and Shutter LA: Concurrent assessment of muscle activity (CAMA): a procedural approach to assess treatment goals, *Phys Ther* 66:218-224, 1986.

111. Wolf SL, LeCraw DE, and Barton LA: Comparison of motor copy and targeted biofeedback training techniques for restitution of upper extremity function among patients with neurologic disorders, *Phys Ther* 69:719-735, 1989.

112. Wolf SL: Electromyographic biofeedback applications to stroke patients: a critical review, *Phys Ther* 63:1448-1459, 1983.

113. Wolf SL: Electromyographic feedback for spinal cord injured patients: a realistic perspective. In Basmajian JV: *Biofeedback principles and practice for clinicians*, ed 3, Baltimore, 1989, Williams & Wilkins.

114. Wolf SL: Use of biofeedback in the treatment of stroke patients, *Stroke* 21 (suppl II):II-22-II-23, 1990.

115. Vodovnik L and others: Recent applications of functional electrical stimulation to stroke patients in Ljubljana, *Clin Orthop* 131:64-69, 1978.

116. Zablotny C: Using neuromuscular electrical stimulation to facilitate limb control in the head injured patient, *J Head Trauma Rehabil* 2(2):28-33, 1987.

CHAPTER 31

Pain Management

Linda Mirabelli-Susens

KEY TERMS

nociceptor
acute pain; chronic pain
pain pathway
fast pain; slow pain
pain modulation: gate
  control theory;
  neurotransmitters;
  endogenous opiates
CNS pain: thalamic pain
ANS pain: causalgia,
  phantom limb pain
Peripheral pain:
  mechanical pain,
  chemical pain
Pain intensity
  measurements: verbal
  rating scale; visual analog
  scale; pain estimate

Pain character measure-
  ments: McGill Pain
  Questionnaire (MPQ)
Thermotherapy: ultrasound;
  phonophoresis
TENS
Iontophoresis
massage
myofascial release
joint mobilization
therapeutic touch
point stimulation
laser
cognitive-behavior methods:
  relaxation exercises;
  hypnosis; biofeedback;
  operant conditioning; body
  scanning

LEARNING OBJECTIVES

After reading this chapter the student/therapist will:
1. Describe the pain pathways.
2. Explain the difference between acute and chronic pain.
3. Explain the difference between fast and slow pain.
4. Describe the role of the gate control theory and of endogenous opiates and neurotransmitters in pain modulation.
5. List the signs and symptoms of CNS, ANS, and peripheral pain and give an example of each.
6. Perform a comprehensive pain evaluation, including taking a pain history, measuring pain intensity, measuring pain character, and examining the client.
7. List at least 12 treatment modalities for pain management with their indications and contraindications.

One of the greatest challenges facing today's therapist is the treatment of pain. This challenge is due, in part, to the multidimensional nature of pain, which presents with both objective and subjective components. The underlying physical cause of pain may be identified, but the sensation is open to interpretation and can well be disproportionate with the magnitude and duration of its cause. Pain tolerances vary among individuals and even within the same individual: What is intolerable to one person may be merely uncomfortable to another; what is tolerable in one instance may be overwhelming when experienced at a different time. In addition curing the cause of pain does not always eliminate the pain.

Thus the challenge in pain management lies not only in identifying and correcting the precipitating injury, but also in addressing other physical, emotional, and psychological factors contributing to its persistence.

PAIN THEORIES

The International Association for the Study of Pain (IASP) defines pain as "an unpleasant sensory and emotional experience associated with actual or potential tissue damage."[28] How this actual or potential tissue damage comes to be perceived as pain has been explained historically by several "pain theories."

The earliest theories were proposed by Weddell,[72] Goldscheider[19] and Gelhard,[19] who associated pain with the summation of impulses to nonspecific receptors and with patterns of impulses travelling along nonspecific nerves from the periphery to the brain. These theories became outdated with the identification of receptor-fiber specialization.

In the late nineteenth century, von Frey proposed specific receptors and neural pathways associated with pain, as well as a specific cortical pain center.[66] His theory was the basis for years of nerve sectioning as a treatment for intractable pain, even though many times the surgical lesions were unsuccessful in abolishing the pain, and occasionally the pain actually increased after surgery.[52]

The current theory identifies stimulus-specific peripheral **nociceptors** that cause pain when activated by mechanical or chemical abnormalities.[69] Woven throughout most human tissue is a continuous tridimensional plexus of unmyelinated fibers called the interstitial nociceptor system. These receptors respond to incision, tearing, laceration, excessive stretching, and compression of the tissues, as well as to the accumulation of abnormally high concentrations of chemical substances including lactic acid, potassium, and histamine.

A similar plexus system, the perivascular nociceptor system, is found in the walls of the peripheral arteries, arterioles, venules, and veins. This system is responsive to the same mechanical and chemical factors, but in addition is stimulated by marked constriction or dilation of the vessels.

The distinction between acute and chronic pain lies in the sensitivity of the nociceptors to stimulation. Acute pain is a warning system. It results when the nociceptors are exposed to intense, potentially damaging noxious stimuli. **Acute pain** is localized, lasts only as long as the nociceptor is being stimulated, and is in proportion to the intensity of the stimulus.[75]

Chronic pain, in contrast, occurs without a clear stimulus to the nociceptors, in response to innocuous stimulation, or in a prolonged exaggerated fashion to noxious stimulation. Chronic pain results from a disruption in the normal sensory mechanism for pain. When a cell is damaged, it spills its contents into the surrounding tissues, summoning inflammatory cells to the area. Along the **pain pathway,** neurotransmitters are released by the transmitting neurons. The combination of these chemicals causes *peripheral sensitization* of the afferent nerves and microcirculation. The nociceptors become hypersensitive and fire in response to innocuous or low-intensity stimulation.[75]

PAIN PATHWAYS

Information from the nociceptors travels into the dorsal gray matter of the spinal cord on A-delta and C fibers, the smallest afferent fibers in the body. In the dorsal gray matter these primary afferent fibers synapse with interneurons, which do one of three things. Some synapse with motoneurons causing reflex movements (i.e., withdrawing the hand from a hot object). Others synapse with autonomic fibers from the sympathetic and sacral parasympathetic systems causing autonomic responses including changes in heart rate and blood pressure and localized vasodilation, piloerection, and sweating. Most fibers travel a multisynaptic route to the higher centers via the anterolateral tract. Information from primary afferent fibers originating caudal to the pelvis ascends on the contralateral side of the body, whereas information from primary afferent fibers originating cranial to the pelvis remains ipsilateral.[14]

The phenomena of fast and slow pain are the result of the size of the conducting fibers, the number of synapses along the neural pathway, and the brain areas to which the neurons project. Fast pain, the sensation first perceived after injury, travels on large myelinated fibers in a fairly direct route from the dorsal gray matter to the thalamus, through the internal capsule to the postcentral gyrus of the cortex. **Fast pain** is accurately localized and qualified, and lasts only as long as the duration of the stimulus.[15]

Slow pain travels a more multisynaptic route on slower conducting nonmyelinated fibers. The primary afferents synapse twice in the dorsal gray matter. The second-order neurons then cross the midline and travel in the anterolateral spinoreticular tracts to the reticular formation, which projects the information to various areas in the midbrain and thalamus. From here it is transmitted to the cortex. Slow pain is poorly localized and outlasts the duration of the stimulus.[15]

The emotional/psychological aspects of pain are due, in part, to the various thalamocortical projections, which provide the perceptual, affective, memory, and hormonal components of the pain experience. The projections from the thalamus to the postcentral gyrus, previously identified with fast pain, are responsible for the perceptual component. It is from this projection that pain can be localized and qualified as to whether it is pricking, throbbing, burning, and so on.[69]

Projections to the frontal lobes and the limbic system are concerned with the emotional component of pain, specifically with identifying pain as an unpleasant experience. It is from this projection that pain hurts.[69] The limbic system's control over motor control can result in more muscle tone and thus more pain (see Chapter 6).

Pain memory results from projections to the memory storage areas of the temporal lobes. This area also receives input from the limbic and sensory cortical areas mentioned previously. From these projections a memory bank of past painful experiences is developed.[69]

The hormonal response to pain is the result of a noncortical projection, from the thalamus to the hypothalamus, which is responsible for global efferent activity in the autonomic system. From this projection the secretion of sympathetic hormones (i.e., epinephrine) takes place.[69]

PAIN MODULATION

Whether stimulation of the nociceptors results in pain depends on several modulating factors. For the intensity of perceived pain varies considerably depending on the individual's mood, the amount of distraction from the pain, and

the positive or negative suggestions of others, as well as on several peripheral and central neurological systems that are capable of modulating transmission at the synapses in the nociceptive pathways.

According to the **gate control theory** proposed by Melzak and Wall,[52] presynaptic inhibition in the dorsal gray matter of the spinal cord blocks pain impulses coming from the periphery. The dorsal gray is laminated. Laminae II, III (substantia gelatinosa), and V (transmission "T" cells) have been implicated in pain impulse transmission by Melzak and Wall in the following manner (Fig. 31-1).

Information entering the dorsal horn via small diameter A-delta and C fibers has a stimulatory effect on T cells, but an inhibitory effect on the substantia gelatinosa. When the substantia gelatinosa is inhibited, the T cells are activated and pain impulses are transmitted to multiple pain centers in the brain including the cerebrum, brainstem, thalamus, and cortex. The gate is, in effect, open.

On the other hand, input from large diameter A-beta fibers (pressoreceptors and mechanoreceptors) stimulates both the T cells and the substantia gelatinosa. Stimulation of the substantia gelatinosa presynaptically inhibits the T cells, and transmission of pain impulses does not occur.[54] In this case, the gate is closed.

Although the gate control theory was widely accepted, it was not without opposition. Opponents[27,53] criticized the theory for failing to explain why pain persists when the small

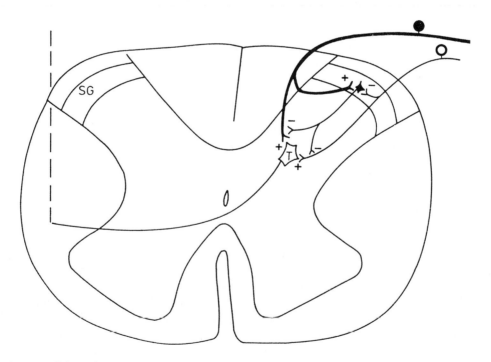

Fig. 31-1. Schematic representation of spinal structures involved in the gate control theory of pain transmission. Afferent input via both large and small diameter fibers is theorized to influence the transmission cell (T) directly and through small internuncial neurons located within the substantia gelatinosa (SG). (From Nolan MF: Anatomic and physiologic organization of neural structures involved in pain transmission, modulation, and perception. In Echternach JL: *Pain*, New York, 1987, Churchill Livingstone.

fibers are destroyed or why pain can be modulated with cognitive measures.

In response, Melzak[51] modified the gate control theory to recognize a descending system, which originated in the higher centers and influenced activity in the dorsal gray matter. He suggested that the limbic system, reticular formation, and neocortex (areas involved with emotions and alertness) all affect pain perception.

Research in the 1970s and 1980s supported Melzak's modified theory;[2,3,23,26] endogenous opiates and other neuromodulating **neurotransmitters** were discovered within the central nervous system (CNS). Receptors for these neurotransmitters were found in high concentrations in areas associated with nociception and the areas identified by Melzak and Wall as significant in presynaptic inhibition of pain impulses: the thalamus, limbic system, periaqueductal gray matter, and substantia gelatinosa.

Endogenous opiates are divided into endorphins, enkephalins, and substance P. Endorphins, long-lasting morphinelike chemicals found primarily in the thalamus, mid-brain, pons, medulla, and hypothalamic-pituitary axis, produce analgesia as well as systemic effects on mood and the gastrointestinal, respiratory, and endocrine systems.[2] Endorphin levels in individuals with chronic pain vary depending on whether the pain is of neurogenic, somatogenic, or psychogenic origin.[67] Endorphins are thought to be significant in activating a central regulatory system that originates in the periaqueductal gray and inhibits transmission by interneurons in the dorsal gray.[2]

Enkephalins mediate a second central pathway in which the descending neurons originate in the reticular formation and inhibit transmission by the interneurons in the dorsal gray. This system is enhanced with diversion (including hypnosis) and increased blood concentrations of catecholamines (epinephrine, norepinephrine, dopamine, etc).[10]

Depolarization of the secondary neurons in the dorsal gray matter is mediated through release of substance P. Increased mechanoreceptor input inhibits the release of substance P, thereby decreasing pain transmission and perception. However, some conflicting evidence suggests that high concentrations of substance P result in excitation of the afferent neurons, thus facilitating pain transmission.[56]

Although serotonin is not classified as an endogenous opiate, it exerts a profound effect on analgesia and enhances analgesic drug potency. High concentrations of serotonin lead to decreased pain,[47] whereas low concentrations result in depression, sleep disturbances, and increased pain.[64] Serotonin also inhibits transmission of nociceptive information within the dorsal horn.[3]

It is now thought that there are two cortical modulating systems, both of which can function as either excitatory or inhibitory, depending on the neurons on which they terminate. The direct cortical modulating system originates in the cortex and travels to the dorsal gray matter in the contralateral motor tract. The indirect cortical modulating

system originates in the cortex and travels to the dorsal gray matter in the contralateral motor tract. The indirect cortical modulating system is a dual mechanism with neurons from the cortex to the reticular formation and neurons from the limbic system to the midbrain. Because the limbic system deals with affect, changes in mood modify the perception of pain intensity and, thereby, alter the pain threshold.[69]

PAIN PERCEPTION

The physical nature of pain is a product of its site of origin. Pain can arise from the CNS, autonomic nervous system (ANS), and the periphery.

Pain from the CNS

Pain from lesions in the CNS is topographical: The site of the lesion determines the location and character of the symptoms, which range from paresthesia to pain. The onset is variable: CNS pain can occur immediately after the insult or much later, and many times pain is the first indicator of a CNS lesion.[10]

Pain from injury to the dorsal horns is felt ipsilateral to the injury in a pattern corresponding to the nerve root distribution. Injury to the ascending anterolateral tracts results in pain below the level of the lesion on the contralateral side of the body. Pain from cortical lesions is referred to regions of the body with the greatest cortical representation, usually areas of the face, hands, and feet.[10]

Thalamic pain is the classic example of central pain. Although thalamic pain is usually concentrated in the contralateral extremities, any region of the contralateral side of the body can be affected, and the pain is frequently migratory. The onset of thalamic pain is easily elicited by movement, skin contact (even air blowing over the skin), heat, cold, and vibration; however, the onset of thalamic pain is frequently spontaneous. It may "develop explosively and spread all over the affected side of the body in floods."[14] Thalamic pain is usually unremitting and irreversible.[10]

Pain from the ANS

Pain from lesions in the ANS is quadratic. Sympathetic and parasympathetic fibers travel in the walls of the blood vessels, and because the major vessels serve quadrants of the body, autonomic pain is spread throughout the involved vessel's distribution. Autonomic pain originating from the sympathetic nervous system is frequently accompanied by other measurable sympathetic disturbances, and because of the sympathetic/parasympathetic connection with emotion, pain originating from the autonomic pathways is far more sensitive to mood changes than is CNS pain.[18] **Causalgia** and **phantom limb pain** are examples of **ANS pain.**

Causalgia is characterized by an intense burning and hyperesthesia throughout the distribution of an incompletely damaged peripheral nerve that has, most commonly, sustained a penetrating wound. Causalgia usually occurs as healing takes place and is so easily elicited by minor tactile stimulation that the individual refuses to move the affected limb for fear of stimulating the pain. Frequently there are concomitant trophic changes. The skin becomes atrophic and scaly. In the acute stage the skin is pink, warm, and glossy; later it becomes cyanotic, mottled, and moist. The muscles can atrophy and the bones can become osteoporotic.[9]

Causalgia is thought to result from the development of "false synapses" between the injured autonomic efferent fibers and the afferents, so that the autonomic impulses divert to sensory fibers providing them with continuous autonomic input. The most common treatment for causalgia is sectioning of the involved nerve with variable results.[14] Sympathetic nerve blocks also have been found to be effective.[3]

Phantom limb sensation, the feeling that a missing limb is still intact, commonly occurs after amputation. Some amputees, however, also experience phantom limb pain, a burning, squeezing sensation accompanied by "pins and needles." Phantom limb pain is thought to result from the formation of a terminal neuroma of nerve fibers and connective tissue at the point of section, creating an abnormal pattern of afferent impulses and leading to interpretation of the incoming impulses as having originated from the missing limb.[14] Both phantom limb pain and phantom limb sensation tend to fade in time. Weakening of the sensations can be expedited with local percussion or vibration to the stump, as well as with other therapeutic modalities including transcutaneous electrical nerve stimulation (TENS) and high voltage galvanic stimulation (HVG).

Pain from the periphery

Peripheral pain results from noxious irritation of the nociceptors. Its character depends on the source of the irritation.

Mechanical pain results from deformation of the receptor and is usually sharp in nature. When there is pressure on a neural structure, there also may be paresthesia and "pins and needles." Mechanical pain lasts only as long as the deformation is present and resolves when the deformation is corrected.[48]

Chemical pain occurs when noxious chemical substances occur in quantities sufficient to irritate the nociceptors. Chemical pain is dull and aching and is relieved only when the concentration of chemicals returns to a subthreshold level.[9]

EVALUATION OF THE CLIENT WITH PAIN

Evaluations of the client with pain are very challenging. Due to the subjectivity of pain recall, it is not always possible to clinically reproduce pain matching the quality and intensity of the original sensation; the client is not always accurate in recall of pain experienced a month, or even a week, previously; and there is no objective way to account for the sensory and affective components or the psychological and cultural contributions to the pain experience. Nevertheless, pain evaluations need to include measurable, reproducible information that identifies the source of the pain, directs the therapist toward appropriate methods of treatment, and assists in establishing attainable goals.

Pain history

Crucial to the evaluation is a comprehensive pain history. It is important to have a standardized format to decrease chances of missing important information and to minimize having the client "lead the interview." The following alphabetic mnemonic device is helpful:

Origin/onset: date and circumstances of the onset of pain. How did the pain start? Gradually or suddenly? Was there a precipitating injury? If so, what was the mechanism of injury? If not, can the client correlate the onset to a particular activity or posture?

Position: location of the pain. Have the client demonstrate where the pain is located rather than relying on description. In addition to being more accurate, demonstration allows observation of the client's ability and willingness to move.

Pattern: pattern of the pain. Is the pain constant or periodic? Does it travel or radiate? Which activities and postures increase the pain? Which decrease the pain? Does medication or time of day have any effect on the pain? Have there been any recent changes in the pattern? Does the client feel that the pain is improving, worsening, or remaining the same?

Quality: characteristics of the pain. Does the client use adjectives indicating mechanical (pressing, bursting, stabbing), chemical (burning), neural (numb, "pins and needles"), or vascular (throbbing) origin?

Quantity: intensity of the pain. Several methods that allow for monitoring change in pain intensity are presented later.

Radiation: characteristics of pain radiation. What causes the pain to radiate? Can the radiation be reversed? How?

Signs/symptoms: functional and psychological components of the pain. Has the pain resulted in any functional limitations? Does the client's personality contribute to the pain or has the pain caused changes in the client's emotional stability? It may be necessary to interview the client's significant others for an accurate picture.

Treatment: previous/current treatment and its effectiveness, including medications and home remedies. It also is important to determine the client's attitude and expectations concerning therapy.

Visceral Symptoms: Physical symptoms of visceral origin that can accompany and be responsible for the pain (see the box on p. 877). Visceral causes for pain require referral to the client's physician for further investigation before the initiation of treatment by a therapist.

Chapter 31 Pain management **877**

Measuring pain intensity

Attempts to quantify pain have varied from relying on the individual's memory of the pain experience to using external stimuli to reproduce pain of the same intensity. Post hoc questioning[41] is not valid for measuring the intensity of chronic pain (which is usually overestimated), but has been of some limited value with acute pain, which is remembered accurately for up to 5 days.

Pain induced by experimental tests utilizing mechanical pressure, temperature, vascular occlusion, and electric

Viscerogenic back pain

General signs and symptoms:
  pain does not increase with spinal stresses/strains
  -pain is not relieved with rest
  -visceral symptoms accompany back pain
Gastrointestinal tract signs and symptoms:
  -pain is accompanied by altered bowel habits
  -pain is related to eating
  -peptic pain is relieved with vomiting
Kidney signs and symptoms:
  increased pain with diuresis indicates hydronephrosis
Pelvic signs and symptoms:
  -low back pain associated with vaginal bleeding or discharge
Prostate signs and symptoms:
  -low back discomfort associated with micturation
Lung signs and symptoms:
  -posterior thoracic pain associated with respiration in chronic obstructive pulmonary disease
Vascular signs and symptoms:
  -deep, boring, pulsating low back pain associated with a palpable abdominal aortic aneurysm AAA
  -back pain with/without calf pain after walking and relieved with standing still; possibly impaired lower extremity pulses and trophic skin changes associated with occlusive disease of the internal iliac artery or its branches

From Makofsky H and Willis GC: Non-mechanical and pathological causes of low back pain, *Phys Therapy Forum* p. 12, May 15, 1989.

stimulation bears little resemblance to the pain produced by disease. In actuality, experimentally induced pain measures only the client's pain threshold and pain ceiling at the time of testing. However, because these parameters are known to change in pathological conditions and be altered by certain analgesics, they may be of value in monitoring changes in the client's medical condition and in assessing the effectiveness of pain medication.[55]

A more accurate approach to objectifying pain intensity involves having the client rate the current level of discomfort in one of the following ways (Fig. 31-2):

1. **Verbal rating scale:** The client rates the pain on a continuum that is subdivided into gradually increasing pain intensities.
2. **Visual analog scale:** The client rates the pain on a continuum that has no subdivisions.
3. **Pain estimate:** The client rates the pain on a scale of 0 to 100, where 0 represents a lack of pain and 100 is the most severe pain possible.

All of these scales are easy to administer, and reliable over time, when used to measure pain that is present at the time of the evaluation.[36] However, because it has more divisions, the numerical rating scale is more sensitive to small changes in pain intensity than either the verbal or visual analog scales.

Measuring the character of pain

Clues about the cause of pain are gathered by examining the characteristics of what the client is experiencing. Pain from muscle, nerve, and the viscera differs in the same way that mechanical and chemical pain differ from each other. It is important to know the cause of pain to treat it as effectively and economically as possible.

One of the leading assessments of pain character is the **McGill Pain Questionnaire (MPQ),** which involves 20 categories of descriptive words covering the sensory, affective, and evaluative properties of pain. Each word has a numerical value. The client selects the one word in each category that best represents his or her immediate pain. If no

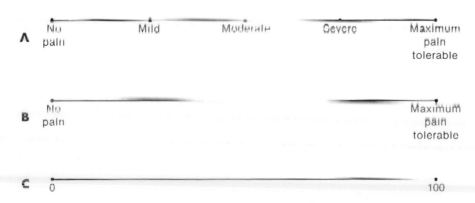

Fig. 31-2. Rating scales for measuring pain intensity. **A,** Verbal rating scale. **B,** Visual analog scale. **C,** Pain estimate.

word in a particular group is suitable, the category is skipped. When completed, the test provides a series of adjectives describing what the client is experiencing as well as a numerical score that can be used to monitor changes in the pain pattern.[48] The MPQ can be completed in 20 minutes. It has been studied extensively and found valid for chronic and acute pain, as well as for a variety of specific pathological states.[8,37,57]

Reliability and validity of this test are based on examiner objectivity. Thus care must be taken to avoid examiner subjectivity which can occur if the client is unfamiliar with some of the words and needs them defined during the test.[49]

Examination of the client

The clinical assessment should begin the moment the client enters the door. Clients frequently change posture and affect when they are being formally evaluated, and it is important to gain an accurate view of pain behavior during nonrequested activities to assess the validity of their complaints.

The formal assessment should include the following:

1. Observation of gait and movement patterns, including the use of assistive devices
2. Notation of body type and anomalies
3. Assessment of sitting and standing posture, including both the normal posture and that assumed because of the pain
4. Inspection of the skin for pliability, trophic changes, scar tissue, and other abnormalities
5. Palpation of the soft tissue structures to identify changes in temperature, swelling, tenderness, and areas of discomfort
6. Palpation of the anatomical structures to determine end feel, the sensation felt at the end of the available movement[12]
   a. Bone-to-bone: hard—normal, for example, at the end range of elbow extension
   b. Spasm: muscular resistance—abnormal
   c. Capsular feel: rubbery—normal at the extreme of full range of motion (ROM); abnormal when encountered before the end of ROM
   d. Springy block: rebound—abnormal
   e. Tissue approximation: soft tissue—normal at the extremes of full passive flexion
   f. Empty feel: no resistance, but client resists movement because of pain
7. Measurement of ROM: active ROM is performed to assess the client's willingness to move and to identify any limitations or painful areas; passive ROM testing is used to further refine the observations[12]
   a. When active and passive movements are painful and restricted in the same direction and the pain appears at the limit of motion, the problem is arthrogenic.

   b. When active and passive movements are painful or restricted in opposite directions, the problem is muscular.
   c. When there is relative restriction of passive movement in the capsular pattern, the problem is arthritic.
   d. When there is no restriction of passive movement but the client cannot perform the movement actively, the muscle is not functioning, either from intrinsic problems within the muscle or interruption in the neural pathway (central or peripheral).
8. Measurement of muscle strength[12]
   a. When the movement is strong and painful, there is a minor lesion in the muscle or tendon.
   b. When the movement is weak and increases the pain, there is a major lesion that needs to be identified with further testing.
   c. When the movement is weak but does not increase the pain, there is the possibility of either complete rupture of the muscle or tendon or a neurological disorder.
   d. When all resisted movements are painful, the pain may be organic or the patient may be emotionally hypersensitive.
   e. When movement is strong and painless, the test is normal.
9. Assessment of bilateral neurological function
   a. Reflexes: Peripheral lesions tend to diminish deep tendon reflexes (DTRs). CNS lesions tend to intensify DTRs, and testing frequently elicits a clonic reaction.[34] Note any asymmetries in response.
   b. Sensation: Test light touch, sharp (noxious) touch and vibration. Pressure on a nerve usually affects conduction on the large, myelinated fibers first. Therefore vibration is the first sensation to be diminished. Where there is decreased perception of touch and noxious stimuli, the lesion is more severe.[34] Note any asymmetries in response.
   c. Coordination.
   d. Stretch and pressure tests to nerve trunks.

The amount of information needed to accurately identify the cause of the client's pain is substantial, and frequently more than one session is needed to perform a full evaluation. It is far better to take several sessions and be accurate than to condense the evaluation into one session and direct treatment at the wrong structures.

TREATMENT OF THE CLIENT WITH PAIN

Successful treatment of pain involves identifying and correcting its cause. As therapists we must first determine the reason for pain and then use our clinical skills to return the tissues to their normal state.

Numerous physical modalities can be applied to the tissues to relieve pain. These include superficial heat, deep heat, cryotherapy, phonophoresis and iontophoresis, laser therapy, TENS, point stimulation, joint mobilization, therapeutic touch, myofascial release, and massage, as well as several effective cognitive measures.

This section reviews the physics and physiology of each of these modalities so that we can knowledgeably select the most appropriate one when establishing a treatment plan. The purpose is to provide an understanding of the mechanism of each so that treatment will be based on sound physiological principles.

Thermotherapy

The physiological effects of therapeutic heat and cold applications are frequently reciprocal, although the end product, relief of pain, is often the same. When selecting heat or cold, it is important to understand the mechanism of each so that the appropriate modality is used.

Heat application. The physiological effects of heat depend on the method of application, the depth of penetration, and the rate and magnitude of temperature change.[16] These physiological effects include the following:

1. Cellular metabolic rate increases with rising temperature until an optimal temperature is reached. If the temperature continues to rise, there is a gradual slowing of metabolic activity until cell death results from denaturation of the protein within the tissue.
2. Speed of skeletal muscle contraction increases until the optimal temperature for metabolic processes is reached; then it, too, gradually decreases.
3. Muscle tension declines, probably because chemical energy is released too rapidly to be converted into mechanical energy.
4. Local blood flow increases. If the area remains below core temperature, increased blood flow results in a transfer of heat from the core. If the area becomes warmer than the core, heat is carried centrally.
5. Capillary permeability, capillary hydrostatic pressure, and capillary filtration rate all increase. There is an escape of protein into the interstitial space, leading to edema.
6. Anastomoses that connect arterioles to venules open and blood is shunted past the capillaries. Because venules are longer than capillaries, blood remains in the area longer, allowing greater time for heat transfer to the tissues.
7. Muscle spasms decrease as a result of decreased activity in gamma motor efferents and decreased muscle spindle excitability.
8. Pain decreases. Ischemic pain is relieved by the influx of oxygen-rich blood into the dilated vessels, and muscle tension pain is decreased by interruption of the pain/spasm cycle.

Because of these effects several precautions are required when using heat as a modality. Heat should be used with caution in very young and elderly individuals because of their inability to thermoregulate adequately. Heat also should be used with caution in individuals with impaired circulation, diminished sensation, or inadequate cardiac or respiratory reserves. Heat application is contraindicated during acute thrombophlebitis because of the increased risk of emboli. It is also contraindicated over a malignancy because the increased blood flow could nourish the tumor and increase the chance of metastases. Heat should not be used where there is hemorrhage or recent trauma.[65]

Heat can be applied by conduction, convection, and radiation. Heat transfer by conduction involves the exchange of heat down a temperature gradient by two objects that are in contact. Heat transferred from one object is dispersed into another at a rate dependent on the thermal conductivity of the objects, the temperature gradients, and the quantity of blood flow (if the object is living tissue). When heat is transferred faster than it can be dissipated, there is a temperature rise in the receiving object, a decrease in the temperature gradient, and a subsequent slowing of the rate of exchange. Eventually, a state of equilibrium is reached and heat exchange stops.[16]

The depth of penetration with conductive heating is usually 1 cm or less.[16] Moist heat packs and paraffin are examples of conductive heating.

In convective heating heat is transferred through the flow of hot fluid. Fluid density decreases as its temperature increases, making warm fluids lighter than cool fluids. Warm fluids rise, cooling as they move upward. Cool fluids sink, warming as they move downward. Heat is exchanged when the moving molecules collide. Objects in the fluid also exchange heat as they come in contact with the moving molecules.[16]

Convective heating is also superficial. Therapeutic convective heating takes place during hydrotherapy.

Molecules with a temperature greater than absolute zero are in an excited state and emit energy, thus creating radiant heat. Objects that are warmed by the energy are heated by radiation.[16] Radiant heat can be superficial, as with infrared and ultraviolet, or deep, as with diathermy and microtherm. Shortwave diathermy involves making the individual part of a circuit that conducts alternating current from a generator, through a capacitor, through the individual to another capacitor, then back to the generator. The systemic ions create friction as they attempt to line up with the continuously reversing polarity, resulting in an increase in tissue temperature deep within the body.

Current density and therefore the magnitude of the temperature increase is dependent on placement of the capacitor. When the capacitor is remote, there is minimal surface heating with a homogenous temperature increase in the deep tissues. When the capacitor is close to the body, there is a greater temperature increase along the current pathway and at the body's surface. Diathermy is indicated where diffuse heating is desired.

In contrast, microtherm converts electrical energy into electromagnetic energy that can be focused on the tissue of choice. Increased temperature results when the electromagnetic waves are absorbed by the tissues. Microwave is far more exact than diathermy and is indicated where heating of individual deep structures is desired.

Deep heating also can be accomplished through the use of **ultrasound.** Unlike the transverse waves of electromagnetic radiation, the ultrasound wave is longitudinal, with alternating areas of compression and expansion that move forward then backward along the line of propagation. The wave is repeatedly refracted as it encounters tissues of differing acoustical resistance while traveling through the skin toward the bone. At each tissue interface it changes directions, and energy is transferred to the tissues (Fig. 31-3).

The areas between the sound head and the coupling agent and the skin also constitute interfaces where energy can be lost to the environment.

Ultrasound cannot travel through air; therefore it requires a coupling agent for effective transmission. Reid and Cummings[58] evaluated various coupling agents for their ability to transmit ultrasound while minimizing energy loss and found the following overall transmission levels: Aquasonic Gel—72.60%; glycerol—67.75%; distilled water—59.38%; Cardio-cream—26.60%; mineral oil—19.06%; air—00.00%. In addition, they determined that, as the dosage increased, a greater percentage of ultrasound energy reached the tissues. They concluded that selection of the appropriate coupling agent and dosage both appear to be important in ensuring that maximum energy is transmitted to the tissues.

Most of the therapeutic value of ultrasound comes from its ability to selectively raise tissue temperature at the interfaces without causing substantial change in the sur-rounding tissues. The amount of heat produced depends directly on the dosage (the amount of energy per unit time). At less than 1.0 W/cm^2 there is a minimal increase in tissue temperature. At 1.5 W/cm^2 the superficial tissues are heated, and at greater than 2.0 W/cm^2 temperature of the deeper tissues is raised.[45]

Dosage is also instrumental in changing the propagation of impulses originating from peripheral nerves. The number of impulses traveling along the nerve decreases at low dosages, but begins to rise slowly beginning at 1.9 W/cm^2. Sounding of C fibers yields pain relief distal to the point of application, whereas sounding of large-diameter A fibers brings relief of spasm by changing gamma fiber activity, making the muscle fibers less sensitive to stretch.[13] Because it is impossible to selectively treat C or A fibers, ultrasound provides both pain relief and relief from muscle spasm, making it effective in the treatment of peripheral neuropathies, neuroma, herpes zoster, and muscle spasm associated with musculoskeletal pathology, including sprains, strains, and contusions.[62]

Ultrasound decreases joint stiffness by changing the viscoelastic properties of joint fluids from a gel to a sol state. In addition, ultrasound increases the extensibility of tendon as a result of thermal depolymerization of protein.[17] These properties make ultrasound effective for treating conditions such as decreased ROM accompanying adhesive capsulitis and joint stiffness and swelling found in arthritis.[60] (Refer to Chapter 8 of Gould: *Orthopaedic and Sports Physical Therapy.*)

The chemical effects of ultrasound are related, in part, to its thermal properties. Raising the tissue temperature accelerates the metabolic processes, including increasing enzyme activity, increasing the rate of ion exchange, increasing cell membrane permeability, and increasing the rate and volume of diffusion across cell membranes. Because of these properties ultrasound can be rendered even more

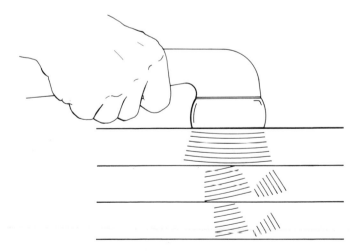

Fig. 31-3. The longitudinal wave of ultrasound is refracted at tissue interfaces where it encounters tissues of differing acoustical resistance. When the wave changes direction, energy is transferred to the tissues, resulting in the production of heat.

effective as a pain reliever with the use of **phonophoresis.** During the process of phonophoresis the ultrasound wave front is used to drive molecules of a pain-relieving chemical into the tissues. Once subcutaneous, the molecules are broken down into ions and taken up into the cells, where they participate in intracellular chemical reactions (Fig. 31-4).

The following pain-relieving chemicals can be administered with phonophoresis:[32]

1. 5% Lidocaine ointment (Xylocaine) for acute conditions where immediate pain relief is the primary goal
2. 1% Hydrocortisone cream or ointment, where pain is the result of inflammation
3. 10% Salicylate cream or ointment, where a combined analgesic-antiinflammatory agent is needed
4. 1%/4% Iodine/salicylate ointment (Iodex with methyl salicylate), where a sclerolytic agent would enhance the analgesic and antiinflammatory effects of salicylate

Following phonophoresis, measurable quantities of these molecules have been found at tissue depths of up to 2 inches.[21]

Phonophoresis cannot be performed subaqueously. The dissipation of the wave front by the intervening water reduces the driving forces, and the usual water-soluble ointments are diluted beyond functional levels. For the same reason phonophoresis cannot be administered with solutions. It is advised that a coupling agent be applied over the chemical before the application of ultrasound to prevent the loss of energy and because many of the ointments used in phonophoresis are too viscous for favorable transmission when used alone.[32]

Cryotherapy. The physiological effects of cold make it superior to heat for acute pain from inflammatory conditions, for the period immediately following tissue trauma, and for treating muscle spasm and abnormal tone. These physiological changes include the following:

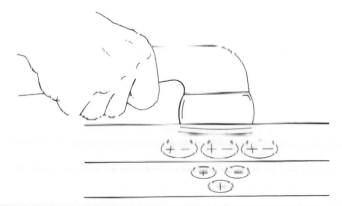

Fig. 31-4. Phonophoresis. Molecules of a substance are driven into the tissues by the ultrasound wave front. They are not free for use by the body until they are broken down into chemical ions.

1. Peripheral nerve conduction velocity in both large myelinated and small unmyelinated fibers decreases 2.4 m/second/° C of cooling. As a result, pain perception and muscle contractability diminish.[68]
2. Peripheral receptors become less excitable.[68]
3. Muscle spindle responsiveness to stretch decreases; as a result, muscle spasm diminishes.[13]
4. Local blood flow first decreases; local edema is decreased, the inflammatory response is diminished, and hemorrhage is minimized. After prolonged cold application, local blood flow increases. Known as the "hunting response," this protective mechanism brings core temperature blood to the surface and prevents tissue injury resulting from prolonged exposure.[16]
5. Cellular metabolic activities slow. The oxygen requirements of the cell decrease.[68]

As with heat, several precautions must be taken when using cold as a therapeutic modality. Cold application is contraindicated in individuals with Raynaud's phenomenon or cold allergy. It should not be used in individuals with rheumatic disease who, with the application of cold, have increased joint pain and stiffness. It should be used with caution in very young or elderly individuals and those with peripheral vascular disease or other circulatory pathologies.[65]

Cryotherapy is applied in three ways. Convective cooling involves movement of air over the skin (fanning) and is rarely used therapeutically. Evaporative cooling results when a substance applied to the skin uses thermal energy to evaporate, thereby lowering surface temperature. Most commonly, this substance is a vapocoolant spray. Conductive cooling uses local application of cold, either by ice packs, ice massage, or immersion. Cooling is accomplished as heat from the higher temperature object is transferred to the colder object down a temperature gradient. Conductive cooling is the most commonly used form of therapeutic cold application.

Because muscles, tendons, and joints respond differently, the best method of cold application depends on which tissues are causing the pain. Muscle spasm is decreased with cold packs and stretching. Trigger points, irritable foci within muscles, are best treated with vapocoolant spray, deep friction massage, and stretching. Tendonitis responds well to ice massage and exercise. Cold packs are many times the only source of pain relief in acute disk pathology. The inflamed joints of rheumatoid arthritis frequently respond to cold packs or ice massage with decreased inflammation, increased function, and long-lasting pain relief.[41,65]

Transcutaneous electrical nerve stimulation

After Melzack and Wall proposed the gate-control theory of pain modulation in 1965, a dorsal column stimulator (DCS) was developed for individuals with intractable pain. In 1970, while screening surgical candidates to determine their suitability for DCS placement, Shealy[62] discovered that, in many candidates, significant pain relief could be obtained with **TENS** alone, and Shealy and others began investigating TENS as a viable treatment alternative.

The exact mechanism by which TENS modulates pain still is not known. It appears that, at a high rate, TENS selectively stimulates the low-threshold, large-diameter A-delta fibers resulting in presynaptic inhibition within the dorsal horns[6] either directly via Melzak and Wall's gate, or indirectly through stimulation of the tonic descending pain inhibiting pathways originating in the periaqueductal gray matter and the brainstem.[71] Research has shown that the neurons in the brainstem fire in synchrony with the TENS stimulation frequency,[73] and although the significance of this is not known at this time, it does indicate that the action of high-rate TENS is not limited to the dorsal columns. TENS delivered at a low rate is thought to facilitate elevation of the level of endorphins in the cerebrospinal fluid. Naloxone, a morphine antagonist, reverses the analgesia obtained through low-rate TENS,[1] indicating that at a low rate the action of TENS includes stimulation of the release of endogenous opiates.[67]

Since their origin in 1970, TENS stimulators have undergone considerable evolution and are now miniaturized, portable, solid-state generators that produce a pulsed current. Depending on the sophistication of the stimulator, the parameters of pulse rate (frequency), pulse width, and amperage (intensity) may be adjustable. Although the wave form (shape) is predetermined and usually cannot be changed, the pattern in which the wave is delivered can be manipulated to change the mode of stimulation.

Stimulation at frequencies between 1 and 250 pulses per second (pps) works to decrease pain. Frequencies between 50 and 100 pps have proven most effective for the majority of individuals receiving high-rate TENS and frequencies between 2 and 3 pps are most effective for the majority of individuals receiving low-rate TENS.[47] Stimulation at exactly 2 pps causes an actual increase in the pain threshold.[24] As the frequency is decreased more time is needed before the onset of relief, but the effects are more long-lasting.[59]

Pulse width duration needs to be appropriate to stimulate the target nerves. Low-threshold fibers are best stimulated at widths between 50 and 100 μs and high-threshold fibers between 150 and 300 μs.[47]

Although stimulus amplitude is set to tolerance, it should be sufficient to cause paresthesia throughout the painful area without stimulating muscle contraction during high-rate TENS and strong enough to result in strong, rhythmic muscle contractions during low-rate TENS. Ten to 30 mA is adequate for high-rate TENS, whereas greater than 30 mA is usually necessary during low-rate TENS.[47]

The output from TENS stimulators can be front-end loaded, back-end loaded, or linear. Front-end loaded stimulators provide greater than 50% of their output in the first half

of the dial range so that the greatest sensory changes will be perceived during early amplitude adjustments. Back-end loaded stimulators provide greater than 50% of their output in the second half of the dial range. Early dial movements may not produce subjective sensory changes, but small changes late in the dial range can result in a sudden (startling) surge of stimulation. Linear stimulators provide equal degrees of subjective sensory change throughout the entire excursion of the amplitude dial.

Some TENS stimulators maintain constant voltage by varying current intensity, whereas others maintain constant current intensity by varying voltage. Because they vary the voltage in response to changes in the stimulation area, constant current stimulators appear to deliver more electrical charge to the neurological structures[42] while avoiding focal areas of hyperstimulation (and potential burns) that can occur when electrodes loosen.

Research has shown that there is no ideal waveform, although some individuals respond better to one form than another. The important factor is that the wave should not have a net direct current (DC) component that causes polar effects under the electrodes, which can cause chemical burns with prolonged application.

Each mode of TENS has a distinct stimulation pattern that appears to modulate pain in a manner different from the other modes. Therefore each mode of TENS is more beneficial for a specific type of pain (although clinically this is not absolute).[47]

Normal TENS. TENS in which the impulses are equally spaced from each other is called normal TENS. Normal TENS is divided into three subcategories: conventional TENS, low-rate TENS, and brief-intense TENS.

When the impulses are generated at a high rate and relatively narrow width, the stimulation is referred to as conventional TENS. Conventional TENS produces mild to moderate paresthesia without muscle contraction throughout the treatment area. There is a relatively fast onset of relief (seconds to 15 minutes), but the duration of relief after stimulation stops is short-lived (at best up to a few hours). Conventional TENS can be worn continuously, although it is recommended that the stimulator be turned off every hour to reassess if TENS is still needed.[47] Conventional TENS is beneficial for acute pain syndromes, including control of postsurgical incision pain and for anesthesia during childbirth. It is also useful for some deep, achy chronic pain syndromes. The main drawback to conventional TENS is neural accommodation, a decrease in perception of the stimulus that occurs as the nerve becomes less excitable with repeated stimulation. This accommodation either can be managed by frequently adjusting the amplitude or avoided by varying (modulating) the stimulus.

When the impulses are generated at a low rate and a relatively wide pulse width, the stimulation is referred to as low-rate TENS. Low-rate TENS produces strong muscle contractions in the treatment area without the perception of paresthesia. The onset of relief is delayed 20 to 30 minutes, presumably the time it takes to deploy the opiates; however, relief frequently lasts hours or days after treatment. Low-rate TENS is beneficial for chronic pain syndromes[47]; however, it is not always well accepted. To be effective, the intensity of the stimulus must cause strong, rhythmical muscle contractions, which are sometimes greater than what can be tolerated in an already painful area. Modulating the stimulus frequently increases comfort. Because stimulation for longer than 1 hour can result in depletion of the body's endorphins, treatment time should be limited to 30- to 45-minute sessions. Sessions can be repeated as pain returns.

Stimulation using high-rate, wide-width impulses is called brief-intense TENS. Brief-intense TENS decreases the conduction velocity of A-delta and C fibers, producing a peripheral blockade to transmission.[47] Brief-intense TENS is beneficial in the clinical setting for use during wound debridement, suture removal, friction massage, joint mobilization, or other painful procedures. Brief-intense TENS should not continue longer than 15 minutes, although sessions can be repeated after a few minutes' rest.

Burst TENS. Stimulation in which the impulses are generated in pulse trains is called burst TENS. The stimulator generates low-rate carrier impulses, each of which contains a series of high-rate pulses. Because burst TENS is a combination of high-rate and low-rate TENS, it provides the benefits of each. The low-rate carrier impulse stimulates endorphin release, and the high-rate pulse trains provide an overlay of paresthesia. The advantage to burst TENS is that muscle contractions occur at a lower, more comfortable amplitude, and accommodation does not occur. Burst TENS is beneficial whenever low-rate TENS cannot be tolerated and conventional TENS is ineffective because of neural accommodation. Treatment time should be limited to 30 to 45 minutes, as with low-rate TENS.[47]

Modulated TENS. Modulating TENS parameters is one way of avoiding the negative aspects of each of the treatment modes. Rate modulation is most beneficial with conventional TENS. By setting the initial pulse rate so that, even with the programed decrement, it will remain within the treatment range, there will be a continuous variation in the impulse rate, thereby avoiding neural accommodation.

Modulating the pulse width changes the amount of energy delivered in each impulse. Width modulation is most beneficial with low-rate TENS. By setting the initial pulse width so that, even with the programed decrement, the impulses are wide enough to recruit all motor units, there will be a continuous variation in strength of the muscle contractions, with a lesser degree of C fiber recruitment making low-rate TENS more tolerable.

Combined modulation makes strong stimulation more tolerable by alternately recruiting high-threshold and low-threshold fibers while inhibiting accommodation. Because of this, combined modulation is effective with either high-rate or low-rate TENS.

Electrode placement sites have to be carefully selected to ensure that the appropriate nerves are being reached and that there is sufficient current to stimulate them. It must be determined whether the pain originates from the superficial or deep structures, whether it is local, whether it is referred or radiated, and whether it is transmitted by the CNS or ANS. Superficial pain is usually well localized and nonradiating and occurs almost immediately after the precipitating incident. Deep pain is usually diffuse, difficult to localize, and perceived at areas other than its point of origin (referred or radiated).[47] Pain of CNS versus ANS origin has been discussed previously.

Electrodes should be the same size. Electrodes with equal surface area will have equal current density beneath them. When electrodes with unequal surface areas are used in the same circuit, there will be greater density beneath the smaller, creating the potential for skin irritation or burns. Current density varies with the distance between electrodes: the closer the electrodes, the greater the density between them. The depth of current penetration varies with the distance between electrodes: the closer the electrodes, the more superficial the current. Current density decreases as it crosses the body.[47]

Various studies and clinical observations have provided a myriad of choices for electrode placement.[32,46,47,62] Site selection depends on the origin of the pain and the mode of stimulation. When using conventional TENS, the best results occur when the area of paresthesia encompasses the pain. The electrodes should be placed around the painful site, with at least one electrode parallel to the involved spinal segment(s). The result of low-rate TENS should be strong, rhythmical muscle contractions in segmentally related myotomes (within or outside of the painful area). Electrodes should be applied over the motor point of the related musculature or over the most superficial point of the mixed or motor nerve(s) serving the muscle(s). Electrode placement during burst TENS depends on which component of the stimulation is being emphasized. If paresthesia is desired the electrodes can be placed as they would be with conventional TENS. If muscle contraction is the goal, the electrode placements used during low-rate TENS can be used.

Other successful stimulation sites include directly over sensory nerves, linear pathways, acupuncture points, related dermatomes, the nerve plexus, trigger points, the contralateral side of the body (when the client cannot tolerate stimulation to the painful side), the upper cervical spine, or a remote area of the body. Stimulation of the ulnar nerve, for example, provides relief to all areas except the head.[47]

Statistics regarding the efficacy of TENS are impressive. The results of various studies[43,62] report that 80% of all clients with acute pain and 25% to 39% of clients with chronic pain no longer needed pain medication, and another 55% to 60% were able to significantly decrease their need for pain medication. Less than 5% found TENS too uncomfortable to wear,[62] and the single reported side effect was skin irritation at the electrode placement site in 1.6% of all individuals wearing TENS.[7] This is directly attributed to allergy to the adhesive used to attach the electrodes to the skin, to improper electrode attachment, or to infrequent electrode changes.

Although the placebo effect is felt to be of some minimal benefit initially, long-range follow-up over a year showed decrease of its influence. Placebo is of short duration, and the general tendency is a reduction in the amount of stimulation needed with longer periods of relief between stimulation sessions.[43]

TENS is of greatest benefit for acute conditions with focal pain, chronic pain syndromes, postoperative incision pain, and during delivery. It is least effective with psychogenic pain[44] and pain of central origin.[50] For additional information on TENS refer to Chapter 30.

Iontophoresis

Iontophoresis is a process in which chemical ions are driven through the skin by a small electrical current. Ionizable compounds are placed on the skin under an electrode that, when polarized by a direct (galvanic) current, repels the ion of like charge into the tissues. Once subcutaneous, the ions are free to combine with the physiological ions or to be transported by the superficial circulation into the systemic blood flow, which carries them to distant areas of the body. In either case, a physiological effect dependent on the characteristics of the ion is obtained (Fig. 31-5).

Ions that are known to be effective analgesics are:[32]

1. 5% Lidocaine ointment (Xylocaine) administered under the positive electrode for an immediate, although short-lived, decrease in pain. Iontophoresis with lidocaine is recommended before ROM, stretching, and joint mobilization, and when immediate relief of acute pain (as in bursitis) is the object of treatment.
2. 1% to 10% Hydrocortisone administered under the positive electrode for relief of inflammatory pain in conditions such as arthritis, bursitis, or entrapment syndromes. Iontophoresis with hydrocortisone has a delayed onset but a prolonged effect, and it frequently eliminates the underlying cause of pain.
3. 2% Magnesium (from Epsom salts) administered

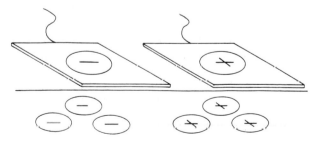

Fig. 31-5. Iontophoresis. Chemical ions are driven into the tissues by a small electrical current. Once subcutaneous they are immediately free to take part in chemical reactions within the body.

under the positive electrode for relief of pain from muscle spasm or localized ischemia. High levels of extracellular magnesium inhibit muscle contraction, including the smooth muscle found in the walls of the vessels, resulting in localized vasodilation.
4. Iodine (from Iodex ointment) administered under the negative pole for relief of pain caused by adhesions or scar tissue. Iodine "softens" fibrotic, sclerotic tissue, thereby increasing tissue pliability.
5. Salicylate (from Iodex with methyl salicylate) administered under the negative pole for relief of pain from inflammation or tissue congestion. Salicylate is effective for arthritic joint inflammation, myalgia, and entrapment syndromes.
6. 2% Acetic acid administered under the negative pole to dissolve calcium deposits.
7. 2% Lithium chloride or lithium carbonate administered under the positive pole to dissolve gouty tophi. In both acetic acid and lithium iontophoresis, the insoluble radicals in the deposits are replaced by soluble chemical radicals so the deposits can be broken down through natural processes.

The contraindication to the use of any ion is an allergy to that ion. Because most clients will not have had iontophoresis previously, it is important to inquire about experiences that might indicate an allergy. For example, an intolerance for shellfish may be the result of an allergy to iodine, and a poor reaction to dental local anesthesia may indicate a problem with lidocaine.

In addition to the potential for allergic reaction to the ions, skin irritation may occur under the electrodes for several reasons. Because the polarity of the electrodes remains constant throughout the treatment, chemical reactions occur directly below each electrode. The tissue under the positive pole (anode) becomes acidic with the formation of hydrochloric acid, while that under the negative pole (cathode) becomes alkaline with the formation of sodium hydroxide. Either chemical in sufficient quantity can injure the tissues, but irritation and burns most commonly occur under the negative electrode.[32]

Electrical burns can occur when the current density or amplitude exceed safe limits. Iontophoresis is administered using a 5-mA current applied for about 15 minutes with the selected ion source under the like pole electrode. When the procedure is too uncomfortable or when marked skin irritation occurs under the electrodes, the current can be decreased and the treatment time increased. To avoid high current densities between the electrodes (the "edge effect"), the indifferent and active electrodes should be separated by at least the width of one electrode.[32]

The negative electrode should always be the larger of the two, regardless of which is the treating electrode, to decrease current density and a high concentration of polarity-induced chemicals under this more irritating pole. The electrodes, the skin below, and the current setting should be checked every 3 to 5 minutes to prevent skin irritation and chemical burns. Proper aftercare of the skin below the electrodes can further decrease skin irritation. The skin should be massaged with an astringent, a witch hazel solution, or carbolated vasoline, then dusted with cornstarch.[32]

Massage

Massage has been recognized as a remedy for pain for at least 3000 years. Evidence of its beneficial effects are first found in ancient Chinese literature, and then in the writings of the Hindus, Persians, Egyptians, and Greeks. Hippocrates advocated massage for sprains and dislocations as well as for constipation.[40]

Massage has both reflex and mechanical effects. Reflex relaxation occurs through changes in muscle tension and circulation brought about by stimulation of the peripheral nerves. Fluid mobilization and intramuscular motion are the result of mechanically compressing and moving the tissues. Massage movements are classified by pressure and the part of the hand that is used.[74]

Stroking involves running the entire hand over large portions of the body. Light stroking involves a very light touch and causes the reflex effects of muscular relaxation and elimination of muscle spasm. Deep stroking, on the other hand, is applied with sufficient pressure to assist in circulation. Both forms of stroking are applied with constant pressure at a constant rate of speed in an even rhythm.

Compression massage, in contrast, is applied with intermittent pressure using lifting, rolling, or pressing movements meant to stretch shortened tissues, loosen adhesions, and assist with circulation. Compression massage is divided into kneading and friction movements. Kneading involves intermittently lifting or compressing a muscle or muscle group so that there is movement within it. Friction massage is performed by using the finger tips to perform circulatory movements that move the superficial tissues over the underlying structures.

Percussion, as it applies to pain management, is performed to stimulate circulation. Hacking involves using the ulnar border of the hand or the fingers to perform a series of brisk, rapid, alternating contacts with the skin. Clapping is done with the palms flat, while cupping is done with the palm formed into a concave surface.

Massage is useful in any condition where pain relief will follow the reduction of swelling or the mobilization of the tissues. These include arthritis, bursitis, neuritis, fibrositis, low-back pain, hemiplegia, paraplegia, quadriplegia, and joint sprains, strains, and contusions. Massage is contraindicated over infected areas, diseased skin, and thrombophlebitic regions.

Myofascial release

Fascia is connective tissue that plays a supportive role within the body. It forms a framework around the viscera, stabilizes articulations, provides a constantly fluctuating biochemical equilibrium to assist in the maintenance of homeostasis in the surrounding tissues, and, in conjunction with muscular activity, assists in the movement of blood and lymph. Fascia contains sensory nerves and tension bands of varying thicknesses.[25]

Ideally, the fascial system is in constant three-dimensional motion: right to left, side to side, and front to back.[25] Under abnormal physical and chemical conditions, such as faulty muscle activity, alteration in the position or relationship of the bones, altered vertebral mechanics, or unnatural postures, the fascial connective tissue can thicken and shorten, creating hypomobile areas with increased tension[71] that can, because the fascia represents one continuous system, affect movement in remote areas of the body by restricting motion of that fascia. Because the fascia contains sensory nerves, areas of increased tension, sudden tension, or traction are painful.[25]

The goal of **myofascial release** techniques is to release the built-in imbalances and restrictions within the fascia and to reintegrate the fascial mechanism. The therapist palpates the various tissue layers, beginning with the most superficial and working systematically toward the deepest, looking for movement restrictions and asymmetry. Areas of altered structure and function are then "normalized" through the systematic application of pressure and stretching applied in specific directions to bring about decreased myofascial tension, myofascial lengthening, and myofascial softening,[71] thereby restoring pain-free motion in normal patterns of movement.

Joint mobilization

Two forms of movement are available to each joint: physiological and accessory. Physiological movement is the gross ROM (defined as flexion, extension, and rotation). Accessory movement is the fine motion that occurs between the surfaces of the opposing bones (defined as distraction, slide, glide, and tilt). Physiological movement can be performed by the individual; accessory movement cannot and requires the application of external force.

Normal accessory movement is necessary for normal physiological movement. When the collagen fibers of the joint capsule become thickened or bound down, accessory movements become restricted, preventing full ROM. Because the joint capsule is richly innervated, pain is produced when the soft tissue structures are stretched in an attempt to produce full gross movement.[61]

Joint mobilization consists of passive oscillations that allow the collagen fibers to rearrange and loosen, thereby restoring normal accessory movements.[61] In addition the rhythmical repetition of the motions provides pain relief via the mechanisms specified in the gate-control theory.[52]

The oscillations involved in joint mobilization are graded as follows.[46]

Grade I: small amplitude movements performed at the beginning of the available ROM

Grade II: larger amplitude movements performed further into the available ROM

Grade III: large amplitude movements performed at the end of the available ROM

Grade IV: small amplitude movements performed at the end of the available ROM

Grade V: high-velocity thrust (manipulation) performed at the end of the available ROM

Grades I and II are performed to maintain joint mobility and for pain relief, making them the choice for subacute conditions where pain and potential loss of motion are the primary considerations. Grades III and IV are performed to increase joint mobility and are indicated for chronic conditions where regaining lost motion is the goal. Grade V thrusts are performed to regain full joint mobility.[61]

Joint mobilization is contraindicated with rheumatoid arthritis, bone disease, advanced osteoporosis, pregnancy (pelvic mobilization), as well as in the presence of malignancy, vascular disease, or infection in the area to be mobilized.[46]

Joint mobilization is covered in Chapter 11 of Gould: *Orthopaedic and Sports Physical Therapy* as well as in several excellent texts addressing musculoskeletal disorders.

Therapeutic touch

Eastern philosophy views human life as one of the many energy forces that coexist and interact with each other within the universe. Ancient Sanskrit writings equate health and illness with an energy called *prana*. According to the writings, health represents an overabundance of prana and illness represents a deficit. One person can heal another by activating their personal prana and transferring it to another at will. Healing through energy exchange is also recorded in the hieroglyphics, cuneiform writings, and pictographs of the earliest literate cultures.[38]

Western philosophy has been slow to accept the view of humanity as interconnected with the universe, preferring, instead, to view us as a distinct entity. However, the treatment technique of **therapeutic touch** (along with the supporting research) has done much to change the view of Western clinicians.

Basic to therapeutic touch is the concept that the healthy human body has an excess of energy, which can be shared with another for the purpose of healing. The healer serves as a conduit, directing personal and environmental energy to a client who then internalizes and directs the energy to restore balance and perform self-healing.[39]

During therapeutic touch the healer contacts the client's energy field by slowly scanning the client's body with his or her own hands. It is not necessary to touch the client to perceive areas of accumulated tension. When tension is encountered, the healer slowly moves his or her hands over the area to redirect the accumulated energy.

Therapeutic touch results first in an energy transfer from the healer to the client, then in a repatterning of the client's energy state comparable to that of the healer.[33] Clients report a subjective sense of heat in the diseased/painful area followed by an overall sense of well-being and relaxation.

Kreiger,[38] who first described and taught therapeutic touch, conducted research on clients receiving the treatment. She compared the posttreatment hemoglobin values in clients receiving therapeutic touch with clients who had been scanned by individuals who let their minds wander. The results were startling: In three different studies clients receiving therapeutic touch showed higher mean hemoglobin values posttreatment than did clients who received placebo treatments. In other studies involving plant growth, plants watered with water treated with therapeutic touch grew larger and faster than plants watered with untreated water.[38] Krieger's research has shown that the technique is effective even if the client does not believe in therapeutic touch, as long as the healer has faith in the technique and is intent on helping the patient heal.

Therapeutic touch has been effective in treating painful conditions resulting from anxiety and tension. Ninety percent of individuals treated with therapeutic touch experienced tension headache relief; 70% had continued relief for greater than 4 hours; only 37% of the placebo group expressed sustained relief.[33]

Point stimulation

The ancient Chinese were the first to become aware of acupuncture points, areas of the skin that become sensitive with internal disease states. Over time they mapped out imaginary lines connecting the points with each other. They believed that energy and nutrients flowed to all parts of the body along these "meridians" and that, when there is disease, the energy flow is interrupted. The most effective sites for treatment, they reasoned, are the acupuncture points.[70]

It is interesting to note that acupuncture points frequently correspond in location to trigger points, tight, elevated bands of tissue that are extremely sensitive when palpated and have a characteristic pattern of radiation to remote regions of the body. Trigger points appear to be areas of "focal irritability" that are myofascial in origin and are usually the site of small aggregations of nerve fibers that produce continuous afferent input when stimulated.

Needling of acupuncture points stimulates the release of endorphins,[70] most probably through the central modulating pathway that originates in the periaqueductal gray matter.[69] Acupressure, finger pressure applied to acupuncture or trigger points, is thought to decrease their sensitivity through the same mechanism. The therapist applies deep pressure in a circular motion to each point for 1 to 5 minutes, until the sensitivity subsides. Pressure must be applied directly to each point for the treatment to be effective. Acupressure can be accompanied by the use of a vapocoolant spray to provide additional sensory stimulation. Acupressure should be followed by full active and passive stretch and rewarming of the muscle in which the trigger point is located.[69]

Sensitive points also can be stimulated using electricity. A point locator is used to identify points along the appropriate meridians that are sensitive to stimulation or more conductive to electricity. Each is then stimulated at the client's level of pain tolerance for 30 to 45 seconds. The points farthest from the site of pain are treated first.

Points that are most sensitive to stimulation are beneficial sites for TENS electrode placement. When pain stimulation alone does not provide sufficient pain relief, TENS can be used between sessions for continuous stimulation for more prolonged relief.

Laser

Laser application to painful tissue can bring about an almost immediate relief of spasm. This is thought to be the result of the physiological properties of the laser that allow it to penetrate and be absorbed by human tissue. These properties are as follows:[35]

1. Monochromatism: Light emitted from the laser has a single wavelength.
2. Coherence: Light emitted from the laser has a high degree of order and a fixed phase relationship.
3. Divergence: Light emitted from the laser has a narrow focus and very little divergence.

Once absorbed, laser energy brings about depolarization and repolarization of abnormally contracted tissues, causes reactive vasodilation in arteriolar spasms, and modifies electron excitability in mitochondria leading to changes in metabolic processes.

Kleinkort[35] found the use of lasers on specific acupuncture points effective where there is not anatomical dysfunction at the base of the pain stimuli. He has used it for myofascial syndromes, inflammatory tendonitis, bursitis, localized arthritis, and painful keloids.

Cognitive-behavioral methods

Chronic pain has effects on all aspects of an individual's life. The functional limitations brought on by pain, as well as the individual's pain behavior, can affect job performance, relationships, recreational pursuits, and aspirations for the future.

Pain perception and, ultimately, pain expression encompass not only the sensation of pain but also the emotional state, expectations, personality, and cognitive view of the person experiencing it. Melzak and Wall[52] proposed that pain has three nonphysical components that can be addressed through cognitive-behavioral measures: sensory/discriminative interpretation of painful inputs, motivational/affective behaviors and attitudes relating to pain and cognitive/

evaluative thoughts, and beliefs concerning the pain experience.

These nonphysical components of pain can be addressed by modifying the interpretation of the sensation of the pain experience with relaxation exercises, hypnosis, biofeedback, operant conditioning, and the relatively new concept of body scanning. Each of these techniques recognizes that the mind is not separate from the body, accepts that there is a mental component to pain, and utilizes the inner resources of the mind to influence the pain experience.

Relaxation exercises. Relaxation exercises help the individual become aware of what tension feels like so that it can be recognized and eliminated. With proper technique, as the muscles relax there is a generalized parasympathetic response including decreased heart rate, decreased respiratory rate, decreased metabolic rate, decreased stomach acid production, increased skin temperature, slowed deep tendon reflexes, and an overall sense of well-being.[29] Benson[4] has named this effect the *relaxation response*. He who also notes that it is accompanied by an increase in alpha brain waves.

Pain relief resulting directly from relaxation is thought to occur in two ways. First, ischemic pain is reduced as normal blood flow to the muscles is reestablished, and there is a rise in oxygen delivery to the tissues. Second, there is a reduction in muscle tension, which aggravates pain.[11]

Deep relaxation can be achieved either by systematically tensing and relaxing the muscles, one region at a time, until the entire body is free of tension, by performing slow, deep breathing while concentrating on an object or word to minimize external and internal distractions, or by visualizing a place where the individual has been able to relax such as by the ocean, or a waterfall.

Once the individual is relaxed, any or all of the following techniques can be used to address the cognitive aspects of their pain experience.

Hypnosis. Hypnosis is an altered state of consciousness during which there is increased receptivity to suggestion. Borysenko[5] defines it as "fixating the attention . . . so that new frames of reference can be established." Clients are instructed in achieving the relaxation response during which they are presented with new paradigms (reinterpretations of reality) concerning their pain. For example clients might be told to disregard their pain or be guided to reframe their pain into a messenger and then be encouraged to listen to its message.

The client with chronic pain frequently develops a pain-supporting behavior because it brings increased attention, because it allows avoidance of distasteful activities and because well behaviors are frequently regarded negatively. In many instances nonspecific feelings are labeled as pain for this reason. Thus many clients have learned the reward of pain expression and continue to experience pain only because there are more positive than negative reinforcing factors.[22]

The aim of hypnotic suggestion is to change what the

client sees as a positive reward. By learning to challenge what they say to themselves, clients can be taught to revise their paradigms and their goals and to gain control over stress, tension, and pain.[22]

Biofeedback. **Biofeedback** is a training process in which the client becomes aware of and learns to selectively change physiological processes with the aid of an external monitor. It has the following three characteristics:[29]

1. Continuous monitoring of the physiological response
2. Continuous feedback of changes in the response either by a light, sound, or gauge (desired performance is rewarded)
3. Motivation on the part of the client to change the response

During biofeedback, the biofeedback instrument is placed on the appropriate area of the body. The machine provides an initial readout. The client is instructed how to change the monitored process, and as change occurs the machine "feeds back" that information. By mentally changing a biological function, the client learns to gain control over it. In time, the client learns to control the process without needing an assist from the instrument. The feedback mechanism becomes feedforward as a procedural process.

Muscle tension, pulse rate, blood pressure, skin temperature, and electromyography (EMG) and electronecephalography (EEG) readings are some of the physiological processes that can be consciously modified with biofeedback.[29]

Biofeedback is proving to be an effective pain management tool with tension headaches, muscle spasms, and other physical dysfunctions that lead to or increase chronic pain (see Chapter 30).

Operant conditioning. **Operant conditioning** addresses the learned (or conditioned) aspects of pain.[17] Individuals with chronic pain express their pain with behaviors that provide them with consistent positive rewards. For example wincing might bring attention from a family member or limping might allow the individual to avoid performing a particular task. Over time the individual with pain becomes conditioned to perform certain behaviors for the behavior's rewards rather than as a reaction to the pain.

Similarly, individuals with chronic pain also can condition their nervous systems through learning. If an individual expects to experience pain as the result of a particular level of activity, the individual will always experience pain at that level of activity.

Operant conditioning involves unlearning or separating the behavior and the response from the pain experience.[17] If the goal of treatment is to lessen social reinforcement of the client's pain behaviors (and thus extinguish those behaviors), the client and the family or other involved individuals are shown how their behaviors and responses provide social reinforcement for the client's reaction to pain. The involved individuals are provided with specific new responses to the client's behavior. Family members might be instructed to ignore wincing, groaning, or the verbal report of pain. They might be told not to perform activities that are the client's responsibility just because the client reports pain. In time, the client will become conditioned to the new response, and pain in those situations will diminish.

If the goal of treatment is to increase the client's painfree activity level, operant conditioning can be utilized to condition the nervous system to a higher level of activity before responding with pain. If the client's usual pattern is to be active until the onset of pain (negative reinforcement for activity) and then rest (positive reinforcement for pain), the client is instructed to be active to just below the pain threshold and then rest (positive reinforcement for activity). In this way the nervous system unlearns the connection between activity and pain, and the client's activity level increases.

Body scanning. Clients with chronic pain frequently become one with their suffering; they do not view themselves as individuals with pain, but, rather, as painful individuals. **Body scanning** is a technique that endeavors to separate the individual from the pain.[31]

The client is taught to achieve a meditative state during which the body scan exercise is performed. Attention is focused on each body area, one at a time. The client is instructed to breathe into and out from each area, relaxing more deeply with each exhalation. When the area is completely relaxed, the client "lets go" of the region and dwells in the stillness for a few breaths before continuing. Painful areas are scanned in an identical manner. The client notes changes in sensation, thoughts, and emotions while scanning each area, but does not judge the changes.

Individuals who practice this technique report new levels of insight and understanding concerning their pain experience. They separate the pain experience into three parts:

1. They become aware of the character of the sensation of pain and their thoughts and feelings about it.
2. They become aware that they are able to objectively examine the sensation and their thoughts and feelings, so these must be separate from each other.
3. They recognize that if they are able to objectively examine the sensation and their thoughts and feelings, then they must be separate from them.

Once clients accept that they are not their pain or their reaction to pain, then they can determine how much influence and control pain has in their lives.

Studies of chronic pain patients at the Stress Reduction Clinic at the University of Massachusetts Medical Center revealed that 72% of patients who used meditation and body scanning along with traditional medical interventions experienced at least a 33% reduction on their McGill-Melzak Pain Rating Index.[31] In addition, at the end of an 8-week training period, they perceived their bodies in a more positive light, experienced an increase in positive mood states, and had major improvements in anxiety, depression, hostility, and the tendency to be overly occupied with their bodily sensations.

Cognitive-behavioral approaches to pain management have two main goals. The first is to activate the descending cortical modulating systems and the second is to teach the client to control, rather than being controlled by, the pain. Used in conjunction with other modalities necessary for immediate relief, these approaches can play a significant role in long-term management and should not be overlooked when seeking a viable pain management alternative.

THE FUTURE

This is an exciting time in the treatment of pain. Research is proving that peoples' thoughts have an effect on their body chemistry. Therapists have noted for years that, within the clinic, most clients who want to improve do, and most clients who do not want to improve do not. Now the scientific community is actually demonstrating that immune cell numbers and activity are influenced by peoples' thoughts, beliefs, and intentions.[5] This discovery has been named psychoneuroimmunology.

Coupled with the changing American health care system, which is providing strict limits on the number of treatments per diagnosis, and the emerging emphasis on prevention, psychoneuroimmunology is opening the scientific door for therapists to approach pain management from a new perspective. Rather than merely applying modalities, future therapists will teach clients to invoke their own healing powers, to use their minds to affect their health and their pain. Proof of the public's willingness to accept this new approach to health is evident in the ever-increasing sale of self-help books. The challenge will come in demonstrating to third-party payers that body-mind techniques have reimbursement value. (A list of suggested readings follow the references.)

CLINICAL EXAMPLES

The following clinical examples demonstrate a problem-solving approach to the treatment of pain.

REFERENCES

1. Abram S and others: Failure of naloxone to reverse analgesia from transcutaneous electrical nerve stimulation in patients with chronic pain, *Anesth Analg* 60:81, 1981.
2. Adler M: Endorphins, enkephalins, and neurotransmitters, *Med Times* 110:32, 1982.
3. Basbaum AI and Fields HL: Endogenous pain control systems, brainstem spinal pathways and endorphin circuitry, *Annu Rev Neurosci* 7:309-338, 1984.
4. Benson H: *The relaxation response,* New York, 1975, Avon Books.
5. Borysenko J: *Minding the body, mending the mind,* Reading, Mass, 1987, Addison-Wesley Publishing Co.
6. Bromage RR: Nerve physiology and control of pain, *Orthop Clin North Am* 4:897, 1976.
7. Burton C: Transcutaneous electrical nerve stimulation to relieve pain, *Postgrad Med* 59:105, 1976.
8. Byrne M and others: Cross-validation of the factor structure of the McGill pain questionnaire, *Pain* 13:193, 1982.

CASE 1 Mrs R.

A 68-year-old female inpatient with a stable compression fracture of the body of T7 is referred to physical therapy for "evaluation and pain control." She reports that the fracture occurred when she fell in the bathtub 3 weeks previously and that her physician had been treating her at home with heat, analgesics, and bedrest; there was no significant decrease in pain. She was admitted to the hospital for more aggressive treatment.

The client describes her pain as a constant dull ache and rates the intensity as "75" on a scale of 1 to 100. The pain is localized to the middorsal spine. It is more intense when the client is upright and relieved slightly when she is supine.

On evaluation, the client is found to have a moderate dorsal kyphosis that is the result of an earlier compression fracture resulting from osteoporosis. There is spasm in the paravertebral dorsal musculature bilaterally, and several trigger points can be located within the back extensors. Palpation of the spine of T7 is exquisitely painful and causes increased spasm in the surrounding musculature. There are no neurological deficits in the trunk or extremities.

The client has previously been fitted with and wears a custom orthosis to stabilize her spine and minimize progression of the kyphosis.

The initial focus of physical therapy for this client is to alleviate her acute pain. Moist heat and phonophoresis with salicylate used in combination twice a day will yield both pain relief and decreased spasm. This can be followed by gentle massage to further induce muscular relaxation. The client should be instructed in proper bed posture that is comfortable and that will maintain the spine as straight as possible.

As the pain and spasm subside and as the client becomes more mobile, she should be evaluated for and receive instruction in proper body mechanics during bed mobility, sitting, transfers, and ambulation. Acupressure can be introduced to treat sensitive trigger points. Strengthening exercises for the back extensors can be initiated with the physician's approval.

As the date of discharge approaches, a home program for pain management needs to be established. If there is still significant pain, the client could be fitted with a TENS unit. Arrangements could be made for her to obtain a moist heating pad for home use. She should be instructed in both a home exercise program to increase strength in her back musculature and in joint preservation measures to minimize further stresses on her spine. The client should return home with an understanding of her injury, with a comprehensive plan for pain management, and with a knowledge of how to lessen the chances of further injury.

CASE 2 ▼ Mrs. L.

A 25-year-old female outpatient with a 5-year history of rheumatoid arthritis is referred to physical therapy for "evaluation and treatment of painful, swollen wrists." The arthritis has been maintained in a chronic state for 2 years with medication and it is felt that this inflammation most probably is the result of isolated trauma rather than a generalized flareup.

Examination of the wrists reveals them to be red, warm, and swollen. Range of motion is limited by about 50% in both flexion and extension. The client reports that movement of the wrists and palation of the soft tissue structures is extremely painful. She rates the pain at "90" on a scale of 1 to 100.

The pain this client is experiencing is the result of inflammation. Therefore treatment should be directed at alleviating the inflammation, which will, in turn, bring about pain relief. Double iontophoresis with one electrode on each wrist can be used to introduce antiinflammatory agents locally into the wrists. Hydrocortisone can be introduced through the positive electrode and salicylate can be introduced through the negative electrode. Since salicylate is also an analgesic, the electrodes can be reversed in each treatment session to provide both wrists with antiinflammatory and analgesic medication.

Following each treatment, the joints should be taken through one full range of motion. Between treatments, the acutely inflamed joints should be immobilized in resting splints. As the inflammation subsides, less time can be spent in the splints and first active, then gentle, resisted exercises can be added to the program. The client should be instructed in joint preservation methods to minimize stress and prolong functional use of her wrists.

CASE 3 ▼ Mr. W.

A 36-year-old paramedic is referred to physical therapy for "evaluation and treatment of left shoulder and arm pain" that developed 3 weeks after he completed therapy for a traction injury to the long head of the biceps tendon in the same shoulder. The original injury occurred while he was lifting an injured person from a wrecked car.

He reports persistent burning pain that developed gradually in the shoulder and is now beginning to affect his hand as well. He states the pain can become so severe that he is reluctant to move the arm for fear of provoking "an episode." He grades the pain as 75 at best and 110 (on a scale of 1 to 100) at worst. He cannot work because of the pain, and he is becoming increasingly anxious about his finances.

While this client waited for therapy, he was observed to cradle his left arm against his body. He used his right arm to open the door, hold a magazine, and assist in standing up from a deep chair.

Evaluation of the left shoulder reveals restricted ROM and diffuse tenderness to palpation that he cannot localize to any individual structure. Examination of the hand reveals mild swelling in the fingers, erythema, and glossy skin. With finger extension he reports that there is a tightness in his palm that is "drawing the fingers into the middle."

This client is developing reflex sympathetic dystrophy (RSD) in the left upper extremity, and treatment must be directed at providing pain relief and preventing further loss of ROM. Prolonged immobilization with this condition leads to fibrosis, articular changes, loss of subcutaneous tissue, and osteoporosis.

This client may benefit from TENS in the conventional mode to provide paresthesia through the painful area. As his pain becomes less severe, low-rate TENS can be instituted to decrease wearing time and to facilitate circulation via the pumping action of the associated muscle contractions.

ROM exercises should be instituted immediately. However, because this client is reluctant to move his arm, movement can be performed using joint mobilization to stretch the capsular structures that are becoming restricted and myofascial release techniques to regain fascial balance in the shoulder complex as well as the entire left upper extremity. Mr. W. may find these procedures more comfortable if they are preceded by the application of cool (not cold) packs. As quickly as possible, an active exercise program emphasizing ROM and stretching should be instituted.

Mr. W.'s anxiety is typical in individuals with RSD, and it is thought to contribute to his physical symptoms. It is important, in treating this condition, to be sympathetic and supportive, but also to reinforce the need for early movement of the extremity to avoid permanent disability. He may also benefit from instruction in several relaxation techniques that he can use to counter the effects of his anxiety concerning his job.

9. Cash J: *Neurology for physiotherapists,* London, 1977, Faber and Faber.
10. Cassini V and Pagne CA: *Central pain: a neurosurgical survey,* Cambridge, Mass, 1969, Harvard University Press.
11. Chapman SL and Shealy CN: Relaxation techniques to control pain. In Brena SF: *Chronic pain: America's hidden epidemic,* New York, 1978, Atheneum Publishers.
12. Cyriax J: *Textbook of orthopaedic medicine,* ed 8, London, 1984, Bailliere Tindall.
13. Eldred E and others: The effect of cooling on mammalian muscle spindles, *Exp Neurol* 2:144, 1960.
14. Evans JH: Neurology and neurological aspects of pain. In Swerdlow M, editor: *Relief of intractable pain: monographs in anesthesiology,* vol 1, New York, 1974, Excerpta Medica.
15. Felton DL and Felton SY: A regional and systemic overview of functional neuroanatomy. In Farber SD: *Neurorehabilitation: a multisensory approach,* Philadelphia, 1982, WB Saunders.
16. Fischer E and Solomon S: Physiological responses to heat and cold. In

Licht S, editor: *Therapeutic heat and cold,* Baltimore, 1972, Waverly Press.

17. Fordyce WE: *Behavioral methods for chronic pain & illness,* St Louis, 1976, Mosby.

18. Gandhavadi B and others: Autonomic pain: features and methods of assessment, *Postgrad Med* 71;85, 1982.

19. Gelhard FA: *The human senses,* New York, 1953, John S. Wiley & Sons.

20. Gorsky BH: *Pain origin and treatment: discussions in patient management,* New Hyde Park, New York, 1982, Medical Examination Publishing Co.

21. Griffin JE: Physiological effects of ultrasonic energy as it is used clinically, *Phys Ther* 46:18, 1966.

22. Grzesiak RC: Cognitive and behavioral approaches to management of chronic pain, *NY State J Med* 82:30, 1982.

23. Hammond DL: Control systems for nociceptive afferent processing: the ascending inhibitory pathway. In Yaksh TL, editor: *Spinal afferent processing,* New York, 1986, Plenum Press.

24. Holmgren E: Increase in pain threshold as a function of conditioning electrical stimulation, *Am J Clin Med* 3:133, 1975.

25. Hubbard RP: Mechanical behavior of connective tissue, handout material from seminar entitled Myofascial Release Concepts. Palpatory and Treatment Skills. E. Lansing, Mich, Sept. 1986.

26. Hughes J and others: Identification of two related pentapeptides from the brain with potent opiate agonist activity, *Nature* 258:577, 1975.

27. Iggo A: Critical remarks on the gate control theory. In Payne JP and Burt RAP, editors: *Pain,* London, 1972, J&A Churchill.

28. International Association for the Study of Pain, Subcommittee on Taxonomy: Pain terms: a list of definitions and notes on usage, *Pain* 6:249-252, 1979.

29. Isele FW: Biofeedback and hypnosis in the management of pain, *NY State J Med* 82:38, 1982.

30. Jacob J: Inflammation revisited: inflammatory pain and mode of action of analgesics, *Agents Actions,* vol. II, 1981.

31. Kabat-Zinn J: *Full catastrophic living,* New York, 1990, Delacorte Press.

32. Kahn J: *Principles and practice of electrotherapy,* ed 2, New York, 1992, Churchill Livingstone.

33. Keller E and Bzdek V: Therapeutic touch and headache, *Nurs Res* 35:101-105, 1986.

34. Kessler R and Hertling D: *Management of common musculoskeletal disorders,* Philadelphia, 1983, Harper & Row.

35. Kleinkort JA: The cold laser, *Clin Manage* 2(4):30, 1982.

36. Kremer E and others: Measurement of pain: patient preference does not confound pain measurement, *Pain* 10:241, 1981.

37. Kremer E and others: Pain measurement: the affective dimensional measure of the McGill pain questionnaire with a cancer pain population, *Pain* 12:153, 1982.

38. Kreiger D: Therapeutic touch: the imprimatur of nursing, *Am J Nurs* 75:784-787, 1975.

39. Krieger D and others: Therapeutic touch: searching for evidence of physiological change, *Am J Nurs* 79:660-662, 1979.

40. Krusen F and others: *Handbook of physical medicine and rehabilitation,* Philadelphia, 1971, WB Saunders.

41. Linton SJ and Melin L: The accuracy of remembering chronic pain, *Pain* 13:281, 1982.

42. Linzen M and Long D: Transcutaneous neural stimulation for relief of pain, *IEEE Trans Biomed Eng* 23:341, 1976.

43. Long D: Cutaneous afferent stimulation for relief of chronic pain, *Clin Neurosurg* 21:257, 1974.

44. Long D: *The comparative efficacy of drugs vs. electrical modulation in the management of chronic pain, current concepts in the management of chronic pain,* Miami, 1977, Symposia Specialists.

45. Madsen PW and Gersten JW: The effect of ultrasound on conduction velocity of peripheral nerve, *Arch Phys Med Rehabil* 42:645, 1961.

46. Maitland G: *Peripheral manipulation,* Ontario, 1976, Butterworth & Scarborough.

47. Mannheimer JS and Lampe GN: Clinical transcutaneous electrical nerve stimulation, Philadelphia, 1984, FA Davis.

48. McKenzie RA: *The lumbar spine,* New Zealand, 1983, Spinal Publications.

49. Melzak R: The McGill pain questionnaire: major properties and scoring methods, *Pain* 1:277, 1975.

50. Melzak R: Prolonged relief of pain by brief, intense transcutaneous somatic stimulation, *Pain* 1:357, 1975.

51. Melzak R: *The gate control theory revisited: current concepts in the management of chronic pain,* Miami, 1977, Symposia Specialties.

52. Melzak R and Wall P: Pain mechanisms: a new theory, *Science* 150:971, 1969.

53. Nathan PW: The gate control theory in pain: a clinical review, *Brain* 99:123, 1976.

54. Nolan MF: Anatomic and physiologic organization of the neural structures involved in pain transmission, modulation and perception. In Echternach JL, editor: *Pain,* New York, 1987, Churchill Livingstone.

55. O'Driscoll SL and Jayson MIV: The clinical significance of pain threshold measurements, *Rheumatol Rehabil* 21:31, 1982.

56. Piercey MF and Folkers K: Sensory and motor functions of spinal cord substance P, *Science* 214:1361, 1981.

57. Reading A: A comparison of the McGill pain questionnaire in chronic and acute pain, *Pain* 13:185, 1982.

58. Reid DS and Cummings GE: Factors in selecting the dosage of ultrasound with particular reference to the use of various coupling agents, *Physiotherapy* 25:5, 1973.

59. Richard RL: Causalgia: a centennial review, *Arch Neurol* 16:339, 1967.

60. Roubal PJ: Ultrasound: clinical observations, *Technic Journal* 5:28, Oct. 1977.

61. Saunders HD: *Evaluation, treatment, and prevention of musculoskeletal disorders,* Eden Prairie, Minn, 1985, author.

62. Shealy C: Transcutaneous electroanalgesia, *Surg Forum* 23:419, 1973.

63. Shealy C and Mauer D: Transcutaneous nerve stimulation for control of pain, *Surg Neurol* 2:45, 1974.

64. Shealy C and others: Effects of transcranial neurostimulation upon mood and serotonin production: a preliminary report, *Pain* 1:13, 1979.

65. Sherman M: Which treatment to recommend? hot or cold, *Am Pharmacol* 20:46, 1980.

66. Sinclair D: *Cutaneous sensation,* New York, 1967, Oxford University Press.

67. Sjolund B and Eriksson M: Electro-acupuncture and endogenous morphines, *Lancet* 2:1085, 1976.

68. Stillwell GK: Therapeutic heat and cold. In Krusen FH and others: *Handbook of physical medicine and rehabilitation,* Philadelphia, 1971, WB Saunders.

69. Swerdlow M: *The therapy of pain,* Philadelphia, 1981, JB Lippincott.

70. Tappan FM: *Healing massage techniques: holistic, classic and emergency methods,* Norwalk, Conn, 1988, Appleton & Lange.

71. Ward RC: The myofascial release concepts. Handout material from course entitled Myofascial Release Concepts, Palpatory and Treatment Skills, Lansing, MI, Sept. 1986.

72. Weddell G: Somesthesis and the chemical senses, *Annu Rev Psychol* 6:119, 1955.

73. Wolf S: Perspectives on central nervous system responsiveness to transcutaneous electrical nerve stimulation, *Phys Ther* 58:1443, 1978.

74. Wood B: *Beard's massage,* Philadelphia, 1974, WB Saunders.

75. Woolf C: Generation of acute pain: central mechanisms, *Br Med Bull* 43(7):523-533, 1991.

ADDITIONAL READINGS (TRADITIONAL)

Barron DH and Matthews BHC: Intermittent conduction in the spinal cord, *J Physiol* 85:73, 1935.

Bowsher D: Pain pathways and mechanisms, *Anaesthesia* 33;935, 1978.

Head H: *Studies in neurology,* London, 1920, Oxford University Press.

Helme RE, Gibson S, and Zeinab K: Neural pathways in chronic pain, *Med J Aust* 153(7):400, 1990.

Noordenboos W: *Pain,* Amsterdam, 1959, Elsevier Science Publishers.

Price D: *Psychological & neural mechanisms of pain,* New York, 1988, Raven Press.

Taylor DC and Pierau F: Nociceptic afferent neurones. In Winslow W, editor: *Studies in neuroscience,* No. 14, St. Martin, 1991, Manchester University Press.

Weddell G and others: Nerve endings in mammalian skin, *Biol Rev* 30:159, 1955.

Williams AR: *Ultrasound: biological effects & potential hazards,* San Diego, 1983, Academic Press.

ADDITIONAL READINGS TO SUPPORT TREATMENT STRATEGIES

Application of TENS in the management of patients with pain, Alexandria, Va, 1985, American Physical Therapy Association.

Barnes JF: *Myofascial release: a search for excellence,* MFR Seminars, Padi, PA, 1990, author.

Mennell JM: *Joint pain: diagnosis & treatment using manipulation techniques,* Boston, 1964, Little, Brown.

Travell JG and Simons DG: *Myofascial pain & dysfunction: the trigger point manual,* Baltimore, 1992, Williams & Wilkins.

Upledger JE and Vredeboogd JD: *Cranial sacral therapy,* ed 12, Seattle, 1983, Eastland Press.

CHAPTER 32

Therapeutic Application of Orthotics

Steven R. Huber

KEY TERMS

orthotics
ankle foot orthosis (AFO)
hip-knee-ankle-foot orthosis (HKAFO)
imprinted casting

LEARNING OBJECTIVES

After reading this chapter the student/therapist will:
1. Identify the therapeutic interaction of exercise and orthotics.
2. Recognize sensory and motor variables to be evaluated before use of an orthotic device.
3. Identify what treatment protocols are important to consider to ensure that orthotic interventions are the most beneficial.

As treatment techniques change and develop, as new and different techniques become proven, and as material options expand, a sound understanding of basic orthotic concepts will prove invaluable to the clinical therapist. Many changes are occurring rapidly in health care technology and in our abilities to deliver quality care.

This chapter attempts to eliminate the "either/or" philosophy of therapeutic exercise and orthotic treatment and introduces the reader to concepts that demonstrate the mutually beneficial relationship between therapeutic exercise and orthotic intervention when treating the neurologically impaired client.

Orthotic treatment may be defined as the application of an external force(s) generated by an appliance worn by a client. These forces, although biomechanically designed, have significant neurological implications related to the input that they provide to the central nervous system (CNS). A well thought out, carefully designed, and properly fitting orthosis often enhances therapeutic treatment. An orthosis can be used as an adjunct to a sound therapeutic exercise program to hasten the desired result of the client's treatment program, but orthotic intervention should never be viewed as a replacement for a sound therapeutic exercise program. To presume that an orthosis can replace the techniques used by a highly skilled therapist is naive at best.

Therapists spend relatively short periods of time with each client; if the client wears an orthosis that successfully duplicates (in part) the support, assist, or CNS input given during a therapeutic exercise session, the client's treatment time is increased by the number of hours he or she uses the orthosis. Realistically, the CNS input offered by an orthosis may be inferior to that offered by the therapist, but for some CNS inputs, for example, prolonged stretch, an orthosis can be more effective than a therapist.

Viewing orthotic intervention as a CNS input requires that it also be viewed as a positive dynamic process when it is applied in a logical manner to obtain a desired result. However, orthotic intervention applied in a careless manner, applied after a less than thorough evaluation, or applied without a specific result in mind can harm the client. It can also negate the effects of a sound therapeutic exercise program. The orthotic treatment and the therapeutic exercise program must address the same or related problems and be directed at the same result, both biomechanically and neurologically. As with any treatment designed to have impact on the CNS, orthotic treatment should be closely monitored to ensure the desirability of the input being provided.

To integrate orthotic management with therapeutic exercise, one can use the following sequential thought process. During any therapeutic evaluation, specific clinical findings are discovered indicating a functional result that is other than normal. The therapist evaluates this result and establishes a functional goal that relates specifically to some activity of daily living. To obtain the functional goal, there are biomechanical options (applications of an external force), and each has a neurological consequence; some consequences are desirable, others are not. In planning the therapeutic integration of orthotics, the therapist must clearly understand the neurological consequence of each biomechanical application. The following example may clarify this further:

A patient in your facility has a simple clinical finding of weak dorsiflexors. The functional result is the inability to clear the foot during the swing phase of gait. The functional goal is to provide the patient with the ability to clear the foot during the swing phase. The biomechanical options include increasing hip flexion, increasing

knee flexion, stopping plantar flexion, increasing dorsiflexion, shortening the relative length of the extremity, positioning the foot in maximum equinus during stance phase to avoid toe stubbing during swing phase, and a number of others. Each option can be accomplished biomechanically; however, each has a significant neurological consequence that should be investigated.

Utilization of the flow sheet seen in the box will assist the therapist in organizing the patients clinical course.

When considering the time constraints placed on a therapist in a clinic or private practice setting or the financial restraints placed on most clients, it seems reasonable to seek out systems that can enhance the effects of individual treatment sessions. Realistically, changing reimbursement guidelines for health care institutions and use of review guidelines necessitate that the practicing therapist evaluate and treat clients in a compressed time frame. The client with a cerebrovascular accident (CVA), who will be discharged from a hospital in 10 days, and who does not have available a rehabilitation setting is a poor candidate for 10 days of mat work in preparation for standing and transfers. Selecting an orthosis that enhances the client's mat and exercise program while encouraging function seems a satisfactory alternative to discharging a person unprepared to perform minimal motoric skills. The client who is unprepared for function and who is not protected orthotically may have an increased tendency to develop poor motor skill habits based on inaccurate sensorimotor input.

The use of a carefully selected and properly fitting orthosis allows the therapist increased flexibility when treating the client, and can, in fact, act as an additional pair of hands. Imagine a therapist working with a client on pelvic and trunk stability in the standing position while trying to control calcaneal valgus and plantar flexion of the foot, which is creating genu valgus and genu recurvatum at the knee. An **ankle foot orthosis (AFO)** that is properly aligned will free the therapist's hands to introduce approximation and/or flexion into the client's system as needed.

The therapist must be aware of specific considerations when orthotically treating a client whose primary disorder is of a neurological nature. These differ significantly from the considerations on which the therapist bases orthotic treatment for the orthopedically impaired client. A partial listing of considerations includes exteroceptive and proprioceptive input. These are discussed in detail later in the chapter.

BASIC CONCEPTS INVOLVED IN ORTHOTICS
Interim care versus definitive care

Orthotic treatment can be categorized in many ways; two major categories are interim care or definitive care. Interim orthotic care is accomplished by using an orthosis that allows variability without major reconstruction of the orthosis. Interim care is seldom maximally cosmetic or the lightest weight option available. Interim orthotics may require more maintenance than definitive orthotics, but they are more

---

Orthotic-therapeutic exercises integration flow sheet

Clinical Finding	1.	2.

Functional Result		

Functional Goal		

Biomechanical Option		

Neurological Consequence		

Neurological Option		

Treatment Plan		

---

valuable to the therapist working with a client with a dynamic, changing neuromuscular system. An example of interim orthotics would be the use of a metal AFO with a solid stirrup and a double-action ankle joint, or a polypropylene AFO with a variable ankle joint. This device allows the treating therapist a large variation of ankle joint options, ranging from a locked ankle to a plantar flexion assist to a dorsiflexion assist. As long as a client demonstrates neuromuscular changes, such as gains or losses in strength, gains or losses in range of motion, or sensory or tonal changes, the orthotic treatment of choice should allow the treating therapist, after recognizing these changes, to accommodate them easily.

Definitive orthotic care, in contrast, should be considered when the client no longer demonstrates neuromuscular change and when the client requires an assistive device for safe, maximally independent functioning. The definitive orthosis should be designed and fabricated to be maximally cosmetic for the client. It should be constructed of the lightest weight yet most durable materials to make it energy efficient while requiring little if any maintenance. For example, a definitive orthosis for a client with extension dominance in the right lower extremity that has responded only partially to therapeutic exercise could be a 4 mm thickness, flesh-colored, polypropylene AFO casted with a solid ankle set in a few degrees of dorsiflexion. The most definitive treatment for this client may be a well-placed, purposely induced contracture—this is definitive but difficult to control.

Dynamic treatment versus static treatment

Along with interim or definitive care, the treating therapist must also choose dynamic or static orthotic treatment. Analysis of a client's gait may reveal talipes equino valgus during swing phase, the inability to clear the toe during the non-weight-bearing phase of gait. This clinical situation can be treated in a number of ways: (1) a metal spring-loaded dorsiflexion assist, (2) a plastic AFO casted into dorsiflexion, (3) a plastic or metal orthosis designed to stop plantar flexion from occurring, or (4) an orthosis stopping plantar flexion at 5 degrees to allow foot flat and providing the option for 15 degrees of dorsiflexion to encourage smooth roll over. Any of the alternatives may be quite appropriate when used under the correct neurological/musculoskeletal circumstances. Options one and four above are clearly dynamic, and option three is static. Option two may be dynamic or static, depending on the configuration of the trim lines about the medial and lateral malleoli.

Protection

An important concept involved with the therapeutic application of orthotics is that of protection. Orthoses can be used quite effectively to protect muscles, ligaments, bony structures, and nervous tissue during periods in which they are changing status and during periods when the systems are stable. A child who is developmentally trained on a severely valgus foot is, in fact, being encouraged into a position of genu valgus and often acquires knee flexion and equinus of the foot secondarily. Yet, that same child, when fitted with shoe inserts that prevent valgus and when provided with therapeutic exercise, can assume postures of lower-extremity abduction and external rotation. Facilitating movement, posture, or tone on a poorly aligned base causes increased ligamentous and muscular damage and inhibits the effects of the therapeutic program. Orthotic treatment can be very effective in protecting the painful muscles of a client recovering from Guillain-Barré syndrome.

Prevention, facilitation, and inhibition

Along with the need for protection goes the opportunity for prevention of deformity or the development of patho-logical motor habits that result from various combinations of muscle weakness, input deficits, and central programming problems. The developing child or the adult hemiplegic client who is allowed to bear weight on a hyperextended knee soon learns to lock the knee to bear weight. The locking pattern, along with a weak gastrocnemius soleus complex and a forward trunk as a result of weak hip extensors, results in stretching of the posterior capsule. The stretched capsule, abnormal weight-bearing forces, muscle weakness, and distorted sensation result in recurvatum deformity at the knee. Faulty proprioception and weak musculature may result in serious deformities, which appear as orthopedic deviations but are in reality neurologically based. Peripheral instability and faulty feedback to inform programmers that feedforward plans are not working lead to adaptations that may not be functional and may do more harm. A simple AFO with a plantar flexion stop can be used to protect the joint and prevent the deformity. This same orthosis can be used as a sensory training device, which is discussed later in this chapter.

When determining the need for orthotic intervention, a skilled therapist should determine whether he or she desires the orthosis to facilitate or inhibit certain muscle groups, sensory inputs, or postural patterns. After determining the desired function of the orthosis, the therapist, in discussion with the fabricating orthotist, can develop a mechanically feasible yet sufficiently effective orthosis that will inhibit or facilitate as desired. Simple examples include shaping a ridge into the cast for an AFO, which when fabricated will apply deep pressure to Achilles tendon to inhibit plantar flexion, or adding a plantar flexion spring assist to an orthosis used by a client with weak dorsiflexors. At each non-weight-bearing phase of gait on the affected extremity, the client's dorsiflexors are given a quick stretch by the antagonistic spring assist. The developing child who postures in flexion can be facilitated toward extension by introducing extension into the CNS. This is easily accomplished by preventing, through the use of a dorsiflexion stop, excessive forward rotation of the tibia on the talus. Although this is a biomechanical answer to excessive knee flexion orthopedi-cally, it is a sensory/proprioceptive input to the neurologi-cally impaired client that results in increased extensor tone throughout the body.

Sensory training

Using orthotic treatment to enhance sensory awareness can be very interesting as well as effective. This technique challenges the thought processes of both the therapist, who determines the desired input, and the orthotist, who must fabricate the orthosis using biomechanical principles and sensory inputs requested by the therapist to assist motor programmers in developing the most appropriate feed-forward plans.

Consider these clinical situations. A 7-year-old boy is unable to assume the vertical position because of multiple problems, including poor foot and leg alignment; the client exhibits tactile defensiveness in the clinic. His therapeutic exercise program may include over-ball activities and kneeling activities, both with deep pressure handling techniques. In preparation for vertical positioning, this child may be fitted with valgus corrective shoe inserts that will reinforce good base alignment. Additionally, textured strips can be placed in the inserts to enhance his sensory retraining program. Starting with coarse strips and progressing to finer fabrics and smaller strips will, along with the deep pressure from weight bearing, help to desensitize the child's feet.

In the next situation, a client with multiple sclerosis with a proprioceptive deficit at the knee that alters her ability to bear weight on extended knees can be fit with AFOs that allow 10 degrees of dorsiflexion and 10 degrees of plantar flexion. By placing stops at the ends of this 20 degrees of available range, the client has standing security and is able to safely practice knee control in weight bearing. The orthosis will abruptly stop knee flexion or recurvatum when the tibia has rotated 10 degrees anterior or 10 degrees posterior from vertical. When the movement stops, the client receives kinesthetic, tactile, and possibly auditory input. The author refers to this technique as "banging."

Alignment

Orthotic selection, whether neurologically, orthopedi-cally, or jointly based, must consider flexible versus fixed deformities. In most cases, early intervention will render most deformities flexible. This is especially true with neurologically induced mechanical abnormalities.

If a deformity or abnormal alignment is flexible, it should be corrected to normal alignment, thus allowing ligaments, muscles, and bones to develop anatomical normalcy. If, on the other hand, the deformity is rigid, it should be supported to minimize stress on the involved, adjacent, or related structures.

A flexible pes planus can be corrected by returning the calcaneus to its proper vertical alignment, thus elevating the longitudinal arch of the foot. A fixed painful pes planus can be supported with a properly fitting scaphoid pad.

When orthotic treatment is considered as an adjunct to the therapeutic exercise program for a neurologically impaired client, it is imperative that the concepts of body alignment be considered. To ensure that the orthotic treatment is enhancing the program and that it is in fact facilitating rather than inhibiting progress toward normalcy, normal body alignment must be understood. This is especially true in the trunk and lower extremities. The normal curves of the spine are (1) cervical lordosis from the apex of the odontoid process to T2, (2) thoracic kyphosis from T2 to the middle of T12, (3) lumbar lordosis from the middle of T12 to the sacrovertebral articulation, and (4) sacral kyphosis.[3] These curves become significant as spinal orthotics and the impact that orthotic treatment of one spinal segment has on another segment are discussed.

The hip joint, because it is a ball-and-socket joint, presents no particular alignment difficulty as related to therapeutic exercise and is placed 6 mm anterior and superior to the proximal tip of the greater trochanter. The knee joint is more difficult to manage because of its polycentric nature. As the client walks, the femur flexes in relation to the tibia and rotates externally approximately 10 degrees about its long axis. The flexion and rotation is certainly a consideration when aligning anatomical and mechanical joints because improper joint placement can provide the neurologically impaired client with inaccurate sensory input.

Because of the complex nature and progressive development of the ankle joint mortice, its rotation is most important. At birth the ankle joint mortice is rotated approximately 2 degrees externally in relation to the knee axis. By age 7, when the child has been upright with a sufficiently narrowed base of support for some time, the mortice is rotated 20 to 30 degrees externally in relation to the knee axis. This rotation allows the center of gravity to progress smoothly during gait. The ankle joint mortice is not perpendicular to the line of progression during gait, but it is parallel to the movement of the center of gravity from heelstrike to midstance. The final alignment in the lower extremity is that of the foot. The long axis of the foot is generally rotated externally, approximately 15 degrees from the line of progression.[2]

Maintenance

During each therapeutic exercise session, specific activities are aimed at a desired end result. It is important that the gains obtained during a specific session be maintained between sessions. The importance of this cannot be overlooked. When trying to increase range of motion, a gain of 10 degrees obtained during a treatment session can easily be lost by the next treatment session. A pattern that is beginning to be functional can be negated if not properly reinforced. The therapist can control hip internal rotation or scapular elevation with his or her hands for the length of a treatment session. An orthosis can reinforce correct patterns until the client's next session.

The client who is no longer changing neurologically or musculoskeletally may have reached his or her maximal potential for function. That limit, however, may be stretched with some external orthotic device. This situation is common

for the client with multiple sclerosis. A client who might be wheelchair bound as a result of the excessive energy required to ambulate against severe lower-extremity extensor tone can be functionally ambulatory by wearing orthoses that inhibit some of the extensor tone while leaving enough for weight support during gait.

EVALUATION

This section discusses general areas to consider when evaluating a client for orthotic intervention. Following the general discussion are specifics related to evaluation of the trunk, upper extremity, and lower extremity.

Range of motion and power

A thorough examination of the passive range of motion available to the patient will provide the therapist with a foundation on which to place information gathered during the evaluation. The passive range evaluation tells the therapist the exact available arc of motion on which external forces can be applied.

Having determined the available range, a determination of power must be made. In an orthotic evaluation, the determination of power is neither a manual muscle test nor a specific test, such as dynomometry. Rather, it is a more general assessment of the client's ability to move a particular joint through a functional range of motion during a specific activity. A muscle grade of fair minus or fair plus in the gastrocnemius muscle or a power grasp of 4 lb will tell the therapist little related to the specific need for orthotic intervention. Specific muscle grades and force values, however, are invaluable when determining the effectiveness of a therapeutic exercise program. Useful information related to power can be obtained by viewing a function and analyzing the reason for deviations from normal in relation to sufficient or insufficient activity in muscle groups performing the function.

For example consider the client who has good grasp and full passive range in the hand and upper extremity but is unable to feed himself or herself. The important facts to determine here are: (1) is there insufficient flexor activity at the elbow? and (2) is there too much extensor activity about the elbow? Answers to these questions will guide the therapist in the direction of appropriate orthotic intervention. A fair muscle grade assigned to the biceps is less useful information. Concurrent with determining the power, the therapist must determine the source of that power. Is it synergy, isolated muscle strength, or reflex? A flexion/extension synergy in the lower extremity that is slightly modified by orthotic intervention can result in an energy efficient, cosmetic gait.

Sensation

When evaluating tactile sensation, it is useful to categorize findings as normal, hyperesthetic, paresthetic, or anesthetic. These categorizations will aid the therapist in determining materials from which the orthosis will be fabricated and may influence the structural design of the orthosis. Standard configurations can be altered to avoid surface areas where tactile input is perceived as discomfort.

Proprioceptive testing produces the most reliable results, in terms of orthotic application, when it is performed with the tested joint in a functional position under the influence of gravity. For example, the sitting position is preferable to the supine position when testing the upper extremity, and standing is preferable to sitting when testing the lower extremity. In these positions, joints and ligaments can be tested in their more normal environment for function.

Tone and obligatory pattern responses

Muscle tone and pattern generator activity are evaluated hand in hand. The therapist needs to determine base tone, fluctuations in that base tone, and causes of the fluctuations if present. Tone is also examined in positions of function. If it appears that a reflex or synergistic pattern is either dampening or facilitating function, further testing should be done using standard test positions. The neurologically impaired child who uses turning of the head (asymmetrical tonic neck reflex) to provide the tonal changes for ambulation may be unable to ambulate if the pattern is completely inhibited. During this child's therapeutic exercise program, an array of neurophysiologically based techniques could be used to integrate the reflex or pattern. A cervical orthosis designed to limit excessive head rotation—hence altering, but not eliminating, the child's mobility—can act to reinforce those techniques used in the therapeutic exercise program.

A child with low tone who demonstrates excessive head, trunk, and lower-extremity flexion when vertical can be gradually facilitated toward extension with the use of AFOs and a neurophysiologically sound therapeutic exercise program.

Skin integrity

Before completing the orthotic evaluation, skin integrity is examined. Clients seen following trauma with multiple injuries often have interruptions in the skin that may have impact on the structural design of an orthosis. Special attention should be paid to the feet of an ambulatory, neurologically impaired child or adult. Bearing weight on an unprotected or poorly aligned foot can result in ulcerations of the navicular and metatarsal heads.

The trunk

When evaluating the neurologically impaired client, the first questions that come to mind are: "What forces can an orthosis apply that will help reinforce the client's treatment program?" and "What patterns or postures are inhibiting the client's progress?" This is especially true when evaluating the client's trunk. Is it realistic to expect 1 hour of therapeutic exercise to improve a client's head control if the client, when seated, has the head flexed forward? The same client may lie supine in bed with a large pillow holding the head in flexion. It will be difficult for the 1 hour of cervical extension, approximation, and cocontraction training to counteract 23 hours of flexion. The cervical musculature, in this case, must surely be biased incorrectly.

Begin the evaluation of the cervical spine by a simple observation of the posture noted when you first see the client. Is the head stationary or mobile? This is a certain clue to the need for stability or mobility. Is the head centered over the body? Are the eyes directed forward? Is the client able to move on command? Is the skin intact? Does movement of the head alter tone in other parts of the body? Are reflexes such as asymmetrical tonic neck reflex (ATNR), symmetrical tonic neck reflex (STNR), neck righting, or optic righting present? Is there visible asymmetry of the face or upper chest secondary to tonal imbalances? See the following evaluation for an example:

1. Describe the client's initial posture. The client is in a wheelchair, the arms are supported, the feet are on footplates, the trunk is stable, and the head is dropped forward with the mandible on the sternum.
2. Is the client's head stationary or mobile? Stationary.
3. Is the client's head centered? No, it is tipped to the right.
4. Are the client's eyes forward? No, they are downcast.
5. Is the client able to move on command? Yes, but the head flops from flexion with rotation to hyperextension.
6. Does movement alter tone? No.
7. Are reflexes detectable? No.
8. Is there visible asymmetry? Slight, the mandible deviates to the left.

Having gathered the previous information, goals are determined and a treatment plan established. If the immediate goal is the development of head control in the sitting position to improve visual input, encourage more normal body tone and work toward advanced mobility training. The therapeutic program may include passive positioning and facilitation to the cervical extensors through techniques such as tapping, brushing, quick icing, reverse tapping, or vibration. To increase stability the therapist may use approximation and attempt to decrease the large arc of motion noted in the evaluation. Prolonged positioning in flexion should be avoided as well.

A program of "cervical stability in neutral training" will be enhanced by the application of the anterior section of a commercially available cervical orthosis, such as a Philadelphia collar. Attaching the orthosis to axillary loops or a figure-of-eight harness will prevent excessive forward flexion, prevent prolonged periods of flexion, and act as a kinesthetic reminder. When the client, at times, simply rests into the collar, the cervical extensors are being protected from overstretching. Should the extension component of movement remain a problem, the posterior section of the orthosis can be loosely applied in the same manner to prevent excessive extension.

This example is in no manner advocating the use of a tightly applied, mobility-eliminating cervical orthosis. On the contrary, it suggests the use of an orthosis that limits or controls excessive movement and that is designed to reinforce a therapeutic principle.

The three most common situations of the cervical spine where orthotics can be beneficial to the neurologically impaired client are poor anteroposterior head control, tonal or postural torticollis, and excessive cervical mobility.

The thoracic spine, by nature of its anatomical configuration, is less suited for problems of excessive mobility than is the cervical spine. It is, as well, less suited for simple evaluation. In the neurologically impaired client, a radiographic examination is invaluable when dealing with the common problem of excessive curves of the thoracic spine. The radiogram provides information as to the vertebral status, and the evaluating therapist must determine the flexibility or rigidity of any pathological curves. The therapist again looks at range of motion. Is there too much or too little movement, or is it simply misdirected? What is the muscular power available? What is the source? Is the tone of the trunk symmetrical? Is it high, low, or fluctuating? Is the sensory system intact or interpreting inadequately? What does the skin look like, and how does it feel? Is it fragile or thick, cold or warm, clear or erupted, dry or moist, or shiny? This information will assist in determining the amount of corrective force that can be applied to the skin. Finally, are there specific reflexes or synergy patterns that seem apparent, such as the ATNR, head on body righting or stereotypical pattern generator responses?

It is important to realize that in most cases of orthotic treatment of the thoracic spine in the neurologically impaired client the goal is increased stability. Stabilizing against asymmetrical or rotary based reflexes may appear to increase the intensity of the reflex. A child who demonstrates a strong neck on body righting reflex may be hindered by an orthosis that stabilizes the thoracic spine, thus causing the spine to move as a unit. The nonstabilized spine is capable of absorbing rotation at various levels of the spine, not only at the ends of the stabilized sections. Few clients with neurological disability require orthotic treatment of the thoracic spine for any reason other than scoliosis. These clients may be treated in the conventional scoliosis systems, or they may benefit from an orthosis that is less conventional and relies on more concepts found in neurophysiology than in pure biomechanics. This is accomplished by inserting flexible panels or by designing corrective pads that create greater sensory inputs. Kyphotic or lordotic curves in the thoracic spine of a neurologically impaired client can often be sufficiently influenced by altering the cervical or lumbar spine.

When evaluating the lumbosacral spine, it is important to evaluate the client in positions of function. In this area, as in the cervical area, the key will be the relationship of stability to mobility. Is there too much mobility? In what direction or directions does the client's spine appear rigid? In what position? Does the spinal alignment look the same regardless of whether the client is in the supine, prone, sitting, or standing position? What is the power of the flexors, extensors, and rotators? What is the power source? Is the muscular tone constant? What is the nature of the skin? Does the lumbosacral area appear affected by specific reflexes?

The available passive range of motion is the major factor influencing the speed with which orthotic treatment will alter the lumbosacral spine in a neurologically impaired client. If the spine is "locked," orthotic treatment may compound the difficulties by reinforcing stability or the results may appear much more slowly. External forces applied to the lumbosacral spine can generally do one of three things: (1) support or hold an existing posture, (2) decrease a lordosis by bridging its apex, placing forces above and below the apex of the curve, or (3) increase a lordosis by placing the major force at the apex of the curve or existing kyphosis. The most significant fact about orthotic treatment of the lumbosacral spine is that forces applied to the lumbosacral spine often have striking effects on the thoracic and cervical spine.

Increasing the lumbar lordosis of a client in the sitting or standing position will generally result in a decreased thoracic kyphosis and an increased cervical lordosis. Increasing the lumbar lordosis with a lumbosacral corset containing rigid stays contoured into extension will often alter the sitting posture of a child who maintains a posterior pelvis. Likewise, a child who maintains an anterior pelvis can be encouraged to rock posteriorly by wearing a corset with stays that bridge the lumbar curve.

When using a spinal orthosis to enhance an established therapeutic exercise program, the treating therapist must be aware of the phenomenon of diaphragmatic alienation. Diaphragmatic alienation occurs when a spinal support is applied in a manner that impedes the downward excursion of the diaphragm during inhalation. The diaphragm, if continually limited in its excursion, loses stretch sensitivity in the shortened range.

The upper extremity

When considering upper extremity possibilities for therapeutic orthotics, evaluators must separate themselves from conventional rationales for uses of orthotic treatment.

The upper extremity is frequently splinted by occupational therapists, physical therapists, and orthotists to allow improved function while the client is wearing the device. Clients may require multiple splints to perform a variety of tasks; this is conventional orthotic care of the upper extremity. Conventional orthotic care is often quite helpful and may be the factor that has the most impact on the client's ability to perform activities of daily living. In many cases conventional orthotic care is the best option, in some cases it is not. These concepts attempt to reinforce the use of orthoses as an adjunct to or as an enhancer of the therapeutic program that is aimed at more normal function with minimal extraneous apparatus. Part of upper-extremity orthotic training needs to address the activities for which the orthosis must be worn and those activities for which it should be removed. The goal of a therapeutic orthotic program is to minimize the client's dependence on a device. There is a fine balance between using an orthosis for training muscles, altering tone, or maintaining status between treatment sessions and learning a splinter skill while wearing an orthosis. Although the latter addresses the immediate tasks at hand, the former will have a greater impact on the long-term activities of a client.

The same areas addressed in the spinal evaluation—passive range, power, sensation, tone, skin integrity, and synergy patterns (reflexive or volitional)—need to be addressed when dealing with the upper extremity. Although the client's visual status is crucial in conventional orthotic management of the upper extremity, it is less important when using concepts of therapeutic orthotics. Training a client how to perform a task with a conventional upper-extremity orthosis generally requires the client to visually attend to the task. When using therapeutic orthotics, the therapist is attempting to have a direct impact on the client's CNS and an indirect impact on the ability to perform a task.

The passive range of motion of the upper extremity should be evaluated in positions of function such as the sitting or standing positions. Information gathered with the supine client will be of little transferable value as related to purposeful movement. Can the client's arm be moved forward and horizontal to the floor? Can the shoulder be fully flexed? Can the client's arm be externally rotated and abducted to 90 degrees? What is the passive range available for internal rotation? How much motion can passively occur at the elbow, forearm, wrist, and fingers?

How much power is available, and from what source is the power derived? For example, a client is able to flex the elbow against gravity to eat finger foods independently, but only by using a mass pattern that includes excessive scapular retraction and elevation. When the scapula is stabilized during a treatment session, the client is able to work through the mass pattern and obtain smoother movement. Is it reasonable to use a chest strap with an anteroposterior shoulder strap to stabilize the scapula and act as a kinesthetic reminder to inhibit scapular retraction and elevation? The orthosis (externally applied forces) will enhance the existing treatment program by inhibiting the mass pattern that the client would use three times a day at meal periods. Collectively, those meal periods may represent more time than the therapist spends during the therapeutic exercise program inhibiting the pattern.

The client's sensation, both tactile and proprioceptive, should be evaluated in terms of normal, hypesthesia, parasthesia, or anesthesia. Areas noted to be hypesthetic or parasthetic may, when orthotic forces are applied to them, amplify abnormal neuromuscular responses. Anesthetic areas should be monitored to minimize or prevent tissue breakdown. Tone is evaluated concurrently with pattern generator activity, as was done in the spinal evaluation and as will be done in the lower-extremity evaluation. Stimulated by head or neck position, recognition of patterns that alter upper-extremity tone is extremely important when determining therapeutic orthotic intervention. Use of an orthosis designed to stop the right elbow from extending would be inappropriate if used with a client who demonstrated a CNS pattern generator problem such as that demonstrated by an ATNR to the right. Clearly, in this example, it is not the elbow that requires treatment.

The upper-extremity evaluation is concluded with assessment of the skin integrity, noting such things as limb color, temperature, texture of skin, presence or absence of hair as compared to the opposite limb, and open areas or scars from previous insults.

When the evaluation is completed, the evaluator determines goals and a treatment plan based on neurophysiological techniques. Compression, traction, tapping, resistance to motion, and tracking techniques can all be enhanced by an upper-extremity orthosis. Most techniques can be satisfactorily simulated with either dynamic or static orthotic treatment. The therapist must determine which techniques are to be simulated.

The lower extremity

The lower extremity, because of its primary purpose as a propeller and its need for stability, is an extremely interesting body part to treat with therapeutic orthotics.[2] As a practicing clinician, it is the author's perception that the majority of lower-extremity pathologies can be influenced from below the knee. To encumber a neurologically impaired client with unnecessary orthoses brings to mind the visualization of a cement balloon. For the minority of clients who require orthotic treatment above the knee, a prime consideration must be the weight of the orthosis and the ease of operation. Unencumbered mobility and adequate stability can be facilitated in the lower extremity by using appropriate orthotic intervention following thorough assessment.

Passive range of motion of the lower extremity may look very different when tested or observed in non-weight-bearing and weight-bearing positions. Leg lengths that appear equal when tested with the client supine or sitting may be grossly different when the client bears weight. Muscle power that previously masked ligamentous laxity may no longer be present in the client who suffers an acquired neurological disability. Valgus or varus deformities at the subtalar joint and valgus, varus, flexion, or recurvatum deformities at the knee can all result in a relative leg length discrepancy. During the evaluation it is important to note variations in passive range related to positioning with respect to gravity. Therapeutic orthotic treatment of the lower extremity requires forces that facilitate mobility or forces that facilitate stability.

The alignment of the calcaneus in weight bearing referred to earlier in this chapter is critical when evaluating the lower extremity of a neurologically impaired client. When viewed posteriorly, the triceps surae tendon should appear perpendicular to the supporting surface. Deviations as slight as 5 to 8 degrees appear to allow sufficient sliding of the talus to permit resultant dropping of the longitudinal arch of the foot. A hallux valgus deformity develops secondary to the pes planus. Progressive genu valgus is seen on occasion.

There is a correlation between valgus of the calcaneus and toe walking in some cases, with the toe walking secondary to the valgus. Anatomically, the wedge-shaped talus that sits between the distal ends of the tibia and the fibula and that rests on the calcaneus is at risk when the calcaneus tips into valgus. The medial lip of the talus, when the calcaneus tips, is pressed against the tibia. The child, unknowingly, raises up on the toes, thus placing the foot in relative plantar flexion, changing the alignment of the talus and reducing the talotibial pressure.

Power of movement in the lower extremity often appears radically different, depending on the position in which it is tested. In the lower extremity, power that is a summation of selected movement, tone, patterns, and reflexology, is easily assessed. Yet the sources of that power are difficult, if not impossible, to quantify individually. Fortunately, it is not necessary initially to quantify those individual components. Careful observation of client responses during the initial treatment sessions will allow the therapist to organize the components in terms of greater to lesser influence. This organization will direct the therapist to the body part requiring treatment if it is, in fact, not the lower extremity.

Therapists who evaluate a large number of clients with neurological disability will recognize specific movements in patterns or synergies. Those patterns may be negligible or quite obvious. They may be complete, involving all lower-extremity joints, or incomplete, affecting an individual segment of the limb. Regardless of whether they are complete or incomplete, the patterns need to be controlled, directed, and hopefully totally integrated to allow smooth, safe, energy efficient movement.

Once power has been assessed, testing for sensation, especially for proprioception, must be completed. Testing with the client in a vertical weight-bearing position will provide information that is most easily applied to functional status. If this is not possible, the ankle and foot should be tested when the client is in a sitting position, and the knee and hip should be tested in the supine position.

At this point, the evaluating therapist should examine the skin integrity, as discussed earlier in the chapter. When evaluating the skin, the therapist should take special note of the sole of the foot. The skin thickness under the metatarsal heads and particularly the area under the second and third metatarsal heads should be examined closely. If the client's

metatarsal arch has dropped, this area may become quite sensitive and may act as a stimulus for tone alteration during weight bearing.

The evaluating therapist has now assessed range, power, tone, obligatory patterns, tactile and proprioceptive status, and skin integrity. Special attention has been paid to the alignment of the foot. Short-term and long-term goals are now established, and a treatment plan is developed. The treatment plan that the therapist designs will determine the appropriate therapeutic application of orthotics. The therapist must determine the neurophysiological impact that the orthosis should produce, and, as examples in the treatment section of this chapter demonstrate, there are numerous options.

TREATMENT GOALS

The basic philosophy for, concepts of, and evaluation techniques used with the application of therapeutic orthotics have been discussed. Before reviewing multiple treatment examples, the goals related to the therapeutic application of orthotics should be evaluated. These goals can be divided into two sets: those directed at the orthotic treatment and those that may result from proper therapeutic application of the orthoses. The principal goals for using orthotics therapeutically are to reinforce a therapeutic exercise program; to hasten a client's progress toward more normal movement, posture, or tone; and to indirectly improve the client's functional abilities. These goals can be accomplished by attempting the following:

1. Minimize the orthotic treatment. Discuss options with the designing orthotist that keep the design as simple as possible. The simpler the orthosis, the more controllable it will be. As the orthosis becomes more complex, there is a greater chance to introduce unwanted inputs to the CNS through unplanned or uncontrolled biomechanical forces. Additionally, the therapeutic exercise program will include exercises that reinforce quality movement and promote a decreased dependence on external devices.

2. Provide options for more movement. Attempt designs that eliminate movement only in cases of excessive motion. With almost every client the therapist works to obtain quality, pain-free mobility of some type. Before eliminating motion in a neurologically impaired limb, the therapist must consider the primary and secondary effects of the elimination of motion. In addition to eliminating motion, we may be eliminating potential progress.

   Consider the client who, when initially evaluated after a CVA, lacks movement distal to the knee. To order a plastic AFO with a rigid ankle designed to eliminate plantar flexion, dorsiflexion, inversion, and eversion for this client is in error. Once applied, the orthosis provides stability but does not provide the option for normal movement. One therapeutic example of orthotic care to clients with CVA is discussed in detail in the treatment section of this chapter.

3. Select orthotic designs that encourage normal movement, tone, or posture and that encourage function. The purpose of the orthosis is to alter movement, tone, or posture and to protect the extremity. The protected, more normalized extremity increases in value to the client as it is used more easily for purposeful activity. Treatments, orthotic or otherwise, that neither directly nor indirectly modulate function are generally inconsistent with the goal of therapeutic intervention. Normal tone and movement should reinforce function, and function should reinforce normal tone and movement.

4. Develop designs that are energy efficient. When construction of the orthosis is discussed with the orthotist, keep in mind the relative weight of the materials from which the orthosis will be constructed as well as the final alignment. Request materials that are lightweight but durable. Material selection is related to the client's height and weight, the expected activity level of the client, and the forces the orthosis is expected to generate. Most important, material selection is secondary in importance to the neuromuscular inputs desired. Desiring a dynamic ankle joint but selecting a rigid plastic design because it is lighter negates the original rationale for therapeutic orthotic intervention. Final alignment is of significant importance when attempting to ensure energy efficiency. Malaligned joint surfaces can create friction on joints intended to be freely mobile. The friction will reduce the energy efficiency of the orthosis and, while actually acting as resistance, may strengthen undesired movement patterns.

5. Consider the cost effectiveness of orthotic treatment. As you begin to develop a rationale for orthotic treatment, consider all alternatives. Consider the expected length of time the orthosis will be used and the cost effects of not using orthotic treatment. A client who is ambulatory with an orthosis may be confined to a wheelchair or bed without the orthosis. The cost to heal skin breakdown is significantly greater than the cost of most orthoses. Consider the cost effectiveness of reducing the number of treatment sessions because neuromuscular changes are being maintained orthotically between treatment sessions. With changes maintained, the therapist can concentrate on progressive treatment without having to use valuable time for maintenance activities.

6. Provide the client with the most cosmetically pleasing orthosis. Seek good cosmesis, but not at the expense of desired function. Clients seem to understand that some orthoses are more noticeable than others. When therapists take the time to explain, patients also seem

to understand that maximal cosmesis may temporarily be sacrificed to obtain maximal neuromuscular results. When the client's neuromuscular status has stabilized, determination of final maximal cosmesis can be made. An orthosis that was used by a client during periods of neuromuscular change may be replaced by a more cosmetic orthosis when the client's neuromuscular status stabilizes. A client with Guillain-Barré syndrome may begin ambulation with metal orthoses that protect the extremities and that allow variability to accommodate muscle strength changes. If deficits remain, this same client may require plastic orthoses, at some point, after muscular return has plateaued.

7. Attempt to minimize maintenance. Consider the stresses that will be applied to the orthosis in relation to its perceived durability. The proximity of the client to the supplying orthotist should also be considered or at least acknowledged before initiating orthotic evaluation and fitting. When complicated schedules or minor fitting problems cause delays, the client and the client's family deal more realistically when the procedures have been clearly outlined from the beginning.

TREATMENT EXAMPLES
Hemiplegia

Clients with hemiplegia secondary to CVA are, in many cases, ideal candidates for therapeutic orthotic management. Some of these clients demonstrate the most changing neuromuscular systems. The CVA client has benefitted greatly from complementary orthotic and therapeutic exercise programs. Brunnstrom[1] has documented six stages of recovery in the lower extremity following CVA. Specific orthotic ankle joint adjustments exist that maximize function in each stage of recovery while facilitating the next stage of recovery. Although this material refers to clients recovering from CVA and to the stages classified by Brunnstrom, its applicability is far greater. Clients with closed-head injury and clients with multiple sclerosis often appear similar clinically. When treating clients who have changing neuromuscular systems, it is imperative that the therapist be alert to changes. For the orthotic technique described here to be maximally effective, the therapist must, in the concurrent exercise program, facilitate and inhibit tone to correspond with noted changes. The therapeutic exercise program is dynamic and so must be the orthotic treatment.

In dealing with a flaccid lower extremity, the goals of therapeutic exercise are to maintain range of motion, protect joints, and stimulate tone in preparation for function. Orthotic treatment is initiated by fitting the client with a training AFO with a solid stirrup and double-action ankle joint. The double-action ankle joint consists of a metal casing with two channels, one anterior and one posterior to the axis of rotation of the joint. The channels are capped by channel screws that exert forces on the contents of the channels.

Springs can be placed in the channels to assist motions, or rods can be placed in the channels to stop motions. A rod placed inside a spring in the channel can act to assist motion in one direction and stop motion in another direction. The training orthosis, readily available in many physical therapy departments, enables the therapist to begin an orthotic program that will, early on, reinforce the therapeutic exercise program. For the client with a flaccid lower extremity, stimulate tone through weight bearing, proprioceptive input from joint approximation, and stimulus to the metatarsal heads by standing the client in an orthosis that protects the ankle and stabilizes the knee in good alignment. This can be accomplished in two ways: (1) an ankle joint fixed in neutral or a few degrees of plantar flexion or (2) a plantar flexion stop and a dorsiflexion assist to a dorsiflexion stop. (NOTE: a fixed joint has no motion and a stop prevents motion in one direction.) When properly adjusted, either option will prevent knee flexion and recurvatum during standing, if the foot is flat on the ground and if the client's trunk is erect or slightly anterior (causing stabilization of the knee biomechanically).

In this situation tone is stimulated in a functional position. With the client in a protected standing position, the therapist can use neurophysiologically based techniques for increasing tone, such as tapping, icing, vibration, and approximation. Concepts of elongation and foreshortening also can be used to stimulate tone for weight bearing.

When, in the therapeutic exercise sessions, the therapist notes an increase in tone or minimal voluntary movement in synergy, the orthotic treatment changes.

This section discusses the two options available for helping the client with a flaccid lower extremity to a standing position using an AFO. If option one, a fixed ankle, was used, there were rods in both anterior and posterior channels. When the client demonstrates minimal voluntary movement, the anterior channel screw is loosened to allow 3 to 5 degrees of dorsiflexion, but the posterior channel is kept tight to prevent plantar flexion. The small amount of dorsiflexion will begin to reinforce the dorsiflexion component of the lower-extremity synergy, and the plantar flexion stop will prevent development of a strong extensor thrust that promotes recurvatum and posterior capsular damage. The sidebars, metal joints, and a well fitting shoe will prevent the development of excessive inversion while guiding the foot into dorsiflexion. The small amount of range available, however, is insufficient to allow the weight line to pass posterior to the knee joint and cause buckling during midstance.

If option two—a plantar flexion stop at neutral and a dorsiflexion assist to a dorsiflexion stop—was used, the assist is removed. This orthotic option, through techniques mentioned previously, has been stimulating tone. In addition, each time the spring-loaded dorsiflexion assist has been activated, the plantar flexors have been provided with a quick stretch. Realizing that, more often than not, extensor tone becomes more powerful than flexor tone in the lower extremity, excessive stimulation is unwarranted.

At this point the orthotic treatment that previously consisted of two options has been consolidated. The client is training in a limited-motion orthosis that allows 3 to 5 degrees of dorsiflexion and that is set in neutral for plantar flexion. This permits motion into flexion at the ankle and knee while discouraging plantar flexion, knee hyperextension, and medial lateral instability at the subtalar joint.

As the therapist notes a continued increase in the synergistic movements in the lower extremity, the ankle joint will require altering. When the client has developed mature synergies, especially the extension synergy, the therapist can completely remove the dorsiflexion stop. This is accomplished by removing the rod from the anterior channel. Although the client is now permitted to dorsiflex using the synergy pattern during the swing phase of gait, he or she is not permitted to bear weight on a hyperextended knee resulting from a mature extension synergy. The inversion component of both patterns is inhibited by the tracking of the mechanical joints. The posterior rod must remain rigid to prevent the development of recurvatum until the client begins to demonstrate in the therapeutic exercise program the ability to deviate from the mass patterns. When hamstring control can be elicited to flex the involved knee past 90 degrees in a sitting position, the therapist may begin to gradually loosen the posterior channel screw and permit more plantar flexion to occur. As the hamstring control increases, the plantar flexion range is increased until there is free plantar flexion.

Fig. 32-1 shows a client with recurvatum uncontrolled by an orthosis that allows too much plantar flexion. Fig. 32-2 shows the same client wearing an orthosis with a plantar flexion stop that is effective in decreasing recurvatum at the knee. As this client's kinesthetic sense improves, more plantar flexion will be eliminated. During ambulation with the AFO pictured in Fig. 32-1, the client demonstrated a relative leg length discrepancy. This did not occur with the orthosis in Fig. 32-2 a **hip-knee-ankle-foot orthosis (HKAFO).**

Even when the client can demonstrate good knee and ankle control in the sagittal plane, there may be medial lateral instability in the coronal plane, especially when the client is ambulatory on uneven terrain. The orthosis, void of channel contents, continues to protect the ankle in the coronal plane while allowing the anterior and posterior leg musculature to be strengthened by uninhibited use.

When it is noted that the client is demonstrating voluntary control of the lower extremity and, specifically, dorsiflexion with knee extension, a spring-loaded plantar flexion assist can be created in the orthosis by placing a spring in the anterior channel. This will, at toe off of each step, provide the dorsiflexors of the ankle with a quick stretch to facilitate contraction. Care must be taken to avoid the application of a force so great as to overpower the returning dorsiflexors.

If the client chooses not to wear the orthosis during

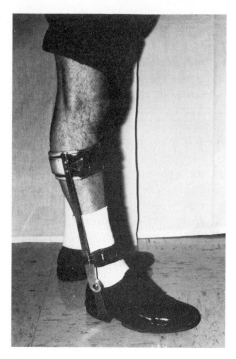

Fig. 32-1. AFO with free plantar flexion. Severe recurvatum resulted in relative leg length discrepancy.

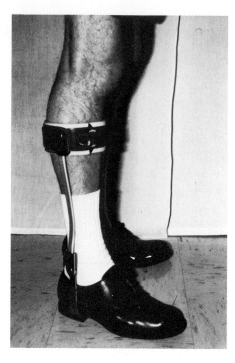

Fig. 32-2. AFO with plantar flexion stop. Recurvation is reduced.

ambulation once voluntary control is demonstrated, it can be set with a stronger plantar flexion assist and used in a home exercise program for dorsiflexor strengthening.

This particular use of orthotics, although discussed here using the example of hemiplegia, can be applied to other neurologically impaired clients, such as those with head injury, multiple sclerosis, or Guillain-Barré syndrome with slight variations.

Spina bifida

CASE 1 ▼ Kenny

Kenny, a 4-year-old child with spina bifida and secondary incomplete paralysis below T6, came to Central Maine Medical Center for orthotic evaluation. Kenny's medical history included shunt controlled hydrocephalus and a developing scoliosis. For the purpose of socialization and physiological standing, the child was seen for fabrication of a "functional stander" type orthosis. Passive range of motion evaluation demonstrated that, when the left leg was adducted past 40 degrees of abduction, the pelvis elevated and created a relative 3-inch leg length discrepancy. This directed the evaluators to the hip to determine a hip abduction contracture of 40 degrees.

Because the child was not a candidate for surgical release because of multiple problems, and because a shoe lift would feed into the hip and spinal problem, an orthosis addressing both problems was designed. The orthosis pictured in Figs. 32-3 and 32-4 resulted. It is designed to allow the child to stand while stabilizing the right hip and creating a prolonged stretch on the left hip abductors. The muscle imbalance and soft tissue contracture must be questioned when there is partial paralysis. The orthosis was adjustable in height to accommodate growth and in abduction range to maintain range gains obtained during therapeutic exercise. Foot wedges were also designed to adjust for proper weight bearing as the legs became positionable in less abduction.

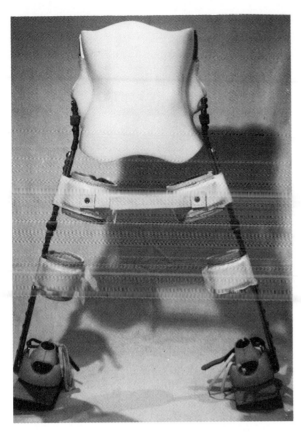

Fig. 32-3. HKAFO with molded body jacket. This orthosis was designed to provide weight bearing and to adjust to eliminate hip abduction contracture.

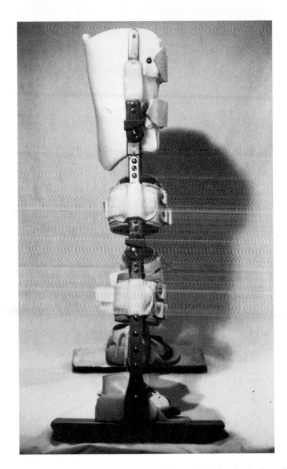

Fig. 32-4. Side view of HKAFO with molded body jacket. Note vertical alignment.

Down syndrome

CASE 2 . ▼ Francine

This 11-year-old client has a primary diagnosis of Down syndrome complicated by a right CVA with resultant left hemiplegia. The client has slight hip and knee flexion contractures and a severe equinus deformity. A leg length discrepancy of plus 4 inches has resulted in ambulation on the great toe and first metatarsal head, under which the skin is thickly calloused. A secondary scoliosis is developing and an ATNR is present.

To improve her gait, decrease energy consumption, inhibit the functional scoliosis, and promote normal ranges of mo-

tion, the child was fitted with the AFO seen in Figs. 32-5 and 32-6. These photographs were taken during the client's initial fitting.

The child's exercise program is aimed at integrating the reflex and obtaining more normal range of motion for a more energy-efficient gait. Ranges gained during therapeutic exercise will be maintained during functional ambulation. Once range gains have stabilized, appropriate footwear with adequate lifts will be constructed.

Osteogenesis imperfecta

CASE 3 ▼ Paul

This child is a 10-year-old boy with a primary diagnosis of osteogenesis imperfecta tarda. Of orthopedic nature, this disease has resulted in over 25 fractures with resultant losses of movement. The child has severe lower-extremity contractures but remains ambulatory with a rolling walker. Multiple upper-extremity fractures inhibited safe use of a walker. The child was experiencing less and less kinesthetic sense resulting

from limited mobility. The orthosis seen in Figs. 32-7 and 32-8 was designed to protect the limb while creating gentle traction to facilitate movement. Single wrist joint construction was desired for control of weight and control of ulnar drift. The circumferential pressure of the forearm and arm cuffs was useful in creating a sense of security for this child to move without fear of fracturing.

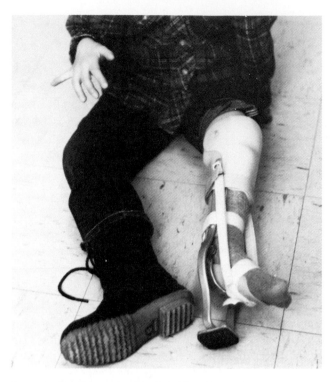

Fig. 32-5. Patellar tendon bearing AFO with polypropelene footplate and adjustable ankle to provide prolonged stretch to posterior leg musculature. Extended bottom equalizes leg length and creates extension force at knee.

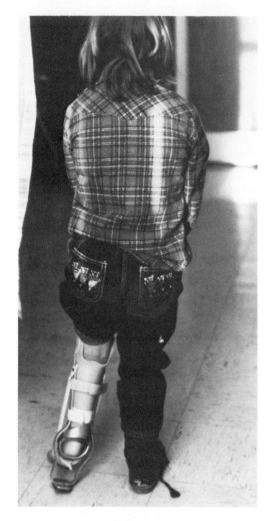

Fig. 32-6. Posterior view of dynamic interim AFO.

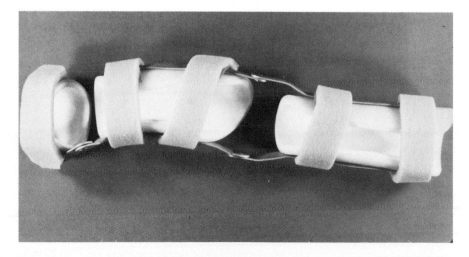

Fig. 32-7. Elbow wrist hand orthosis designed to protect extremity and facilitate movement through traction.

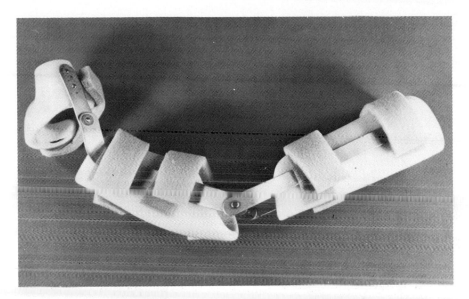

Fig. 32-8. View of ranges available at time of initial fit.

Multiple pathologies

CASE 4 ▼ Mr. P

The orthosis shown in Fig. 32-9 was designed as an interim orthosis for a 67-year-old client with Paget's disease, a CVA, and third-degree burns on the sole and instep of the foot. This demonstrates simple management of multiple pathologies. The client was independently ambulatory with a cane.

AFO for hemiplegia

CASE 5 ▼ Mrs. T

Fig. 32-10 shows the orthosis fabricated for a 64-year-old client to replace a conventional knee-ankle-foot orthosis (KAFO) that the client was fit with after a CVA. Three years following the insult she had equino varus during swing phase, extreme valgus during weight bearing, and genu recurvatum. After the client was fit with a polypropylene AFO with a rigid ankle set in slight dorsiflexion and a valgus corrective flare, her mobility skills improved significantly. The AFO pictured replaced a KAFO with a dorsiflexion assist and a valgus corrective strap.

IMPRINTING THROUGH CASTING: A NEW TREATMENT CONCEPT

This section describes a technique that incorporates the use of casting with various therapeutic techniques that are applied for a specified time to produce a specific result to modulate CNS activity and ultimately influence over-motor generators. It is based on the philosophy that CNS learning occurs through consistency and repetition. The neurophysiology of the technique is drawn from earlier chapters in this book. The basic assumption of the casting concept is that many of the effects of certain techniques can be preserved—or **"imprinted"**—if the treated limb or body part is set in a cast while the therapeutic procedure is being performed. These techniques may include traction, approximation, rotation, deep tendon pressure, prolonged stretch, the option for movement, single component elimination, foreshortening, or elongation.

Definitions/differentiation

Casting can be categorized into the following four types:

1. *Conventional casting* uses material, such as plaster or fiberglass, applied to various body parts to repair osseous or ligamentous tissue. Such casts inhibit motion in the injured part, allowing it to heal. The normal time of cast application is 4 to 6 or more weeks.
2. *Serial casting* uses one or more well-padded plaster or fiberglass casts to increase or occasionally decrease range of motion over a period of time. The body part

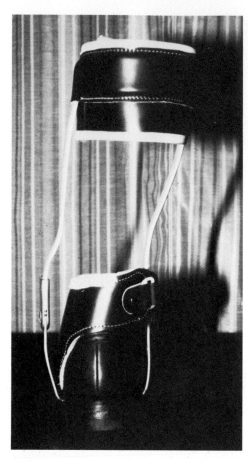

Fig. 32-9. Interim AFO for a client with Paget's disease, cerebrovascular accident, and burns on the foot.

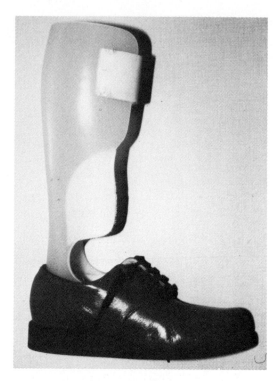

Fig. 32-10. Definitive polypropylene AFO with valgus corrective flare for stabilized client with cerebrovascular accident with valgus on weight bearing and equino varus during swing phase of gait.

is taken to the end of the available range, decreased a few degrees, and the cast is applied for 7 to 10 days. At the end of this period, the cast is removed and the process is repeated, with an increase or decrease in the range of motion.

3. *Inhibitory casting* uses casting material applied with specific techniques that attempt to reduce muscle tone and alter range of motion.
4. *Facilitory casting* uses casting materials applied with techniques that increase muscle tone in a specific group and increase or decrease a specific range of motion.

These cast types can be used in an interactive manner. Facilitory and inhibitory techniques, for example, can be used within the same cast.

Facilitory or inhibitory casting techniques use casts with minimal padding and for a duration of 48 hours only. The most significant features of these casting techniques are their subtlety. With minimal padding present, forces must be gentle and pressures on the tissue must be evenly distributed. Use of forces that are too harsh may result in skin breakdown.

If one assumes that imprinting the CNS occurs through consistent repetition, then techniques that produce desired results during a treatment session can produce dramatic results when applied for prolonged periods of time (48 hours).

To effectively use casting techniques, the following procedures must be strictly followed. The patient must be handled before attempting casting so the therapist can clearly identify exactly which techniques elicit a response from the patient's CNS. For example if the person responds to deep tendon pressure, then that technique may well be used in the cast. However, if traction, compression, rotation, or elongation—or any combination of these techniques—seem to have little effect and do not produce a desired outcome, then those techniques will be of little value if applied for the prolonged period of time.

The client to be put in a cast, the family or support system, and any health care provider who will come in contact with the client during the casting period must be well informed regarding specifics of the technique. A well-informed team will undoubtedly enhance the client's chances of having a successful experience with the cast.

The following indications must be clearly defined for those involved in the casting process:

1. Desired increase in range of motion
2. Desired decrease in range of motion
3. Desired increase in muscle tone
4. Desired decrease in muscle tone

5. Desired modulation over pattern generators
6. Desired provision of a more normal sensory feedback system to help modulate more normal motor responses

Contraindications to this technique include the following:

1. Uninformed support systems
2. Open wounds
3. Heterotopic bone as evidenced by a solid end feel

Special caution should be taken with a sensory-impaired limb resulting from circulatory problems or diabetes. This is clearly a consideration, although not necessarily a contraindication.

Technique

The casting procedure involves two therapists, one working as the "holder" and the other as the "caster." The two work together to prepare the patient. The therapist who is more skilled in modulating the state of the motor pool, or who has a better mastery of the CNS techniques, is assigned the task of the holder. The therapist with lesser skills in the manual and therapeutic arena is given the task of the caster. The caster applies the plaster or fiberglass while the holder facilitates or inhibits those responses previously determined by handling the patient clinically.

Once the roles of holder and caster have been established, the following technique can be performed. A single layer of cotton stockinette is rolled over the extremity to be casted. Enough material is applied to allow a 4- to 6-inch end proximal and distal to the proposed cast trimlines. Cast padding is wrapped circumferentially at the proximal and distal points where the cast is to be terminated. Various pads, such as metatarsal or scaphoid pads or pads that have been cut earlier, are applied in specific areas. One thickness of cast padding is placed over bony prominences. After this, a second layer of stockinette is applied to cover all padding as well as the first layer of stockinette. A length of surgical tubing is now applied to the extremity to make a channel for cast removal. The surgical tubing should extend approximately 3 inches past the point where the cast will end. It is positioned to encourage easy cast removal. Three layers of elastic plaster are now applied distally to proximally, with the caster using no excess tension and simply unrolling the elastic plaster onto the extremity or body part. Ridging or causing a gapping around the tubing must be avoided because this creates a pressure area under the tubing. Once the elastic plaster has been applied, three layers of standard plaster are added for reinforcement. It is crucial that the holder apply the predetermined facilitory or inhibitory technique while the plaster is still wet. Once the casting material has hardened, which usually takes 5 to 8 minutes, the caster turns down the excess length of surgical tubing, turns the excess stockinette back onto the cast, and then tapes the loose ends in place. As a rule, the author pulls an additional piece of stockinette over the entire cast to keep

any plaster from scratching or harming the client. If possible, weight bearing on the lower-extremity casts should be avoided for the 48 hours. In addition, the therapist should inspect exposed portions of extremities to ensure that circulation is adequate and swelling has not occurred. If swelling or discoloration becomes a problem, the cast should be removed immediately by simply pulling the surgical tubing from the cast and using cast scissors to cut and remove the cast. As a rule, the author does not use mechanical cast saws, because of the negative auditory and vibratory stimulation to the client. The cast is allowed to remain intact for 48 hours. If no problems have arisen at the end of that time, it is removed and the situation is assessed. If appropriate, a second cast may be applied, but this is generally not necessary. When the cast is removed, appropriate splinting should be provided to avoid loss of the desired result until the client is properly instructed in harnessing the new-found tone, range, or motor response.

Therapists using this technique must take care to avoid the possibility of unwanted motion within the cast. A cast may piston or slide up and down if it is applied to a cylindrical body part with no appropriate purchase. The purchase can be obtained with the elastic plaster by gently molding the plaster to the body part. If the limb is particularly conicular, then harnessing can be wrapped into the cast, such as figure-of-eight harnessing for the shoulder or waist-belt type harnessing for the lower extremity. If the upper extremity is to be casted and the hand allowed to be free, it is crucial the wrist opening be oval and not circular, which allows the extremity to rotate within the cast. Rotation within the cast will almost certainly cause chafing and skin breakdown. Pressures applied within the cast should be subtle: they should not exceed 4 psi (pounds per square inch).

Again, once the treating therapist has determined those techniques to which the client responds clinically, she or he can determine those which may realistically be incorporated into casting. Having established the techniques and applied the cast (after instructing the client, the family or support system, and the associated health care providers), the therapist must develop appropriate follow-up for harnessing the newly accomplished goal.

The limitations of this technique are created by the therapist's understanding of the spectrum of techniques available. Thorough evaluation of the client, and well-planned application of casts can greatly enhance established therapy treatment programs. Functional activities can then be practiced. The client may have stabilization peripherally and modulation centrally to practice feedforward plans in many different environments.

SUMMARY

Materials and fabrication techniques will continue to change rapidly in the field of orthotics. Advances will continue to improve the options available to therapists. Most important, thorough evaluations of neurologically impaired clients are necessary. Remembering that short-term goals and immediate responses must be weighed against long-term results, will assist the therapist develop accurate orthotic intervention plans. Open and ongoing communications between therapists and fabricating orthotists will allow all parties involved to benefit maximally from the orthotic experience. The client, who is the primary concern, should then achieve the most favorable result. Realizing that an orthosis can reinforce sound therapeutic exercise programs and introduce various neurological inputs to the CNS encourages physicians, therapists, and orthotists to add well-thought out orthotic treatments to the list of therapeutic options available to the neurologically impaired client.

REFERENCES

1. Brunnstrom S: *Movement therapy in hemiplegia,* New York, 1970, Harper & Row.
2. Lehneis HR: Principles of orthotic alignment in the lower extremity. In *American Academy of Orthopaedic Surgeons, Instructional course lectures,* vol 20, St Louis, 1971, Mosby.
3. Pansky B and House E: *Review of gross anatomy,* New York, 1969, Macmillan.

ADDITIONAL READINGS

Adams R and Victor M: *Principles of neurology,* ed 2, New York, 1981, McGraw-Hill Book Co.

American Academy of Orthopaedic *Surgeons: Atlas of orthotics: biomechanical principles and application,* St Louis, 1975, Mosby.

Bobath K and Bobath B: An analysis of the development of standing and walking patterns in patients with cerebral palsy, *Physiotherapy* 48(6):144-153, June 1962.

Brunnstrom S: *Clinical kinesiology,* ed 3, Philadelphia, 1972, FA Davis.

Carpenter M and Sutin J: *Human neuroanatomy,* ed 8, Baltimore, 1983, Williams & Wilkins.

Cailliet R: *Foot and ankle pain,* Philadelphia, 1975, FA Davis.

Duncan WR: Tonic reflexes of the foot: their orthopedic significance in normal children and in children with cerebral palsy, *J Bone Joint Surg* 42A:859, 1960.

Lehneis H and others: Energy expenditure with advanced lower limb orthoses and with conventional braces, *Arch Phys Med Rehabil* 57:20, 1976.

Prensky A and Palkes H: *Care of the neurologically handicapped child,* New York, 1982, Oxford University Press.

Redford J: *Orthotics etcetera,* ed 2, Baltimore, 1980, Williams & Wilkins.

Salek B: *The significance of structural and functional development in the normal foot and therapeutic implications thereof in the child with neuromotor disorder,* New York, 1977, Suffolk Rehabilitation Center.

CHAPTER 33

An Overview of Pharmaceutical Agents and the Implications for Therapists

Timothy J. Smith and Howell Runion

OUTLINE

The role of the pharmacist
The importance of drug disposition
Adverse drug effects and physical or occupational therapy
Drug classes relevant to physical therapy
    Cardiovascular-renal agents
    Nonsteroidal antiinflammatory agents and aceta-
      minophen
    The endocrine agents
    Chemotherapeutic agents
    Central and peripheral nervous system agents
    Drugs used in the treatment of respiratory disease
Conclusion
    Case 1 A.W.
    Case 2 C.K.

LEARNING OBJECTIVES

After reading this chapter the student/therapist will:

1. Understand the role of the pharmacist in assisting the physical therapist with medication-related problems.
2. Recognize the factors influencing the differences in drug response among various patient groups.
3. Obtain an increased awareness of the impact of adverse effects of drugs with respect to cognitive and motor function.
4. Identify the various classes of drugs that may have an impact on physical therapy with respect to cognitive and motor function.
5. Acknowledge the limitations of drug and physical therapy.

KEY TERMS

pharmacist	chemotherapeutic agents
drug disposition	central nervous system agents
adverse drug reactions	
cardiovascular agents	anxiolytic agents
antiinflammatory agents	sedative-hypnotic
endocrine agents	respiratory disease

The main purpose of this chapter is to familiarize the therapist with the common problems and adverse effects seen with the major classes of therapeutic agents that may complicate or augment effective physical and occupational therapy. This chapter is *not* a comprehensive overview, but rather a guide sufficient in scope to aid the therapist in consultation with physicians, pharmacists, nurses, and other health professionals.

THE ROLE OF THE PHARMACIST

The **pharmacist** provides several valuable services in the delivery of effective health care. With reference to inquiries by the physical and occupational therapist, these include the following (not an inclusive list):

1. Identification of drug dosage forms
2. Counseling on the management of drug side effects
3. Resolving problems regarding duplicate medications (especially with regard to multiple physicians and prescriptions)
4. Identification and resolution of drug interactions, including over-the-counter drugs with prescription medications
5. Recognition of drug abuse problems
6. Monitoring the effectiveness of drug therapy

Although a detailed discussion of these factors is not possible within the context of this chapter, they should be kept in mind when dealing with the problems of patients which may or may not be drug-related. In view of the thousands of available pharmaceutical preparations, the therapist should recognize that providing the pharmacist with a trade name or generic name for a product may not always result in a positive identification and resolution of the problem. This situation commonly occurs when the drug preparation in question is not associated with a prescription or if the original package is missing. In any inquiry, the pharmacist may be interested in patient-related factors such as age, sex, weight, disease states, nutrition, environment, and race/genetic factors, depending on the agent in question. Nevertheless, the services of the pharmacist are currently underutilized, which is a major factor for the inappropriateness and ineffectiveness of drug therapy. In the following sections, the drug-related factors that may adversely influence cognitive and motor function, as well as other major problems associated with each class of pharmaceutical agents, are examined.

THE IMPORTANCE OF DRUG DISPOSITION

Drugs may be administered either enterically (placed into the gut through oral or rectal administration) or parenterally (routes other than the enteric route, such as transcutaneous, subcutaneous, intravenous, etc.). Most drugs follow a few common processes after they are administered. These processes are known as absorption, distribution, metabolism, and elimination. Absorption is a process of transfer of drug through a tissue barrier into the systemic circulation. After absorption, the drug may be distributed to various tissues, including the target tissue or site of action. Many drugs may undergo chemical changes (metabolism) due to interactions with cellular enzymes, which may result in increased activity, decreased activity, or no change in activity. Metabolism may also influence the way that the body eliminates the drug, such as excretion of the drug through the urine, feces, or lungs. Ethanol is totally metabolized and utilized by the body for energy.

Factors influencing the processes of absorption, distribution, metabolism, and excretion include age, sex, disease states, concurrently administered drugs, nutrition, environmental factors, exercise, and racial/genetic background (and family history). The preceding factors are important considerations for each of the classes of pharmaceutical agents discussed below. This chapter focuses on **adverse drug reactions.** A discussion of these and other properties of the drugs may be found in the general references listed at the end of the chapter. References are listed for specific cases of interest.

ADVERSE DRUG EFFECTS AND PHYSICAL OR OCCUPATIONAL THERAPY

As a physical or occupational therapist, it is important to note that adverse drug effects can interfere with effective therapy. We can divide drugs into two major actions: (1) drugs that adversely affect cognitive function and (2) drugs that affect motor function. In most cases there is always significant overlap such that one may not clearly be able to separate the two groups. When reviewing the different classes of agents, this will become apparent. Drugs affecting cognitive function include those that cause drowsiness, confusion, and behavioral disorders. These adverse effects impede not only the instructional ability of the therapist, but also the ability of the patient to cooperate, learn, and accommodate motor control skills. Drug classes that pre-

---

Classes of drugs that may directly or indirectly affect cognitive and motor function

Cardiovascular-renal agents

Nitrates
Calcium channel blockers
Antiarrhythmic agents
Digoxin
Antihypertensive agents
Diuretics

Chemotherapeutic agents

Antitubercular agents
Aminoglycosides
Quinolines
Antiviral agents

Central and peripheral nervous system agents

Anticonvulsant medications
Drugs used to treat basal ganglia dysfunction
Agents for disorders of muscle tone
Sedative-hypnotics and anxiolytic agents
Antipsychotic agents
Lithium carbonate
Antidepressant drugs
Narcotic analgesics
Drugs used in the treatment of motion sickness and vertigo

dominantly affect motor control, either directly or indirectly are included in the boxes on p. 912 and 913. In view of these major adverse effects as applied to physical or occupational therapy, it is necessary to focus on each drug class.

DRUG CLASSES RELEVANT TO PHYSICAL THERAPY

Cardiovascular-renal agents

Pharmaceuticals used in the management of cardiovascular disease are among the most important in the therapeutic arena. This class includes drugs used for angina, arrhythmias, circulatory failure, hypertension, edema, and hyperlipidemias. Although patients with heart disease may be taking these drugs, they are not the only patients receiving them. These **cardiovascular agents** may be divided into the following categories.

Nitrates. These agents are used in the management of angina and include nitroglycerin (Nitro-Dur), erythrityl (Cardilate) and pentaerythritol tetranitrate (Peritrate), and amyl nitrite. These agents often cause headache soon after administration and may cause postural hypotension in elderly persons sufficient to result in syncope.[5]

Calcium channel blockers. Diltiazem (Cardizem), nicardipine (Cardene), nifedipine (Procardia), and verapamil (Calan) are often used in the management of angina. They may cause dizziness, headache, and hypotension.[2]

Antiarrhythmic agents. Although these agents are used to treat patients with abnormalities in heart rhythm, they may cause other rhythm disturbances. In addition to cardiac conduction abnormalities, the adverse effect profile of these agents may vary widely due to their diversity.[10] Quinidine (Quinidex) may be associated with headache, tinnitus, vertigo, visual disturbances, and syncope. Procainamide (Pronestyl) overdose may result in confusion and lethargy. Disopyramide (Norpace) may be associated with confusion and hallucinations in elderly persons. Lidocaine (Xylocaine), mexiletine (Mexitil), tocainide (Tonocard), encainide (Enkaid), and flecainide (Tambocor) may share effects such as dizziness, headache, syncope, confusion, and hallucinations. Amiodarone (Cordarone) administration has been associated with paresthesias, tremor, ataxia, and headache.

Digoxin. Many drugs used in the management of congestive heart failure (CHF) have been used in the treatment of other diseases; however, digoxin (Lanoxin) and other digitalis glycosides are specifically used in the treatment of CHF and related disorders. Digoxin is very toxic and several central nervous system (CNS) effects have been associated with this drug, including visual disturbances, confusion, and hallucinations.[6,10] These side effects may be associated with overdose situations, and their presence may be considered a medical emergency.

Antihypertensive agents. Management of high blood pressure involves a very diverse class of agents. These include the diuretics, sympatholytics, beta-blockers, alpha-blockers, vasodilators, and angiotensin-converting enzyme inhibitors. Administration of beta-blockers, such as propranolol (Inderal), have been associated with sedation, depression, sleep disturbances, lethargy, and impotence. Methyldopa (Aldomet), a centrally mediated antihypertensive agent, may share the effects of the beta-blockers and rarely CNS effects may include reactions such as choreoathetosis. Clonidine (Catapres), guanabenz (Wytensin), and guanfacine (Tenex) produce an antihypertensive effect centrally. Adverse effects of these agents may include drowsiness, sleep disturbances, and in overdose (in the case of clonidine), seizures, delirium, and hallucinations.[7,10,19] Older antihypertensive drugs such as reserpine (Serpasil) may precipitate depression. Reserpine and guanethidine (Ismelin) may produce syncope. Guanethidine may impair ejaculation. With regard to alpha-blocking agents, prazosin (Minipress) may produce a first-dose syncope. Although this problem is unlikely with subsequent physical therapy, the dizziness and headache may be troublesome during initiation of antihypertensive therapy. Phenoxybenzamine (Dibenzyline), which has an unlabelled use for prostatic hypertrophy, may precipitate orthostatic hypotension and impair ejaculation.

Diuretics. These agents are used as antihypertensives and in the treatment of edema. The thiazides—hydrochlorothiazide (HydroDIURIL), indapamide (Lozol), metolazone (Zaroxolyn), and others—may produce light-headedness, vertigo, weakness, restlessness, insomnia, and fatigue. The loop diuretics such as furosemide (Lasix) may produce orthostatic hypotension, syncope, vertigo, headache, blurred vision, paresthesias, and xanthopsia.[10,23] Some of these effects may be shared by the potassium-sparing diuretics such as spironolactone (Aldactone), amiloride (Midamor), and triamterene (Dyrenium). The carbonic anhydrase inhibitor acetazolamide (Diamox), although classified as diuretic, is used for other disorders. Paresthesias, tremor, drowsiness, confusion, and ataxia have been associated with the use of this agent.[8]

Hypolipidemic agents. Within the context of this chapter, one of the most important adverse effects of the hypolipidemic class of agents is the myopathy that occurs with the hydroxymethylglutaryl CoA reductase inhibitors.[27] This class includes lovastatin (Mevacor). This myopathy may be reversible, although it may be increased with exercise.

Classes of drugs that may directly or indirectly affect motor function

Cardiovascular-renal agents
Hypolipidemic agents
Glucocorticoids
Chemotherapeutic agents
Antitumor agents
Drugs used in the treatment of respiratory disease

Nonsteroidal antiinflammatory agents and acetaminophen

This class of agents is used for the treatment of pain associated with inflammation, which commonly occurs with arthritis and injury. This class includes aspirin, indomethacin (Indocin), and ibuprofen (Advil). The major adverse effect of these agents is the exacerbation or induction of peptic ulcer disease.[15] It must be understood that although the analgesic acetaminophen (Tylenol) reduces pain, it does not reduce the inflammation that is associated with arthritis or musculoskeletal injury.

The endocrine agents

Among the agents commonly used to modify endocrine systems include glucocorticoids (as antiinflammatory agents), insulin (for diabetes), thyroid hormone (hypothyroidism), and oral contraceptives. Of these, the most pertinent to problems encountered in physical and occupational therapy are the glucocorticoids. These **endocrine agents** include dexamethasone (Decadron), prednisone, cortisone, and prednisolone (Delta-Cortef) used in the management of inflammatory disorders. These agents, when used chronically at high doses, may cause muscle wasting and bone resorption, which may increase muscle weakness and result in bone fractures.[16,21]

Chemotherapeutic agents

Although CNS and neuromuscular disorders are not common with the antimicrobial, antiviral, and antitumor **chemotherapeutic agents,** there are notable exceptions.

Antitubercular agents. Isoniazid, one of the most widely used agents for prophylaxis and treatment of tuberculosis, may produce a peripheral neuropathy that may respond to pyridoxine. Ethambutol (Myambutol) may cause a reversible loss of visual acuity.[18] The effects of streptomycin are listed with the aminoglycosides.

Aminoglycosides. These agents are used for treatment of severe bacterial infections. This class includes amikacin (Amikin), gentamicin (Garamycin), kanamycin (Kantrex), and streptomycin. Aminoglycosides may induce confusion, disorientation, ototoxicity, tremor, weakness, and muscle paralysis.[14]

The quinolines. Ciprofloxacin (Cipro) and norfloxacin (Noroxin) are used to treat bacterial infections and may cause dizziness, headache, and light-headedness.[12,22] In high doses or in combination with other agents, seizures have been noted.

Antiviral agents. Amantadine (Symmetrel), an agent used in elderly persons to prevent influenza A infection (as well as an adjunct in the management of Parkinson's disease), can produce behavioral changes and orthostatic hypotension.[7]

Antitumor agents. Agents used in the treatment of cancer are very toxic. Major adverse effects of the antitumor agents include hematological and gastrointestinal toxicity.

Neurotoxicity is the major adverse effect of vincristine (Oncovin). Neurotoxicity may include peripheral neuropathies, which may increase muscle weakness and associated incoordination.[20]

Central and peripheral nervous system agents

Of greatest concern to the physical and occupational therapist are agents that influence motor control and learning. Although the preceding drugs have adverse effects that may influence these factors, agents that affect the CNS and peripheral nerves directly are of immediate importance. These agents may be divided into nine major categories: 1) anticonvulsant drugs, 2) drugs used to treat basal ganglia dysfunction, 3) drugs used to treat disorders of muscle tone and myasthenia gravis, 4) sedative-hypnotic and antiolytic drugs, 5) antipsychotic drugs, 6) drugs used to treat manic-depressive illness, 7) antidepressant drugs, 8) narcotic analgesics, and 9) drugs used to treat motion sickness and vertigo.

Anticonvulsant medications. Drugs used in the treatment of absence, tonic-clonic, and other seizure disorders differ substantially in the adverse effects profile. They may be administered to all ages and to individuals with other disorders. Ethosuximide (Zarontin), valproic acid (Depakene), clonazepam (Klonopin), phenytoin (Dilantin), carbamazepine (Tegretol), and primidone (Mysoline) may cause headache, drowsiness, ataxia, confusion, and in some cases, nystagmus, hallucinations, and euphoria.[29]

Drugs used to treat basal ganglia dysfunction. In view of the ability of levodopa (often in combination with carbidopa as Sinemet) to modify central dopaminergic pathways, both motor and cognitive functions are affected. Adverse effects include dystonias, choreiform movements, confusion, agitation, anxiety, hallucinations, and behavioral changes.[1] Another troublesome aspect of motor control is the development of an "on-off phenomenon," whereby patients may experience extreme rigidity and difficulty with initiating movement between periods of reasonably normal motor function. As an adjunct in the management of "on-off phenomenon," bromocriptine (Parlodel) may be used; however this agent may produce headache, dizziness, dyskinesias, and behavioral changes. Many anticholinergic agents, such as trihexyphenidyl (Artane) and benztropine (Cogentin), have been used in the management of parkinsonism; however, adverse effects of this class of agents includes depression, disorientation, agitation, psychosis, hallucinations, and mental confusion, especially in elderly persons. These effects may be added to autonomic effects such as mydriasis, blurred vision, and urinary retention. Although some of these agents have been used for the management of other disorders of the basal ganglia, they are of limited effectiveness.

Drugs used to treat disorders of muscle tone and myasthenia gravis. Disorders of muscle tone may occur as the result of several disease processes such as spinal injury, cerebral palsy, stroke, multiple sclerosis, and polio. Although several other drugs are currently under investigation, baclofen (Lioresal), dantrolene (Dantrium), and diazepam (Valium) are the most common. Because these drugs produce muscle relaxation, they may also produce weakness.[28] Baclofen acts primarily at the level of the spinal cord. Dantrolene predominantly reduces muscle contraction within skeletal muscle. Diazepam may influence peripheral muscle contraction through central GABAnergic systems, nerves which utilize gamma-aminobutyric acid. Because all of these agents may also affect CNS pathways, drowsiness, ataxia, and dizziness are common. Older drugs such as carisoprodol (Soma), cyclobenzaprine (Flexeril), and metaxalone (Skelaxin) generally do not produce muscle relaxation without a significant degree of CNS depression (i.e., drowsiness, dizziness).[17] Although rarely encountered in practice, anticholinesterase agents are generally drugs of choice in the management of the weakness associated with myasthenia gravis. Excessive cholinergic discharge at the neuromuscular junction, however, may produce muscle fasciculations and paralysis.[26]

Sedative-hypnotic and anxiolytic agents. These agents produce sleep and reduce anxiety. In several instances, they have been used to reduce hyperactivity (primarily in adults and in association with other disorders). Although dozens of these agents are available, with a few exceptions they differ very little in their side effect profile. Examples of commonly used agents are shown in the box below. All of these agents may cause significant hangover when used as sleep-inducing agents,[3] particularly in elderly patients, where improper balance due to lack of sensory-motor responsiveness may lead to falls and severe injury. Many of the benzodiazepines may be used as **anxiolytic agents** (see the box at right). In combination with alcohol and other CNS depressants,

dangerous CNS depression can result with the use of either the **sedative-hypnotics** or anxiolytic agents. A newer agent, zolpidem (Ambien), may be much safer with regard to hangover effects when used as a sleep-inducing agent.[4] The anxiolytic agent buspirone (BuSpar) does not appear to induce as severe a CNS depression with ethanol as do the other agents listed in the boxes. Although the amphetamine class of agents is not a sedative-hypnotic agent, many of them such as methylphenidate (Ritalin), can reduce hyperactivity in children, although they are clearly CNS stimulants in adults.

Antipsychotic agents. Most of the medications currently used for the treatment of psychoses (including agents used in the management of schizophrenia) are dopaminergic antagonists and affect both cognitive and motor functions.[24] A partial list is shown in the bottom box below. These effects depend on the agent used, may be dose-specific, and may be seen when used as antiemetics. In view of the dopaminergic antagonism, acute effects such as dystonias and akathesia may be seen. The acute parkinsonism-like effects can be

---

Drugs (of the benzodiazepine class) used to reduce anxiety (anxiolytics)

Lorazepam (Ativan)
Prazepam (Centrax)
Chlordiazepoxide (Librium)
Halazepam (Paxipam)
Oxazepam (Serax)
Clorazepate (Tranxene)
Diazepam (Valium)
Alprazolam (Xanax)

Examples of drugs used to produce sleep (sedative-hypnotics)

Benzodiazepines

Lorazepam (Ativan)
Flurazepam (Dalmane)
Quazepam (Doral)
Triazolam (Halcion)
Temazepam (Restoril)

Barbiturates

Amobarbital (Amytal)
Pentobarbital (Nembutal)
Secobarbital (Seconal)

Miscellaneous

Glutethimide (Doriden)
Methyprylon (Noludar)
Ethchlorvynol (Placidyl)
Ethinamate (Valmid)

Examples of drugs used to treat psychoses (antipsychotics)

Phenothiazine

Prochlorperazine (Compazine)
Thioridazine (Mellaril)
Fluphenazine (Permitil)
Mesoridazine (Serentil)
Trifluoperazine (Stelazine)
Chlorpromazine (Thorazine)
Acetophenazine (Tindal)
Perphenazine (Trilafon)
Triflupromazine (Vesprin)

Others

Haloperidol (Haldol)
Clozapine (Clozaril)
Loxapine (Loxitane)
Molindone (Moban)
Thiothixene (Navane)
Chlorprothixene (Taractan)

antagonized by anticholinergics such as diphenhydramine (Benadryl), which is useful in emergency dyskinesias. Long-term use of most antipsychotics may result in a syndrome known as "tardive dyskinesia," which is not readily revers-ible. These drugs may precipitate seizures in those with a history of epilepsy or other convulsive disorders.

Manic-depressive illness. Lithium carbonate is the drug of choice for management of this disorder. Blood levels must be monitored frequently because the drug has a low therapeutic index.[13] Due to the ability of lithium to influence ion channels in the CNS, adverse effects relative to motor function are common. These include dizziness, ataxia, and fine tremor. Severe drowsiness and muscle weakness may indicate intoxication.

Antidepressant drugs. The box below lists commonly used antidepressant agents. Most of these agents block the reuptake of neurotransmitters at the synapse, which in part explains both their therapeutic and adverse effects.[25] Many of the agents belong to the class designated *tricyclic antide-pressants.* The tricyclic agents tend to have a high degree of anticholinergic actions. The adverse effects are much like those of the anticholinergics used in the management of Parkinson's disease. In addition, incoordination, ataxia, and tremor may be seen. The more selective serotonin reuptake inhibitors fluoxetine (Prozac) and paroxetine (Paxil) are rela-tively free of these effects in most patients.

Narcotic analgesics. The use of strong analgesic agents are necessary for injury and several disease processes. Among these are the drugs related to morphine or "narcotic analgesics" as listed in the box at right. Most of these agents may produce drowsiness, dizziness, vertigo, and headache in

the usual dosages.[11] In higher doses or rarely with standard doses, nervousness, depression, euphoria or dysphoria, and several cognitive disorders may result.

Drugs used in the treatment of motion sickness and vertigo. Travel in aircraft or in watercraft commonly results in vestibular problems, nausea, and vomiting. Agents used predominantly for antiemetics are related to the antipsy-chotic phenothiazines. However, many of the antihistamines, anticholinergics, and related agents are commonly used as motion sickness remedies and antivertigo agents. These include buclizine (Bucladin), cyclizine (Marezine), dimen-hydrinate (Dramamine), meclizine (Antivert), and scopola-mine (Transderm-Scop). Among the most common side effects are drowsiness and blurred vision.

Drugs used in the treatment of respiratory disease

Among the drugs used for management of asthma and seasonal allergy are sympathomimetic drugs (epinephrine and ephedrine), theophylline, and antihistamines. Epineph-rine (Medihaler-Epi), ephedrine, and theophylline (Theo-Dur) have CNS stimulant effects and often cause tremor.[7,19] Many antihistamines may cause sedation, although the incidence is less for many of the newer agents.[9]

CONCLUSION

As stated earlier, specific drugs used for specific di-agnosis can have adverse effects on a variety of CNS functions. If a clinical problem, whether cognitive, af-fective, or motor, does not seem to match the disability or seems to be increasing disproportionately to what would be the clinical problem and the therapist thinks it may be drug related, the therapist needs to immediately seek assistance. It is recommended that the therapist contact the pharmacist and physician to eliminate the possibility that

Drugs used to treat depression (antidepressants)

Tricyclic antidepressants

Clomipramine (Anafranil)
Amoxapine (Asendin)
Nortriptyline (Aventyl)
Amitriptyline (Elavil)
Desipramine (Norpramin)
Doxepin (Sinequan)
Imipramine (Tofranil)
Protriptyline (Vivactil)

Monoamine oxidase inhibitors

Isocarboxazid (Marplan)
Phenelzine (Nardil)
Tranylcypromine (Parnate)

Others

Trazodone (Desyrel)
Maprotiline (Ludiomil)
Fluoxetine (Prozac)

Narcotic analgesics and related agents for pain

Alfentanil (Alfenta)
Morphine sulfate
Buprenorphine (Buprenex)
Propoxyphene (Darvon)
Meperidine (Demerol)
Hydromorphone (Dilaudid)
Methadone (Dolophine)
Levorphanol (Levo-Dromoran)
Nalbuphine (Nubain)
Oxymorphone (Numorphan)
Oxycodone (Roxicodone)
Butorphanol (Stadol)
Fentanyl (Sublimaze)
Dihydrocodeine (Synalgos-DC)
Pentazocine (Talwin)

drugs are causing the difficulty or creating additional problems and decreasing the client's quality of life. The therapist and family members are often the first to recognize these problems. In many causes early recognition and a change in medication may eliminate the problem and prevent any possibility for permanent problems.

Two case presentations have been included to help the reader understand the interactive nature of drugs and therapy and their overall influence on function more easily. Drugs may be counterproductive to physical management of life activities. In some cases no matter the drug or the therapy, the client will not benefit.

CASE 1 ▼ A.W.

Complications of Drug Therapy, Degenerative Pathology, Cognitive Function, and Accidental Trauma to Successful Physiotherapy.

A.W. is an 83-year-old male Parkinson's patient with concurrent degenerative right hip joint and spinal column disease. He was initially referred to our clinic for management of his Parkinson's disease. A.W. had been active until a recent fall from a ladder. The fall left him with compression deformities at T12 and L2. He already had significant vertebral column osteopenia, which has been aggravated by degenerative changes in his right trochanter. A.W. was a professional builder and master carpenter. He is married and has a 37-year-old son. For the past 35 years he and his wife shared their home with a woman who was designated as a pseudo aunt to their son. The aunt recently died after a prolonged, agonizing illness. The aunt's illness and recent death correlate with A.W.'s history of increased skeletal muscular pain and mild dementia.

A.W.'s other medical problems include moderately well-managed gout, a prolonged history of intermittent peptic ulcer disease, chronic constipation, impaired hearing, and significant progressive osteopenia. The osteopenia is clinically significant, as it involves his right hip and vertebral column. The degenerative processes have left him with significant kyphosis, mild scoliosis, compromised respiratory function, and chronic pain.

Management of A.W.'s osteopenic pain and recent compression fractures has presented a unique therapeutic challenge. Initially, nonsteroidal antiinflammatory drugs (NSAIDs) were used to moderate his pain. Several compounds were tried; however, the NSAIDs only aggravated his intermittent peptic ulcer disease, which was treated with ranitidine (Zantac). Failure of the NSAID therapy lead to therapeutic trials of several analgesic compounds containing codeine. The levels required to lower his pain threshold decreased his cognitive functions and aggravated his GI tract by their constipation-producing side effects. To relieve both the cognitive and GI motility problems from high doses of codeine he was switched to hydrocodone bitartrate acetaminophen (Vicodin). Vicodin provided mild pain relief, and lowered his cognitive impairment. It still aggravated his chronic constipation problem. It is important to keep in mind, however, that constipation is not only a problem frequently encountered in elderly persons but is a part of the natural history of his Parkinson's disease and its relationship to GI function.

A.W.'s current drug regimen includes carbidopa/levodopa (Sinemet) 25/100 1 and $\frac{1}{2}$ Tabs QID, selegiline hydrochloride (Eldepryl) 5 MG 1 QD (at the current levels of Sinemet if he takes Eldepryl 5 MG Bid as generally prescribed, he will hallucinate; thus he takes $\frac{1}{2}$ of the recommended daily dose), hydrocodone bitartrate acetaminophen (Vicodin) 1 QID, ranitidine hydrochloride (Zantac) 150 MG 1 HS; over-the-counter compounds include Tylenol Extra Strength PRN and Docolax, a stool softener. Clearly his cognitive functions will be related not only to dose levels of Vicodin, his chronic pain level from the compression fractures, osteopenia, kyphosis, and scoliosis, but also to his primary condition of Parkinson's disease. It is generally accepted that 50% of Parkinson's patients go on to demonstrate some degree of dementia. This only underscores the importance of obtaining a complete patient history.

A.W. clearly needed some form of pain management other than soporific or cognitive disruptive drugs. He was referred to a physical therapist for transcutaneous electrical nerve stimulation (TENS) evaluation and thoracic taping trial. The thoracic taping was successful in providing spinal column support. However, taping is an impractical daily modality; thus he was sent for body casting to have a back brace fabricated. This has helped by his history and clinical observation that have also been confirmed by his family. The TENS unit was also effective in relieving some of his pain, allowing for a reduction in Vicodin use to prn as opposed to qid. In the absence of chronic pain he has once again become verbal and interactive with his family.

COMMENTS: This case highlights some of the problems inherent in providing effective therapy to patients with multiple problems. The patient's gradual loss of cognitive functions has made directing his day-to-day therapy management sometimes difficult. Unfortunately the prognosis for A.W. remains poor. The biggest factors mitigating against his recovery are his age and the degenerative nature of Parkinson's disease. Adding to his already poor prognosis, are the recently acquired spinal compression fractures and subsequent compression of his chest. There is no doubt, however, about the major contribution therapy has played in improving the quality of life via the fitting of a spinal column brace and the introduction of the TENS unit. The interaction of physical or occupational therapy with drug therapy creates the greatest potential for maintaining his existing functional skills and quality of life. Working in close communication between disciplines and with the client helps to guarantee that the therapies together interact to create a positive effect.

C.K. is a 38-year-old obese woman who was involved in a rear-end auto accident 6 years ago and continues to complain of unremitting cervical pain at C-5-6 and 7 and point muscular tenderness in her left shoulder. Pain still can be evoked on palpation of the levators scapulae and distal region of the rhomboid major and minor muscles. C.K. works as a nursing aid in a board and care facility. She is responsible for bathing patients and moving them from bed to chairs. C.K. has attempted to remain employed throughout much of the past 6 years.

After the car accident, she was initially seen by her family practitioner and given a course of naproxen (Naprosyn) and offered physical therapy (PT). She declined the PT. On follow-up, she reported that the naproxen, a NSAID, was moderately effective in relieving her neck and shoulder pain. In comparing her initial visit, the Naprosyn did allow for a measurable increasing her range of motion. C.K.'s physician placed her on disability for 2 weeks and sent her home to rest. Several weeks later she returned complaining of increased cervical and left shoulder pain. To manage her increased pain level, she was given Tylenol with 30 MG of codeine bid. Within 2 months she had increased her Tylenol codeine use to four or five per day. She now complained of constipation. Her doctor recognized the codeine was probably responsible for her constipation and elected to use a combination analgesic. He ordered hydrocodone bitartrate and acetaminophen (Vicodin) 1 twice a day. In less than 2 months she had increased her Vicodin use to 5 per day with no apparent pain relief. C.K. now demanded the PT that had been initially offered post injury. However, she found PT to be of little benefit. The PT staff notes report "she winces and complains of pain whenever she is touched." She returned to her primary care physician and now demanded a referral to an orthopedist.

She was subsequently seen by an orthopedist who examined her and ordered a spinal computed tomography (CT) and eventually a magnetic resonance imaging (MRI) of her neck. All imaging was reported as essentially normal except for slight disk bulging at C-6-7. However, MRI enhancement with contrast media showed no impingement on the spinal cord or roots emanating from the foramen.

Shortly before she requested her primary physician refer her to an orthopedist, she began complaining of bilateral lumbar-sacral pain at L-4-5 and S1. The lumbar pain initially did not radiate in a clearly defined dermatome distribution. Her back examination was clinically nonconclusive; MRIs were normal. Nevertheless, C.K. was now totally dependent on narcotic analgesics. She next began to develop daily headaches. Her family practitioner on recommendation of the orthopedist referred her to a neurologist to evaluate the possibility of neural impingement not seen in the CT or MRI and to evaluate her new chief complaint of headaches.

The headaches were immediately treated by ordering a withdrawal from the Vicodin and refusing any further codeine compounds. To manage her depression, she was given amitriptyline (Elavil). She has been subsequently tried on several other NSAIDs, as she would periodically complain of gastrointestinal distress. She was next given diflunisal (Dolobid) followed by ketorolac tromethamine (Toradol).

In the interim, electromyograms (EMG) and nerve conduction studies were conducted to rule out nerve root compression. The findings were normal for all muscle and peripheral

nerves tested. Again PT was ordered and some advantages realized from modality treatments of heat, ultrasound, and traction. The working diagnosis at this point was now myofacial pain.

C.K. was next given amitriptyline (Elavil), a tricyclic antidepressant. Some improvement was reported in her myofascial pain as well as her depression. However, C.K. continued to claim to be in "constant pain" and dependent on NSAID therapy. PT was ordered but did not produce significant relief. She now began each office visitation with "when are you going to fix my pain?"

At this point she discovered that intramuscular (IM) ketorolac tromethamine 60 mg IM (Toradol) offered help for the neck, shoulder, and low back pain while relieving her HAs.

In investigating the cause of her new chief complaint of headache, she inadvertently volunteered she had filed a law suit against the driver that "rear ended her." She had been advised that a careful medical record of her injury detailing her pain and suffering would be needed for a successful trial. She did not inform her physicians that she had filed a law suit. The lawsuit was subsequently thrown out before it went to court; however, almost 2½ years had elapsed. The court found she had backed into the car while claiming she had been hit from behind.

C.K. had lived up to her expectations. Once the law suit had been filed she needed to document her pain and suffering. Unfortunately, as the facts of the case were uncovered, she had no legal case but she still had the pain.

She continued to insist that there was a physiological basis for her pain and demanded a second MRI, EMG, and additional nerve conduction studies. The studies confirmed that there was no structural damage that could be addressed surgically and that her chronic pain was attributable to acute awareness of her discomfort, which then became the focus of her life.

The consequence of these problems has left a legacy of myofacial pain. Psychiatric assistance will be required to alleviate her pain and resolve her anger at not being able to pursue a law suit for her pain and suffering. She has steadfastly refused any psychiatric or psychological counseling to help her deal with her pain.

COMMENTS: In reviewing the practitioner/client relationship, it becomes obvious that C.K.'s dishonest dealings with her primary care and consulting physicians prevented an acceptable outcome. Her self-deceptive relationship with her physicians would have been missed by most people because C.K. set out to defeat any and all therapy recommended or offered. C.K. subsequently perceived failure in her drug therapy with NSAIDs despite the initial evidence to the contrary. She suffered no mental impairment from the drug therapy, but it continued to be ineffective in reducing the pain. Pain did give her a potential secondary gain through initiation of litigation, and she may have adapted her CNS to feel and attend to pain. Physical therapy may have been beneficial had she accepted it when first offered. However with her hidden agenda of litigation, it was not in her best interest to succeed when it was again offered and tried. Today C.K. is left with an unresolved soft tissue irritation that may be more mental than physical. Without patient receptivity neither PT/OT or drug therapy will probably be effective regardless of treatment.

REFERENCES

1. Abbott R and others: Comparisons of the therapeutic effects of levodopa, levodopa and selegiline, and bromocriptine in patients with early, mild Parkinson's disease: three year interim report, *Br Med J* 307(6902):469-472, 1993.

2. Arstall MA and others: Incidence of adverse events during treatment with verapamil for suspected acute myocardial infection. *Am J Cardiol* 70(2):1611-1612, 1992.

3. Ballinger BR: Hypnotics and anxiolytics, *Br Med J* 300(6722):456-458, 1990.

4. Berlin I and others: Comparison of the effects of zolpidem and triazolam on memory function, psychomotor performance, and postural sway in healthy subjects, *J Clin Psychopharmacol* 13(2):100-106, 1993.

5. Bonema JD and Maddens ME: Syncope in elderly patients: why their risk is higher, *Postgrad Med* 91(1):129-144, 1992.

6. Bressler R, Katz M, and Conrad K: Side effects in a man taking digoxin, *Drug Ther* 19(3):101-104, 1989.

7. Bullinger M: Psychotropic effects of non-psychotropic drugs, *Adv Drug React Ac Pois Rv* 6(3):141-167, 1987.

8. Dimsdale JE: Reflections on the impact of antihypertensive medications on mood, sedation, and neuropsychologic functioning, *Arch Intern Med* 152(1):35-39, 1992.

9. Donoghue PD and Tuttle CB: Non-sedating antihistamines, *Can Pharm J* 120(6):378-383, 1987.

10. Einarson TR: Drug-related hospital admission, *Ann Pharmacother* 27(8):832-840, 1993.

11. Ench RE: Pain control in the ambulatory elderly, *Geriatrics* 46(3):49-60, 1991.

12. Fass RJ: The quinolines, *Ann Intern Med* 102(3):400-402, 1985.

13. Gelenberg AJ: Lithium efficacy and adverse effects, *J Clin Psychiatry* 49(11S):8-9, 1988.

14. Gleckman RA and Czachor JS: Reviewing the safe use antibiotics in the elderly, *Geriatrics* 44(7):33-39, 1989.

15. Jaszewski R, Calzada R, and Dhar R: Persistence of gastric ulcers caused by plain aspirin or non-steroidal antiinflammatory agents in patients treated with a combo of cimetidine, antacids, and enteric coated aspirin, *Dig Dis Sci* 34(9):1361-1364, 1989.

16. Lear J and Daniels RG: Muscle cramps related to corticosteroids, *Br Med J* 306(6886):1169, 1993.

17. Littrell RA, Hayes LR, and Stillner V: Carisoprodol (SOMA): a new and cautious perspective on an old agent, *South Med J* 86(7):753-756, 1993.

18. Nariman S: Adverse reactions to drugs used in the treatment of tuberculosis, *Adv Drug React Ac Pois Rev* 7(4):207-227, 1988.

19. Nicholson AN and Pascoe PA: Drug-induced impairment of performance. *Adv Drug React Tox Rev* 11(3):193-204, 1992.

20. Nudleman KL: Preventing chemotherapy-induced neuropathy, *West J Med* 155(1):70, 1991.

21. Olbricht T and Benker G: Glucocorticoid-induced osteoporosis pathogenesis, prevention, and treatment, with special regard to the rheumatic diseases, *J Intern Med* 234(3):237-244, 1993.

22. Paton JH and Reeves DS: Adverse reaction to the fluoroquinolines, *Adv Drug React Bull* 153:575-578, 1992.

23. Polkey M: Hypertension guidelines. beware diuretics in elderly patients, *Br Med J* 306(6888):1337, 1993.

24. Raskind MA and Risse SC: Antipsychotic drugs and the elderly, *J Clin Psychiatry* 47(5S):17-22, 1986.

25. Settle EC: Managing antidepressant side effects, *Drug Ther* 23(7):17-30, 1993.

26. Shemesh I and others: Chlorpyrifos poisoning treated with ipratropium and dantrolene: a case report, *J Toxicol Clin Toxicol* 26(7):495-498, 1988.

27. Smellie WAS and Lorimer AR: Adverse effects of the lipid-lowering drugs, *Adv Drug React Tox Rev* 11(2):71-92, 1992.

28. Smith CR and others: High dose oral baclofen: experience in patients with multiple sclerosis, *Neurology* 41(11):1829-1831, 1991.

29. Trimble MR: Anticonvulsant drugs and cognitive function: a review of the literature, *Epilepsia* 28(S3):S37-S43, 1987.

ADDITIONAL READINGS

Clark WG, Brater DC, and Johnson AR: *Goth's Medical Pharmacology*, ed 13, St Louis, 1992, Mosby.

Gillman AG and others: *Goodman and Gilman's The Pharmacological Basis of Therapeutics*, ed 8, New York, 1990, Pergamon Press.

Katzung BG: *Drug Therapy*, ed 2, San Mateo, 1991, Appleton and Lange.

McEvoy GK: *AHFS Drug Information 93*, Bethesda, 1993, American Society of Hospital Pharmacists.

Wingard LB and others: *Human Pharmacology, Molecular to Clinical*, St Louis, 1991, Mosby.

CHAPTER 34

Health Education

Key to an enriched environment

Donna El-Din

KEY TERMS

wholistic model
health education
provider-patient relationship

empowerment
patient/client education
patient/client satisfaction

LEARNING OBJECTIVES

After reading this chapter the student/therapist will:

1. Identify the importance of a client-based decision making health care system.
2. Discuss reasons for the philosophical shift from medical based to community based health care delivery.
3. Value the tenet that client education and empowerment will lead to the highest quality of life and often the best health care recovery.

A conceptual model is presented in Chapter 1 of this text. Umphred states, "The question arises as to why the sequence worked effectively with one therapist one day and not on the next day with the other therapist." Later she notes that "When two people are interacting as in a client-therapist relationship, each person is responding to the moment-to-moment changes occurring within the environment." The author of these phrases has taken a snapshot of the dilemma facing practitioners. If in fact each client has a right to health care, can such care be delivered in the same way by every health care practitioner? Should we, or could we, standardize care?

OVERVIEW

Disability is more likely to be dramatically reduced through preventive programs than advances in biomedical technology. The notion that we should begin here and not after the fact of trauma seems sensible, yet we are faced with innumerable variables of human nature. Decisions made before catastrophic or complex events are often thought to be made on the basis of soft data, whereas the decisions made after catastrophic or complex events appear to be based on logical, hard data. Medicine has been better equipped to deal with the latter.

How would society deal with funding prevention programs over biomedical programs? Whose responsibility is health? Do people have a right to health? Is there a moral obligation instead to preserve one's own health? How would we measure outcome or progress?

Health is universally revered, and a healthy population ultimately means a productive nation. But can any government or agency, no matter how benevolent or wealthy, promise to deliver health to all people? The term "health" refers to a momentary state. Neither individuals nor societies are stagnant; they are ever changing. The appropriate time to measure health and to influence the state and the worth of the health of the individual is always the same—the moment of attention to it.

The health of the client changes with changing practitioners, environments, cultures, times of day, and political structures. The client's state of health, from the practitioner's point of view, is influenced by the client's professional education and the person he or she is. The extent to which the client's state of health can be influenced, whether at the prospective or retrospective end of the health continuum, depends on the practitioner and the client's current status. The purpose of the relationship between the practitioner and the client is to share information. It is an opportunity for the client to learn about the practitioner's expectations and for the practitioner to learn about the client's expectations. The learning environment facilitates or inhibits the process.

Several factors determine the overall situation in which the client and practitioner operate. There is the internal environment of the client already alluded to. The lesion is one part of that internal environment. There is the internal environment of the practitioner, whose skills are but one part of his or her internal environment. There is an external environment as interpreted by the client, and an external environment as interpreted by the practitioner. These come together through the learning environment. The principles presented in Chapter 1 deliver a strong message. Individuals need to solve problems and must want to solve the problem given a chance that the solutions will be successful. Unless the task fits the individual's current capability, it will be approached by lower-level problem-solving methods. Learning is taking place in all aspects of the client's and practitioner's world, and the client must ultimately take responsibility for the means to solve the problem.

The current curriculums of physical therapy education are including skill areas of education methods. The curricula are influenced, however, by many variables. The resources of the institution of higher education vary, students come with varying backgrounds, requirements of preprofessional programs differ, support services vary, and, of course, the faculty have distinct philosophies of the importance of teaching educational methods. There is no argument that we should prepare practitioners for the important role of education, but the extent to which teaching and learning are emphasized in professional schools varies from very little to moderately important.

Active participation in life and in relationships promotes learning. Rogers[47] defines significant learning as learning that makes a difference, that affects all parts of a person. We have spoken of a relationship—educational in nature and centered on an individual's health. Additionally, one of the individuals involved in the relationship has knowledge that is to be imparted or skills to be practiced on the other. The relationship "works" if the learning environment facilitates exchange. The concept of equal partners is crucial. The issue and practice of informed consent is not just political or ethical; it is central to client care. Voluntariness has to be practiced by both practitioner and client alike. Each has a moral obligation to facilitate the process of health care within the moment. The Western world of medicine has steadily climbed a mountain toward the peak of excellence in medical technology. Why has it taken us so long to recognize the client's need to assume an equal role or for the practitioner to seek the client's help?

Now we pause to reflect. The pause is thrust upon us by diminishing funds for biomedical research, and equally as much by an honest appraisal by practitioners of the issue of quantity versus quality of life. However, the time allotted allows us to look at other health care systems in the world. As we look down from the peak of Western world medicine, our eyes drift to peaks around us, some at the same level of health care, some higher, and many are peaks of mountains that have stood for centuries. What has brought us to this place and where our journey will lead are questions to be dealt with in coming decades.

MEDICAL MODEL OF HEALTH CARE

The medical model is the dominant model of health care in Western society.[34] It forms the conceptual basis for health care in America. The model assumes that illness has an organic base that can be traced to discrete molecular elements. The origin of disease is found at the molecular level of the individual's tissue. The first step toward alleviating the disease is to identify the pathogen that has invaded the tissue and, after proper identification, to apply appropriate treatment techniques.

It is implicit in the model that specialists who are professionally competent have the sole responsibility for the identification of the cause of the illness and for the judgment as to what constitutes appropriate treatment. The medical knowledge required for these judgments is thought to be the domain of the professional medical specialists and therefore inaccessible to the public.

Western medicine is often viewed as having developed from Greek medicine. The Greeks philosophized that humans and nature were inexplicably intertwined, the mind and the body each influencing the health of the other. Diagnosis and cataloging of diseases became more rational during this period of history, which may be a reason for tracing medicine's beginnings to the Greco-Roman era. However, the theory of the interrelationships of the mind and the body is not true of the present medical model of health care. Disease is now viewed in society as a battle between microbes and humans.

Two developments may be more directly responsible for the establishment of today's model of medical practice: the practice of human anatomical dissection and the development of the germ theory of disease. Increasing sophistication in dissection and cellular research formed the basis for scientific medicine as we know it today. The procedure followed is to locate the cells responsible for the disease and eradicate those cells. The health care professional who fails to locate and eradicate the disease is considered by society in general to have failed in his or her responsibility. In the quest to avoid failure, the health care professional therefore welcomes, encourages, and demands technological advances that promise more accurate diagnosis and treatment. Letting nature take its course and allowing the myriad of unmeasurable environmental influences to enter this scientific process are considered a waste of time, money, and resources. The health care professional considers health his or her business only after disease has occurred or stabilized and health has to be restored.[35]

Perhaps the fact that mental illness is now considered a disease in the Western world is further indication of the extent to which medicine focuses on pathology. At any moment a specific pathogen is expected to be found in the tissue of mentally ill patients. Following such an identification, treatment will be possible. Medicine pits technology against nature rather than concentrating on their harmonious coexistence.

Medical science has developed a body of knowledge that the public does not share. It has given the physician and other health professionals, including the therapist, an authority over the public. The knowledge is transmitted from professional to professional in select university settings. The control of the dissemination of knowledge is reinforced by exclusive professional organizations of physicians and other health professionals. The organizations set educational standards for their members, support restricted licensure laws, and enforce a code of ethics. They also monitor, and in some cases control, the practices of groups whose health care activities are related to the particular health profession or impinge on what they consider their particular area of health care.[11]

Health care professionals, on the other hand, are relatively free of control by the public. They have developed a clear professional autonomy over the years. Professionalism has been fostered by rigid admission criteria for students, research-oriented academic departments, and early specialization of practice. The result is that a health care professional who becomes part of such a system embraces its high ideals and then views someone outside the system as having lower status. This approach to professionalism has led to an increasingly narrowed view of dysfunction and its impact on the individual. Such an attitude works against establishing cooperative relationships with the other health professionals who have recently begun to challenge the control that a physician holds over their practices. Extreme professional attitudes that a health care worker may hold regarding the practices of medicine might encourage the professional to see himself or herself as the decision maker in the process of health care. These attitudes would work against the possibility of sharing the role of decision making with the consumer of health care, and they would reflect the model of decision making that was instituted by physicians.[12]

Purtillo and Cassel[43] list three general characteristics of a profession. The first characteristic is that the members claim to have "maximal competence and/or knowledge in a specific area." The second is that a profession "offers a service which is of some significant social value." The third requires that the profession "control its own work": in other words that it have recognized autonomy as a result of its specialized expertise. Physical therapy, for example, is a health profession that has been in existence long enough to see a pattern of professional growth. Physical therapy meets these criteria though it does not have complete autonomy of practice. In most cases, physician's referral is required before a patient can be treated by a therapist, but it is not required for patient evaluations, nor is the actual care monitored on site by the physician.

The health care provided by a physical therapist to the client is based on a medical model. The therapist is trained in medical school environments, licensed by the state following graduation, and has established a national professional organization, the American Physical Therapy Association (APTA).

The APTA[2] accredits physical therapy and physical therapy assistant schools. Individual states license physical therapists, and a physical therapy assistant must, by law, work under the direction of a physical therapist. In the process of this training, a therapist acquires attitudes toward the practice of the profession much like those acquired by a physician. As a result, health professionals continue to seek control of health care through insistence on delivery of health care through the medical model and strengthening of professional organizations. Although the medical model continues to be perpetuated, consumers are now seeking to play a more active role in their health care.

Clients, or consumers of health care, are becoming aware of the impact of medicine's control over their lives. This awareness has been fueled by the price they are paying for that health care. The Surgeon General's report confirms that expenditures for health are increasing.

In addition, preventive care assumes major importance in view of the fact that 75% of all deaths today are the result of degenerative diseases, such as heart disease, cerebrovascular accidents, and cancer. Like other major causes of death, accidents (cited as the most frequent cause of death in persons under age 49) are increasingly linked to life-styles.

The average consumer does not know what medicine can

and cannot do for him or her. The physician and patient therefore must be candid with one another. Personal experience with rising hospital costs, depersonalization as a result of technology, and the exposure to national health problems via mass media have encouraged the consumer to take a more active role in his or her health care. Insurance companies also advocate consumer involvement in hope of reducing payments for health care. Levin[27] points out that there is a lot that consumers can do for themselves. Most people can assume responsibility to care for minor health problems. Use of nonpharmaceutical methods to control pain, (e.g., hypnosis, biofeedback, meditation, and acupuncture) are becoming common. The recognition of the value of approaching illnesses in a wholistic approach is receiving increasing attention in society. Treatment of emotional needs as well as physical needs during illness has been advocated as a way to help individuals regain some control over their lives.

WHOLISTIC MODEL

A **wholistic model** of health care seeks to involve the patient in the process and take the mystery out of health care for the consumer. Successful outcome measures are shifting from the traditional measure of whether the person lives or dies as the outcome indicator of success in health care to the quality of a person's life. The use of the phrase "quality of life" or living implies more than physical health. It implies that the individual is mentally and emotionally healthy as well. It is a holistic (*holos* is the Greek word meaning whole) model of health care that takes the other dimensions of a person's being into consideration regarding health. Hippocrates emphasized treatment of the person as a whole. He emphasized the influence of society and the environment on health. But, as humanity progressed through the ages, the influence of technology and the germ theory of disease moved health care toward a distinct approach based on scientific causation.

A wholistic approach to health care acknowledges that multiple factors are operating in disease, trauma, and aging and that there are many interactions among the factors. Social, emotional, environmental, political, economic, psychological, and cultural factors are all acknowledged to influence health. An approach that takes this perspective centers its philosophy on the individual. The individual with this orientation is less likely to have the physician look only for the chemical basis of his or her difficulty and ignore the psychological factors that may be present.

The wholistic model contains concepts of health care for both the individual and the health care provider. Pelletier[39] mentions six ideas that form the basis for the theory of wholistic health. The first is that all diseases are psychosomatic. All diseases consist of an element that is physical and an element that is emotional or psychological. An individual who is emotionally stressed may trigger onset of disease when infected with a pathogen, whereas another might not. Some stresses can be identified before illness results. Obesity

stresses the cardiovascular system. Preventive care that reduces the stress may also reduce chances of illness: this is a prospective outlook on disease. Another concept relates to the importance of people as individuals. An individual exists within the environment in a unique way and responds to stresses in an infinite variety of ways, not in a stereotyped manner. A third concept is that wholistic health care employs not only conventional but also nontraditional methods (such as acupuncture, massage, and biofeedback) to treat disease. It also uses methods that depart from traditional, scientifically proven ones, such as the Eastern practice of meditation, music, and dance. The fourth concept departs from the negative connotation of disease and illness by suggesting that illness may provide an opportunity for an individual to learn more about himself or herself. An individual may use disease as a chance to get to know personal values and look on it as a time to grow and change. The fifth concept is that of keeping human needs central to health care. Humanness is central to the wholistic philosophy; individual needs should determine a course of care. The sixth concept of wholistic care is central to this study. The health professional and the client should interact in a relationship in which each assumes some responsibility for the process of health care and where each respects the other. The traditional approach fosters dependency, with the professional assuming an authoritative role and the client a passive role. An approach that includes the client in the process has the potential to foster an informed, satisfied client who can take more responsibility for his or her health care. A cooperative relationship develops in programs where the client and the health professional, physician, nurse, or physical therapist, for example, form a partnership. A closer relationship between health professionals and clients, one that involves the client in the process, is advocated.

Individuals in health professions internalize values during their training that reinforce the traditional professional attitude alluded to earlier. Many of these values do not support a partnership relationship with the client. Although society is beginning to question the traditional role of the health professional as the expert, the professional training and organizations resist the pressure to change the image. The professions still hold the image of great authority given to them by the public and fostered through increased political activity.

The major purpose of the patient's relationship with the health professional is to exchange information useful to both in the health care of the client. McNerney[34] calls **health education** of the client the missing link in health care delivery. As the gap grows between technology and the users of that technology, client health education becomes more important than ever. McNerney[34] notes that although health care providers are now making efforts to educate their clients, they are doing so with little consistency, enthusiasm, theoretical base, imagination—and often with little coordination with other services. The health professional continues to receive training and embrace professional organizational membership that places a premium on control of information and control of the decision making. There should be a special effort to introduce health education concepts into the basic educational programs of health care professionals.

When patients are given more information about their illnesses, and retain the information, they express more satisfaction with their caregivers. A study by Bertakis[4] tested the hypothesis that patients with greater understanding and retention of the information given by the physician would be more satisfied with the doctor-patient relationship. The experimental group received feedback and retained 83.5% of the information given them by the doctor. The control group received no feedback and retained 60.5% of the information. Not surprisingly, the experimental group was more satisfied with the doctor-patient relationship.

If the client is to be informed and included in the treatment process, client health education will have to go beyond the present styles of information giving. If the client is to assume some of the responsibility for his or her therapy, the therapist will have to facilitate that involvement. The attitude of the therapist toward educating clients about their health could affect his or her ability to facilitate client involvement in the care process.

The more the professional sees himself or herself as the expert, the less likely he or she will be to see the client as capable of responsibility or expertise in the care process. If communication skills and health education were a part of medical school and the other health professional school curricula, perhaps the health care professionals would temper their assumption of the "expert" professional role. Payton[38] points out that it is the client alone who can ultimately decide whether a goal is worth working for. Careful planning can be influential in helping all providers include the client in the process.

The health care delivery system in America has to serve all of the citizens. That is no easy task. The United States is a society of great pluralism. It is a free society. It is a society that is used to being governed by persuasion, not coercion. Given the variety of economic, political, cultural and religious forces at work in American society, education of the people in regard to their health care is probably the only method that can work in the long run. The future task of health education will be to "cultivate people's sense of responsibility toward their own health and that of the community." Health education is an effective approach with perhaps the most potential to move us toward a concept of preventive care.

Generation of a new model

Carlson[7] thinks that pressure to change to wholistic thinking in medicine continues as a result of a societal change in its perspective of the rights of individuals. A concern to keep the individual central in the care process will continue to grow in response to continued technological growth that threatens to dehumanize care even more. The wholistic model takes into account each person's unique psychosocial, political, economic, environmental, and religious needs as they affect the individual's health.

Engel[12] sees a need to broaden the approach to disease and include the psychosocial aspects without sacrificing the advantages of the biomedicine model. He accepts Von Bertalanffy's theory that all life events are linked to each other in an ascending order of complexity, from molecules to organs to individuals to families to communities, to society to the universe, and that a change in any of these ultimately affects another element of the chain. With this interdependence in mind, a new medical model that has the following characteristics is suggested: (1) a biochemical defect does not have to be present for a human to experience illness, (2) behavioral processes would be related to the biochemical changes, (3) other variables of life would be taken into account as they interact with somatic function, (4) the patient's view of his or her illness would be taken into account, (5) treatment would be directed at the psychosocial aspects of illness as well, and (6) the relationship of the provider and the client would be recognized as it influences the outcome of the disease process.

Fink[14] also views health as a hierarchy of systems and supports a wholistic model of care. He includes the provider and patient relationship as a major variable in health care delivery. Fink envisions a continuum from the point when the patient is a passive recipient of the provider's care to a point where the provider and the patient each contribute to the relationship to the final point of patient self-care.

The unique religious nature of human beings makes health not an end in itself, but an important means to better experience life and allow individuals to accomplish what they strive for. Pastoral counselors who observed patients visiting their physician too late in their illness appealed to the American Medical Association's Committee on Medicine and Religion to use pastoral counseling as a complementary service to the physician, and the first holistic health center was established in 1970. As a result, pastoral counselors met the patient when he or she came in, established a friendly atmosphere, and administered a personal health inventory scale. The patient participates in an internal planning conference, explaining what kind of help he or she wants and participating in selecting alternatives for care.

Life-style/stress

One of the assumptions practitioners of wholistic health commonly make is that a person with a physically or mentally self-abusive life-style is not free of pathology. This statement is made more credible in light of Breslow's findings.[5] Breslow looked at 7000 Californians' health habits of: (1) no smoking, (2) moderate drinking, (3) 7 or 8 hours sleep each night, (4) regular meals with no snacks, (5) breakfast each day, (6) maintenance of normal weight, and

(7) regular exercise. He concluded that if a person followed all seven of the habits, his or her health was significantly better than that of a person who followed only six, and so on. He was able to relate the findings with longevity figures to further substantiate his findings.

The most significant cause of all the illness or disorders that cannot be explained at the molecular level is stress. Migraine headache and hypertension have not been found to be convincingly explained by the presence of a pathogen. Rather they develop over a period of time, and stress is thought to play a major role. Selye[51] has done the primary scientific research in this area, and has described a formal syndrome, the general adaptation syndrome. It consists of three stages: (1) an alarm reaction when the anterior pituitary gland secretes adrenocorticotrophic hormone, (2) a stage of resistance when physiological secretion ceases, and (3) a stage of exhaustion when the body loses capacity to respond to further stress. If the stage of exhaustion continues, the animal dies. Psychological problems can stress the body. Selye conceptualizes that an organ has a certain capacity for tolerating stress; if this capacity is exceeded, the organism will break down.

In Brown's work[6] with biofeedback, she observed the activity of subconscious action during stress. She reasoned that if subconscious centers are responsible for stress and if stress accounts for a large proportion of illness, an intervention that acts through those centers similar to biofeedback is reasonable. It provides an opportunity for the individual to become aware of his or her internal state and thus to take a first step toward changing it.

Kreiger[25] researched the effects of the sensation of touching on decreasing stress. She studied nurses in New York, half of whom used a lot of touching in their patient care and a control group who did not. The patients in the experiment had blood samples drawn before and after treatment. Kreiger hypothesized that if touch had an effect, it could be found physiologically in a hemoglobin change in the patient and that the mean hemoglobin values of the experimental group would be higher after treatment. The experimental group did show a significant increase in their hemoglobin mean value, though the increase may only have been part of a larger unidentified response. Kreiger has been the first to define this aspect of human interaction in physiological terms.

Holmes and Rahe[22] hypothesized that an event is probably as stressful as the person perceives it to be. They attempted to quantify events in the social environment that can be classed as stressful, for example, death of a loved one or a change of jobs. The events they chose theoretically required some kind of adaptation by the individual. They listed the events and assigned points for each. It appeared that, when a certain number of such events occurred in a person's life within a prescribed time, that person's chances of becoming physically ill increased.

Friedman and Rosenman[17] classified people who are described as type A and type B. Type As are hard-driving, aggressive people and Bs are more easy going. They found a significant number of cardiovascular problems occurring in type A people as opposed to type B.

Stein and others[53] reviewed the effect of hypothalamic lesions on the immune processes of the body. The condition of hypothalamus has been identified as a good indicator to the body's reaction to psychosocial stress. They saw corresponding changes in both the autonomic nervous system and in neuroendocrine activity. They recorded further studies to evaluate the immune processes response to stress.

Hough[23] reminds us that we are often faced with situations in physical therapy in which we can offer little professional skilled help, but that the offer of autonomy for clients, by allowing them some control of events can reduce feelings of helplessness and resultant stress.

Client participation

Becker and Maiman[3] discussed Rosenstock's Health Belief model as a framework to account for the individual's decision to use preventive services or engage in preventive health behavior. They cite noncompliance with a physician's recommendation in about one third of all patients. Action taken by the individual, according to the model, depends on the individual's perceived susceptibility to the illness, his or her perception of the severity of the illness, the benefits to be gained from taking action, and a "cue" of some sort that triggers action. The cue could be advice from a friend, reading an article about the illness, a television commercial, and so on. In some way, the person is motivated to do something.

Split-brain research, research in the functions of the left and right halves of the brain, seems to be a pertinent area of mind-body research. The left hemisphere of the brain processes experiences in a factual, logical, and analytical way, whereas the right half appears to process the same experiences in the form of images and impressions. The recognition that one half of the brain may be designed to record the impressionistic part of an experience gives further credibility to including the individual's accounts of his feelings and emotions as a part of the input for diagnosis of illness.

Travis[55] considers the responsibility the client takes for his or her own health care to be at the heart of the wholistic health model. Travis is a physician who set up a Wellness Resource Center in California and developed a wellness inventory to assess the individual's present state of health. He recognizes three distinct phases in promoting the health of the client: (1) an assessment (the wellness inventory), (2) education of the client to learn the options available and to participate in choice of treatment, and (3) growth toward wellness. Growth toward wellness includes trying some of the options and reevaluating them after a period of time. He reasons that each person has responsibility for his or her own health and that no one can change anyone unless that person wants to be changed. Wellness is a lifelong process. Travis views health as client-oriented and emphasizes wholistic thinking as opposed to the reductionist thinking of biomedicine.

Two articles have appeared in reputable medical journals written by patients experiencing a serious illness who have taken responsibility for their own health care. The first article is an account by Norman Cousins[9] Cousins was stricken with ankylosing spondolitis. Bedridden and given 1 chance in 500 to survive, he analyzed his situation. He had been suffering exhaustion, and remembering what he had read about exhaustion and the influence of stress on chemical changes in the glands, he decided that if negative reactions produced stresses, positive ones might halt the process. He had the full support of his doctor. He placed himself in a pleasant environment, reduced his medication, increased his intake of vitamin C, and watched a lot of funny movies to keep his spirits high. He found that the nodules in his hands shrank, he moved with less pain, and he began to walk again. Cousins said that the placebo effect is demonstrated here and that the will to live was translated somehow into a physical reality of healing.

Fiore,[16] a psychologist, wrote of his experience in surviving cancer. He came to a point where he felt that he was taking drugs more to please his oncologist and support a research project than for his own health's sake. He actively sought to regain some control that he felt he had lost by insisting that a hospital tumor board review his case. Because the specialized physician is too busy, he advocated the use of ancillary personnel to provide emotional and psychological support. They can conduct nutrition, fitness, and relaxation classes and help patients communicate their feelings. Fiore encourages patients to become more independent to enhance the quality of their lives. He advocates that patients be viewed as experts about their own feelings.

Glickman and colleagues,[19] responded with letters to the editor after publication of Fiore's article. Glickman's comment was that a team approach tends to deflect responsibility from the physician who can "best perform those tasks"; Manson thought Fiore was wrong to implicate life-style as responsible for cancer or its cure, and that entering the process as he did is a cause of more harm than help. The last of the three to respond, Ellison, supported Fiore's ideas. He suggested, in particular, that words like "terminal" and phrases like "nothing else can be done" be omitted from conversation between patients and physicians since they form mental images that the patient finds hard to forget or escape from. He supports the active involvement of the patient.

Dubos[10] stated that even though societal and environmental conditions may be harmful to a client in the long run and even though medical experts think they understand and can anticipate what is best for the client, that does not give them the license to decide what is best for the client. The role of medicine, Dubos cautioned, is to help people achieve a healthy state so they can make their own decisions.

Issues

So far, there are no data on comparative studies between the traditional medical model approach to health care and the wholistic model of health care. A few authors have discussed the approaches.[15,36] They list the benefits of a wholistic approach as broadening the perspectives on illness, potentially affecting chronic disease, lowering costs, demystifying health care, making health care more democratic, making clients aware of our current health care delivery system problem, and improving patient-provider relationships. There are limitations of the wholistic approach as well. Limitations include bringing inappropriate areas of living into the health care problem, the fact that people may deal too subjectively with their problems, and that acceptability of the health problem would vary with the social class of the individual.[36] Self-help may ultimately benefit people who already have a better chance for survival. It is also unrealistic to expect changes in health care if societal problems of employment, housing, income, and racism are not dealt with at the same time. The medical profession's power and vested financial interest are societal problems to be dealt with in this context.[15]

Hayes-Bautista and Harveston[20] pointed out that for the person to cooperate and work on the health problem with the provider, the problem does have to be well defined. Many of the daily problems of health care that could respond to wholistic approach are multifaceted and have more than one possible approach or solution. They are often handled at present by community health clinics, which are set up in traditional modes and are not equipped in terms of knowledge, manpower, and resources to deal with health problems in a wholistic way.

Freymann[18] sees a problem getting health care workers excited about preventive care. A successful case of preventive care would mean that no medical action would have to be taken. Clinical medicine involving active intervention, such as surgery, evaluation of complex laboratory tests, and the problem-solving approach to diagnosis, is what excites health care workers today. Freymann ponders the strange logic of traditional medicine, which rewards the specialist who confines his or her practice to a very few and shows little concern for a public health physician whose field is broad and who treats so many. Dramatic traditional medicine does not result in many health benefits for large numbers of people.

McKay[33] asks to what extent health providers are willing to commit themselves to explore and implement alternative forms of health care. The provider-client relationship becomes very important to a successful therapeutic outcome, as does health education and promotion of positive health behaviors. Health providers seem to forget that well-being calls for wellness of the mind, body, and environment. Though they may talk about supporting a focus on health they continue to focus on disease. The training that health providers receive makes disease more interesting than wellness.

Saward and Sorenson[48] observe that the mass media has promoted the technology of health care. The consumer thus has a heightened expectation of the quality of care he or she will receive. However, we should avoid excesses in the other extreme. If society adheres to inappropriate life-styles, the health professional cannot turn around and blame the victim for bringing on the illness and absolve himself or herself from responsibility. Wholistic health care carried to an extreme might result in "blaming the victim." Saward and Sorenson see that in the extremes, the medical model and the wholistic model of health care have different objectives; evolve from different historical, philosophical and economic perspectives; and use practitioners with essentially different training and outlook on health care. Perhaps, they suggest, two health care systems should be available to people instead of one.

Szasz and Hollender[54] described five basic relationships between providers and clients on a continuum from a provider-dominated relationship, consistent with the medical model, through a mutual participation relationship, to a relationship where the client accepts the larger share of responsibility, which is consistent with the wholistic model. Whether the client takes some responsibility for his or her care depends a great deal on whether the health provider gives some to him or her.

Fink[14] also recognized the importance of the **provider-patient relationship** and made three points about it. The first is that a relationship between them is given. The second is that what the relationship becomes is mutually agreed on, consciously or not. Third, whatever the form of the relationship, it should meet the needs and health care requirements of the particular patient.

Trends

Monaco[37] claims that despite the difficulty in identifying all the elements of the wholistic model, the wholistic health advocates are multiplying. They are coming from all walks of life, and their very enthusiasm may produce a rift in the health care field with traditional medicine on one side and wholistic medicine on the other. As the wholistic movement begins to gather data, there will be a more realistic basis for blending the models or for separating them. Monaco thinks it will be the consumer who decides which it will be. Maer[31] sees the technological gains of the past 25 years slowing and biomedical research retrenching. He urges that research in the human sciences be promoted to a point of excellence. Strong support will come from the younger generation with its natural optimism and differing points of view.

One of the issues consumers and society will have to deal with is that standards of care have been traditionally linked to licensure. Wholistic health practitioners are usually unlicensed, and many physicians avoid associating with them in order to protect their image. Yahn[58] urges that standards of care be part of the future for wholistic practitioners and that regulations be set for direction.

Health education has been mentioned by nearly all of the proponents of wholistic care. Sechrist[50] cautioned the health educator not to get on the bandwagon. He feels that wholistic health care's education goals are still very nebulous. To prove its value, health education should address more well-defined problems. Though the wholistic health care goals are in tune with health education, joining the trend might result in disruption within the field just as it is beginning to establish an identity.

Which model will result in better health care? McDermott[32] advocates regularly identifying the variables in whichever model is used, measuring their effect, and taking corrective actions necessary to assure quality care. An important corrective action he suggests is to educate the health provider at the level of the school curriculum. Two major variables present in every health care setting are the attitudes the provider has toward the practice of his or her profession and the attitudes he or she holds toward educating clients and involving them in the process.

CLIENT HEALTH EDUCATION
Client/provider relationship

The relationship between the provider and the client is a major variable in quality of care in every health-related setting. The extent to which the care given is biomedical or wholistic can be traced to that intimate encounter and the attitudes, values, and beliefs that each of the participants bring to it.

Leopold[26] called the relationship of the therapist and client "the emotional bridge over which the more mechanical forms of treatment are conducted." The psychological makeups of the therapist and of the client have an impact on the relationship that is established. The psychological development of both of them during their growth stages of dependency, aggressiveness, and ability to subordinate personal gratification must be acknowledged as having an effect on the relationship.

The illness or trauma of the client that represents a disintegrating force in his or her life may represent an opportunity for the therapist to grow professionally. The client and the therapist may have different psychological backgrounds, and though the client is usually there because of the medical crisis, the therapist may be there for purposes of personal growth, financial gain, prestige, and unconscious gratification in influencing the lives of others through professional skill.

Awareness of the importance of these factors would

enable the therapist to approach the relationship with better understanding.

Pratt[42] recognized the large amount of time a physical therapist spends in face-to-face patient contact. In this respect, the therapist has an advantage over most other health practitioners who see the patient at infrequent intervals and who seldom touch the patient as a physical therapist does. The physical contact itself may provide psychological support and promote a close relationship between the therapist and the patient. It is important then that the therapist be aware of the importance of the relationship itself. The therapist's attitudes and values can affect the expectations of patients regarding the outcome of treatment. The patient's expectations can be made realistic if he or she is an active participant in care from the start. Any process that involves personal commitment and purports to effect change should focus on the person seeking help. An attitude of acceptance of the patient as an equal in the process may be of healing value by itself and referred to as **empowerment.**

Ramsden[44] discussed the reality that transference (i.e., the client incorporating some of the therapist's qualities) takes place during physical therapy treatments as it does whenever human contact takes place. Though physical therapy purports to recognize the importance of the whole patient, there is still a major focus on the physical aspect of patient care and little on the psychological aspects. Professional responsibility in therapy extends to the development of maximal efficiency in interpersonal communication. Enough is known about the area of communication to teach it to practitioners rather than allowing it to develop by chance.

Conine[8] noted that there are reports that therapists spend nearly one quarter of their time with patients listening or talking. However, therapists have had little training in listening attentively or tolerating silence in conversation. In their own education they also have had too little experience of being listened to in order to appreciate the importance of doing that for others. If listening to a patient can relieve that patient's anxieties, the patient might be more motivated to channel energy into working to help himself or herself. Conine conjectured that much of the superficial conversation that goes on during treatment sessions may be an attempt on the part of the therapist to avoid release of the patient's deep-seated thoughts. The therapist may not feel capable of dealing with those thoughts. Listening to the patient is particularly important if the therapist wants to understand the patient's needs to formulate treatment programs and instruct the patient.

A role common to all therapists is that of educator. **Patient/client education** is receiving more emphasis, particularly in areas of chronic disease. Patient education programs have to be evaluated to determine how much this contributes to quality care and cost containment. Clients with chronic disease of a certain type may react in a manner influenced by the disease. For example, a client in chronic pain from arthritis may become used to the pain and deny its

presence at times. In such cases, it may be difficult to separate the disease's influence on the client's commitment to involvement in the healing process from the provider's influence on involving the client. Rand[45] pointed out how rarely patient education programs are evaluated. She advocated a comprehensive evaluation model including listing of needs, goals, criteria for success, plans, and outcomes. The therapist in an educator's role would want to evaluate the patient education program to see if the objectives were met to establish the worth of the program, and to get information to help with decision making.

The scientific foundation of physical therapy relates movement and exercise to pathological conditions. Hislop[21] describes the major role of the therapist as that of a pathokinesiologist. She acknowledges that the interpersonal relationships with patients may characterize a major area of a therapist's work, but she cautions that the profession must focus on its scientific role if it wants to survive. Basic and applied scientific research supplied by our own professionals, is necessary. Although she recognizes the humanistic and social responsibility that any profession must have, Hislop stresses our lack of a strong base of scientific knowledge and urges that therapists take on the research role to add to our body of scientific knowledge. She adds that science must be balanced with humanistic care and does not believe that a sharper scientific focus would obscure our roles as humanistic care givers.

Long[28] suggests that the consumers become as knowledgeable as possible about their condition, find out the level of the therapist's professional education, question the therapist about the equipment used, be aware of treatments that go on too long or treatments with little result. He also advocates that consumers ask for detailed instructions and demonstrations, use logic, and practice thinking for themselves.

As the consumer becomes more involved, so should the family. The family is seldom brought into the practice. Sasano and others[49] described a patient program that includes the family. They made some comments relative to therapy's inclusion of the family in the care process. Patients were happier with the family involved; the family itself felt less anxious and could be more supportive. All of these factors facilitate the work of the therapist. The therapist, however, must be willing to facilitate the family involvement and help them learn to take responsibility for some of the care and decision making. Most health professionals are not conditioned to the patient assuming greater authority. The family cannot take responsibility for the care unless the therapist allows the family to assume that role.

Lopopola and others[29] formed a comprehensive care team for arthritic patients. The departments of internal medicine, orthopedics, physical therapy, and occupational therapy worked closely with the patient and family. Intensive training and education were carried out, and a follow-up program was established. A stated goal was to produce an atmosphere to encourage the patient to take responsibility for his or her care. To compare program effectiveness and cost of care, 20 patients were studied in a conventional way and 20 cared for by the team concept. Results of the program showed that for the group that had been cared for by the team concept: (1) length of stay had shortened; (2) communication between the professional departments involved had improved; (3) program planning had become a team effort and included the patient and the family; and (4) patients felt less confused about their program of care. The authors believed they had found a way to increase quality of care and decrease costs for arthritic patients using a team approach. Versloot and others[57] looked at the client enrolled in a back school in a longitudinal controlled field study. They concluded that studies conducted to date indicate that even simple health educational programs are capable of deversing absenteeism, which, by nature reflects cost savings.

A multidisciplinary pain management center was the setting for a program described by Roesch and Ulrich.[46] Physical therapy has traditionally focused on the pain reported by the patient. In this center, the therapists applied behavior modification techniques to attempt to extinguish the patient's pain behavior. Education was carried out including assertiveness training and awareness of the dynamics of the chronic pain syndrome. Physical therapy exercises were done in groups and lectures were conducted on body mechanics, exercise, and gait. Self-motivation was encouraged by giving the patient options to increase activity and participate in establishing a schedule to eliminate assistive devises such as braces. The patient and family participated in the home program planning. Therapists felt that with this overall approach the patients became less anxious and more knowledgeable and thus less susceptible to reinjury. They encouraged the therapists to create an atmosphere that allows the patient to change and gradually move from a focus on treatment of the pain to a focus on activity in the treatment of chronic pain.

The therapist is caught up in the same problems of the health care system as other health professionals. Inflation has caused profit to become a more important motive for setting priorities in our clinics than human considerations. Research is heavily focused on technical procedures, yet the relationship with patients in the care process is vital. Singleton[52] labeled this phenomenon a paradox in physical therapy. Despite the commitment to humanistic service on which the profession was founded, the service rendered is mechanistic.

Is the patient approached like a machine? Has scientific technology captured the therapist's attention to the extent that he or she ignores patient care procedures that cannot or have not been scientifically analyzed? Alexander[1] sees the necessity of reorganizing the education and work of the therapist to encourage a humanistic approach to care. To what degree, Alexander[1] asks, are we "masters or servants to our patients?" The educational programs could emphasize whole-patient treatment, increase communication skills and interdisciplinary awareness, video-tape students as they

interact with others, and encourage role-playing. Finally, he proposes that although restructuring educational experiences is useful, selection procedures also have to be considered.

If medicine succeeds in bringing humanistic medicine into focus and shifting some emphasis from a scientific technology approach, it is conceivable that some people currently suited to practicing therapy would find it intolerable to do so in the future.

The community role

Today's complex world of health care goes beyond the one-to-one health care relationship. To achieve quality care for a neurologically disabled individual, the community must be utilized. Prevention of head injuries can be the focus of many community groups. Prevention programs in the community can address both the chemical and mechanical standards of that community's environment. The employers in the area should have safe working environments and programs should exist for stress reduction, counseling, and family-related concerns. Traffic problems, regulations for safe recreational pursuits—everything, in short, that affects our living from day to day—involves our community and that community's willingness to create as hazard-free an environment as possible.

One task of communication is to reduce risk-taking decisions for the client. The responsibility falls first on the shoulders of the health care professional dealing with the patient, but the success of that undertaking is also directly related to the support the client receives from the community in which the client lives. All activities that relate to achieving that goal are under consideration for any client, but particularly for the neurologically involved individual whose disability spans the continuum of need for support.

Questions to be considered are the following: (1) How comprehensive should the services be? (2) How much continuity of service is available? (3) Are creative solutions sought to the problems within the community? (4) Does a rational planning process exist that gathers input from all citizens and sets priorities? (5) Is there a commitment of the community to follow through with the necessary budget support?

Criticisms of community services include lack of commitment to such programs, focus on individual problems of the client as opposed to setting broader goals and putting in place programs that benefit many, failure to integrate such services, placing low priority on educating both community lay people and the health care workers in all aspects of the problem, neglecting nontraditional methods of care, and placing low priority on planning and evaluation. The results of research studies that are well controlled and conducted seldom find their way into the publications read or utilized by planners or users of such systems.

Appropriate efforts that could be undertaken by communities to provide support to the neurologically disabled individual include: (1) moving from an emphasis on clinical intervention to a use of community funds for education programs aimed at prevention of, for example accidents and risk-taking behaviors; (2) involving individuals in the community; (3) developing councils of agencies on such matters; (4) sponsoring seminars and workshops for families and peers of clients to help them deal with the stress, anger, and guilt, as well as workshops on care giving and utilizing available resources; (5) clarifying roles of care within the community by making a realistic master plan for the care within the community; (6) educating and training those people who provide the care and not leaving it entirely up to the specific agency or professional group to do it in isolation; (7) bringing in experts in the field to disseminate the latest findings; (8) establishing a reference guide through the library and creating ready access to materials needed by clients and their families; (9) gathering community support for the volunteer services needed by nursing homes in the area and maintaining lines of communication with those homes and the community at large (especially to make clear lines of communication possible in such areas as zoning and housing regulations and transportation within the community); (10) establishing a center in town where clients and/or families can gather, discuss common interests, socialize, and find information, or if such a center cannot be funded, using volunteers trained to man such a center; (11) motivating the leaders of the community to get involved, including the philanthropic and church groups; and (12) as services proliferate, helping the community keep track of them, keeping records becomes increasingly important. Computerization may help coordinate and create access to services. As in all programs run by a collective group, to be successful the group has to want success. Even one well-run service for the client can be a major breakthrough.

A WHOLISTIC APPROACH TO THE NEUROLOGICAL CLIENT

Neurological clients interact with the medical community for short or long periods of time. They present neurological problems of all types that are sudden or insidious in nature. All aspects of human function are represented in the variety of problems. If individual beliefs and values energize and motivate physical behavior, think of the possibilities for stimulating wellness.

Ida Rolf[41] and Feldenkrais[13] put forth dramatic, new ways of approaching well-being. Research has just begun on naturally occurring opiates within the brain and on the ability to control body functions through sensory feedback. Perhaps the art and science of care are coming closer together. Many areas of therapeutic intervention once ignored by health professionals are watched with more than intellectual curiosity. Flynn[15] states that this new interest quite possibly signals the beginning of a paradigm shift in health care. The shift to a new model should make use of current knowledge, dispose of outdated information, and incorporate new information.

That new information is becoming available. Additionally, some information that has been available is becoming visible.[15] As health care practitioners, our therapeutic choices have widened. Reasons include a heightened awareness of "the Heisenberg Uncertainty Principle," in which Heisenberg hypothesized that if you are specific about the exact location of an electron at any one point of time, you cannot also specify its momentum or velocity. The transfer to therapeutic intervention has been stated in such a way that if you observe or look at an object, that object is changed. It is no longer the object it was before the observation. Thus certain aspects of an object or individual will always remain undefinable. We become part of the person we observe or touch.

Pribham, a neurophysiologist, has demonstrated the brain as a holographic model.[15] Gabor received a Nobel Prize in 1947 for his work in holography, whose idea is that the waveform of light scattered by an object is recorded on a plate as an interference pattern. When the photographic record, hologram, is subjected to a laser beam, the original wave pattern creates a three-dimensional image of the photographed object. A piece of the hologram, when exposed to the laser beam, gives a representation of the whole object. Pribham has proposed, with substantiating evidence, that the brain works that way with long-term memory. The whole of a memory is contained or retrieved from each of millions of fragmented parts. In other words, each of the fragments or parts contains the whole, making it possible, as William Blake wrote, "to see the world in a grain of sand."[15]

It is important to recall that the entire nervous system begins with the formation of one embryonic disc. Each cell is derived from its parent cells in methodical fashion. Once complete, however, the system attains a complexity of communication that remains little understood. Physical laws have been applied to explain the function. For example, Muller's law of specific energies states that specific sensations are activated by specialized nerve endings for that sensation. The cornea, however, has shown responses of touch, cold, warmth, and pain though only bare nerve endings exist on that surface.

Prigigine, a physical chemist, proposed a theory of dissipative structures. In general, the theory states that certain fluctuations can be the means used by fluid, self-organizing systems to change. The fluctuations or mechanisms that cause the fluctuation are often a result of altered states of consciousness, such as meditation. These changes in energy fields of neurons have been demonstrated by electroencephalogram. These energy fields create fluctuation in areas of the brain, and the theory states that in this way systems such as the human mind can reorder and reorganize patterns of thinking and feeling. Music, imagery, rhythmic breathing, moving, and relaxation are implicated.[15]

It is beyond the scope of this chapter to begin an exploration of each tool that could be used therapeutically. Some have received more attention than others. A partial list includes biofeedback, acupressure, acupuncture, hypnosis, herbal nutrition, transactional analysis, yoga, Feldenkrais, rolfing, martial arts, occult sciences, transcendental meditation, homeopathic medicine, imaging, awareness of roles of stress, laughter, and relaxation.

The effects of neural activity have been shown to last for tens of minutes through release of synaptic transmitters. Time probably plays a major role in effecting permanent change in the nervous system. The systems mentioned above (i.e., music, breathing) are potentially reinforcing phenomena with their regular, rhythmical influence. In such cases, perhaps, rhythmic influence over time creates permanent change.

CURRENT ISSUES
Health care reform

The nation faces significant social change in the area of health care. The coming years will change the access to health care for our citizens, the benefits, the reimbursement process for providers, and the delivery system.

Health care providers have a major role in the success of the final product. The Pew Health Professions Commission[40] identified issues that must be addressed as any new system is developed, implemented, and addressed. Most, if not all, of the issues involve close interactions of the provider and client. Issues include: (1) the need of the provider to stay in step with client needs, (2) need for flexible educational structures to address a system that reassigns certain responsibilities to other personnel, (3) need to redirect national funding priorities away from narrow, pure research access to include broader concepts of health care, (4) the licensing of health care providers, (5) the need to address the issues of minority groups, (6) the need to emphasize general care with less concentration on educating specialists, (7) the issue of promoting teamwork, and (8) the need to emphasize the community as the focus of health care. There are other important issues, but the last to be included here is mentioned in more detail because it is relevant to the consumer.

The Pew Commission[40] concludes that the public has not been educated about the health care workforce and the consumer's role in it. Without the consumer's understanding during development of a new system, the system could omit several opportunities for enrichment of design. Without the understanding of the consumer during implementation of a new system, the consumer might block delivery systems due to lack of knowledge.

All of the information about health care reform conveys with certainty the role of the client as the center of the focus of care. The client will assume greater involvement, greater responsibility, and greater control of the personal care process.

Providers will be more willing to include the client; will design care for the client; and be better able to educate the client, address the issues of minority clients, and become proactive team caregivers. The influence of such methods will extend to the community and lead to greater **patient/client satisfaction.**

Health care for the year 2000

Neurological rehabilitation will take place in a conceivably changed environment and with a changed delivery system in the year 2000. The balance between visionary and pragmatist must be maintained.

Client-centered care is a reality. As visionaries we will find new ways of sharing information with our client; computers will aid in this effort. The provider will set functional outcomes and work to accomplish performance goals. More people will be involved in the care process, and the process will extend on a continuum from acute care, through to the home setting. As a pragmatist, the provider must continue to enhance health care on a daily basis for each client. The case can be made that the most powerful tool for successful outcome is education.

SUMMARY

The responsibility for the well-being of our clients may well rest within our capability more than we know. This chapter has postulated that, with increased understanding of the client-provider relationship and elements of human nature, we can enhance the client's physical function. Quality of life may be influenced as much by programs of prevention within the community as by biomedical research advances day by day. Much of the environment within our reach can be used to create change for the client. The relationships between the client and the health care provider are influential. Patterns of support systems and belief and value systems are also powerful vehicles of change. Perhaps the art and science of health care are moving closer together. The illness-to-wellness continuum is really a circle. One never just backs up or goes forward on the line. One is changed forever from moment to moment. The therapeutic relationship involves two people, changed forever by and within the relationship, circling along the continuum of health, each teaching and each learning.

REFERENCES

1. Alexander DA: Yes, but what about the patient? *Physiotherapy* 59:391-394, 1973.
2. American Physical Therapy Association: Progress Report 9, July/August, 1980.
3. Becker M and Maiman L: Sociobehavioral determinants of compliance with health and medical care recommendation, *Med Care* 13:10-24, 1975.
4. Bertakis K: The communication of information from physician to patient: a method for increasing patient practice, *J Fam Pract* 5:217-222, 1977.
5. Breslow L: A positive strategy for the nation's health, *JAMA* 242:2093-2095, 1979.
6. Brown BB: *Stress and the art of biofeedback*, New York, 1977, Harper & Row.
7. Carlson RJ: Holism and reductionism as perspectives in medicine and patient care, *West J Med* 131:466-470, 1979.

8. Conine T: Listening in the helping relationship, *Phys Ther* 56:159-162, 1976.

9. Cousins N: Anatomy of an illness (as perceived by the patient), *N Eng J Med* 295:1458-1463, 1976.

10. Dubos R: The state of health and the quality of life, *West J Med* 25:8-9, 1976.

11. Duffy J: *The healers: the rise of the medical establishment,* New York, 1976, McGraw-Hill.

12. Engel GL: The need for a new medical model: a challenge for biomedicine, *Science* 196:129-133, 1977.

13. Feldenkrais M: *Awareness through movement,* New York, 1972, Harper & Row.

14. Fink D: Holistic health: the evolution of western medicine. In Flynn P, editor: *The healing continuum,* Bowie, Md, 1980, Robert J Brady Co.

15. Flynn P: *Holistic health,* Bowie, Md, 1980, Robert J Brady Co, Prentice-Hall Pub. Co.

16. Fiore N: Fighting cancer: one patient's perspective, *N Engl J Med* 300:284-289, Feb 1979.

17. Friedman M and Rosenman RH: Type A behavior pattern: its association with coronary heart disease, *J Clin Res* 3:300-312, 1971.

18. Freymann JG: Medicine's great schism, prevention vs. cure: an historical interpretation, *Med Care* 13:525-536, 1975.

19. Glickman L, Manson A, and Ellison NM: Letter to the editor, *N Engl J Med* 12:1219-1220, 1979.

20. Hayes-Bautista D and Harveston DS: Holistic health care, *Soc Policy* 7:7-13, 1977.

21. Hislop HJ: The not-so-impossible dream, *Phys Ther* 55:1069-1080, 1975.

22. Holmes TH and Rahe RH: The social readjustment rating scale, *J Psychosom Res* 11:213-218, 1967.

23. Hough A: Communication in health care 73:2, Feb. 1987, pp. 56-59.

24. Jensen GM and others: The novice versus the experienced clinician: insights into the work of the physical therapist, *Phys Ther* 70:314-332, 1990.

25. Kreiger D: Therapeutic touch: the imprimatur of nursing, *Am J Nurs* 75:784-787, 1975.

26. Leopold RL: Patient-therapist relationship: psychological considerations, *Phys Ther* 34:8-13, 1954.

27. Levin L: Forces and issues in the revival of interest in self-care impetus for redirection in health, *Health Educ Monogr* 5:115, Summer 1977.

28. Long RW: Physical therapy and the consumer, *Health Educ* 6:18-21, 1975.

29. Lopopolo RB and others: Minimal care concept, *Phys Ther* 58:700-703, 1978.

30. Mahew LB and others: *The quest for quality.* San Francisco, 1990, Jossey-Bass Pub., pp. 136-137.

31. Masi LA: A wholistic concept of health and illness: a tricentennial goal for medicine and public health, *J Chron Dis* 31:563-572, 1978.

32. McDermott W: Evaluating the physician and his technology. In Knowles JH, editor: *Doing better and feeling worse,* New York, 1977, WW Norton Co.

33. McKay S: Holistic health care: challenge to providers, *J Allied Health,* 9:194-201, 1980.

34. McNerney WJ: The missing link in health services, *J Med Educ* 50:11-23, 1975.

35. Mechanic D: *Medical sociology,* New York, 1978, The Free Press.

36. Menke WG: Medical identity: change and conflict in professional roles, *J Med Educ* 46:58-63, 1971.

37. Monaco AJ: Coming of wholistic medicine, *Hosp Top* 56:10-11, July-Aug 1978.

38. Payton OD: *Patient participation in program planning: a manual for therapists.* Philadelphia, 1990, FA Davis.

39. Pelletier KR: *Mind as healer, mind as slayer,* New York, 1977, Dell.

40. Pew Health Professions Commission: Healthy America: *Practitioners for 2005.* San Francisco, 1991, the University of California.

41. Pierce R: Rolfing. In Bauman E and others, editors: *The holistic health handbook,* Berkeley, 1978, And/Or Press.

42. Pratt JW: A psychological view of the physiotherapist's role, *Physiotherapy* 64:241-242, 1978.

43. Purtillo RB and Cassel CK: *Ethical dimensions in the health professions,* Philadelphia, 1981, WB Saunders.

44. Ramsden EL: Interpersonal communications in physical therapy, *Phys Ther* 48:1130-1132, 1968.

45. Rand PH: Evaluation of physical therapy education programs, *Phys Ther* 58:851-856, 1978.

46. Roesch R and Ulrich D: Physical therapy management in the treatment of chronic pain, *Phys Ther* 60:53-57, 1980.

47. Rogers C: A humanistic concept of man. In Farsom R, editor: *Science and human affairs,* Palo Alto, Calif 1965, Science and Behavior Books.

48. Saward E and Sorenson A: The current emphasis on preventive medicine, *Science* 200:889-894, 1978.

49. Sasano E and others: The family in physical therapy, *JAPTA* 57:153-159, 1977.

50. Sechrist WC: Total wellness and wholistic health—a bandwagon we cannot afford to jump onto! *Health Educ* 10:27, 1979.

51. Selye H: *The stress of life,* New York, 1976, McGraw-Hill.

52. Singleton M: Profession—a paradox? *JAPTA* 60:439, 1980.

53. Stein M, Schiavi PC, and Camerino M: Influence of brain and behavior on the immune system, *Science* 191:435-440, 1976.

54. Szasz TS and Hollender MH: A contribution to the philosophy of medicine, *Arch Intern Med* 97:585-592, May 1956.

55. Travis JW: Wellness education: a new model for health. In Flynn P, editor: *The healing continuum,* Bowie, Md, 1980, Robert J Brady Co.

56. US Dept. of Health and Human Services: *Healthy people 2000.* Washington DC, 1990, US Gov't Printing Office.

57. Versloot JM and others: The cost-effectiveness of a back school program in industry, *Spine* 17:1, 1992.

58. Yahn G: The impact of holistic medicine, medical groups and health concepts, *JAMA* 242:2202-2205, 1979.

ADDITIONAL READINGS

Cai J: Toward a comprehensive evaluation of alternate medicine, *Soc Sci Med* 25:659-667, 1987.

Coombs R: *Mastering medicine: professional socialization in medical school,* New York, 1978, The Free Press.

Hancock T: The soft health path: a healthier future for physician? *Can Med Assoc J* 112:1019, 1982.

Harrison M and Cotanch P: Pain: advances and issues in critical care, *Nurs Clin North Am* 22:691-697, 1987.

Keller E and Bzdek V: Effects of therapeutic touch on tension headache pain, *Nurs Res* 35:101-106, 1986.

LaPatria J: *Healing: the coming revolution in holistic medicine,* New York, 1978, McGraw-Hill.

Pownall M: Holistic nursing: all in the mind's eye, *Nurs Times* 82:26-27, 1986.

Sarkis J and Skonor M: An analysis of the concept of holism in nursing literature, *Holist Nurs Pract* 2:61-69, 1987.

Shealy C: Holistic management of chronic pain, *Clin Nurs* 2:1-8, 1980.

Standardized Evaluation Tools Discussed and Presented Within the Body of the Text Along with Screening Tools

Visual pursuit
Saccades
Near point of convergence
Near cover test
Far cover test
Depth perception
Visual field screening

CHAPTER 28

Discussed and/or shown in entirety:
Quiet Standing
   Romberg
   One-legged-stance-test
   Postural sway
   Nudge/push test
   Postural stress test
   Motor control test
Active Standing
   Functional Reach test
   Limits of Stability test
   Rhythmic Weight Shift test
Sensory Manipulation Test
   Sensory Organization test

Clinical Test for Sensory Interaction on Balance
   (Foam & Dome)
Vertigenous Positions tests
Hallpik-Dix test
Vestibular-ocular reflex test
Ocular-motor test
Fukuda Stepping test
Functional Scales
   4 Mobility scales
      Berg Balance scale
      Mobility Skills Assessment
      Get-Up-and-Go
      Tinetti Performance Oriented Assessment of
         Balance
2 Gait Scales
   Tinetti Performance Oriented Assessment of Gait
   Gait Assessment Rating scale
Combination test batteries
   Fregley-Graybiel Ataxia Test Battery
   Fugl-Meyer Sensorimotor Assessment of Balance
      Performance
   Physical Therapy Checklist

Glossary

abulia A loss or deficiency of will power.

ACTH (adrenocorticotropic hormone) A hormone released by the adenohypophysis, which stimulates the adrenal cortex to secrete its entire spectrum of hormones. Thought to be immunosuppressive and antiinflammatory in treating multiple sclerosis.

acute That period of time immediately following spinal cord injury when the management of all primary injuries and the prevention of further complications are the emphasis of care.

acute pain Pain that arises from stimulation of the nociceptors and functions as a warning system of impending or actual tissue injury.

adaptive response An appropriate response to an environmental demand. Adaptive responses require good sensory integration; they also allow the sensory integrative process to progress.

adjustment The ongoing process of responding to the world with a positive adaptive response that allows the person and significant others to grow and mature in regard to all aspects of life.

agraphia Loss of ability to write.

alcoholism A disease characterized by chronic, heavy consumption of alcohol which may lead to peripheral nerve disease, cerebellar degeneration, as well as other systemic and psychiatric symptoms which impair health and function.

alexia Word blindness: inability to recognize or comprehend written or printed words.

Alzheimer's disease A term used as a diagnosis when, based on the symptoms of confusion and impaired intellectual functioning, all other possible causes have been eliminated. It is not possible to ascertain if a client has this disease until an autopsy or brain biopsy has been done. At present, there is no known cause or treatment for Alzheimer's disease, but clients and families *can be helped* to cope better with the presenting losses of intellectual functioning.

amblyopia Dimness of vision not caused by refractive error or organic disease of the eye.

Amigo A scooterlike, battery operated vehicle.

amniocentesis A procedure in which a needle is passed through the mother's abdomen into the amniotic sac of the fetus. Amniotic fluid is withdrawn and analyzed to detect a variety of abnormalities.

amygdala A nuclear mass within the anterior portion of the temporal lobe involved with limbic function, especially arousal, motivation, and declarative learning.

angiography The visualization of blood vessels by injection of a nontoxic radiopaque material.

ankle/foot orthosis (AFO) An external device which controls the foot and ankle complex, and can be utilized to generate forces about the knee.

ANS pain Pain arising from injuries within the sympathetic or parasympathetic nervous systems.

anterograde amnesia The inability to establish new memories.

anticholinergic Blocking the passage of impulses through the parasympathetic nerves; also an agent that so acts.

anticipatory responses The use of information about the environment and from past experience in order to plan and program intended actions for the immediate future.

anxiolytic An agent that reduces anxiety.

aphasia An impairment caused by brain damage, which interferes with the ability to process language symbols. It is disproportionate to impairment of other intellectual functions and is not caused by dementia, sensory loss, or motor dysfunction.

apraxia of speech An articulatory disorder resulting from the inability to program the position of speech muscles and the sequence of muscle movements in order to volitionally produce speech. The disorder results from an impairment arising from brain damage.

Arnold-Chiari malformation A deformity in which the medulla and pons are reduced in size, and the cerebellum herniates into the spinal canal.

ASHA American Speech, Language and Hearing Association, which certifies audiologists and speech pathologists with the Certificate of Clinical Competence (CCC).

aspiration The act of inhaling fluids or substances into the lungs or the removal of fluids and gases from a cavity by suction.

asthenia Chronic lack of strength and energy.

ataxia Loss of muscular coordination.

ataxia telangiectasia An inherited disorder characterized by progressive ataxia, oculocutaneous dilation of terminal arteries and capillaries, sinopulmonary disease, and abnormal eye movements.

athetosis From the Greek origin of the word: "without posture". An dyskinetic condition that includes inadequate timing, force, accuracy, and coordination of movement in the limbs and trunk.

autism A disorder that in childhood is characterized by withdrawal behavior, reduced socialization, perseveration, bizarre behavior, lack of purposeful verbal communication, and echolalia.

autogenic movement patterns (AMP) Movements of body segments (e.g., head, limbs and/or trunk) which are the result of spontaneous activity of 'motor neurons'; in contrast to reflexive or volitional (voluntary) movements.

autoimmunity Disease in which the body produces a disordered immunological response against its own tissue. Antibodies against normal parts of the body are produced to an extent that causes tissue injury.

automatic postural responses Functionally-organized, long-loop responses that produce muscle activation to bring the body's center-of-gravity into a state of equilibrium. Examples: ankle strategy, hip strategy, etc.

automatic speech Words or phrases spoken without voluntary control, such as curse words, expletives, and greetings.

autonomic dysfunction A massive uncompensated cardiovascular reaction of the sympathetic division of the autonomic nervous system to noxious stimuli, usually visceral, below the level of the lesion.

axonotmesis Interruption of the axon with subsequent Wallerian degeneration; connective tissue of the nerve, including the Schwann cell basement membrane, remains intact.

babbling A stage in speech development characterized by the production of strings of speech sounds in vocal play.

balance The ability to control the center-of-gravity (COG) over the base-of-support in a given sensory environment.

ballistic movement High-velocity movement, such as a tennis serve or boxer's punch, requiring reciprocal organization of agonistic and antagonistic synergies.

basal ganglia A collection of nuclei at the base of the cerebral cortex. They include the caudate nucleus, putamen, globus pallidus, and functionally include the substantia nigra and subthalamic nucleus.

base-of-support The surfaces of the body which experience pressure as a result of body weight and gravity, and the projected area between them.

Betaseron (Beta Interferon) A drug distributed by Berlex Labs, (Richmond, CA) licensed by the Federal Drug Administration in 1993 for the treatment of relapsing/remitting MS. The drug is based on Interferon (beta), which is a protein formed by the body when cells are exposed to viruses. The drug has an immuno-modulatory effect and in clinical trials reduced disease activity in relapsing/remitting MS.

biasing motor generators Modulatory influence through synaptic excitation and inhibition over the resting state of the motor generators.

biofeedback A cognitive treatment technique in which the client becomes aware of and learns to selectively change physiological processes with the aid of an external monitor.

bite reflex This pathological reflex is a swift biting action produced by stimulation of the oral cavity. The bite may be difficult to release in some cases when an object such as a spoon or tongue depressor has been introduced into the mouth.

body scanning A cognitive treatment technique in which clients are taught to view their pain objectively in order to separate themselves from their pain.

bonding The process of creating a connection that results in trust and respect between two or more individuals.

brain abscess A localized collection of pus in a cavity formed by the disintegration of brain tissue.

Caregiver Training and Support (1) Organizing educational experiences to assist caregivers to be better able to assist or perform needed tasks for patient. (2) Organizing experiences (group or individual) to assist caregivers to cope with the challenges of performing as a caregiver. The support can be in the form of physical assistance or psychosocial activities.

causalgia ANS pain characterized by intense burning and hyper-aesthesia throughout the distribution of an incompletely dam-aged peripheral nerve.

center-of-gravity (COG) An imaginary point in space about which the sum of the forces and moments equals zero (equilibrium).

cerebellar atrophy (spinocerebellar degeneration) A general term for several familial disorders in which the cerebellum deteriorates.

cerebral evoked potentials (EPs) Study of potentials evoked from the cortex, including *visually evoked potentials* (VEPs) stimu-lated by light, *auditory evoked potentials* (AEPs) stimulated by sound, and *somatosensory evoked potentials* (SEPs) stimulated by electrical stimulation of the peripheral sensory nerves.

cerebral palsy A diagnostic term applied principally to a history of anoxia for a variety of reasons shortly before, during, or after the birth process, up to two years of age. The same conditions or experiences are often labeled with alternate diagnostic terms that vary with the geographic area and the clinic policy.

chewing reflex Pathological signs elicited in brain-damaged adults when the mouth is stimulated and repetitive "chewing" motions ensure.

childhood aphasia A disturbance of the capacity to process language resulting from brain dysfunction in childhood.

chorea Involuntary movements of the face and extremities which are of short duration, spasmodic, irregular; frequently involve a component of rotation.

chronic pain Pain that occurs without a clear stimulus to the nociceptors, in response to innocuous stimulation or in a prolonged exaggerated fashion to noxious stimulation.

climbing fibers One of two fiber types carrying input to cerebellar cortex; terminates in 1:1 relationship on a Purkinje cell.

clinical electromyography An electrophysiologic evaluation en-compassing the observation, recording, analysis, and interpreta-tion of bioelectric muscle and nerve potentials detected by means of needle electrodes inserted into the muscles, for the purpose of evaluating the integrity of the neuromuscular system.

clinical problem solving A method of analyzing specific questions that are difficult or perplexing, whose solution will be founded on actual observation and treatment of a patient as distinguished from data or facts obtained by experimentation or pathology.

closure Visualization of the whole figure when only a portion is visible.

CNS pain Pain arising from CNS lesions.

cognition The mind processes that allow the individual to perceive and be aware of the self, objects, and others in a persons internal or external environment.

cognitive-behavior methods Treatment methods which deal with the sensory/discriminative, motivation/affective, and cognitive/evaluative aspects of pain.

cold application The use of cooling modalities to accomplish a therapeutic goal.

coma A complete paralysis of cerebral function, a state of unresponsiveness. Clients do not obey commands, speak, or open their eyes.

communication A reciprocal act of social interaction and sending/receiving information through conventional symbol systems (e.g., language) and affective messages (e.g., smiling). Customary rules of communication are established within individual social cultures.

complete A lesion in which there is absence of sensory and motor function in the lowest sacral segment.

complex spatial relations Relationship of one figure or part of a figure to another.

computed axial tomography (CT or CAT scan) An x-ray technique designed to show detailed images of structures on separate planes of tissue. When combined these images can often detail multiple sclerosis lesions and other neurological deficits.

concentric contraction Controlled shortening of the muscle.

conceptual disorders A disturbance in thought processes, in cognitive activities, or in the ability to formulate concepts.

configuration Overall shape or enclosure of a figure.

constancy The invariant quality of distinctive features in spite of valuation in location rotation, size, or color.

contrecoup injury Injury to the brain produced distant to the part sustaining the blow.

coping Behaviors used to respond to positive or negative stressors in a person's environment in an effort to overcome or deal with them.

Copolymer 1 (Copaxone) A drug under study by TEVA Pharmaceuticals (Kulpsville, PA) which, in clinical trials is reported to reduce the frequency of exacerbations in early exacerbating/remitting MS.

Cor pulmonale Heart disease due to pulmonary hypertension secondary to lung disease with right benricular hypertrophy.

cortisone, prednisone Synthetic adrenal glucocorticoids, used in multiple sclerosis to reduce edema and other aspects of inflammation. They are immunosuppressive and also been shown to be useful in improving nerve conduction in demyelinated fibers.

coup injury Injury to the brain at the site of the impact.

cryosurgery Technique of exposing tissues to extreme cold to produce well demarcated areas of cell destruction. The cold is usually produced by use of a probe containing liquid nitrogen. In rare cases, used to destroy thalamic tissue in persons with multiple sclerosis to control severe tremor and other involuntary movements.

declarative memory The mental registration, retention, and recall of past experiences, sensations, ideas, knowledge, and thoughts. This memory has a high cognitive basis to it. The original data must relay either through the amygdala or hippocampal nuclear structures before long-term storage is possible.

decorticate rigidity A term derived from animal transections, sometimes used to describe abnormal posturing in humans, that is characterized by exaggerated flexor responses in the upper extremities and exaggerated extensor responses in the lower extremities. In reporting, it is preferable to describe the posture observed.

decubitus ulcer An ulcer resulting from pressure to an area of the body, usually from a bed or chair; the heels, sacrum, ischia, and trochanters are most prone to the development of these ulcers.

deep vein thrombosis The existence of a blood clot within a deep vein.

Deiter's nucleus One of the vestibular nuclei, also known as the lateral vestibular nuclei; located in the brainstem.

delayed language Failure of language to develop at the expected

age because of any number of causes such as hearing loss, emotional disturbance, or brain injury.

delirium A delirious person shows both a change in intellectual function *and* in the level of consciousness. The client is less alert than normal and may be confused, disoriented, forgetful, and/or sleepy. Other commonly used terms to describe this condition are acute brain syndrome or reversible brain syndrome. If the underlying medical or emotional problem(s) are treated in a timely fashion, the level of alertness and intellectual functions will return to normal.

dementia Dementia is an impairment in some or all aspects of intellectual functioning in a person who is clearly awake. Other terms used to describe this condition are organic brain syndrome, senility, senile dementia, hardening of the arteries, and shrinking of the brain. Some diseases that can cause dementia are treatable. In these diseases the distortion of intellectual capacity is reversed when treatment is given and/or the intellectual functioning is prevented from becoming worse.

demyelination The process of breakdown or destruction of the myelin sheath surrounding the axons of nerve tissue.

dentate nucleus One of the deep cerebellar nuclei; found lateral to the emboliform nucleus in man, within the cerebellar hemisphere; receives fibers from the lateral zone of the cerebellar cortex; fibers leave nucleus via brachium conjunctivum; is considered part of the neocerebellum.

developmental dyspraxia A disorder of sensory integration characterized by an impairment in the ability to plan skilled nonhabitual movement.

developmental handling Moving a child through part or all of the developmental sequence to enhance the expression of normal movement patterns (i.e., righting and equilibrium reactions).

dioptric power Unit of measurement of the refractive power of an optic lens.

diplopia Double vision.

direct intervention Hands-on therapy to alter the possibility for new motor learning when movement and postural control is inadequate.

disability Any restriction or lack of ability to *perform an activity* in a normal manner or within the normal range. Examples: requires a cane to walk, requires assistance to transfer, etc.

disablement model An evaluation and treatment model based on the specific impairment, functional loss, and quality of life attainable not on the medical diagnosis of the injury or disease process.

distal sparing The spinal cord below the congenital lesion remains intact. The reflex arc through the spinal cord therefore remains but is unmodified by supraspinal influences. This results in spastic movements distal to the level of the lesion.

drug disposition Refers to the absorption, distribution, metabolism, and excretion of a drug.

ductions Movements of each single eye from the primary position into the secondary or tertiary positions of gaze.

dynamic equilibrium Ability of clients to adjust to displacements of their center of gravity by appropriately changing their base of support.

dysarthria A disorder of articulation resulting from impairment of the central or peripheral nervous system in the control of the muscles of speech—errors in articulation of speech sounds.

dysdiadochokinesia Inability to perform rapidly alternating motion.

dysethesias Impaired sensation, but not absent. Often used when referring to "pins and needles" sensation.

dyskinesia A defect in voluntary movements.

dysmetria An inability to position the limbs accurately with respect to another object.

dysphagia A disorder of swallowing or deglutition.

dystonia An abnormal involuntary sustained movement or posture involving the contraction of a group of muscles.

dystrophin Protein that is missing or defective in DMD which is localized to the sarcolemma of the muscle cell membrane. Its absence results in abnormal cell permeability which may lead to cell destruction.

eccentric contraction Controlled lengthening of a muscle.

echolalia Automatic reiteration of words or phrases that have been heard.

ecology Study of the environmental relations of organisms.

ego-dystonic Destructive to self-enhancement.

ego-syntonic Supportive of self-enhancement.

electrical stimulation Study of muscle response to electrical currents including reaction of degeneration (RD), rheobase and chronaxie, strength-duration (SD), and galvanic-tetanus ratio tests.

electroencephalography (EEG) Study of the electrical activity of the brain.

electroglottography Process of measuring changes in electrical potential across membrane of the glottial tissue.

electromyographic biofeedback (EMGBF) Use of electronic instrumentation to elevate normally subconscious electromyographic potentials to a conscious level through auditory or visual signals, so that muscle contractions may be facilitated, inhibited, or coordinated for neuromuscular activity.

electroneuromyography (ENMG) The electrical activity of the muscles and their associated motor and sensory nerves.

electronystagmography Study of eye movements to evaluate vestibular function.

electrophoresis The movement of charged particles through the medium in which they are dispersed as a result of changes in electric potential; useful in analysis of protein mixtures because protein particles move with different velocities.

electroretinography Study of the potentials produced by the light-sensitive tissues of the retina.

emboliform nucleus One of the deep cerebellar nuclei in man; receives input from intermediate zone of the cerebellum; involved in control of posture and voluntary movement.

emotional behavior Motor behavior activated by chemical reactions induced by emotional responses. The motor patterns activated by specific emotions elicit specific pattern generators.

empowerment The process by which power or authority over all aspects of self is reassumed by the client.

encephalitis Inflammation of the brain tissue.

encephalomeningitis Inflammation of the meninges and the brain substance.

end-feel Sensation experienced by therapist at the end of a patient's passive range of motion. May be springy or an abrupt halt, bone to bone, capsular, or tissue approximation.

endogenous opiates Naturally occurring substances which produce opiate-like effects including analgesia.

endoscopy Examination of organs accessible to observation through endoscope (small tube with light camera), which is inserted through the mouth.

epicritic Pertaining to the somatic sensations of fine discriminative touch, vibration, two-point discrimination, sterognosis, and conscious and unconscious proprioception.

ergotropic Combinations of cortical alpha rhythm, sympathetic nervous system activity, and somatic muscle activation. Activity or work state.

evoked potentials The electrical manifestation of the brain's reception of and response to an external stimulus; a way of measuring efficiency in the CNS.

exacerbating-remitting An unpredictable disease course characterized by episodes of symptom appearance or worsening followed by partial or complete recovery.

experimental autoimmune encephalomyelitis (EAE) An induced, laboratory model of multiple sclerosis characterized by inflammation and demyelination.

exteroceptive Receptors activated primarily by stimuli from the external environment.

extrafusal muscle Striated muscle tissue found outside the muscle spindle.

extrinsic ophthalmoplegia Paralysis of the extrinsic ocular muscles.

eye diseases Any systemic or local disease which affects visual function; may cause a reduction in visual acuity (being able to see clearly with central vision), or some type of visual field defect.

F²ARV continuum This continuum begins with fear or frustration and proceeds to anger, rage, and violence in that sequential order. This is a highly volatile emotional reaction and escalates as the emotions mount.

family involvement The interactions of significant others in a person's life that relate to an individual's development and coping.

family priorities Importance of services and intervention goals based on family values and preferences.

fast pain The sensation first perceived after injury; it is localized, easily qualified, and lasts as long as the duration of the stimulus.

fastigial nucleus One of the deep cerebellar nuclei; receives input from the medial zone of the cerebellum; involved in the control of equilibrium and posture.

fine motor coordination Motor behaviors involving manipulative, discrete finger movements, and eye-hand coordination.

flaccidity The absence of voluntary, postural, and reflex movements resulting in muscle laxity and lack of resistance to passive stretch; this condition results from destruction of all or practically all peripheral motor fibers supplying a muscle.

functional electrical stimulation (FES) Use of electrical stimulation of the peripheral nervous system to activate muscle contractions to assist in functional activities, such as walking or upper extremity function.

functional skills Ability to accomplish necessary daily activities.

functional visual skills These include eye aiming, eye alignment or eye posture, oculomotilities, and depth perception.

gag reflex Also known as the pharyngeal reflex, this involuntary contraction of the pharynx and elevation of the soft palate is elicited in most normal individuals by touching the pharyngeal wall or back of the tongue.

gate control theory The pain modulation theory developed by Melzak and Wall who proposed that presynaptic inhibition in the dorsal gray matter of the spinal cord results in blocking of pain impulses from the periphery.

gaze-evoked nystagmus Abnormal oscillation of the eyes when attempting to fixate gaze on an object.

Gestalt Form, space, concept; the configuration of separate units into a pattern that itself seems to function as a unit or a whole.

gliosis An excess of astroglia in damaged areas of the central nervous system.

globose nucleus One of the four deep cerebellar nuclei in man; receives input from intermediate zone of the cerebellar cortex; involved in control of posture and voluntary movement.

goal-oriented movements These used to be called voluntary movements in contrast to reflexive movements. These are movements which are organized around behavioral goals, environmental context, and task specificity.

gross motor coordination Motor behaviors concerned with posture and locomotion, ranging from early developing behaviors to finely tuned balance.

habilitation To supply with the means to develop maximum independence that has never been obtained.

handling In this context refers to physical contact with the client's body to guide directly the movement and postural adaptation to a more normal pattern. Usually refers to functional movement patterns used in daily care.

heat application The use of heating modalities to accomplish a therapeutic goal.

higher cortical processing Refers to the functions of the many association areas of the cerebral cortex. This includes memory, learning, and associating multiple information from a variety of sensory and motor sources. Outcomes of this processing include something as relatively simple as stereognosis or complex as mathematical processing, abstract thinking, or art. Simply stated, higher cortical processing results in gnosis (knowing).

Hip/knee/ankle/foot orthosis (HKAFO) Essentially a device to control all lower extremity segments.

hippocampus A nuclear complex forming the medial margin of the cortical mantle of the cerebral hemisphere. It forms part of the limbic system and projects by way of the fornix to the septum, anterior nucleus of the thalamus, and the mamillary body.

holistic The spiritual dimension of a health care model.

homeostasis The maintenance of a steady state, in particular, the maintenance of the internal (physiological milieu) and the maintenance of safety or viability in the external environment.

homonymous hemianopsia Loss of the same side of the field of vision in both eyes.

humoral Pertaining to any fluid or semifluid of the body.

Huntington's disease An inherited disease with degeneration of the basal ganglia and cerebral cortex; characterized by choreiform movements and loss of cognitive functions.

hyperbaric oxygen Oxygen under greater pressure than at normal atmospheric pressure (usually at 1½ to 3 times absolute atmospheric pressure). Thought to be immunosuppressive in treating multiple sclerosis.

hypermetria Distortion of target-directed voluntary movement, in which the limb moves beyond the target.

hypesthesias Abnormally decreased sensitivity to stimulation.

hypnosis A cognitive treatment technique that involves changing pain perception while the client is deeply relaxed.

hypometria Distortion of target directed voluntary movement, in which the limb falls short of reaching the target.

hypotonicity Reduced resistance to passive stretch; displayed as inability to hold resting posture against gravity; limp, "floppy" extremities during passive movement.

immunoglobulins Any one of several proteins that are capable of acting as antibodies. May be found in plasma, urine, and cerebrospinal fluid, for example, IgG is an immunoglobulin.

impairment Any loss or abnormality of psychological, physiological, or anatomical structure or function. Examples: loss of joint mobility, weakness, sensory loss.

imprinting casting The application of casting material to subject the body part to consistent input for a specified period of time. This allows the central nervous system to "learn" the warranted response.

incomplete A lesion in which partial preservation of sensory and/or motor function is found below the neurological level and includes the lowest sacral segment.

indirect intervention Instruction of parents and other caregivers to modify their daily care of the child or individual to open new possibilities for motor learning and preventing expression of abnormal movement patterns.

inferior olivary nucleus A large nucleus in the anterolateral medulla; origin of climbing fibers to the cerebellum.

inpatient Services delivered to the patient during the hospitalization.

input systems or modalities The ways specific information enters into the nervous system to inform the brain about the external world.

intention tremor An abnormal tremor of 4 to 6 Hz that occurs during voluntary, goal-directed movement.

interferon A protein formed when cells are exposed to viruses. Noninfected cells exposed to interferon are protected against viral infection. Thought to be of use in treating multiple sclerosis.

intermediate region of the cerebellum cortex A longitudinal zone of the cerebellar cortex; located on either side of the median zone; involved in the control of posture and voluntary movement; projects to globose and emboliform nucleus in man and the interpositus nucleus in lower animals.

internal ophthalmoplegia Paralysis of the intrinsic muscles of the eye—those of the iris and ciliary body.

interoceptive Receptors activated by stimuli from within visceral tissues and blood vessels.

interpositus nucleus One of the deep cerebellar nuclei in lower animals (globose and emboliform in humans); receives input from intermediate region of the cerebellar cortex; involved in the control of posture and voluntary movement.

intrafusal muscle Striated muscle tissue found within the muscle spindle.

iontophoresis The use of electricity to drive chemical ions into the body for therapeutic purposes.

isometric contraction Muscle tension without shortening.

isotonic contraction Contraction associated with shortening or lengthening of the muscle tissue can be either concentric or eccentric.

jaw jerk Closure of the mouth caused by striking the lower jaw while it hangs passively open. This reflex is rare in normal individuals.

joint mobilization Graded passive oscillations at a joint for the purpose of increasing range of motion.

kinesiological electromyography Study of the muscle activity produced on motion.

knowledge of results Augmented information provided about success or errors in achieving environmental goals.

kyphosis The exaggeration or angulation of the normal posterior curve of the spine.

language A code for representing feelings and ideas about the world through a conventional system of signals (such as sign language) or symbols (such as spoken or written words). Language includes understanding and producing the conventional symbols and the rules for combining and using symbols.

language disorder A complete or partial disruption in the ability to understand and produce the conventional symbols or words which comprise one's native language, not directly attributable to sensory loss (e.g., blindness, hearing loss) or motor impairments.

laser A device that produces a coherent, monochromatic beam of light that can be used therapeutically for pain management, as well as for surgical procedures.

lateralization The tendency for certain processes to be more highly developed on one side of the brain than on the other. In most people, the right hemisphere develops the processes of spatial and musical thoughts, and the left hemisphere develops the areas for verbal and logical processes.

lateral region of the cerebellar cortex A longitudinal zone of the cerebellar cortex; located lateral to intermediate zone; comprises bulk of cerebral hemispheres; involved in the control of skilled voluntary movement; receives projection from motor cortex and has output to dentate nucleus.

learning disabilities A disorder in one or more of the basic physiological processes involved in understanding or using spoken or written language. This may be manifested in disorders of listening, thinking, talking, reading, writing, spelling, or doing arithmetic. They include conditions that have been referred to as, for example, perceptual handicaps, brain injury, minimal brain dysfunction, dyslexia, and developmental aphasia. They do not include learning problems that are primarily caused by visual, hearing, or motor handicaps, to mental retardation or emotional disturbance, or to environmental disadvantage.

learning environment All the conditions (internal and external), circumstances, and influences surrounding and affecting the learning of the client.

learning theory The theoretical basis used to describe changes in behavior or performance.

leptomeningitis Inflammation of the arachnoid and pia mater layers of the meninges. The same condition may be referred to as meningitis.

ligation Application of a ligature (a ligature being any material used for tying a vessel or to constrict a part).

limbic system A group of brain structures which include amygdala, hippocampus, dentate gyrus, cingulate gyrus, and their interconnections with hypothalamus, septal areas and brainstem.

limits-of-stability The boundary or range which is the furthest distance in any direction a person can lean away from vertical (midline) without changing the original base of support (stepping, reaching, etc.) or falling.

lipofuscin Any of a class of fatty pigments formed by the solution of a pigment in fat.

long-loop stretch reflex Stretch reflex mediated through the brain.

loss and grief The process of dealing with the removal of function or roles in a person's life.

magnetic resonance imaging (MRI) A scanning technique using magnetic fields and radio frequencies to produce a precise image of the body tissue; used for diagnosis and monitoring of disease.

massage Manipulation of the soft tissues of the body for the purpose of affecting the nervous, muscular, respiratory, and circulatory systems.

McGill pain questionnaire A pain character measurement tool in which clients are asked to select words that describe their pain from a series of word categories.

medial zone of cerebellar cortex The longitudinal zone of the cerebellar cortex, which includes the vermis and the flocculonodular lobe; involved in control of equilibrium and posture; projects to fastigial and vestibular nuclei.

meningitis Acute inflammation of the meninges covering the brain and spinal cord.

metencephalon The cephalic part of the rhombencephalon, giving rise to the cerebellum and pons.

minimal brain dysfunction A mild or minimal neurological abnormality that causes learning difficulties in the child with average intelligence.

modulation A variation in levels of excitation and inhibition over sensory and motor neural pools.

morphogenesis The morphological transformation including growth, alterations of germinal layers, and differentiation of cells and tissues during development.

mossy fibers One of two fiber types carrying information to the cerebellar cortex.

motor control The ability of the central nervous system to regulate and/or direct the musculoskeletal system in purposeful acts.

motor coordination Functions that are traditionally defined as motoric. Includes gross motor, fine motor, and motor planning functions.

motor dysfunction, motor deficit, motor disorder, motor disturbance Generic terms for any type of disorder found in learning disabled children that has a motor component.

motor lag A prolonged latent period between the reception of a stimulus and the initiation of the motor response.

motor learning The acquisition of skilled movement based on previous experience.

motor learning stages The process through which a learner acquires, refines, and retains a new motor skill, where performance of the skill occurs with diminishing errors and greater efficiency and flexibility.

motor planning (praxis) The ability to plan and execute skilled nonhabitual tasks.

motor skill The ability to execute coordinated motor actions with proficiency.

movement decomposition Distortion of voluntary movement in which the movement occurs in a distinct sequence of isolated steps, rather than in a normal, smooth, flowing pattern.

movement speed The time elapsed between the initiation of a movement and its completion.

multiple sclerosis A chronic disease of the white matter of the central nervous system characterized by inflammation, demyelination, and the development of hardened plaques. The symptoms and signs are numerous; the course is erratic; its etiology appears to be autoimmune.

myelencephalon The lower part of the embryonic hindbrain from which the medulla oblongata develops.

myelin A fatlike substance forming the principal component of the sheath of nerve fibers in the CNS.

myelin basic protein (MBP) A protein component of myelin which has been the subject of considerable study in MS research. An injection of MBP can induce a demyelinating condition reminiscent of MS in animals called Experimental Allergic Encephalomyelitis (EAE).

myelination The process of forming the 'white' lipid covering of nerve cell axons; myelin increases the conduction velocity (speed) of the neuronal impulse; forms the 'white matter' of the brain and spinal cord (as opposed to the 'gray matter').

myelography Radiographical inspection of the spinal cord by use of a radiopaque medium injected into the intrathecal space.

myasthenia gravis A disorder of neuromuscular function, thought to be due to the presence of antibodies to acetylcholine receptors at the neuromuscular junction. Clinically, there is fatigue and exhaustion of the muscular system with a tendency to fluctuate in severity and without sensory disturbance of atrophy.

myofascial release Manipulation of the soft tissues of the body for the purpose of interrupting built-in imbalances and restrictions within the fascia and reintegrating the fascial mechanism.

natural environments All integrated community settings.

neocerebellum Those parts of the cerebellum that receive input via the corticopontocerebellar pathway.

neologism A new, meaningless word, often spoken by fluent aphasic clients.

nerve conduction tests Measurement of the electrical conductivity of motor and sensory nerves by application of an external electrical stimulus to the nerve and evaluation of parameters such as nerve conduction time, velocity, amplitude, and shape of the resulting response as recorded from another site on the nerve or from a muscle supplied by the nerve.

neurapraxia Interruption of nerve conduction without loss of continuity of the axon.

neurography Study of the action potentials of nerves.

neuromechanism A neurologic system whose component parts work together to produce central nervous system function.

neuronal sprouting The process of regrowing a neuronal process, e.g., axon, in an injured neuron attempting to re-establish innervation with a target structure.

neuropathy Any disease or dysfunction of the nerves.

neurotmesis Damage to the axon and the endoneurial tube with the nerve remaining macroscopically intact, or complete transection of the nerve. Regeneration is less successful than in axonotmesis.

neurotransmitter A specific chemical agent that is released from presynaptic cells and travels across the synapse to stimulate or inhibit postsynaptic cells, thereby facilitating or inhibiting neural transmission.

neurotrophic Nutrition and maintenance of tissues as regulated by nervous influence.

nociceptor A peripheral nerve ending which appreciates and transmits painful or injurious stimuli.

nosocomial Hospital acquired.

nuchal rigidity Reflex spasm of the neck extensor muscles resulting in resistance to cervical flexion.

nystagmus A series of automatic, back and forth eye movements. Different conditions produce this reflex. A common way of producing them is by an abrupt stop following a series of rotations of the body. The duration and regularity of postrotary

nystagmus are some of the indicators of vestibular system efficiency.

ocular dysmetria The eyes are unable to fix gaze on an object or follow a moving object with accuracy.

oligoclonal banding A process by which cerebrospinal fluid IgG is distributed, following electrophoresis, in discrete bands. Approximately 90% of clients with multiple sclerosis show oligoclonal banding.

oligodendroglia Myelin-producing cells in the CNS.

operant conditioning A cognitive treatment technique in which a voluntary, nonautomatic behavior is paired with a new stimulus through reinforcement or punishment.

ophthalmoplegia Paralysis of ocular muscles.

opisthotonus Position of extreme hyperextension of the vertebral column caused by a tetanic spasm of the extensor musculature.

optokinetic nystagmus Nystagmus induced by watching stripes on a drum revolving around one's face.

oral myelin (Myloral) An oral bovine myelin therapy for MS currently under study by Autoimmune, Inc. (Lexington, MA) which is based on the theory of 'oral tolerance' to reduce immune activity against myelin. Oral tolerance refers to the ability of the immune system associated with the digestive tract to protect against immune reactions to foreign proteins that are ingested.

orthostatic hypotension A dramatic fall in the blood pressure when a patient assumes an upright position, usually caused by a disturbance of vasomotor control decreasing the blood supply returning to the heart.

orthotic An external device utilized to apply forces to a body part to limit movement, increase the velocity or power of a movement, stop movement, or hold the body part in a particular position. Previously called braces.

orthotics External devices used to support and correct deformities or add stability to enhance control and function.

outpatient Services provided to the patient following discharge from the inpatient hospitalization, or services provided to a patient referred to the therapist directly from the physician.

pachymeningitis Acute inflammation of the dura mater.

pain character measurements Any of the tools used to define the character of a client's pain.

pain estimates A pain intensity measurement in which clients rate pain on a scale of 0 to 100.

pain intensity measurements Any of the scales used to quantify pain intensity.

pain modulation Variation in the intensity and appreciation of pain secondary to CNS and ANS affects on the nociceptors and along the pain pathways, as well as secondary to external factors such as distraction and suggestion.

pain pathway The route along which nerve impulses arising from painful stimuli are transmitted from the nociceptor to the brain, including transmission within the brain itself.

papilledema Edema of the optic disc.

parallel talk A form of speech used during play therapy with children in which the clinician verbalizes actions such as what is happening or what the child is doing without requiring "answers" from the child. For instance, "I'm making a cake. Mine is good. You're making a cake, too." The clinician often repeats utterances of the child correctly and parallels the child's activities.

paranodal myelin intussusception The ultrastructural change that occurs at Ranvier's node because of acute focal compression of a nerve, resulting in a neuropraxic lesion.

paraplegia The impairment or loss of motor and/or sensory function in the thoracic, lumbar, or sacral (but not cervical) segments of the spinal cord, secondary to damage of neural elements within the spinal canal.

paraxial Lying near the axis of the body.

paresthesia An abnormal spontaneous sensation such as burning, pricking, tickling, or tingling.

Parkinson's disease; parkinsonism A degenerative disease of the substantia nigra; cause is unknown for ideopathic parkinsonism; disease is characterized by a slow movements, rigidity, a resting tremor, and postural instability.

patterned responses The programs either preprogrammed or created by the motor system to succeed at the presented task in the most efficient and integrated response possible at that moment in time.

pendular knee jerk Upon elicitation of the deep tendon reflex of the knee; the lower leg oscillates briefly like a pendulum after the jerk, instead of returning immediately to resting position.

perceptual-motor The interaction of the various channels of perception with motor activity, including visual, auditory, tactual, and kinesthetic channels.

perceptual-motor match The process of comparing and collating the input data received through the motor system and through perception.

peripheral pain Pain arising from injury to a peripheral structure.

phantom limb pain Paresthesia or severe pain felt in the amputated part of a limb.

phenol block An injection of phenol (hydroxybenzene) into individual nerves. Used as a topical anesthetic and produces a selective block of these nerves. Sometimes used to control severe spasticity in specific muscle groups.

phonophoresis The use of ultrasound waves to drive chemical molecules into the tissues for therapeutic purposes.

physical therapy Treatment of injury and disease by mechanical means, as heat, light, exercise, massage, and mobilization.

physiological flexion The excessive amount of flexor tone that is *normally* present at birth because of the existing level of CNS maturation and fetal positioning in utero.

plaque A multiple sclerosis lesion characterized by loss of myelin and hardening of tissue.

plasmapheresis A process by which blood is removed from the client; plasma is discarded and replaced by normal plasma or human albumin. Reconstituted blood is then returned to the client. In treating multiple sclerosis this process is believed to rid the blood of antibodies or substances that are damaging to myelin or that impair nerve conduction.

plasticity Anatomical and electrophysiological changes in the central nervous system.

pneumoencephalogram Radiographical examination of ventricles and subarachnoid spaces of the brain following withdrawal of cerebrospinal fluid and injection of air or gas via lumbar puncture.

point stimulation The stimulation of sensitive areas of skin using electricity, pressure, laser, or ice for the purpose of relieving pain.

polyradiculopathy Inflammation of multiple nerve roots.

polysomnography Study of sleep.

position in space Direction in which figures point, relationship of one body part to another, or the entire body's relationship to objects or others in space.

posttraumatic amnesia The time elapsed between a brain injury and the point at which the functions concerned with memory are determined to have been restored.

postural background movements The subtle, spontaneous body adjustments that make overt movements of the hands easier, for example, reaching for a distant object. These postural adjustments depend on good vestibular and proprioceptive integration.

postural tremor A pathological tremor of 3 to 5 Hz that appears in a limb or the trunk when either is working against the pull of gravity.

posture In the strictest sense, the position of the body or body part in relation to space and/or to other body parts. Functionally, the anticipation of and response to displacement of the body's center of mass.

pragmatics The study of language as it is used in context.

problem solving The process of logically or intuitively overcoming barriers in an individuals environment.

proprioceptive Receptors that respond to stimuli originating primarily from muscle spindles, Golgi tendon organs, and joints.

protopathic Pertaining to the somatic sensations of fast, localized pain, slow, poorly localized pain, and temperature.

Pro-Ven A processed mixture of cobra, krait, and water moccasin venoms developed by Florida physicians to treat multiple sclerosis. The FDA has banned the sale of Pro-Ven until it is tested for safety and effectiveness.

pulmonary embolism An obstruction of the pulmonary artery or one of its branches usually caused by an embolus from a lower extremity thrombosis.

Purkinje cells Large neurons found in the cerebellar cortex, which provide the only output from the cerebellar cortex after the cortex processes sensory and motor signals from the rest of the nervous system.

reaction of degeneration The condition in which a short duration electrical stimulus (usually less than 1 msec.) applied to a motor nerve results in a sluggish or absent muscle response, rather than the normally brisk contraction. The reaction may be partial or complete, depending on the extent of neuropathology. This electrophysiologic reaction can be used as a screening assessment of peripheral nerve integrity.

rebound phenomenon Inability to stop a resisted muscle contraction, such that movement of the limb occurs when the resistance is unexpectedly withdrawn from the limb.

red nucleus Large, vascular nucleus found in mesencephalon, involved in transmission of cerebellar communications to the motor cortex and thalamus.

reflux Back flow of urine from bladder to ureters.

refractive error Nearsightedness (myopia), farsightedness (hyperopia), astigmatism, or presbyopia. All conditions are improved with corrective lenses.

rehabilitation The restoration of a disabled individual to maximum independence commensurate with his or her limitations.

relaxation techniques A cognitive treatment technique that addresses muscle tension accompanying pain.

response speed The time elapsed between presentation of a stimulus and the client's initiation of movement.

retardation A retarded person has had some degree of mental impairment all his or her life. A retarded person can also develop a delirium or dementia. A delirium or dementia differs from retardation in that there has been a change from what was normal for that person.

retrograde amnesia The inability to recall events that have occurred during the period immediately preceding a brain injury.

reverberating loops or circuits A process by which closed chains of neurons when excited by a single impulse will continue to discharge impulses from collateral neurons back onto the original neuronal pool. The end result may produce a higher level of excitation than the original input itself.

rhizotomy A neurosurgical intervention at the level of the caudus equinus, or the lumbar level of the spine, to interrupt abnormal sensory feedback that appears to maintain hypertonus. The procedure was developed in 1908 and has been modified by a series of neurosurgeons, with the objective of reducing hypertonus associated with CNS dysfunction to allow the expression of functional postural control.

rigidity Resistance to passive range of motion which is not velocity dependent and affects the muscles on both sides of the joint.

rooting reflex This normal reflex in infants up to 4 months of age consists of head turning in the direction of the stimulus when the cheek is stroked gently.

saccadic eye movement An extremely fast movement of the eyes, allowing the eyes to accurately fix on a still object in the visual field.

saccadic fixations A rapid change of fixation from one point in a visual field to another.

scanning speech An abnormal pattern of speech characterized by regularly recurring pauses.

scoliosis Lateral curvature of the spine; this usually consists of two curves, the original abnormal curve and a compensatory curve in the opposite direction.

sensorimotor therapy Therapy planned to enhance the integration of reflex phenomena and the emergence of voluntary motor behaviors concerned with posture and locomotion.

sensory conflict Situations in which sensory signals that are *expected* to match ("agree") do NOT match, either between systems (vision, somatosensory or vestibular) or within a system (left versus right sides).

sensory deprivation An enforced absence of the usual repertoire of sensory stimuli. The continued absence of adequate, normal stimuli can produce severe mental changes, including hallucinations, anxiety, depression, and insanity.

sensory environment The conditions which exist in the real world around us which impact balance, i.e., darkness, visual movement, compliant surfaces, etc.

sensory integration The organization of sensory input for use, a perception of the body or environment, an adaptive response, a learning process, or the development of some neural function.

sensory integrative dysfunction A disorder or irregularity in brain function that makes sensory integration difficult. Many, but not all, learning disorders stem from sensory integrative dysfunctions.

sensory integrative therapy Therapy involving sensory stimulation and adaptive responses to it according to a child's neurological needs. Treatment usually involves full body movements that provide vestibular, proprioceptive, and tactile stimulation. It usually does not include desk activities, speech training, reading lessons, or training in specific perceptual or

motor skills. The goal is to improve the brain's ability to process and organize sensations.

sensuality Responding to sensory input in a positive manner resulting in the person deriving pleasure from the body.

septicemia Systemic disease associated with the presence and persistence of pathogenic microorganisms or toxins in the blood.

serial speech Overlearned speech involving a series of words such as counting and reciting the days of the week.

sexuality The behaviors that relate psychological, cultural, emotional, and physical responses to the need to reproduce.

slow pain The second sensation perceived after injury; it is poorly localized and outlasts the duration of the stimulus.

smooth pursuit movement of the eyes When the eyes are following a slowly moving object, they move together at a steady velocity, not in saccades.

soft neurological signs Mild or slight neurological abnormalities that are difficult to detect.

spastic diplegia An increase in postural tonus that is distributed primarily in the lower extremities and the pelvic area.

spastic quadriplegia An increase in postural tonus that is distributed throughout all four extremities. These findings are often coexistent with relatively lower tone in the trunk and severe difficulty in controlling posture.

spasticity A motor disorder characterized by a velocity-dependent increase in tonic stretch reflexes with exaggerated tendon-jerks, resulting from hyperexcitability of the stretch reflex. Spasticity is one component of the upper motor neuron syndrome.

speech The meaningful production and sequencing of sounds by the speech sensorimotor system (e.g. lips, tongue, etc.) for the transmission of spoken language.

spinal cord injury An insult to the spinal cord which results in neurological deficits.

spirometry (Pneumatometry) The measurement of air inspired and expired.

static equilibrium Ability of an individual to adjust to displacements of his or her center of gravity while maintaining a constant base of support.

stereognosis The ability to recognize the sizes, shapes, and weights of familiar objects without the use of vision.

stereopsis Quality of visual fusion.

strabismus Oculomotor misalignment of one eye.

sudomotor Stimulating the sweat glands.

synaptogenesis The process of forming 'synaptic connections' between nerve cells, or between nerve cells and muscle fibers; the basis of neuronal communication.

synergy Fixed set of muscles contracting with a present sequence and time of contraction.

systems interactions The ways the various CNS systems effect or interact with each other in order to provide a more integrative and functional nervous system.

systems model A conceptual representation which incorporates a set of major functional divisions or systems within the CNS which interlock and interrelate to create the functional whole. Although each division may be considered a whole in and of itself with multiple subsystems interlocking to form its entire division, each major component or division influences and is influenced by all others and thus the totality of the CNS is based on the summation of the interactions, not individual function.

systems model/approach A cyclical framework for understanding postural control which includes (1) environmental stimuli,

(2) sensory reception, perception, and organization, and (3) motor planning, execution, and modification.

systems theory A theory describing movements emerging as a result of an interaction among many peripheral and central nervous system components with influence changing depending on the task.

tactile defensiveness A sensory integrative dysfunction characterized by tactile sensations that cause excessive emotional reactions, hyperactivity, or other behavior problems.

telereceptive The exteroceptors of hearing, sight, and smell that are sensitive to distant stimuli.

tenotomy Surgical section of a tendon used in some cases to treat severe spasticity and contractures.

TENS Transcutaneous electrical nerve stimulation; the use of electricity for pain management.

tetraplegia Impairment or loss of motor and/or sensory function in the cervical segments of the spinal cord due to damage of neural elements within the spinal canal.

thalamic pain CNS pain caused by injury to the thalamus and characterized by contralateral and sometimes migratory pain brought on by peripheral stimulation.

therapeutic environment Organizing all aspects of the environment in a systematic way so that they enhance a patients' abilities to perform desired tasks and activities (mental, emotional, functional).

therapeutic touch The exchange of energy from one person to another for the purpose of healing.

thermotherapy The use of heat or cold for therapeutic purposes.

thrombophlebitis Inflammation of a vein associated with thrombus formation.

thyrotropin-releasing hormone A hormone of the anterior pituitary gland having an affinity for and specifically stimulating the thyroid gland.

tongue-thrust swallow An immature form of swallowing in which the tongue is projected forward instead of retracted during swallowing.

topognosis The ability to localize tactile stimuli.

total lymphoid irradiation (TLI) Radiation therapy targeted to the body's lymph nodes; in the treatment of multiple sclerosis, the goal is to suppress immune system functioning (reduce the number of lymphocytes in the blood).

transcutaneous nerve stimulation (TNS) A procedure in which electrodes are placed on the surface of the skin over specific nerves and electrical stimulation is carried out. Stimulation of the CNS in this manner is thought to improve CNS function, reduce spasticity, and control pain.

traumatic head injury An insult to the brain caused by an external physical force, that may produce a diminished or altered state of consciousness, which results in impairment of cognitive abilities or physical functioning.

treatment Application of or involvement in activities/stimulation to effect improvement in abilities for self-directed activities, self-care or maintenance of the home.

trophotropic Combination of parasympathetic nervous system activity, somatic muscle relaxation, and cortical beta rhythm synchronization. Resting or sleep state.

truncal ataxia Uncoordinated movement of the trunk.

ultrasound A therapeutic modality using sound waves.

universal cuff An adaptive device worn on the hand to hold items such as utensils, shaver, or pencil, allowing an individual with weak grasp to participate in self-care activities.

verbal rating scale A pain intensity measurement in which clients rate pain on a continuum that is subdivided from left to right into gradually increasing pain intensities.

vergences Movements of the two eyes in the opposite direction.

vermis Forms the unpaired medial region of the cerebellum.

versions Movements of the two eyes in the same direction.

vestibular-bilateral disorder A sensory integrative dysfunction characterized by shortened duration nystagmus, poor integration of the two sides of the body and brain, and difficulty in learning to read or compute. The disorder is caused by under-reactive vestibular responses.

vestibuloocular reflex A normal reflex in which eye position compensates for movement of the head, induced by excitation of vestibular apparatus.

visual analogue scale A pain intensity measurement in which clients rate pain on a continuum that is without subdivisions.

visual analytical problem-solving The ability to look at a complex array of visual stimuli, identify the critical attributes, and then use appropriate strategies to solve simple to complex problems.

visual-motor coordination The ability to coordinate vision with the movements of the body or parts of the body.

visual-motor function The ability to draw or copy forms or to perform constructive tasks.

visual perceptual dysfunction May include deficits in any of the areas of visual perception: figure-ground, form constancy, or size discrimination. Distinct from deficits in functional visual skills and tested separately.

vision screening Can include distance and near visual acuities, oculomotilities, eye alignment or posture, depth perception, and visual fields.

volitional postural movements Movement patterns under volitional control that relate specifically to controlling the center-of-gravity, as in skating, ballet, gymnastics, etc.

wallerian degeneration The physical and biochemical changes that occur in a nerve because of the loss of axonal continuity following trauma.

wholistic A model or approach to health care that takes into account all internal and external influences during the process.

zero-to-three infant stimulation groups Groups that provide therapeutic services for children from birth to 3 years of age, since this age-group is not yet eligible for public school placement.

Index